# CANCER
## of the
# SKIN

*Commissioning Editors:* Claire Bonnett and Russell Gabbedy
*Development Editor:* Rachael Harrison
*Project Manager:* Jess Thompson
*Design:* Kirsteen Wright
*Illustration Manager:* Merlyn Harvey
*Illustrator:* Ethan Danielson
*Marketing Manager:* Gaynor Jones and Helena Mutak

# CANCER of the SKIN

## Second Edition

**Darrell S. Rigel** MD
Clinical Professor of Dermatology
New York University Medical Center
New York, NY, USA

**June K. Robinson** MD
Professor of Clinical Dermatology
Feinberg School of Medicine
Northwestern University
Chicago, IL, USA

**Merrick Ross** MD
Professor of Surgery
Chief, Melanoma Section
Department of Surgical Oncology
University of Texas
MD Anderson Cancer Center
Houston, TX, USA

**Robert J. Friedman** MD, MSc (Mcd)
Clinical Professor
Department of Dermatology
New York University School of Medicine
New York, NY, USA

**Clay J. Cockerell** MD
Clinical Professor, Dermatology and Pathology;
Director, Cockerell and Associates Dermpath
Diagnostics;
Director, Division of Dermatopathology
University of Texas Southwestern Medical Center
Dallas, TX, USA

**Henry W. Lim** MD
Chairman and C. S. Livingood Chair
Department of Dermatology
Henry Ford Hospital
Senior Vice President for Academic Affairs
Henry Ford Health System
Detroit, MI, USA

**Eggert Stockfleth** MD, PhD
Professor of Dermatology
Head of Skin Cancer Center Charité
Vice-chair of Department of Dermatology, Venereology
and Allergy
Charité – University Medical Center Berlin
Berlin, Germany

**John M. Kirkwood** MD
Usher Professor of Medicine, Dermatology,
and Translational Science
University of Pittsburgh School of Medicine
Director, Melanoma and Skin Cancer Program
University of Pittsburgh Cancer Institute
Pittsburgh, PA, USA

For additional online content visit
**www.expertconsult.com**

Expert | CONSULT

ELSEVIER
SAUNDERS

## ELSEVIER
### SAUNDERS

SAUNDERS an imprint of Elsevier Inc.

First edition 2005
Second edition 2011

**Notices**
Knowledge and best practice in this field are constantly changing. As new research and
experience broaden our understanding, changes in research methods, professional practices,
or medical treatment may become necessary. Practitioners and researchers must always rely
on their own experience and knowledge in evaluating and using any information, methods,
compounds, or experiments described herein. In using such information or methods they should
be mindful of their own safety and the safety of others, including parties for whom they have a
professional responsibility.

With respect to any drug or pharmaceutical products identified, readers are advised to check
the most current information provided (i) on procedures featured or (ii) by the manufacturer of
each product to be administered, to verify the recommended dose or formula, the method and
duration of administration, and contraindications. It is the responsibility of practitioners, relying
on their own experience and knowledge of their patients, to make diagnoses, to determine
dosages and the best treatment for each individual patient, and to take all appropriate safety
precautions.

To the fullest extent of the law, neither the Publisher nor the authors, contributors, or editors,
assume any liability for any injury and/or damage to persons or property as a matter of products
liability, negligence or otherwise, or from any use or operation of any methods, products,
instructions, or ideas contained in the material herein.

**ISBN:** 978-1-4377-1788-4

**Cancer of the skin. – 2nd ed.**
**1. Skin–Cancer.**
**I. Rigel, Darrell S.**
**616.9′9477-dc22**

**Library of Congress Cataloging in Publication Data**
A catalog record for this book is available from the Library of Congress

Printed in China
Last digit is the print number:   9  8  7  6  5  4  3  2  1

# CONTENTS

Foreword   viii
Preface   ix
List of Contributors   x
Dedication & Acknowledgements   xv

## Part 1: Basic skin cancer biology and epidemiology

1. The Biology of Skin Cancer Invasion and Metastasis - *Ricardo L. Berrios and  Jack L. Arbiser*   1
2. Genetics of Skin Cancer - *Oscar R. Colegio and David J. Leffell*   12
3. The Biology of the Melanocyte - *Julie V. Schaffer and Jean L. Bolognia*   23
4. Skin Cancer: Burden of Disease - *Abrar Qureshi*   40
5. Epidemiology of Skin Cancer - *Melody J. Eide and Martin A. Weinstock*   44
6. Etiological Factors in Skin Cancers: Environmental and Biological - *Luigi Naldi, Drusilla Hufford, and Luke Hall-Jordan*   56
7. The Importance of Primary and Secondary Prevention Programs for Skin Cancer - *June K. Robinson*   66
8. Chemoprevention of Skin Cancers - *Marie-France Demierre and Michael Krathen*   73
9. Current Concepts in Photoprotection - *Christopher T. Burnett, Darrell S. Rigel, and Henry W. Lim*   80

## Part 2: Non-melanoma

10. Actinic Keratoses and Other Precursors of Keratinocytic Cutaneous Malignancies - *Christina L. Warner and Clay J. Cockerell*   89
11. Basal Cell Carcinoma - *Clay J. Cockerell, Kien T. Tran, John Carucci, Emily Tierney, Pearon Lang, John C. Maize Sr., and Darrell S. Rigel*   99
12. Squamous Cell Carcinoma - *Sanjay Bhambri, Scott Dinehart, and Avani Bhambri*   124
13. Adnexal Carcinomas of the Skin - *Sarah N. Walsh and Daniel J. Santa Cruz*   140
14. Paget's Disease - *Gagik Oganesyan, S. Brian Jiang, and Dirk M. Elston*   150
15. Sarcomas of the Skin - *Tawnya L. Bowles, Merrick I. Ross, and Alexander J. Lazar*   157
16. Kaposi's Sarcoma - *Miguel Sanchez*   168
17. Merkel Cell Carcinoma - *Jayasri G. Iyer, Renee Thibodeau, and Paul Nghiem*   179
18. Malignant Neoplasms: Vascular Differentiation - *Omar P. Sangueza and Luis C. Requena*   186
19. Cutaneous Neoplastic Disorders Related to HPV and HIV Infection - *Kien T. Tran, Jane M. Grant-Kels, and Clay J. Cockerell*   196
20. Pseudolymphomas of the Skin - *Lorenzo Cerroni and Helmut Kerl*   207
21. Cutaneous T-cell Lymphoma: Mycosis Fungoides and Sézary Syndrome - *Brittany A. Zwischenberger, Amit G. Pandya, and Joan Guitart*   217

# Part 3: Melanoma and related melanocytic neoplasms

**22.** Dysplastic Nevi - *Holly Kanavy, Jennifer A. Stein, Edward Heilman, Michael K. Miller, David Polsky, and Robert J. Friedman* 231

**23.** Congenital Melanocytic Nevi - *Julie V. Schaffer, Harper N. Price, and Seth J. Orlow* 246

**24.** The Many Faces of Melanoma - *Darrell S. Rigel* 262

**25.** The Importance of Early Detection of Melanoma, Physician and Self-Examination - *Julie E. Russak, Darrell S. Rigel, and Robert J. Friedman* 272

**26.** Prognostic Factors and Staging in Melanoma - *Jeffrey E. Gershenwald* 282

**27.** Pathology of Melanoma: Interpretation and New Concepts - *Carlos Ricotti, Jennifer Cather, and Clay J. Cockerell* 295

**28.** Management of the Patient with Melanoma - *Jacqueline M. Goulart and Allan C. Halpern* 318

**29.** Pregnancy and Melanoma - *Marcia S. Driscoll and Jane M. Grant-Kels* 327

**30.** Genetic Testing for Melanoma - *Wendy Kohlmann and Sancy A. Leachman* 334

# Part 4: Other cancers of the skin and related issues

**31.** Spitz Nevus - *Philip E. LeBoit* 341

**32.** Cutaneous Carcinogenesis Related to Dermatologic Therapy - *Rebecca Kleinerman, Allison P. Weinkle, and Mark G. Lebwohl* 349

**33.** Genetic Disorders Predisposing to Skin Malignancy - *Courtney Schadt and Jo-David Fine* 357

**34.** Dermatologic Manifestations of Internal Malignancy - *Diana D. Antonovich, Bruce H. Thiers, and Jeffrey P. Callen* 367

**35.** Dermatologic Manifestations of Systemic Oncologic Therapy of Cutaneous Malignancies - *Beth McLellan, Caroline Robert, and Mario E. Lacouture* 379

# Part 5: New approaches

**36.** The Dermoscopic Patterns of Melanoma and Non-Melanoma Skin Cancer - *Steven Q. Wang, Margaret C. Oliviero, and Harold S. Rabinovitz* 386

**37.** Computer-Aided Diagnosis for Cutaneous Melanoma - *Sallyann Coleman King, Clara Curiel-Lewandowski, and Suephy C. Chen* 400

**38.** Confocal Microscopy in Skin Cancer - *Verena Ahlgrimm-Siess, Harold S. Rabinovitz, Margaret Oliviero, Rainer Hofmann-Wellenhof, Ashfaq A. Marghoob, Salvador González, and Alon Scope* 407

**39.** Clinical Genomics for Melanoma Detection - *William Wachsman* 429

# Part 6: Therapeutic considerations in the management of patients with cancer of the skin

**40.** Biopsy Techniques - *Joseph F. Sobanko, Justin J. Leitenberger, Neil A. Swanson, and Ken K. Lee* 434

**41.** Curettage and Electrodesiccation - *Samuel F. Almquist, Oliver J. Wisco, and J. Michael Wentzell* 443

**42.** Cryosurgery - *Paola Pasquali* 450

**43.** Topical Treatment of Skin Cancer - *Victoria Williams, Theodore Rosen, Roger I. Ceilley, James Q. del Rosso, and Eggert Stockfleth* 462

**44.** Immune Response Modulators in the Treatment of Skin Cancer - *Brian Berman, Martha Viera, Sadegh Amini, and Whitney Valins* 477

**45.** Photodynamic Therapy in Skin Cancer - *Colin A. Morton* 497

**46.** Surgical Excision for Non-Melanoma Skin Cancer - *Sherrif F. Ibrahim and Marc D. Brown* 508

**47.** Mohs Surgery - *Edward Upjohn and R. Stan Taylor* 515

**48.** Treatment of Disseminated Non-Melanoma Skin Cancers - *Kathryn A. Gold and Merrill S. Kies* 526

**49.** Surgical Excision of Melanoma - *Robert H.I. Andtbacka* 532

**50.** Regional Lymph Node Surgery in Melanoma Patients - *Merrick I. Ross* 544

**51.** Reconstructive Surgery for Skin Cancer - *Justin M. Sacks, Kriti Mohan, and Donald Baumann* 559

**52.** Radiation Therapy in the Treatment of Skin Cancers - *Jay S. Cooper* 576

**53.** Adjuvant Therapy for Cutaneous Melanoma - *Ahmad A. Tarhini, Stergios J. Moschos, and John M. Kirkwood* 589

**54.** Vaccine Therapy for Melanoma - *Amod A. Sarnaik, Nasreen Vohra, Shari Pilon-Thomas, and Vernon K. Sondak* 606

**55.** Targeted Therapy for Melanoma - *Stergios Moschos* 613

**56.** Imaging Work-up of the Patient with Melanoma - *Hussein Tawbi and John M. Kirkwood* 623

**57.** Treatment of Disseminated Melanoma - *Jason L. Chang, Patrick A. Ott, and Anna C. Pavlick* 629

**58.** Management of Skin Cancer in the Immunocompromised Patient - *Thomas Stasko, Allison Hanlon, and Anna Clayton* 634

## Part 7: Other aspects of skin cancer

**59.** Indoor Tanning - *James M. Spencer and Darrell S. Rigel* 644

**60.** Vitamin D and UV: Risks and Benefits - *Henry W. Lim, Wenfei Xie, and Darrell S. Rigel* 650

**61.** Photography in Skin Cancer Treatment - *Bill Witmer and Peter Lebovitz* 657

**62.** Psychological Responses and Coping Strategies in Skin Cancer Patients - *Nadine Angele Kasparian and Phyllis Nancy Butow* 662

**63.** Medical and Legal Aspects of Skin Cancer Patients - *Abel Torres, Clay Cockerell, Jamison Strahan, and Tanya Nino* 668

Index 677

 Additional video content can be found at expertconsult.com

# FOREWORD

It is now over two decades ago that several of the editors and myself (Robert J. Friedman, Darrell S. Rigel and Alfred W. Kopf) published the seminal comprehensive text entitled *Cancer of the Skin*. The current text is an update on the enormous progress that has been made on all levels, including clinical, therapeutic, epidemiologic, genetic and histopathologic, and on all levels of basic sciences with emphasis on neoplastic cellular biology.

Cancers of the skin in the United States of America have the highest incidence of malignancies of any organ system – and the incidence keeps rising inexorably. In addition to the over 2,000,000 non-melanoma skin cancers anticipated in 2010, it is expected there will be over 68,000 new invasive melanomas diagnosed and over 8700 deaths from melanomas. This translates to a lifetime risk for melanoma of 1 in 37 for men and 1 in 56 for women!

A broad array of cancers of the skin is included in this comprehensive work. Special emphasis is placed on those cutaneous cancers that are particularly prevalent (e.g. basal cell carcinoma) and those which are responsible for the highest number of fatalities (e.g. melanoma and squamous cell carcinoma).

In order to relay to the reader in the most vivid way, all of the clinical images are published in full color. Every attempt has been made to provide clinical and histologic images of the highest quality.

Major emphasis in this text is on the diagnosis and management of cutaneous malignancies so that the reader is provided with the most advanced diagnostic and therapeutic measures available to date for each type of skin cancer. Thus, the editors and authors have made every effort to provide not only the commonly used therapeutic approaches, but also those modalities considered on the 'cutting edge' of our present therapeutic armamentaria.

The backbone of *Cancer of the Skin* is the remarkable productivity of the many authors who have been selected by the editors because of their interest and recognition of the specific malignant neoplasm dealt with in each of the chapters. Their broad experience in cutaneous etiology and the therapeutic guidelines they have documented are valuable assets to any individual involved in the multi-disciplinary needs of these patients. Thus, *Cancer of the Skin* serves as a valuable resource not only to physicians but also to all others who deal with the consequences of malignant tumors of the skin.

It is our aspiration that you will find this comprehensive textbook a valuable summary of the current knowledge gleaned by the literally thousands of years of combined clinical and therapeutic experience coupled with extensive reviews of literature by the multiple authors who have so arduously presented in written and pictorial form the very best of what is known today.

**Alfred W. Kopf MD**

# PREFACE

Skin cancer rates are rising dramatically. In the United States each year there are over 2 million newly diagnosed cases – more than all other cancers combined! One in five Americans will develop at least one skin cancer during their lifetime and similar rates are found in many other countries worldwide. This continued increase in skin cancer incidence is even more dramatic as it is occurring at a time when most other cancers are either stable or decreasing in rate.

The public health ramifications of these facts are profound. Skin cancer, once viewed as a relatively uncommon disease limited to dermatologists and surgeons, is now being seen on a daily basis by primary care physicians, oncologists and other healthcare professionals. The resulting need to educate all of these groups on recognizing and managing patients with this cancer is also increasing.

In addition, the advances that have occurred even in the past decade alone in our understanding of the basic biology, genetics, diagnosis, and treatment of skin cancer have been staggering. In sitting down to review the layout of this text, we were amazed at the multitude of topics that had changed extensively or did not even exist for inclusion in our prior textbook 12 years ago. The advent of dermoscopy, confocal microscopy, computer-aided diagnosis, digital photographic documentation, topical immune response modulators, and advances in immunotherapy, lymph node biopsies, photoprotection agents and our understanding of the biologic basis of this cancer all demonstrate the incredible dynamism of this field. Social issues that have arisen such as genetic testing and the deleterious effects of tanning salons also emphasize our need to understand this cancer within a broader context. All of these topics are covered in depth in this textbook to facilitate a wide-ranging understanding of skin neoplasms.

Primary prevention efforts are also becoming increasingly important. Skin cancer is one of the few cancers where we know the cause of the vast majority of neoplasms – excess ultraviolet exposure whether from the sun or artificial sources. Simple behavioral changes can lead to a significant decrease in a person's chance of developing skin cancer. An understanding of the mechanisms and risk factors of skin cancer are critical in counseling patients to facilitate prevention. Skin cancer is also one of the most clear-cut cases of a disease where early detection and treatment are critical. Skin cancers treated early are virtually 100% curable with simple therapies, while lesions that are advanced often have no effective treatment available. Therefore, the need for medical practitioners to be able to recognize and treat skin cancer in its earliest phase cannot be overstated.

The changing demographics of skin cancer have also led to a need to focus prevention efforts on subsets of the population and to alter therapy for these groups. We have tried to meet this need through providing information on such topics as the management of melanoma in the pregnant patient. To develop an inclusive understanding of skin cancer, one must remember that there are more than basal and squamous cell carcinoma and melanoma. This text has been designed to provide an inclusive review of precursor lesions, other non-melanoma skin cancers and cutaneous neoplasms related to other disorders.

*Cancer of the Skin* has been designed to meet the aforementioned needs in a format that is conducive to effectively transmitting relevant data to the reader. Through the use of representative color clinical images, photomicrographs and flow diagrams, information on diagnosing and treating skin cancer is portrayed in an easy-to-understand manner.

We hope that you will find *Cancer of the Skin* useful in the treatment of your patients with skin cancer and a help in reaching the goal that we all strive for – lowering the morbidity and mortality from this disease.

Darrell S. Rigel MD
June K. Robinson MD
Merrick Ross MD
Robert J. Friedman MD
Clay J. Cockerell MD
Henry Lim MD
Eggert Stockfleth MD
John Kirkwood MD
Robert J. Friedman MD

# LIST OF CONTRIBUTORS

**Verena Ahlgrimm-Siess MD**
Department of Dermatology
Medical University of Graz
Graz, Austria

**Samuel Fehring Almquist MD**
Dermatology Resident
Wilford Hall Medical Center/
Brooke Army Medical Center
San Antonio, TX, USA

**Sadegh Amini MD**
Senior Clinical Research
Fellow
Department of Dermatology
and Cutaneous Surgery
University of Miami
Miller School of Medicine
Miami, FL, USA

**Robert H.I. Andtbacka MD, CM, FRCSC**
Assistant Professor of Surgery
Department of Surgery,
Surgical Oncology
The Huntsman Cancer
Institute
University of Utah
Salt Lake City, UT, USA

**Diana D. Antonovich MD**
Assistant Professor
Department of Dermatology
and Dermatologic Surgery
Medical University of South
Carolina
Charleston, SC, USA

**Jack L. Arbiser MD, PhD**
Professor
Department of Dermatology
Emory University School of
Medicine
Atlanta Veterans Affairs
Medical Center
Atlanta, GA, USA

**Donald Baumann MD**
Department of Plastic
Surgery
The University of Texas MD
Anderson Cancer Center
Houston, TX, USA

**Brian Berman MD, PhD**
Professor of Dermatology
and Internal Medicine
Department of Dermatology
and Cutaneous Surgery
University of Miami Miller
School of Medicine
Miami, FL, USA

**Ricardo L. Berrios MD**
Post-Doctoral Research
Fellow
Department of Dermatology
Emory University School of
Medicine
Atlanta, GA, USA

**Avani Bhambri MD**
Dermatopathology Fellow
The University of Texas
MD Anderson Cancer
Center
Houston, TX, USA

**Sanjay Bhambri DO**
Procedural Dermatology
Fellow
Arkansas Skin Cancer
Center
Little Rock, AR, USA

**Jean L. Bolognia MD**
Professor of Dermatology
Department of Dermatology
Yale Medical School
New Haven, CT, USA

**Tawnya L. Bowles MD**
Clinical Assistant Professor of
Surgery
University of Utah/
Intermountain Medical Center
Salt Lake City, UT, USA

**Marc David Brown MD**
Professor of Dermatology
and Oncology
University of Rochester
Rochester, NY, USA

**Christopher T. Burnett MD**
Resident
Department of Dermatology
Henry Ford Hospital
Detroit, MI, USA

**Phyllis Nancy Butow BA(Hons), DipEd, MClinPsych, MPH, PhD**
Professor and NHMRC
Principal Research Fellow
Centre for Medical
Psychology and Evidence-
Based Decision-Making
and Chair, National Psycho-
Oncology Co-operative
Research Group, PoCoG
School of Psychology
University of Sydney
Sydney, NSW, Australia

**Jeffrey P. Callen MD**
Professor of Medicine
(Dermatology)
Chief, Division of
Dermatology
University of Louisville
School of Medicine
Louisville, KY, USA

**John A. Carucci MD, PhD**
Chief, Mohs Micrographic
and Dermatologic Surgery,
Weill Medical College of
Cornell,
New York Presbyterian
Hospital,
New York, NY, USA

**Jennifer Clay Cather MD**
Medical Director,
Modern Dermatology
and Modern Research
Associates,
Dallas, TX, USA

**Roger I. Ceilley MD**
Clinical Professor,
Department of Dermatology,
The University of Iowa Carver
School of Medicine,
Iowa City, IA, USA

**Lorenzo Cerroni MD**
Associate Professor of
Dermatology,
Department of Dermatology,
Medical University of Graz,
Graz, Austria

**Jason Chang MD**
Medical Oncology Fellow,
New York University School
of Medicine,
New York, NY, USA

**Suephy C. Chen MD, MS**
Associate Professor
Department of Dermatology
Emory University
School of Medicine
Division of Dermatology,
Atlanta VA Medical Center
Atlanta, GA, USA

**Melissa Chiang MD, JD**
Dermatopathology Fellow
Department of Dermatology
University of Texas
Southwestern
Dallas, TX, USA

**Anna Sancho Clayton MD**
Assistant Professor of
Dermatology
Vanderbilt University
Nashville, TN, USA

**Clay J. Cockerell MD**
Clinical Professor,
Dermatology and Pathology
Director, Cockerell and
Associates Dermpath
Diagnostics
Director, Division of
Dermatopathology
University of Texas
Southwestern Medical
Center
Dallas, TX, USA

**Oscar R. Colegio MD, PhD**
Assistant Professor of
Dermatology
Department of Dermatology
Yale School of Medicine
New Haven, CT, USA

**Sallyann M. Coleman King MD, MSc**
Department of Dermatology
Emory University School of
Medicine
Atlanta, GA, USA

**Jay S. Cooper MD**
Chair
Department of Radiation
Oncology
Maimonides Medical Center
Director
Maimonides Cancer Center
Brooklyn, NY, USA

**Clara Curiel-Lewandowski
MD**
Assistant Professor of
Dermatology
Clinical Director
Skin Cancer Institute Arizona
Cancer Center
University of Arizona
Tucson, AZ, USA

**James Q. Del Rosso DO**
Dermatology Residency
Director
Valley Hospital Medical
Center
Las Vegas, NV, USA

**The late Marie-France
Demierre MD, FRCPC**
Formerly Professor of
Dermatology and Medicine
Director, Skin Oncology
Program
Department of Dermatology
Boston University School of
Medicine
Boston, MA, USA

**Scott Dinehart MD**
Director
Arkansas Skin Cancer Clinic
Clinical Professor of
Dermatology
University of Arkansas for
Medical Sciences
Little Rock, AR, USA

**Marcia S. Driscoll MD,
PharMD**
Clinical Associate Professor
Department of Dermatology
University of Maryland School
of Medicine
Baltimore, MD, USA

**Melody J. Eide MD, MPH**
Staff Physician Scientist
Henry Ford Hospital
Departments of Dermatology
and Biostatistics & Research
Epidemiology
Detroit, MI, USA

**Dirk M. Elston MD**
Director
Department of Dermatology
Geisinger Medical Center
Danville, PA, USA

**Jo-David Fine MD, MPH,
FRCP**
Professor of Medicine
(Dermatology) and Pediatrics
Vanderbilt University School
of Medicine
Head of National
Epidermolysis Bullosa Registry
Nashville, TN, USA

**Robert J. Friedman MD,
MSc, (Med)**
Clinical Professor
New York University School
of Medicine
New York, NY, USA

**Jeffrey E. Gershenwald
MD, FACS**
Professor of Surgery,
Department of Surgical
Oncology
Professor, Department of
Cancer Biology
The University of Texas MD
Anderson Cancer Center
Houston, TX, USA

**Kathryn A. Gold MD**
Medical Oncology Fellow
The University of Texas MD
Anderson Cancer Center
Houston, TX, USA

**Jacqueline M. Goulart BA**
Dermatology Service
Memorial Sloan-Kettering
Cancer Center
New York, NY, USA

**Jane M. Grant-Kels MD**
Assistant Dean of Clinical
Affairs
Professor and Chair,
Department of Dermatology
Director, Dermatopathology
Laboratory
Director, Cutaneous
Oncology Center and
Melanoma Program
Dermatology Residency Director
University of Connecticut
Health Center
Farmington, CT, USA

**Joan Guitart MD**
Professor of Dermatology
and Pathology
Northwestern University
Chicago, IL, USA

**Luke Hall-Jordan BA**
Outreach and Education
Specialist
US Environmental Protection
Agency
Washington, DC, USA

**Allan C. Halpern MD, MS**
Chief
Dermatology Service
Memorial Sloan-Kettering
Cancer Center
New York, NY, USA

**Allison Hanlon MD, PhD**
Assistant Professor
Department of Dermatology
Yale University
New Haven, CT, USA

**Edward Heilman MD**
Clinical Associate Professor
Department of Dermatology
and Pathology
State University of New York
Downstate Medical Center
Brooklyn, NY, USA

**Rainer Hofmann-Wellenhof
MD**
Professor of Dermatology
Department of Dermatology
Medical University of Graz
Graz, Austria

**Drusilla Hufford MBA**
Director
Stratospheric Protection Division
US Environmental Protection
Agency
Washington, DC, USA

**Sherrif F. Ibrahim MD, PhD**
Assistant Professor
Department of Dermatology
Division of Dermatologic Surgery
University of Rochester
Rochester, NY, USA

**Jayasri G. Iyer MD**
Acting Instructor in Dermatology
Department of Dermatology/
Medicine
University of Washington
Seattle, WA, USA

**S. Brian Jiang MD**
Associate Clinical Professor of
Medicine and Dermatology
Director, Dermatologic and
Mohs Micrographic Surgery
University of California
San Diego School of Medicine
La Jolla, CA, USA

**Holly Kanavy DO**
Melanoma Research Fellow
New York University Langone
Medical Center
New York, NY, USA

**Nadine Angele Kasparian
BA, (Psych, Hons I), PhD, MAPS**
Head, Psychological Research
and Supportive Care

Heart Centre for Children,
The Children's Hospital at
Westmead
NHMRC Postdoctoral Clinical
Research Fellow
University of New South
Wales
Sydney, Australia

**Helmut Kerl MD**
Professor of Dermatology
Department of
Dermatology
Medical University of Graz
Graz, Austria

**Merrill S. Kies MD**
Professor of Medicine
University of Texas MD
Anderson Cancer Center,
Houston, TX, USA

**John M. Kirkwood MD**
Professor of Medicine and
Dermatology
Director, Melanoma and Skin
Cancer Program
University of Pittsburgh
School of Medicine and
University of Pittsburgh
Cancer Institute
Pittsburgh, PA, USA

**Rebecca Kleinerman MD**
Chief Resident
Department of Dermatology
Mount Sinai Hospital
New York, NY, USA

**Wendy Kohlmann MS, CGC**
Genetic Counselor
University of Utah Huntsman
Cancer Institute
Salt Lake City, UT, USA

**Michael Krathen MD**
Resident Physician
Department of Dermatology
Boston University Medical
Center
Boston, MA, USA

**Mario E. Lacouture MD**
Dermatology Service
Department of Medicine
Memorial Sloan-Kettering
Cancer Center
New York, NY, USA

**Pearon G. Lang Jr. MD**
Professor of Dermatology,
Pathology, Otolaryngology
and Communicative
Sciences
Medical University of South
Carolina
Charleston, SC, USA

**Alexander J. Lazar MD, PhD**
Associate Professor of
Pathology & Dermatology
Director of Sarcoma
Molecular Diagnostics
Sarcoma Research Center
The University of Texas MD
Anderson Cancer Center
Houston, TX, USA

**Sancy Leachman MD, PhD**
Associate Professor
Department of Dermatology
Director
Melanoma and Cutaneous
Oncology Program at
Huntsman Cancer Institute
University of Utah Health
Sciences Center
Salt Lake City, UT, USA

**Philip E. LeBoit MD**
Professor
Departments of Pathology
and Dermatology
University of California
San Francisco - School of
Medicine
San Francisco, CA, USA

**Peter J. Lebovitz BS, MBA**
Canfield Imaging Systems
Fairfield, NJ, USA

**Mark G. Lebwohl MD**
Professor and Chairman
Department of Dermatology
Mount Sinai School of
Medicine
New York, NY, USA

**Ken K. Lee MD**
Associate Professor
Department of Dermatology
Oregon Health & Science
University
Portland, OR, USA

**David J. Leffell MD**
David Paige Smith Professor
of Dermatology & Surgery
Deputy Dean for Clinical
Affairs
CEO, Yale Medical Group
Yale School of Medicine
New Haven, CT, USA

**Justin J. Leitenberger MD**
Resident
Department of Dermatology
Oregon & Health Science
University
Portland, OR, USA

**Henry W. Lim MD**
Chairman and C. S.
Livingood Chair

Department of Dermatology
Henry Ford Hospital
Detroit, MI, USA

**John C. Maize Sr. MD**
Professor of Dermatology,
Pathology, Laboratory
Medicine
Chairman
Department of Dermatology
Medical University of South
Carolina
Charleston, SC, USA

**Ashfaq A. Marghoob MD**
Associate Member
Memorial Sloan-Kettering
Cancer Center
Associate Professor of
Dermatology
State University of New York
at Stony Brook
New York, NY, USA

**Beth McLellan MD**
Resident in Dermatology
Henry Ford Health System
Detroit, MI, USA

**Michael K. Miller MD**
Associate Pathologist
Dermpath Diagnostics
New York, NY, USA

**Kriti Mohan BS**
Baylor College of Medicine
Houston, TX, USA

**Colin A. Morton MBChB,
MD, FRCP(UK)**
Consultant Dermatologist,
NHS Forth Valley
Department of Dermatology
Stirling Royal Infirmary
Stirling, UK

**Stergios J. Moschos MD**
Assistant Professor of
Medicine
Department of Medicine,
Division of Hematology/
Oncology
University of Pittsburgh
Medical Center
Pittsburgh, PA, USA

**Luigi Naldi MD**
Director
Centro Studi GISED
Department of Dermatology
Ospedali Riuniti
Bergamo, Italy

**Paul Nghiem MD, PhD**
Associate Professor of
Medicine/Dermatology and
Pathology (Adjunct)

University of Washington
Medical Center
Affiliate Investigator
Fred Hutchinson Cancer
Research Center
Seattle, WA, USA

**Tanya Nino MD**
Resident Physician
Loma Linda University
Department of Dermatology
Corona, CA, USA

**Gagik Oganesyan MD,
PhD**
Resident Physician
Division of Dermatology
University of California
Rady Children's Hospital
San Diego, CA, USA

**Margaret C. Oliviero MSN,
ARNP-C**
Skin and Cancer Associates/
ADM
Plantation, FL, USA

**Seth J. Orlow MD, PhD**
Chairman, The Ronald O.
Perelman Department of
Dermatology
Samuel Weinberg Professor
of Pediatric Dermatology
Professor of Cell Biology and
Pediatrics
New York University School
of Medicine
New York, NY, USA

**Patrick A. Ott MD, PhD**
Assistant Professor of
Medicine
New York University School
of Medicine
New York, NY, USA

**Amit G. Pandya MD**
Professor
Department of Dermatology
University of Texas
Southwestern Medical Center
Houston, TX, USA

**Paola Pasquali MD**
Coordinator Dermatology
Department
Department of Dermatology
Pius Hospital de Valls,
Tarragona, Spain

**Anna C. Pavlick MS, MD**
Director, New York University
Melanoma Program
Associate Professor of
Medicine and Dermatology
New York University School of
Medicine, New York, NY, USA

**Shari Pilon-Thomas PhD**
Assistant Professor
Immunology Program
Moffitt Cancer Center
Tampa, FL, USA

**David Polsky MD, PhD**
Associate Professor of
Dermatology and Pathology
Director, Pigmented Lesion
Clinic
Director, Dermatology
Residency Training Program
New York University Langone
Medical Center
New York, NY, USA

**Harper N. Price MD**
Pediatric Dermatology
Phoenix Children's Hospital
Phoenix, AZ, USA

**Abrar A. Qureshi MD,
MPH**
Vice Chair, Department of
Dermatology, Brigham and
Women's Hospital
Assistant Professor, Harvard
Medical School
Boston, MA, USA

**Harold S. Rabinovitz MD**
Voluntary Clinical Professor of
Dermatology
Department of Dermatology
Miller School of Medicine
University of Miami
Miami, FL, USA

**Luis Requena MD**
Department of Dermatology
Fundación Jiménez Díaz
Universidad Autónoma de
Madrid
Madrid, Spain

**Carlos Ricotti MD**
Clinical Instructor
University of Texas
Southwestern
Department of Dermatology
Dallas, TX, USA

**Darrell S. Rigel MD**
Clinical Professor of
Dermatology
New York University Medical
Center
New York, NY, USA

**Caroline Robert MD, PhD**
Head of the Dermatology Unit
Institute Gustave Roussy
Villejuif, France

**June K. Robinson MD**
Professor of Clinical
Dermatology
Northwestern University
Feinberg School of Medicine
Chicago, IL, USA

**Theodore Rosen MD**
Professor of Dermatology
Baylor College of Medicine
Chief of Dermatology Services
Michael E. DeBakey VA
Medical Center
Houston, TX, USA

**Merrick Ross MD**
Professor of Surgery
Chief, Melanoma Section
Department of Surgical
Oncology
The University of Texas MD
Anderson Cancer Center
Houston, TX, USA

**Julie E. Russak MD, FAAD**
Clinical Instructor
Department of Dermatology
Mount Sinai School of Medicine
New York, NY, USA

**Justin M. Sacks MD**
Assistant Professor
Department of Plastic and
Reconstructive Surgery
The Johns Hopkins School
of Medicine
Baltimore, MD, USA

**Miguel Sanchez MD**
Associate Professor
Department of Dermatology
New York University School
of Medicine
Director of Dermatology
Bellevue Hospital Center
New York, NY, USA

**Omar P. Sangueza MD**
Departments of Pathology
and Dermatology
Wake Forest University
School of Medicine
Winston Salem, NC, USA

**Daniel J. Santa Cruz MD**
Dermatopathologist
Cutaneous Pathology
WCP Laboratories
St Louis, MO, USA

**Amod A. Sarnaik MD**
Department of Cutaneous
Oncology
Moffitt Cancer Center
Assistant Professor of
Oncologic Sciences
University of South Florida
Tampa, FL, USA

**Courtney R. Schadt MD**
Resident Physician
Division of Dermatology
Vanderbilt University School
of Medicine
Nashville, TN, USA

**Julie V. Schaffer MD**
Assistant Professor of
Dermatology and Pediatrics
Director of Pediatric
Dermatology
Department of Dermatology
New York University School
of Medicine
New York, NY, USA

**Alon Scope MD**
Attending Dermatologist
Department of Dermatology
Sheba Medical Center
Ramat Gan, Israel

**Joseph F. Sobanko MD**
Clinical Instructor
Department of Dermatology
Oregon & Health Science
University
Portland, OR, USA

**Vernon K. Sondak MD**
Department Chair, Cutaneous
Oncology
Moffitt Cancer Center
Professor of Surgery and
Oncologic Sciences
University of South Florida
Tampa, FL, USA

**James M. Spencer MD, MS**
Professor of Clinical
Dermatology
Mount Sinai School of
Medicine
St Petersburg, FL, USA

**Thomas Stasko MD**
Professor of Medicine
(Dermatology)
Vanderbilt University
Nashville, TN, USA

**Jennifer Stein MD, PhD**
Assistant Professor of
Dermatology
Associate Director
Pigmented Lesion Clinic
New York University Langone
Medical Center
New York, NY, USA

**Eggert Stockfleth MD, PhD**
Professor of Dermatology
Head of Skin Cancer Center
Charité
Vice-chair of Department of
Dermatology, Venereology
and Allergy
Charité – University Medical
Center Berlin
Berlin, Germany

**Jamison Strahan MD**
Attending Physician and
Mohs Surgery Fellow
Loma Linda University
Loma Linda, CA, USA

**Neil A. Swanson MD**
Professor and Chair
Department of Dermatology
Oregon Health & Science
University
Portland, OR, USA

**Ahmad Tarhini MD, MSc**
Assistant Professor of
Medicine
Clinical and Translational
Science
University of Pittsburgh
School of Medicine
Pittsburgh, PA, USA

**Hussein Tawbi MD, MSc**
Assistant Professor of
Medicine, Clinical &
Translational Science
Co-Leader, UPCI Sarcoma
Program
Director, UPCI-CTRC
University of Pittsburgh
Cancer Institute
Pittsburgh, PA, USA

**R. Stan Taylor MD**
Professor of Dermatology
University of Texas
Southwestern
Dallas, TX, USA

**Renee Thibodeau BA**
Research Scientist
Department of Medicine/
Dermatology
University of Washington
Seattle, WA, USA

**Bruce H. Thiers MD**
Professor and Chairman
Department of Dermatology
and Dermatologic Surgery
Medical University of South
Carolina
Charleston, SC, USA

**Emily Tierney MD**
Assistant Professor of
Dermatology
Boston University School of
Medicine
Boston, MA, USA

**Abel Torres MD, JD**
Chairman
Department of Dermatology
Loma Linda University School
of Medicine
Loma Linda, CA, USA

**Kien T. Tran MD, PhD, FAAD**
Dermatopathology Fellow
Department of Dermatology
University of Texas
Southwestern Medical Center
Dallas, TX, USA

**Edward Upjohn MBBS, MMed, FACD**
Consultant Dermatologist
The Royal Melbourne
Hospital
Parkville, Victoria, Australia

**Whitney Elizabeth Valins BS**
Clinical Research Fellow
University of Miami School of
Medicine
Miami, FL, USA

**Martha H. Viera MD**
Senior Clinical Research
Fellow
Department of Dermatology
and Cutaneous Surgery
University of Miami Miller
School of Medicine
Miami, FL, USA

**Nasreen Vohra MD**
Fellow in Surgical Oncology,
Moffitt Cancer Center,
Tampa, FL, USA

**William Wachsman MD, PhD**
Associate Professor of
Clinical Medicine
Division of Hematology-
Oncology and Moores
Cancer Center
University of California
San Diego Research Service
Veterans Affairs
San Diego Healthcare System
La Jolla, CA, USA

**Sarah N. Walsh MD**
Dermatopathologist
Cutaneous Pathology
WCP Laboratories, Inc.,
St. Louis, MO, USA

**Steven Q. Wang MD**
Dermatology Service
Memorial Sloan-Kettering
Cancer Center
New York, NY, USA

**Christina L. Warner MD**
Dermatopathology Fellow
University of Texas
Southwestern Medical Center
Dallas, TX, USA

**Allison Weinkle**
Summer Research Associate
Department of Dermatology
Mount Sinai School of Medicine
New York, NY, USA

**Martin A. Weinstock MD, PhD**
Dermatoepidemiology Unit
Providence V A Medical
Center
Departments of Dermatology
and Community Health
Brown University
Providence, RI, USA

**J. Michael Wentzell MD**
Surgical Fellowship Director
Billings Clinic
Billings, MT, USA

**Victoria Williams MD**
Department of Dermatology
Baylor College of Medicine
Houston, TX, USA

**Oliver J. Wisco DO, FAAD, Maj, USAF, MC, FS**
Staff Dermatologist
Wilford Hall Medical Center
Lackland AFB, TX, USA

**William K. Witmer BS**
Director
DermaTrak Skin Imaging
Centers, a division of Canfield
Scientific, Inc
Fairfield, NJ, USA

**Wenfei Xie MD**
Resident Physician
Department of Dermatology
University of Michigan
Ann Arbor, MI, USA

**Brittany A. Zwischenberger MD**
University of Texas
Southwestern Medical Center
Dallas, TX, USA

# DEDICATION & ACKNOWLEDGEMENTS

Because of the magnitude of the public health problem associated with cutaneous neoplasms, there are millions of people each year worldwide that are diagnosed with skin cancer. This text is dedicated to all who develop skin cancer and to those thousands who sadly succumb to its effects. In addition, we also dedicate this textbook to those who are working tirelessly to hopefully provide the key to more effective diagnostic techniques and treatment modalities that will lower future morbidity and mortality from skin cancer.

A textbook of this magnitude could not be produced at the level that has been achieved without the help of many. I would like to thank my co-editors and academic collaborators over many years: June Robinson, MD, Merrick Ross, MD, Robert Friedman, MD, Clay Cockerell, MD, Henry Lim, MD, Eggert Stockfleth, MD, and John Kirkwood, MD. Their incredibly detailed efforts and review significantly contributed to the successful outcome.

In addition, the efforts of the clinicians and researchers across multiple disciplines who generously provided their time and energy are reflected in the high quality of the chapters they wrote. They were particularly helpful in submitting their chapters in a very rapid timeframe so that the most recent up-to-date information could be provided. Also, the New York University Department of Dermatology Skin and Cancer Photography Unit graciously supplied a number of clinical photos of many of the disorders presented in this textbook.

However, the successful culmination of a textbook depends on more than the editors and writers. We could not have reached the level of excellence that was achieved without the help of many others. My staff, Carol Gunther, Susan Rothman and Carolyn Gumpel, provided innumerable hours of coordination and logistics. The Elsevier team including Claire Bonnett, Rachael Harrison, Jess Thompson and Rus Gabbedy were equally committed to a successful outcome.

Finally, I want to thank my wife Beth and children, Ethan, Adam and Ashlee, for their love and encouragement and for allowing me all the time away from them while working on this textbook.

**Darrell S. Rigel MD**

# The Biology of Skin Cancer Invasion and Metastasis

*Ricardo L. Berrios and Jack L. Arbiser*

## Key Points

- Malignant tumors are characterized by biologic heterogeneity, made of cells with different metastatic potentials.

- Metastasis is a sequential and selective process involving the tumor cell and the surrounding stroma (or microenvironment).

- Skin cancer deaths are mainly due to chemoresistant metastases.

- The role of cancer stem cells is becoming increasingly important in understanding the metastatic process.

- Therapy of metastasis should be directed against the unique metastatic cells and the organ microenvironment of metastatic organs.

## INTRODUCTION

According to National Cancer Institute estimates, more than one million cases of cutaneous malignancies were diagnosed in 2009 in the United States (US) with basal cell carcinoma representing the vast majority of cases (80–90%).[1] Other estimates suggest that the number of cases in the US exceeds 3 million annually.[2] While incidence rates for most major cancers in the US are falling, that the rate of melanoma continues to rise is of utmost concern, considering that the 5-year survival rate for patients with metastatic melanoma is less than 10%.[3]

Deaths from cutaneous malignancies are most often due to recurrent metastases that are chemoresistant and unrelenting. While metastatic potential is far from equal across the three major neoplasms, their relatively high and rising (in the case of melanoma) incidence should put consideration and evaluation for metastasis on the checklist of all healthcare providers as they diagnose and treat each patient.

In particular, the resistance of metastatic melanoma to conventional therapy can be attributed to the biologic heterogeneity present not only in the primary tumor but in subsequent metastatic foci as well. The once dominant perception that neoplasms are nothing more than monoclonal, homogenous collections of cells characterized predominantly by unregulated growth has been replaced by a seemingly more sinister and complex understanding.

What is now readily apparent is that tumors are collections of many distinct cell populations with varied growth rates, metastatic potentials, karyotypes, immunogenicities, and treatment sensitivities; the inherent genomic instability accounts for the variation in capacities, and a fully capable metastatic cell is actually a rare clone within a larger tumor.[4] Moreover, stromal microenvironments surrounding the primary tumor and its end-organ metastatic targets also play critical roles in the acceptance, maintenance and propagation of these unique cell types. Resistance to current therapeutic modalities is most likely due to the aggregate of myriad cell types and stromal milieus.

Only continued investigation into the mechanisms underlying the development and sustainability of this phenomenon will permit the breakthroughs necessary for the ultimate treatment strategy to emerge.

## MECHANISMS OF CANCER GROWTH AND METASTASIS

The process of cancer metastasis is dynamic, complex and consists of a large series of interrelated steps. While the complete picture is yet to emerge, a growing narrative demonstrates consistent principles and conditions absolutely necessary for invasion and metastasis across all cancer types. To produce a clinically relevant lesion, metastatic cells must survive all the steps of the process. If a cell or subset of cells fails to develop any one of these 'steps' and/or the surrounding microenvironment is inhospitable, it is rendered impotent and cannot successfully propagate outside of the primary tumor site.

In essence, cellular aggregates capable of metastasis are selected for through a series of rigorous and stringent conditions that may not be present entirely throughout the tumor or the target organ but at specific locations within them. A general scheme for metastatic selection can be thought of as a process that follows the following order (Figs 1.1 and 1.2):

1. Initial transformation and propagation
2. Neoplastic angiogenesis and lymphangiogenesis
3. Local extension
4. Entry into venolymphatic channels
5. Detachment and embolization of tumor cell aggregates
6. Immune system evasion and survival in the general circulation
7. Arrest in capillary or lymphatic beds
8. Extravasation into secondary target sites
9. Proliferation within secondary target sites

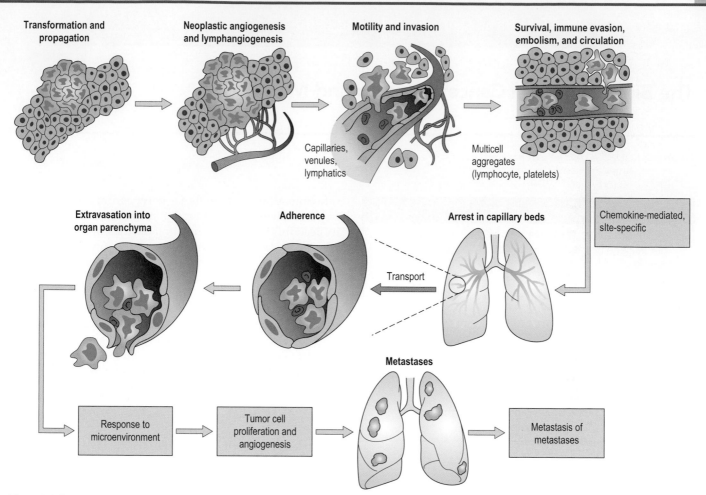

**Figure 1.1** Schematic representation of the process of metastasis. Metastatic cells must complete all the steps of the process. If a disseminating tumor cell fails to survive any one of these steps, it will fail to produce a metastasis.

## Initial transformation and propagation

Like most neoplastic processes, metastatic melanoma does not develop from a single genomic hit but from a progression of successive and varied hits in the context of environmental factors and familial predisposing genes (see Fig. 1.3). The most prominent risk factors for the development of melanoma are a positive family history, previous personal history, and multiple benign or atypical nevi.

At a molecular level, two genes have been associated with familial melanomas: cyclin-dependent kinase inhibitor 2A (*CDKN2A*) and cyclin-dependent kinase 4 (*CDK4*). Both of these are tumor suppressor genes, but homozygous deletions of chromosome 9p21 and subsequent loss of *CDKN2A* gene products are associated with a larger fraction of the familial cases (25–40%).[5–8] Phenotypically, patients with loss of *CDKN2A* exhibit melanomas at an earlier age, multiple atypical moles, multiple primary melanomas, multiple melanomas in the family, and a higher incidence of pancreatic cancer.[9]

Specifically, *CDKN2A* encodes two distinct products as a result of alternative splicing: inhibitor of kinase 4A (*INK4A* or *p16*[INK4A]) and alternate reading frame (*ARF* or p14[ARF]). Together, these gene products bridge the retinoblastoma (Rb) and *p53* pathways. *INK4A* inhibits a series of cyclin-dependent kinases, including *CDK4*, thus blocking the cell

cycle at the G$_1$–S checkpoint. While other mutations are necessary to develop melanomas outright, a murine model lacking *INK4A* demonstrates increased sensitivity to carcinogens and propensity to form tumors.[10] *ARF*, the other gene product of *CDKN2A*, also acts to stop the cell cycle if too much DNA damage has occurred; it is responsible for binding and inactivating mouse double minute 2 (*MDM2*), whose activity, in turn, is to ubiquinate *p53* for destruction. Therefore, absence of *ARF* leads to unrestricted *MDM2* activity, subsequent destruction of *p53*, and eventual accumulation of DNA damage.[11,12] Animal models lacking *ARF* and exposed to ultraviolet light developed melanoma over a shorter time frame.[13] Interestingly, it has been suggested that the absence of *ARF* and subsequent destruction of *p53* may explain the low frequency of mutations observed in *p53* and melanoma.[14,15]

Although rarer, cases of familial melanoma have been associated with mutations in *CDK4* as well. As alluded to earlier, *CDK4* is a downstream target of *INK4A*; mutations in *CDK4* render *INK4A* incapable of suppressing it, thus allowing for progression of the cell cycle despite DNA damage.[16]

In addition to family history, a personal history of atypical moles is also a risk factor for the development of melanoma. There are a variety of lesions considered predisposing, and they include atypical, congenital, Spitz,

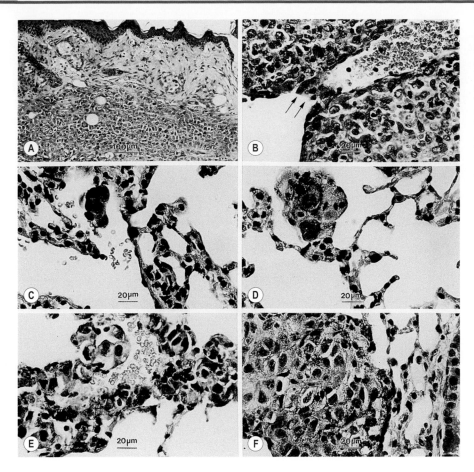

**Figure 1.2** The pathogenesis of a mouse K-1735 melanoma metastasis: histologic studies. A) Mouse K-1735 melanoma growing in the external ear of a syngeneic mouse. Note that tumor cells do not invade into cartilage. B) Note the fibrous capsule surrounding the subcutaneous tumor, which is well vascularized. C) Melanoma cell arrested in the microvasculature of the lung 1 day after intravenous injection. Proliferation of melanoma cells in lungs of mice D) 10 and E) 14 days after the tumor cells were injected intravenously. These are micrometastases. F) 45 days after intravenous injection of K-1735 cells, large melanoma metastases replace normal lung parenchyma. (Courtesy of Dr. IJ Fidler.)

and blue nevi. As shown in Figure 1.3, melanoma can be thought of as a molecular progression of successfully more aggressive mutations; however, they begin as a proliferation of benign melanocytes secondary to unique genomic alterations that precede mutations in *CDKN2A*.

Atypical moles have been found to contain mutations in *BRAF*, which result in upregulation of the mitogen-activated protein kinase (MAPK) pathway by way of constitutive activation of participating serine-threonine kinases. This pathway, also known as the extracellular-related kinase (ERK) pathway, can also be activated by mutations in N-RAS, often found in congenital nevi. Spitz nevi have been shown to contain alterations in H-RAS, a GTPase proto-oncogene, while mutations in GNAQ, a *q* class G-protein α-subunit involved in mediating interactions between G-protein-coupled receptors (GPCRs) and downstream signaling, have been found in blue nevi.[17,18]

Given that these clinically benign lesions already contain growth-promoting mutations, what prevents them from becoming malignant? The answer is thought to lie in a concept known as oncogene-induced cell senescence. Oncogenic stress, the result of the alterations such as BRAF and N-RAS, is recognized by the cell as potentially dangerous. Senescence, a cellular fail-safe mechanism marked by factors such as senescence-associated β-galactosidase, is brought on in attempts to contain the aberrant proliferation in damaged or aged cells.[19] This has also been shown by Peeper et al., who demonstrated the cessation of DNA synthesis in BRAF-mutated melanocytes via an SA-h-gal–positive growth arrest.[20]

Oncogene-induced cell senescence can be maintained for decades; however, if a subgroup of melanocytes develops additional alterations, senescence can be bypassed and they may potentially advance on to malignant transformation. Three molecular pathways have been associated with the development of dysplastic nevi, the next step in progression: loss of *CDKN2A* (discussed above) and PTEN and increased telomerase activity.

Lost mainly through homozygous deletion of chromosome 10q23.3, PTEN is responsible for controlling levels of intracellular phosphatidylinositol phosphate ($PIP_3$), an integral component used by several growth factors. When PTEN is absent, $PIP_3$ becomes readily available, activating AKT (also known as protein kinase B or PKB). AKT, in turn, inactivates a series of proteins responsible for arresting the cell cycle and inducing apoptosis. Thus, absence of PTEN and subsequent activation of AKT allows for damaged cells to escape senescence. The importance of PTEN in melanoma progression was evident when Stahl et al. demonstrated that restoration of PTEN function significantly reduced the capacity of cultured melanoma cells to form tumors.[21]

Recently, telomerase activity has been shown to correlate with melanoma progression. Normally, each round of DNA replication results in shortening of the terminal regions of a chromosome, known as the telomere; the more times a cell has divided, the shorter the telomere, and the 'older' the cell. Once the length of the telomeric region has been exhausted, the cell is signaled to undergo senescence, apoptosis, or cell death. This is true in most

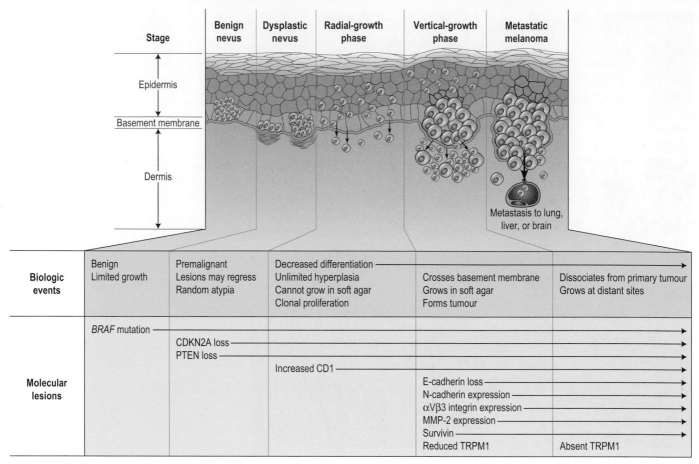

**Figure 1.3** Progression of melanoma. Beginning with benign nevi, lesions accumulate genetic hits over time, gaining abilities or losing restrictions as they become fully metastatic. (Adapted from Miller AJ, Mihm MC. Melanoma. *N Engl J Med*. 2006;355(1):51-65.)

somatic cells; however, telomerase, a ribonucleoprotein DNA polymerase, is responsible for maintenance of the telomere. Experiments by Batinac et al. have demonstrated the upregulation of telomerases independent of increased *bcl-2* expression in melanoma, suggesting that, like other cancers, melanoma cells, too, preserve their telomeres; a mechanism that, in addition to other genomic insults, aids in progression to immortality.[22]

## Neoplastic angiogenesis and lymphangiogenesis

Because oxygen can diffuse only a short distance (150–200 μm) beyond a capillary, in order to escape nutrient deprivation and thus continue expanding, a neoplasm must develop additional blood supply if it is to grow beyond approximately 1 mm in size.[23] In normal tissues, vascular supply is a function of the balance between proangiogenic and antiangiogenic factors elaborated by a variety of cells and adjacent stroma; which is altered from time to time depending on the changing needs of the tissue, e.g. response to injury.

Angiogenesis is, in itself, a complex process involving degradation of a capillary's basement membrane, recruitment of endothelial and supporting cells and invasion into the tissue; it is coordinated by a series of factors that guide and direct new vessel growth through concentration gradients. Recent evidence from various investigators suggests that the source material for neoangiogenesis comes from

multiple sites, including local endothelial cells as well as bone marrow-derived collections; they include endothelial progenitor cells, pericyte progenitor cells, myeloid progenitor cells, and a population of CXCR4+ VEGFR1+ hematopoietic progenitor cells, also known as hemangiocytes.[24-28]

Many proangiogenic factors have been identified in melanoma, elaborated both by the malignant cells and by surrounding cells, including neutrophils and platelets (see Fig. 1.4). Vascular endothelial growth factor (VEGF), a proangiogenic chemokine, is produced by melanoma cells, but it and its receptor are further upregulated in the presence of matrix metalloproteinase-9 (MMP-9), a factor secreted by infiltrating neutrophils.[28,29] Other chemokines elaborated by tumor cells include fibroblast growth factor-β (FGF-β), interleukin-8 (IL-8), placental growth factor (PlGF), and platelet-derived growth factor (PDGF).[30] A set of factors are also responsible for organizing the architecture of newly formed vessel; in tumors grown in angiopoietin-2-deficient mice, for example, diameters of intratumoral microvessels were smaller and the vasculature had an altered pattern of pericyte recruitment and maturation, especially in the early phases of B16F10 melanoma growth.[31] Nonetheless, they are all controlled by a series of complex pathways that include interactions with surrounding keratinocytes, in a paracrine fashion.

Recruitment of progenitor cells from the bone marrow implies that these factors act in an endocrine fashion as well. A subset of Gr1+ CD11b+ myeloid progenitor cells,

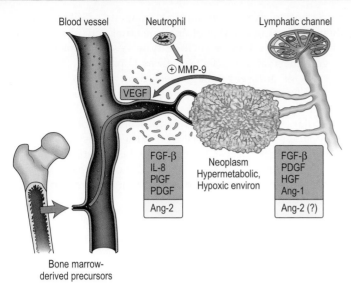

**Figure 1.4** Process of tumor angiogenesis and lymphangiogenesis.

in response to MMP-9, releases soluble Kit ligand (sKitL), which, in turn, mobilizes additional endothelial progenitor cells and hemangiocytes from the bone marrow in a feed-forward cycle.[27,29] Secondly, prokinectin-2 (also known as Bv8), a factor also expressed by Gr1+ CD11b+ myeloid progenitor cells, following stimulation by tumor- or stromal-derived granulocyte colony-stimulating factor (G-CSF), goes on to mobilize additional cells from the bone marrow.[32] Thirdly, stroma-derived factor-1 (SDF-1), a platelet chemokine stimulated by sKitL, has been shown to mobilize hemangiocytes as well.[33] Thus, tumor angiogenesis depends on multiple factors, elaborated by tumor cells, infiltrating cells, and surrounding stroma.

The role of tumor lymphangiogenesis has just recently begun to be elucidated through the discovery of specific lymphangiogenic markers such as VEGF-C and VEGF-D and their corresponding receptor, VEGF-receptor 3 (VEGF-R3), located on lymphatic endothelium.[34–37] Tumor lymphangiogenesis proceeds much in the same way as angiogenesis, with the exception that bone marrow-derived cells are yet to be identified as participating in the formation of new lymphatic vessels.[38] Several pro-angiogenic factors have also demonstrated lymphangiogenic properties, including FGF-β and PDGF, in addition to the recently identified properties of hepatocyte growth factor (HGF) and angiopoietin-1 (ang-1);[39–45] the contribution of angiopoietin-2 (ang-2) is still unclear but that its deficiency results in a series of lymphatic abnormalities suggests a potential role.[46]

## Local extension and entry into venolymphatic channels

In order to gain access to newly formed blood and lymph vessels, tumor cells must first gain the ability to surmount the natural confining architecture of tissues and organs, from basement membranes to fascial planes. Several molecular mechanisms exist by which cells accomplish this, but it may begin with sheer tumor volume. As the tumor grows, it begins to exert physical pressure, allowing for extension

to occur along tissue planes of least resistance. But, in order to go beyond invasion through simple forces, cells must gain the abilities to separate from neighboring cells, actively move, and degrade normal anatomical barriers. These abilities are particularly important in melanoma as the depth of invasion (Breslow thickness) is critical to assessing metastatic potential and eventual prognosis.[47]

Several factors have been identified in the transition of radial- to vertical-growth phases in melanoma, including alterations in cadherins and integrins, cell adhesion molecules. Epithelial cadherin (E-cadherin) is downregulated, via factors such as T-box transcription factors 2 and 3, in poorly differentiated and aggressive carcinomas, indicating loss of cell–cell connections;[48] whereas overexpressed E-cadherin has recently been shown to inhibit chemokine-mediated invasion via p190RhoGAP/p120ctn-dependent inactivation of RhoA.[49] Similar results have been demonstrated with other members of the cadherin family, namely H-cadherin.[50] Integrins, cell surface molecules that mediate a cell's attachment to the surrounding stroma, have also been implicated in the transition to local invasion. Namely, αVβ3 integrin upregulates MMP-2, a collagen-degrading enzyme that helps melanoma cells overcome the basement membrane;[51–53] additionally, Tzukert et al. have shown that αVβ3 integrin also imparts partial protection from anoikis following dynamic matrix detachment, an important factor in survival once invasive cells have detached.[54]

Our group has shown that overexpression of AKT can also convert melanoma from radial- to vertical-growth phase through a series of novel mechanisms. We demonstrated that its overexpression in the WM35 melanoma cell line led to upregulation of VEGF, increased production of superoxide reactive oxygen species (ROS), and the switch to a more pronounced glycolytic metabolism.[55] The mechanism by which ROS is increased may be twofold: stabilization of cells with extensive mitochondrial DNA damage, and/or upregulation of NOX4, a ROS-generating enzyme. ROS, in turn, are responsible for a series of changes, including oxidation of the inhibitor of κ-B (I-κB). Oxidized I-κB can no longer inhibit NF-κB, whose overexpression has been associated with vertical growth progression and directed migration.[56]

Once the malignant cell detaches from the primary site, it must develop means of locomotion to advance to and beyond the basement membrane. Several factors promote motility, mainly via concentration gradients, one of which is phosphoglucose isomerase (or autocrine motility factor, AMF). Araki et al. demonstrated that the proangiogenic factor IL-8 also promotes AMF expression via the ERK 1 and 2 pathways in an autocrine fashion.[57] Melanoma chondroitin sulfate proteoglycan (MCSP) also induces motility by the ERK pathway via changes in cell morphology and enhanced expression of HGF via c-Met upregulation.[58]

To date, two modes of motility have been described: mesenchymal and ameboid (see Fig. 1.5). Mesenchymal motility involves cell membrane elongations called lamellipodia (or filopodia, invadopodia) and movement dependent on extracellular proteolysis at the leading edges. Ameboid motility, on the other hand, describes more rounded cells that move via actomyosin-mediated blebbing, with blebs defined as spherical hyaline outpouches that form when

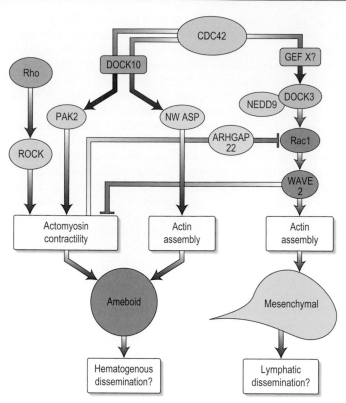

**Figure 1.5** Modes of metastatic motility and their molecular pathways. (Adapted from Sanz-Moreno V, Marshall CJ. Rho-GTPase signaling drives melanoma cell plasticity. *Cell Cycle*. 2009;8(10):1484-1487.)

the cell membrane detaches from its cytoskeleton. It is important to realize that these modes of motility are interchangeable and that metastatic cells frequently switch from one mode to the other, depending on the surrounding environment. At a molecular level, the production of Rho-GTPases has proven fundamental to the interplay between modes and to cellular motility in general.[59] Activation of Rac1, a GTPase member of the Rho family, promotes mesenchymal differentiation while at the same time inhibiting ameboid differentiation by way of WAVE2, a downstream effector molecule that inhibits actomyosin contraction.[60] Conversely, RhoA activation promotes ameboid motility and production of ARHGAP22, an inhibitor of Rac1 and downstream actin assembly.[59] They both, however, depend on CDC42, a Rho member that is affected by different guanine nucleotide exchange factors, or GEFs; for example, DOCK10 is a GEF that acts on CDC42 to promote ameboid motility.[59,61] The GEF that acts on CDC42 to promote mesenchymal motility is yet to be identified.

Each mode of motility may have its own advantages; Sanz-Moreno and Marshall propose that the spherical morphology of ameboid movement may offer protection from sheer stress during vessel travel.[59] Mesenchymal motility may, in turn, offer greater benefit during tissue penetration via proteolysis. Ultimately, as has been suggested by several authors, these distinct modes of locomotion may end up playing a role in the eventual targets of metastasis, lymph nodes versus solid organs.[62,63]

Now mobile, tumor cells must gain the ability to disrupt and cross normal barriers. They do so by binding to components of the surrounding extracellular matrix and

basement membrane (laminin, collagen, or fibronectin), then expressing a series of enzymes that actively degrade them.[64] These enzymes include type IV collagenases such as gelatinase and MMPs as well as heparinase. The sheer number of different collagenases directly correlates with metastatic potential: the higher the number, the more metastatic the cell.[65] Newly formed or thinly walled vessels (vascular or lymphatic) as well as local areas of necrosis or hemorrhage offer little resistance to these cells, where they can readily gain access to the general circulation. Once in the vessel lumen, the loose intercellular cohesion already established allows them to easily detach and embolize, either singularly or in aggregate.

## Immune system evasion and survival in the general circulation

Why the immune system does not effectively recognize, target, and eliminate aggressive tumor cells has been a focus of intense study. The small response rates to melanoma vaccine trials despite laboratory evidence of adequate CD8+ T-cell formation, in addition to appropriate T-cell formation following cancer implantation in several models, all point to immune system failures somewhere down the line from initial T-cell priming.[66-77] Several studies indicate that chemotaxis (via production of multiple factors) and T-cell infiltration into tumors are detectable but their effectiveness, i.e. the effector phase, is directly inhibited by the tumor microenvironment.

T cells require costimulation via interaction with B7 in order to become fully active; if this does not occur, anergy (hyporesponsiveness) is induced in the T cell. Gajewski et al.[100] have demonstrated that B7-1 and B7-2 are minimally expressed in the tumor microenvironment despite mRNA evidence of the same; they have also demonstrated a lack of appropriate cytokine production upon T-cell receptor/CD28 stimulation. Together, they indicate that CD8+ T-cell anergy is at play in melanoma immune evasion.[78-82]

There is also evidence to suggest extrinsic inhibition of T-cell activity as well. Gajewski et al. also successfully demonstrated the presence of CD4+ CD25+ regulatory T cells (Tregs) that were also positive for forkhead box protein 3 (Foxp3), a subset of cells from cancer patients that has been shown to suppress activation of CD8+ T cells (Gajewski unpublished data).[83-85] Myeloid suppressor cells, another subset of cells present in the melanoma microenvironment, have also been shown to suppress CD8+ T-cell activity via the production of inducible nitric oxide synthase (iNOS) and transforming growth factor-β (TGF-β), two well-described T-cell inhibitors.[86-91] Tumor cells also elaborate T-cell inhibitory molecules, the most notable of which is programmed death ligand-1 (PD-L1). This compound interacts with the receptor programmed death-1 (PD-1) on T cells and directly inhibits activity.[92,93] Two other factors have also been identified in other cancers, PD-L2 and B7.x, but their role in melanoma is still unclear.[94-96]

The tumor microenvironment also includes products of metabolism that have been shown to inhibit T-cell function, one of which is indoleamine-2,3-dioxygenase (IDO), produced mainly by stromal cells. Induced by IFN-γ and IFN-α, IDO depletes T cells of tryptophan and generates kynurenine metabolites, known proapoptotic compounds.[97-99] The availability of glucose is also an important factor that is beginning to be studied. Constantly growing and in need of it, tumor cells are local sinks for glucose; relative T-cell deprivation of cellular fuel may ultimately exhibit itself as decreased effector function.[100]

Ultimately evading apoptosis through well-established pathways (NF-κB, bcl-2), metastatic cells that have gained access to the general circulation are not likely to survive there. It is estimated that 99.9% of tumor cells that make it to the circulation do not survive. Most are killed because of simple mechanical forces such as shear; however, through mechanisms including ameboid morphology, immune system evasion, and aggregation with platelets and lymphocytes, there are still 0.1% of cells that survive and go on to produce successful metastases.[101-103]

## Arrest, extravasation, and proliferation within metastatic sites

If metastatic cells survive the general circulation, they then must reverse the process and enter hospitable tissues to set up sites of metastasis. The first step involves non-specific mechanical interactions with the microcirculation (such as simple lodgment) and specific receptor–ligand interactions with the vascular or lymphatic endothelium. Similar to leukocyte chemotaxis, circulating tumor cells first adhere loosely to the endothelium by way of selectins, specifically E-selectin. Tighter adhesion is mediated by integrins (a5b1, a6b1, and a6b4) and hyaluronate receptor CD44, as well as galactoside-binding galectin-3.[104,105] Once adhered, they then extravasate into the surrounding stroma by proteolytic mechanisms similar to those employed during local invasion.

But, what accounts for the organ-specific proclivity of certain cancers? As mentioned earlier, during angiogenesis and lymphangiogenesis, tumor cells secrete chemoattractants that act on a variety of tissues, both local and removed, including the bone marrow. The ability of these cells to secrete factors that mobilize bone marrow-derived cells raises the possibility that they may be able to act in reverse, i.e. metastatic tumor cells may be attracted to the bone marrow by way of receptors for the same. Breast cancer, which commonly metastasizes to the bone, can express CXCR4 and CCR7, chemokine receptors for SDF-1 and CCL21, respectively, whose highest expression (outside of the tumor itself) is in bone;[106] apart from in bone, CCL21 is also expressed by lymphatic endothelium, which promotes dissemination there. Melanoma cells express CCR10, whose ligand is CCL27 (or CTACK), a compound that is specifically found in skin and plays a role in skin-to-skin spread;[106] additionally, uveal melanoma, which preferentially spreads to the liver, has been shown to express receptors for hepatocyte growth factor (HGF) and insulin-like growth factor-1 (IGF-1).[107] Altogether, these linkages illustrate potential pathways for organ-specific metastasis of many types of cancer (see Fig. 1.6).

Apart from site-specific metastasis, this is increasing evidence that cancer cells, via secretion of chemokines, may also prepare a 'premetastatic niche' prior to actual arrival at their target organ. For example, it has been demonstrated that VEGF-A, a chemokine important in neoplastic

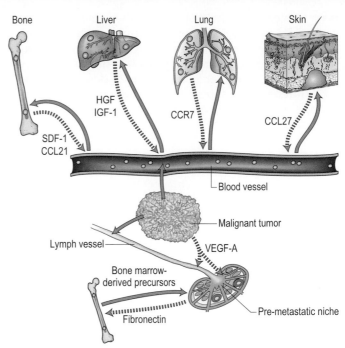

**Figure 1.6** Schematic illustrating potential pathways in tissue-specific metastasis.

lymphangiogenesis, also induces new vessel growth in draining lymph nodes prior to actual metastasis.[38,108] Presumably, this allows for easier entry and a higher likelihood of survival. Once metastatic cells arrive at the 'prepared' sentinel node, overexpression of VEGF-A there can induce lymphangiogenesis in subsequent draining lymph nodes, thereby creating the potential for widespread and distant nodal metastasis.[109]

Evidence for premetastatic niches has also been demonstrated in solid tumor spread. Hematopoietic precursor cells (HPCs), important in neoplastic angiogenesis, are also vital to initiating the premetastatic niche; they home to favorite metastatic sites of lung cancer and melanoma by way of VEGF-R1 and VLA-4 (or integrin α4β1) expression.[110] Furthermore, niche fibroblasts, in an endocrine response to tumor-derived factors, increase their expression of fibronectin, another ligand for VLA-4, providing another substrate for bone marrow-derived precursor cells to home to.[110] Upon arrival, these precursor cells begin to prepare the stromal environment for later tumor cell arrival by expressing MMP-9, which degrades normal architecture and allows for further influx of HPCs and tumor cells.[111] The altered environment of the premetastatic niche also induces production of integrins and chemokines, such as SDF-1, which will later promote attachment and survival of metastatic cells.[111]

Once they have extravasated into their prepared target sites, metastatic cells then go on to re-establish a hospitable environment, and they do so by employing the entire series of capacities selected for at the primary site: increasing genetic instability, unregulated growth and invasion, neoangiogenesis, continued immune evasion, and further metastatic spread ('metastasis from metastases'). However, not all metastatic foci are the same. Be it a result of homing to different sites or eventual differences in the stromal microenvironments, metastatic cells display what has been termed clonal heterogeneity – the same biologic heterogeneity present in the primary tumor and responsible for metastatic selection ultimately manifesting as unique tumor cell types proliferating at each site of metastasis. This process, then, accounts for well-described behavioral differences in antigenicity, immunogenicity, receptor expression, and sensitivities to chemotherapeutic agents of each metastatic focus.[112]

## CANCER STEM CELLS AND PROLIFERATION

An emerging concept in cutaneous oncology is the cancer stem cell (CSC) and its role in metastasis. CSCs are so termed because their properties resemble those of physiologic stem cells; they undergo asymmetric division, are capable of self-renewal, and can develop into any cell in the tumor population.[113] CSCs represent a portion of the overall tumor population, and they exist in localized niches within the tumor. Their role, however, is to provide a constant pool of cells that drive continued growth and expansion, both of the primary tumor and of metastatic foci.

The origin of CSCs remains unclear. One possibility is that they arise from somatic cells undergoing de-differentiation and regaining stem cell properties. A second possibility is that stem cells already present in the tissue (e.g. follicular stem cells) may acquire genetic hits that transform them into CSCs, so-called transdifferentiation. A third explanation centers on the roles of bone marrow-derived progenitor cells in the metastatic process; upon reaching the tumor microenvironment, they could conceivably transdifferentiate into CSCs given the appropriate chemokine milieu. Genetically, evidence exists for deregulations in the Bmi-1, Notch, Wnt, and sonic hedgehog (Shh) pathways – the same ones that play active roles in embryogenesis and maintenance of normal stem cell populations (see Figs 1.7 and 1.8).[114–120]

Whatever their source, the role of CSCs in clinical aggressiveness also remains unclear. La Porta suggests it may be an issue of quantity and/or quality.[113] There are studies to suggest that the overall percentage of CSCs within a tumor correlates negatively with survival and positively with tumorigenicity, but the inherent biological properties of CSCs may play a role in resistance to therapy as well.[121–123] Under normal conditions, the ABCB5 drug transporter

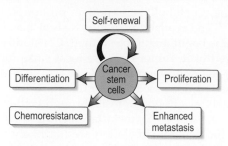

**Figure 1.8** Proposed roles for cancer stem cells in cancer biology. (From Schatton T, Frank MH. Cancer stem cells and human malignant melanoma. *Pigment Cell Melanoma Res.* 2008;21(1):39-55.)

(a member of the multi-drug resistance P-glycoprotein family) serves to control cell differentiation via alterations in cell membrane polarity; however, Frank et al. have demonstrated that the same transporter is responsible for doxorubicin exchange and subsequent chemoresistance in CD133+ G3361 melanoma cells (CD133 is a general marker associated with CSCs).[124] This suggests that CSCs present in melanoma may be partly responsible for generalized tumor chemoresistance which ultimately drives recurrence and further metastasis.

A more definitive role for melanoma CSCs in metastasis is still being investigated, but their unique properties certainly lend them to being suspect. Relative to primary lesions, cells of metastatic foci have increased expression of several CSC markers, including CD133, CD166, nestin, and Notch family members, suggesting a role for CSCs in metastatic disease.[125–128] Also, the pluripotent nature of CSCs may explain why the overwhelming majority of melanoma cells that reach circulation do not result in successful metastases; Schatton and Frank suggest that the plasticity present in CSCs and absent in regular melanoma cells offers CSCs a selective advantage once they reach a premetastatic niche.[129]

Furthermore, the undifferentiated CSC, upon arrival and exposure to the stromal milieu, can then transform into what best suits the local environment – another possible explanation for clonal heterogeneity. Whatever their eventual role, CSCs will undergo further investigation, not only for characterization but for potential therapeutic targets as well.

## FUTURE OUTLOOK

The process of metastasis depends on multiple favorable interactions of metastatic cells with host homeostatic mechanisms. Interruption of one or more of these interactions can lead to the inhibition or eradication of cancer metastasis. For many years, all of our efforts to treat cancer have concentrated on the inhibition or destruction of tumor cells. Strategies both to treat tumor cells (e.g. chemotherapy and immunotherapy) and to modulate the host microenvironment (e.g. tumor vasculature) should provide additional approaches for cancer treatment. Building upon the recent advancements in our understanding of the biological basis of cancer metastasis will present unprecedented possibilities for translating basic research in cancer growth and metastasis to the clinical reality of more effective cancer therapies.

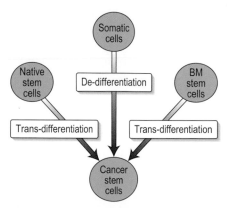

**Figure 1.7** Potential origins of cancer stem cells. (Adapted from La Porta CAM. Cancer stem cells and skin cancer. In: Majumder S, ed. *Stem Cells and Cancer.* New York, NY: Springer Science; 2009:251-267.)

# REFERENCES

1. National Cancer Institute. *Skin cancer*. http://www.cancer.gov/cancertopics/types/skin. Accessed 20.10.09.

2. Rogers HW, Weinstock MA, Harris AR, et al. Incidence estimate of nonmelanoma skin cancer in the United States, 2006. *Arch Dermatol*. 2010;146(3):283–287.

3. Balch CM, Soong SJ, Gershenwald JE, et al. Prognostic factor analysis of 17,600 melanoma patients: validation of the American Joint Committee on Cancer melanoma staging system. *J Clin Oncol*. 19:3622–3634.

4 Chiang AC, Massagué J. Molecular basis of metastasis. *N Engl J Med*. 359(26):2814–2823.

5. Kamb A, Shattuck-Eidens D, Eeles R, et al. Analysis of the p16 gene (CDKN2) as a candidate for the chromosome 9p melanoma susceptibility locus. *Nat Genet*. 1994;8:23–26.

6. Hussussian CJ, Struewing JP, Goldstein AM, et al. Germline p16 mutations in familial melanoma. *Nat Genet*. 1994;8:15–21.

7. Pollock PM, Trent JM. The genetics of cutaneous melanoma. *Clin Lab Med*. 2000;20:667–690.

8. Thompson JF, Scolyer RA, Kefford RF. Cutaneous melanoma. *Lancet*. 2005;365:687–701.

9. Santillan AA, Cherpelis BS, Glass LF, et al. Management of familial melanoma and nonmelanoma skin cancer syndromes. *Surg Oncol Clin N Am*. 2008;18:73–98.

10. Serrano M, Lee H, Chin L, et al. Role of the INK4a locus in tumor suppression and cell mortality. *Cell*. 1996;85:27–37.

11. Pomerantz J, Schreiber-Agus N, Liegeois NJ, et al. The Ink4a tumor suppressor gene product, p19Arf, interacts with MDM2 and neutralizes MDM2's inhibition of p53. *Cell*. 1998;92:713–723.

12. Harris SL, Levine AJ. The p53 pathway: positive and negative feedback loops. *Oncogene*. 2005;24:2899–2908.

13. Recio JA, Noonan FP, Takayama H, et al. Ink4a/arf deficiency promotes ultraviolet radiation-induced melanomagenesis. *Cancer Res*. 2002;62:6724–6730.

14. Sharpless E, Chin L. The INK4a/ARF locus and melanoma. *Oncogene*. 2003;22:3092–3098.

15. Miller AJ, Mihm MC. Melanoma. *N Engl J Med*. 2006;355(1):51–65.

16. Zuo L, Weger J, Yang Q, et al. Germline mutations in the p16INK4a binding domain of CDK4 in familial melanoma. *Nat Genet*. 1996;12:97–99.

17. Bastian BC, LeBoit PE, Pinkel D. Mutations and copy number increase of HRAS in Spitz nevi with distinctive histopathological features. *Am J Pathol*. 2000;157(3):967–972.

18. Van Raamsdonk CD, Bezrookove V, Green G, et al. Frequent somatic mutations of GNAQ in uveal melanoma and blue naevi. *Nature*. 2009;457(7229):599–602.

19. Michaloglou C, Vredeveld LC, Soengas MS, et al. BRAFE600-associated senescence-like cell cycle arrest of human naevi. *Nature*. 2005;436(7051):720–724.

20. Peeper DS, Dannenberg JH, Douma S, et al. Escape from premature senescence is not sufficient for oncogenic transformation by Ras. *Nat Cell Biol*. 2001;3:198–203.

21. Stahl JM, Cheung M, Sharma A, et al. Loss of PTEN promotes tumor development in malignant melanoma. *Cancer Res*. 2003;63:2881–2890.

22. Batinac T, Hadzisejdić I, Brumini G, et al. Expression of cell cycle and apoptosis regulatory proteins and telomerase in melanocytic lesions. *Coll Antropol*. 2007;31(suppl 1):17–22.

23. Folkman J. How is blood vessel growth regulated in normal and neoplastic tissue? GHA Clowes Memorial Award Lecture. *Cancer Res*. 1986;46:467–473.

24. Peters BA, Diaz LA, Polyak K, et al. Contribution of bone marrow-derived endothelial cells to human tumor vasculature. *Nat Med*. 2005;11:261–262.

25. Greenberg JI, Shields DJ, Barillas SG, et al. A role for VEGF as a negative regulator of pericyte function and vessel maturation. *Nature*. 2008;456:809–813.

26. Stockmann C, Doedens A, Weidemann A, et al. Deletion of vascular endothelial growth factor in myeloid cells accelerates tumorigenesis. *Nature*. 2008;456:814–818.

27. Yang L, DeBusk LM, Fukuda K, et al. Expansion of myeloid immune suppressor Gr1CD11b1 cells in tumor-bearing host directly promotes tumor angiogenesis. *Cancer Cell*. 2004;6:409–421.

28. Jin DK, Shido K, Kopp HG, et al. Cytokine-mediated deployment of SDF-1 induces revascularization through recruitment of CXCR41 hemangiocytes. *Nat Med*. 2006;12:557–567.

29. Heissig B, Hattori K, Dias S, et al. Recruitment of stem and progenitor cells from the bone marrow niche requires MMP-9 mediated release of kit-ligand. *Cell*. 2002;109:625–637.

30. Marneros AG. Tumor angiogenesis in melanoma. *Hematol Oncol Clin N Am*. 2009;23:431–446.

31. Nasarre P, Thomas M, Kruse K, et al. Host-derived angiopoietin-2 affects early stages of tumor development and vessel maturation but is dispensable for later stages of tumor growth. *Cancer Res*. 2009;69(4):1324–1333.

32. LeCouter J, Zlot C, Tejada M, et al. Bv8 and endocrine gland-derived vascular endothelial growth factor stimulate hematopoiesis and hematopoietic cell mobilization. *Proc Natl Acad Sci U S A*. 2004;101:16813–16818.

33. Jin DK, Shido K, Kopp HG, et al. Cytokine-mediated deployment of SDF-1 induces revascularization through recruitment of CXCR41 hemangiocytes. *Nat Med*. 2006;12:557–567.

34. Joukov V, Pajusola K, Kaipainen A, et al. A novel vascular endothelial growth factor, VEGF-C, is a ligand for the Flt4 (VEGFR-3) and KDR (VEGFR-2) receptor tyrosine kinases. *EMBO J*. 1996;15:1751.

35. Orlandini M, Marconcini L, Ferruzzi R, et al. Identification of a c-fos-induced gene that is related to the platelet-derived growth factor/vascular endothelial growth factor family. *Proc Natl Acad Sci U S A*. 1996;93:11675–11680.

36. Yamada Y, Nezu J, Shimane M, et al. Molecular cloning of a novel vascular endothelial growth factor, VEGF-D. *Genomics*. 1997;42:483–488.

37. Achen MG, Jeltsch M, Kukk E, et al. Vascular endothelial growth factor D (VEGF-D) is a ligand for the tyrosine kinases VEGF receptor 2 (Flk1) and VEGF receptor 3 (Flt4). *Proc Natl Acad Sci U S A*. 1998;95:548–553.

38. Rinderknecht M, Detmar M. Tumor lymphangiogenesis and melanoma metastasis. *J Cell Physiol*. 2008;216(2):347–354.

39. Kubo H, Cao R, Brakenhielm E, et al. Blockade of vascular endothelial growth factor receptor-3 signaling inhibits fibroblast growth factor-2-induced lymphangiogenesis in mouse cornea. *Proc Natl Acad Sci U S A*. 2002;99:8868–8873.

40. Chen Z, Varney ML, Backora MW, et al. Down-regulation of vascular endothelial cell growth factor-C expression using small interfering RNA vectors in mammary tumors inhibits tumor lymphangiogenesis and spontaneous metastasis and enhances survival. *Cancer Res*. 2005;65:9004–9011.

41. Shin JW, Min M, Larrieu-Lahargue F, et al. Prox1 promotes lineage-specific expression of fibroblast growth factor (FGF) receptor-3 in lymphatic endothelium: A role for FGF signaling in lymphangiogenesis. *Mol Biol Cell*. 2006;17:576–584.

42. Cao R, Bjorndahl MA, Religa P, et al. PDGF-BB induces intratumoral lymphangiogenesis and promotes lymphatic metastasis. *Cancer Cell*. 2004;6:333–345.

43. Kajiya K, Hirakawa S, Ma B, et al. Hepatocyte growth factor promotes lymphatic vessel formation and function. *EMBO J*. 2005;24:2885–2895.

44. Morisada T, Oike Y, Yamada Y, et al. Angiopoietin-1 promotes LYVE-1-positive lymphatic vessel formation. *Blood*. 2005;105:4649–4656.

45. Tammela T, Saaristo A, Lohela M, et al. Angiopoietin-1 promotes lymphatic sprouting and hyperplasia. *Blood*. 2005;105:4642–4648.

46. Gale NW, Thurston G, Hackett SF, et al. Angiopoietin-2 is required for postnatal angiogenesis and lymphatic patterning, and only the latter role is rescued by angiopoietin-1. *Dev Cell*. 2002;3:411–423.

47. Payette MJ, Katz 3rd M, Grant-Kels JM. Melanoma prognostic factors found in the dermatopathology report. *Clin Dermatol*. 2009;27(1):53–74.

48. Rodriguez M, Aladowicz E, Lanfrancone L, et al. Tbx3 represses E-cadherin expression and enhances melanoma invasiveness. *Cancer Res*. 2008;68(19):7872–7881.

49. Molina-Ortiz I, Bartolomé RA, Hernández-Varas P, et al. Overexpression of E-cadherin on melanoma cells inhibits chemokine-promoted invasion involving p190RhoGAP/p120ctn-dependent inactivation of RhoA. *J Biol Chem*. 2009;284(22):15147–15157.

50. Kuphal S, Martyn AC, Pedley J, et al. H-cadherin expression reduces invasion of malignant melanoma. *Pigment Cell Melanoma Res*. 2009;22(3):296–306.

51. Brooks PC, Stromblad S, Sanders LC, et al. Localization of matrix metalloproteinase MMP-2 to the surface of invasive cells by interaction with integrin alpha v beta 3. *Cell*. 1996;85:683–693.

52. Felding-Habermann B, Fransvea E, O'Toole TE, et al. Involvement of tumor cell integrin alpha v beta 3 in hematogenous metastasis of human melanoma cells. *Clin Exp Metastasis*. 2002;19:427–436.

53. Hofmann UB, Westphal JR, Waas ET, et al. Coexpression of integrin alpha(v)beta3 and matrix metalloproteinase-2 (MMP-2) coincides with MMP-2 activation: correlation with melanoma progression. *J Invest Dermatol*. 2000;115:625–632.

54. Tzukert K, Shimony N, Krasny L, et al. Human melanoma cells expressing the alphavbeta3 integrin are partially protected from necrotic cell death induced by dynamic matrix detachment. *Cancer Lett*. 2010;290(2):174–181.

55. Govindarajan B, Sligh JE, Vincent BJ, et al. Overexpression of Akt converts radial growth melanoma to vertical growth melanoma. *J Clin Invest*. 2007;117(3):719–729.

56. Hodgson L, Henderson AJ, Dong C. Melanoma cell migration to type IV collagen requires activation of NF-kappaB. *Oncogene*. 2003;22(1):98–108.

57. Araki K, Shimura T, Yajima T, et al. Phosphoglucose isomerase/autocrine motility factor promotes melanoma cell migration through ERK activation dependent on autocrine production of interleukin-8. *J Biol Chem*. 2009;284(47):32305–32311.

58. Yang J, Price MA, Li GY, et al. Melanoma proteoglycan modifies gene expression to stimulate tumor cell motility, growth, and epithelial-to-mesenchymal transition. *Cancer Res*. 2009;69(19):7538–7547.

59. Sanz-Moreno V, Marshall CJ. Rho-GTPase signaling drives melanoma cell plasticity. *Cell Cycle*. 2009;8(10):1484–1487.

60. Sanz-Moreno V, Gadea G, Ahn J, et al. Rac activation and inactivation control plasticity of tumor cell movement. *Cell*. 2008;135(3):510–523.

61. Gadea G, Sanz-Moreno V, Self A, et al. DOCK10-mediated Cdc42 activation is necessary for amoeboid invasion of melanoma cells. *Curr Biol*. 2008;18(19):1456–1465.

62. Clark EA, Golub TR, Lander ES, et al. Genomic analysis of metastasis reveals an essential role for RhoC. *Nature*. 2000;406(6795):532–535.

63. Ferraro D, Corso S, Fasano E, et al. Pro-metastatic signaling by c-Met through RAC-1 and reactive oxygen species (ROS). *Oncogene*. 2006;25(26):3689–3698.

64. Ruoslahti E. Fibronectin and its a5b1 integrin receptor in malignancy. *Inv Metastasis*. 1994–1995;14:87–94.

65. Morikawa K, Walker SM, Nakajima M, et al. The influence of organ environment on the growth, selection, and metastasis of human colon cancer cells in nude mice. *Cancer Res*. 1988;48:6863–6871.

66. Davis ID, Chen W, Jackson H, et al. Recombinant NY-ESO-1 protein with ISCOMATRIX adjuvant induces broad integrated antibody and CD4(+) and CD8(+) T cell responses in humans. *Proc Natl Acad Sci U S A*. 2004;101:10697–10702.

67. Peterson AC, Harlin H, Gajewski TF. Immunization with Melan-A peptide-pulsed peripheral blood mononuclear cells plus recombinant human interleukin-12 induces clinical activity and T-cell responses in advanced melanoma. *J Clin Oncol*. 2003;21:2342–2348.

68. Rosenberg SA, Yang JC, Schwartzentruber DJ, et al. Immunologic and therapeutic evaluation of a synthetic peptide vaccine for the treatment of patients with metastatic melanoma. *Nat Med*. 1998;4:321–327.

69. Rosenberg SA, Sherry RM, Morton KE, et al. Tumor progression can occur despite the induction of very high levels of self/tumor antigen-specific CD8+ T cells in patients with melanoma. *J Immunol*. 2005;175:6169–6176.

70. Fallarino F, Uyttenhove C, Boon T, et al. Improved efficacy of dendritic cell vaccines and successful immunization with tumor antigen peptide-pulsed peripheral blood mononuclear cells by coadministration of recombinant murine interleukin-12. *Int J Cancer*. 1999;80:324–333.

71. Blank C, Brown I, Kacha AK, et al. ICAM-1 contributes to but is not essential for tumor antigen cross-priming and CD8+ T cell-mediated tumor rejection in vivo. *J Immunol*. 2005;174:3416–3420.

72. Spiotto MT, Yu P, Rowley DA, et al. Increasing tumor antigen expression overcomes "ignorance" to solid tumors via crosspresentation by bone marrow-derived stromal cells. *Immunity*. 2002;17:737–747.

73. Velicu S, Han Y, Ulasov I, et al. Cross-priming of T cells to intracranial tumor antigens elicits an immune response that fails in the effector phase but can be augmented with local immunotherapy. *J Neuroimmunol*. 2006;174:74–81.

74. Drake CG, Doody AD, Mihalyo MA, et al. Androgen ablation mitigates tolerance to a prostate/prostate cancer-restricted antigen. *Cancer Cell*. 2005;7:239–249.

75. Nguyen LT, Elford AR, Murakami K, et al. Tumor growth enhances cross-presentation leading to limited T cell activation without tolerance. *J Exp Med*. 2002;195:423–435.

76. Valmori D, Dutoit V, Liénard D, et al. Naturally occurring human lymphocyte antigen-A2 restricted CD8+ T-cell response to the cancer testis antigen NY-ESO-1 in melanoma patients. *Cancer Res*. 2000;60:4499–4506.

77. Jager E, Stockert E, Zidianakis Z, et al. Humoral immune responses of cancer patients against "cancer-testis" antigen NY-ESO-1: correlation with clinical events. *Int J Cancer*. 1999;84:506–510.

78. Van den Hove LE, Van Gool SW, Van Poppel H, et al. Phenotype, cytokine production and cytolytic capacity of fresh (uncultured) tumour-infiltrating T lymphocytes in human renal cell carcinoma. *Clin Exp Immunol*. 1997;109:501–509.

79. Roussel E, Gingras MC, Grimm EA, et al. Predominance of a type 2 intratumoural immune response in fresh tumour-infiltrating lymphocytes from human gliomas. *Clin Exp Immunol*. 1996;105:344–352.

80. Nakagomi H, Pisa P, Pisa EK, et al. Lack of interleukin-2 (IL-2) expression and selective expression of IL-10 mRNA in human renal cell carcinoma. *Int J Cancer*. 1995;63:366–371.

81. Fields P, Fitch FW, Gajewski TF. Control of T lymphocyte signal transduction through clonal anergy. *J Mol Med*. 1996;74:673–683.

82. Fields PE, Gajewski TF, Fitch FW. Blocked Ras activation in anergic CD4+ T cells. *Science*. 1996;271:1276–1278.

83. Zhou G, Drake CG, Levitsky HI. Amplification of tumor-specific regulatory T cells following therapeutic cancer vaccines. *Blood*. 2006;107:628–636.

84. Viguier M, Lemaître F, Verola O, et al. Foxp3 expressing CD4+ CD25(high) regulatory T cells are overrepresented in human metastatic melanoma lymph nodes and inhibit the function of infiltrating T cells. *J Immunol*. 2004;173:1444–1453.

85. Curiel TJ, Coukos G, Zou L, et al. Specific recruitment of regulatory T cells in ovarian carcinoma fosters immune privilege and predicts reduced survival. *Nat Med*. 2004;10:942–949.

86. Kryczek I, Zou L, Rodriguez P, et al. B7-H4 expression identifies a novel suppressive macrophage population in human ovarian carcinoma. *J Exp Med*. 2006;203:871–881.

87. Blesson S, Thiery J, Gaudin C, et al. Analysis of the mechanisms of human cytotoxic T lymphocyte response inhibition by NO. *Int Immunol*. 2002;14:1169–1178.

88. Bingisser RM, Tilbrook PA, Holt PG, et al. Macrophage-derived nitric oxide regulates T cell activation via reversible disruption of the Jak3/STAT5 signaling pathway. *J Immunol*. 1998;160:5729–5734.

89. Ekmekcioglu S, Ellerhorst JA, Prieto, et al. Tumor iNOS predicts poor survival for stage III melanoma patients. *Int J Cancer*. 2006;119:861–866.

90. Gorelik L, Flavell RA. Immune-mediated eradication of tumors through the blockade of transforming growth factor-beta signaling in T cells. *Nat Med*. 2001;7:1118–1122.

91. Peng Y, Laouar Y, Li MO, et al. TGF-beta regulates in vivo expansion of Foxp3-expressing CD4+CD25+ regulatory T cells responsible for protection against diabetes. *Proc Natl Acad Sci U S A*. 2004;101:4572–4577.

92. Zha YY, Blank C, Gajewski TF. Negative regulation of T-cell function by PD-1. *Crit Rev Immunol*. 2004;24:229–238.

93. Dong H, Strome SE, Salomao DR, et al. Tumor-associated B7-H1 promotes T-cell apoptosis: a potential mechanism of immune evasion. *Nat Med*. 2002;8:793–800.

94. Tseng SY, Otsuji M, Gorski K, et al. B7-DC, a new dendritic cell molecule with potent costimulatory properties for T cells. *J Exp Med*. 2001;193:839–846.

95. Zang X, Loke P, Kim J, et al. B7x: a widely expressed B7 family member that inhibits T cell activation. *Proc Natl Acad Sci U S A*. 2003;100:10388–10392.

96. Sica GL, Choi IH, Zhu G, et al. B7-H4, a molecule of the B7 family, negatively regulates T cell immunity. *Immunity*. 2003;18:849–861.

97. Uyttenhove C, Pilotte L, Théate I, et al. Evidence for a tumoral immune resistance mechanism based on tryptophan degradation by indoleamine 2,3- dioxygenase. *Nat Med*. 2003;9:1269–1274.

98. Fallarino F, Grohmann U, Vacca C, et al. T cell apoptosis by tryptophan catabolism. *Cell Death Differ*. 2002;9:1069–1077.

99. Grohmann U, Fallarino F, Puccetti P. Tolerance, DCs and tryptophan: much ado about IDO. *Trends Immunol*. 2003;24:242–248.

100. Gajewski TF, Meng Y, Blank C, et al. Immune resistance orchestrated by the tumor microenvironment. *Immunol Rev*. 2006;213:131–145.

101. Fidler IJ. Metastasis: quantitative analysis of distribution and fate of tumor emboli labeled with 125I-5-iodo-2'-deoxyuridine. *J Natl Cancer Inst*. 1970;45:773–782.

102. Gasic GJ. Role of plasma, platelets and endothelial cells in tumor metastasis. *Cancer Metastasis Rev*. 1984;3:99–114.

103. Fidler IJ, Bucana C. Mechanism of tumor cell resistance to lysis by syngeneic lymphocytes. *Cancer Res*. 1977;37:3945–3956.

104. Nesbit M, Herlyn M. Adhesion receptors in human melanoma progression. *Inv Metastasis*. 1994–1995;14:131–138.

105. Ruoslahti E. Fibronectin and its α5β1 integrin receptor in malignancy. *Inv Metastasis*. 1994–1995;14:87–94.

106. Muller A, Homey B, Soto H, et al. Involvement of chemokine receptors in breast cancer metastasis. *Nature*. 2001;410:50–56.

107. Economou MA, All-Ericsson C, Bykov V, et al. Receptors for the liver synthesized growth factors IGF-1 and HGF/SF in uveal melanoma: intercorrelation and prognostic implications. *Acta Ophthalmol*. 2008;86 Thesis 4: 20–25.

108. Hirakawa S, Kodama S, Kunstfeld R, et al. VEGF-A induces tumor and sentinel lymph node lymphangiogenesis and promotes lymphatic metastasis. *J Exp Med*. 2005;201:1089–1099.

109. Hirakawa S, Brown LF, Kodama S, et al. VEGF-C-induced lymphangiogenesis in sentinel lymph nodes promotes tumor metastasis to distant sites. *Blood*. 2007;109:1010–1017.

110. Kaplan RN, Riba RD, Zacharoulis S, et al. VEGFR1-positive haematopoietic bone marrow progenitors initiate the pre-metastatic niche. *Nature*. 2005;438:820–827.

111. Kaplan RN, Rafii S, Lyden D. Preparing the "soil": the premetastatic niche. *Cancer Res*. 2006;66(23):11089–11093.

112. Fidler IJ, Talmadge JE. Evidence that intravenously derived murine pulmonary melanoma metastases can originate from the expansion of a single tumor cell. *Cancer Res*. 1986;46(10):5167–5171.

113. La Porta CAM. Cancer stem cells and skin cancer. In: Majumder S, ed. Stem Cells and Cancer. New York, NY: Springer Science; 2009:251–267.

114. Niemann C, Watt FM. Designer skin: lineage commitment in postnatal epidermis. *Trends Cell Biol*. 2002;12:185–192.

115. Owens DM, Watt FM. Contribution of stem cells and differentiated cells to epidermal tumors. *Nat Rev Cancer*. 2003;3:444–451.

116. Fuchs E, Tumbar T, Guash G. Socializing with the neighbours: stem cells and their niche. *Cell*. 2004;166:769–778.

117. Hutchin ME, Kariapper MS, Grachtchouk M, et al. Sustained Hedgehog signaling is required for basal cell carcinoma proliferation and survival: conditioning skin tumorigenesis recapitulates the hair growth cycle. *Genes Dev*. 2005;19:214–223.

**118.** Grabber C, van Boehmer H, Look AT. Notch 1 activation in the molecular pathogenesis of T cell acute lymphoblastic leukemia. *Nat Rev Cancer*. 2006;6:347–359.

**119.** Taipale NJ, Beachy PA. The hedgehog and Wnt signaling pathways in cancer. *Nature*. 2001;411:349–354.

**120.** Jacobs JJ, Scheijen B, von Cken JW, et al. Bmi-1 collaborates with c-Myc in tumorgenesis by inhibiting c-Myc induced apoptosis via INK-4alpha/ARK. *Gene Dev*. 1999;13:2678–2690.

**121.** van Rhenen A, Feller N, Kelder A, et al. High stem cell frequency in acute myeloid leukemia at diagnosis predicts high minimal residual disease and poor survival. *Clin Cancer Res*. 2005;11:6520–6527.

**122.** Bao S, Wu Q, McLendon RE, et al. Glioma stem cells promote radioresistance by preferential activation of the DNA damage response. *Nature*. 2006;444:756–760.

**123.** Fang D, Nguyen TK, Leishear K, et al. A tumorigenic subpopulation with stem cell properties in melanomas. *Cancer Res*. 2005;65:9328–9337.

**124.** Frank NY, Margaryan A, Huang Y, et al. ABCB5-mediated doxorubicin transport and chemoresistance in human malignant melanoma. *Cancer Res*. 2005;65(10):4320–4333.

**125.** Klein WM, Wu BP, Zhao S, et al. Increased expression of stem cell markers in malignant melanoma. *Mod Pathol*. 2007;20:102–107.

**126.** Van Kempen LC, Van Den Oord JJ, Van Muijen GN, et al. Activated leukocyte cell adhesion molecule /CD166, a marker of tumor progression in primary malignant melanoma of the skin. *Am J Pathol*. 2000;156:769–774.

**127.** Balint K, Xiao M, Pinnix CC, et al. Activation of Notch1 signaling is required for beta-catenin-mediated human primary melanoma progression. *J Clin Invest*. 2005;115:3166–3176.

**128.** Massi D, Tarantini F, Franchi A, et al. Evidence for differential expression of Notch receptors and their ligands in melanocytic nevi and cutaneous malignant melanoma. *Mod Pathol*. 2006;19:246–254.

**129.** Schatton T, Frank MH. Cancer stem cells and human malignant melanoma. *Pigment Cell Melanoma Res*. 2008;21(1):39–55.

# Genetics of Skin Cancer

*Oscar R. Colegio and David J. Leffell*

## Key Points

- Specific genes implicated in causing each major form of skin cancer have been identified through genetic studies on hereditary and/or sporadic skin cancer. Their role in promoting cutaneous neoplasia is supported and confirmed by functional studies in animal model systems.

- Defects in the *CDKN2A* tumor suppressor locus are associated with both familial and sporadic cutaneous malignant melanoma and may cooperate with *RAS* or *RAF* proto-oncogene activation to promote tumor formation.

- Mutations resulting in *RAS* proto-oncogene activation may cooperate with inactivation of either *CDKN2A* or *p53* tumor suppressor genes in causing cutaneous squamous cell carcinoma.

- Defects in the *PTCH* gene have been implicated in both hereditary and sporadic basal cell carcinoma and mutations in genes encoding other components of the SHH signaling pathway have been associated with sporadic tumors. Defects in the *p53* tumor suppressor gene are common in basal cell carcinoma as well.

- Although significant advances have been made in identifying genes associated with skin cancers, additional yet-to-be-identified genes likely contribute to the pathogenesis of each major form of skin cancer.

## INTRODUCTION

Tumorigenesis is a multi-staged process that derives from a series of genetic alterations, some of which are acquired and others inherited. Genetic aberrations that result in tumor formation alter basic cellular processes, including cell differentiation, cell cycle regulation and cell death. Significant progress has been made over the past two decades in identifying genes associated with specific cancers. The study of hereditary and sporadic skin cancers has led to the identification of numerous genes critical to tumorigenesis. Functional studies using in-vitro and in-vivo models have verified the critical role these genes play in tumor formation.

Cancer-associated genes fall into two general categories: proto-oncogenes and tumor suppressor genes (Fig. 2.1). Proto-oncogenes, such as *RAS* and *RAF*, normally regulate cell proliferation or survival. However, upon mutation, proto-oncogenes may be activated to become oncogenes, which allows them to bypass regulatory mechanisms that normally prevent their function in an uncontrolled manner. An activating mutation in just one allele is typically sufficient to contribute to tumorigenesis. By contrast, tumor suppressor genes, such as those encoded in the *CDKN2A* locus and the *TP53* gene, normally inhibit cell cycle progression and proliferation. Inactivation of both alleles of such genes, through mutation, deletion or silencing, is typically required to lose suppressor function and permit tumor formation.

Another form of regulation of both proto-oncogenes and tumor suppressor genes is epigenetic modification that results in the enhancement or silencing of gene expression. These modifications do not change the DNA sequence of the genes but rather affect their expression by covalently modifying either DNA-associated proteins, such as histones, or the DNA itself. Patterns of epigenetic changes linked with specific cancer-associated genes are being established.[1]

In addition, mRNA stability can further be regulated by microRNAs, single-stranded RNA molecules that are 21 to 23 nucleotides in length. MicroRNAs are predicted to regulate the mRNA stability of up to 33% of all genes. They function by encoding complementary sequences to their target genes such that upon binding, the target mRNA is either degraded or its translation to protein is inhibited.[2] MicroRNAs associated with specific cancers are beginning to be identified and functionally characterized. This chapter reviews and summarizes the current understanding of the genetic basis of the three predominant forms of skin cancer: basal cell carcinoma, squamous cell carcinoma, and melanoma.

## BASAL CELL CARCINOMA

The most common human malignancies are non-melanoma skin cancers, and among these cancers, basal cell carcinoma (BCC) is the most common type. Insights into the molecular pathogenesis of basal cell carcinomas were originally derived from the genetic analysis of kindreds with basal cell nevus syndrome (BCNS; Gorlin syndrome, OMIM 109400). This syndrome is inherited in an autosomal dominant manner and is characterized by the development of hundreds of BCCs, which can be generalized but are often concentrated in sun-exposed areas. Further, individuals with BCNS demonstrate an increased sensitivity to ionizing radiation, with BCCs developing within radiation ports. Other features of BCNS include palmoplantar pits, odontogenic cysts, calcification of the falx cerebri, skeletal abnormalities, and the development of medulloblastoma.

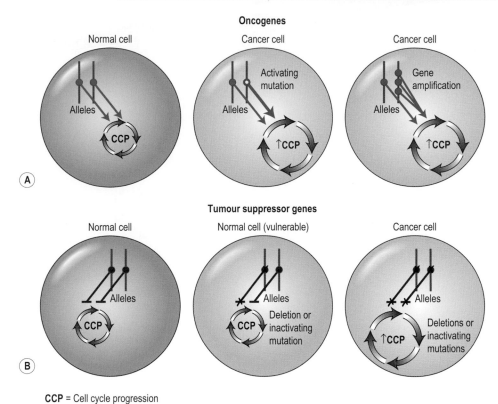

Oncogenes

Tumour suppressor genes

CCP = Cell cycle progression
↑CCP = Increased cell cycle progression

**Figure 2.1** Oncogenes versus tumor suppressor genes. **A)** Proto-oncogenes control the rate of cell cycle progression under physiologic conditions (left cell). Proto-oncogenes can become oncogenes upon acquiring an activating mutation (represented by the yellow dot on the right allele in the center cell) or through gene number amplification (represented by the acquisition of several alleles on the right chromosome in the right cell). As a result of these genetic aberrations, cell cycle progression can be increased in a dominant manner. **B)** Tumor suppressors often control cell proliferation (left cell), functioning in a recessive manner as a brake on cell cycle progression (center cell). Loss of both alleles of tumor suppressor genes through deletions or mutations is typically required for their complete loss of function (right cell). (Adapted from Ponten F, Lundeberg J, Asplund A. Principles of tumor biology and pathogenesis of BCCs and SCCs. In: Bolognia J, Jorizzo J, Rapini R, eds. *Dermatology*. 2nd ed. Philadelphia; Elsevier; 2008.)

Linkage analysis of BCNS identified a chromosomal locus at 9q22.3,[3] a locus also found to be deleted in sporadic BCCs.[4] Subsequently, mutations in *PTCH1*, the human homolog of the *Drosophila patched* gene located at 9q22.3, were identified.[5,6] *PTCH1* encodes a transmembrane receptor for the hedgehog family of soluble effector proteins.

## The hedgehog pathway

The hedgehog signaling pathway is critical to tissue development and homeostasis. First identified in the fruit fly *Drosophila melanogaster*, hedgehog was found to be one of a set of genes critical to establishing anterior and posterior polarity within the developing fly;[7] flies without hedgehog were found to be shorter than wild-type flies. In vertebrates, hedgehog plays a role in neural tube development.[8] Hedgehog is a secreted lipoprotein that has three mammalian orthologs: sonic hedgehog, Indian hedgehog, and desert hedgehog. Sonic hedgehog signals through the patched family of receptors.

The *PTCH1* gene encodes the 12-span transmembrane protein patched that is the receptor for sonic hedgehog. When sonic hedgehog binds patched, the constitutive inhibition of the G-protein receptor smoothened is released, resulting in the release of the Gli (glioma-associated oncogene) transcription factors (Gli1, Gli2, Gli3) from a cytosolic inhibitory complex. This leads to nuclear localization of Gli and a subsequent signaling cascade, which includes a feed-forward induction of *PTCH1* (Fig. 2.2). Gli proteins are members of the Kruppel family of zinc finger transcription factors and have been found to mediate activation (Gli1, Gli2) and inhibition (Gli3) of transcription of numerous

genes. Tumor-promoting Gli targets include *PDGFRα*, *WNT* and *IGF2*. Recent studies using small alkaloid molecules that bind smoothened and inhibit the downstream activation of the hedgehog pathway have demonstrated significant antitumor effects against BCCs and may be useful therapeutic agents for treating patients with BCNS or locally advanced BCCs.[9]

The protein that holds Gli in an inhibitory complex is SUFU, a human homolog of the *Drosophila* suppressor of fused. As would be predicted, loss of SUFU results in a phenotype consistent with constitutive Gli activation. Mice that are *Sufu+/−* develop odontogenic cysts and basaloid epidermal proliferations.[10,11] In human studies, mutations in *SUFU* have been found in children with medulloblastomas;[12] SUFU mutations have not yet been identified in BCCs.

The hedgehog pathway has been found to rely on the primary cilium during development. Primary cilia are cellular organelles that are present on most cells of the body and play a critical role in intercellular and environmental communication. When hedgehog is present, PTCH1 relocates from the primary cilium to endosomes; conversely, smoothened relocates from intracellular vesicles to the primary cilium. Intriguingly, recent studies in murine models of tumorigenesis have demonstrated that when the primary cilium is absent in cells, activated SMO fails to induce expression of hedgehog target genes and to generate tumors.[13,14]

*PTCH2* encodes a homolog of *PTCH1* with ~73% amino acid similarity to *PTCH1*. The role of *PTCH2* remains undefined; a murine knockout of *Ptch2* results in mice with no increased susceptibility to developing tumors. However,

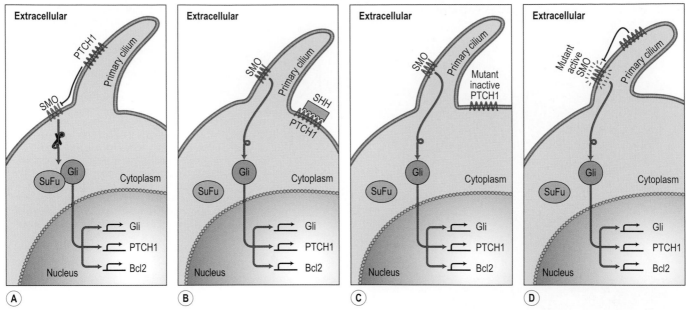

**Figure 2.2** The hedgehog signaling pathway. **A)** Patched-1 that is not bound to its ligand, hedgehog, inhibits smoothened signaling. **B)** Upon binding hedgehog, patched-1-mediated repression of smoothened signaling is removed, resulting in the release of activating Gli transcription factors (Gli1, Gli2) from a cytosolic inhibitory complex with SuFu. The Gli transcription factors induce a cascade of gene expression in the nucleus. **C)** Inactivating mutations in patched-1 results in loss of smoothened repression and constitutive expression of Gli gene targets. **D)** Activating mutations in smoothened result in constitutive expression of Gli gene targets despite attempted repression by patched-1.

crossing *Ptch1+/−* with *Ptch2−/−* mice resulted in a higher incidence of tumors and a broader spectrum of types of tumors than in *Ptch1+/−* mice, suggesting that patched-2 may complement the tumor suppressor role of patched-1.[15] In support of this hypothesis, *Ptch2* expression levels have been found to be increased in medulloblastomas in which *Ptch1* expression is reduced. In humans, mutant *PTCH2* was found to be associated with nevoid basal cell carcinoma syndrome in a Han Chinese kindred.[16]

Like BCCs, medulloblastomas have been found to develop as a result of mutations within the hedgehog signaling pathway. Recently, a microRNA family, the miR-17~19 cluster family, was found to be overexpressed in human medulloblastomas, and forced expression of these microRNAs in *Ink4c−/− ; Ptch1+/−* mice resulted in the development of medulloblastomas. Whether these microRNAs or others will play a role in the pathogenesis of BCCs remains unknown.

The pathways through which hedgehog signaling induces tumorigenesis remain unclear. Forced expression of *SHH* was demonstrated to downregulate the expression of p21CIP1, a cell cycle inhibitor.[17] In a murine model, elimination of *Ptch1* from mouse skin resulted in basal cell-like tumors that were found to have accumulated the cell cycle regulators cyclin D1 and B1 within their nuclei.[18] Further, patched-1 has been demonstrated to bind directly to cyclin B1 and thus prevent its translocation in the nucleus. This leads to mitogenic progression, suggesting that patched-1 may have cell cycle gatekeeper functions.[19]

## p53 tumor suppressor

Mutations in the gene encoding the p53 tumor suppressor have been found in more than half of sporadic BCCs. The inactivating mutations usually bear evidence of UV induction, bearing CC → TT and C → T substitutions produced by the photoproducts of adjacent pyrimidines. In one study of the prevalence of *TP53* and *PTCH1* mutations in sporadic BCCs, it was found that among 18 BCCs, 61% demonstrated loss of 9q markers (*PTCH1*), 61% had acquired *TP53* mutations, and 39% had alterations in both genes.[4] In subsequent studies, 38% of early onset BCCs were found to have mutations in both *TP53* and *PTCH1*[20] and 75% of all BCCs were found to have allelic loss of 9q and a *TP53* mutation.[21]

## Other syndromes

In addition to BCNS, non-syndromic multiple basal cell carcinomas (OMIM 605462) have been described in several families, one in which male-to-male transmission was noted and three which were strictly unilateral.[22] Whether these presentations represented mutations in genes known to be associated with BCC in a mosaic pattern has not been determined. More recently, a family was described in which numerous BCCs developed in a generalized distribution, most likely in an autosomal dominant fashion.[23,24]

In Rombo syndrome (OMIM 180730), multiple basal cell carcinomas are accompanied by vermiculate atrophoderma, milia, hypotrichosis, telangiectasias and acral erythema. Bazex syndrome (Bazex–Dupre–Christol syndrome, OMIM 301845) is characterized by the triad of multiple basal cell carcinomas, congenital hypotrichosis, and follicular atrophoderma. Whereas the gene defects which give rise to these syndromes have yet to be determined, the X-linked mode of inheritance of Bazex syndrome suggests that additional genes within the same pathway or novel pathways have yet to be determined.

## SQUAMOUS CELL CARCINOMA

Squamous cell carcinoma (SCC) is a common type of skin cancer, which has incidence rates that greatly vary according to environmental sun exposure, from 5 per 100,000 per year in Finland for females to 1035 per 100,000 per year in Australia for males.[25] In contrast to BCC and melanoma, specific associations of hereditary syndromes with SCC have not been described. In the absence of such an associated syndrome, identification of genes specific to the development of SCC has been complex.

Most genetic analyses of cutaneous SCC have focused on oncogenes and tumor suppressor genes known to contribute to the development of other forms of cancers when altered. Studies have focused predominantly on *RAS* proto-oncogenes or the *CDKN2A* or *p53* tumor suppressor genes. A variety of mutation analysis studies on sporadic SCCs and functional studies forcing aberrant gene expression have provided considerable insight into the molecular pathogenesis of SCC.

## *RAS* gene defects in SCC

The *RAS* family genes (*H-RAS, K-RAS, N-RAS and R-RAS*) encode membrane-associated GTPases that signal downstream of activated cell surface receptors, such as tyrosine kinase receptors, G-protein-coupled receptors, and integrin cell adhesion receptors. *RAS* proteins regulate signaling from the cell surface to the nucleus to alter patterns of gene expression and regulate cell proliferation and differentiation (Fig. 2.3).[26] Activating mutations in the *RAS* family of proto-oncogenes are among the most common genetic abnormalities identified in human cancers. These mutations result in constitutive activation of signaling pathways downstream of *RAS* which affect numerous cellular activities, including progression through the cell cycle and resistance to programmed cell death or apoptosis.[26] A variety of activating *RAS* mutations has been reported. These mutations occur at a wide range of different frequencies in SCCs. For example, a common mutation in which a valine is substituted for a glycine at position 12 of *H-RAS* was found in 35% to 46% of SCCs of skin.[27,28] Mutations in the related genes *K-RAS* and *N-RAS* were not found to exist in the same frequencies. Importantly, genetic analysis of actinic keratoses (AKs), precursor lesions of SCCs, has revealed that 16% of AKs have *H-RAS* or *K-RAS* mutations. This suggests that mutations in *RAS* may be an early event in the pathogenesis of cutaneous SCCs.[29]

In support of the human disease genetic correlates, studies in mouse keratinocytes have revealed that *RAS* activation is an important early event in the development of cutaneous SCCs. Primary murine keratinocytes that are forced to express the oncogene *v-ras Ha* develop into benign squamous papillomas when grafted onto immunodeficient mice. Activated *RAS* has been demonstrated to circumvent apoptosis, or programmed cell death, through multiple downstream pathways,[30,31] which may be one of its effects that result in tumorigenesis.

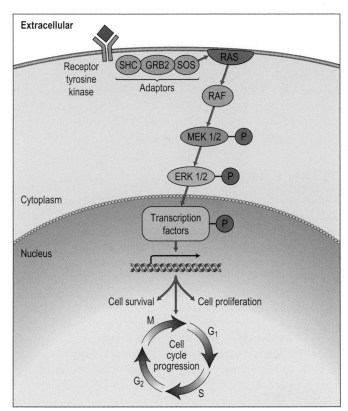

**Figure 2.3** *RAS* signaling pathway. The *RAS* family of genes encode small GTPases that become activated upon stimulation by receptor tyrosine kinases, G-protein-coupled receptors or integrins. *RAS* proteins signal to the RAF family of serine/threonine kinases which begins the MAP kinase signaling cascade. Shown in the figure, RAF phosphorylates MEK1/2, and MEK1/2 phosphorylates ERK1/2, which accumulates in the nucleus where it activates numerous transcription factors through phosphorylation. These transcription factors lead to cell cycle progression, cell proliferation and cell survival. Oncogenic activating mutations in *RAS* and *RAF* genes result in constitutive activation of the *RAS* signaling pathway.

However, *RAS* activation alone is not sufficient for SCC tumorigenesis, indicating that additional genetic lesions or alterations in gene expression are required for transformation to the premalignant and malignant lesions in which cell proliferation is unregulated. Forced expression of activated H-*RAS* in primary human keratinocytes induces growth arrest, presumably as a means of protecting against unregulated *RAS* activity.[32,33] This growth arrest appears to be mediated by *RAS*-induced expression of CDK inhibitors and suppression of *CDK4* expression, resulting in blockade of the cell cycle in G1, prior to DNA synthesis. To bypass this blockade in the cell cycle, forced co-expression of both activated *RAS* and either CDK4 or IκBα in primary human keratinocytes results in tumors resembling invasive SCCs when grafted onto immunodeficient mice.[32,33] IκBα is an inhibitor of NF-κB, a transcription factor that inhibits the proliferation of primary human keratinocytes.[34] IκBα was found to induce the expression of the cell cycle activator *CDK4* to bypass *RAS*-induced growth arrest, thus leading to cell proliferation. These studies of tumor models demonstrate how alterations in the *RAS* and CDK4 pathways may cooperate to circumvent apoptosis and bypass growth arrest leading to cell proliferation, respectively, to promote SCC tumorigenesis.

## CDKN2A gene defects in SCC

Chromosomal deletions have been found to be prevalent in SCCs. Specifically, deletions in 9p are common, and have been reported in 30% to 50% of SCCs.[35,36] The tumor suppressor CDKN2A is encoded at 9p21, and mutations at this locus have been found in 9% to 42% of SCCs. And like the RAS mutations, deletions in the CDKN2A locus have been found in approximately 21% of AKs.[37]

## p53 gene defects in SCC

Mutations in TP53, which encodes the tumor suppressor p53, have been described in a variety of human cancers, including SCC of the skin. p53 has been termed 'guardian of the genome' as it functions to control cell cycle progression and apoptosis in response to DNA damage. With mild DNA damage, p53 blocks cell cycle progression at the G1 stage by inducing the expression of p21CIP1, which inhibits cyclin-dependent kinases (CDK) 2 and 4. This G1 blockade allows for DNA repair prior to DNA replication in S phase. If the DNA damage is severe, p53 mediates a programmed cell death known as apoptosis by inducing the expression of BAX, an inhibitor of the anti-apoptotic protein Bcl-2. Therefore, without p53, cells that acquire DNA damage are unable to stall DNA replication so as to repair the acquired damage. Some of these damaged cells persist, out-compete their neighboring cells and form tumors.

The high frequency with which mutations in TP53 have been found in SCCs provides evidence supporting the critical role p53 plays in the pathogenesis of cutaneous SCC. The reported rate of TP53 mutations in SCCs ranges between 41% and 69%. The precancerous AKs also acquire TP53 mutations at a frequency of 50% to 60%.[38–40] Many of the genetic lesions in TP53 bear the UV signature CC → TT or C → T tandem transition mutations. These genetic findings suggest that mutations in TP53 may represent early events in the pathogenesis of SCC and that UV irradiation contributes to these genetic lesions.

Experimental models using UV irradiation support a role for p53 in the development of AKs and SCCs. Early insights into the critical role of p53 in SCCs came from studies in which mice deficient in p53 were irradiated with UV light. In normal mice, UV radiation-induced p53 mediates cell cycle arrest and, with increasing levels, apoptosis of keratinocytes. The apoptotic 'sunburn cells' develop after UVB irradiation in an attempt to abort the aberrant cell. Significantly fewer sunburn cells were detected in the skin of UV-irradiated keratinocytes lacking p53, and this correlated with the development of AKs and SCCs.[41] Additional studies have verified that mice deficient in p53 develop the full spectrum of premalignant AKs, SCCs in situ and invasive SCCs upon UV irradiation.[42,43]

The combinatorial effects of multiple gene pathways may play a role in SCC tumorigenesis. Primary murine keratinocytes that are p53-deficient and are forced to express the oncogene v-rasHa develop SCCs when grafted onto immunodeficient mice. Murine keratinocytes expressing oncogenic RAS do not spontaneously develop SCCs; however, when challenged with UV irradiation, they develop SCCs, possibly because of the loss of p53. Similarly, when keratinocytes lacking p19ARF (murine equivalent of the human p14ARF) are forced to express oncogenic RAS, invasive SCCs develop. As expression of p19ARF is known to result in the stabilization of p53, tumor formation upon the loss of p19ARF represents an alternative pathway to disrupt the function of p53. Taken together, these studies provide parallel lines of experimental evidence that cooperation between the RAS and p53 pathways is sufficient for SCC tumorigenesis.

## Alternative genetic loci in SCC

Despite advances in identifying the genes that contribute to the pathogenesis of SCC, it is likely that many genes important in the pathogenesis of SCCs have not yet been identified. Evidence for this derives from identification of recurrent chromosomal aberrations through genome-wide analysis of SCC tumors, which revealed that loss of DNA markers mapping to several chromosomes was common.[35] In addition to loss of heterozygosity at 9p (41%), as discussed previously, frequent losses at 3p (23%), 13q (46%), 17p (33%) and 17q (33%) were observed.[35] Deletion of DNA markers at 17p, 17q and 13q were commonly observed in AKs as well, suggesting that loss of potential tumor suppressor genes that map to these regions may contribute to the pathogenesis of both AKs and SCCs.[44] While the p53 gene maps to 17p and may represent a target for deletion in some tumors, potential novel tumor suppressor genes may localize to other areas that are often deleted. More recent studies also found evidence for chromosomal losses at 13q, in addition to other regions of gain or loss, using the technique of comparative genomic hybridization.[45] Further studies evaluating larger numbers of tumors may permit more refined mapping and identification of a putative 13q tumor suppressor gene and possibly other genes that contribute to squamous neoplasia.

In addition to the genetic aberrations, post-transcriptional modification of gene expression may be tumor promoting. Recently, miRNA-205 was determined to be overexpressed in head and neck SCC cell lines. Although the targets of miRNA-205 have not been clearly defined, knock-down of miRNA-205 resulted in inhibition of the tumor-promoting AKT pathway and an increase in apoptosis of SCC cells.[46] Given that approximately one-third of human genes are predicted to be targets of miRNAs, post-transcriptional regulation genes critical to tumor progression may provide novel diagnostic and therapeutic targets.

## CUTANEOUS MALIGNANT MELANOMA

### CDKN2A and CDK4 gene defects

Familial melanomas represent approximately 10% of all cases of melanoma. Early studies on the genetics of melanoma linked the deletion of DNA markers at the short arm of chromosome 9 in both primary melanomas and melanoma cell lines. Subsequently, a putative melanoma tumor suppressor gene was predicted to be located at region 9p21.[47] CDKN2A was shown to be the significant melanoma susceptibility locus associated with familial melanoma. CDKN2A mutations have been estimated to account for

10% to 40%[48-50] of familial melanomas, with the remaining families bearing mutations in *CDK4*[51] and unidentified genes. In addition to melanoma, inactivating mutations in the *CDKN2A* locus result in an increased susceptibility to pancreatic adenocarcinoma.[52,53]

The *CDKN2A* locus is unusual in that it encodes two unique proteins, p16[INK4A] and p14[ARF], utilizing overlapping alternative codons (Fig. 2.4). Although distinct in sequence and structure, p16[INK4A] and p14[ARF] both play a role in regulating the cell cycle and thus cell proliferation.

Advancement through the G1 phase of the cell cycle is controlled by the tumor suppressor retinoblastoma (RB1). In its native state, RB1 is not phosphorylated and can bind to the transcription factor E2F. Binding of E2F prevents it from inducing a series of genes essential for the transition from G1 to S phase. RB1 is phosphorylated by the protein complex of cyclin D1 and CDK4. Formation of the cyclin D1 and CDK4 complex is regulated by the relative amount of

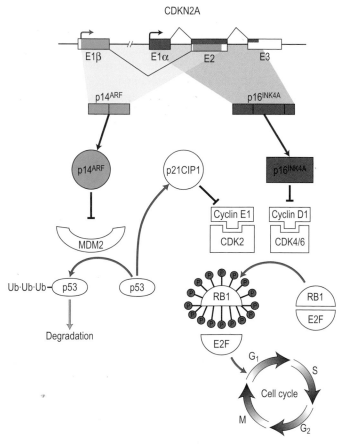

**Figure 2.4** *CDKN2A* locus and signaling pathway. p16[INK4A] and p14[ARF] are both encoded in the *CDKN2A* locus. These genes use alterative promoters and first exons; their second exons are encoded using alternative reading frames of the same coding segment of DNA yet share no amino acid sequence homology. Both p16[INK4A] and p14[ARF] are tumor suppressors that function as negative regulators of cell cycle progression. p16[INK4A] inhibits activation of CDK4 and -6 by cyclin D1, resulting in inhibition of RB1 hyperphosphorylation. When RB1 is not phosphorylated, it sequesters the transcription factor E2F, thereby preventing cell cycle progression. p14[ARF] inhibits the function of MDM2, a ubiquitin ligase that targets p53 for degradation. Therefore, p14[ARF] indirectly stabilizes p53, which induces the cell cycle inhibitor p21CIP1; this inhibitor prevents the activation of CDK2 and cyclin E, resulting in RB1 hyperphosphorylation, sequestration of E2F and inhibition of cell cycle progression. Adapted from Sekulic A, Haluska P Jr, Miller AJ, et al. Malignant melanoma in the 21st century; the emerging molecular landscape. *Mayo Clin Proc.* 2008;83(7):825-846.)

p16[INK4A] such that high levels of p16[INK4A] inhibit formation of the complex. Therefore, when p16[INK4A] is missing, as would be the case through an inactivating mutation, the cyclin D1 and CDK4 complex forms, resulting in the phosphorylation of RB1 and the subsequent release of the E2F transcription factor, and ultimately leads to the expression of genes essential for cell cycle progression. In short, p16[INK4A] functions as a brake of the cell cycle.

The tumor suppressor p14[ARF] is also encoded in the *CDKN2A* locus. However, it utilizes a different first exon (1β) and alternative reading frames of codons for exon 2 (thus the acronym ARF). p14[ARF] plays a role in regulating cell cycle progression through the p53 signaling pathway. Elevated levels of p53 result in the expression of the tumor suppressor p21CIP1, which functions in a manner analogous to p16[INK4A]. p21CIP1 inhibits the formation of the cyclin E and CDK2 complex and thus RB1 phosphorylation; therefore, E2F remains bound to RB1 and cannot activate cell cycle progression. MDM2 is a negative regulator of p53 and functions by binding to p53 and targeting its destruction by tagging it with ubiquitin moieties. p14[ARF] inhibits the function of MDM2. Therefore, in the absence of p14[ARF], MDM2 is not inhibited from ubiquitinating p53, resulting in the degradation of p53 and therefore removing the cell cycle break induced by the downstream pathways of p21CIP1.

Most germline *CDKN2A* mutations in familial melanoma interfere with the ability of p16[INK4A] to bind with CDK4.[54] Abrogation of the interaction with CDK4 renders p16[INK4A] non-functional as a brake of the cell cycle. Conversely, mutations in *CDK4* that interfere with p16[INK4A] binding have been identified in melanoma-prone families.[55] All *CDK4* mutations identified to date cause an amino acid substitution for the arginine at residue 24, which is required for the interaction of CDK4 and p16[INK4A]. Although *CDK4* mutations in melanoma-prone families are rare, their identification further underscores the importance of the role of the p16[INK4A] pathway in the pathogenesis of melanoma. Further, familial melanoma patients have usually been characterized as having only one mutation in either the *p16INK4A* or *CDK4* gene, suggesting that a single mutation in this pathway is sufficient for the activation of this cell cycle progression pathway. Additional kindreds of familial melanoma have demonstrated linkage to chromosome 9p yet lack mutations in the *p16INK4A* gene, suggesting that other melanoma susceptibility genes map to this area. One candidate gene is *p14ARF* as it shares a locus with *p16INK4A*. However, given that deletions of the *CDKN2A* locus commonly result in loss of expression of both *p16INK4A* and *p14ARF*, the specific role played by p14[ARF] as a tumor suppressor remained undefined until a series of melanomas were characterized with mutations in the *CDKN2A* locus limited to *p14ARF*. Most of these mutations are insertions or deletions in the first exon (1β) of *p14ARF* and result in premature termination of translation.[56-58]

As in familial melanoma, genetic aberrations within the *CDKN2A* locus and in *CDK4* have been characterized in cultured and sporadic melanomas. In addition to mutations and deletions, alterations to the promoter region of genes can affect the gene's function. Methylation of promoters is associated with reduced expression or silencing of genes. In cultured melanomas, nearly all clones have altered CDKN2A function either through mutations or promoter methylation. Approximately half of all sporadic melanomas have deletions of DNA markers within the *CDKN2A* locus. However, upon sequence analysis, only 8% have intragenic mutations in *CDKN2A*, and only 6% are inactivated through *CDKN2A* promoter methylation.[59]

The presence of stromal and inflammatory cells in tumor samples may obscure detection of gene defects specific to melanoma cells, and homozygous deletions may be difficult to detect. Furthermore, culturing tumor cells may select for cells that have acquired *CDKN2A* mutations. Nevertheless, these studies provide support for the association between alterations to the *CDKN2A* locus and the pathogenesis of melanoma. Similarly, mutations in the *CDK4* gene have been identified in sporadic melanomas. Two cases of sporadic melanomas revealed mutations in *CDK4* in which arginine was substituted with cysteine at position 24, which interferes with p16$^{INK4A}$ binding to CDK4.[60] Despite these reports, *CDK4* mutations in sporadic melanoma are exceedingly rare.[61] In contrast, no mutations specific to the first exon of *p14ARF*, resulting in its inactivation independently of *p16INK4A*, have been identified as of yet in melanoma.[62]

## Experimental studies of *CDKN2A* and *CDK4* genes in mouse models of melanoma

Experimental murine models verify the findings from mutation analysis of familial and sporadic melanomas and directly implicate genetic aberrations in *CDKN2A* and *CDK4* in the pathogenesis of melanoma. Mice with a deletion in the murine equivalent of the human *CDKN2A* locus that disrupts both the expression of p16$^{INK4A}$ and p19$^{ARF}$ (the murine homolog of human p14$^{ARF}$) undergo normal development but they develop spontaneous tumors early in life and are highly susceptible to tumorigenesis in response to UV irradiation and chemical mutagens. However, the tumors they develop are mostly fibrosarcomas, sarcomas and lymphomas.[63] In contrast, targeting expression of an oncogenic *H-RAS* gene in melanocytes in *Cdkn2a*-deficient mice specifically induces melanoma with a short latency and a high penetrance.[64] This study provides direct support for a causal and cooperative relationship between oncogenic *H-RAS* and defects at the *CDKN2A* locus and development of melanoma in humans. Similarly, mice that express oncogenic *H-RAS* in melanocytes and are deficient for either *p16INK4A* or *p19ARF* also develop melanoma; however, these mice develop melanoma with a greater latency compared with mice lacking both genes.[65] In addition, mice that express a mutation in *Cdk4* that prevents binding to p16$^{INK4A}$ develop invasive melanomas in response to treatment with topical carcinogens.[66] Thus, mouse models with mutations or deletions in each class of genes identified through analysis of melanoma-prone kindreds have been developed. Each faithfully recapitulates the human susceptibility to melanoma and provides functional proof for the association of alterations in these genes with the development of melanoma.

## *PTEN* gene defects in melanoma

DNA markers at chromosome 10q are frequently deleted in melanoma, and recently, mutations in the tumor suppressor gene *PTEN* (phosphatase and tensin homolog), which maps to 10q23, have been detected. Mutations and deletions in *PTEN* are associated with a wide variety of human cancers. Germline mutations in *PTEN* cause Cowden's syndrome, which is associated with the development of hamartomatous lesions and malignancies in the breast, thyroid and uterus. PTEN functions as a phosphatase and influences several cellular processes, including cell cycle regulation by inducing p27$^{KIP1}$ (a cyclin-dependent kinase inhibitor), which suppresses the formation of the cyclin E/CDK complex.[67] As with the p16$^{INK4A}$ inhibition of the cyclin D1 and CDK4 complex, RB1 remains unphosphorylated and sequesters the E2F transcription factor, resulting in G1 cell cycle arrest. Deletion and mutation of the *PTEN* gene in sporadic melanomas has been examined in a number of studies and *PTEN* gene defects have been observed in approximately 30% to 50% of melanoma cell lines and approximately 5–20% of primary melanomas.[67] Recently, an experimental murine model clearly demonstrated the critical role PTEN can have in development of melanoma. When mice that harbor a melanocyte-specific activating mutation of BRAF$^{V600E}$, a downstream target of *RAS*, lose expression of *PTEN*, metastatic melanomas develop with complete penetrance and short latency.[68] The genetic associations in combination with the functional models support a critical role for the loss of *PTEN* expression in the pathogenesis of melanoma.

## *RAS* and *RAF* gene defects in melanoma

*RAS* proteins transduce signaling from the cell surface to the nucleus to alter patterns of gene expression and regulate cell proliferation and differentiation.[27] As discussed earlier, expression of activated oncogenic *RAS* can cooperate with inactivation of the *CDKN2A* locus to promote progression of melanoma in a murine model.[64] These experimental studies correlate well with findings of *RAS* mutations in familial melanomas. Activating *N-RAS* mutations were detected in 95% of primary hereditary melanomas from patients with germline *CDKN2A* mutations.[69] In contrast, *RAS* gene mutations were detected in only 4% to 31% of sporadic melanomas and melanoma cell lines.[70,71] Nearly all melanomas with *RAS* mutations have an activating mutation of *N-RAS* at codon 61. The discrepancy between the high rate of *RAS* mutations in familial melanomas and the paucity of *RAS* mutations observed in sporadic melanomas may be explained, in part, by the prevalence of *BRAF* mutations in a high proportion of sporadic melanomas.[72]

RAF family proteins are serine/threonine kinases that function downstream of *RAS* proteins in the MAPK (mitogen-activated protein kinase) signal transduction pathway.[26] RAF proteins localize to the plasma membrane through interaction with *RAS* proteins, and are activated through dimerization and phosphorylation. Activated RAF proteins initiate phosphorylation events that precipitate a cascade of signal transduction. RAF proteins phosphorylate MEK1/2, which then phosphorylates ERK1/2.

This kinase cascade results in the phosphorylation of transcription factors that promote cell proliferation, survival, motility and invasion. As RAF proteins are immediately downstream of *RAS* signaling, mutations that activate *RAF* could have an effect similar to that of activated *RAS*. Mutations in either *RAS* or *RAF* genes may be important in the pathogenesis of melanoma.

Mutations in *BRAF* have been reported in as high as 70% of melanomas, whereas mutations in *ARAF* and *RAF1*, other RAF isoforms, have not been reported. All activating mutations in *BRAF* are located in the kinase domain and 80% are characterized by a substitution of glutamic acid for valine at residue 600 (V600E). Mutant BRAF is essential for melanoma growth and functions through persistent MAPK-mediated proliferation and survival. In addition to melanomas, BRAF signaling is exceedingly common in benign melanocytic nevi, with the BRAF[V600E] mutation being detected in 82% of nevi.[73] This finding suggests that activation of MAPK signaling may be a critical early event in melanocytic neoplasia; however, additional genetic aberrations, such as inactivation of the *CDKN2A* locus, may be required for development of melanoma.

## Emerging melanoma susceptibility loci

Melanocortin-1 receptor (MC1R) is a G-protein-coupled receptor expressed on melanocytes. Upon binding its ligand, alpha-melanocyte stimulating hormone, MC1R activates adenylate cyclase, resulting in cyclic AMP production. Increased levels of cyclic AMP lead to an increase in pigment synthesis in melanocytes. *MC1R* variants are associated with red hair and a two- to fourfold increased risk of developing melanoma.[74-77] The increased risk of melanoma with variants of *MC1R* has been determined primarily in association with other melanoma-associated mutations. The relationship between *MC1R* variants and the *p16INK4A* tumor suppressor gene was elucidated in kindreds with mutations in *p16INK4A*. Patients who harbored both a *MC1R* mutation and a *p16INK4A* mutation developed melanoma at an earlier age than those with only a *p16INK4A* mutation.[77,78] The association between *MC1R* variants and *BRAF* mutations was investigated in the context of chronic sun-damaged versus non-chronic sun-damaged skin. In two different Caucasian populations, variants of *MC1R* were found to be strongly associated with activating *BRAF* mutations in melanomas found on non-chronic sun-damaged skin but not in chronic sun-damaged skin, suggesting a UV light-independent or indirect mechanism for *BRAF* mutagenesis.[79,80]

KIT is a receptor tyrosine kinase critical for melanocyte development. KIT activation upon binding its ligand, stem cell factor, results in receptor dimerization and subsequent autophosphorylation. This activation is required for the development of melanocytes and other types of cells. Although immunohistochemical studies have associated a decrease in KIT levels with progression of melanoma, genetic analysis of melanomas from different anatomic sites and different levels of sun exposure showed that activating mutations in KIT were associated with a subset of melanomas. An increase in copy number and activating mutations in KIT was found in 39% of mucosal melanomas, 36% of acral melanomas, and 26% of melanomas on chronically

sun-damaged skin but not non-chronically sun-damaged skin.[81] Preliminary studies suggest that a subset of patients with activating KIT mutations may benefit from therapy with imatinib, a competitive inhibitor of KIT.[82]

GNAQ is a G-protein α-subunit that mediates signals from numerous G-protein-coupled receptors and downstream effectors. GNAQ was identified in a forward genetic screen of mice with diffuse skin hyperpigmentation. Activating mutations in *GNAQ* were subsequently detected in 46% of uveal melanomas and 83% of blue nevi.[83] The mutations were all in a Ras-like domain and resulted in constitutive activation of GNAQ. In-vitro functional studies revealed that although the mutations in *GNAQ* were activating, they were not sufficient for progression to melanoma – similar to activating mutations in *BRAF* and *NRAS*. Of note, GNAQ mediates signaling from endothelin, which is essential for melanocyte survival during development. Further, the same activating mutations in *GNAQ* were detected in nevi of Ota, a known risk factor for the development of uveal melanoma.

*Golgi phosphoprotein 3* (*GOLPH3*) was identified as a novel oncogene that is frequently amplified in several tumors, including melanomas (32%), breast (32%), prostate (37%), ovarian (38%) and non-small cell lung carcinomas (56%).[84] GOLPH3 localizes to the *trans*-Golgi network, where it activates the mammalian target of rapamycin (mTOR), enhancing growth factor-induced mTOR signaling and increasing cell size. Cells in which GOLPH3 confers a growth advantage are sensitive to rapamycin inhibition of mTOR and thus cell growth; amplification of *GOLPH3* may be a positive predictor for rapamycin sensitivity.

Micro-ophthalmia-associated transcription factor (MITF) is a transcription factor that is a master regulator of melanocyte development, differentiation and survival. In single-nucleotide polymorphism array-based analysis, *MITF* was amplified in 15% to 20% of metastatic melanomas, and its amplification correlated with overall decreased patient survival.[85] However, MITF amplification is not sufficient to result in melanoma development; rather, in-vitro studies revealed that MITF can transform immortalized melanocytes in cooperation with activated BRAF[V600E].[85]

NEDD9 – or neural precursor cell expressed, developmentally downregulated 9 – is a cytoplasmic adaptor protein that is important in regulating migration of cells. In a screening of genes that increased the metastatic potential of melanomas, copies of *NEDD9* were found to be amplified.[86] Immunohistochemical analysis verified that NEDD9 was overexpressed in metastatic melanomas, and functional studies demonstrated that NEDD9 promoted invasion and metastasis.

## Alternative genetic loci in melanoma

In addition to *CDKN2A* and *CDK4* genes, there is substantial evidence that several other genes likely contribute to the pathogenesis of melanoma. Aberrations involving the *CDKN2A* locus have been documented in 25% to 40% of melanoma-prone families.[45] Of those families that do not harbor *CDKN2A* defects, many nevertheless show genetic linkage to markers on chromosome 9p. One obvious candidate was the *CDKN2B* gene, which encodes a cell cycle inhibitory protein (CDKN2B, formerly referred to as p15[INK4B]) similar to p16[INK4A]. The *CDKN2B* gene lies in close proximity to the *CDKN2A* locus, and both are commonly deleted together in melanomas. However, mutation analysis failed to reveal any germline *CDKN2B* mutations in subjects from 154 families.[87] Additional evidence suggesting the presence of other melanoma-associated loci on chromosome 9p derives from studies demonstrating the loss of DNA markers in regions distinct from the *CDKN2A* locus in sporadic melanomas.[88] However, no alternative tumor suppressor genes in these regions have been identified as of yet.

Similarly, linkage analysis of additional melanoma-prone families and loss of heterozygosity, cytogenetic, and comparative genomic hybridization studies in sporadic melanomas have defined several other genetic loci that may harbor genes that play some role in melanoma development. Included among these are loci at chromosomes 1p, 3p, 6q, 6p, 10q, 11q and 17p.[89-92] Notably, a locus at 1p36 was the first to be identified by linkage analysis of families susceptible to melanoma.[93] However, the inclusion of dysplastic nevi as a clinical feature of affected subjects may have clouded these studies, and no subsequent studies have shown linkage of familial melanoma to 1p36.[94] Loss of DNA markers from the 1p36 region has been observed in sporadic melanomas, providing support for the presence of a putative melanoma-associated tumor suppressor gene in this region.[95] More recently, linkage analysis of 49 Australian melanoma families that lack *CDKN2A* or *CDK4* mutations revealed a novel susceptibility locus associated with early onset melanoma at chromosomal region 1p22.[96] A familial melanoma candidate gene within this region has not yet been identified.

## FUTURE OUTLOOK

Significant progress has been made in identifying oncogenes and tumor suppressor genes that cause BCC, SCC and melanoma. Identification of such genes has permitted characterization of the molecular pathways in which they participate and how mutations in different genes may interact cooperatively to alter the balance between cell proliferation, cell death and cell differentiation in favor of tumorigenesis. However, our understanding of the genetic and molecular mechanisms underlying these cancers is far from complete. There is substantial evidence indicating that additional genes may contribute to the development of BCC, SCC and melanoma. The various screening studies discussed in this chapter have detected gene defects in only some of the tumors examined. Although this, in part, may reflect limitations of techniques used to identify gene defects, it is likely that a number of tumors derive from alterations in genes not yet identified. In addition, many tumor types carry recurrent, non-random genomic aberrations that may activate proto-oncogenes through DNA amplification or inactivate tumor suppressor genes through gene deletion. Such aberrations frequently occur in regions distinct from those of known cancer genes, suggesting that they might harbor novel genes that promote tumorigenesis. Lastly, specific germline gene defects have not been identified in the majority of melanoma-prone families, and the various genetic disorders that increase susceptibility to BCC do not appear to involve the *PTCH* gene.

In the course of future study and with application of increasingly sophisticated technology, novel skin cancer genes will be identified. Subsequent experimentation will elucidate the function of these genes, the consequences of altering them, and how they interact with other known cancer genes and pathways to promote tumorigenesis. As novel skin cancer genes are identified and studied, a more comprehensive understanding of the genetic and molecular basis of skin cancer will be achieved. Ultimately, knowledge of these central oncogenic pathways may permit the development of novel therapies that target specific genes and their molecular pathways in the treatment of skin cancer.

## REFERENCES

1. Esteller M. Cancer epigenomics: DNA methylomes and histone-modification maps. *Nat Rev Genet*. 2007;8(4):286–298.
2. Sun BK, Tsao H. Small RNAs in development and disease. *J Am Acad Dermatol*. 2008;59(5):725–737; quiz 38–40.
3. Gailani MR, Bale SJ, Leffell DJ, et al. Developmental defects in Gorlin syndrome related to a putative tumor suppressor gene on chromosome 9. *Cell*. 1992;69(1):111–117.
4. Gailani MR, Leffell DJ, Ziegler A, et al. Relationship between sunlight exposure and a key genetic alteration in basal cell carcinoma. *J Natl Cancer Inst*. 1996;88(6):349–354.
5. Johnson RL, Rothman AL, Xie J, et al. Human homolog of patched, a candidate gene for the basal cell nevus syndrome. *Science*. 1996;272(5268):1668–1671.
6. Hahn H, Wicking C, Zaphiropoulous PG, et al. Mutations of the human homolog of Drosophila patched in the nevoid basal cell carcinoma syndrome. *Cell*. 1996;85(6):841–851.
7. Nusslein-Volhard C, Wieschaus E. Mutations affecting segment number and polarity in Drosophila. *Nature*. 1980;287(5785):795–801.
8. Jessell TM. Neuronal specification in the spinal cord: inductive signals and transcriptional codes. *Nat Rev Genet*. 2000;1(1):20–29.
9. Von Hoff DD, LoRusso PM, Rudin CM, et al. Inhibition of the hedgehog pathway in advanced basal-cell carcinoma. *N Engl J Med*. 2009;361(12):1164–1172.
10. Lee Y, Kawagoe R, Sasai K, et al. Loss of suppressor-of-fused function promotes tumorigenesis. *Oncogene*. 2007;26(44):6442–6447.
11. Svard J, Heby-Henricson K, Persson-Lek M, et al. Genetic elimination of Suppressor of fused reveals an essential repressor function in the mammalian Hedgehog signaling pathway. *Dev Cell*. 2006;10(2):187–197.
12. Taylor MD, Liu L, Raffel C, et al. Mutations in SUFU predispose to medulloblastoma. *Nat Genet*. 2002;31(3):306–310.
13. Wong SY, Seol AD, So PL, et al. Primary cilia can both mediate and suppress Hedgehog pathway-dependent tumorigenesis. *Nat Med*. 2009;15(9):1055–1061.
14. Toftgard R. Two sides to cilia in cancer. *Nat Med*. 2009;15(9):994–1946.
15. Lee Y, Miller HL, Russell HR, et al. Patched2 modulates tumorigenesis in patched1 heterozygous mice. *Cancer Res*. 2006;66(14):6964–6971.
16. Fan Z, Li J, Du J, et al. A missense mutation in PTCH2 underlies dominantly inherited NBCCS in a Chinese family. *J Med Genet*. 2008;45(5):303–308.
17. Fan H, Khavari PA. Sonic hedgehog opposes epithelial cell cycle arrest. *J Cell Biol*. 1999;147(1):71–76.
18. Adolphe C, Hetherington R, Ellis T, et al. Patched1 functions as a gatekeeper by promoting cell cycle progression. *Cancer Res*. 2006;66(4):2081–2088.
19. Barnes EA, Kong M, Ollendorff V, et al. Patched1 interacts with cyclin B1 to regulate cell cycle progression. *EMBO J*. 2001;20(9):2214–2223.
20. Zhang H, Ping XL, Lee PK, et al. Role of PTCH and p53 genes in early-onset basal cell carcinoma. *Am J Pathol*. 2001;158(2):381–385.
21. Ping XL, Ratner D, Zhang H, et al. PTCH mutations in squamous cell carcinoma of the skin. *J Invest Dermatol*. 2001;116(4):614–616.
22. Happle R. Nonsyndromic type of hereditary multiple basal cell carcinoma. *Am J Med Genet*. 2000;95(2):161–163.
23. Coquart N, Meyer N, Lemasson G, et al. A new non-syndromic type of familial carcinomas? *J Eur Acad Dermatol Venereol*. 2009;23(2):223–224.
24. Itin PH, Happle R. Non-syndromic hereditary basal cell carcinomas: a reduplicated discovery. *J Eur Acad Dermatol Venereol*. 2009;23(10):1219–1220; author reply 1220.

**25.** Stern RS. The mysteries of geographic variability in nonmelanoma skin cancer incidence. *Arch Dermatol.* 1999;135:843–844.

**26.** Shields JM, Pruitt K, McFall A, et al. Understanding Ras: 'it ain't over 'til it's over'. *Trends Cell Biol.* 2000;10(4):147–154.

**27.** Pierceall WE, Goldberg LH, Tainsky MA, et al. Ras gene mutation and amplification in human nonmelanoma skin cancers. *Mol Carcinog.* 1991;4(3):196–202.

**28.** Kreimer-Erlacher H, Seidl H, Back B, et al. High mutation frequency at Ha-ras exons 1-4 in squamous cell carcinomas from PUVA-treated psoriasis patients. *Photochem Photobiol.* 2001;74(2):323–330.

**29.** Spencer JM, Kahn SM, Jiang W, et al. Activated ras genes occur in human actinic keratoses, premalignant precursors to squamous cell carcinoma. *Arch Dermatol.* 1995;131(7):796–800.

**30.** Bonni A, Brunet A, West AE, et al. Cell survival promoted by the Ras-MAPK signaling pathway by transcription-dependent and -independent mechanisms. *Science.* 1999;286(5443):1358–1362.

**31.** Stambolic V, Mak TW, Woodgett JR. Modulation of cellular apoptotic potential: contributions to oncogenesis. *Oncogene.* 1999;18(45):6094–6103.

**32.** Dajee M, Lazarov M, Zhang JY, et al. NF-kappaB blockade and oncogenic Ras trigger invasive human epidermal neoplasia. *Nature.* 2003;421(6923):639–643.

**33.** Lazarov M, Kubo Y, Cai T, et al. CDK4 coexpression with Ras generates malignant human epidermal tumorigenesis. *Nat Med.* 2002;8(10):1105–1114.

**34.** Seitz CS, Lin Q, Deng H, et al. Alterations in NF-kappaB function in transgenic epithelial tissue demonstrate a growth inhibitory role for NF-kappaB. *Proc Natl Acad Sci U S A.* 1998;95(5):2307–2312.

**35.** Quinn AG, Sikkink S, Rees JL. Delineation of two distinct deleted regions on chromosome 9 in human non-melanoma skin cancers. *Genes Chromosomes Cancer.* 1994;11(4):222–225.

**36.** Saridaki Z, Liloglou T, Zafiropoulos A, et al. Mutational analysis of CDKN2A genes in patients with squamous cell carcinoma of the skin. *Br J Dermatol.* 2003;148(4):638–648.

**37.** Mortier L, Marchetti P, Delaporte E, et al. Progression of actinic keratosis to squamous cell carcinoma of the skin correlates with deletion of the 9p21 region encoding the p16(INK4a) tumor suppressor. *Cancer Lett.* 2002;176(2):205–214.

**38.** Bolshakov S, Walker CM, Strom SS, et al. p53 mutations in human aggressive and nonaggressive basal and squamous cell carcinomas. *Clin Cancer Res.* 2003;9(1):228–234.

**39.** Nelson MA, Einspahr JG, Alberts DS, et al. Analysis of the p53 gene in human precancerous actinic keratosis lesions and squamous cell cancers. *Cancer Lett.* 1994;85(1):23–29.

**40.** Brash DE, Rudolph JA, Simon JA, et al. A role for sunlight in skin cancer: UV-induced p53 mutations in squamous cell carcinoma. *Proc Natl Acad Sci U S A.* 1991;88(22):10124–10128.

**41.** Ziegler A, Jonason AS, Leffell DJ, et al. Sunburn and p53 in the onset of skin cancer. *Nature.* 1994;372(6508):773–776.

**42.** Li G, Tron V, Ho V. Induction of squamous cell carcinoma in p53-deficient mice after ultraviolet irradiation. *J Invest Dermatol.* 1998;110(1):72–75.

**43.** Jiang W, Ananthaswamy HN, Muller HK, et al. p53 protects against skin cancer induction by UV-B radiation. *Oncogene.* 1999;18(29):4247–4253.

**44.** Rehman I, Quinn AG, Healy E, et al. High frequency of loss of heterozygosity in actinic keratoses, a usually benign disease. *Lancet.* 1994;344(8925):788–789.

**45.** Hayward NK. Genetics of melanoma predisposition. *Oncogene.* 2003;22(20):3053–3062.

**46.** Yu J, Ryan DG, Getsios S, et al. MicroRNA-184 antagonizes microRNA-205 to maintain SHIP2 levels in epithelia. *Proc Natl Acad Sci U S A.* 2008;105(49):19300–19305.

**47.** Fountain JW, Karayiorgou M, Ernstoff MS, et al. Homozygous deletions within human chromosome band 9p21 in melanoma. *Proc Natl Acad Sci U S A.* 1992;89(21):10557–10561.

**48.** Eliason MJ, Larson AA, Florell SR, et al. Population-based prevalence of CDKN2A mutations in Utah melanoma families. *J Invest Dermatol.* 2006;126(3):660–666.

**49.** Goldstein AM, Chan M, Harland M, et al. Features associated with germline CDKN2A mutations: a GenoMEL study of melanoma-prone families from three continents. *J Med Genet.* 2007;44(2):99–106.

**50.** Newton Bishop JA, Gruis NA. Genetics: what advice for patients who present with a family history of melanoma? *Semin Oncol.* 2007;34(6):452–459.

**51.** Goldstein AM, Chidambaram A, Halpern A, et al. Rarity of CDK4 germline mutations in familial melanoma. *Melanoma Res.* 2002;12(1):51–55.

**52.** Hussussian CJ, Struewing JP, Goldstein AM, et al. Germline p16 mutations in familial melanoma. *Nat Genet.* 1994;8(1):15–21.

**53.** Kamb A, Shattuck-Eidens D, Eeles R, et al. Analysis of the p16 gene (CDKN2) as a candidate for the chromosome 9p melanoma susceptibility locus. *Nat Genet.* 1994;8(1):23–26.

**54.** Ranade K, Hussussian CJ, Sikorski RS, et al. Mutations associated with familial melanoma impair p16INK4 function. *Nat Genet.* 1995;10(1):114–116.

**55.** Zuo L, Weger J, Yang Q, et al. Germline mutations in the p16INK4a binding domain of CDK4 in familial melanoma. *Nat Genet.* 1996;12(1):97–99.

**56.** Randerson-Moor JA, Harland M, Williams S, et al. A germline deletion of p14(ARF) but not CDKN2A in a melanoma-neural system tumour syndrome family. *Hum Mol Genet.* 2001;10(1):55–62.

**57.** Rizos H, Puig S, Badenas C, et al. A melanoma-associated germline mutation in exon 1beta inactivates p14ARF. *Oncogene.* 2001;20(39):5543–5547.

**58.** Hewitt C, Lee Wu C, Evans G, et al. Germline mutation of ARF in a melanoma kindred. *Hum Mol Genet.* 2002;11(11):1273–1279.

**59.** Castellano M, Pollock PM, Walters MK, et al. CDKN2A/p16 is inactivated in most melanoma cell lines. *Cancer Res.* 1997;57(21):4868–4875.

**60.** Wolfel T, Hauer M, Schneider J, et al. A p16INK4a-insensitive CDK4 mutant targeted by cytolytic T lymphocytes in a human melanoma. *Science.* 1995;269(5228):1281–1284.

**61.** Guldberg P, Kirkin AF, Gronbaek K, et al. Complete scanning of the CDK4 gene by denaturing gradient gel electrophoresis: a novel missense mutation but low overall frequency of mutations in sporadic metastatic malignant melanoma. *Int J Cancer.* 1997;72(5):780–783.

**62.** Peris K, Chimenti S, Fargnoli MC, et al. UV fingerprint CDKN2a but no p14ARF mutations in sporadic melanomas. *J Invest Dermatol.* 1999;112(5):825–826.

**63.** Serrano M, Lee H, Chin L, et al. Role of the INK4a locus in tumor suppression and cell mortality. *Cell.* 1996;85(1):27–37.

**64.** Chin L, Pomerantz J, Polsky D, et al. Cooperative effects of INK4a and ras in melanoma susceptibility in vivo. *Genes Dev.* 1997;11(21):2822–2834.

**65.** Sharpless E, Chin L. The INK4a/ARF locus and melanoma. *Oncogene.* 2003;22(20):3092–3098.

**66.** Sotillo R, Garcia JF, Ortega S, et al. Invasive melanoma in Cdk4-targeted mice. *Proc Natl Acad Sci U S A.* 2001;98(23):13312–13317.

**67.** Wu H, Goel V, Haluska FG. PTEN signaling pathways in melanoma. *Oncogene.* 2003;22(20):3113–3122.

**68.** Dankort D, Curley DP, Cartlidge RA, et al. Braf(V600E) cooperates with Pten loss to induce metastatic melanoma. *Nat Genet.* 2009;41(5):544–552.

**69.** Eskandarpour M, Hashemi J, Kanter L, et al. Frequency of UV-inducible NRAS mutations in melanomas of patients with germline CDKN2A mutations. *J Natl Cancer Inst.* 2003;95(11):790–798.

**70.** Albino AP, Nanus DM, Mentle IR, et al. Analysis of ras oncogenes in malignant melanoma and precursor lesions: correlation of point mutations with differentiation phenotype. *Oncogene.* 1989;4(11):1363–1374.

**71.** Demunter A, Stas M, Degreef H, et al. Analysis of N- and K-ras mutations in the distinctive tumor progression phases of melanoma. *J Invest Dermatol.* 2001;117(6):1483–1489.

**72.** Davies H, Bignell GR, Cox C, et al. Mutations of the BRAF gene in human cancer. *Nature.* 2002;417(6892):949–954.

**73.** Pollock PM, Harper UL, Hansen KS, et al. High frequency of BRAF mutations in nevi. *Nat Genet.* 2003;33(1):19–20.

**74.** Valverde P, Healy E, Jackson I, et al. Variants of the melanocyte-stimulating hormone receptor gene are associated with red hair and fair skin in humans. *Nat Genet.* 1995;11(3):328–330.

**75.** Valverde P, Healy E, Sikkink S, et al. The Asp84Glu variant of the melanocortin 1 receptor (MC1R) is associated with melanoma. *Hum Mol Genet.* 1996;5(10):1663–1666.

**76.** Kennedy C, ter Huurne J, Berkhout M, et al. Melanocortin 1 receptor (MC1R) gene variants are associated with an increased risk for cutaneous melanoma which is largely independent of skin type and hair color. *J Invest Dermatol.* 2001;117(2):294–300.

**77.** Box NF, Duffy DL, Chen W, et al. MC1R genotype modifies risk of melanoma in families segregating CDKN2A mutations. *Am J Hum Genet.* 2001;69(4):765–773.

**78.** van der Velden PA, Sandkuijl LA, Bergman W, et al. Melanocortin-1 receptor variant R151C modifies melanoma risk in Dutch families with melanoma. *Am J Hum Genet.* 2001;69(4):774–779.

**79.** Flaherty KT, Puzanov I, Kim KB, et al. Inhibition of mutated, activated BRAF in metastatic melanoma. *New Engl J Med.* 2010;363:809–819.

**80.** Landi MT, Bauer J, Pfeiffer RM, et al. MC1R germline variants confer risk for BRAF-mutant melanoma. *Science.* 2006;313(5786):521–522.

**81.** Curtin JA, Busam K, Pinkel D, et al. Somatic activation of KIT in distinct subtypes of melanoma. *J Clin Oncol.* 2006;24(26):4340–4346.

**82.** Garrido MC, Bastian BC. KIT as a therapeutic target in melanoma. *J Invest Dermatol.* 2010;130(1):20–27.

**83.** Van Raamsdonk CD, Bezrookove V, Green G, et al. Frequent somatic mutations of GNAQ in uveal melanoma and blue naevi. *Nature.* 2009;457(7229):599–602.

**84.** Scott KL, Kabbarah O, Liang MC, et al. GOLPH3 modulates mTOR signalling and rapamycin sensitivity in cancer. *Nature.* 2009;459(7250):1085–1090.

**85.** Garraway LA, Widlund HR, Rubin MA, et al. Integrative genomic analyses identify MITF as a lineage survival oncogene amplified in malignant melanoma. *Nature.* 2005;436(7047):117–122.

**86.** Kim M, Gans JD, Nogueira C, et al. Comparative oncogenomics identifies NEDD9 as a melanoma metastasis gene. *Cell.* 2006;125(7):1269–1281.

**87.** Pollock PM, Trent JM. The genetics of cutaneous melanoma. *Clin Lab Med.* 2000;20(4):667–690.

**88.** Holland EA, Beaton SC, Edwards BG, et al. Loss of heterozygosity and homozygous deletions on 9p21-22 in melanoma. *Oncogene.* 1994;9(5):1361–1365.

**89.** Walker GJ, Nancarrow DJ, Walters MK, et al. Linkage analysis in familial melanoma kindreds to markers on chromosome 6p. *Int J Cancer.* 1994;59(6):771–775.

**90.** Healy E, Rehman I, Angus B, et al. Loss of heterozygosity in sporadic primary cutaneous melanoma. *Genes Chromosomes Cancer.* 1995;12(2):152–156.

**91.** Thompson FH, Emerson J, Olson S, et al. Cytogenetics of 158 patients with regional or disseminated melanoma. Subset analysis of near-diploid and simple karyotypes. *Cancer Genet Cytogenet.* 1995;83(2):93–104.

**92.** Bastian BC, LeBoit PE, Hamm H, et al. Chromosomal gains and losses in primary cutaneous melanomas detected by comparative genomic hybridization. *Cancer Res.* 1998;58(10):2170–2175.

**93.** Bale SJ, Dracopoli NC, Tucker MA, et al. Mapping the gene for hereditary cutaneous malignant melanoma-dysplastic nevus to chromosome 1p. *N Engl J Med.* 1989;320(21):1367–1372.

**94.** Piepkorn M. Melanoma genetics: an update with focus on the CDKN2A(p16)/ARF tumor suppressors. *J Am Acad Dermatol.* 2000;42 (5 Pt 1):705–722 quiz 723–726.

**95.** Poetsch M, Woenckhaus C, Dittberner T, et al. An increased frequency of numerical chromosomal abnormalities and 1p36 deletions in isolated cells from paraffin sections of malignant melanomas by means of interphase cytogenetics. *Cancer Genet Cytogenet.* 1998;104(2):146–152.

**96.** Gillanders E, Juo SH, Holland EA, et al. Localization of a novel melanoma susceptibility locus to 1p22. *Am J Hum Genet.* 2003;73(2):301–313.

# The Biology of the Melanocyte

*Julie V. Schaffer and Jean L. Bolognia*

## Key Points

- The major determinant of human skin color and sensitivity to ultraviolet radiation (UVR) is the activity of melanocytes, i.e. the quantity and quality of pigment production, not the density of melanocytes.

- Melanocytes contain a unique lysosome-related intracytoplasmic organelle, the melanosome, which is the site of melanin biosynthesis.

- Compared with lightly pigmented skin, darkly pigmented skin has more numerous, larger melanosomes that contain more melanin; once transferred to keratinocytes, the melanosomes of darkly pigmented skin are singly dispersed and degraded more slowly.

- Tyrosinase is the key enzyme in the melanin biosynthetic pathway.

- Two major forms of melanin are produced by melanocytes: brown-black, photoprotective eumelanin and yellow-red, photolabile pheomelanin.

- In humans, binding of melanocyte-stimulating hormone (MSH) to the melanocortin-1 receptor (MC1R) stimulates eumelanogenesis, most notably as a protective response to UVR.

- Loss-of-function variants of the MC1R largely account for the red hair phenotype in humans, are associated with fair skin even in those without red hair, and confer a risk of melanoma and non-melanoma skin cancer shown to be independent of pigmentary phenotype.

## INTRODUCTION

Pigmentation of the hair and skin is not only one of the most striking visible human traits, it also represents a major determinant of sensitivity to ultraviolet radiation (UVR) and risk of both melanoma and non-melanoma skin cancer (NMSC). An appreciation of the biology of the melanocyte is required in order to understand the physiology of normal constitutive and facultative pigmentation, as well as the biology of melanoma and the pathophysiology of disorders of pigmentation that predispose affected individuals to the development of skin cancer.[1,2] A classic example of the latter is type 1 oculocutaneous albinism (OCA), a genodermatosis in which pigmentary dilution of the skin, hair and eyes due to absent or decreased tyrosinase activity results in a markedly increased risk of UVR-induced squamous cell carcinoma. With regard to melanoma, knowledge of melanosomal proteins such as tyrosinase, gp100/Pmel17 and

MelanA/MART1 is critical to the use of immunohistochemical methods of diagnosis, the understanding of immune responses such as melanoma-associated leukoderma, and the development of vaccine therapies. Furthermore, the elucidation of signaling pathways for proliferation and differentiation in normal melanocytes is fundamental to the understanding of melanoma tumorigenesis and progression.

Within the realm of physiologic pigmentation, the melanocyte melanocortin-1 receptor (MC1R), via interactions with melanocyte-stimulating hormone (MSH), plays a key role in the determination of skin type and hair color. Loss-of-function variants of the *MC1R* gene, which result in increased production of pheomelanin rather than eumelanin, have been shown to largely account for the red hair phenotype in humans and to have a strong association with fair skin and a decreased ability to tan even in individuals without red hair. These MC1R variants also confer a risk of melanoma and NMSC that is independent of pigmentary phenotype.[3]

## HISTORY

Although human epidermal melanocytes were first observed by Riehl in 1884, the cytologic basis of human pigment production was not yet known in the early twentieth century when Raper and others defined the metabolic pathway converting tyrosine to melanin in invertebrates. In 1917, research in human melanocyte biology began when Bloch developed a technique to stain pigment-producing cells by using dihydroxyphenylalanine (DOPA) as a substrate for melanin formation. Tyrosinase was identified in human melanocytes several decades later and in 1961, Seiji et al.[4] isolated and characterized the melanosome, the subcellular localization of melanin biosynthesis. Since that time, advances in molecular biology have facilitated the discovery of many genes, proteins and regulatory pathways important to melanogenesis.

## STRUCTURE AND FUNCTION OF THE MELANOCYTE

Melanocytes are pigment-producing dendritic cells derived from the neural crest. During embryogenesis, pluripotent neural crest cells develop into lineage-restricted melanocyte precursors (melanoblasts) as they migrate along the dorsolateral pathway between the somite and overlying ectoderm to the dermis, eventually reaching their final destinations in the epidermis and hair follicles. Cutaneous melanocytes

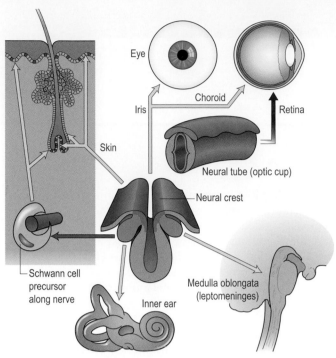

**Figure 3.1** Migration of melanocytes from the neural crest. Melanocytes migrate to the uveal tract of the eye (iris and choroid), the cochlea of the inner ear, and the leptomeninges, as well as to the epidermis and the hair follicle. Cutaneous melanocytes can also arise from Schwann cell precursors located along nerves in the skin, which also originate from the neural crest. The retina actually represents an outpouching of the neural tube. (Adapted from Bolognia JL, Jorizzo JJ, Rapini RP, eds. *Dermatology*. 2nd ed. Philadelphia: Elsevier; 2008.)

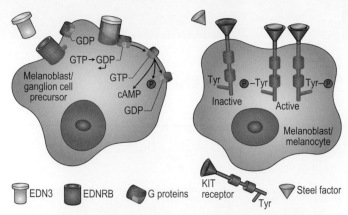

**Figure 3.2** Receptor–ligand interactions required for the survival and migration of neural crest cells. In the developing neural crest, G-protein-coupled endothelin B receptors (EDNRB) on melanoblast-ganglion cell precursors are activated by endothelin-3 (EDN3) (see also Fig. 3.17). In the mesenchyme and final destination sites, binding of steel factor to KIT tyrosine kinase receptors on melanoblasts and melanocytes induces activation via dimerization and autophosphorylation. (Adapted from Bolognia JL, Jorizzo JJ, Rapini RP, eds. *Dermatology*. 2nd ed. Philadelphia: Elsevier; 2008.)

can also arise from Schwann cell precursors located along nerves in the skin, which originate from the neural crest via the ventral pathway.[5] In addition, melanoblasts migrate to the uveal tract of the eye (choroid, ciliary body and iris), the inner ear (stria vascularis of the cochlea) and the leptomeninges (pia mater; Fig. 3.1). This distribution of melanocytes accounts for the melanocytosis and risk of developing melanoma in the eye (e.g. choroid) and leptomeninges that is seen in patients with nevus of Ota and the occurrence of neurocutaneous melanocytosis in patients with large and/or multiple congenital melanocytic nevi.

The study of patients with inherited pigmentary disorders and animal models of such has led to insights into critical signaling pathways in melanocyte development and homeostasis. The survival and migration of neural crest-derived cells during embryogenesis depend upon interactions between specific receptors on the cell surface and their extracellular ligands. For example, steel factor (KIT ligand [KITLG], stem cell factor) binds to and activates the KIT transmembrane tyrosine kinase receptor on melanoblasts and melanocytes (Fig. 3.2). Heterozygous germline mutations in the *KIT* gene that result in receptors with decreased function cause human piebaldism, while loss-of-function mutations in either the KIT gene or the *steel* gene can lead to dominant white spotting in mice.[6] Recently, a heterozygous gain-of-function germline mutation in the human *steel* (*KITLG*) gene was found to underlie a form of familial progressive hyperpigmentation with autosomal dominant inheritance.[7] On the other hand, somatic activating mutations in the human *KIT* gene are often found in lesional

tissue from adult patients with mastocytosis/mast cell leukemia and melanomas of the mucous membranes, acral sites, or chronically sun-damaged skin.[8] The steel/KIT signaling pathway can also stimulate melanocyte proliferation and dendricity in normal adult human skin, where it has a role in UVR-induced pigmentation.[9] In the developing neural crest, interactions also occur between endothelin-3 (EDN3) and the endothelin B receptors (EDNRB) found on melanoblast-ganglion cell precursors (Fig. 3.2). Mutations in both alleles of the *EDN3* gene or the *EDNRB* gene can produce a combination of Waardenburg syndrome (WS) and Hirschsprung disease (type IV WS).

Downstream of these receptor–ligand interactions, several transcription factors (i.e. proteins with the ability to bind to DNA and influence the activity of other genes) have important functions in melanocytes and their precursors. Microphthalmia-associated transcription factor (MITF), the earliest known marker of commitment to the melanocytic lineage, has been implicated as the 'master gene' for melanocyte survival as well as a key regulator of the promoters of the genes encoding tyrosinase and other major melanogenic proteins.[10] MITF activity is modulated both through a cAMP-dependent pathway of transcriptional upregulation (which can be induced by α-MSH, see below) and via mitogen-activated protein kinase (MAPK)-dependent phosphorylation of MITF itself. The latter, which can be stimulated by the KIT signaling pathway, increases the intrinsic activity of MITF but also targets it to the proteasome for degradation. Heterozygous mutations in the *MITF* gene result in type II WS. Furthermore, MITF has been shown to mediate UVR-induced pigmentation and to promote viability of melanoma cells as well as melanocytes by upregulating the expression of the anti-apoptotic protein Bcl2.[11] Other transcription factors expressed in melanocytes include paired box gene-3 (*PAX3*) and SRY box-containing gene 10 (*SOX10*), both with roles in regulating the expression of MITF. Heterozygous mutations in the *PAX3* gene or the *SOX10* gene can result in types I and III WS or type IV WS, respectively.[6]

As predicted by their migratory pathway, melanocytes are present throughout the dermis during intrauterine development. Dermal melanocytes first appear in the head and neck region, and they begin to produce pigment at a gestational age of approximately 10 weeks. However, by the time of birth, active dermal melanocytes have disappeared with the exception of three anatomic sites – the head and neck, the dorsal aspects of the distal extremities, and the presacral area.[12] Although a fraction of the 'lost' dermal melanocytes can be accounted for by migration to the epidermis, it is clear that cell death (presumably apoptotic) has also occurred. Of note, the three locations of persistent dermal melanocytes correspond to the most common locations for dermal melanocytosis and blue nevi, with the scalp representing a site of predilection for malignant blue nevi. Interestingly, hepatocyte growth factor (HGF), which binds and activates the MET tyrosine kinase receptor, has been shown to promote the survival, proliferation and differentiation of dermal melanocytes when it is overexpressed in transgenic mice, resulting in a 300-fold increase compared with normal mice in the number of active dermal melanocytes seen after birth. With autocrine HGF signaling in a similar transgenic mouse model, the development of cutaneous and metastatic melanomas was also observed.[13]

In the epidermis of the human fetus, melanocytes can be identified by immunohistochemical staining as early as 50 days' gestational age.[14] By the fourth month of gestation, melanin-containing melanosomes can be recognized within the epidermal melanocytes via electron microscopy. With the exception of benign and malignant neoplasms, melanocytes reside in the basal layer of the epidermis, accounting for approximately 10% of the cells in this location (Fig. 3.3). Although the cell bodies of melanocytes rest on the basal lamina, their dendrites reach keratinocytes as far away as the mid stratum spinosum. Each melanocyte supplies melanosomes to approximately 30–40 neighboring keratinocytes, an association referred to as the epidermal melanin unit.[15] As melanocytes represent intruders into the epidermis, they do not form desmosomal connections with surrounding keratinocytes.

The basal layer of the hair matrix and the outer root sheath of hair follicles are additional sites to which melanocytes migrate during development (Fig. 3.1). While melanocytes in the matrices of pigmented anagen hairs actively produce melanin and are therefore easily recognized, those in the outer root sheath are usually amelanotic, less differentiated, and more difficult to identify.[16] It has been suggested that melanocytes in the epidermis and the hair follicle represent two antigenically distinct populations,[17] explaining the preferential destruction of the former in vitiligo. A population of melanocyte stem cells exists in the lower permanent portion of mouse hair follicles throughout the hair cycle, with activation at early anagen to supply progeny to the hair matrix.[18]

When DOPA-stained epidermal sheets from various anatomic sites are analyzed, regional differences are observed in the density of epidermal melanocytes, ranging from ~2000/mm$^2$ on the face and in the genital area to ~800/mm$^2$ on the trunk. However, despite the wide variation in pigmentation seen among humans, when the same anatomic site is examined there are no significant differences in melanocyte density between those with light and those with dark constitutive skin pigmentation. For example, a person who has extremely fair skin and an inability to tan has a density of epidermal melanocytes similar to that of a person whose natural skin color is dark brown to black. Even individuals with OCA type 1A, the most severe form of OCA, have a normal number of melanocytes. Nonetheless, melanocyte density does appear to decline with age, with a decrease of approximately 5–10% per decade during adulthood.[19]

The major determinant of human skin color is therefore not the density of melanocytes, but rather the activity of melanocytes.[20] In comparison with lightly pigmented skin, the melanocytes of darkly pigmented skin have increased dendricity and produce larger, more numerous melanosomes that are higher in melanin content. The quantity and quality of pigment production depend on constitutive (baseline, genetically programmed) and facultative (stimulated, e.g. by UVR) activity levels of the enzymes involved in melanin biosynthesis as well as the characteristics of

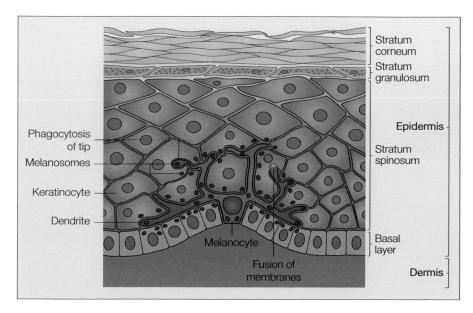

Phagocytosis of tip
Melanosomes
Keratinocyte
Dendrite
Melanocyte
Fusion of membranes

Stratum corneum
Stratum granulosum
Epidermis
Stratum spinosum
Basal layer
Dermis

Figure 3.3 A melanocyte residing in the basal layer of the epidermis. In normal skin, approximately every tenth cell in the basal layer is a melanocyte. Melanosomes are transferred from the dendrites of the melanocyte to approximately 30–40 neighboring keratinocytes, an association referred to as the epidermal melanin unit. (Adapted from Bolognia JL, Jorizzo JJ, Rapini RP, eds. *Dermatology*. 2nd ed. Philadelphia: Elsevier; 2008.)

individual melanosomes (e.g. diameter and ultrastructure). Interactions between the melanocyte MC1R and extracellular ligands such as α-MSH have important influences on both constitutive and facultative melanocytic activity (see below).

## STRUCTURE AND FUNCTION OF THE MELANOSOME

Melanosomes are lysosome-related, membrane-bound intracytoplasmic organelles that specialize in the synthesis and storage of melanin.[21] Both melanocytes and retinal pigment epithelial cells produce melanosomes. However, while the latter cells retain the melanosomes within their own cytoplasm, the transfer of mature melanosomes to keratinocytes is an important function of epidermal and hair matrix melanocytes. By providing compartmentalization, melanosomes protect the remainder of the cell from reactive melanin precursors (e.g. phenols, quinones) that can oxidize lipid membranes; this is analogous to the protection conferred by sequestration of proteases and other degradative enzymes within lysosomes. Melanosomes contain both specific matrix proteins that provide a striated scaffolding upon which melanin is deposited and enzymes that regulate melanin biosynthesis.

During their synthesis by ribosomes, proteins destined for melanosomes are targeted to the lumen of the rough endoplasmic reticulum (ER; Fig. 3.4) by an N-terminal signal sequence. In both normal melanocytes and melanoma cells, misfolded tyrosinase and aberrant tyrosinase-related protein 1 (TYRP1; see Fig. 3.11) produced from an alternate reading frame are 'sorted' via ER quality-control mechanisms for degradation in the cytosol by proteasomes (Fig. 3.4),

resulting in the presentation of antigenic peptides to the immune system by MHC class I molecules. In amelanotic melanoma cell lines, wild-type tyrosinase is retained in the ER due to factors such as abnormal acidification of organelles and decreased expression of TYRP1 (which facilitates tyrosinase processing in the ER), resulting in accelerated degradation of the enzyme and contributing to the dedifferentiated phenotype.[22]

The targeting of proteins to intracytoplasmic organelles versus the plasma membrane and the sorting of specific proteins to the correct type of organelle (e.g. melanosome versus lysosome) are complex processes. Most melanogenic enzymes are glycoproteins that must undergo post-translational modification (i.e. the attachment of sugars) in the ER and Golgi apparatus; they are then transferred from the trans-Golgi network (TGN) via clathrin-coated vesicles to join matrix proteins in endosomes or maturing melanosomes (Fig. 3.5).[23] This triaging from the TGN requires the equivalent of 'traffic police' within the cell, an example of which is the heterotetrameric adaptor protein-3 (AP-3). The binding of AP-3 to a di-leucine-based motif in the cytoplasmic domain of tyrosinase may facilitate this protein-sorting process. Mutations in the gene that encodes the β3A subunit of AP-3 can cause type 2 Hermansky–Pudlak syndrome (HPS), a disorder in which melanosomes and other intracytoplasmic organelles are defective, and the resultant pigmentary dilution can increase the risk of NMSC (Fig. 3.6; Table 3.1). Additional forms of HPS result from mutations in genes that encode components of *b*iogenesis of *l*ysosome-related *o*rganelle *c*omplexes (BLOCs; Fig. 3.7).[24]

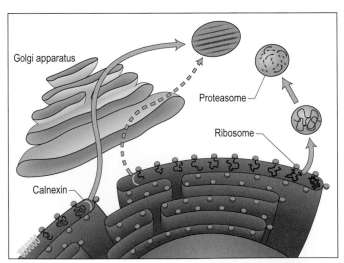

Figure 3.4 Synthesis and processing of glycoproteins destined for melanosomes. As they are synthesized by ribosomes, tyrosinase and other melanogenic enzymes are translocated into the lumen of the rough endoplasmic reticulum (ER), where co- and post-translational glycosylation begins and molecular chaperones (e.g. calnexin and calreticulin) bind the nascent glycoproteins and promote efficient folding. Properly folded proteins are exported from the ER to melanosomes via the Golgi apparatus (left), while misfolded proteins are targeted for degradation by the ubiquitin-dependent proteasome pathway (right). The latter process results in degradation of mutant tyrosinase in many patients with oculocutaneous albinism types 1A and 1B.

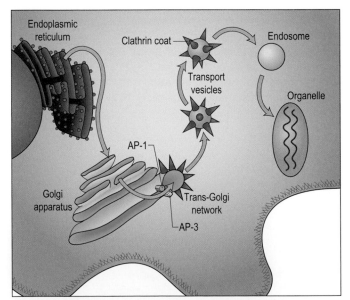

Figure 3.5 Shuttling of proteins within the cell following translation and post-translational processing. After modifications such as the attachment of sugar residues in the endoplasmic reticulum and Golgi apparatus, proteins must be triaged to the correct cellular location, either a specific organelle or the plasma membrane. Heterotetrameric adaptor proteins, AP-1 and AP-3, regulate this protein-sorting process. The latter binds to a di-leucine-based motif in the cytoplasmic tail of tyrosinase, facilitating its transfer via clathrin-coated vesicles from the trans-Golgi network to maturing melanosomes. Mutations in the gene that encodes the β3A subunit of AP-3 can cause Hermansky–Pudlak syndrome. (Adapted from Bolognia JL, Jorizzo JJ, Rapini RP, eds. *Dermatology*. 2nd ed. Philadelphia: Elsevier; 2008.)

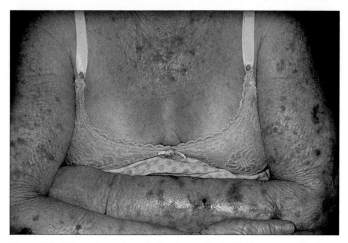

**Figure 3.6** Diffuse pigmentary dilution in a patient with Hermansky–Pudlak syndrome. In addition to abnormal formation of melanosomes, defective protein trafficking results in a bleeding diathesis due to an absence of platelet dense granules. Note the development of multiple actinic keratoses and squamous cell carcinomas in sun-exposed areas.

The progression of a melanosome from an organelle that lacks melanin to one that is fully melanized has been divided into four morphologic stages (Fig. 3.8). Cleavage and refolding of the matrix protein gp100/Pmel17 (the protein detected by the HMB45 immunohistochemical stain) into an amyloid core accompanies the transition from a spherical, amorphous stage I melanosome (structurally similar to an early multivesicular endosome) to an elliptical, fibrillar, highly organized stage II melanosome.[25,26] At the same time, stabilization of melanogenic enzymes allows biosynthesis of melanin (eumelanin in particular) to begin. In the setting of pheomelanin rather than eumelanin production (see below), pheomelanogenic melanosomes retain a spherical shape and an unstructured matrix with vesicular bodies.

As melanin is deposited within them, melanosomes migrate along microtubules from the cell body into the dendrites in preparation for transfer to neighboring keratinocytes (Fig. 3.9). Myosin Va is a dimeric molecular motor that

## Table 3.1 Disorders Characterized by Diffuse Pigmentary Dilution in Which the Genetic Defect is Known

| Disorder | Gene | Protein | Clinical phenotype* | Pathogenesis |
|---|---|---|---|---|
| **Oculocutaneous albinism (OCA)** | | | | |
| Type 1A | *TYR* | Tyrosinase | White hair, pink skin and gray eyes | Complete absence of tyrosinase activity and melanin production<br>Retention of tyrosinase protein within the ER |
| Type 1B | *TYR* | Tyrosinase | Same as Type 1A at birth, but develop yellow to red hair with age ('yellow albinism') | Decreased tyrosinase activity; can produce pheomelanin<br>Retention of tyrosinase protein within the ER<br>Variant with temperature-sensitive tyrosinase – activity normal at 35°C, but diminished at 37°C |
| Type 2 | *OCA2 (P)* | P protein | Born with lightly pigmented hair (not white), skin and eyes<br>Large, jagged lentigines<br>Brown albinism in Africa | Transmembrane protein found in the ER as well as in melanosomes<br>Possible functions include regulating organelle pH, facilitating vacuolar accumulation of glutathione, and processing/trafficking of tyrosinase |
| Type 3 (rufous/ red) | *TYRP1* | Tyrosinase-related protein 1 | Reddish hair and skin ('rufous') | TYRP1 stabilizes tyrosinase in mice and humans, and it also functions as a DHICA oxidase in mice<br>Both mutant TYRP1 and tyrosinase are retained in the ER and degraded |
| Type 4 | *SLC45A2 (MATP)* | Membrane-associated transporter protein | Variable, with hair ranging from white to yellow-brown<br>Pigment may increase over time<br>Most common in Asians | Transmembrane transporter with a role in tyrosinase processing and intracellular trafficking to the melanosome |
| **Hermansky–Pudlak syndrome (HPS)†** | | | | |
| 1 | *HPS1* | HPS1 | Pigmentary dilution of hair, skin and eyes<br>Bleeding diathesis<br>Pulmonary fibrosis and granulomatous colitis due to ceroid lipofuscin deposits | Defective trafficking of organelle-specific proteins to melanosomes, lysosomes and cytoplasmic granules (including platelet dense granules)<br>Proteins interact in biogenesis of *lysosome*-related organelle complexes (BLOCs 1–3; Fig. 3.7) |
| 2 | *AP3B1* | Adaptor protein 3, β3A subunit | | |
| 3 | *HPS3* | HPS3 | | |
| 4 | *HPS4* | HPS4 | | |
| 5 | *HPS5* | Ruby-eye 2 (ru2) | | |
| 6 | *HPS6* | Ruby-eye (ru) | | |
| 7 | *DTNBP1* | Dysbindin | | |
| 8 | *BLOC1S3* | BLOC1S3 | | |

*(Continued)*

## Table 3.1 Disorders Characterized by Diffuse Pigmentary Dilution in Which the Genetic Defect is Known—Cont'd

| Disorder | Gene | Protein | Clinical phenotype* | Pathogenesis |
|---|---|---|---|---|
| **Chédiak–Higashi syndrome** | | | | |
| | CHS1 (LYST) | Lysosomal trafficking regulator | Mild pigmentary dilution Slivery hair Bleeding diathesis Neurologic abnormalities Recurrent infections Accelerated phase‡ | Abnormal vesicle trafficking results in giant organelles (e.g. melanosomes, neutrophil granules [lysosomes], platelet dense granules) |
| **Griscelli syndrome** | | | | |
| 1 | MYO5A | Myosin Va | Mild pigmentary dilution Silvery hair Neurologic abnormalities | Defective attachment of organelles to the actin cytoskeleton; this normally occurs by linkage of myosin Va (via melanophilin) to RAB27A, a GTPase present in melanosomes Melanocytes are 'stuffed' with melanosomes due to failure of transfer to keratinocytes |
| 2 | RAB27A | RAB27A | Mild pigmentary dilution Silvery hair Recurrent infections Accelerated phase‡ | |
| 3 | MLPH MYO5A | Melanophilin Myosin Va F-exon deletion | Mild pigmentary dilution Silvery hair | |

*All types of OCA and HPS result in an increased risk of ultraviolet-induced non-melanoma skin cancers, particularly squamous cell carcinoma.

†As there are ≥15 known loci for HPS-like phenotypes in mice, additional genes may be discovered in humans with this disorder.

‡Characterized by pancytopenia and lymphohistiocytic infiltrates of the liver, spleen and lymph nodes.

ER, endoplasmic reticulum; DHICA, 5,6-dihydroxyindole-2-carboxylic acid

captures the melanosomes when they reach the cell periphery, attaching them to the actin cytoskeleton beneath the plasma membrane.[23] Melanophilin links myosin Va with RAB27A, a GTPase that is present in mature melanosomes. Mutations in the MYO5A, RAB27A or MLPH genes cause different forms of Griscelli syndrome (Table 3.1), a disorder in which diffuse pigmentary dilution results from a lack of melanosome transfer to keratinocytes. In this condition, failure to securely attach the melanosomes to the actin cytoskeleton within the dendrites causes them to 'slip back' and accumulate in the center of the melanocyte, reminding us, as do other disorders (e.g. hypopigmented mycosis fungoides), that normal cutaneous pigmentation depends on an orderly transfer of melanosomes from melanocytes to keratinocytes.

It is the activity of melanocytes, not their density, that determines skin color and sensitivity to UVR. The number and size of melanosomes produced, their degree of melanization, and the ability to transfer them efficiently to keratinocytes are all indicators of melanocyte activity. For example, stage II melanosomes predominate in lightly pigmented skin, whereas primarily stage IV melanosomes are seen in darkly pigmented skin (Table 3.2). Additional factors include the distribution and rate of degradation of the melanosomes after they are transferred to keratinocytes. The smaller melanosomes of lightly pigmented skin are clustered in groups of two to ten within secondary lysosomes, and are degraded by the time they reach the mid stratum spinosum. In contrast, the larger melanosomes found in darkly pigmented skin are singly dispersed and are

**Figure 3.7** Regulation of protein trafficking by adaptor protein 3 (AP-3) and *b*iogenesis of *l*ysosome-related *o*rganelle *c*omplexes (BLOCs). Various mouse phenotypes are in light purple-colored boxes. Lysosome-related organelles include melanosomes, platelet dense granules, and lytic granules of cytotoxic lymphocytes and natural killer cells. HPS, Hermansky–Pudlak syndrome. (Reproduced with permission from Bolognia JL, Jorizzo JJ, Rapini RP, eds. *Dermatology*. 2nd ed. Philadelphia: Elsevier; 2008.)

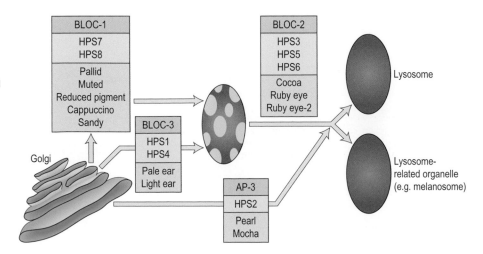

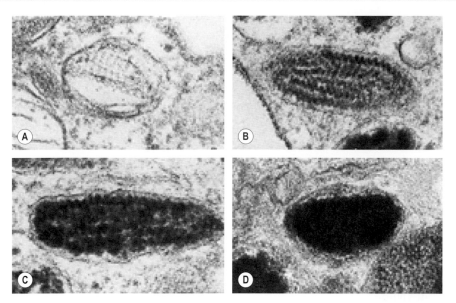

**Figure 3.8** Descriptions and electron photomicrographs of the four major stages of eumelanogenic melanosomes. (Reproduced with permission from Bolognia JL, Jorizzo JJ, Rapini RP, eds. *Dermatology*. 2nd ed. Philadelphia: Elsevier; 2008.)

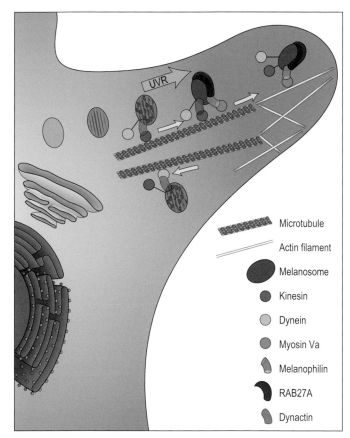

Microtubule

Actin filament

Melanosome

Kinesin

Dynein

Myosin Va

Melanophilin

RAB27A

Dynactin

**Figure 3.9** Movement of melanosomes into dendrites. As melanin is deposited within melanosomes, they migrate along microtubules from the cell body into dendrites in preparation for transfer to keratinocytes. Kinesin and dynein serve as molecular motors for microtubule-associated anterograde and retrograde melanosomal transport, respectively, and UVR results in augmented anterograde transport via increased kinesin and decreased dynein activity. Myosin Va, which is linked to the melanosomal RAB27A GTPase by melanophilin, captures mature melanosomes when they reach the cell periphery and attaches them to the actin cytoskeleton. (Adapted from Bolognia JL, et al. Dermatology, 2nd edn. Philadelphia: Elsevier; 2008).

### Table 3.2 Variation in Types of Melanosomes Within Melanocytes and Keratinocytes With Level of Cutaneous Pigmentation

| Pigmentation of Skin | Predominant Melanosomal Stages | |
|---|---|---|
| | Melanocytes | Keratinocytes |
| Fair | II, III | Occasional III |
| Medium | II, III, IV | III, IV |
| Dark | IV > III | IV |

(Courtesy of Ray Boissy PhD. Reproduced with permission from Bolognia JL, et al. Dermatology. Philadelphia: Elsevier; 2003.)

| | Lightly pigmented skin | Darkly pigmented skin |
|---|---|---|
| Melanization | Stages II, III | Stage IV |
| Size (diameter) | 0.3–0.5 µm | 0.5–0.8 µm |
| Number per cell | <20 | >200 |
| Distribution within lysosomes in keratinocytes | Groups of 2–10 | Single |
| Degradation | Fast | Slow |

**Figure 3.10** Differences between melanosomes in lightly pigmented and darkly pigmented skin. (Reproduced with permission from Bolognia JL, Jorizzo JJ, Rapini RP, eds. *Dermatology*. 2nd ed. Philadelphia: Elsevier; 2008.)

## MELANIN BIOSYNTHESIS AND ITS REGULATION

The functions of melanin in the skin and hair range from camouflage in animals to protection from UVR via photo-absorption and free-radical scavenging in humans. Melanin represents a group of complex polymeric pigments that exist in two basic forms in human skin, brown-black eumelanin

degraded much more slowly, often remaining intact in the stratum corneum (Fig. 3.10).[20] Furthermore, mature eumel-anogenic melanosomes form supranuclear melanin 'caps' that help shield the nuclei of keratinocytes from UVR.

and yellow-red pheomelanin. These types of melanin differ in their biochemical and photoprotective properties as well as the architecture of the melanosomes within which they are produced (see above). For example, the eumelanin found in elliptical, highly structured eumelanosomes is less soluble and has a higher molecular weight than the cysteine-rich pheomelanin found in spherical, unstructured pheomelanosomes. Moreover, pheomelanin is photolabile, generating oxidative stress and resulting in photosensitivity, whereas eumelanin may have some inherent cytotoxicity but confers substantial photoprotection.[27]

## The melanin biosynthetic pathway

The amino acid tyrosine is the starting material for the production of both eumelanin and pheomelanin. Tyrosinase, the key enzyme in the melanin biosynthetic pathway, catalyzes the initial rate-limiting conversion of tyrosine to DOPA. It is a copper-dependent enzyme with two copper-binding sites. This explains the diffuse pigmentary dilution seen in rare cases of copper deficiency and in patients with Menkes kinky hair syndrome who have defects in the ATP7A transporter that delivers copper to melanosomes.[28] In addition to its essential role as a tyrosine hydroxylase, human tyrosinase has DOPA oxidase, 5,6-dihydroxyindole (DHI) oxidase, and perhaps 5,6-dihydroxyindole-2-carboxylic acid (DHICA) oxidase activities that regulate several other steps in the pathway (Fig. 3.11). The total lack of melanin in the skin, hair and eyes of patients with OCA type 1A underscores the importance of

tyrosinase in melanin biosynthesis. In this and other types of OCA (Table 3.1), the decreased production of photoprotective melanin results in increased susceptibility to the development of UVR-induced NMSC, in particular squamous cell carcinomas which can metastasize and lead to premature death, especially in those who reside in the tropics.

Once produced via tyrosinase activity, DOPA can spontaneously oxidize and cyclize to form melanin. However, although tyrosinase was initially thought to be the sole enzyme involved in melanin biosynthesis, by the late 1970s it became clear that there were additional regulators in the pathway. These include two tyrosine-related proteins (TYRPs) that have roles in eumelanogenesis, each a transmembrane protein with approximately 40% amino acid sequence homology with tyrosinase. The major function of TYRP1 is to stabilize tyrosinase; in mice, TYRP1 also acts as a DHICA oxidase, while in humans tyrosinase itself may have this catalytic capacity (Fig. 3.11).[29] Mutations in the TYRP1 gene result in OCA type 3, which is typically associated with a 'rufous' phenotype of reddish-colored hair and skin.[6] TYRP2 serves as a DOPAchrome tautomerase, converting DOPAchrome to DHICA (Fig. 3.11). In the absence of TYRP2, a carboxylic acid group is spontaneously lost and black, insoluble DHI-melanin that has cytotoxic effects as well as photoprotective properties is formed. With TYRP2 activity and the utilization of gp100/Pmel17 as a solid-phase substrate for polymerization, DHICA-melanin is produced. This brown, slightly soluble pigment provides photoprotection with minimal cytotoxicity.

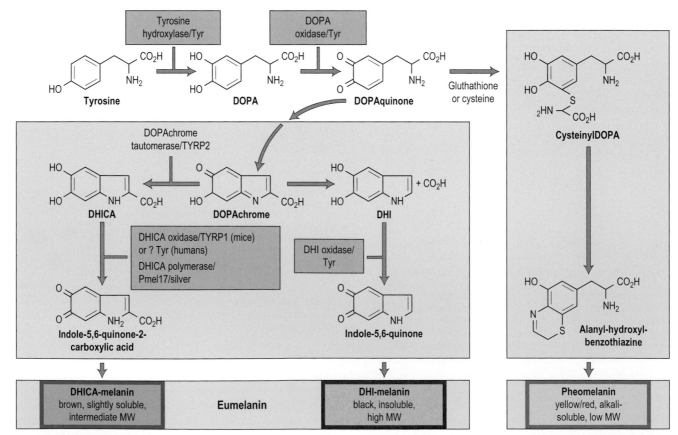

**Figure 3.11** The melanin biosynthetic pathway. The pathway includes the sites of dysfunction in OCA1 (tyrosinase) and OCA3/rufous OCA (TRP1). The two major forms of melanin in the skin and hair are brown-black eumelanin and yellow-red pheomelanin. DHI, 5,6-dihydroxyindole; DHICA, 5,6-dihydroxyindole-2-carboxylic acid; DOPA, dihydroxyphenylalanine; MW, molecular weight; Tyr, tyrosine; TYRP, tyrosinase-related protein. (Courtesy of Dr Vincent Hearing.)

The eumelanin and pheomelanin biosynthetic pathways diverge early on, following the formation of DOPAquinone (Fig. 3.11). At this point, the production of pheomelanin entails the addition of a cysteinyl group that accounts for its yellow-red color. Whereas eumelanin synthesis is associated with increased tyrosinase activity and involves additional melanogenic proteins such as TYRP1 and TYRP2, pheomelanin synthesis in murine melanocytes is associated with a reduction in tyrosinase and a marked reduction to absence of TYRP1, TYRP2, and the P protein (see below).[30] The formation of pheomelanin is therefore regarded as a default pathway.

The P protein, encoded at the *pink-eyed dilution* locus in mice, is a transmembrane protein with an important role in eumelanogenesis (Fig. 3.12),[31] although its exact function is not currently known. Mutations in the *P* gene in humans lead to OCA type 2 (Table 3.1).[32] Because its amino acid sequence is homologous to that of transmembrane transporters of small molecules and high concentrations of tyrosine can increase pigment production in P-null melanocytes, it was initially predicted that the P protein might serve to transport tyrosine across the melanosomal membrane. However, kinetic studies showed no difference between the melanosomes of wild-type and P-null melanocytes in the rate of tyrosine uptake. A second hypothesis is that the P protein regulates the pH of melanosomes and/or other organelles, potentially mediating neutralization of pH to optimize the activity and/or folding of tyrosinase.[33] The restoration of pigment production in P-null cells by vacuolar $H^+$-ATPase inhibitors (e.g. bafilomycin A1) that are known to alkalinize (i.e. neutralize) organelles supports this theory. More recently, it was shown that the majority of the P protein in melanocytes is actually located in the ER rather than in melanosomes, and that abnormal processing and trafficking of tyrosinase occurs when the P protein is absent.[34] In addition, it was observed that the P protein facilitates vacuolar accumulation of glutathione, a major redox buffer that is required for the folding of cysteine-rich proteins such as tyrosinase. The P protein may thus regulate the processing of tyrosinase via control of glutathione. It has been speculated that the resistance of melanoma cells to chemotherapeutic agents detoxified by glutathione-dependent mechanisms (e.g. cisplatin and doxorubicin) could be related to decreased sequestration of glutathione due to a lack of P protein activity.

## Melanogenesis-related proteins and other melanoma-associated antigens

A number of melanoma-associated antigens (MAAs) have been identified and shown to induce both cytotoxic T-lymphocyte and antibody responses in melanoma patients, providing the basis for the development of vaccine therapies (e.g. utilizing tumor lysates, peptides, peptide-loaded dendritic cells, or DNA plasmids expressing peptides). There are two major types of MAA proteins (Table 3.3): (1) melanocyte-differentiation antigens and (2) tumor/testis-specific antigens.

The pathogenesis of melanoma-associated leukoderma (MAL) has important implications with regard to tumor

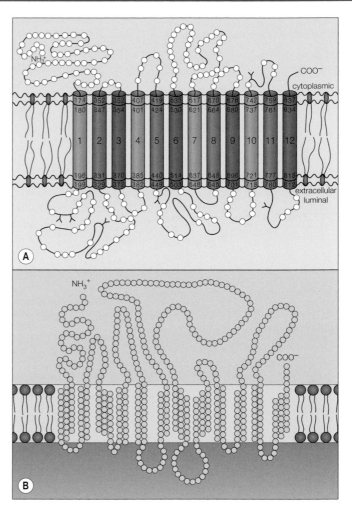

**Figure 3.12** Proposed models for the arrangements of the P protein and membrane-associated transporter protein (MATP) within the lipid bilayer. **A)** The P protein, which is defective in OCA type 2, has 12 putative transmembrane domains. (Reprinted with permission from Rinchik EM, et al. A gene for the mouse pink-eyed dilution locus and for human type II oculocutaneous albinism. Nature 1993;361:72–76. Copyright © 1993 Macmillan Magazine Ltd.) **B)** The membrane-associated transporter protein, which is defective in OCA type 4, also has 12 transmembrane domains. (Reproduced with permission of the University of Chicago from Newton JM, Cohen-Barak O, Hagiwara N, et al. Mutations in the human orthologue of the mouse underwhite gene (uw) underlie a new form of oculocutaneous albinism, OCA4. Am J Hum Genet. 2001;69:981-988. Copyright © 2001 American Society of Human Genetics.)

immunity. Like vitiligo, it is associated with the presence of autoreactive T cells and antibodies directed against melanocyte-differentiation antigens (Fig. 3.13). The development of MAL can herald spontaneous disease regression in a small subset of patients with metastatic melanoma and is seen in responders to immunotherapy (e.g. IL-2, peptide vaccines, anti-CTLA-4 antibody).[35]

The presence of melanocyte-differentiation antigens also serves as a diagnostic marker for melanoma. In addition to the use of immunohistochemical stains, reverse transcriptase–polymerase chain reaction (PCR)-based assays have been developed to detect melanoma cells in tumor-draining lymph nodes and in the circulation. However, it is important to be aware of the variable sensitivities and specificities of PCR-based tests, as well as other potential diagnostic pitfalls such as nodal nevi.

### Table 3.3  Selected Melanoma-Associated Antigens

| Gene | Protein (Immunohistochemical Stain) | Functions |
|---|---|---|
| **Melanocyte-differentiation antigens** – melanogenesis-related proteins specific to melanocytes and melanoma cells | | |
| TYR | Tyrosinase (T311) | Tyrosine hydroxylase, DOPA oxidase, e and, in humans, possibly DHICA oxidase |
| TYRP1 | TYRP1/gp75 (MEL-5) | Stabilizes tyrosinase; in mice, also functions as DHICA oxidase |
| TYRP2 (DCT) | TYRP2/DCT | DOPAchrome tautomerase |
| OCA2 (P) | P protein | Regulates organelle pH, glutathione accumulation, and/or processing/trafficking of tyrosinase |
| SILV | gp100/Pmel17/silver (HMB45) | Generates fibrillar matrix of melanosomes; stabilizes melanogenic enzymes/intermediates and acts as a substrate for DHICA polymerization; marker for cellular activation |
| MART1 | MelanA/MART1 (A103) | Membrane protein required for Pmel17 function and melanosome maturation |
| MC1R | MC1R | Stimulates eumelanin production, melanocyte proliferation and dendricity |
| MITF | MITF | Regulates transcription of TYR, TYRP1 and TYRP2; also upregulates expression of the anti-apoptotic protein Bcl2 |
| **Tumor/testis-specific antigens*** – proteins encoded by genes that are expressed in various tumors including melanomas, but are silent in normal adult tissues other than the testis | | |
| MAGE1 | MAGE1/MZ2-E | |
| MAGE3 | MAGE3/MZ2-D | |
| BAGE | BAGE/Ba | |
| GAGE1/2 | GAGE1/2/MZ2-F | |
| NY-ESO1 | NY-ESO1 | |
| **Other types of tumor-specific antigens that result from mutated or aberrantly expressed genes** | | |
| Antigens that result from mutations (unique to each patient, with the exception of CDC27) | | |
| MUM1–3 | MUM1–3 | |
| CDK4 | Cyclin-dependent kinase 4 | |
| CTNNB1 | β-catenin | |
| MART2 | MART2 | |
| CDC27 | CDC27 | |
| Antigens that result from alternative transcription and/or splicing | | |
| TYRP2 | TYRP2-6b, TYRP2-INT2, others | |
| GNT-V | NA17-A (encoded by an intronic region in the N-acetylglucosaminyl-transferase V gene) | |
| Antigens reflecting selective overexpression in melanomas, other tumors, and leukemias of genes that are expressed at a low level in a variety of tissues | | |
| PRAME | PRAME | |
| P15 | p15 | |

OCA2, oculocutaneous albinism 2; TYRP, tyrosinase-related protein; MART, melanoma antigen recognized by T cells; MC1R, melanocortin-1 receptor; MITF, microphthalmia-associated transcription factor; MUM, melanoma-ubiquitously mutated; PRAME, preferentially expressed antigen in melanoma.

*In general, lower immunogenicity than melanocyte-differentiation antigens. For a more complete list, see www.cancerimmunity.org/peptidedatabase/tumorspecific.htm.

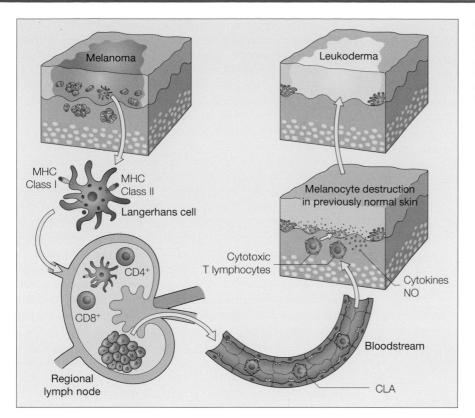

**Figure 3.13** Model for the pathogenesis of melanoma-associated leukoderma. Sensitization to melanocyte-differentiation antigens expressed by melanoma cells can result in immunologic attack on normal melanocytes, producing vitiligo-like patches of depigmentation. CLA, cutaneous lymphocyte antigen; NO, nitric oxide.

## Regulation of melanin biosynthesis

The ratio of eumelanin to pheomelanin, as well as the total melanin content, is higher in skin types V to VI than in skin types I to II. Pheomelanin levels are greatest in 'fire' red hair, while eumelanin predominates in most human hair colors other than red.[36] The amount and type of melanin produced is determined by a complex interplay of the activity levels of the enzymes, transporters, and enzyme-stabilizing or structural proteins that are involved in melanogenesis. The factors known to influence the activity of these key proteins and control the eumelanin/pheomelanin switch include α-MSH, agouti signaling protein (ASIP), endothelin-1, basic fibroblast growth factor (bFGF), and UVR (Fig. 3.14).

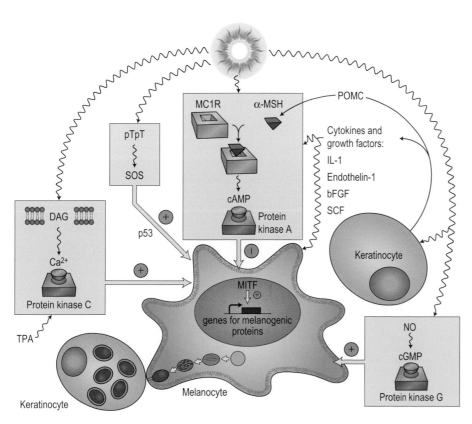

**Figure 3.14** Mechanisms of UVR-induced melanogenesis. These include an increase in one or more of the following: (1) expression of POMC and its derivative peptides by keratinocytes, melanocytes and other cells in the skin; (2) the number of MC1R on melanocytes; (3) the release of diacylglycerol (DAG) from the plasma membrane, which activates protein kinase C; (4) the induction of an SOS response to UVR-induced DNA damage; (5) nitric oxide (NO) production, which activates the cGMP pathway; and (6) production of cytokines and growth factors by keratinocytes. As a result, there is enhanced transcription of the genes that encode MITF and melanogenic proteins including tyrosinase, TYRP1, TYRP2, gp100/Pmel17, and P. In addition, melanocyte dendricity and transfer of melanosomes to keratinocytes is stimulated via increased activity of RAC1 (involved in dendrite formation), ratio of kinesin to dynein, and expression of protease-activated receptor-2 (PAR2; involved in melanosome transfer). TPA, tetradecanoyl phorbol acetate. (Adapted from Bolognia JL, Jorizzo JJ, Rapini RP, eds. *Dermatology*. 2nd ed. Philadelphia: Elsevier; 2008.)

The melanocortin peptides (including α-, β- and γ-MSH as well as adrenocorticotropic hormone [ACTH]), β-endorphin and β-lipotropic hormone are all cleavage products of a single precursor protein, pro-opiomelanocortin (POMC; Fig. 3.15). Although POMC-derived peptides were originally identified as pituitary hormones, POMC is also synthesized and differentially processed in the hypothalamus, other regions of the brain, and a variety of peripheral tissues, including the gastrointestinal tract, gonads and, of particular interest to us, the skin. In humans, α-MSH (the major type of MSH) and ACTH have similar potencies in activating the melanocyte MC1R,[37] and the relative contribution of centrally and peripherally derived forms of each to baseline melanogenesis in vivo has yet to be determined. Nevertheless, it is clear that centrally produced melanocortins can dramatically influence cutaneous pigmentation, as evidenced by the generalized hyperpigmentation seen in disorders such as Addison's disease that are characterized by pituitary hypersecretion of ACTH and/or α-MSH.

Likewise, melanocortins produced peripherally by the skin can have a prominent role in promoting melanogenesis, most notably as a protective response to UVR. POMC is expressed by a variety of epidermal and dermal cell types, including melanocytes, keratinocytes, fibroblasts, endothelial cells and antigen-presenting cells. Both UVR and the epidermally derived, UVR-induced cytokine interleukin-1 (IL-1) stimulate increased synthesis and enzymatic processing of POMC by melanocytes and keratinocytes, providing autocrine as well as paracrine regulation of cutaneous pigmentation (Fig. 3.14).

In addition to their well-known roles in pigmentation and adrenocortical steroidogenesis, melanocortin peptides serve other important functions by binding to the various melanocortin receptors (MCRs) present in different tissues (Table 3.4). These biologic activities range from suppression of inflammation to regulation of body weight to stimulation of lipid production in sebaceous glands. A phenotype of severe early onset obesity, adrenal insufficiency and red hair has been described in individuals with mutations in the *POMC* gene.[38] It is therefore not surprising that mutations in the genes that encode the receptors to which the POMC-derived peptides bind can produce similar clinical manifestations. For example, *MC4R* mutations result in morbid obesity, *MC2R* mutations cause adrenal insufficiency, and *MC1R* mutations are associated with red hair (see below).

To date, five MCRs (MC1R–MC5R) have been identified, each with distinctive tissue distribution, relative affinities for melanocortin ligands, and physiologic roles (Table 3.4). The MCRs represent a subfamily of G-protein-coupled receptors, all with seven transmembrane domains (Fig. 3.16) and signal transduction via an associated protein complex that binds guanosine triphosphate (GTP) and guanosine diphosphate (GDP). Upon ligand binding to an MCR, the α-subunit of the receptor-coupled stimulatory G-protein ($G_s\alpha$) activates adenylate cyclase, which increases production of the second messenger cyclic adenosine monophosphate (cAMP; Fig. 3.17).[39]

The key MCR in the skin, the MC1R, is found on many types of cells, including keratinocytes, fibroblasts, endothelial cells and antigen-presenting cells; however, melanocytes clearly have the highest MC1R density.[40] Melanocyte MC1R expression has a central role in the induction of photoprotective melanization in response to UV exposure,

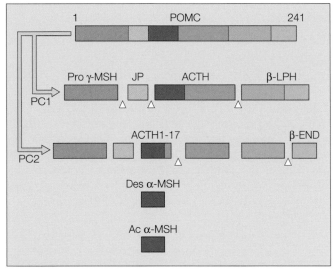

**Figure 3.15** Post-translational processing of the pro-opiomelanocortin (POMC) precursor protein. Ac, acetylated; ACTH, adrenocorticotropic hormone; Des, desacetyl; END, endorphin; JP, joining peptide; LPH, lipotropic hormone; MSH, melanocyte-stimulating hormone; PC, prohormone-converting enzyme. (Adapted from Bolognia JL, Jorizzo JJ, Rapini RP, eds. *Dermatology*. 2nd ed. Philadelphia: Elsevier; 2008.)

## Table 3.4 Melanocortin Receptors

| Receptor | Distribution | | Ligands |
| --- | --- | --- | --- |
| | **Major** | **Minor** | **Ligands** |
| MC1R* | Melanocytes | Keratinocytes, fibroblasts, endothelial cells, antigen-presenting cells | α-MSH, ACTH >> β-MSH |
| MC2R | Adrenal cortex | Adipocytes | ACTH |
| MC3R† | Brain | Gut, placenta | α-, β-, γ-MSH, ACTH |
| MC4R† | Brain | | α-, β-MSH, ACTH |
| MC5R | Peripheral tissues | Fibroblasts, adipocytes, sebaceous glands | α-, β-MSH, ACTH |

*Agouti protein (mouse) and agouti signaling protein (ASIP; human) are the major antagonistic ligands.

†Agouti-related protein (AGRP) is the major antagonistic ligand.

(Reproduced with permission from Bolognia JL, et al. Dermatology, 2nd edn. Philadelphia: Elsevier; 2008.)

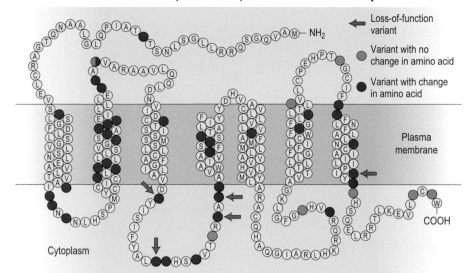

**Melanocortin-1 receptor within the plasma membrane of a melanocyte**

Loss-of-function variant

Variant with no change in amino acid

Variant with change in amino acid

Plasma membrane

Cytoplasm

**Figure 3.16** Melanocortin-1 receptor (MC1R) within the plasma membrane of a melanocyte. The red dots indicate the locations of amino acid changes (compared to the wild type) in MC1R variants that have been reported. Some of the variants are due to partial or complete loss-of-function mutations (i.e. the generation of cAMP in response to α-MSH binding is impaired), whereas others have no effect on function. Loss-of-function variants, e.g. Arg151Cys, Arg160His, and Asp294His, are associated with red hair, fair skin, and increased risk of melanoma and non-melanoma skin cancers. The tan dots represent synonymous variants where there is no change in amino acid sequence. (Adapted from Bolognia JL, Jorizzo JJ, Rapini RP, eds. *Dermatology*. 2nd ed. Philadelphia: Elsevier; 2008.)

and is stimulated by α-MSH, ACTH, UVR, and a variety of UVR-induced, keratinocyte-derived cytokines and growth factors such as IL-1, endothelin-1 and bFGF (Fig. 3.14). When the melanocyte MC1R is activated by ligand binding, elevated intracellular cAMP results in melanocyte proliferation, increased dendricity, and stimulation of the expression and activity of tyrosinase and other melanogenic proteins, which leads to eumelanin production.[41] If the MC1R is dysfunctional and ligand binding fails to induce cAMP production, pheomelanogenesis is favored (Fig. 3.18).

Although human pigmentation is genetically complex, the *MC1R* gene plays a major role in physiologic variation of hair and skin color.[42] The *MC1R* gene is highly polymorphic, with approximately 50% of individuals in white populations carrying at least one of more than 50 variant alleles reported to date (Fig. 3.16). Homozygous or compound heterozygous loss-of-function *MC1R* mutations (i.e. resulting in impaired cAMP generation in response to α-MSH) have been shown to largely account for the red hair phenotype in humans, which approximates an autosomal recessive trait and increases the risk of developing melanoma over fourfold.[43] In addition, these loss-of-function *MC1R* mutations have a strong association with fair skin, a decreased ability to tan, and freckling, resulting in a significant heterozygote effect in individuals without red hair.

Moreover, loss-of-function *MC1R* mutations also confer a significantly increased risk of melanoma (approximately doubled for each variant allele carried) and NMSC (two- to threefold increase with two variant alleles) that is independent of pigmentary phenotype.[3] In the setting of familial melanoma, *MC1R* genotype modifies melanoma risk in individuals carrying mutations in the cyclin-dependent kinase inhibitor gene *CDKN2A*, with the presence of a variant *MC1R* allele significantly increasing raw penetrance (from 50% to 80%) and decreasing mean age of onset (from 58 years to 37 years; Fig. 3.19).[44] Loss-of-function *MC1R* mutations markedly increase the sensitivity of melanocytes to the cytotoxic effects of UVR and, in melanoma

cells, reduce α-MSH-induced effects such as suppression of proliferation and decreased binding to fibronectin.[45] The *MC1R* genotype may thus serve as a marker of susceptibility to skin cancer beyond its visible effects on pigmentary phenotype. Other pigmentation gene polymorphisms that have been shown to contribute to physiologic variation in skin, hair or eye color and (in some instances) risk of melanoma or NMSC are presented in Table 3.5.[46–49]

The switch between eumelanin and pheomelanin synthesis is regulated not only by the binding of melanocortin ligands that activate the MC1R, but also by a physiologic antagonist known as the agouti protein.[50] The latter is a soluble paracrine factor synthesized by dermal papilla cells within the hair follicle that acts as a competitive inhibitor of α-MSH binding to the MC1R and also reduces basal MC1R activity in the absence of α-MSH, likely by functioning as an inverse agonist or effecting MC1R desensitization. Binding of agouti protein to the MC1R thus blocks eumelanin production and induces pheomelanin synthesis (Fig. 3.18). The term 'agouti' refers to the presence of a subapical band of yellow pheomelanic pigment in an otherwise black eumelanic hair shaft; this pattern results from transient 'turning on' of agouti protein production during the mid phase of the hair growth cycle, and it is seen in mice, dogs and foxes. In mice with a dominant mutation at the agouti locus, excessive synthesis of agouti protein throughout the body results in a uniformly yellow coat and obesity, the latter caused by antagonism of the hypothalamic MC4R.

In addition to signaling via the MC1R, pigment production can be enhanced by exposure of melanocytes to agents that increase cytoplasmic levels of cAMP, such as isobutyl-methylxanthine (Figs 3.13 and 3.16). The activation of protein kinase A (PKA) by cAMP leads to the phosphorylation of many substrates, one of which is the cAMP responsive element binding protein (CREB), a transcription factor that regulates the expression of multiple genes, including those with pivotal roles in melanogenesis.[41] For example, CREB binds and activates the *MITF* promoter, and increased production of MITF (see above) in turn results in upregulation of *TYR*, *TYRP1* and *TYRP2* gene expression.

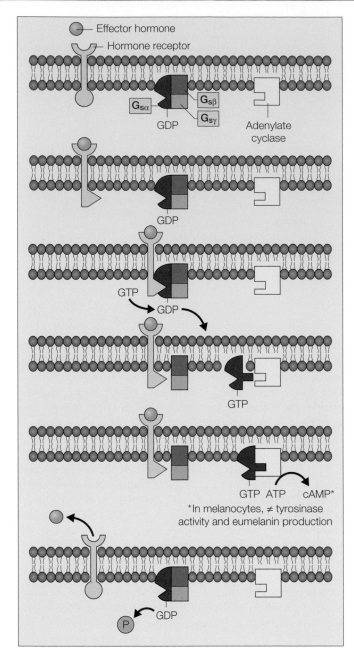

Figure 3.17 Activation of a G-protein-coupled receptor such as the melanocortin-1 receptor (MC1R). Binding of a ligand to the receptor results in activation of adenylate cyclase via the α-subunit of the receptor-coupled stimulatory G-protein (G$_{s\alpha}$). This produces an elevation in the intracellular concentration of cyclic adenosine monophosphate (cAMP), which, in the case of the MC1R, leads to an increase in tyrosinase activity and eumelanin production. GDP, guanosine diphosphate; GTP, guanosine triphosphate; P, phosphate group; ATP, adenosine triphosphate. (Adapted from Alberts B, Johnson A, Lewis J, et al. Molecular biology of the cell, 3rd edn. New York, NY: Garland; 1994.)

## Effects of ultraviolet radiation

Stimulation of melanogenesis by UVR (i.e. tanning) is a well-known phenomenon (Fig. 3.14). Considering that the MCIR plays a central role in the process, it is not surprising that it closely resembles the pigmentary response of melanocytes to α-MSH.[30] Following either a single erythemal exposure or several suberythemal exposures to UVR, an increase in the size, dendricity and number of active melanocytes as well as enhanced tyrosinase function and melanin

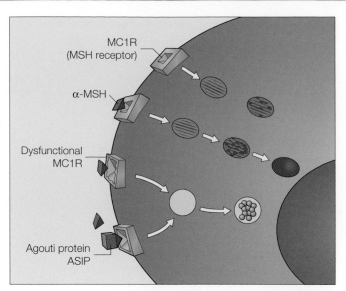

Figure 3.18 Interaction of α-melanocyte stimulating hormone (α-MSH) and agouti signaling protein (ASIP) with the melanocortin-1 receptor (MC1R). There is some baseline activity of the MC1R; this is enhanced by α-MSH-binding, resulting in increased eumelanogenesis. Dysfunction of the MC1R (as in the case of humans with red hair) or binding of ASIP, a physiologic antagonist, leads to pheomelanogenesis.

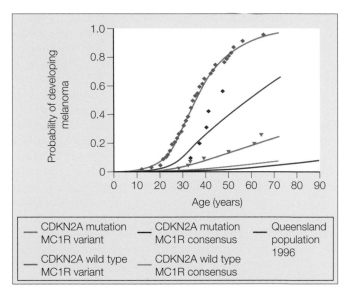

Figure 3.19 Modification of melanoma risk by the presence of a variant *MC1R* allele in individuals carrying mutations in the cyclin-dependent kinase inhibitor gene *CDKN2A*. (Reproduced by kind permission of the University of Chicago. Box NF, Duffy DL, Chen W, et al. MC1R genotype modifies risk of melanoma in families segregating CDKN2A mutations. *Am J Hum Genet*. 2001;69:765-773. Copyright © 2001. American Society of Human Genetics.)

production can be observed.[51] Repeated exposures to UVR lead to increased formation of stage IV melanosomes and their efficient transfer to keratinocytes, while treatment with psoralens plus UVA (PUVA) also leads to an alteration in the size and aggregation pattern of melanosomes, which become larger and singly dispersed (i.e. similar to those found in darkly pigmented skin; Fig. 3.10). Chronically sun-exposed sites (e.g. the outer upper arm) have an up to twofold higher density of melanocytes than adjacent sun-protected sites (e.g. the inner upper arm).[19] As melanocytes normally have a low mitotic rate, it is not clear whether the increased number of pigment-producing melanocytes results from a higher mitotic rate or an activation of

**Table 3.5 Genes Associated with Physiologic Variation in Human Pigmentation[46-49]**

| Gene | Protein | Selected Variant(s): Amino Acid Alteration (if applicable) or SNP | Skin Color, Sun Sensitivity, and Freckles | Hair Color | Eye Color | Skin Cancer Risk* | Population Frequencies of Variant Haplotype | | |
|---|---|---|---|---|---|---|---|---|---|
| | | | | | | | European | East Asian | African |
| TYR | Tyrosinase | Ser192Tyr | Freckles | -- | -- | SCC Melanoma, BCC | 0.4 | 0 | 0 |
| | | Arg402Gln | Fair, sun sensitive | Light (weak) | Blue (vs green) | BCC | 0.4 | 0 | 0.07 |
| TYRP1 | TYRP1 | rs1408799 C>T | Sun sensitive | Light | Blue | Melanoma | 0.7 | 0.02 | 0.2 |
| | | rs2733832 C>T | -- | Light | Blue | -- | 0.6 | 0.02 | 0.07 |
| OCA2 (P) | P protein | Arg305Trp | -- | -- | Brown | -- | 0.07 | 0.04 | 0.02 |
| | | Arg419Gln | -- | -- | Green/hazel Brown | Melanoma, BCC | 0.07 | -- | 0 |
| | | His615Arg | -- | -- | Blue | -- | 0 | 0.5 | 0 |
| | | rs12913832 T>C in HERC2† | Fair | Light | | Melanoma (weak) | 0.75 | -- | -- |
| SLC45A2 | MATP | Glu272Lys | Dark | Dark | Non-blue | -- | 0 | 0.4 | 0.05 |
| | | Leu374Phe | Fair | Light | Blue | Melanoma, NMSC | 0.95 | 0.01 | 0 |
| SLC24A5 | NCKX5 | Ala111Thr | Light | -- | -- | -- | 0.99 | 0.01 | 0.02 |
| SLC24A4 | SLC24A4 | rs12896399 G>T | Sun sensitive | Light | Blue (vs green) | -- | 0.6 | 0.5 | 0.01 |
| MC1R | MC1R | R alleles‡ | Fair, sun sensitive, freckles | Red/light | -- | Melanoma, NMSC | 0.3 | 0 | 0 |
| | | r alleles§ | Variable | Variable | -- | Melanoma, NMSC | 0.3 | 0.4 | 0.01 |
| ASIP | ASIP | g.8818 A>G | Dark | Dark | Brown | -- | 0.15 | -- | 0.6 |
| | | ASIP haplotype‖ | Fair, sun sensitive, freckles | Red/light | Light | Melanoma, NMSC | 0.1-0.3 | 0-0.2 | 0-0.1 |
| KITLG | KIT ligand | rs642742 A>G | Fair | -- | -- | -- | 0.85 | 0.8 | 0.07 |
| | | rs12821256 T>C | -- | Light | -- | -- | 0.15 | 0 | 0 |
| TPCN2 | TPCN2 | Met484Leu | -- | Light | -- | -- | 0.2 | 0 | 0 |
| | | Gly734Gln | -- | Light | -- | -- | 0.4 | 0.2 | 0.02 |
| IRF4 | Interferon regulatory factor 4 | rs12203592 C>T | Fair, sun sensitive | Dark | Blue | -- | 0.8 | 0 | 0 |
| | | rs1540771 G>A | Sun sensitive, freckles | Dark (weak) | -- | -- | 0.5 | 0.2 | 0.05 |

ASIP, agouti signaling protein; BCC, basal cell carcinoma; MATP, membrane-associated transporter protein; MC1R, melanocortin-1 receptor; NCKX5, Na-Ca-K exchanger 5; NMSC, non-melanoma skin cancer; SCC, squamous cell carcinoma; SLC24A4/5, solute carrier family 24, member 4/5; SLC45A2, solute carrier family 45, member 2; TPCN2, two-pore segment channel 2; TYRP1, tyrosinase-related protein 1.

Gray highlight = polymorphism associated with darker pigmentation

*Independent of pigmentary phenotype.

†Intronic regulatory region that determines expression of the OCA2 gene; other intronic polymorphisms in the HERC2 gene have also been linked to decreased pigmentation, with the same proposed mechanism.

‡High-penetrance, loss-of-function 'red hair color' alleles, e.g. Asp84Glu, Arg151Cys, Arg160Trp, and Asp294His.

§Low-penetrance alleles, e.g. Val60Leu, Val92Met, and (especially in East Asians) Arg163Gln.

‖Single long (~1.8 Mb) haplotype that includes multiple single nucleotide polymorphisms (SNPs; e.g. rs4911414 G>T and rs4911442 A>G) and encompasses several smaller haplotype blocks.

'dormant' melanocytes or melanocyte precursors. UVR exposure has been shown to induce KIT+ melanocyte precursors in mouse epidermal sheets to proliferate and differentiate into mature melanocytes.[52]

In human skin, the pigmentary response to UVR has two phases. Immediate pigmentary darkening occurs within minutes of exposure to UVA radiation and fades over 6–8 hours. Most prominent in darkly pigmented skin, it is thought to result from photo-oxidation of pre-existing melanin or melanin precursors. The second phase, delayed tanning, is clinically apparent within 48–72 hours of exposure to UVA and/or UVB radiation and represents de novo melanogenesis via an increase in tyrosinase activity. Of note, oxygen dependence is a feature particular to UVA-induced erythema and pigment production, explaining the lack of tanning over dorsal pressure points in those who use UVA tanning 'beds'.

Melanin defends the skin from UVR-induced damage not only by absorbing and scattering incident light, but also by scavenging reactive oxygen species. However, paradoxically, pheomelanin itself is photolabile, generating free radicals and oxidative stress upon UVR exposure. Individuals with increased pheomelanin production due to the presence of two *MC1R* variant alleles have significantly steeper dose–response curves for UVB radiation-induced erythema than those with one or no variant allele. In addition, the presence of certain pheomelanin derivatives in the hair has been shown to serve as a marker for individuals with extremely low minimal erythemal dose values.[36] The level of photoprotection thus depends both on the total content of melanin and the eumelanin:pheomelanin ratio. Although constitutive pigmentation has been estimated to provide the equivalent of a sun protection factor (SPF) of 10–15 in individuals with dark brown to black skin, with five times more UVR reaching the papillary dermis of Caucasian than black skin,[20,27] the 'induced' SPF provided by a tan is only 2–3 in those with skin types II–IV.[53]

## FUTURE OUTLOOK

Overwhelming epidemiologic evidence implicates solar radiation as a major cause of skin cancer in humans. The photoprotective or photosensitizing properties of melanin pigment itself, which are largely determined by the functional status of the MC1R, represent critical factors in the development of both cutaneous melanoma and NMSC. In the future, characterization of the chemical nature of the melanin produced as well as the status of the *MC1R* gene, which appear to have effects on susceptibility to tumor development beyond the visible phenotype, may provide a more accurate method for assessment of an individual's risk for skin cancer.

## REFERENCES

1. Lin JY, Fisher DE. Melanocyte biology and skin pigmentation. *Nature.* 2007;445:843–850.
2. Yamaguchi Y, Brenner M, Hearing VJ. The regulation of skin pigmentation. *J Biol Chem.* 2007;282:27557–27561.
3. Raimondi S, Sera F, Gandini S, et al. MC1R variants, melanoma and red hair color phenotype. *Int J Cancer.* 2008;122:2753–2760.
4. Seiji M, Fitzpatrick TB, Birbeck MSC. The melanosome: a distinctive subcellular particle of mammalian melanocytes and the site of melanogenesis. *J Invest Dermatol.* 1961;36:243–252.
5. Adameyko I, Lallemend F, Aquino JB, et al. Schwann cell precursors from nerve innervations are a cellular origin of melanocytes in skin. *Cell.* 2009;139:366–379.
6. Bolognia JL. Molecular advances in disorders of pigmentation. *Adv Dermatol.* 1999;15:341–365.
7. Wang ZQ, Si L, Tang Q, et al. Gain-of-function mutation of KIT ligand on melanin synthesis causes familial progressive hyperpigmentation. *Am J Hum Genet.* 2009;84:672–677.
8. Curtin JA, Busam K, Pinkel D, et al. Somatic activation of KIT in distinct subtypes of melanoma. *J Clin Oncol.* 2006;24:4340–4346.
9. Hachiya A, Kobayashi A, Ohuchi A, et al. The paracrine role of stem cell factor/c-kit signaling in the activation of human melanocytes in ultraviolet-B-induced pigmentation. *J Invest Dermatol.* 2001;116:578–586.
10. Goding CR. Mitf from neural crest to melanoma: signal transduction and transcription in the melanocyte lineage. *Genes Dev.* 2000;14:1712–1728.
11. McGill GG, Horstmann M, Widlund HR, et al. Bcl2 regulation by the melanocyte master regulator Mitf modulates lineage survival and melanoma cell viability. *Cell.* 2002;109:707–718.
12. Zimmerman AA, Becker Jr SW. Precursors of epidermal melanocytes in the Negro fetus. In: Cordon M, ed. *Pigment Cell Biology.* New York, NY: Academic Press; 1959:159–170.
13. Kunisada T, Yamazaka H, Hayashi S. Ligands for receptor tyrosine kinases expressed in the skin as environmental factors for melanocyte development. *J Invest Dermatol Symp Proc.* 2001;6:6–9.
14. Holbrook KA, Underwood RA, Vogel AM, et al. The appearance, density and distribution of melanocytes in human embryonic and fetal skin revealed by the anti-melanoma monoclonal antibody, HMB-45. *Anat Embryol.* 1989;180:443–455.
15. Jimbow K, Quevedo Jr WC, Fitzpatrick TB, et al. Some aspects of melanin biology: 1950-1975. *J Invest Dermatol.* 1976;67:72–89.
16. Horikawa T, Norris DA, Johnson TW, et al. DOPA-negative melanocytes in the outer root sheath of human hair follicles express premelanosomal antigens but not a melanosomal antigen or the melanosome-associated glycoproteins tyrosinase, TRP-1, and TRP-2. *J Invest Dermatol.* 1996;106:28–35.
17. Tobin DJ, Bystryn JC. Different populations of melanocytes are present in hair follicles and epidermis. *Pigment Cell Res.* 1996;9:304–310.
18. Nishimura EK, Jordan SA, Oshima H, et al. Dominant role of the niche in melanocyte stem-cell fate determination. *Nature.* 2002;416:854–860.
19. Gilchrest BA, Blog FB, Szabo G. Effects of aging and chronic sun exposure on melanocytes in human skin. *J Invest Dermatol.* 1979;73:41–43.
20. Bolognia JL, Pawelek JM. Biology of hypopigmentation. *J Am Acad Dermatol.* 1988;19:217–255.
21. Orlow SJ. Melanosomes are specialized members of the lysosomal lineage of organelles. *J Invest Dermatol.* 1995;105:3–7.
22. Watabe H, Valencia JC, Yasumoto KI, et al. Regulation of tyrosinase processing and trafficking by organellar pH and by proteasome activity. *J Biol Chem.* 2004;279:7971–7981.
23. Marks MS, Seabra MC. The melanosome: membrane dynamics in black and white. *Nat Rev Mol Cell Biol.* 2001;2:1–11.
24. Wei ML. Hermansky-Pudlak syndrome: a disease of protein trafficking and organelle function. *Pigment Cell Res.* 2006;19:19–42.
25. Kushimoto T, Basrur V, Valencia J, et al. A model for melanosome biogenesis based on the purification and analysis of early melanosomes. *Proc Natl Acad Sci U S A.* 2001;98:10698–10703.
26. McGlinchey RP, Shewmaker F, McPhie P, et al. The repeat domain of the melanosome fibril protein Pmel17 forms the amyloid core promoting melanin synthesis. *Proc Natl Acad Sci U S A.* 2009;106:13731–13736.
27. Ortonne J-P. Photoprotective properties of skin melanin. *Br J Dermatol.* 2002;146:7–10.
28. Setty SR, Tenza D, Sviderskaya EV, et al. Cell-specific ATP7A transport sustains copper-dependent tyrosinase activity in melanosomes. *Nature.* 2008;454:1142–1146.
29. Olivares C, Jiminez-Cervantes C, Lozano JA. The 5,6-dihydroxyindole-2-carboxylic acid (DHICA) oxidase activity of human tyrosinase. *Biochem J.* 2001;354:131–139.
30. Hearing VJ. Biochemical control of melanogenesis and melanosomal organization. *J Invest Dermatol Symp Proc.* 1999;4:24–28.
31. Newton JM, Cohen-Barak O, Hagiwara N, et al. Mutations in the human orthologue of the mouse underwhite gene (uw) underlie a new form of oculocutaneous albinism, OCA4. *Am J Hum Genet.* 2001;69:981–988.
32. Rinchik EM, Bultman SJ, Horsthemke B, et al. A gene for the mouse pink-eyed dilution locus and for human type II oculocutaneous albinism. *Nature.* 1993;361:72–76.
33. Ancans J, Tobin DJ, Hoogduijn MJ, et al. Melanosomal pH controls rate of melanogenesis, eumelanin/phaeomelanin ratio and melanosome maturation in melanocytes and melanoma cells. *Exp Cell Res.* 2001;268:26–35.
34. Chen K, Manga P, Orlow SJ. Pink-eyed dilution protein controls the processing of tyrosinase. *Mol Biol Cell.* 2002;13:1953–1964.
35. Rosenberg SA, White DE. Vitiligo in patients with melanomas: normal tissue antigens can be targets for cancer immunotherapy. *J Immunother Emphasis Tumor Immunol.* 1996;19:81–84.

36. Prota G. Melanins, melanogenesis and melanocytes: looking at their functional significance from the chemist's viewpoint. *Pigment Cell Res.* 2000;13:283–293.

37. Abdel-Malek Z, Swope VB, Suzuki I, et al. Mitogenic and melanogenic stimulation of normal human melanocytes by melanotropic peptides. *Proc Natl Acad Sci U S A.* 1995;92:1789–1793.

38. Krude H, Biebermann H, Luck W, et al. Severe early-onset obesity, adrenal insufficiency and red hair pigmentation caused by POMC mutations in humans. *Nat Genet.* 1998;19:155–157.

39. Alberts B, Johnson A, Lewis J, et al. *Molecular Biology of the Cell.* 3rd ed. New York, NY: Garland; 1994.

40. Luger TA, Scholzen T, Grabbe S. The role of alpha-melanocyte stimulating hormone in cutaneous biology. *J Invest Dermatol Symp Proc.* 1997;2:87–93.

41. Busca R, Ballotti R. Cyclic AMP as key messenger in the regulation of skin pigmentation. *Pigment Cell Res.* 2000;13:60–69.

42. Sturm RA, Teasdale RD, Box NF. Human pigmentation genes: identification, structure and consequences of polymorphic variation. *Gene.* 2001;277:49–62.

43. Schaffer JV, Bolognia JL. The melanocortin-1 receptor: red hair and beyond. *Arch Dermatol.* 2001;137:1477–1485.

44. Box NF, Duffy DL, Chen W, et al. MC1R genotype modifies risk of melanoma in families segregating CDKN2A mutations. *Am J Hum Genet.* 2001;69:765–773.

45. Robinson SJ, Healy E. Human melanocortin 1 receptor (MC1R) gene variants alter melanoma cell growth and adhesion to extracellular matrix. *Oncogene.* 2002;21:8037–8046.

46. Sturm RA. Molecular genetics of human pigmentation diversity. *Hum Mol Genet.* 2009;18:R9–R17.

47. Gudbjartsson DF, Sulem P, Stacey SN, et al. *ASIP* and *TYR* pigmentation variants associate with cutaneous melanoma and basal cell carcinoma. *Nat Genet.* 2008;40:886–891.

48. Nan H, Kraft P, Hunter DJ, et al. Genetic variants in pigmentation genes, pigmentary phenotypes, and risk of skin cancer in Caucasians. *Int J Cancer.* 2009;125:909–917.

49. Duffy DL, Zhao ZZ, Sturm RA, et al. Multiple pigmentation gene polymorphisms account for a substantial proportion of risk of cutaneous malignant melanoma. *J Invest Dermatol.* 2010;130(2):520–528.

50. Lu D, Willard D, Patel IR, et al. Agouti protein is an antagonist of the melanocyte-stimulating hormone receptor. *Nature.* 1994;371:799–802.

51. An HT, Yoo J, Lee MK, et al. Single dose radiation is more effective for the UV-induced activation and proliferation of melanocytes than fractionated dose radiation. *Photodermatol Photoimmunol Photomed.* 2001;17:266–271.

52. Kawaguchi Y, Mori N, Nakayama A. Kit+ melanocytes seem to contribute to melanocyte proliferation after UV exposure as precursor cells. *J Invest Dermatol.* 2001;116:920–925.

53. Sheehan JM, Cragg N, Chadwick CA, et al. Repeated ultraviolet exposure affords the same protection against DNA photodamage and erythema in human skin types II and IV but is associated with faster DNA repair in skin type IV. *J Invest Dermatol.* 2002;118:825–829.

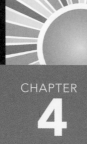

# Skin Cancer: Burden of Disease

*Abrar Qureshi*

**Key Points**

- The burden of skin cancer is measured by incidence and cost, and by newer approaches such as non-traditional measures that take into account the impact of skin cancer on the psychological, social, and economical aspects on an affected individual's life.

- Costs associated with treatment significantly increase with advanced disease.

- With the rising rates of skin cancer, the burden of this disease will continue to increase.

## INTRODUCTION

The burden of a skin disease is defined as the effect of the disease on the overall welfare of a population, which encompasses the adverse impact of skin diseases on physical health, psychological health, social functioning, quality of life (QoL), and economic well-being. Skin diseases are among the most common health problems worldwide, with over 3000 known diseases classified,[1] and they are associated with a considerable burden. Moreover, burden of disease can be assessed from the viewpoints of the individual, the family, and society.[2] Chronic and incurable skin diseases, such as psoriasis and eczema, are associated with significant morbidity in the form of physical discomfort and impairment of patients' quality of life; whereas skin cancers, such as malignant melanoma, can carry a substantial mortality.

Although the traditional epidemiological measures of burden of disease remain important in the assessment of the public health burden of skin cancer, they do not indicate the overall degree of impairment and cost associated with the skin malignancies. In this era of economic concerns, skin cancer expenses have become an important measure. The total cost of skin cancer in Sweden in 2005 was estimated at euro 142.4 million (euro 15/inhabitant), of which euro 79.6 million (euro 8/inhabitant) was spent on health services and euro 62.8 million (euro 7/inhabitant) was due to loss of production.[3] The main cost driver was resource utilization in outpatient care, amounting to 42.2% of the total cost. Melanoma was the most costly skin cancer diagnosis. Non-melanoma skin cancer was, however, the main cost driver for health services alone.

In addition, in attempts to more thoroughly describe the burden of disease, recent focus has been on non-traditional measures that take into account the impact of skin cancer on the psychological, social, and economical aspects of an affected individual's life, notably financial costs and the impact on patients' QoL. With the availability of a wide range of health status and quality-of-life measures, the effects of skin cancer on patients' lives can be measured efficiently. This chapter will focus on the overall burden of disease of skin cancers in order to highlight the magnitude of the associated problem and also to suggest ways to better quantify this issue.

## MELANOMA

### Epidemiology

Important epidemiologic measures of the burden of melanoma include incidence and mortality. The Surveillance, Epidemiology and End Results (SEER) registries maintained by the National Cancer Institute since the 1970s provide epidemiologic data on melanoma.[4] Melanoma is one of the fastest growing cancers worldwide; studies from Europe,[5–8] Singapore,[9] Canada,[10] and the United States (US)[11–13] suggest that its incidence is continuing to increase, especially amongst light-skinned racial groups, by 3–7% annually.[14] The highest incidence rates overall are observed among white males 65 years of age and over (120.6 per 100,000), followed by white females 65 and over (46.9 per 100,000). The lowest incidence is among African Americans, with a rate of 1.0 per 100,000. Thus, in the US, melanoma is more than 20 times more common among whites than among blacks.[15] As a group, ethnic minorities represent <5% of all diagnosed cases. Men carry a larger proportion of the burden of disease, with a male:female ratio of 3:2.[14] From 2002 to 2006, the median age at diagnosis for melanoma of the skin was 59 years, reflecting a relatively long latent period of the disease (see Chapter 5 for further analysis).

In terms of prevalence, in 2006 in the US there were approximately 758,688 men and women alive who had a history of melanoma of the skin, 367,925 men and 390,763 women, which is roughly 0.25% of the US population.

Although melanoma accounts for only 4% of diagnoses of skin cancer, it accounts for 80% of skin cancer-related deaths. According to data from the SEER registry, the age-adjusted death rate was 2.7 per 100,000 men and women per year based on patients who died in 2002–2006 in the Unites States, with a median age at death of 68 years.[4] Lesser increases in mortality rates in the face of dramatic increases in incidence are not thought to be attributable to improvements in treatment but may be due in part to earlier detection.[16–18]

For men and women over 65 years of age, mortality increased by 3.0% annually, reaching 13.0 deaths per

100,000 in 2006. Men over 65 years had the fastest increase in mortality over this period (APC 3.9%), reaching 20.8 deaths per 100,000 in 2004. Melanoma in the elderly may have a different biology and altered host immune response, both of which could contribute to increased incidence and mortality.[16] According to these trends, melanoma will soon become an increasingly major concern for the aging population and their healthcare providers and warrants public health attention.[14]

## Costs

### Direct costs

In 2004, the estimated total direct cost associated with treatment of melanoma was $291 million annually, of which $213 million was attributable to care provided in hospitals, physicians' offices, and emergency rooms. According to data from the National Ambulatory Medical Care Survey (NAMCS), there were 603,800 visits to physicians' offices, 57,000 visits to hospital outpatient departments, and 6000 visits to emergency rooms made for melanoma diagnosis and/or treatment in 2004. Hospital inpatient costs for an estimated 10,400 inpatient hospital stays totaled $35 million, and prescription drugs specifically prescribed for the treatment of melanoma accounted for $78 million of the total direct costs of the disease.[19]

The direct costs of melanoma rise sharply as disease severity progresses. There is a dramatic incremental total cost associated with progressively higher initial stages of the disease, ranging from a total of $4648.48 for in-situ tumors to $159,808.17 for stage IV melanoma (Fig. 4.1).[20] There is a significant cost decrement when melanoma is diagnosed at an earlier stage, with a T4b lesion being approximately 2200 percent more expensive to diagnose and treat than an early in-situ melanoma and 1000 percent more expensive than a stage T1a tumor. An increase in surveillance costs from $3759.00 to $50,566.44 is seen from in-situ melanoma to clinical stage IIIC (Fig. 4.2). Another study reported the 20% most severe cases were responsible for 90% of the direct costs of care for melanoma.[19] This study also reported that the average total cost of care for a patient with stage 1 disease (localized, non-invasive melanoma) was approximately $1310 (in 1997 US dollars), versus $42,410 for a patient with stage 4 disease (distant metastases and lymphatic involvement) during the same

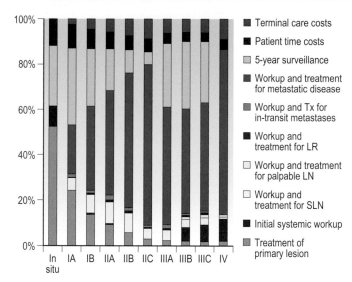

**Figure 4.2** Distribution of costs per clinical stage. (Adapted from Alexandrescu.[20])

time period. Terminal care for patients with advanced melanoma accounted for the largest portion (approximately 35%) of the total direct cost of melanoma.[19]

### Indirect costs

The indirect costs associated with melanoma are also significant, with an estimated $2.9 billion in annual lost productivity alone. Since melanoma affects relatively younger individuals, it is also important in terms of lost years of potential life due to premature death and a subsequent loss of future earnings.[12] Studies have reported melanoma is now the second leading cause of lost productive work years due to cancer. As many as 45% of melanoma deaths occur prior to retirement age, and the average loss in future earnings due to premature death is approximately $364,000 in the US.[19] In Belgium, an individual dying of melanoma would die approximately 6–8 years before the age of 65 years, in Denmark 14–15 years before the age of 65,[21,22] and in the US almost 17 years before the age of 65.[23]

### Quality of life (QoL)

In 1994, the World Health Organization (WHO) defined quality of life as 'the personal perception of an individual's situation in life, within the cultural context and the values of life in which we live, and in regard to individual objectives, expectations, values and interests'.[24] QoL comprises functional status, social functioning, physical well-being, psychological well-being, and health perceptions.[25] The physical, social, and emotional consequences of skin cancers are myriad and substantial. Numerous health status and quality-of-life measures have been developed to more effectively measure the effect of skin cancer on patients' lives.[26] Several of these instruments assess health-related quality of life (HRQOL), which refers to patients' level of function and perceptions of their physical and mental health over time.

Melanoma has been shown to have a significant impact on patients' quality of life. In terms of assessing QoL in melanoma patients, several instruments have been

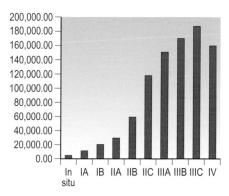

**Figure 4.1** Melanoma overall costs per patient by clinical TNM stage. (Adapted from Alexandrescu.[20])

developed, some of which are melanoma-specific and others of which are not. Because for 75% of melanoma patients local surgical excision is an effective form of treatment, HRQOL impairment in melanoma is predominantly in the form of psychosocial impairment. The psychosocial issues that patients with highly curable, early stage melanoma have to deal with are significantly different from those of patients with more advanced stage disease.[27,28] The emotional impact of melanoma can be long-lasting and profound, with the most common reactions to the disease being depression and anxiety, with a subsequent deterioration in quality of life.[29] Some research has found differences in emotional reactions to melanoma by sex, with women reporting higher levels of anxiety, depression, tiredness and sleep disturbance compared with men.[30]

Studies examining HRQOL in melanoma patients have reported three distinct periods in the melanoma experience during which HRQOL is differentially impacted: diagnosis, treatment, and follow-up.[31,32]

The acute survival phase, or the immediate period following diagnosis, is most often associated with high levels of HRQOL impairment. Patients reported more pain, less energy, and more physical and emotional stressors. They also gave worse evaluations of overall personal health.[33,34] Patients with a recent diagnosis of melanoma exhibit the same levels of psychological distress as patients diagnosed with other cancers.[35] During the diagnostic process, insomnia increased, while emotional functioning and global health status deteriorated, for patients ultimately diagnosed with melanoma.[33] The period following immediate diagnosis is the extended survival phase, during which patients report experiencing fears of recurrence. Physical limitations due to the cancer or its associated therapies were less of an issue during this phase.[32] Three months after surgical intervention, approximately a fifth of melanoma patients reported clinically high levels of anxiety, and depressive symptoms were more evident amongst patients with metastatic melanoma.[36] Upon initial diagnosis, patients with metastatic melanoma have a high level of functioning, but these patients progress quickly and have a decline in almost all of the major functional areas assessed by the QoL scales and an increase in the symptoms of their disease and the adverse effects of the therapies used to treat the illness.[36]

To describe the effects of melanoma in a monetary context, a willingness-to-pay approach can also be applied. In this type of analysis, the QoL effects of a particular condition are quantified by assessing the amount of money individuals affected by the condition are willing to pay for symptomatic relief. Thus, the more substantial the effects of the condition on quality of life, the more an individual affected by the condition would be willing to pay. The average amount that an individual with melanoma was willing to pay for symptom relief was estimated to be $1005 per year. This amount was not reflective of how much an individual with melanoma would be willing to pay to be cured of the disease, which is estimated to be substantially higher given the mortality rate of melanoma. When adjusted for disease severity and applied to the entire population of individuals with melanoma, the collective willingness-to-pay for symptom relief for this condition was determined to be $370 million per year.[19]

## NON-MELANOMA SKIN CANCER

### Epidemiology

Squamous cell and basal cell carcinomas (SCC, BCC; also known as non-melanoma skin cancers or NMSCs) of the skin together are the most frequent malignant tumors in Caucasian populations. Incidence data on basal and squamous cell skin cancers, however, are not reported or collected by most cancer registries in the US. Thus, all incidence data for NMSCs are an estimate. In the US, reports have estimated the crude prevalence of NMSC to be approximately 450 cases per 100,000 individuals.[19] Applying this rate to the 2009 US population yields an estimated 1.4 million individuals with NMSC per year.

The estimated incidence of NMSCs has increased steadily since the 1970s. This rise in incidence can be attributed to increases in sun exposure as well as the use of artificial tanning lamps. The average increase in NMSCs in Caucasian populations in the US, Australia, Canada, and Europe is estimated to be 3–8% per year.[19]

The incidence of BCC in the US is approximately 146 per 100,000 people. In Australia, where the average amount of UV exposure is among the highest on the planet due to depleted ozone, the incidence of BCC is approximately 788 per 100,000. In the US, approximately 200,000 new SCCs are diagnosed annually. Similar to BCC, the risk for developing SCC is highest among Caucasian males, who have an estimated lifetime chance of 9–14% of developing this disease[19] (see Chapter 5).

### Costs

#### Direct costs

The direct cost associated with treatment for NMSC in the Unites States is estimated to be $1.5 billion annually, of which $1.2 billion is allocated to care received in a physician's office. There were 1.8 million physician office visits for NMSCs in 2004, making it the most frequent option for obtaining care for NMSC. Hospital outpatient departments were visited 63,000 times, with an associated cost of $162 million. There were also 22,500 inpatient hospital stays reported for NMSC. The total cost of these stays was $65 million, or roughly 4% of the total direct cost associated with NMSC in the Unites States. On the contrary, prescription drugs for NMSC only amounted to slightly more than 1% of the total direct cost, indicating that the current treatment for this disease is largely procedural. However, these data are not entirely comprehensive as they do not include costs associated with drugs sold through specialty pharmacies.[19]

#### Indirect costs

The indirect costs associated with NMSC are substantial: an estimated $961 million was lost in 2004 due to loss in productivity. Of this, $893 million was allocated to future earnings lost due to premature death secondary to skin cancer.[19]

## Quality-of-life impact

The anatomical location of NMSCs on cosmetically sensitive areas such as the face, head and neck may give rise to psychological and social consequences. The situation is compounded by the fact that most of the available treatments mean that patients are left with scars mostly on visible areas and sometimes with significant disfigurement.

When patients were evaluated using the Dermatology Life Quality Index, giving a range from 0 (no impairment) to 30 (maximum impairment), the average score reported for individuals with NMSC was 4.8, compared with a score of 3.5 for actinic keratosis and 5.5 for cutaneous fungal infections. Translated into willingness-to-pay, this score indicates that an individual with NMSC is willing to pay approximately $1005 per year for symptomatic relief.[19]

## FUTURE TRENDS

The burden of disease of skin cancer is a multidimensional concept that has a significant impact on society. It includes traditional measures such as epidemiological data as well as non-traditional measures such as financial costs and impact on quality of life. If trends in incidence and mortality continue as they have in recent years, it appears that the burden of disease of skin cancer will also continue to increase. For that reason, it will be necessary for better metrics and more information to become available in order to more accurately assess this burden.

## REFERENCES

1. Bickers DR, Lim HW, Margolis D, et al. The burden of skin diseases: 2004: a joint project of the American Academy of Dermatology Association and the Society of Investigative Dermatology. *J Am Acad Dermatol*. 2006;55:490–500.
2. Chren MM, Weinstock MA. Conceptual issues in measuring the burden of skin diseases. *J Invest Dermatol*. 2004;9:97–100.
3. Tinhög G, Carlsson P, Synnerstad I, et al. Societal cost of skin cancer in Sweden in 2005. *Acta Derm Venereol*. 2008;88(5):467–473.
4. Surveillance Research Program, Cancer Statistics Branch. Surveillance, Epidemiology and End Results (SEER) Program. Washington DC: National Cancer Institute; 2006.
5. Mansson-Brahme E, Johansson H, Larsson O, et al. Trends in incidence of cutaneous malignant melanoma in a Swedish population 1976-1994. *Acta Oncol*. 2002;41(2):138–146.
6. de Vries E, Coebergh JW. Cutaneous malignant melanoma in Europe. *Eur J Cancer*. 2004;40(16):2355–2366.
7. Lasithiotakis K, Kruger-Krasagakis S, Manousaki A, et al. The incidence of cutaneous melanoma on Crete, Greece. *Int J Dermatol*. 2006;45(4):397–401.
8. Stang A, Pukkala E, Sankila R, et al. Time trend analysis of the skin melanoma incidence of Finland from 1953 through 2003 including 16,414 cases. *Int J Cancer*. 2006;119(2):380–384.
9. Koh D, Wang H, Lee J, et al. Basal cell carcinoma, squamous cell carcinoma and melanoma of the skin: analysis of the Singapore Cancer Registry data 1968-97. *Br J Dermatol*. 2003;148(6):1161–1166.
10. Ulmer MJ, Tonita JM, Hull PR. Trends in invasive cutaneous melanoma in Saskatchewan 1970-1999. *J Cutan Med Surg*. 2003;7(6):433–442.
11. Dennis LK. Analysis of the melanoma epidemic, both apparent and real: data from the 1973 through 1994 surveillance, epidemiology, and end results program registry. *Arch Dermatol*. 1999;135(3):275–280.
12. Hall HI, Miller DR, Rogers JD, et al. Update on the incidence and mortality from melanoma in the United States. *J Am Acad Dermatol*. 1999;40(1):35–42.
13. Geller AC, Miller DR, Annas GD, et al. Melanoma incidence and mortality among US whites, 1969-1999. *JAMA*. 2002;288(14):1719–1720.
14. Linos E, Swetter SM, Cockburn MG, et al. Increasing burden of melanoma in the United States. *J Invest Dermatol*. 2009;129(7):1666–1674.
15. Rajagopalan R, Sherertz EF, Anderson R, eds. Care Management of Skin Disease: Life Quality and Economic Impact. New York, NY: Marcel Dekker; 1998.
16. Swerlick RA, Chen S. The melanoma epidemic: more apparent than real? *Mayo Clin Proc*. 1997;72(6):559–564.
17. Lamberg L. "Epidemic" of malignant melanoma: true increase or better detection? *JAMA*. 2002;287(17):2201.
18. Florez A, Cruces M. Melanoma epidemic: true or false? *Int J Dermatol*. 2004;43(6):405–407.
19. The Lewin Group, Inc. The burden of skin diseases. 2004. http://www.sidnet.org/pdfs/Burden%20of%20Skin%20Diseases%202004.pdf. Accessed 15.07.09.
20. Alexandrescu DT. Melanoma costs: a dynamic model comparing estimated overall costs of various clinical stages. *Dermatol Online J*. 2009;15(11):1.
21. Brochez L, Myny K, Bleyen L, et al. The melanoma burden in Belgium; premature morbidity and mortality make melanoma a considerable health problem. *Melanoma Res*. 1999;9(6):614–618.
22. Osterlind A. Epidemiology on malignant melanoma in Europe. *Acta Oncol*. 1992;31(8):903–908.
23. Albert VA, Koh HK, Geller AC, et al. Years of potential life lost: another indicator of the impact of cutaneous malignant melanoma on society. *J Am Acad Dermatol*. 1990;23(2 Pt 1):308–310.
24. Casado J, González N, Moraleda S, et al. Calidad de vida relacionada con la salud en pacientes ancianos en atención primaria. *Aten Primaria*. 2001;28:167–173.
25. Gill TM, Feinstein AR. A critical appraisal of the quality of life measurements. *JAMA*. 1994;272(8):619–625.
26. Basra MKA, Shahrukh M. Burden of skin diseases. *Expert Rev Pharmacoecon Outcomes Res*. 2009;9:271–283.
27. Francken AB, Bastiaannet E, Hoekstra HJ. Follow-up in patients with localised primary cutaneous melanoma. *Lancet Oncol*. 2005;6:608–621.
28. Cornish D, Holterhues C, van de Poll-Franse LV, et al. A systematic review of health-related quality of life in cutaneous melanoma. *Ann Oncol*. 2009;20(suppl 6):vi51–vi58.
29. Crosby T, Fish R, Coles B, et al. Systemic treatments for metastatic cutaneous melanoma. *Cochrane Database Syst Rev*. 2000;(2) CD001215.
30. Barth A, Wanek LA, Morton DL. Prognostic factors in 1521 melanoma patients with distant metastases. *J Am Coll Surg*. 1995;181:193–201.
31. Trask PC, Paterson AG, Hayasaka S, et al. Psychosocial characteristics of individuals with non-stage IV melanoma. *J Clin Oncol*. 2001;19:2844–2850.
32. Boyle DA. Psychological adjustment to the melanoma experience. *Semin Oncol Nurs*. 2003;19:70–77.
33. Al-Shakhli H, Harcourt D, Kenealy J. Psychological distress surrounding diagnosis of malignant and nonmalignant skin lesions at a pigmented lesion clinic. *J Plast Reconstr Aesthet Surg*. 2006;59:479–486.
34. Ko CY, Maggard M, Livingston EH. Evaluating health utility in patients with melanoma, breast cancer, colon cancer, and lung cancer: a nationwide, population-based assessment. *J Surg Res*. 2003;114:1–5.
35. Fawzy FI, Cousins N, Fawzy NW, et al. A structured psychiatric intervention for cancer patients. I. Changes over time in methods of coping and affective disturbance. *Arch Gen Psychiatr*. 1990;47:720–725.
36. Brandberg Y, Bolund C, Sigurdardottir V, et al. Anxiety and depressive symptoms at different stages of malignant melanoma. *Psychooncology*. 1992;2:71–78.

CHAPTER

# 5

# Epidemiology of Skin Cancer

*Melody J. Eide and Martin A. Weinstock*

> ## Key Points
>
> - Melanoma is 20 times more common today than it was 60 years ago.
> - Melanoma incidence continues to increase.
> - Overall melanoma mortality is increasing in the United States, especially for older men, but is declining in younger generations.
> - Keratinocyte carcinoma is the most common malignancy in the United States.

## INTRODUCTION

Skin cancer is the most common malignancy in the United States (US)[1] and in many other nations worldwide, and consequently has substantial public health significance. Malignant melanoma (MM), keratinocyte carcinoma (KC) including basal cell carcinoma (BCC) and squamous cell carcinoma (SCC), and other cutaneous malignancies such as cutaneous lymphoma have increased in incidence over the last several decades. Monitoring trends in disease, identifying risk factors for disease, and modifying these risks to reduce disease impact are a few of the many critical roles served by epidemiology. This chapter will discuss key issues in the descriptive, analytic, and interventional aspects of the dermatoepidemiology of cutaneous malignancies.

## HISTORY

Epidemiology has a rich history in relation to skin diseases. Percival Pott's suspicion of the association between soot and scrotal cancer in British chimney sweeps in the 18th century eventually led to recognition of this occupational risk.[2] In 1956, it was H. O. Lancaster's classic report of the distribution of melanoma mortality that was pivotal in the recognition of the role of sun exposure in melanoma etiology.[3] Today, cancer registries of countries worldwide routinely include melanoma and other cutaneous malignancies. In the US, the longest record of melanoma incidence is provided by the Connecticut Tumor Registry which has kept a record of malignant melanoma diagnosed since 1935, and continues to be an important source of information on melanoma incidence today.[4,5] In 1973, the National Cancer Institute (NCI) initiated a system of population-based registries to track most cancers, including melanoma. The Surveillance, Epidemiology, and End Results (SEER) program is the broadest system of cancer registration in the US. Originally, SEER included information representing about 10% of the

US, utilizing nine population-based cancer registries: the metropolitan areas of Atlanta, Detroit, San Francisco and Seattle, and the states of Connecticut, Iowa, New Mexico, Utah and Hawaii. The registry has expanded to include 17 registries ('SEER-17') and approximately 26% of the US population, including 23% of Caucasians, 23% of African Americans, 40% of Hispanics, 32% of American Indians and Alaska Natives, 53% of Asians, and 70% of Hawaiian/ Pacific Islanders.[6]

## DESCRIPTIVE EPIDEMIOLOGY

### Melanoma incidence

Melanoma incidence has increased rapidly over the past 65 years. Between 1935 and 1939, the incidence of melanoma in Connecticut was 1.0 per 100,000 (age-standardized, 1970).[7] In 2006, melanoma incidence had increased to 20.9 per 100,000 (age-standardized, 1970)[5] (Fig. 5.1). Similar trends have been noted in the SEER registry. In 1973, the melanoma incidence rate was 6.8 per 100,000, but by 2006, this rate had climbed to 21.1 per 100,000.[8] It is estimated that in the US in 2010, there will be 68,130 new cases of melanoma diagnosed and an additional 46,770 cases of melanoma in situ.[1] The increase in invasive melanoma incidence was 6.1% per year between 1973 and 1981, and 1.6% per year between 1997 and 2006 (based on rates age-adjusted to 2000 US standard population).[8] It is currently estimated that melanoma will be the fifth most common cancer (other than keratinocyte carcinoma) diagnosed in men, with 38,870 cases (5%), behind prostate, lung, colon, and urinary bladder. In women it is estimated to be the seventh most common cancer, with 29,260 cases (4%), behind breast, lung, colon, uterine, thyroid, and non-Hodgkin lymphoma.[1] Melanoma is the fourth most common cancer in Australia, New Zealand and Sweden, the tenth most common in Scandinavia, and the eighteenth most common cancer in most of the United Kingdom (England, Scotland and Wales) (other than keratocyte carcinoma).[9-11]

Studies continue to examine incidence and mortality trends to further determine the contribution of increasing age or birth cohort (all individuals born within a specific time period, and who subsequently may share similar early exposures and experiences). There have been attempts to distinguish a 'cohort' from a 'period' effect ( time trends are influenced by more recent exposures or events, such as changes in diagnostic criteria or cancer screening). Melanoma incidence, however, has generally been found to follow cohort patterns of changes. For example, assume incidence started to increase. With a cohort effect, this

44

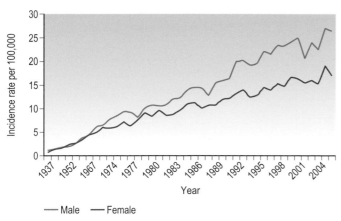

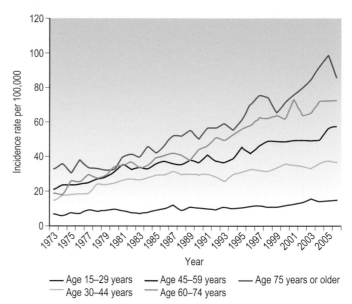

**Figure 5.1** Melanoma incidence in Connecticut, 1937–2006. Data source: Connecticut Tumor Registry Cancer Inquiry System. http://www.cancerates.info/ct/.

**Figure 5.3** Age-adjusted melanoma incidence by age in females, United States, 1973–2006. Data source: SEER program. http://seer.cancer.gov/.

change would be noted first among more recent birth cohorts (younger people) and would not be observed in prior birth cohorts (older people). A change in middle-age incidence first would be noted when these more recent birth cohort populations reached middle-age.

It has been suggested that a 'leveling off' of the melanoma incidence is occurring in many countries. In the US, more recent generations of men have similar incidence rates compared to prior generations, even though these rates are still increasing in these older generations of men. However, incidence appears to be increasing in more recent generations of women. This is consistent with a cohort effect[12] (Figs 5.2 and 5.3). Incidence also appears to have leveled off in Australia, especially in younger cohorts born after 1960, supportive of a birth cohort effect.[13] Incidence appears to even have fallen significantly in the last 20 years in young women (age groups 15–34 and 35–49) in New South Wales (annual percent change −3% and −0.9% respectively).[13] Trends in melanoma incidence in Europe (1953–1997) show a plateauing of incidence rates in younger age groups in Scandinavian countries, whose rates are expected to remain

stable or decrease further in the future, though these trends in incidence were less distinct in young people in other areas of northern and western Europe.[14]

The stabilization of melanoma incidence in recent cohorts may be related to the educational programs implemented in the last 35 years. Increased quality and potency of sunscreens in common use, albeit at times ineffective use, might suggest reduced exposures. However, the prevalence of sunburns, at least in the US, appears to be increasing and there is continued migration to sunnier climates and exposures to indoor tanning as well. Regardless of the apparent recent trend toward stabilization in the US and several other countries, the incidence rate of melanoma has increased faster than the mortality rate. Improved surveillance may have increased detection and resulted in the potential surgical removal of earlier 'cancers' that may never have progressed to become lesions of clinical significance, or may have increased removal of potentially fatal lesions at a curable point in their evolution, or a combination of both.

Because the frequency of skin cancer is significantly lower in non-white populations, epidemiological information is more limited. SEER provides detailed estimates of incidence by race only for blacks.[15] In 2006, SEER data showed an incidence rate in whites of 25.6 and in blacks of 0.9 per 100,000 (age-standardized, 2000). Melanoma incidence from 2002 to 2006 was: white Hispanic, 4.6 cases per 100,000; Asian/Pacific Islander, 1.4 cases per 100,000; American Indian/Alaskan native, 3.3 cases per 100,000; and black, 1.0 cases per 100,000 (age-standardized, 2000).

SEER incidence data indicate that melanoma incidence in the US trends upward with age (Fig. 5.4). Melanoma incidence peaks at 80–84 years of age at a rate of 82.2 cases per 100,000. Similar age-trends have been seen in other countries, including Australia, Italy and the Netherlands.[16,17]

In the US, melanoma is more common in men than in women. In 1973, the incidence rates were 7.3 per 100,000 in males and 6.4 per 100,000 in females. In 2006, the incidence rate had risen in men and women, to 26.1 and 17.6 cases per 100,000, respectively (Fig. 5.5). Gender differences have

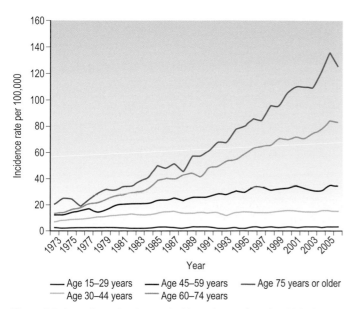

**Figure 5.2** Age-adjusted melanoma incidence by age in males, United States, 1973–2006. Data source: SEER program. http://seer.cancer.gov/.

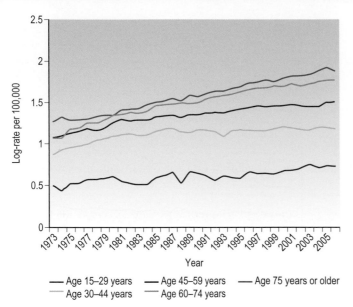

Figure 5.4 Trends in melanoma incidence by age, United States.

Age 15–29 years — Age 45–59 years — Age 75 years or older
Age 30–44 years — Age 60–74 years

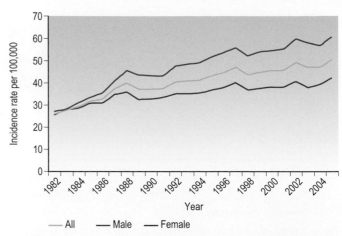

All — Male — Female

Figure 5.6 Age-adjusted incidence of melanoma in Australia, 1982–2005. Data source: National Health Priority Areas, Cancer Indicators: http://www.aihw.gov/au/hhpa/cancer. Age-standardized to the 2001 Australian population.

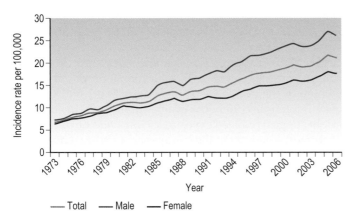

Total — Male — Female

Figure 5.5 Age-adjusted incidence of melanoma in the United States, 1973–2006. Data source: SEER program. http://seer.cancer.gov/. Age-standardized to 2000 US Census.

## Table 5.1 Age-standardized Incidence of Melanoma in Selected Countries of the World

| Country | Incidence Rate Per 100,000 | |
| --- | --- | --- |
| | Male | Female |
| Brazil, Sao Paulo | 6.5 | 5.7 |
| Columbia, Cali | 3.5 | 2.9 |
| Canada | 10.9 | 9.3 |
| United States, SEER-14 non-Hispanic, white | 19.4 | 14.4 |
| United States, SEER-14 Hispanic, white | 3 | 3.2 |
| United States, SEER-14 black | 0.9 | 0.6 |
| India, Mumbai (Bombay) | 0.3 | 0.2 |
| Israel, Jew | 12.2 | 10.5 |
| Israel, non-Jew | 1.4 | 0.8 |
| Japan, Hiroshima | 0.5 | 0.7 |
| China, Hong Kong | 0.7 | 0.6 |
| Czech Republic | 9.9 | 8.8 |
| Denmark | 11.9 | 14.1 |
| Iceland | 9.3 | 19 |
| Germany, Saarland | 8.1 | 7.8 |
| The Netherlands | 10 | 12.9 |
| Poland, Warsaw City | 4.4 | 4.6 |
| Spain, Murcia | 6.5 | 7 |
| Sweden | 11.9 | 12.1 |
| UK, England, South and Western Region | 10.7 | 11.9 |
| UK, Scotland | 8.4 | 10.1 |

(Continued)

been noted in other countries, including Australia, where in 2005, the age-adjusted incidence in males was 60.9 cases per 100,000 population while the female incidence was 42.5 cases per 100,000 (age-standardized, Australia, 2001)[18] (see Fig. 5.6).

Gender differences appear to vary with age as well. In 2002 to 2006, in SEER registrants under age 45, melanoma incidence was higher in women, whereas after age 45, men had higher incidence rates.[8] Between 2002 and 2006 in the US, the age-adjusted incidence in males over age 65 was 105.5 per 100,000 while the incidence in elderly females was 41.0 per 100,000 (age-standardized, 2000).[8]

Incidence rates vary substantially worldwide (Table 5.1). New Zealand and Australia have the highest incidence. In Queensland, Australia, the incidence rate is 41.1–55.8 cases per 100,000, more than four times that in the US SEER-14 program (10.5–14.8 cases per 100,000) (age-standardized, world population).[19] These high rates have led to a large public health and economic burden which has motivated extensive and successful public health campaigns. Incidence in European nations ranges from 2.4–2.6 cases per 100,000 in Bulgaria to 11.5–19.6 per 100,000 in Switzerland. In Africa

## Table 5.1 Age-Standardized Incidence of Melanoma in Selected Countries of the World—cont'd

| Country | Incidence Rate Per 100,000 | |
| --- | --- | --- |
| | Male | Female |
| Ireland | 7.4 | 11 |
| Italy, North-East Cancer Surveillance Network | 9.5 | 10.6 |
| Switzerland, Geneva | 18.5 | 19 |
| Australia, New South Wales | 38.5 | 26.5 |
| Australia, Queensland | 55.8 | 41.1 |
| New Zealand | 34.8 | 31.4 |
| Uganda | 0.9 | 1.4 |

Information source: *Cancer Incidence in Five Continents, Volume IX.* Lyon: IARC Scientific Publications; 2008. Age-standardized to the 2000 world population.

and Central and South America, incidence is low. It is also low in Asia, with India and China reporting less than one case per 100,000. In Israel, incidence varies with ancestry and place of birth. It is higher in Israeli Jews (10.5–12.2 cases per 100,000) than non-Jews (0.8–1.4 cases per 100,000).[19]

Trends in international incidence suggest that melanoma is continuing to increase.[20] Between the mid 1960s and the mid 1980s, the average annual percent increase in melanoma incidence generally ranged from 3% to 6%, with the highest rate of increase noted in white residents of Hawaii, who had over a 9% increase.[20] Kricker and Armstrong examined international data for trends in age-specific rates, and found that incidence rates have stabilized or begun to fall in young people (less than age 55) in some populations, including Denmark, Canada, the US, Australia, New Zealand, Norway and the UK, but are continuing to rise in other countries such as Poland, Spain and Yugoslavia.[20] There is evidence suggesting a latitudinal effect world wide in melanoma incidence, with generally higher incidence reported nearer the equator. In New Zealand data from 1968 to 1989, a latitudinal trend from north to south existed for each gender and across time. New Zealanders living in the northern region of the country may have at least a 37% higher incidence than those living in the south.[21] There is a higher incidence in Scandinavian compared to Mediterranean countries, which is attributable to gradients in sun sensitivity in these populations.[22]

### Melanoma mortality

Nearly 75% of skin cancer deaths in the US are attributable to melanoma.[23] Melanoma mortality has increased substantially in the US over the last 30 years, although it is now stabilizing. Mortality increased 4.3% annually in the white population between 1973 and 1977, 1.5% annually between 1977 and 1990, and 0.2% annually between 1990 and 1999 and from 1997 to 2006.[6,24] It is estimated that in 2010, 8700 Americans will die of the disease.[1]

An analysis of World Health Organization (WHO) Cancer Mortality Data Bank data (examining Australia, Canada, Czechoslovakia, France, Italy, Japan, UK, US, and a combined Denmark, Finland, Sweden and Norway) examined mortality rates and recent trends from 1960 to 1994. In 1960, some of the lowest mortality rates for the 30–59 age group were seen in France, Italy and Czechoslovakia (fewer than 0.5 deaths per 100,000 (world standard population)). However, over the last 30 years the highest rates of increase in mortality were found in these same three countries, with death rates increasing annually by 9–16%. Age-adjusted mortality in Japan remained low (less than one death per 100,000 in all age groups) over the entire time period.[25]

There are marked differences in mortality with increasing age in the US. The mortality rate in 2002–2006 for men and women younger than age 65 was 1.7 and 0.9 deaths per 100,000 respectively. However, for those aged 65 and older, the mortality rate for men was 19.5 per 100,000 and for women was 7.6 per 100,000. The highest mortality is seen in men over age 80: 128.9–134.9 cases per 100,000.[8]

There is a higher mortality rate in men compared with women of the same age in the US.[8] In men, there was a significant increase in annual percent change in melanoma mortality of 2.4% between 1975 and 1987, 0.7% from 1987 to 1998, and 2.0% from 2002 to 2006, with no significant change during 1998–2002. In women, the annual percent change in melanoma mortality was 0.8% between 1975 and 1988; however, in recent years (1988–2006) it appears to be decreasing (−0.6%) significantly[8] (Fig. 5.7). It is estimated that there will be almost twice as many deaths in men (5670) as in women (3030) in the US in 2010.[1] The mortality rate in Australia is also higher for men than for women (Fig. 5.8).

The age-adjusted death rate from melanoma in 2006 was 3.1 per 100,000 for the white population and 0.4 per 100,000 in the black population.[8] The 5-year relative survival rate of melanoma is subsequently lower in blacks compared to whites (all stages: 77% vs. 91%).[8] Examination of stage of diagnosis reveals that a higher percentage of blacks diagnosed with melanoma between 1999 and 2005 had regional or distant disease-stage than did the white population (34% vs. 12%).[8]

The mortality rate appears to be stabilizing in portions of the world, including the US, Australia and parts of Europe. Unlike incidence, US mortality has declined in

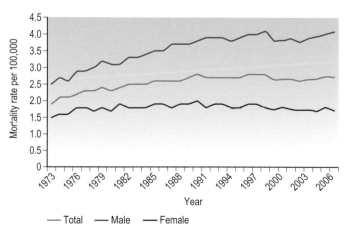

**Figure 5.7** Age-adjusted melanoma mortality by gender in the United States, 1973–2006. Data source: SEER program. http://seer.cancer.gov/. Age standardized to 2000 US Census.

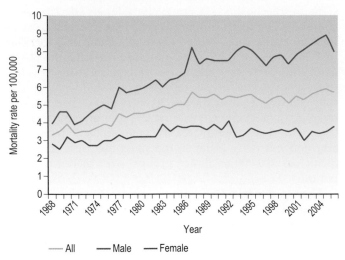

**Figure 5.8** Age-adjusted melanoma mortality by gender in Australia, 1968–2006. Data source: National Health Priority Areas, Cancer Indicators: http://www.aihw.gov/au/hhpa/cancer. Age-standardized to the 2001 Australian population.

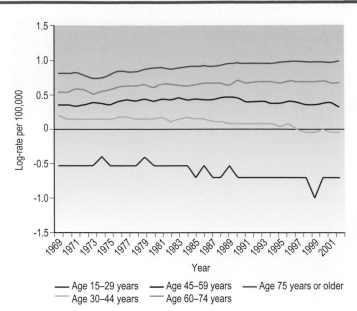

**Figure 5.10** Trends in melanoma mortality in females by age, United States. Data source: SEER program. http://seer.cancer.gov/.

more recent birth cohorts. Death certificate or histopathology criteria changes are not felt to have a significant impact on this trend.[26] The stabilization of melanoma mortality in more recent cohorts may be the result of a combination of a slower increase in melanoma incidence and a lower case-fatality, presumably due at least in part to earlier detection (Figs 5.9 and 5.10).

Cohort analysis of WHO mortality data have demonstrated several different patterns. In Australia, the US, and the Scandinavian countries, there appears to be an increasing mortality rate for the generation born prior to 1940, followed by a decrease in mortality in younger cohorts. In the UK and Canada, the rates increase in generations born between 1920 and 1950, with a stabilization in more recent cohorts. In France, Czechoslovakia and Italy, there has been a step increase in melanoma mortality that appears linear with little change in trend.[25] In Sweden, mortality has plateaued in men in the last 10–15 years and slightly

decreased in women (−2.3%). Mortality has decreased in women among all age groups but in men only for those younger than 60, and analysis of trends has been suggestive of a period effect.[27]

## Cutaneous malignancies other than melanoma

Keratinocyte carcinoma (KC) includes both basal cell (BCC) and squamous cell carcinoma (SCC).[28,29] The term 'nonmelanoma skin cancer' (NMSC) is commonly used to refer to KC, but also includes other cutaneous malignancies. The fundamental problem with the term NMSC, beyond its ambiguity, is that it defines the most common malignancy by what it is *not*, thereby impeding its proper study and demeaning its significance. The more specific term of keratinocyte carcinoma has been recommended as an alternative.

### Keratinocyte carcinomas

It is estimated that in 2009 there will be over one million cases of keratinocyte carcinoma (BCC and SCC) diagnosed in the US alone.[1] The ICD9-CM code of 173 covers not only the more common BCC and SCC but also other skin cancers including Merkel cell carcinoma, angiosarcoma, sebaceous carcinoma and many others;[22] thus, precise incidence rates are typically unavailable (Table 5.2 and Fig. 5.11). In the few registries that include KC, there is concern that, because of their high incidence, generally excellent prognosis, and potential for outpatient treatment without histologic evaluation, these cancers may be subject to significant under-registration.

Other sources have been used to evaluate the occurrence of KC, including using information from large health maintenance organizations (HMOs) and self-reported surveys. Regardless of data source, there are several complicating factors. Some investigators enumerate KC by individual person while others prefer counting all incident cancers as unique measures, regardless of multiplicity in a single person. The former method is the one most accepted by the

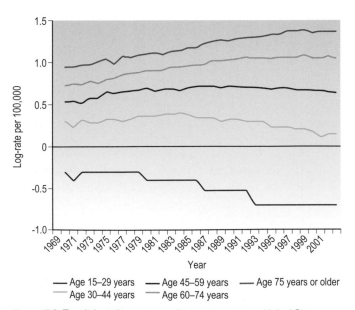

**Figure 5.9** Trends in melanoma mortality in males by age, United States. Data source: SEER program. http://seer.cancer.gov/.

## Table 5.2 Incidence Rate of Basal Cell And Squamous Cell Carcinoma of the Skin in Available Countries of the World

| Country | Standard Population | Year(s) of Study | Year Published | Incidence Rate Per 100,000 Population | | | |
| | | | | SCC | | BCC | |
| | | | | Male | Female | Male | Female |
|---|---|---|---|---|---|---|---|
| United Kingdom, South Wales[44] | World | 1998 | 2000 | 25 | 9 | 128 | 105 |
| United Kingdom, Scotland[37] | World | 2001–2003 | 2007 | 24 | 9 | 61 | 47 |
| United Kingdom, Northern Ireland[51] | European Standard | 1993–2002 | 2007 | 46 | 23 | 94 | 72 |
| Germany, Northrhine-Westphalia[35] | World | 1998–2003 | 2007 | 17 | 10 | 64 | 54 |
| Germany, Schleswig-Holstein[40] | World | 1998–2001 | 2003 | 11 | 5 | 54 | 44 |
| Canada, New Brunswick[39] | World | 1992–2001 | 2007 | 34 | 16 | 87 | 68 |
| Canada, Manitoba[31] | World | 2000 | 2005 | 26 | 12 | 94 | 77 |
| Australia[18] | World | 2002 | 2008 | 561 | 323 | 1151 | 825 |
| Jordan, Northern* | Jordan | 1997–2001 | 2006 | 14 | 4 | 20 | 23 |
| Norway[35] | World | 2000 | 2007 | 7 | 3 | 83 | 87 |
| United States, New Mexico[33] | US 2000 | 1998–1999 | 2003 | 356 | 150 | 930 | 486 |
| The Netherlands, Eindhoven[56] | World | 1998–2000 | 2004 | NA | NA | 63 | 58 |
| United Kingdom[50] | World | 1996–2003 | 2007 | NA | NA | 69 | 53 |
| Croatia† | World | 2003–2005 | 2009 | NA | NA | 34 | 25 |

For relevant studies published prior to 2003, please see corresponding Chapter 4, 'Epidemiology of skin cancer' in Rigel DS, Friedman RJ, Dzubow LM, eds. *Cancer of the Skin*. 1st ed. London: Saunders; 2005.

*Omari AK, Khammash MR, Matalka I. Skin cancer trends in northern Jordan. *Int J Dermatol*. 2006;45(4):384-388.

†Celic D, Lipozencic J, Toncic RJ, et al. The incidence of basal carcinoma in Croatia: an epidemiological study. *Acta Dermatovenerol Croat*. 2009;17(2):108-112.

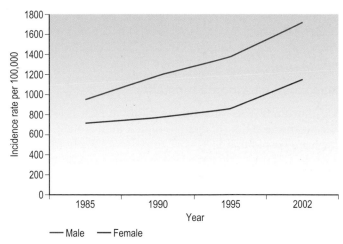

**Figure 5.11** Age-adjusted incidence of basal cell and squamous cell carcinomas, Australia, 1985 2001. Data source: National Health Priority Areas, Cancer Indicators: http://www.aihw.gov/au/hhpa/cancer. Age standardized to the 2000 World population.

scientific community and utilized in this chapter. However, when counting only first cancer, the observation interval may vary significantly between reports. Furthermore, sometimes SCC and BCC are considered and studied together, despite the clinical and epidemiological differences. Hence, reports of incidence rates must be carefully scrutinized.

## Squamous cell carcinoma incidence

The incidence of SCC has been rising worldwide over the last several decades at an estimated 3–10% per year.[7,30,31] It was estimated that in 1994 there were between 135,000 and 250,000 cases of SCC diagnosed in the US.[32] An NCI-funded survey by the New Mexico Tumor Registry suggests that from 1978–79 to 1998–99 the incidence of SCC increased 90% in men and 109% in women.[33] A Canadian study comparing 1960 through 2000 SCC incidence showed an increase of more than 200% during the time period.[31]

In general, SCC incidence is higher in the elderly and in men.[34,35] The incidence rate of SCC in New Mexico in 1999 was estimated in men and women respectively at 356 and 150 cases per 100,000.[33] The incidence of SCC in Australia was estimated in 2002 for men and women respectively at 561 and 323 cases per 100,000.[18,36] The majority of SCC occurs on sun-exposed areas such as the head and neck.[31,37,38] Anatomic site differences by gender have been reported, with significantly higher rates on the ear in men and lower leg in women, and these differences may be due to fashion differences, including clothing and hairstyle.[37,39,40] Another contributor to increases in SCC may be higher organ transplant rates and improved transplant patient survival and subsequent duration of immunosuppression.

In darker-skinned populations, the etiology of SCC may be unrelated to sun exposure, but may be associated with chronic irritation or injury, while there is evidence to suggest that sun exposure is related to SCC development in lighter-skinned populations.[7] Human papillomavirus (HPV) antibodies, especially HPV-5, have been associated with SCC (see Chapter 19).[41]

In the US there appears to be a higher incidence of SCC with lower latitudes, with an approximate doubling when compared to northern areas.[2] A similar trend has been seen in Australia, with higher rates in the north (closer to the equator).[36] Incidence rates in Australia have shown that the odds of developing SCC are higher among persons born in Australia.[42] The incidence rate has also been shown to increase with decreasing latitude in Norway.[43] However, this gradient may not be true in all of Europe.[19,22]

Trends in SCC do not appear to be consistent across populations. In North America, a significant change in incidence was seen in New Mexico from 1978 to 1999 and in Manitoba from 1960 to 2000, whereas the rate remained stable in Scotland between 1992 to 2003, with the exception of a small increase in men over age 60.[31,33,37] In South Wales, no significant difference was seen in the standardized incidence rate from 1988 to 1998;[44] however, the trend in Finland between 1956 and 1995 suggests a steady increase in SCC incidence.[45] In Singapore, SCC incidence rates have decreased by 0.9% per year for both genders between 1968 and 1997.[46] There are several possible reasons for these ambiguities. SCC incidence may be affected by diagnostic accuracy (i.e. misclassification of actinic keratoses and SCC in situ) or changes in histologic criteria. Furthermore, some physicians may treat SCC without histologic confirmation of the diagnosis.

## Squamous cell carcinoma mortality

While melanoma among whites is responsible for 90% of skin cancer deaths before 50 years of age, in adults over 85 years of age the majority of skin cancer deaths are attributable to SCC.[23] It is estimated that 70% of deaths from nonmelanoma skin cancer may be attributed to SCC.[38] Though Australian death certificate information has been demonstrated to be reasonably accurate, inaccuracies in death certificate information in the US have limited direct epidemiologic study.[38,47] In the Western Australian Cancer Registry, age-adjusted SCC mortality rates for 2002 were 1.2 deaths per 100,000 for men and 0.3 deaths per 100,000 for women, while in Scotland the 2002 mortality rate was 0.7 and 0.3 deaths per 100,000 for men and women respectively.[38] The age-adjusted mortality rate (1970 US standard) for SCC in Rhode Island has also been reported at 0.3 deaths per 100,000.[47] Men have higher death rates from SCC than women (further amplified with age-adjustment). The age-adjusted mortality rate ratio for men compared to women is 3.9. SCC mortality is higher in whites and with increasing age. Case-fatality also appears to be higher in certain locations, including the head (face, scalp and ear).[38,47] SCC mortality appears to be declining for decades based on the observed decrease in NMSC mortality, which declined by another 19% during the period from 1985–1994 to 1995–2000.[48]

## Basal cell carcinoma incidence

Basal cell carcinoma (BCC) is the most common skin cancer and is three to five times more common than SCC in many Caucasian populations.[33,35,39,44] Men generally have higher rates of BCC than women, with a ratio of almost 2:1 in North America.[2,33] Like SCC, BCC commonly occurs on the head and neck in both genders.[31,49] Changes have been noted in the anatomic site over the last 20 years, with a larger increase in lesions located in anatomic sites other than head, including the trunk and limbs.[49,50] An increased incidence of BCC has also been reported in more affluent residents of Northern Ireland.[51]

In the last 30 years, BCC incidence rates have been estimated to have risen between 20% and 80% in the US, with higher increases seen in men.[7,33] In Manitoba, Canada, the percent change in incidence of BCC was 180% between 1960 and 2000 and in Singapore that incidence rate more than tripled between 1968 to 2006.[31,52] BCC was estimated in Finland to have doubled from the late 1960s until the early 1990s, with a similar doubling reported in Switzerland in 1998 over the preceding 20 years.[53,54]

Recent studies have found substantial increases in BCC amongst younger women.[50,55,56] In Olmstead County, Minnesota, the incidence of BCC in women rose from 13.4 cases per 100,000 in 1976–1979 to 31.6 cases per 100,000 in 2000–2003.[55] In the Netherlands, while the overall BCC incidence rate has increased 2.4% annually, it has increased more than 3.9% in young women, especially for BCC on the trunk (5.7% increase), with increasing rates in younger cohorts, suggestive of a cohort effect.[56] In the UK from 1996 to 2003, there has also been more than a 3% increase in BCC incidence for women aged 30–49 years.[50] This has raised concern that behaviors such as sunbathing or indoor tanning by young women may be driving the increase in cancer incidence in this group. In Australia, which has been targeting youth over the last two decades through public health campaigns and messages on skin cancer prevention, there has been no change in BCC incidence noted in young adults.[36]

## Basal cell carcinoma mortality

Death from BCC is rare. The mortality of BCC is lower and the mean age at time of death is higher than with SCC. It has been suggested that SCC is 12 times more likely to be fatal than BCC. From 1996 to 2005, 365 deaths from NMSC were reported to the Western Australia Cancer Registry; no cases were attributed to BCC. The age-adjusted mortality rate for BCC has been estimated at 0.12 per 100,000.[47] Higher mortality is seen with increasing age, male gender, and in the white population. Age-adjusted rate ratios, which correct for the higher proportion of elderly females, suggested that mortality among men may be over twice that of women.[47]

## Social impact

Disability and disfigurement may result from these malignancies and their treatment, with resultant economic and psychosocial implications, though it is difficult to quantify the morbidity impact. In an investigation of patient and health system delay factors and associated keratinocyte carcinoma morbidity, the size of defect from Mohs micrographic surgery (MMS) was used as a proxy for size of malignancy. After controlling for anatomic site, histologic subtype, age and gender, a delay from first examination by a physician until having MMS of more than 1 year resulted in a doubling in size of the defect. Examination of contributors to delay included initial misdiagnosis, initial provider treatment, and number of prior surgical treatments, suggesting that attention to the process of care delivery for KC may have an impact on morbidity.[57]

## Other cancers of the skin

The epidemiology of other cutaneous malignancies is often obtained from defined populations or using cumulative cases from large registries such as the SEER registry.[58,59]

### Cutaneous T-cell lymphoma

Incidence of cutaneous T-cell lymphoma (CTCL) in the US has been estimated at between 0.4 and 1.0 cases per 100,000 population.[58-60] The estimated age-adjusted incidence in the US from 1973 to 2002 was estimated at 0.64 cases per 100,000.[60] The annual incidence of CTCL has been increasing over time, with an estimated increase of $2.9 \times 10^{-6}$ per decade, and the most recent incidence for the years 1996–2002 is estimated at 0.96 cases per 100,000.[60] Between 3% and 5% of these cases are classified as Sézary syndrome.[60] Incidence of CTCL is higher with increasing age, male gender and in the black population. The age-adjusted (US 2000) incidence per 100,000 in the United States from 1973 to 2002 for men and women respectively was 0.87 and 0.46 while the incidence for black compared to white population was 0.9 and 0.6 respectively.[60] The etiology of CTCL remains unclear.[59,61]

The age-adjusted estimated mortality from 1991 SEER registry data was 0.055 cases per 100,000. There is evidence, however, that this mortality rate substantially underestimates the true rate.[62,63] In the US SEER program, mortality underestimation is high, with more than a 50% underestimate.[63] Higher CTCL mortality is seen in older adults, males, and in the black population.[61] In the US between 1973 and 1992, the relative survival in CTCL patients was approximately 77% at 5 years and 69% at 10 years.[62] The mortality rate for CTCL has decreased more than 20% since the early 1980s. This decline has been seen regardless of gender or race (see Chapter 21).

### Primary cutaneous B-cell lymphoma

The age-adjusted incidence of primary cutaneous B-cell lymphoma (PCBCL) has been estimated at 0.39 cases per 100,000 in the US from 1973 to 2001.[64] Incidence increases with age, with the highest rate of PCBCL reported in those over 80 years old (1.08 cases per 100,000).[64] PCBCL incidence was found to be higher in men than women (0.23 and 0.16 ).[64] Racial differences in incidence of PCBCL are inconsistent, with reports of higher incidence in the black population as compared with the white population (0.9 and 0.2 per 100,000 respectively)[64] as well as higher rates in non-Hispanic whites (0.35 per 100,000) compared to Hispanic whites (0.28 per 100,000) and blacks (0.15 per 100,000).[65] The 5-year survival rate from more indolent histologic types in favorable locations is 94% while survival from immunoblastic and unfavorable sites (leg, trunk, disseminated disease) is only 34%.[64]

There were more than 5900 cutaneous lymphomas reported to the SEER-9 program between 1980 and 2005, with an increasing incidence over time.[65] They found that the incidence rate rose from 5.0 cases per 1,000,000 person-years during 1980–1982 to 12.7 during 2004–2005, with increases in most racial and ethnic groups, especially non-Hispanic whites. Peaks in the incidence of both CTCL and CBCL were noted between 2001 and 2003 (14.3 cases per 1,000,000). However, this may not represent the true peak as delays in reporting may be responsible for the slightly lower rate in the last period of 2004–2005. CBCL was increasing more rapidly than CTCL during the time periods of 1992–1996 to 2001–2005.[65]

### Merkel cell carcinoma

While the SEER registry officially added Merkel cell carcinoma (MCC [see Chapter 17]) to its list of surveillance cancers in 1986, between 1973 and 1982 21 cases (2%) were reported to SEER with the numbers reported expanding with time to 255 cases between 1983 and 1991 (25%) and an additional 758 cases (73%) between 1992 and 1999.[66,67] The incidence of MCC in the US per 100,000 from 1973 to 1999 was estimated at 0.24, increasing over time with an estimated annual percent change of 8% per year between 1986 and 2001.[66,68] US incidence of MCC for 2001 was estimated at 0.44 per 100,000.[68] MCC incidence between 1980 and 2004 in eastern France has been estimated at 0.13 cases per 100,000.[69] MCC incidence is 11-fold higher in Caucasians compared to blacks and it is estimated that 94–97% of SEER reported cases were white.[66,67] MCC incidence in the US per 100,000 has been estimated at 0.23 in whites and 0.01 in blacks.[67] MCC incidence in the US is 0.34–0.65 per 100,000 in men and 0.15–0.26 per 100,000 in women.[66-68] There is a higher incidence of MCC after approximately age 50, with more than 76% of cases reported in those over age 65.[66] MCC is often diagnosed at a more advanced stage, and less than half of all cases of MCC reported to the US SEER program are classified as localized disease.[66] An increase in MCC incidence has been noted in patients with other neoplasms and in organ transplant recipients.[66,67]

Deaths from MCC account for roughly 17% of all NMSC deaths in Western Australia (WA).[38] The 5-year mortality rate of MCC in WA has been estimated at 0.25 and 0.09 cases per 100,000 respectively for men and women. The 5-year observed and relative survival rates in the US are 45% and 62% respectively. Survival varies by stage at diagnosis, with 5-year MCC survival for stage I disease estimated at 75% compared to 25% for stage III disease.[66]

### Dermatofibrosarcoma protuberans

The age-adjusted US incidence rate of dermatofibrosarcoma protuberans (DFSP [see Chapter 15]) has been estimated at 0.42 per 100,000.[70] The incidence rate of DFSP has increased in the US by 43% between 1973 and 2000 as reported to the US SEER program. In the US, the incidence of DFSP is slightly higher in women (0.44 per 100,000) compared to men (0.42 per 100,000) and is most commonly reported on the trunk (42% of all tumors).[70] The incidence of DFSP peaks during the fourth and fifth decades, and the incidence in blacks is almost double that of whites (0.65 vs. 0.39 per 100,000). Five-year relative survival is favorable and is estimated to be more than 99%.[70]

## Kaposi sarcoma

There are several types of Kaposi sarcoma (KS [see Chapter 16]): epidemic or HIV-associated, iatrogenic or transplant-associated, endemic African, and classical. KS was a rare tumor among Western populations prior to 1981, occurring in only 0.02–0.06 per 100,000 people per year. It was classically seen in people of Mediterranean or Ashkenazi descent, often between age 40 and 70, and almost 10 times more often in men than women. With the arrival of acquired immunodeficiency syndrome (AIDS), the incidence of KS increased dramatically. In the early years of the epidemic, it is estimated that 15–25% of men affected with human immunodeficiency virus (HIV) in the United States were diagnosed with KS. The endemic African type of KS occurs in blacks in equatorial Africa, such as Uganda, where it accounts for 3–9% of malignancies. The endemic type is seen in middle-aged adults and children, again more often in males than females. The immunosuppressive therapies necessary for organ-transplant success are responsible for the iatrogenic variant. Recent reviews of iatrogenic KS note that incidence in immunosuppressed patients is approximately 80 to 500 times that of the non-immunosuppressed population, and that it is seen in transplant patients of all ages, though two to three times more frequently in males than females.[71,72]

## ANALYTIC EPIDEMIOLOGY

Skin cancer has many causes. In 2002, ultraviolet light was added to the list of carcinogens reported in the Tenth Report on Carcinogens released by the National Institute of Environmental Health Sciences, because of its association with cutaneous malignancies.[73] Size, type and multiplicity of nevi, personal and family history of melanoma, and early, intense and intermittent exposure are important risk factors for melanoma. Other risk factors include eye color, hair color, facultative skin color, and ethnicity. Immunosuppression and photochemotherapy also appear to have a role.[74] Many of these potential etiological factors have been identified through analytical epidemiology.

Both case–control and cohort investigations have led to improved knowledge about the etiology of melanoma. Cohort study design was used to identify the increased risk of melanoma in those who have a family history of the disease as well as the suggested association between dysplastic nevi and melanoma. Cohort studies have also been used to quantify these associations.[2] Studies of twins have also contributed. In the Finnish Twin Cohort, almost 26,000 twins were linked prospectively to the Finnish Cancer Registry and followed for 22 years. The incidence of cutaneous malignancies in this cohort reflected that of the general population. There were no twin pairs in which both of the twins developed melanoma, and only one pair in which both developed SCC.[75]

In case–case study, researchers examined melanoma patients in Queensland, Australia to explore their hypothesis that melanomas in different anatomic locations may arise through different causal pathways. Patients with lentigo maligna melanoma and melanomas on the head and neck were significantly more likely to have more actinic keratoses and significantly fewer nevi than those patients who had melanoma on the trunk. This study was supportive of a divergent pathway for melanoma induction suggesting that in people who have a low tendency to develop nevi, more sunlight exposure is needed to induce melanoma than in those people with multiple nevi.[29] This is now supported by studies of correlates of somatic mutations found in melanomas.[76,77]

Case–control studies have made major contributions to our knowledge of skin cancer. Case–control studies helped establish the link between melanoma and several factors: severe sunburns, extent of youth sun exposure, and intense intermittent sun exposure.[2] In a case–control study conducted in Belgium, France and Germany, ultraviolet exposure in childhood and adulthood were both associated with an increased risk of melanoma, and an interaction between early and later life exposure further magnified the risk.[78]

Other risk factors for keratinocyte carcinoma have also surfaced using the analytic type of study design, such as cigarette smoking and squamous cell carcinoma.[79] Ultraviolet exposure is a major contributor to the risk of developing basal cell and squamous cell carcinoma of the skin. People with evidence of solar damage, including elastosis, telangiectasia and solar keratosis, appear to be at higher risk. In a case–control study of SCC in Australia, the role of sun exposure was investigated through the Geraldton Skin Cancer Prevention Survey. A large positive relationship with SCC was seen with hours of bright sunlight accumulated over the course of a lifetime. Also, a strong association was noted for sunlight exposure with the specific anatomic site of the carcinoma, and this site-specific exposure risk was greater for exposure early in life. There was also a significant association between the number of blistering sunburns of the anatomic site and SCC. Investigators found little evidence that use of sunscreen or hats was associated with SCC risk in this study.[34]

Inherited factors play a role in the development of these cancers. Individuals with xeroderma pigmentosa have a significantly higher incidence of melanoma, BCC, and SCC. Familial risk for SCC was examined using the national Swedish Family Cancer database from 1961 to 1998. Evidence of family clustering was found, with a standardized incidence ratio of 2.72 for invasive SCC in offspring of parents with skin cancer. No correlation of SCC was found between spouses, suggesting that heritable factors may be more significant than adult environmental exposure.[11] Potential genetic risk factors include racial origin, skin type, and eye and hair color. Inherited genes that have been linked to skin cancer include CDKN2 and MC1R for melanoma, p53 for SCC, and PTCH for BCC.[80–82]

## INTERVENTIONAL EPIDEMIOLOGY

Interventional studies provide the potential for a higher degree of validity of the findings of the study, and potentially a more definitive result. Goals of interventional epidemiology include establishing reliable evidence on which public health policy and resources can be focused.[83] Interventional epidemiologic design has played a more limited role in the study of cutaneous malignancies.

Trial evidence suggests that sunscreen use is important in skin cancer prevention.[7] In the Nambour trial, in which patients were randomly assigned to daily sunscreen use versus discretionary use, and simultaneously to beta-carotene versus placebo tablets independently of sunscreen assignment, investigators found a significant association with regular sunscreen use but not with beta-carotene. Comparing 1994 to 1992, the estimated increase in the number of solar keratoses (SK) in the regular sunscreen users was 20% compared to an increase of 57% in the control group, which is the equivalent of one additional SK per person over that time.[84] The Nambour Skin Cancer Prevention Trial also investigated the effectiveness of daily sunscreen use on the prevention of BCC and SCC. Daily sunscreen use had no effect on overall risk of BCC but did decrease SCC incidence by 40%.[85,86] Sunscreen use and the development of melanocytic nevi has also been investigated in a randomized controlled trial. White schoolchildren aged 6–10 years in British Columbia, Canada were randomly assigned to a group that was given a supply of sunscreen and application instruction or to a control group that received neither advice nor sunscreen. Children in the sunscreen group developed significantly fewer new nevi than the control group children in the 3-year study period.[87]

Clinical trials can provide additional evidence to support or to help reject suggested associations that arise from descriptive and analytic epidemiology reports. Findings from the Nutritional Prevention of Cancer Trial, a multicenter, randomized clinical trial of selenium supplementation in areas of the Southeastern US, were consistent with no association between selenium and melanoma, contradicting the previous associations from analytical studies that led the authors to investigate this area.[88] In the Nambour trial, no difference was seen in solar keratoses development or skin cancer in those receiving beta-carotene versus placebo.[84]

## FUTURE OUTLOOK

For the past several decades we have been able to measure melanoma incidence and mortality, and the picture has been clear and concerning: a meteoric rise in both incidence and mortality. The future situation will be more complex.

There are pressures to shift diagnostic criteria for skin cancers. Pathologists' fear of legal liability may lead to an artificial increase in incidence, particularly for melanoma because of the associated risk of fatality.

The impact of the various diagnostic categories including dysplastic nevi, atypical nevi, Clark's nevi, lentigo maligna, and others that have been used for melanocytic dysplasias may also affect future melanoma incidence, although no such effect has been documented to date.

Publicity around skin cancer issues has increased in recent years, and this may be causing more people to present to their physician with concern about a skin lesion, which may lead to more skin cancer diagnoses and an artifactual increase in skin cancer incidence.

Changes in the healthcare system in the future will have an uncertain effect on the degree of under-registration of skin cancer in established registries. For the past 30 years there has been a cycle of health system changes in the locus of skin cancer diagnosis followed by some cancer registry attempts to capture cases that might otherwise be missed due to these changes.

Beyond these artifactual impacts on skin cancer incidence, these rates are likely to show real impacts of several trends. First, access to sites of natural intense ultraviolet exposure may have reached a plateau in light-skinned populations worldwide. There may even be a decreasing trend among some segments of youth more enamored with video games than stickball. In either case, the resulting trends in population-based incidence may not be manifest for quite some time for melanoma and BCC because of the long lag time between exposure and the cancer diagnosis.

The most important issues for anticipating future trends in melanoma, SCC, and BCC are the impacts of behavioral changes and of public health campaigns and awareness around skin cancer issues. Tanning salon usage may have a major future impact[89,90] and epidemiologic evidence has linked such exposures to skin cancers (see Chapter 59).[91-93] Sunscreens are considerably more effective in blocking ultraviolet radiation than those from earlier decades (see Chapter 9). Sunscreens can reduce the risk of at least some of the adverse consequences of excessive exposure to ultraviolet radiation with appropriate application before the exposure. However, their use is often inadequate, so their impact on future incidence is not yet known.[94]

Finally, the widespread campaigns aimed at skin cancer prevention do seem to be associated with improved prognosis and perhaps reduced incidence (Chapter 7). It is clear that properly constructed campaigns can have an effect on sun-related behavior,[95] and can be associated with effects observable at the population level and sustainable over time.[42,96] Secondary prevention through improved screening for skin cancers is also key to reducing disease burden, at least for melanoma. Epidemiologic investigations across all of these factors are critical to pointing the way forward to a better future.

## REFERENCES

1. Jemal A, Siegel R, Xu J, et al. Cancer statistics, 2010. *CA Cancer J Clin.* 2010;60(5):277–300.
2. Weinstock MA. Ultraviolet radiation and skin cancer: epidemiologic data from the United States and Canada. In: Young AR, Bjorn LO, Moan J, et al., eds. Environmental UV *Photobiology.* New York, NY: Plenum Press; 1993:295–344.
3. Lancaster HO. Some geographical aspects of the mortality from melanoma in Europeans. *Med J Aust.* 1956;1:1082–1087.
4. *The Connecticut Tumor Registry.* Hartford: State of Connecticut Department of Public Health; July 2001.
5. *Connecticut Tumor Registry Cancer Inquiry System.* <http://www.cancer-rates.info/ct/>. Accessed 14.08.09.
6. *SEER program.* <http://seer.cancer.gov/registries/data.html>. Accessed 17.08.09.
7. Mikkilineni R, Weinstock MA. Epidemiology. In: Sober AJ, Haluska FG, eds. *Atlas of Clinical Oncology: Skin Cancer.* London: BC Decker; 2001:1–15.
8. Horner M, Ries L, Krapcho M, et al. SEER *cancer statistics review, 1975-2006 based on November 2008 SEER data submission, posted to the SEER web site,* 2009. <http://seer.cancer.gov/csr/1975_2006/>. Accessed 17.08.09.
9. Marks R. Epidemiology of melanoma. *Clin Exp Dermatol.* 2000;25:459–463.
10. National Health Priority Areas: Cancer Indicators. <http://www.aihw.gov.au/hhpa/cancer>. Accessed 21.08.09.

11. Hemminki K, Zhang H, Czene K. Familiar invasive and in situ squamous cell carcinoma. *Br J Cancer.* 2003;88:1375–1380.

12. Weinstock MA, Skin cancer I. Melanoma and nevi. In: Williams HC, Strachan DP, eds. *The Challenge of Dermato-Epidemiology.* Boca Raton: CRC Press; 1997:191–207.

13. Marrett LD, Nguyen HL, Armstrong BK. Trends in the incidence of cutaneous malignant melanoma in New South Wales, 1983-96. *Int J Cancer.* 2001;92:457–462.

14. De Vries E, Bray FI, Coebergh JWW, et al. Changing epidemiology of malignant cutaneous melanoma in Europe 1953-1997: rising trends in incidence and mortality but recent stabilizations in western Europe and decreases in Scandinavia. *Int J Cancer.* 2003;107:119–126.

15. For this chapter, racial and ethnic groups are discussed as they are classified by SEER: white, black, Hispanic, and Asian/Pacific Islander

16. Boi S, Cristofolini M, Micciolo R, et al. Epidemiology of skin tumors: data from the cutaneous cancer registry in Trentino, Italy. *J Cutan Med Surg.* 2003;7(4):300–305.

17. de Vries E, Schouten LJ, Visser O, et al. Rising trends in the incidence of and mortality from cutaneous melanoma in the Netherlands: a Northwest to Southeast gradient? *Eur J Cancer.* 2002;39:1439–1446.

18. *Australian Cancer Statistics Update.* <http://www.aihw.gov.au/cancer/index.cfm>. Accessed 21.08.09.

19. Curado MP, Edwards B, Shin HR, et al, eds. *Cancer Incidence in Five Continents.* Vol. IX. Lyon: International Agency for Research on Cancer (IARC); 2008.

20. Kricker A, Armstrong BK. International trends in skin cancer. *Cancer Forum.* 1996;20:192–195.

21. Bulliard J-L, Cox B, Elwood M. Latitude gradients in melanoma incidence and mortality in the non-Maori population of New Zealand. *Cancer Causes Control.* 1994;5(3):234–240.

22. Parkin DM, Whelan SL, Ferlay J, et al, eds. Cancer Incidence in Five Continents. Vol. VII. Lyon: International Agency for Research on Cancer (IARC); 1997.

23. Weinstock MA. Death from skin cancer among the elderly: epidemiologic patterns. *Arch Dermatol.* 1997;133:1207–1209.

24. Ries LAG, Eisner MP, Kosary CL, et al. SEER *Cancer Statistics Review, 1973-1999.* Bethesda, MD: National Cancer Institute; 2002.

25. Severi G, Giles GG, Robertson C, et al. Mortality from cutaneous melanoma: evidence for contrasting trends between populations. *Br J Dermatol.* 2000;82(11):1887–1891.

26. van der Esch EP, Muir CS, Nectoux J, et al. Temporal change in diagnostic criteria as a cause of the increase of malignant melanoma over time is unlikely. *Int J Cancer.* 1991;47(4):483–489.

27. Cohn-Cedermark G, Mansson-Brahme E, Rutqvist LE, et al. Trends in mortality from malignant melanoma in Sweden, 1970–1996. *Cancer.* 2000;89:348–355.

28. Weinstock MA, Bingham SF, Cole GW, et al. Reliability of counting actinic keratoses before and after brief consensus discussion. *Arch Dermatol.* 2001;137:1055–1058.

29. Whiteman DC, Watt P, Purdie DM, et al. Melanocytic nevi, solar keratoses and divergent causal pathways to cutaneous melanoma. *J Natl Cancer Inst.* 2003;95(11):806–812.

30. Cook J, Zitelli JA. Mohs micrographic surgery: a cost analysis. *J Am Acad Dermatol.* 1998;39(5 Pt 1):698–703.

31. Demers AA, Nugent Z, Mihalcioiu C, et al. Trends of nonmelanoma skin cancer from 1960 through 2000 in a Canadian population. *J Am Acad Dermatol.* 2005;53(2):320–328.

32. Miller DL, Weinstock MA. Nonmelanoma skin cancer in the United States: incidence. *J Am Acad Dermatol.* 1994;30(5 Pt 1):774–778.

33. Athas WF, Hunt WC, Key CR. Changes in nonmelanoma skin cancer incidence between 1977-1978 and 1998-1999 in Northcentral New Mexico. *Cancer Epidemiol Biomarkers Prev.* 2003;12(10):1105–1108.

34. English DR, Armstrong BK, Kricker A, et al. Demographic characteristics, pigmentary and cutaneous risk factors for squamous cell carcinoma of the skin: a case-control study. *Int J Cancer.* 1998;76:628–634.

35. Stang A, Ziegler S, Buchner U, et al. Malignant melanoma and nonmelanoma skin cancers in Northrhine-Westphalia, Germany: a patient-vs. diagnosis-based incidence approach. *Int J Dermatol.* 2007;46(6):564–570.

36. Staples MP, Elwood M, Burton RC, et al. Non-melanoma skin cancer in Australia: the 2002 national survey and trends since 1985. *Med J Aust.* 2006;184(1):6–10.

37. Brewster DH, Bhatti LA, Inglis JH, et al. Recent trends in incidence of nonmelanoma skin cancers in the East of Scotland, 1992-2003. *Br J Dermatol.* 2007;156(6):1295–1300.

38. Girschik J, Fritschi L, Threlfall T, et al. Deaths from non-melanoma skin cancer in Western Australia. *Cancer Causes Control.* 2008;19(8):879–885.

39. Hayes RC, Leonfellner S, Pilgrim W, et al. Incidence of nonmelanoma skin cancer in New Brunswick, Canada, 1992 to 2001. *J Cutan Med Surg.* 2007;11(2):45–52.

40. Katalinic A, Kunze U, Schafer T. Epidemiology of cutaneous melanoma and non-melanoma skin cancer in Schleswig-Holstein, Germany: incidence, clinical subtypes, tumour stages and localization (epidemiology of skin cancer). *Br J Dermatol.* 2003;149(6):1200–1206.

41. Karagas MR, Nelson HH, Sehr P, et al. Human papillomavirus infection and incidence of squamous cell and basal cell carcinomas of the skin. *J Natl Cancer Inst.* 2006;98(6):389–395.

42. Staples M, Marks R, Giles G. Trends in the incidence of non-melanocytic skin cancer (NMSC) treated in Australia 1985-1995: are primary prevention programs starting to have an effect? *Int J Cancer.* 1998;78:144–148.

43. Moan J, Dahlback A. The relationship between skin cancers, solar radiation and ozone depletion. *Br J Cancer.* 1992;65(6):916–921.

44. Holme SA, Malinovszky K, Robert DL. Changing trends in non-melanoma skin cancer in South Wales, 1988-98. *Br J Dermatol.* 2000;143:1224–1229.

45. Hannuksela-Svahn A, Pukkala E, Karvonen J. Basal cell skin carcinoma and other nonmelanoma skin cancers in Finland from 1956 through 1995. *Arch Dermatol.* 1999;135:781–786.

46. Koh D, Wang H, Lee J, et al. Basal cell carcinoma, squamous cell carcinoma and melanoma of the skin: analysis of the Singapore Cancer Registry data 1968-97. *Br J Dermatol.* 2003;148(6):1161–1166.

47. Weinstock MA, Bogaars HA, Ashley M, et al. Nonmelanoma skin cancer mortality. *Arch Dermatol.* 1991;127:1194–1197.

48. Lewis KG, Weinstock MA. Trends in nonmelanoma skin cancer mortality rates in the United States, 1969 through 2000. *J Invest Dermatol.* 2007;127(10):2323–2327.

49. Karagas MR, Greenberg ER, Spencer SK, et al. Increase in incidence rates of basal cell and squamous cell skin cancer in New Hampshire, USA. New Hampshire Skin Cancer Study Group. *Int J Cancer.* 1999;81(4):555–559.

50. Bath-Hextall F, Leonardi-Bee J, Smith C, et al. Trends in incidence of skin basal cell carcinoma. Additional evidence from a UK primary care database study. *Int J Cancer.* 2007;121(9):2105–2108.

51. Hoey SE, Devereux CE, Murray L, et al. Skin cancer trends in Northern Ireland and consequences for provision of dermatology services. *Br J Dermatol.* 2007;156(6):1301–1307.

52. Sng J, Koh D, Siong WC, et al. Skin cancer trends among Asians living in Singapore from 1968 to 2006. *J Am Acad Dermatol.* 2009;61(3):426–432.

53. Hannuksela-Svahn A, Pukkala E, Karvonen J. Basal cell skin carcinoma and other non melanoma skin cancers in Finland from 1956 through 1995. *Arch Dermatol.* 1999;135:781–786.

54. Levi F, Erler G, Te V-C, et al. Trends in skin cancer in Neuchatel, 1976-98. *Tumori.* 2001;87(5):288–289.

55. Christenson LJ, Borrowman TA, Vachon CM, et al. Incidence of basal cell and squamous cell carcinomas in a population younger than 40 years. *JAMA.* 2005;294(6):681–690.

56. de Vries E, Louwman M, Bastiaens M, et al. Rapid and continuous increases in incidence rates of basal cell carcinoma in the southeast Netherlands since 1973. *J Invest Dermatol.* 2004;123(4):634–638.

57. Eide MJ, Weinstock MA, Dufresne Jr RG, et al. Relationship of treatment delay with surgical defect size from keratinocyte carcinoma (basal cell carcinoma and squamous cell carcinoma of the skin). *J Invest Dermatol.* 2005;124(2):308–314.

58. Chuang T-Y, Su WPD, Sigfrid AM. Incidence of cutaneous T cell lymphoma and other rare skin cancers in a defined population. *J Am Acad Dermatol.* 1990;23(2):254–256.

59. Weinstock MA, Horm JW. Mycosis fungoides in the United States. *JAMA.* 1988;260(1):42–46.

60. Criscione VD, Weinstock MA. Incidence of cutaneous T-cell lymphoma in the United States, 1973-2002. *Arch Dermatol.* 2007;143(7):854–859.

61. Weinstock MA, Gardstein B. Twenty-year trends in the reported incidence of mycosis fungoides and associated mortality. *Am J Public Health.* 1999;89(8):1240–1244.

62. Weinstock MA, Reynes JF. The changing survival of patients with mycosis fungoides. *CA Cancer J Clin.* 1999;85(1):208–212.

63. Barzilai DA, Weinstock MA. Deaths due to cutaneous T-cell lymphoma: bias of certification and a revised estimate of national mortality. *Epidemiology.* 2008;19(5):761–762.

64. Smith BD, Smith GL, Cooper DL, et al. The cutaneous B-cell lymphoma prognostic index: a novel prognostic index derived from a population-based registry. *J Clin Oncol.* 2005;23(15):3390–3395.

65. Bradford PT, Devesa SS, Anderson WF, et al. Cutaneous lymphoma incidence patterns in the United States: a population-based study of 3884 cases. *Blood.* 2009;113(21):5064–5073.

66. Agelli M, Clegg LX. Epidemiology of primary Merkel cell carcinoma in the United States. *J Am Acad Dermatol.* 2003;49(5):832–841.

67. Miller RW, Rabkin CS. Merkel cell carcinoma and melanoma: etiological similarities and differences. *Cancer Epidemiol Biomarkers Prev.* 1999;8:153–158.

68. Hodgson NC. Merkel cell carcinoma: changing incidence trends. *J Surg Oncol.* 2005;89(1):1–4.

69. Riou-Gotta MO, Fournier E, Danzon A, et al. Rare skin cancer: a population-based cancer registry descriptive study of 151 consecutive cases diagnosed between 1980 and 2004. *Acta Oncol.* 2009;48(4):605–609.

70. Criscione VD, Weinstock MA. Descriptive epidemiology of dermatofibrosarcoma protuberans in the United States, 1973 to 2002. *J Am Acad Dermatol.* 2007;56(6):968–973.

71. Aboulafia DM. Kaposi's sarcoma. *Clin Dermatol.* 2001;19:269–283.

72. Euvrard S, Kanitakis J, Claudy A. Skin cancers after organ transplantation. *N Engl J Med.* 2003;348:1681–1691.

**73.** Twonbly R. New carcinogen list includes estrogen, UV radiation. *J Natl Cancer Inst.* 2003;95(3):185–186.

**74.** Weinstock MA. Issues in the epidemiology of melanoma. *Hematol Oncol Clin North Am.* 1998;12(4):681–698.

**75.** Milan T, Verkasalo PK, Kaprio J, et al. Malignant skin cancers in the Finnish twin cohort: a population-based study, 1976-1997. *Br J Dermatol.* 2002;147:509–512.

**76.** Curtin JA, Fridlyand J, Kageshita T, et al. Distinct sets of genetic alterations in melanoma. *N Engl J Med.* 2005;353(20):2135–2147.

**77.** Thomas NE, Edmiston SN, Alexander A, et al. Number of nevi and early-life ambient UV exposure are associated with BRAF-mutant melanoma. *Cancer Epidemiol Biomarkers Prev.* 2007;16(5):991–997.

**78.** Autier P, Dore J-F. Influence of sun exposure during childhood and during adulthood on melanoma risk. *Int J Cancer.* 1998;77:533–537.

**79.** Boyd AS, Shyr Y, King LE. Basal cell carcinoma in young women: an evaluation of the association of tanning bed use and smoking. *J Am Acad Dermatol.* 2002;46(5):706–709.

**80.** de Gruijl FR, van Kranen HJ, Mullenders LH, UV-induced DNA damage, repair, mutations and oncogenic pathways in skin cancer. *J Photochem Photobiol B.* 2001;63(1–3):19–27.

**81.** Bataille V. Genetic epidemiology of melanoma. *Eur J Cancer.* 2003;39(10):1341–1347.

**82.** Giglia-Mari G, Sarasin A. TP53 mutations in human skin cancers. *Hum Mutat.* 2003;21(3):217–228.

**83.** Hennekens CH, Buring JE. *Epidemiology in Medicine.* 1st ed Philadelphia: Lippincott Williams and Wilkins; 1987.

**84.** Darlington S, Williams G, Neale R, et al. A randomized controlled trial to assess sunscreen application and beta carotene supplementation in the prevention of solar keratoses. *Arch Dermatol.* 2003;139:451–455.

**85.** Green A, Williams G, Neale R, et al. Daily sunscreen application and beta-carotene supplementation in prevention of basal-cell and squamous-cell carcinomas of the skin: a randomised controlled trial. *Lancet.* 1999;354:723–729.

**86.** van der Pols JC, Williams GM, Pandeya N, et al. Prolonged prevention of squamous cell carcinoma of the skin by regular sunscreen use. *Cancer Epidemiol Biomarkers Prev.* 2006;15(12):2546–2548.

**87.** Gallagher RP, Rivers JK, Lee TK, et al. Broad-spectrum sunscreen use and the development of new nevi in white children. *JAMA.* 2000;283(22):2955–2960.

**88.** Duffield-Lillico AJ, Reid ME, Turnbull BW, et al. Baseline characteristics and the effect of selenium supplementation on cancer incidence in a randomized clinical trial: a summary report of the Nutritional Prevention of Cancer Trial. *Cancer Epidemiol Biomarkers Prev.* 2002;11(7):630–639.

**89.** Cokkinides VE, Weinstock MA, O'Connell MC, et al. Use of indoor tanning sunlamps by US youth, ages 11-18 years, and by their parent or guardian caregivers: prevalence and correlates. *Pediatrics.* 2002;109(6):1124–1130.

**90.** Demko CA, Borawski EA, Debanne SM, et al. Use of indoor tanning facilities by white adolescents in the United States. *Arch Pediatr Adolesc Med.* 2003;157:854–860.

**91.** Swerdlow AJ, Weinstock MA. Do tanning lamps cause melanoma? An epidemiologic assessment. *J Am Acad Dermatol.* 1998;38(1):89–98.

**92.** Karagas MR, Stannard VA, Mott LA, et al. Use of tanning devices and risk of basal cell and squamous cell skin cancers. *J Natl Cancer Inst.* 2002;94(3):224–226.

**93.** Gallagher RP, Spinelli JJ, Lee TK. Tanning beds, sunlamps, and risk of cutaneous malignant melanoma. *Cancer Epidemiol Biomarkers Prev.* 2005;14(3):562–566.

**94.** Davis KJ, Cokkinides VE, Weinstock MA, et al. Summer sunburn and sun exposure among US youths ages 11 to 18: national prevalence and associated factors. *Pediatrics.* 2002;110(1):27–35.

**95.** Dietrich AJ, Olson AL, Sox CH, et al. Persistent increase in children's sun protection in a randomized controlled community trial. *Prev Med.* 2000;31:569–574.

**96.** van der Pols JC, Williams GM, Neale RE, et al. Long-term increase in sunscreen use in an Australian community after a skin cancer prevention trial. *Prev Med.* 2006;42(3):171–176.

# Etiological Factors in Skin Cancers: Environmental and Biological

*Luigi Naldi, Drusilla Hufford, and Luke Hall-Jordan*

## Key Points

- Exposure to ultraviolet radiation plays a major role in the causation of squamous cell carcinoma, basal cell carcinoma, and melanoma.

- The timing and character of exposure to ultraviolet radiation may affect differently the risk of different skin cancers and of the same cancer at different body locations.

- Interaction with several other factors, including host-related factors, e.g. skin phenotype, and environmental factors, such as viruses, ionizing radiation, chemical agents, and concomitant chronic inflammatory conditions, may further increase risks.

- Genome-wide association studies and analyses of genetic–environmental interactions will probably help elucidating the impact on skin cancer risk of external factors

## INTRODUCTION

There are several types and subtypes of skin tumors which are induced by different exogenous and endogenous factors. Exposure to sunlight plays a major role in many of them. Additional factors include ionizing radiations, infectious agents, various chemical carcinogens, and chronic inflammation. Among host-related factors, gender, aging and skin phenotype are all important risk modifiers in squamous cell carcinoma (SCC) and basal cell carcinoma (BCC), collectively grouped under the label 'non-melanoma skin cancer' (NMSC), and in melanoma.

## HISTORY

One of the earliest published observations about carcinogens was made in the 1750s by Percival Potts, who showed that chimney sweeps developed skin cancer of the scrotum from soot. By 1934, the link between ionizing radiation and skin cancer was already suspected when the International Congress of Radiology, a commission to assess the occurrence of cancers among medical users of radioactive chemicals, was created. In 1945, work documenting a dose–response relationship for the induction of skin tumors in mice by ultraviolet (UV) radiation demonstrated that UVB was the causative portion of the solar spectrum. Other factors have subsequently been shown to be related to skin cancer risk.

## RISK FACTORS (Table 6.1)

### Ultraviolet radiation

UV radiation, visible light, infrared radiation, gamma rays, and X-rays are all part of the electromagnetic spectrum (Fig. 6.1). Visible, UV, and infrared radiation do not ionize molecules and are thus referred to collectively as non-ionizing radiation. Such radiation travels as three-dimensional waves in a vacuum and acts as discrete 'packets' of energy or photons when interacting with matter. In order for such radiation to have an effect in biologic systems, it must be absorbed by the molecules of such systems. The energy of a photon of non-ionizing radiation defines its ability to interact with a given molecule. The energy of a photon varies inversely with its wavelength.

The effects of non-ionizing radiation on human cells rely on complex cellular interactions. Specifically, when radiation is absorbed, molecules become raised to an excited state. As molecules return to the resting state through a process of dissipating the absorbed energy, the energy may be converted to chemical change, which in turn results in biologic alterations. UV radiation, emitted both by the sun and by artificial sources, is a well-accepted cause of skin cancer recognized by both the Food and Drug Administration (FDA) and the World Health Organization (WHO) as a significant carcinogen.[1]

The spectrum of UV radiation is conventionally divided into three bands, defined in ranges of nanometers: UVA, UVB, and UVC. Approximately 90–95% of the UV radiation spectrum reaching the Earth's surface is longer-wave radiation, or UVA, the remaining 5–10% being represented by UVB. Several factors influence the intensity of UV exposure, including altitude, latitude, position of the sun, local conditions like weather, health of the ozone layer, and human behavior.

*Latitude* – Locations that are closer to the equator experience higher levels of UV radiation because the sun is directly overhead. Thus, UV radiation has a shorter distance to travel through the atmosphere, giving less opportunity for attenuation. In addition, the ozone layer, which reduces the amount of UVB radiation available at the ground, is naturally thinner over the equatorial region year round.[2]

*Altitude* – As altitude increases, UV exposure also increases. Again, this has to do with the lesser distance through the Earth's atmosphere that UV travels before reaching the Earth's surface. UV radiation intensity increases by 8–12% for every 1000 meters in elevation gained.[3,4]

## Table 6.1 Summary of Risk Factors for Skin Cancer

| Risk Factor | Melanoma | Non-Melanoma Skin Cancer (NMSC) |
|---|---|---|
| Age | Age-related incidence rises with increasing age | More common with increasing age |
| Family history | Occurrence of melanoma in a first- or second-degree relative confers increased risk. Familial atypical mole melanoma syndrome (FAMMS) confers even higher risk | Family history is associated with increased risk for BCC but not SCC |
| Gender | Slight male predominance | Substantially more common in males |
| Race | More common in whites | More common in whites |
| Skin type/ethnicity | Increased incidence in those with fair complexions and red headed, those who burn easily, tan poorly and freckle | Increased incidence in those with fair complexions |
| Nevi | A large number of melanocytic nevi, and giant pigmented congenital nevi confer increased risk | Limited influence on risk |
| Occupation | Higher incidence in indoor workers, as well as those with higher education and income | Higher incidence in outdoor workers for SCC |
| Sun exposure | | |
| Cumulative | May influence risk in the head/neck region | Single greatest risk factor for SCC; may influence risk of BCC in the head/neck region |
| Episodic | Intense, intermittent exposure and blistering sunburns in childhood and adolescence are associated with increased risk | Intense, intermittent exposure and blistering sunburns in childhood and adolescence are associated with increased risk of BCC, especially on the trunk, but not SCC |
| Artificial UV light | PUVA therapy and tanning devices probably increase risk | PUVA therapy, UVB therapy, and tanning devices increase risk |
| Ionizing radiations | Possible association | Definite association with BCC, and probable association with SCC |
| Chemicals and pollutants | Possible association with arsenic exposure | Arsenic and several other chemicals increase risk. Cigarette smoking probably increases SCC risk |
| Diet and nutrients | Elevated BMI may increase risk | No evidence of protective effect from beta-carotene supplementation |

*Position of the sun* – UV radiation levels vary by time of day and time of year. On any given day, assuming clear rather than overcast conditions, UV radiation levels are highest at solar noon during the middle of the day. On an annual basis, UV radiation levels peak during the Summer Solstice, and are at their lowest during the Winter Solstice.

*Local conditions* – Cloud cover is the most significant factor influencing UV. A very dense continuous cloud cover can effectively block UV. However, under some conditions,

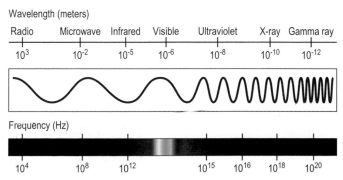

Wavelength (meters)

Radio | Microwave | Infrared | Visible | Ultraviolet | X-ray | Gamma ray

$10^3$   $10^{-2}$   $10^{-5}$   $10^{-6}$   $10^{-8}$   $10^{-10}$   $10^{-12}$

Frequency (Hz)

$10^4$   $10^8$   $10^{12}$   $10^{15}$   $10^{16}$   $10^{18}$   $10^{20}$

**Figure 6.1** Diagrammatic representation of the electromagnetic spectrum. The longer the wavelength, the smaller the frequency of the electromagnetic wave. UV radiation is usually classified as UVC (<290 nm), UVB (290–320 nm), UVA2 (320–340 nm) and UVA1 (340–400 nm).

50% or more may penetrate cloud cover. There are also meteorological conditions of scattered clouds that may actually enhance exposure levels, because incoming UV can even reflect off scattered and wispy clouds. Other local conditions that affect the amount of UV radiation people may be exposed to include reflective surfaces like snow, light-colored sand, pavement and water. Reflective surfaces can increase UV exposure dramatically. For example, clean snow may raise exposure levels by up to 80%, while dry beach sand can increase exposure by 15%.[3] Local factors like pollution and aerosols also affect UV radiation levels. In these cases, the effect can be to decrease exposure levels by blocking UV radiation from reaching the Earth's surface.

*Ozone layer status* – The ozone layer plays a vital role in absorbing UVB radiation entering the Earth's atmosphere (Fig. 6.2). In the 1970s and 1980s, scientists discovered that chlorofluorocarbons (CFCs) – then a common propellant in aerosol cans and commonly used as refrigerants, solvents and foam-blowing agents – were damaging the ozone layer. CFCs were used widely in many industrial and consumer applications, and were highly valued for their low reactivity and chemical stability. Unfortunately, as theorized by US scientists Sherwood Rowland and Mario Molina in 1975, that very chemical stability made these chemicals ideal 'transport mechanisms' for ozone-damaging chlorine.

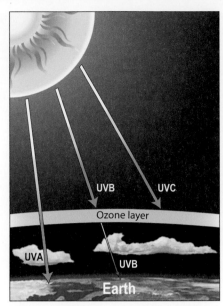

**Figure 6.2** Filtering of UV by the ozone layer. Virtually all UVC and most of the UVB radiation is filtered by the ozone layer in the stratosphere. Most UVA and a limited proportion of UVB reaches the Earth's ground.

Once emitted, CFCs maintain their chemical structure intact through all atmospheric transport processes until they reach the stratosphere, where UVC breaks the bonds binding molecules of CFCs together. This frees the chlorine contained in these molecules to react with the ozone ($O_3$) in the Earth's ozone layer. The resulting chemical reactions enhance natural ozone destruction processes already existing in the stratosphere; before the anthropogenic emission of CFCs, these natural destruction processes were balanced by natural mechanisms that also create ozone.

While scientists have loosely used the term 'ozone hole', the occurrence is actually more like an extreme thinning of ozone at the South Pole, caused by chlorine released from CFCs and other ozone-damaging compounds, such as brominated chemicals used as fire extinguishers and agricultural fumigants. As the austral spring ends, ozone-poor air from the Antarctic region then mixes with the atmosphere generally, decreasing the amount of $O_3$ available to screen out UVB radiation worldwide. As a result, 'average erythemal UV radiation levels increased by up to a few percent per decade between 1979 and 1998'.[2] The largest increases in UV radiation levels have occurred in mid to high latitudes as a result of stratospheric ozone layer depletion.

In response to this problem, the international treaty to control chemicals that deplete the ozone layer – the Montreal Protocol on Substances that Deplete the Ozone Layer – was opened for signature in 1987 and signed thereafter by all the 196 United Nation members. This level of international cooperation has proved remarkably successful: annual world use of ozone-depleting substances has been reduced over 90%. Still, due to the long atmospheric residence time of these chemicals, ozone damage continues. Scientists do not expect the ozone layer to recover to 1980 levels until 2065 at the earliest (Fig. 6.3). Using daily measures of UV intensity at stations around the world (a measure known as

**Figure 6.3** The ozone hole is the region over Antarctica with total ozone of 220 Dobson Units or lower. This map shows the ozone hole on September 24, 2006.

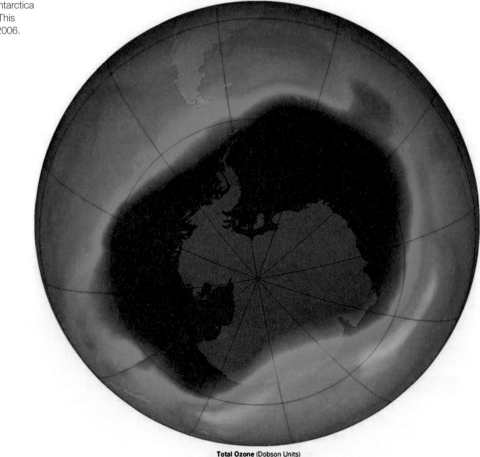

**Total Ozone** (Dobson Units)
110   220   330   440   550

the Global Solar UV Index), it has been projected that, in the absence of global action on ozone-damaging compounds, for mid-latitudes in the northern hemisphere (30°–50° N latitude), the UV Index on an average summer day would have risen from 6–7 (high) to 15 (extreme) by 2040, and to 30 (extreme) by 2065.[5]

Ozone depletion may already be making an impact on skin cancer rates. Incidence and mortality rates are disproportionally rising in Southern Chile[6] (in populated areas significantly impacted by ozone depletion) and should current losses continue, it has been estimated that there will be an additional 5000 cases of skin cancer annually in the UK by mid century.[7]

*Individual behavior* – Individual behavior plays a key role in exposure to UV radiation, and, in fact, is likely much more influential in shaping lifetime risk than is damage to the ozone layer. As an example of current population-wide sun-protective behavior, surveys in the US found that up to one-third of Americans are using any one form of sun protection, including wearing sunscreen, hats, sunglasses, and shirts, and seeking shade. Trend data from the US National Cancer Institute show that while sun protection practices have increased since the early 1990s, they seem to have leveled off or even fallen since 2000.[8]

Both UVA and UVB have been documented to be related to skin cancer risk and the action spectra for the development of SCC and melanoma in mammalians have been developed (Fig. 6.4).[9] UV causes mutations and immunosuppressive effects that are essential to photocarcinogenesis.[10] DNA is a major epidermal chromophore

with an adsorption spectrum that is highest in UVC range and decreases steadily in UVB and UVA. The absorption of UV photon energy can result in its dissipation by the rearrangement of electrons to form new bonds which result in structural alterations. When UV radiation strikes the skin, it is absorbed by pyrimidine bases in DNA and induces the formation of cis-syn cyclobutane pyrimidine dimer and pyrimidine(6-4)pyrimidone photoproduct (Fig. 6.5). The pyrimidone ring of the (6-4) photoproduct is subjected to further modification by UV irradiation to a product called Dewar valence isomer. These photoproducts result in the covalent association of adjacent pyrimidines and usually occur in areas of consecutive pyrimidine residues, which are preferential areas for mutation. Unrepaired or incorrectly repaired pyrimidine dimers lead to mutations that are very specific to UVB. In such mutations, cytosine (C) is changed to thymine (T). These specific types of mutations, that is C to T or CC to TT transitions, are referred to as the 'signature' or 'fingerprint' of the effect of UVB on DNA. Sequencing data from a large number of tumors show that *p53* is mutated in more than 90% of SCCs with C to T transition in about 70% of the cases. That these mutations are an early event and play a critical role in the development of skin cancer is supported by the observation that most actinic keratoses also contain mutations with patterns similar to those of SCC, and that chronically sun-exposed skin contains larger numbers of *p53*-mutated clones than sun-protected skin.[11] In the skin, UV irradiation leads to the formation of 'sunburn cells' that are apoptotic keratinocytes. Inactivation of *p53* in mouse skin reduces the appearance of sunburn cells. BCC have also been found to contain UV signature mutations in *p53* and in the *PTCH1* gene.[12] The mechanism of cancerogenesis linked with UV exposure in melanoma is far less understood.

While most studies point to UVB as a causative factor in skin cancer, UVA is also carcinogenic, but not as efficient, probably by orders of magnitude. UVA is important, however, since it represents the largest proportion of UV reaching human skin. UVA penetrates window glass and exposure may not be blocked by sunscreen usage. UVA radiation affects both epidermal and dermal chromophores. Although indirect DNA damage from ROS becomes relatively more important going from UVB to UVA wavelengths, the dominant DNA lesions induced by UVA are cyclobutane-pyrimidine dimers.[13]

UVA and UVB exposure can come from sources other than sunlight. UVB used therapeutically has a low risk of producing cutaneous cancers. One systematic review

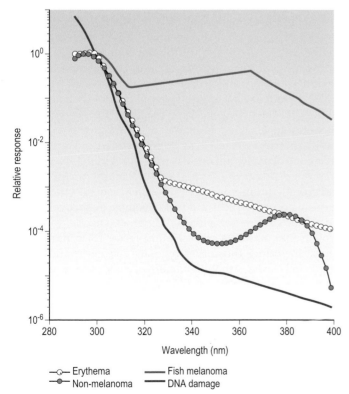

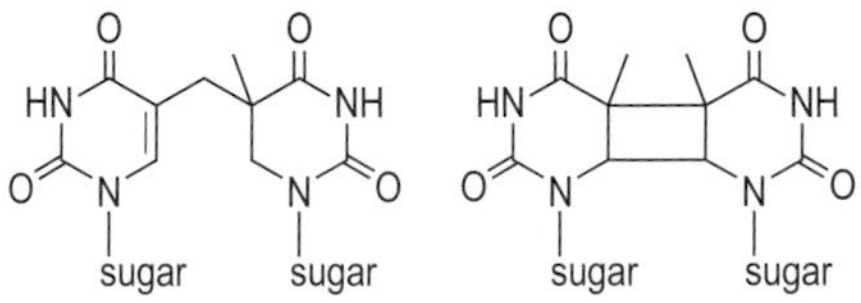

**Figure 6.4** Action spectra for selected UV-related effects. The curve for NMSC shows a rapid decline in relative response as the UV wavelength increases and a more limited sine-like wavelength dependency between 340 and 400 nm. The relevance of the fish melanoma curve for human melanoma has been challenged.

**Figure 6.5** Pyrimidine dimers, induced by UV light. result from bond formation between adjacent pyrimidines, thymine (T) or cytosine (C), within one DNA strand. These dimers distort the DNA structure and interfere with base pairing during DNA replication. The most prevalent photoproduct is cyclobutane pyrimidine dimer (right in the figure), followed by pyrimidine-pyrimidone (6-4) photoproduct (left in the figure).

estimated that the excess annual risk of NMSC associated with UVB radiation was likely to be less than 2%.[14] Photosensitizers can play an important role in UVA carcinogenesis. Dose-dependent increased risks of SCC, BCC, and possibly malignant melanoma have been documented with the therapeutic combination of oral psoralen and UVA (PUVA), with particularly high risk in people with skin type I and II.[15] Recent studies suggest that the use of tanning devices that mainly emit UVA radiation, such as tanning lamps and tanning beds, may be associated with a significant increase in BCC, SCC and melanoma[16,17] (see Chapter 59).

The timing and character of sun exposure may affect differently the risk of different skin cancers and of the same cancer at different body locations. SCC is associated with total lifetime sun exposure[18,19] and with occupational exposure.[20] Late-stage solar exposure may play an important role in the development of SCC since sunlight exposure just prior to diagnosis is associated with an increased risk of the tumor and of its precursor, actinic keratosis (AK). AKs may spontaneously disappear in people who limit solar exposure, and their progression to malignancy seems to require continued exposure to relatively high doses of solar radiation.[21]

BCC and melanoma have been most significantly linked to sun exposure early in life. Intermittent sun exposure and sunburn history are more important than cumulative dose in predicting adult risk for these tumors.[18,22,23] However, variations in risk profiles have been proposed at different body locations and with different clinicopathological variants. Chronic sun exposure may be an etiologic factor for nodular BCC in the head/neck region, while intermittent sun exposure plays a role in superficial lesions on the trunk.[24,25] Similarly, heterogeneity of risk by anatomical site has been proposed for melanoma, with chronic sun exposure influencing the risk of melanoma of the head and neck and intermittent sun exposure, associated with a nevus-prone phenotype, influencing the risk of melanoma elsewhere.[26]

Melanocytic nevi, whose total count overall represent the single greatest predictor of melanoma risk,[27] are a complex exposure variable combining constitutional and environmental effects.[28,29] Boys develop more nevi than girls. While the number of nevi increases with age up to 18–20 years, nevus density (i.e. number per square meter of body surface area) reaches a plateau earlier in life, at age 9–10 years, suggesting a genetic influence for such a variable. Nevi are more common in children with lighter phenotype who burn and do not tan easily in the sun, and with freckling and a history of sunburns. However, red-haired subjects have fewer nevi than other children. These subjects have a higher melanoma risk, suggesting different pathways to melanoma development.

Among other skin cancers, Merkel cell carcinoma (MCC) has also been linked with sun exposure.[30]

## Ionizing radiation

Ionizing radiation has electromagnetic forms (X-rays and gamma rays) and particulate forms (electrons, protons, alpha particles, and neutrons). X-rays, gamma rays, and electrons are classified as sparsely ionizing, whereas alpha particles (such as those associated with radon) and neutrons are densely ionizing. Ionizing radiation can produce ionizations in target molecules, such as DNA, directly or indirectly by interactions with water molecules that result in ROS formation. Besides effects on directly irradiated cells, changes in un-irradiated cells neighboring or co-cultured with exposed cells have been documented ('bystander effects').[31]

Ionizing radiations mainly affect BCC risk.[32] An association with SCC and melanoma is less firmly established. The incidence of BCC is related and proportional to the total dose of radiation and influenced by age at radiation. Patients suffering from basal cell nevus syndrome are abnormally susceptible to ionizing radiation. Skin cancer that occurs after exposure to ionizing radiation has a latency of several months to several decades, with most cases occurring 20 years after initial exposure. The finding of fewer excess skin cancers among irradiated African-Americans as compared to Caucasians with a comparable dose indicates that there may be an interaction of radiation with skin susceptibility to UV exposure. In one study, radiation therapy was a risk factor for SCC mainly among those with a sun-sensitive skin type.[33] In another study of radiation technologists, melanoma risk was increased among those who first worked before 1950, particularly among those who worked five or more years, when radiation exposures were likely highest.[34]

## Genetic influences and molecular mechanisms

The hallmark of malignant cells is that they grow in the absence of appropriate extracellular signals such as growth factors and cytokines. Extracellular signals are transmitted by a signal transduction cascade. The cascade involves tyrosine-specific and serine/threonine-specific kinases, GTPases, and several transcription factors such as NF-κB and c-*myc*. The genes encoding for these proteins may turn into oncogenes when mutated or overexpressed. Hence, these genes are referred to as proto-oncogenes. The intracellular control of the cell cycle is mainly regulated by cyclins, cyclin-dependent kinases (CDK), CDK inhibitors (p21, p27), and so-called tumor suppressor proteins such as the retinoblastoma protein (pRb) and p53. The most extensively studied tumor suppressor gene is *p53*, which encodes a 53-kDa protein that acts as a transcription factor for a number of genes, including those that regulate cell cycle and apoptosis. Cell stress situations, such as exposure to carcinogens, lead to activation of *p53*, which results in a transient cell-cycle arrest to allow DNA repair before entry into the S phase and to avoid irreversible mutations generated by replication of damaged DNA. In cases of extensive damage, p53 induces apoptosis to eliminate the affected cell by caspase activation. Such a pathway has been termed as 'cellular proofreading' because it aborts the aberrant cell rather than restoring its genome. Most of the key regulators of the cell cycle and apoptosis, such as p53, are mutated in various combinations in human cancers. Dysregulation of cell cycle and apoptotic mechanisms leads to a further increase in mutation rates and genomic instability.[35] Tumor progression is accompanied by escape of the cancer cell from immunological surveillance and by acquisition of additional properties favorable for tumor growth and invasion such as increased angiogenesis.[36] An in-depth discussion of the biochemistry behind cancerogenesis can be found in Chapter 1.

The occurrence of germinal (inherited) mutations associated with skin cancer propensity has helped understanding some of the molecular events involved in the development of BCC, SCC and melanoma. Loss-of-function germline mutations of PTCH1, the human homolog to the Drosophila patched gene, are present in patients with the basal cell nevus syndrome (BCNS).[37] The PTCH1 gene encodes a transmembrane protein that represses the signaling activity of the membrane-bound proto-oncogene smoothed (SMOH). In the presence of hedgehog proteins (HH), the inhibitory effect of PTCH on SMOH is relieved. Usually, BCNS patients inherit one mutated copy of PTCH1 and inactivation of the other copy is required for tumor development. Mutations of PTCH1 and activating mutation of the gene SMOH have been detected in variable proportions of sporadic BCC.[38] Next to the mutation of the HH pathway, the most common genetic change in BCC is found in the p53 gene, which may correlate with increase of tumor growth and aggressive course.[39] Early molecular events in the development of SCC include mutations of p53, mainly represented by UV signature mutations. Normally, damage to DNA in epidermal cells due to UV light exposure and leading to formation of pyrimidine dimers, is repaired by a process entailing nucleotide excision. Patients with xeroderma pigmentosum (XP), an autosomal recessive disorder associated with defects in the DNA repair mechanisms, are at a remarkably increased risk of skin cancer, especially SCC. Moreover, some DNA repair polymorphisms have been associated with SCC in epidemiologic studies.[40] Susceptibility genes for the development of melanoma have been identified by studying families with a high incidence of the tumor. These genes were represented by CDKN2A encoding the cyclin-dependent kinase inhibitor p16[INK4a] and the tumor suppressor p14[ARF], and genes CDK4 and CDK6 encoding cyclin-dependent kinases 4 and 6.[41] Variants of melanocortin-1 receptor (MC1R) are also associated with an increased risk of melanoma.[42] A role for p53 in inducing pro-opiomelanocortin (POMC) gene activation and transient pigmentation has been recently documented together with an association of the p53 Pro/Pro genotype with melanoma risk.[43] Distinct sets of genetic alterations suggesting distinct pathways in tumor development have been documented in melanoma lesions from different body areas.[44]

## Constitutional variables: gender, age, skin phenotype

SCC and BCC are substantially more common in males. There is also a slight male predominance for melanoma. Reasons for these gender differences have been explored in animals models but are still poorly understood.[45]

Incidence rates of melanoma and NMSC rise steadily with age, at least up to 80 years. A simple dose-duration effect of carcinogenic exposures may play a role. However, aging-related processes are also likely to be involved.

Senescent fibroblasts can stimulate the growth and tumorigenic transformation of premalignant epithelial cells in culture and in vivo.[46]

Variations in skin, eye and hair color have been consistently linked to the risk of skin cancer, with lighter phenotypes being at higher risk. Light skin complexion (especially light skin and blond-red hair), freckling, and tendency to burn, not tan, after sun exposure, are constitutional variables related to UV sensitivity which affect the risk of SCC, BCC and melanoma.[47,48] People from Southern European ethnic origin are at a significantly lower risk than those from English, Celtic and Scandinavian origin. Those who migrate early in their life from such regions to lower latitudes increase their exposure levels to sunlight and show a higher risk of developing skin cancer.[49]

Inability to tan also portends an increased risk. Melanin contained in melanosomes is the key contributor to pigmentation. There are two main types of melanin: red/yellow pheomelanin and brown/black eumelanin. Pigmentation differences can arise from variation in the number, size, composition and distribution of melanosomes, whereas melanocyte numbers typically remain relatively constant. Despite the identification of more than 100 loci involved in vertebrate pigmentation, the MC1R is consistently a major determinant of pigment phenotype (see Chapter 30 for genetic clinical considerations). Agonists of human MC1R include α-melanocyte-stimulating hormone (α-MSH) and adrenocorticotropic hormone (ACTH), and these cause an increase in eumelanin production through elevated cAMP levels. The human MC1R coding region is highly polymorphic, with at least 30 allelic variants, most of which result in a single amino-acid substitution. Certain substitutions, such as R151C, R160W and D294H, are associated with red hair. The 'red-head' phenotype is defined not only by hair colour but also by fair skin, inability to tan, a propensity to freckle, and high levels of pheomelanin.[50]

Pro-opiomelanocortin (POMC) is the precursor for both α-MSH and ACTH, as well as for other bioactive peptides, including β-endorphin. Although originally identified in the pituitary gland, POMC production is now known to occur in skin as well, and α-MSH is secreted by both keratinocytes and melanocytes. In humans, mutations in POMC result in a red-haired phenotype (like that of MC1R alleles), as well as metabolic abnormalities such as adrenal insufficiency and obesity.[50] There is evidence that DNA damage in itself might be important to the triggering of pigment production, the molecular mechanism being possibly linked to p53 activation.[51]

## Viruses

Human papillomaviruses (HPV) are small epitheliotropic DNA viruses, comprising more than 100 different types (Fig. 6.6). Although the carcinogenetic role of high-risk mucosal HPV in cervical cancer is well established, the evidence for the involvement of beta-HPVs in skin carcinogenesis is less straightforward.[52] The association of beta-HPV and SCC first originated from patients with epidermodysplasia verruciformis (EV), a rare autosomal recessive genetic disease, characterized by abnormal susceptibility to widespread beta-HPV infections of the skin, pityriasis

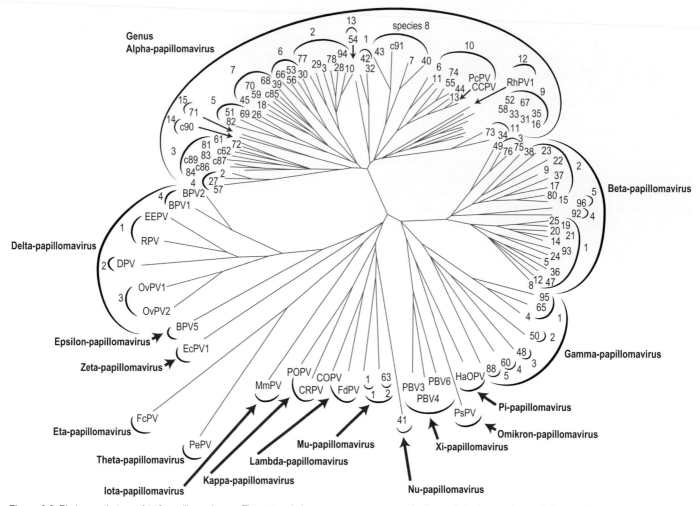

**Figure 6.6** Phylogenetic tree of 118 papillomaviruses. The outer circle encompasses genera, the inner circle the species, and the numbers at the ends of the branches identify type. C-numbers refer to candidate HPV types (from De Villiers 2004).[53]

versicolor-like lesions, and development of numerous SCCs on sun-exposed areas. At variance with alpha-HPV in cervical cancer, beta-HPVs occur in episomal rather than integrated forms, and encode E6 proteins which are unable to target *p53* for ubiquitin-mediated degradation. Beta-HPVs are very common in most people, the reservoir probably being within epidermal stem cells of the hair bulge, and they can persist long term. While the infection in immune-competent people remains subclinical, organ transplant recipients (OTRs) often develop extensive warts and hyperkeratotic lesions linked to beta-HPV infection. The number of these keratotic skin lesions is a strong indicator of the risk of skin cancer in OTRs.[54] HPV might act as a co-factor together with UV exposure in tumor initiation.

Other viruses play important roles in skin carcinogenesis. Human herpesvirus 8 (HHV8) is a double-stranded DNA gamma herpesvirus which has been consistently associated with all the varieties of Kaposi sarcoma (KS). HHV8 reactivation is probably mandatory at early phases of HHV8-associated proliferation. HHV8 v-cyclin is expressed in most KS spindle cells and probably drives cells to uncontrolled progression from the G1 to S phase of the cell cycle. The latent nuclear antigen (LANA), which binds viral DNA to host chromatin during cell mitosis, is also involved

in the cell cycle and binds *p53*, blocking p53-mediated apoptosis.[55]

Polyomaviruses are a growing family of small DNA viruses. Recently, a novel polyomavirus, Merkel cell polyomavirus (MCPyV), was discovered and isolated in approximately 75% of MCCs.[56]

## Immunosuppression and iatrogenic factors

An excess risk of skin cancer is documented in several conditions associated with immunosuppression. Loss of immune competence facilitates the frequency and persistence of viral infection causal to the development of some tumors, and may reduce eradication of precancerous lesions. In OTRs, there is a disproportionate increase in the incidence of NMSC, post-transplant lymphoma/lymphoproliferative disorders (PTLD), anogenital dysplasia, and Kaposi sarcoma.[57,58] The relative importance of each individual cancer depends on the ethnic group considered, on geographic location, and on age at transplantation. In Caucasians, NMSC is the main cancer in adults and in renal-transplanted children. NMSC in OTRs is mainly SCC, which frequently occurs as multiple tumors, with a reversal of the BCC to SCC ratio of approximately 3:1 seen in the general population. Age at transplantation, gender (male) and duration of transplantation are all established risk factors. UV light exposure, skin phenotype, and number of HPV-related keratotic lesions also affect the risk. The immunosuppressive load is probably an important variable; however, there is no satisfactory method to quantify it. Besides NMSC, an increased risk for melanoma, MCC, and other rarer skin cancers have been documented in OTRs.

The weakened cellular immune system of HIV-infected patients resembles in some ways the iatrogenic immunosuppression in solid-organ transplant recipients. Apart from Kaposi sarcoma, non-Hodgkin lymphoma, and cervical cancer, which are considered as AIDS-defining, several additional cancers, referred to as 'non-AIDS-defining cancers', including NMSC and MCC, are also statistically increased in HIV-infected persons.[58,59] People treated for cancer when younger than 21 years have a three- to sixfold increased risk of developing second malignancies, including NMSC and melanoma, compared to the general population.[60] Radiotherapy is usually considered as a risk factor in these patients; however, concomitant use of cytotoxic agents such as alkylating agents may contribute. Interestingly, children treated for hematological malignancies develop an increased number of melanocytic nevi compared to untreated control groups irrespective of the radiotherapy they receive.[61] Some cancers in adults, e.g. chronic myeloid leukemia (CML) and chronic lymphocytic leukemia (CLL), and selected chemotherapeutic agents, such as fludarabine, nitrogen mustards, and hydroxyurea, are also associated with increased risk of NMSC.

Some immune-related inflammatory conditions, such as systemic lupus erythematosus (SLE), rheumatoid arthritis (RA), and sarcoidosis, have been associated with increased risk of cancer, including NMSC. Reasons for these associations are unclear and may involve multiple factors such as treatment modalities and increased surveillance and detection rates. Ciclosporin used alone for conditions other than organ transplantation, e.g. psoriasis, is associated with increased risk of NMSC.[62] A few studies found increased risk for BCC, SCC and melanoma, among users of oral glucocorticoids for indications other than organ transplantation.[63] A meta-analysis of randomized clinical trials of RA patients treated with anti-tumor necrosis factor (anti-TNF) antibodies indicated a short-term threefold increase in the risk of malignancies, including skin cancer, in treated patients compared with placebo.[64] Longer-term cohort studies provide conflicting results on cancer risk in anti-TNF-treated patients.

## Chemicals and pollutants

Among the best-known skin carcinogens are polycyclic aromatic hydrocarbons (PAHs) contained in tars, mineral oils, and phorbol esters. In PAHs, substituted 3- and 4-ring polycyclic aromatic compounds probably induce cancers by causing DNA adducts.[65] Phorbol esters are the classic tumor promoters used in the development of the multistage model for murine skin cancer; their activity as promoters is linked to dysregulation of protein kinase C.

So-called 'heavy metals' are frequently encountered pollutants. Among them, arsenic is a well-recognized skin carcinogen. Long-term exposure to inorganic arsenic from drinking water has been documented to induce cancers in lung, bladder, kidney, liver and skin (mainly Bowen's disease) in a dose–response relationship. Arsenic may act as a skin carcinogen by enhancing the effects of UV radiation. In-vitro studies have demonstrated that arsenic inhibits the ligation and incision steps of nucleotide excision repair, even at low concentrations. Polymorphisms in nuclear excision repair genes may modify the association between NMSC and arsenic.[66] Other chemical carcinogens are listed in Table 6.2.

## Smoking

Cigarette smoke is a cocktail of over 4000 chemicals, classified operationally as 'particulate' and 'vapour' phases. PAHs, nicotine and phenol are examples of components of the particulate phase, while carbon monoxide is the main component of the vapour phase. Smoking and other types of tobacco use are clearly associated with SCC of the lip. The association with SCC at other cutaneous sites is less firmly established.[67]

## Table 6.2 Chemical Agents Associated with Skin Cancer

| Substance | Exposure Route | Activities at Risk |
|---|---|---|
| Polycyclic aromatic hydrocarbons | Topical, systemic | Timber proofing (creosote oil), brick and pottery production, aluminum production, coal gasification, coke production, iron and steel foundries, tar distillation, shale oil extraction, wood impregnation, roofing, road paving, carbon black production, carbon electrode production, chimney sweeping, calcium carbide production, transport industry |
| Mineral oils | Topical | Mule spinner's disease represents the occurrence of scrotal cancer in cotton textile workers exposed to mineral oils on a long-term basis while working on a machine called 'the mule'. |
| Hexachlorobenzene | Systemic | It has been banned in several countries |
| Polychlorinated biphenyls (PCBs) | Topical, systemic | They have been banned in several countries |
| Arsenic | Topical, systemic | Drinking water in some regions, pesticides, mining activities, combustion of fuel oil |

## Diet and nutrients

The relationship between skin cancer and diet has been investigated in a limited number of studies. A high intake of n-3 fatty acids was associated with a lower risk of SCC in a case–control study.[68] The incidence of SCC was not influenced by beta-carotene supplementation in a large-scale interventional study.[69] A number of studies indicate that increased body mass index (BMI), which may be influenced by caloric intake, is associated with an increased risk of cutaneous melanoma, and a lower caloric intake during development has been associated with a decrease in the future incidence of malignancy in some animal models.[70]

The role of vitamin D in relation to skin cancer prevention has been the focus of substantial debate in recent years (see Chapter 60). A meta-analysis has suggested a possible significant role of VDR *FokI* and *BsmI* polymorphisms in cutaneous melanoma and NMSC risk.[71] It should be noted that cutaneous synthesis of vitamin D is self-limited and in light-skinned people it fades away after 5 to 10 minutes of sun exposure. Longer durations will not further increase vitamin D, but will increase skin cancer risk.

## Chronic inflammation and wounds

A variety of chronic inflammatory disorders, such as lichen sclerosus et atrophicus and cutaneous tuberculosis, are associated with increased risk of developing skin cancer. Inflammatory conditions may facilitate cancer development through induction of genetic instability leading to accumulation of random genetic alterations.[72] Long-term thermal stress may be responsible for the development of SCC, as documented by the association between SCC and erythema ab igne (Fig. 6.7). In spite of a long-lasting belief and several case reports, recent cohort studies failed to document any association between burn scars and skin cancer. Improvement in burn care in the last decades leaving limited scar sequelae may explain these negative findings.[73]

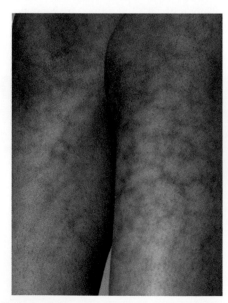

**Figure 6.7** Erythema ab igne, a pruritic, non-blanching discoloration which results from long-lasting exposure to heating sources such as heating pads.

## Previous history of skin cancer as a risk factor

Once a person has developed a first NMSC there is a significantly increased risk of developing subsequent primary NMSC and selected other cancers, including melanoma, non-Hodgkin lymphoma, and cancer of the salivary glands.[74] The reasons for these increased risks may involve both genetic background and shared environmental factors. The concept of 'field cancerization' has been proposed to explain the development of clusters of multiple primary cancers of epithelial origin, in limited areas.[75]

## FUTURE OUTLOOK

Complexity and synergy underlie the etiological factors that are related to the development of skin cancer. In the not-distant future, genome-wide association studies, analyses of genetic–environmental interactions, and profiling of gene expression by microarray technologies, will probably help in elucidating pathomechanisms.

## REFERENCES

1. El Ghissassi F, Baan R, Straif K, et al. A review of human carcinogens. Part D: radiation. *Lancet Oncol.* 2009;10:751–752.
2. Fahey DW. *Twenty Questions and Answers About the Ozone Layer: 2006 Update. Geneva.* Switzerland: World Meteorological Organization; 2007.
3. World Health Organization. *Global Solar UV Index: A Practical Guide. Geneva.* Switzerland: WHO; 2002.
4. Rigel DS, Rigel EG, Rigel AC. Effects of altitude and latitude on ambient UVB radiation. *J Acad Dermatol.* 1999;40(1):114–116.
5. Newman PA, Oman LD, Douglass AR, et al. What would have happened to the ozone layer if chlorofluorocarbons (CFCs) had not been regulated? *Atmos Chem Phys.* 2009;9:2113–2128.
6. Alonso FT, Garmendia ML, Bogado ME. Increased skin cancer mortality in Chile beyond the effect of ageing: temporal analysis 1990 to 2005. *Acta Derm Venereol.* 2010;90(2):141–146.
7. Diffey B. Climate change, ozone depletion and the impact of ultraviolet exposure of human skin. *Phys Med Biol.* 2004;49(1):R1–R11.
8. National Institutes of Health, U.S. Department of Health and Human Services. *Cancer trends progress report – 2007 update.* < http://progressreport.cancer.gov >. Accessed 21.09.09.
9. De Fabo EC. Initial studies on an in vivo action spectrum for melanoma induction. *Prog Biophys Mol Biol.* 2006;92:97–104.
10. Beissert S, Loser K. Molecular and cellular mechanisms of photocarcinogenesis. *Photochem Photobiol.* 2008;84:29–34.
11. Ziegler A, Jonason AS, Leffell DJ, et al. Sunburn and p53 in the onset of skin cancer. *Nature.* 1994;372:773–776.
12. Reifenberger J, Wolter M, Knobbe CB, et al. Somatic mutations in the PTCH, SMOH, SUFUH and TP53 genes in sporadic basal cell carcinomas. *Br J Dermatol.* 2005;152:43–51.
13. Mouret S, Baudouin C, Charveron M, et al. Cyclobutane pyrimidine dimers are predominant DNA lesions in whole human skin exposed to UVA radiation. *Proc Natl Acad Sci U S A.* 2006;103:13765–13770.
14. Pieternel CM, Pasker-de-Jong M, Wielink G, et al. Treatment with UV-B for psoriasis and nonmelanoma skin cancer. A systematic review of the literature. *Arch Dermatol.* 1999;135:834–840.
15. Stern RS, Nichols KT, Vakeva LH. Malignant melanoma in patients treated for psoriasis with methoxsalen (psoralen) and ultraviolet A radiation (PUVA). The PUVA Follow-Up Study. *N Engl J Med.* 1997;336:1041–1045.
16. Karagas MR, Stannard VA, Mott LA, et al. Use of tanning devices and risk of basal cell and squamous cell skin cancers. *J Natl Cancer Inst.* 2002;94:224–226.
17. Clough-Gorr KM, Titus-Ernstoff L, Perry AE, et al. Exposure to sunlamps, tanning beds, and melanoma risk. *Cancer Causes Control.* 2008;19:659–669.
18. Rosso S, Zanetti R, Martinez C, et al. The multicentre south European study 'Helios'. II: Different sun exposure patterns in the aetiology of basal cell and squamous cell carcinomas of the skin. *Br J Cancer.* 1996;73:1447–1454.
19. Gallagher RP, Hill GB, Bajdik CD, et al. Sunlight exposure, pigmentation factors, and risk of nonmelanocytic skin cancer. II. Squamous cell carcinoma. *Arch Dermatol.* 1995;131:164–169.

20. Vitasa BC, Taylor HR, Strickland PT, et al. Association of nonmelanoma skin cancer and actinic keratosis with cumulative solar ultraviolet exposure in Maryland watermen. *Cancer.* 1990;65:2811–2817.

21. Harvey I, Frankel S, Marks R, et al. Non-melanoma skin cancer and solar keratoses. II Analytical results of the South Wales Skin Cancer Study. *Br J Cancer.* 1996;74:1308–1312.

22. Gallagher RP, Hill GB, Bajdik CD, et al. Sunlight exposure, pigmentary factors, and risk of nonmelanocytic skin cancer. I. Basal cell carcinoma. *Arch Dermatol.* 1995;131:157–163.

23. Gandini S, Sera F, Cattaruzza MS, et al. Meta-analysis of risk factors for cutaneous melanoma: II. Sun exposure. *Eur J Cancer.* 2005;41:28–44.

24. Bastiaens MT, Hoefnagel JJ, Bruijn JA, et al. Differences in age, site distribution, and sex between nodular and superficial basal cell carcinoma indicate different types of tumors. *J Invest Dermatol.* 1998;110:880–884.

25. Lovatt TJ, Lear JT, Bastrilles J, et al. Associations between ultraviolet radiation, basal cell carcinoma site and histology, host characteristics, and rate of development of further tumors. *J Am Acad Dermatol.* 2005;52:468–473.

26. Siskind V, Whiteman DC, Aitken JF, et al. An analysis of risk factors for cutaneous melanoma by anatomical site (Australia). *Cancer Causes Control.* 2005;16:193–199.

27. Gandini S, Sera F, Cattaruzza MS, et al. Meta-analysis of risk factors for cutaneous melanoma: I. Common and atypical naevi. *Eur J Cancer.* 2005;41:28–44.

28. English DR, Armstrong BK. Melanocytic nevi in children. I. Anatomic sites and demographic and host factors. *Am J Epidemiol.* 1994;139:390–401.

29. Carli P, Naldi L, Lovati S, et al, Oncology Cooperative Group of the Italian Group for Epidemiologic Research in Dermatology (GISED). The density of melanocytic nevi correlates with constitutional variables and history of sunburns: a prevalence study among Italian schoolchildren. *Int J Cancer.* 2002;101:375–379.

30. Miller RW, Rabkin CS. Merkel cell carcinoma and melanoma: etiological similarities and differences. *Cancer Epidemiol Biomarkers Prev.* 1999;8:153–158.

31. Mancuso M, Pasquali E, Leonardi S, et al. Oncogenic bystander radiation effects in Patched heterozygous mouse cerebellum. *Proc Natl Acad Sci U S A.* 2008;105:12445–12450.

32. Karagas MR, McDonald JA, Greenberg ER, et al. Risk of basal cell and squamous cell skin cancers after ionizing radiation therapy. For The Skin Cancer Prevention Study Group. *J Natl Cancer Inst.* 1996;88:1848–1853.

33. Karagas MR, Nelson HH, Zens MS, et al. Squamous cell and basal cell carcinoma of the skin in relation to radiation therapy and potential modification of risk by sun exposure. *Epidemiology.* 2007;18:776–784.

34. Freedman DM, Sigurdson A, Rao RS, et al. Risk of melanoma among radiologic technologists in the United States. *Int J Cancer.* 2003;103:556–562.

35. Loeb LA, Bielas JH, Beckman RA. Cancers exhibit a mutator phenotype: clinical implications. *Cancer Res.* 2008;68:3551–3557.

36. Hanahan D, Weinberg RA. The hallmarks of cancer. *Cell.* 2000;100:57–70.

37. Hahn H, Wicking C, Zaphiropoulous PG, et al. Mutations of the human homolog of Drosophila patched in the nevoid basal cell carcinoma syndrome. *Cell.* 1996;85:841–851.

38. Xie J, Murone M, Luoh SM, et al. Activating Smoothened mutations in sporadic basal-cell carcinoma. *Nature.* 1998;391:90–92.

39. Bolshakov S, Walker CM, Strom SS, et al. p53 mutations in human aggressive and nonaggressive basal and squamous cell carcinomas. *Clin Cancer Res.* 2003;9:228–234.

40. Han J, Hankinson SE, Colditz GA, et al. Genetic variation in XRCC1, sun exposure, and risk of skin cancer. *Br J Cancer.* 2004;91:1604–1609.

41. Meyle KD, Guldberg P. Genetic risk factors for melanoma. *Hum Genet.* 2009;126:499–510.

42. Scherer D, Nagore E, Bermejo JL, et al. Melanocortin receptor 1 variants and melanoma risk: a study of 2 European populations. *Int J Cancer.* 2009;125:1868–1875.

43. Nan H, Qureshi AA, Hunter DJ, et al. Interaction between p53 codon 72 polymorphism and melanocortin 1 receptor variants on suntan response and cutaneous melanoma risk. *Br J Dermatol.* 2008;159:314–321.

44. Curtin JA, Fridlyand J, Kageshita T, et al. Distinct sets of genetic alterations in melanoma. *N Engl J Med.* 2005;353:2135–2147.

45. Mancuso M, Gallo D, Leonardi S, et al. Modulation of basal and squamous cell carcinoma by endogenous estrogen in mouse models of skin cancer. *Carcinogenesis.* 2009;30:340–347.

46. Finkel T, Serrano M, Blasco MA. The common biology of cancer and ageing. *Nature.* 2007;448:767–774.

47. Gandini S, Sera F, Cattaruzza MS, et al. Meta-analysis of risk factors for cutaneous melanoma: III. Family history, actinic damage and phenotypic factors. *Eur J Cancer.* 2005;41:2040–2059.

48. Zanetti R, Rosso S, Martinez C, et al. The multicentre south European study 'Helios'. I: Skin characteristics and sunburns in basal cell and squamous cell carcinomas of the skin. *Br J Cancer.* 1996;73(11):1440–1446.

49. Whiteman DC, Green AC. Melanoma and sun exposure: where are we now? *Int J Dermatol.* 1999;38:481–489.

50. Lin JY, Fisher DE. Melanocyte biology and skin pigmentation. *Nature.* 2007;445:843–850.

51. Cui R, Widlund HR, Feige E, et al. Central role of p53 in the suntan response and pathologic hyperpigmentation. *Cell.* 2007;128:853–864.

52. Pfister H. Human papillomavirus and skin cancer. *J Natl Cancer Inst Monogr.* 2003;31:52–56.

53. De Villiers EM, Fauquet C, Broker TR, et al. Classification of papillomaviruses. *Virology.* 2004;324:17–27.

54. Bouwes Bavinck JN, De Boer A, Vermeer BJ, et al. Sunlight, keratotic skin lesions and skin cancer in renal transplant recipients. *Br J Dermatol.* 1993;129:242–249.

55. Jarviluoma A, Ojala PM. Cell signaling pathways engaged by KSHV. *Biochim Biophys Acta.* 2006;1766:140–158.

56. Feng H, Shuda M, Chang Y, et al. Clonal integration of a polyomavirus in human Merkel cell carcinoma. *Science.* 2008;319:1096–1100.

57. Proby CM, Wisgerhof HC, Casabonne D, et al. The epidemiology of transplant-associated keratinocyte cancers in different geographical regions. *Cancer Treat Res.* 2009;146:75–95.

58. Lanoy E, Costagliola D, Engels EA. Skin cancers associated with HIV infection and solid organ transplant among elderly adults. *Int J Cancer.* 2010;126(7):1724–1731.

59. Stebbing J, Duru O, Bower M. Non-AIDS-defining cancers. *Curr Opin Infect Dis.* 2009;22:7–10.

60. Meadows AT, Friedman DL, Neglia JP. Second neoplasms in survivors of childhood cancer: findings from the Childhood Cancer Survivor Study cohort. *J Clin Oncol.* 2009;27:2356–2362.

61. Naldi L, Adamoli L, Fraschini D, et al. Number and distribution of melanocytic nevi in individuals with a history of childhood leukemia. *Cancer.* 1996;77:1402–1408.

62. Paul CF, Ho VC, McGeown C, et al. Risk of malignancies in psoriasis patients treated with cyclosporine: a 5 y cohort study. *J Invest Dermatol.* 2003;120:211–216.

63. Jensen AØ, Thomsen HF, Engebjerg MC, et al. Use of oral glucocorticoids and risk of skin cancer and non-Hodgkin's lymphoma: a population-based case-control study. *Br J Cancer.* 2009;100:200–205.

64. Bongartz T, Sutton AJ, Sweeting MJ, et al. Anti-TNF antibody therapy in rheumatoid arthritis and the risk of serious infections and malignancies: systematic review and meta-analysis of rare harmful effects in randomized controlled trials. *JAMA.* 2006;295:2275–2285.

65. Baudouin C, Charveron M, Tarroux R, et al. Environmental pollutants and skin cancer. *Cell Biol Toxicol.* 2002;18:341–348.

66. Applebaum KM, Karagas MR, Hunter DJ, et al. Polymorphisms in nucleotide excision repair genes, arsenic exposure, and non-melanoma skin cancer in New Hampshire. *Environ Health Perspect.* 2007;115:1231–1236.

67. De Hertog SA, Wensveen CA, Bastiaens MT, et al. Relation between smoking and skin cancer. *J Clin Oncol.* 2001;19:231–238.

68. Hakim IA, Harris RB, Ritenbaugh C. Fat intake and risk of squamous cell carcinoma of the skin. *Nutr Cancer.* 2000;36:155–162.

69. Green A, Williams G, Neale R, et al. Daily sunscreen application and beta-carotene supplementation in prevention of basal-cell and squamous-cell carcinomas of the skin: a randomised controlled trial. *Lancet.* 1999;354:723–729.

70. Renehan AG, Tyson M, Egger M, et al. Body-mass index and incidence of cancer: a systematic review and meta-analysis of prospective observational studies. *Lancet.* 2008;371:569–578.

71. Köstner K, Denzer N, Müller CS, et al. The relevance of vitamin D receptor (VDR) gene polymorphisms for cancer: a review of the literature. *Anticancer Res.* 2009;29:3511–3536.

72. Colotta F, Allavena P, Sica A, et al. Cancer-related inflammation, the seventh hallmark of cancer: links to genetic instability. *Carcinogenesis.* 2009;30:1073–1081.

73. Lindelöf B, Krynitz B, Granath F, et al. Burn injuries and skin cancer: a population-based cohort study. *Acta Derm Venereol.* 2008;88:20–22.

74. Marcil I, Stern RS. Risk of developing a subsequent nonmelanoma skin cancer in patients with a history of nonmelanoma skin cancer: a critical review of the literature and meta-analysis. *Arch Dermatol.* 2000;136:1524–1530.

75. Braakhuis BJ, Tabor MP, Kummer JA, et al. A genetic explanation of Slaughter's concept of field cancerization: evidence and clinical implications. *Cancer Res.* 2003;63:1727–1730.

CHAPTER
7

# The Importance of Primary and Secondary Prevention Programs for Skin Cancer

*June K. Robinson*

## Key Points

- As the US population of adults 65 and older increases, the number of people developing and dying from new skin cancers will rise.

- Skin self-examination (SSE) with the assistance of a partner may achieve some reduction in the estimated 8400 deaths from cutaneous melanoma (CM) and reduce the physical and emotional burden of non-melanoma skin cancer (NMSC) and CM.

- Technologic advances, such as computer-assisted screening of the high-risk population, improve physician detection of early melanoma.

- The role of parents in adolescent health and disease prevention is very influential. Parents may reframe the sun protection health promotion message with their children to, 'Daily sun protection now means fewer or no painful burns. Tanning now means loss of the skin's health and beauty; you may get wrinkles in your 20s.'

## INTRODUCTION

Skin cancer, the most common malignancy in the United States (US), is an important public health concern with an incidence rate that will continue to increase as the US population of adults 65 and older increases. The incidence of invasive cutaneous melanoma (CM) has nearly tripled in the US between 1975 and 2004,[1] making melanoma the sixth most common cancer in men and women in the US, with more than 68,000 cases of invasive melanoma diagnosed and almost 8700 deaths in 2010.[2] Primary prevention programs are related to encouraging behavioral changes to lower subsequent skin cancer risk. Secondary prevention efforts focus on enhancing early detection of skin cancer. Primary prevention influences incidence while secondary prevention impacts on morbidity and mortality. While secondary prevention with early detection is an effective strategy for those who sustained unprotected sun exposure in youth, primary prevention by effective sun protection throughout life for those at risk to develop skin cancer may reduce the development of skin cancer over a lifetime.

## HISTORY

The relevance of effective primary and secondary skin cancer prevention programs is becoming increasingly important as the numbers of these cancers continue to rise. Although melanoma is less common than basal cell carcinoma (BCC) and squamous cell carcinoma (SCC), the much higher mortality of melanoma makes it a major concern as the incidence continues to increase globally by 3–7% annually.[3] Melanoma age-adjusted incidence rates have increased by 4.1% per year since 1981. The increasing incidence of melanoma is also associated with an increased mortality in both the US and Europe. Mortality rates in the US have continued to increase from 1985 to 2004. In 2010, in the US 8700 people died of melanoma when the disease progressed to stage IV with organ metastases. In 2000, 8300 European men died out of the approximately 26,100 diagnosed with melanoma and, of 33,000 European women diagnosed with melanoma, 7600 died.[4]

In the US, non-melanoma skin cancer (NMSC) is the most common malignant neoplasm in the Caucasian population.[5] The incidence of NMSC is 18–20 times greater than melanoma and is increasing.[6] Since NMSCs are usually treated in outpatient settings and are not reported to cancer registries, exact US incidence rates are not available. The crude prevalence of NMSC in the US is roughly 450 cases per 100,000 individuals.[7] An estimated 2300 people in the US will die annually from NMSC, primarily due to metastatic cutaneous SCC. While NMSC is likely to claim fewer lives than melanoma, considerable morbidity results from treatment. Since many NMSCs arise on the frequently sun-exposed areas of the head and neck, surgical resection may result in significant disfigurement with impaired quality of life and social interaction.

## TARGETING PREVENTION EFFORTS

### Personal risk factors

For prevention programs to have the greatest impact, a focus on those at greater risk must be achieved. Older age is associated with higher risk of developing NMSC. There is a rapid rise in incidence after age 40, with SCC increasing more rapidly than BCC. While the incidence for men and women are similar at early ages, after age 45, men develop NMSC two to three times more frequently than women.

In the Surveillance, Epidemiology and End Results (SEER) program, 75% of the thicker melanomas with poor prognosis were in patients older than 50. Scalp/neck melanoma represented 6% of melanoma from 1992 to 2003, but 10% of deaths from melanoma.[8] It is expected that the US population of adults 65 and older will increase as much as 20% between 2010 and 2030; therefore, the number of people with skin cancer and the number of deaths it causes can be expected to continue to rise.

Skin cancer is more common in people with immunosuppressive diseases or with diseases that are controlled by chronic immunosuppressive therapy, e.g. survivors of non-Hodgkin lymphoma, organ transplant patients, and those with rheumatoid arthritis. Among transplant recipients, the incidence of SCC is markedly increased in those with sun-sensitive skin, a history of sun exposure, and clinical signs of photoaging. NMSCs usually appear 3 to 7 years after the onset of chronic immunosuppressive therapy. Renal transplant patients with a functioning graft for more than 5 years have a relative risk of 6.5 of developing NMSC, which increases to 20 after more than 15 years.[9] There is a 75% increased risk of CM among non-Hodgkin lymphoma survivors, and a two- to fourfold higher incidence in organ transplant recipients undergoing immunosuppressive regimens.

The considerable variability in genetic susceptibility to developing skin cancer is attributed to the melanin content of skin and the skin's ability to tan in response to ultraviolet radiation (UVR) exposure. Pale complexion, freckling, inability to tan, past severe sunburns and cumulative sun exposure, light eye color, northern European or Celtic heritage, and red or blonde hair are strong predictors of developing NMSC, and all are related to the melanin content of the individual's epidermal cells. A family history or personal history of melanoma or NMSC is associated with an increased risk of developing other skin cancers. While families with multiple affected members account for about 10% of melanoma cases, the relative contributions of genetic and shared environmental risk factors are unknown.

The familial tendency to develop NMSC is probably related to the gene *MC1R* (melanocortin-1 receptor), leading to red hair and sun sensitivity. For example, *MC1R* may identify people of color with a darker skin type that are at increased risk for melanoma.[10] The rates of NMSC for non-Hispanic whites were approximately 11 times greater than for Hispanics, who do not share the same phenotype. NMSCs in Caucasians have a log-linear increasing incidence with age, which may be due to cumulative environmental UVR exposure (Fig. 7.1).

## Environmental risk factors

When occupational and recreational patterns of ultraviolet light (UVL) exposure place those with genetic susceptibility in harm's way, NMSCs occur. There is a clear latitudinal gradient in incidence of NMSC. NMSCs occur more frequently in residents of areas with high solar radiation such as Australia, than in areas of low solar radiation like parts of the US. While the incidence of BCC in the US is approximately 146 per 100,000 people, the incidence is 788 cases per 100,000 people in Australia, where the average amount of sun exposure is much greater than in other parts of the world.[11] Over the past 10–30 years, the age-adjusted incidence of cutaneous SCC has increased by 50% to 200% due to increasing long-term overexposure to UVL.[12,13] SCCs occur on sun-exposed body locations with maximum exposure, such as the head and neck, and in outdoor workers more commonly than in indoor workers.

CM and BCC have a more complex relationship with sun exposure and appear to be associated with a history of sunburns, particularly in childhood. Migration studies show a higher rate of CM in those who migrate to a sunnier climate than those who remain in their own country, particularly if migration occurs in childhood. The risk of CM is higher in indoor workers than in outdoor workers. CM is more common in body areas with intermittent light exposure. BCC has a similar distribution pattern in the trunk and lower limbs, i.e. areas not so frequently exposed.

Both NMSC and CM occur in people with actinic keratoses, sun-related precancerous lesions. Actinic keratoses can be considered a marker of past excessive sun exposure. The indoor or outdoor UVL exposure sustained by an adult in their youth places them at risk to develop melanoma and NMSC several decades later. For adults with a genetic predisposition to develop skin cancer who sustained unprotected sun exposure or deliberate tanning, death and disfigurement from surgical resection may be modified by secondary prevention.

## PRIMARY PREVENTION OF SKIN CANCER: PROTECTION FROM ULTRAVIOLET RADIATION

### Interventions to modify sun protection behaviors

Reduction of UV exposure and deterrence of intentional tanning through knowledge-based educational programs has been attempted with mixed success. High-risk youths are described relative to others in terms of demographic variables, personality variables, general attitudinal variables, and topic knowledge. Since individual attitudes and beliefs about sun-risk and sun-safe behaviors have a major influence on their intentional sunbathing and sunbathing consequences, research focusing on modifying attitudes was the next logical step.[14,15]

Mahler et al. used a randomized controlled protocol with 146 volunteer college students with a UV facial photograph of the participant's face and a brief videotape describing the causes and consequences of photoaging. The effects of the photoaging information/UV photographic intervention only, the intervention plus use of sunless tanning lotion, and a control condition were tested. The intervention resulted in significantly stronger sun protection intentions ($P<0.001$) and greater sun protection behaviors ($P<0.05$) relative to controls. Those using sunless tanning lotion tended to engage in greater sun protection behaviors than the group that received the intervention alone.[16] Olson et al. demonstrated that a brief educational intervention that emphasizes risk-to-appearance by viewing sun damage was effective among middle-school students.[17]

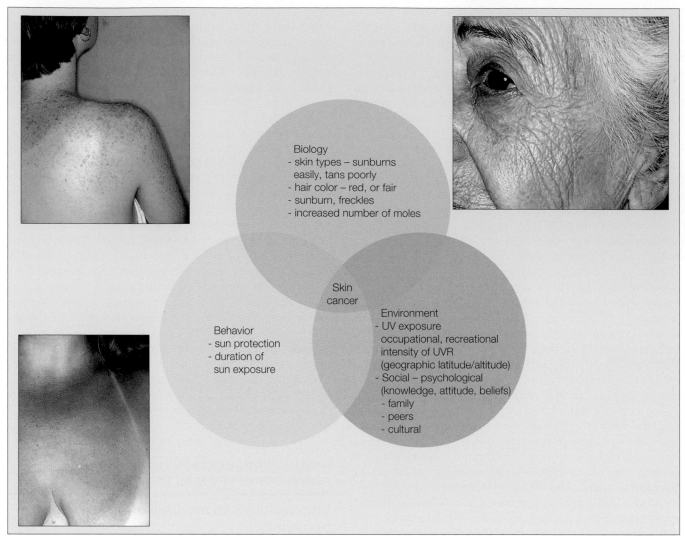

**Figure 7.1** The biologic inherited traits of the person (such as the adolescent girl with freckles over her back and shoulders) form the base upon which the individual's occupation, intensity of ultraviolet radiation in their geographic location, as well as their social and family normative beliefs regarding sun protection (such as the 90-year-old woman with a lifetime of sun protection having no freckles) are laid to establish their sun exposure behavioral patterns. After repetitive events of sunburns (young adult woman with sunburn of the chest) or chronic tanning over a period of years, skin cancer develops.

## School curriculum

Several interventions have in-depth school curricula and thorough methodology examining short-term, long-term and process-based effects.[18] With few minor exceptions, these studies report positive effects on attitudes and behavioral tendencies in their sample populations. Despite this, studies examining the quantity and frequency of youth sun-risk activities continue to report widespread rates of intentional sun exposure and low sun protection among young people. It is doubtful that the variables that are important predictors of tanning and other sun-risk behaviors will be amenable to change with short-term school-based interventions. Attitudes toward sunbathing, sun protection, appearance, and risk of UVL exposure paired with normative beliefs and the social reinforcement of tanning are critical variables predicting numerous sun-risk and sun-safe behavioral outcome variables.

## Parental role

From infancy until about age 8 to 9, young children have their sun protection provided by their parents. During this period, parents who have good communication patterns with their children may guide their children through initiating conversations about skin cancer and high-risk behaviors, and frame the sun protection health promotion message for their children. Parents serve as role models of sun protection for their children and may identify sports figures, musicians, and other media figures with untanned skin as role models for the children.

Young people often tend to discount health-related information, particularly when that information pertains to long-term consequences. This effect is further bolstered by the adolescent's tendency to view people who worry about such things as future skin cancer as too passive, careful, non-adventurous, and not cool. Young people also have a well-documented sense of personal invulnerability, and a tendency to misperceive true risk when it goes against the desired behavior (tanning). The message from parents can shift the emphasis from the long-term benefits of sun protection decreasing the chance of getting skin cancer to talking about using daily sun protection now to have fewer or no painful burns. For teen women, a message that tanning now means loss of the skin's health and beauty, and the chance of getting wrinkles in their 20s, is often effective. Enhanced sun protection in adolescence holds great potential to reduce the incidence of skin cancer.

## Tanning

Behaviors such as intentional tanning with indoor ultraviolet light (tanning lamps/salons) or sunlight, and inadequate sun protection (e.g. lack or misuse of sunscreen/block and protective clothing) by young individuals contribute to the increasing incidence of skin cancer. Despite laboratory, case–control, and prospective studies all pointing toward a positive relation between youthful indoor tanning (IT) and CM and SCC, approximately 10% of US adolescents under age 15 have used IT in the past year, with the prevalence among older adolescent females estimated at 25% to 40%.[19-21] Children begin IT as early as 9 years old, with the majority reporting their first exposure by high school (see Chapter 59).

Widespread IT among young people is clearly a potential health risk because there is an 8.1 odds ratio for developing malignant melanoma for individuals younger than 36 years old who regularly indoor tan versus those who never do. The majority of the case–control studies have documented some form of dose–response relationship. There is consistent evidence suggesting that the younger the age of exposure, the greater the risk for melanoma.

### Tanning attitudes and beliefs

The rank order of predictive factors for IT use is the belief that being tan improves appearance, social factors, perceived susceptibility to skin damage, and dependence on UVL exposure.[22] Tanning behavior almost always begins in childhood as an unintentional byproduct of outdoor activity. Although there is evidence that some children begin to tan intentionally at relatively young ages, it is more typically initiated during the early teens. By adolescence, the majority of young people report finding a tan attractive both in themselves and others. They also report the desire to be attractive as a critical variable in their decisions to tan. In theory, the perception that tanning is attractive occurs due to social learning and prior experience. In childhood, the child is socialized to view tanned skin as healthy-looking and untanned skin as unhealthy. By adolescence, this initial socialization is reinforced by the reactions of others. Their experience, in terms of others' comments and physical response to them, is that a tan is perceived as more desirable. This experience is further reinforced by the reaction that others within their peer group receive, as well as by the tanned image often portrayed by media role models.

Skin is a critical element of self-image.[23] Some of the IT variability comes from differences in the actual versus ideal self-image and social self-concept. Adolescents who define themselves as a 'tanned person', desire to be like a 'tanned person' or belong to social reference groups that define being tanned as part of group membership will be much more likely to tan. Generally, tanned individuals are perceived as athletic, outdoor-loving, adventurous, popular, assertive, confident, and having more sexually appealing bodies, while pale individuals are rated as non-athletic, passive, uncertain, and having less sexually appealing bodies. Adolescents perceive tanned skin as more attractive, perceive positive personal correlates of tanned skin, and frequently develop fantasies about what tanning will do for themselves socially, sexually, etc. Therefore, it is not surprising that the initiation of tanning behavior typically begins during this time.

For adolescents, tanning is associated with experiences at the beach, poolside, and tanning salon. All of these experiences are socially sanctioned environments where members of the opposite sex can mingle wearing minimal clothing. Most adolescents engage in tanning with their friends, at fun, socially arousing locations. Lying in the sun is also a relaxing, physically pleasurable activity for many people. For some people, UVL exposure has mood-enhancing effects. Thus, while people cognitively recognize that tanning is not the 'best' overall choice, they base their decision to tan on more affective, non-cognitive factors.

Our group (Drs. Hillhouse, Robinson, and Turrisi) took a different approach to modifying attitudes about IT by positive reinforcement of decision-making regarding enhancing the appearance of college women with alternatives to IT. The appearance-focused intervention demonstrated strong effects on IT behavior and intentions in young indoor tanners. Appearance-focused approaches to skin cancer prevention need to present alternative behaviors as well as alter IT attitudes.[22]

## SECONDARY PREVENTION OF SKIN CANCER: EARLY DETECTION

Early detection is achieved by enhanced surveillance by the person who is at risk and their physicians.

### Skin self-examination and partner-assisted skin examination

Skin self-examination (SSE) was first described in 1985 as a method to enhance early CM detection.[24] Since most melanomas are discovered by the patient or a partner, SSE with the assistance of a partner has the potential to improve long-term survival,[25-27] and could reduce mortality by as much as 64%.[28] Training in how to conduct SSE was significantly enhanced when delivered to patients with their partners relative to patients alone.[29] Body maps and total body baseline photographs of moles given to patients help them perform SSE more effectively.[30, 31] Demonstrating border irregularity and color variation of a person's moles can improve patients' confidence in their ability to perform SSE.[32]

Factors that can influence the performance of SSE include: 1) individual host factors such as gender, age, sun sensitivity, vision; 2) cognitive factors such as perception of risk, importance of skin cancer, and knowledge of the warning signs of skin cancer; 3) social factors such as peer group norms, social norms, and social interactions; and 4) environmental factors such as skin cancer health promotion messages delivered by the media. In those at risk of developing melanoma, the strongest predictors of SSE performance were attitude, having dermatology visits with skin biopsies and at least one skin cancer in the previous 3 years, and confidence in SSE performance.[33] Other predictors of SSE performance were younger age (40–59 years of age), being a woman, asking a partner for help, and physician recommendation to perform SSE.[34]

For SSE, the partner assists with checking the skin in locations that are difficult to see, e.g. back of scalp, back of legs or below the buttocks. Once skin examination is initiated, the partner provides social reinforcement. Fulfillment of expectations by finding a worrisome lesion also reinforces SSE. Skin examination by a partner may be limited by privacy concerns, availability of a partner, or relationship with the partner (Fig. 7.2).

Partners are encouraged to perform SSE more frequently (monthly on average) than screening by a physician, and to alert their physicians to a changing lesion. While there is general agreement about the need to check all skin surfaces of the body, there is little consensus about the frequency of SSE. Regular thorough self-examinations, preferably once a month, are recommended by the American Cancer Society.[35] Monthly SSEs are recommended with the intention of making the behavior a personal habit and to establish familiarity with the appearance of moles in order to be able to identify suspicious changes. The importance of changes of size, shape, symptoms, surface (especially bleeding) and shades of color was recently recognized by revising the criteria for the visual inspection of pigmented lesions to include evolving (E).[36] Change in the Asymmetry, Border irregularity, Color variation, and Diameter (A, B, C, D) is likely to occur

over a period of 6 months to 1 year.[37] The caveat is that for people whose melanoma progresses to the advanced stage of the disease (stage IV), there has been very little improvement in the survival rate over the last 20 years.

## Physician surveillance

### Aids for physician surveillance

The difficulty with performing melanoma surveillance is that although this cancer is relatively uncommon, the benign counterpart, the nevus, is extremely frequent in the population. Thus, many benign nevi are excised to detect melanoma early enough to prevent the consequences of metastatic disease. The aim of tools to assist physician surveillance is to maximize early detection of melanoma while minimizing the unnecessary excision of benign skin tumors.

The desire to improve diagnostic accuracy, especially for melanocytic skin lesions, led to the development of non-invasive diagnostic imaging tools, such as dermoscopy, reflectance confocal microscopy (RCM), and computer-assisted diagnosis. At this time, the only imaging method to emerge from the research arena into general use in clinical dermatology is dermoscopy. By reducing light reflection, refraction and diffraction, dermoscopy (epiluminescence microscopy) permits visualization of subsurface structures not discernible to the unaided eye by rendering the epidermis translucent.[38] Dermoscopy is an established tool which has been demonstrated to improve the clinical recognition of melanoma (see Chapter 36).

### Initiating physician surveillance

While the median age for developing melanoma is in the early 50s, the age for someone with a family history of melanoma and atypical moles is earlier.[39] Screening for those with atypical mole syndrome gives the physician the opportunity to educate the patient and the family about the importance of periodic SSE and of avoiding unnecessary UVL exposure.

### Primary care physicians and skin cancer detection

There are opportunities for case finding during the annual examination provided by primary care physicians; however, since the prevalence of melanoma is low, most physicians rarely have the opportunity to detect a melanoma. This hampers diagnostic accuracy and does not provide adequate reinforcement to physicians to perform skin cancer screening for their patients. Because of lack of confidence in their ability to detect skin cancers, primary care physicians may not routinely perform skin cancer screening. Aids that enhance the confidence of primary care physicians and provide reinforcement for performing skin cancer screening might be expected to be effective in increasing case finding because primary care physicians reach patients – especially elderly men, who have a higher mortality from melanoma than others. After a 1-day training course, dermoscopy improved the accuracy of primary care physicians performing triage of clinically suspicious skin tumors by 25% in comparison to unaided visual examination, without a

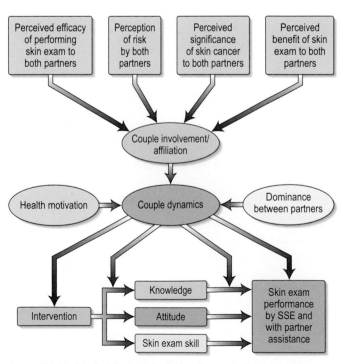

**Figure 7.2** Model of reinforcement of skin self-examination by couples.

concomitant decrease in specificity.[40] An additional benefit of digital dermoscopy is the ability to exchange the image with an expert and obtain a second opinion.

Controversy about screening for skin cancer exists. While the American Cancer Society and the American College of Preventive Medicine support selected skin cancer screening, the US Preventive Service Task Force (USPSTF), which uses an evidence-based approach, concluded that there is insufficient evidence to assess the balance of benefits and harms of screening by primary care physicians or by patient SSE.[41] This recommendation is largely due to the lack of evidence from randomized controlled trials. Importantly, the USPSTF recommendation does not consider the circumstances of selected skin cancer screening that was endorsed by other national organizations, e.g. patients with a history of premalignant or malignant skin lesions, those with a familial syndrome, or screening performed by dermatologists or screening using tools such as dermoscopes.

## FUTURE OUTLOOK

Primary and secondary prevention programs for skin cancer can make a significant difference in the mortality and morbidity from skin cancer. Strategies that enable change in the behaviors of those at risk to develop skin cancer are being developed. Promising approaches include: 1) improving the personal risk perception of people, 2) providing written materials that serve as a reference to enhance early detection, 3) developing improved parental skills to engage their children in conversations about sun protection, and 4) better identification of those at risk for developing melanoma and encouraging the use of SSE in that group.

Tanning attitudes are influencing the sun exposure and indoor tanning habits of our youth and young adults. Since tanning is largely an affective driven decision in which the tanners often ignore or discount the cognitive-based information such as skin cancer risk and premature aging of the skin, societal attitude change promoting the appearance and healthy look of natural skin tones may set the stage for individual change. Legislation and regulation may influence cultural attitudes and effectively impact public health. An example of legislation changing behaviors in the US is the use of seat belts. Only 10–15 % of the US population used seat belts in the early 1980s. After seat-belt legislation enactment and enforcement of mandatory seat-belt use and public education campaigns, the use in 1993 was 70%.[42,43] Enacting youth access IT laws may spark societal changes that foster positive behavioral modifications.

## ACKNOWLEDGEMENT

Robert J Turrisi, PhD, Director of Biobehavioral Health and Prevention Research Center, The Pennsylvania State University, University Park, and Joel J Hillhouse, PhD, Professor of Psychology, East Tennessee State University, Johnson City, Tennessee, have worked with Dr. Robinson in formulating the behavioral models of primary and secondary skin cancer prevention. The collaboration of the group is represented in this work.

## REFERENCES

1. Ries LAG, Melbert D, Krapcho M, et al. *SEER Cancer Statistics Review, 1975-2004, National Cancer Institute.* < http:// seer.cancer.gov/csr/1975_2004/ > (November 2006 SEER data submission); Accessed 04.08.09.
2. Cancer Facts and Figures 2010. American Cancer Society. <http:// cancer.org/acs/groups/content/@epidemiologysurveilance/documents/ documents/document/acspc-026238.pdf. Accessed September 27, 2010.
3. Lens MB, Dawes M. Global perspectives of contemporary epidemiological trends of cutaneous malignant melanoma. *Br J Dermatol.* 2004;150:179–185.
4. Ferlay J, Bray F, Pisani P, et al. *GLOBOCAN 2002: Cancer Incidence, Mortality, and Prevalence Worldwide.* IARC Cancer Base No 5, version 2.0. Lyon, France: IARC Press; 2004.
5. Joseph AK, Mark TL, Mueller C. The period prevalence and costs of treating nonmelanoma skin cancers in patients 65 years of age covered by Medicare. *Dermatol Surg.* 2001;27:955–959.
6. Diepgen TL, Mahler V. The epidemiology of skin cancer. *Br J Dermatol.* 2002;146(suppl 61):1–6.
7. Bickers DR, Lim HW, Margolis D, et al. The burden of skin diseases: 2004 a joint project of the American Academy of Dermatology Association and the Society for Investigative Dermatology. *J Am Acad Dermatol.* 2006;55(3):490–500.
8. Lachiewicz AM, Berwick M, Wiggins CL, et al. Survival differences between patients with scalp or neck melanoma and those with melanoma of other sites in the Surveillance, Epidemiology, and End Results (SEER) program. *Arch Dermatol.* 2008;144:515–521.
9. Jensen P, Hansen S, Moller B, et al. Skin cancer in kidney and heart transplant recipients and different long-term immunosuppressive therapy regimens. *J Am Acad Dermatol.* 1999;40:177–186.
10. Goldstein AM, Chaudru V, Ghiorzo P, et al. Cutaneous phenotype and MC1R variants as modifying factors for the development of melanoma in CDKN2A G101W mutation carriers from 4 countries. *Int J Cancer.* 2007;121(4):825–831.
11. Wong CS, Strange RC, Lear JT. Basal cell carcinoma. *BMJ.* 2003;327(7418):794–798.
12. Gray DT, Suman VJ, Su WP, et al. Trends in the population based incidence of squamous cell carcinoma of the skin first diagnosed between 1984-1992. *Arch Dermatol.* 1997;133:735–750.
13. Rudoph R, Zelac D. Squamous cell carcinoma of the skin. *Plast Reconstr Surg.* 2004;114:82–94.
14. Turrisi R, Hillhouse J, Gebert C. Examination of cognitive variables relevant to sunbathing. *J Behav Med.* 1998;21(3):299–311.
15. Robinson JK, Rademaker AW, Sylvester J, et al. Summer sun exposure: knowledge, attitudes, and behaviors of Midwest adolescents. *Prev Med.* 1997;26:364–372.
16. Mahler HIM, Kulik JA, Harrell J, et al. Effects of UV photographs, photoaging information, and use of sunless tanning lotion on sun protection behaviors. *Arch Dermatol.* 2005;141:373–380.
17. Olson AL, Gaffney CA, Starr P, et al. The impact of an appearance-based educational intervention on adolescent intention to use sunscreen. *Health Educ Res.* 2008;23(5):763–769.
18. Buller DB, Borland R. Public education projects in skin cancer prevention: childcare, school and college-based. *Clin Dermatol.* 1998;16:447–459.
19. Geller AC, Colditz G, Oliveria S, et al. Use of sunscreen, sun burning rates, and tanning bed use among more than 10,000 US children and adolescents. *Pediatrics.* 2002;109:1009–1014.
20. IARC. The association of use of sun beds with cutaneous malignant melanoma and other skin cancers: a systematic review. *Int J Cancer.* 2006;120:1116–1122.
21. Westerdahl J, Ingvar C, Masback A, et al. Risk of cutaneous malignant melanoma in relation to use of sun beds: further evidence for UV-A carcinogenicity. *Br J Cancer.* 2000;82:1593–1599.
22. Hillhouse JJ, Turrisi R, Stapleton J, et al. A randomized controlled trial of an appearance-focused intervention to prevent skin cancer. *Cancer.* 2008;113:3257–3266.
23. Hillhouse J, Turrisi R, Holwiski F, et al. An examination of psychological variables relevant to artificial tanning tendencies. *J Health Psychol.* 1999;4(4):507–516.
24. Friedman RJ, Rigel DS, Kopf AW. Early detection of malignant melanoma: the role of physician examination and self-examination of the skin. *CA Cancer J Clin.* 1985;35:130–151.
25. McPherson M, Elwood M, English DR, et al. Presentation and detection of invasive melanoma in a high-risk population. *J Am Acad Dermatol.* 2006;54:783–792.
26. Carli P, De Giorgi V, Pallli D, et al. Dermatologist detection and skin self- examination are associated with thinner melanomas; results from a survey of Italian multidisciplinary group on melanoma. *Arch Dermatol.* 2003;139:607–612.
27. Brady MS, Oliveria SA, Christos PJ, et al. Patterns of detection in patients with cutaneous melanoma. Implications for secondary prevention. *Cancer.* 2000;89:342–347.

**28.** Berwick M, Begg CM, Fine JA, et al. Screening for cutaneous melanoma by skin self-examination. *J Natl Cancer Inst.* 1996;88:17–23.

**29.** Robinson JK, Turrisi R, Stapleton J. Efficacy of a partner assistance intervention designed to increase skin self-examination performance. *Arch Dermatol.* 2007;143:37–41.

**30.** Chiu V, Won E, Malik M, et al. The use of mole-mapping diagrams to increase skin self-examination accuracy. *J Am Acad Dermatol.* 2006;55:245–250.

**31.** Oliveria SA, Chau D, Christos PJ, et al. Diagnostic accuracy of patients in performing skin self-examination and the impact of photography. *Arch Dermatol.* 2004;140:57–62.

**32.** Robinson JK, Nickoloff BJ. Digital epiluminescence microscopy monitoring of high-risk patients. *Arch Dermatol.* 2004;140:49–56.

**33.** Robinson JK, Fisher SG, Turrisi RJ. Predictors of skin self-examination performance. *Cancer.* 2002;95:135–146.

**34.** Robinson JK, Rigel DS, Amonette RA. What promotes skin self-examination? *J Am Acad Dermatol.* 1998;39:752–757.

**35.** American Cancer Society. *Can melanoma be found early?* < http://www.cancer.org/docroot?CRI/content?CRI_2_4_3X_Can_melanoma_be_found_early_50.asp?sitearea >; 2006. Accessed 05.08.09.

**36.** Abbasi NR, Shaw HM, Rigel DS, et al. Early diagnosis of cutaneous melanoma. *JAMA.* 2004;292:2771–2776.

**37.** Liu W, Dowling JP, Murray WK, et al. Rate of growth in melanoma characteristics and associations of rapidly growing melanoma. *Arch Dermatol.* 2006;142:1551–1558.

**38.** Stoltz W, Braun-Falco O, Bilek P, et al. Basis of dermatoscopic and skin surface microscopy. In: *Color Atlas of Dermoscopy.* Cambridge: Blackwell; 1994:7–10.

**39.** Tiersten AD, Grin CM, Kopf AW, et al. Prospective follow-up for malignant melanoma in patients with atypical-mole (dysplastic-nevus) syndrome. *J Dermatol Surg Oncol.* 1991;17(1):44–48.

**40.** Argenziano G, Puig S, Zalaudek I, et al. Dermoscopy improves the accuracy of primary care physicians to triage lesions suggestive of skin cancer. *J Clin Oncol.* 2006;24:1877–1882.

**41.** Federman DG, Concato J, Kirsner RS. Screening for skin cancer: absence of evidence? *Arch Dermatol.* 2009;145:926–927.

**42.** US Department of Transportation National Highway Traffic Safety Administration. Legislative Fact Sheet. < http://www.nhtsa.dot.gov/people/injury/airbags/buckleplan/buckleup/legfact.html >. Accessed 008.08.09.

**43.** Nelson DE, Bolen J, Kresnow M. Trends in safety belt use by demographics and by type of state safety belt law, 1987 through 1993. *Am J Public Health.* 1998;88:245–249.

# Chemoprevention of Skin Cancers

*Marie-France Demierre and Michael Krathen*

## Key Points

- Interest in chemoprevention strategies for skin cancer is increasing.
- Retinoids may play a significant role.
- Oral agents are more effective for melanoma than are topicals.
- As cell and cancer biology in the skin continues to be explored, it is likely that there will be an even greater interest in the study of chemopreventative therapies.

## INTRODUCTION

Skin cancers account for half of all cancers in the United States (US).[1] In a review of Medicare claims data from 1992 to 1995 in the US, non-melanoma skin cancer (NMSC) was the fifth most costly cancer to treat overall, despite the relatively low per patient cost of treatment.[1] The burden of melanoma has also continued to increase, with the lifetime risk of getting melanoma in 2009 being about 1 in 50 for whites,[2] and, more concerning, a significantly increased number of melanomas since the 1990s among women, with thicker melanomas, truncal melanomas, and later-stage disease in general.[3] Successful primary prevention (prevention of disease onset) of NMSC or melanoma could dramatically reduce this burden. As a result, there has been growing interest in additional prevention approaches. In NMSCs, chemoprevention strategies have become standard in clinical practice, while in melanoma, chemoprevention is a growing area of research. We review the current data on chemoprevention strategies for NMSCs and highlight evolving areas of research in melanoma chemoprevention.

## HISTORY OF CHEMOPREVENTION

The concept of chemoprevention, originated by Sporn et al. in 1976, has been defined as the use of specific natural or synthetic chemical agents to reverse, suppress, or prevent progression to invasive cancer.[4] This concept fundamentally changed ideas about cancer, allowing the exploration of interventions that could prevent disease progression. Lippman and Hong further refined the concept of chemoprevention, emphasizing the importance of cancer delay; for example, 'Chemopreventive success will be measured in part by periods of delayed cancer development, morbidity, and mortality.'[5]

## PRINCIPLES AND RATIONALE FOR CHEMOPREVENTION OF NON-MELANOMA SKIN CANCERS

The most important risk factor in the development of NMSC is sun exposure.[6] Characteristic gene mutations in p53 and the Patched/Smoothened pathway are often noted in lesions of squamous cell carcinoma (SCC) and basal cell carcinoma (BCC), respectively. Whereas SCC is linked to cumulative sun exposure, BCC is related to intermittent and possibly childhood sun exposure.[6] Thus, primary prevention of NMSC at the most basic level includes limiting total sun exposure and responsible behavioral modifications during episodes of intermittent exposure. Application of sunscreen with combined UVA and UVB protection, avoiding sun exposure during peak hours, and wearing protective clothing are all essential elements in reducing one's exposure to damaging ultraviolet radiation. The data supporting such recommendations, unfortunately, are weak and sometimes contradictory.[7] Nonetheless, sunscreen use and responsible sun exposure are considered beneficial in reducing skin cancer risk.[7]

Once DNA photodamage has already been established, preventing progression to NMSC theoretically depends on removing premalignant cells, preventing additional oncogenic mutations, repairing existing DNA damage, inhibiting downstream effects of oncogenes, or restoring functionality to lost tumor suppressor genes.

Treatment of actinic keratoses (AKs; see Chapter 10), the most clinically evident premalignant lesion of NMSC, is an important focus of skin cancer prevention. Recent data from the Department of Veterans Affairs Topical Tretinoin Chemoprevention Trial suggest that the risk of progression of AK to primary SCC (invasive or in situ) increases slowly over time, being 0.60% at 1 year and 2.57% at 4 years.[8] Of note, approximately 65% of all primary SCCs and 36% of all primary BCCs diagnosed in the study cohort arose in lesions that previously were diagnosed clinically as AKs.

Although grossly abnormal and altered cells can be detected clinically (AKs, NMSC), 'normal-appearing' skin adjacent to such lesions likely shares at least some of the same oncogenic mutations. The concept of field cancerization explains how a field of genetically altered cells, within which one or more cells acquire further mutations and progress to form a unique NMSC, may develop from a single mutant cancer stem cell.[9] Treatment of the AK or NMSC which develops within this field may serve more as

## Table 8.1 Interventions in Prevention After DNA Damage Established (Secondary Prevention)

| Encourage cellular maturation and growth arrest | Retinoids (oral and topical) |
|---|---|
| Enhance host response/immunity | Imiquimod |
| Selective destruction of pre-malignant cell clones | Photodynamic therapy, topical 5-fluorouracil |
| Improvement in endogenous repair mechanisms | T4 endonuclease |
| Inhibiting downstream effects of mutated genetic pathways | Inhibitors of hedgehog signaling (GDC-0449) |
| Restoration of lost tumor-suppressor genes | No mechanisms to date |

a temporizing measure than a cure. As we learn more about cancer biology in the skin, focusing on field therapy may become even more important (Table 8.1).

## Cellular maturation and growth arrest

**Retinoids** The role of vitamin A in malignancy was first hypothesized in the 1920s when the relationship between hypovitaminosis A, epithelial changes, and stomach cancer was noted in rats.[10] Since the 1950s, oral – and, years later, topical – retinoids have been evaluated for their role in cancer treatment and prevention. Numerous studies since have investigated the role for retinoids in cancer chemoprevention, including skin and head and neck cancer. It is not fully understood how retinoids function in chemoprevention; nonetheless, retinoids are thought to promote cellular differentiation, maturation, and growth arrest.[10]

One landmark study in 1988 evaluated the prospective use of oral isotretinoin in patients with xeroderma pigmentosum (XP), a rare autosomal recessive disorder of the nucleotide excision repair (NER) pathway.[10] Five of seven patients were treated with isotretinoin (2 mg/kg/day) for 2 years and exhibited a 63% reduction in NMSC in comparison with baseline. Other studies investigating low-dose (10 mg/kg) isotretinoin have not shown efficacy.[11]

The effect of retinoids in transplant patients has also been studied.[10] A randomized controlled trial in renal transplant recipients demonstrated a 37% reduction in the development of new SCCs while taking acitretin 30 mg/day for 6 months.[12] A 20% relative reduction in SCC was reported in psoriasis patients using retinoids after exposure to PUVA; BCC rates, in contrast, were unaffected.[13] Other high-risk patient groups considered good candidates for oral retinoid (isotretinoin or acitretin) therapy include patients with basal cell nevus syndrome or chronic lymphocytic leukemia, organ transplant recipients, and those patients with high incidence of cutaneous neoplasia for unclear reasons.

The use of retinoids (vitamin A [retinol]) has also been investigated in patients with moderate skin cancer risk. A randomized controlled trial of approximately 2300 patients with a history of at least 10 actinic keratoses but no more than either two SCCs or BCCs demonstrated a 26% relative risk reduction in developing subsequent SCC when treated

with vitamin A 25,000 IU daily.[14] There was no effect on development of BCC. Interestingly, when this same regimen was applied to high-risk patients (as defined by having greater than four BCCs or SCCs) no benefit was seen.[11] The administration of retinol at these doses in the moderate-risk treatment group was well tolerated; nonetheless, leucopenia, anemia, hypercholesterolemia, abnormal liver enzymes, and anemia were noted.[14]

Despite beneficial responses while on therapy, oral retinoid chemoprevention does not seem to last beyond the treatment period.[10] Risks of therapy acutely include hepatic transaminitis and hepatitis, hyperlipidemia, cheilitis, eczematous cutaneous reactions, and epistaxis. Osteoporosis is the main chronic risk of therapy with retinoids.

Topical retinoids have also been examined in detail in the chemoprevention of NMSC. Most recently, an increase in all-cause mortality in patients treated with topical tretinoin was reported in the Veterans Affairs Topical Tretinoin Chemoprevention Trial.[15] In this multi-site, prospective, blinded, randomized, controlled study, 1131 veterans were randomized to either topical tretinoin 0.1% or vehicle creams with twice daily application. The implications of this study are unclear, especially since endogenous levels of retinoids are mostly unaffected by topical tretinoin application.[15] Future studies are required to address these surprising results. Meanwhile, the Veterans Affairs have initiated another chemoprevention trial (CSP 562), focusing on the effect of topical 5-FU treatment (compared to a vehicle control treatment) on reducing surgeries for NMSCs on the face and ears.

## Miscellaneous pathways

Numerous pathways are likely involved in development and progression of NMSC. Several classes of drugs have been investigated in chemoprevention of NMSC, including cyclo-oxygenase (COX) inhibitors, angiotensin-converting enzyme (ACE) inhibitors, and mTOR pathway inhibitors.

**Cyclo-oxygenase inhibition** Diclofenac gel is a COX-2 inhibitor that is approved for treatment of actinic keratoses in the US. In a case–control study of non-steroidal anti-inflammatory drugs (NSAIDs), modest, non-significant reductions in the number of BCCs and SCCs were noted with NSAID use.[16] A small number of non-randomized, retrospective studies in humans have shown some benefit of oral NSAIDs on prevention of NSMC.[17]

**Angiotensin-converting enzyme pathway** The use of ACE inhibitors or angiotensin receptor blockers (ARBs) may be protective against development of SCCs and BCCs in high-risk patients (with at least two BCCs or SCCs in previous 5 years).[18] Again, prospective, randomized, controlled studies need to be performed.

**mTOR pathway** Immunosuppression required after solid organ transplantation elevates the risk of skin cancer dramatically. Several studies have demonstrated dramatic reduction in incidence of new NMSCs after switching to an immunosuppression regimen containing an inhibitor (either sirolimus or everolimus) of the mammalian target of rapamycin (mTOR) pathway.[19] In patients with a strong personal history of skin cancer who will be having or already have had a solid organ transplant, an immunosuppression regimen with an mTOR inhibitor should strongly be considered.

**Hedgehog pathway** Inhibition of the hedgehog pathway with a novel oral agent (GDC-0449) showed clinical responses among patients with locally advanced BCC.[20] For patients at risk of multiple BCCs, such as in the basal cell nevus syndrome, this new agent could have a role in chemoprevention.

## Destructive modalities

**Intrinsic: enhancement of host-initiated cellular destruction** The premise of tumor immunology rests on the body's ability to launch a successful immune response against malignant cells via recognition of altered tumor antigens. Imiquimod's efficacy in treating actinic keratoses and superficial NMSCs likely performs in this manner. Theoretically, the notion of a cancer vaccine could also reduce incidence of NMSC if common tumor antigens are used. Nonetheless, there are no studies which evaluate vaccination and NMSC prevention to date.

**Extrinsic: exogenously directed destruction** Delayed onset of new actinic keratoses and SCC has been shown in small studies of immunosuppressed transplant patients after both methyl aminolevulinate (MAL) and aminolevulinic acid (ALA) photodynamic therapy (PDT). PDT for BCC prevention is supported by mouse models as well.[21] Hairless skin mouse models indicate that direct phototoxicity of premalignant cells is unlikely why PDT may prove beneficial in NMSC prevention; rather, host-response and cellular-specific immunity after PDT-induced cell death may explain delayed onset of NMSC after treatment.[21]

## Improvement in endogenous repair mechanisms

T4 endonuclease V is a bacterial DNA repair enzyme which has been shown to accelerate human DNA repair when delivered intracellularly.[11] In principle, repair of cyclobutane pyrimidine dimers and pyrimidine-pyrimidinone photo-products could essentially restore host DNA back to baseline before more serious genome disruption occurs. A randomized, double-blind, controlled trial in 30 patients with xeroderma pigmentosum showed promising initial results in reducing incidence of BCC and actinic keratoses.[11,22]

## Ineffective agents

Several agents have been shown to have no effect on the prevention of NMSC. These include several antioxidants (beta-carotene, vitamin E, selenium)[11] and statins[23] (Table 8.2).

## PRINCIPLES AND RATIONALE FOR MELANOMA CHEMOPREVENTION

To reduce the burden of morbidity and mortality and for melanoma chemoprevention to be a valid strategy, certain principles are relevant. In addition to a strong scientific rationale, a systematic approach to chemoprevention agent development with rigorous chemoprevention designs has been emphasized[29] as well as careful selection of surrogate endpoint biomarkers. Several potential agents exist (Table 8.3). The information for those candidate agents with the greatest amount of data and undergoing investigation is reviewed.

Similar to other cancers, UV-induced melanoma is recognized as a multi-step process.[30] Ideally, specific steps can be targeted. Alterations of *ras* pathway genes are critically

| Table 8.2 Selected Potential Future Clinical Targets for NMSC Prevention | | |
|---|---|---|
| **Pathway** | **Agent** | **Comments** |
| PPAR pathway | None to date | |
| Ornithine decarboxylase pathway | DFMO ($\alpha$-difluoromethyl-DL-ornithine) | Irreversible ornithine decarboxylase (ODC) inhibitor targeting ODC and polyamine pathway[11] |
| PTEN pathway[24] | None to date | |
| Cyclo-oxygenase (COX) pathway | Nimesulide | Blocks COX-2: reduced tumor burden and progression to SCCs in nbUVB-exposed mice;[25] ODC expression also reduced |
| Antioxidants | Polyphenolic antioxidants: black and green tea, grape seed ((-)-epigallocatechin gallate)[11] Vitamin C[26] Phytochemical antioxidants: isoflavones (genistein)[11] Lycopene[11] | Oral and topical forms studied in mice |
| Apoptosis pathway | Silymarin[27] | |
| EGFR pathway[28] | None to date | |
| Miscellaneous | Caffeine[26] Perillyl alcohol[26] Isothiocyanates[26] Vitamin D[26] Curcumin[11] | |

## Table 8.3 Examples of Candidate Agents for Melanoma Chemoprevention

| Agent | Mechanism(s) | Melanoma Data – Epidemiologic/Preclinical/Clinical |
|---|---|---|
| Apomine | Induces apoptosis | Preclinical (murine data), clinical |
| Carotenoids (β-carotene, lycopene) | Increase intercellular communication | Epidemiologic |
| ASA/NSAIDs/COX-2 inhibitors | Induce apoptosis<br>Restore immune function | Epidemiologic, preclinical (in vitro), clinical phase IIa (ongoing) |
| Curcumin | Induces apoptosis<br>Antioxidant<br>COX and LOX inhibition | Preclinical (in vitro), clinical topical phase I (ongoing) |
| DFMO | Inhibits polyamine metabolism | Preclinical (in vitro and murine data), clinical |
| Flavonoids (genistein) | Induce apoptosis | Preclinical (in vitro, murine data) |
| L-ascorbic acid (vitamin C) | Induces apoptosis | Epidemiologic (negative data), preclinical (in vitro) |
| Perillyl alcohol | Induces apoptosis | Preclinical (murine data), clinical topical phase I |
| Resveratrol (found in grapes and red wine) | Induces apoptosis<br>Scavenges free radicals | Preclinical (in vitro) |
| Retinoids | Inhibit polyamine synthesis<br>Induce terminal differentiation<br>Induce apoptosis<br>Increase intercellular communication | Preclinical (in vitro, murine data), clinical |
| Statins | Induce apoptosis<br>Inhibit angiogenesis | Epidemiologic, preclinical (in vitro, murine data), clinical phase IIa (ongoing) |
| Selenium | Induces apoptosis<br>Restores immune response | Epidemiologic (conflicting data), preclinical (murine data) |
| Tea (polyphenols) | Antimutagenesis<br>Induce apoptosis<br>Restore immune functions<br>Scavenge free radicals | Preclinical (in vitro, murine data) |
| Alpha-tocopherol (vitamin E) | Restores immune response | Epidemiologic (conflicting data), preclinical (conflicting murine data) |
| Vitamin D | Antiproliferative<br>Pro-differentiation | Preclinical (in vitro, murine), epidemiologic (conflicting) |
| N-acetylcysteine | Antioxidant | Clinical oral phase I |

important in the pathogenesis of sporadic melanoma.[30] N-ras and BRAF mutations represent alternative genetic changes that result in the activation of the same signaling pathway, the Ras/ERK/MAPK cascade, driving tumorigenesis. There has been a proven rationale for targeting ras signaling in metastatic melanoma patients. Thus, there has been a thrust towards targeting this same signaling in chemoprevention. Three candidate chemoprevention agents have fulfilled a scientific rationale for investigation in melanoma: apomine, a bisphosphonate ester; perillyl alcohol, a monoterpene isolated from essential oils; and statins.[30] Among those agents, both apomine and perillyl alcohol are topical. A topical approach has its challenges as it may not be sufficient to achieve a biological effect. Thus, most melanoma prevention interventions are given orally so that the drug can be adequately delivered to the organ or tissue of interest. In assessing the level of evidence supporting the role of an agent in melanoma chemoprevention, both experimental and epidemiologic levels of evidence have been examined (Fig. 8.1).[29]

There have been growing data on the potential role of statins in chemoprevention.[31] While a meta-analysis of randomized controlled trials of statins in cardiovascular disease, with patients receiving therapy for at least 4 years, revealed no significant difference between statin and observation groups with regard to the secondary outcome of melanoma incidence,[32] others have found evidence for a protective role. Farwell et al.[33] found an apparent dose–response relationship between statin use and both incidence of total cancers (p<0.001) and melanoma (p = 0.004), with fewer cancers with increased statin dosage, among a cohort of 45,105 patients. In the same cohort, for biopsy-proven melanoma, there was a statistically significant decreased risk for invasive melanoma (RR = 0.61 [0.39, 0.94]) but not melanoma in situ (RR = 0.82 [0.48, 1.40]) among patients taking a statin compared to patients taking an antihypertensive medication. A statistically significant decreased risk for melanoma was also found with increasing statin dose (p<0.02) (Farwell W, et al., personal communication, Melanoma Prevention Working Group, October 22, 2009,

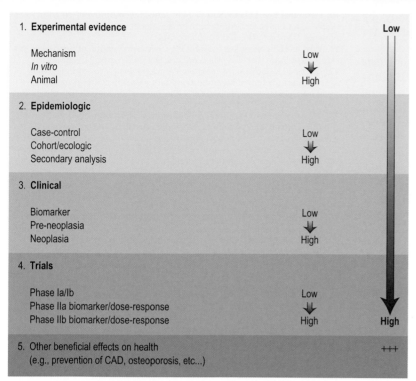

1. **Experimental evidence**

    Mechanism                        Low
    *In vitro*
    Animal                          High

2. **Epidemiologic**

    Case-control               Low
    Cohort/ecologic
    Secondary analysis       High

3. **Clinical**

    Biomarker                  Low
    Pre-neoplasia
    Neoplasia                  High

4. **Trials**

    Phase Ia/Ib                Low
    Phase IIa biomarker/dose-response
    Phase IIb biomarker/dose-response   High

5. Other beneficial effects on health    +++
   (e.g., prevention of CAD, osteoporosis, etc...)

**Figure 8.1** Criteria of evidence to move chemopreventive agents to large randomized trials.[29]*

The authors have also proposed a point system to ensure that evidence from multiple weak studies would not have more weight that the evidence from one stronger study.

Chicago, IL). Similarly, in a Dutch pharmacoepidemiological database, among 1318 cases and 6786 controls, statin use was associated with a reduced Breslow thickness (p = 0.03).[34] However, Curiel et al. did not find a protective effect for statins on the development of melanoma with a statin length of exposure greater than 5 years (Curiel C, personal communication, Melanoma Prevention Working Group, November 15, 2008). Currently, one phase II randomized study is evaluating the effects of lovastatin on various endpoints (clinical, histological, molecular) of melanoma patients with clinical atypical nevi (NCI.clinical trials.gov).

Results of laboratory studies and a few case–control studies have suggested that NSAIDs[35] or COX-2 inhibitors[36] might have chemopreventive activity and therapeutic efficacy against melanoma. Asgari et al. examined whether NSAID use was associated with melanoma risk among 63,809 men and women in the Vitamins and Lifestyle (VITAL) cohort study. No melanoma risk reduction was detected for any NSAID dose (RR = 1.12, 95% CI = 0.84–1.48), for any NSAID excluding low-dose aspirin (RR = 1.03, 95% CI = 0.74–1.43), for regular- or extra-strength aspirin (RR = 1.10, 95% CI = 0.76–1.58), or for non-aspirin NSAIDs (RR = 1.22, 95% CI = 0.75–1.99). That authors concluded that overall, based on their data, NSAIDs do not appear to be good candidates for the chemoprevention of melanoma.[37] However, Joosse et al. found that continuous use of low-dose aspirin was associated with significant reduction of melanoma risk in women (adjusted OR = 0.54, 95% CI = 0.30–0.99), but not in men.[38] A significant trend (p = 0.04) from no use, non-continuous use to continuous use was observed in women. Interestingly, Curiel et al. found that extended use of NSAIDs (>5 years)

decreases the risk of melanoma development (OR = 0.66, 95% CI = 0.5–0.9, p = 0.004) with the observed effect primarily limited to the use of ASA (OR = 0.56, 95% CI = 0.4–0.8, p = 0.001) (Curiel C, personal communication, Melanoma Prevention Working Group, November 15, 2008). As a result of these data, Curiel et al. have initiated a phase II study of oral sulindac among patients with clinical atypical nevi (NCI/UAZ Chemoprevention Consortium) evaluating clinical, histologic, and molecular changes in nevi.

Curcumin, the major yellow pigment extracted from turmeric, a commonly used spice, is another potential agent. It has long been used as a treatment for inflammation, skin wounds, and tumors in India and Southeast Asia. The clinical efficacy of curcumin has yet to be confirmed, but its cancer chemopreventive potential is demonstrated by its anticarcinogenic effects in cell culture and animal models of breast, gastrointestinal, and skin (including UV-induced) carcinogenesis.[39] Numerous mechanisms of anti-carcinogenesis have been identified[39] with apoptosis in human melanoma cells induced by curcumin through inhibition of the NF-κB cell survival pathway and the Fas receptor/caspase 8 pathway, and through suppression of the apoptotic inhibitor XIAP. Several preclinical models have confirmed activity.[39] To date, when taken orally, curcumin has shown excellent tolerance, up to 12 g as a single dose and 8000 mg in repeated oral doses.[40] A phase I study of topical curcumin has been initiated.

Another strategy is to protect a person's melanocytes from UV-induced oxidative stress/damage and prevent the development of UV-induced melanoma. In in-vivo murine models, oral N-acetylcysteine protected melanocytes against oxidative stress/damage and delayed onset of UV-induced melanoma in mice.[41] Grossman et al. are investigating the chemopreventive potential of oral N-acetylcysteine for UV-induced melanoma among at-risk subjects.

Adequate vitamin D levels may also be relevant (see Chapter 60). In a UK case–control study, among 1043 incident cases from the first Leeds case–control study, a single estimation of serum 25-hydroxyvitamin $D_3$ level taken at recruitment was inversely correlated with Breslow thickness (p = 0.03 for linear trend).[42] These data suggest that vitamin D and vitamin D receptors (VDR) may have a small but potentially important role in melanoma susceptibility, and possibly a greater role in disease progression.[42] The same group found that higher 25-hydroxyvitamin $D_3$ levels, at diagnosis, were associated with both thinner tumors and better survival from melanoma, independent of Breslow thickness.[43] However, a study of supplemental vitamin D intake and melanoma risk among 68,611 men and women, participants of the VITAL cohort study, did not find an association between vitamin D intake and melanoma risk.[44] Vitamin D and VDR may have a role in melanoma susceptibility, and possibly in disease progression. Thus, ensuring adequate vitamin D levels among melanoma patients or those at risk for melanoma with supplementation may possibly be protective.

## FUTURE OUTLOOK

Many interventions have been studied in the chemoprevention of NMSC. Despite the efficacy noted in small trials, case reports, and animal studies, there are no large randomized trials demonstrating effective prevention of NMSC (outside of treating actinic keratoses). Several candidate agents are under investigations in melanoma. Similarly to other cancers, surrogate endpoint biomarkers (histologic and/or molecular) are needed to facilitate research. The future for chemoprevention appears bright, but will require additional research and rigorous chemoprevention design. As cell and cancer biology in the skin continues to be explored, we are likely to see an even greater interest in the study of preventative therapies.

## REFERENCES

1. Housman TS, Feldman SR, Williford PM, et al. Skin cancer is among the most costly of all cancers to treat for the Medicare population. *J Am Acad Dermatol*. 2003;48(3):425–429.
2. American Cancer Society. *Cancer facts & figures*. 2009. <http://www.cancer.org>. Accessed 29.09.09.
3. Purdue MP, Freeman LE, Anderson WF, et al. Recent trends in incidence of cutaneous melanoma among US Caucasian young adults. *J Invest Dermatol*. 2008;128(12):2905–2908.
4. Sporn MB, Dunlop NM, Newton DL, et al. Prevention of chemical carcinogenesis by vitamin A and its synthetic analogs (retinoids). *Fed Proc*. 1976;35:1332–1338.
5. Lippman SM, Hong WK. Cancer prevention science and practice. *Cancer Res*. 2002;62:5119–5125.
6. Cleaver JE, Crowley E. UV damage, DNA repair and skin carcinogenesis. *Front Biosci*. 2002;7:d1024–d1043.
7. Koh HK. Preventive strategies and research for ultraviolet-associated cancer. *Environ Health Perspect*. 1995;103(suppl 8):255–257.
8. Criscione VD, Weinstock MA, Naylor MF, et al. Actinic keratoses: natural history and risk of malignant transformation in the Veterans Affairs Topical Tretinoin Chemoprevention Trial. *Cancer*. 2009;115(11):2523–2530.
9. Braakhuis BJ, Tabor MP, Kummer JA, et al. A genetic explanation of Slaughter's concept of field cancerization: evidence and clinical implications. *Cancer Res*. 2003;63(8):1727–1730.
10. Campbell RM, DiGiovanna JJ. Skin cancer chemoprevention with systemic retinoids: an adjunct in the management of selected high-risk patients. *Dermatol Ther*. 2006;19(5):306–314.
11. Wright TI, Spencer JM, Flowers FP. Chemoprevention of nonmelanoma skin cancer. *J Am Acad Dermatol*. 2006;54(6):933–946 quiz 947–950.
12. Bavinck JN, Tieben LM, Van der Woude FJ, et al. Prevention of skin cancer and reduction of keratotic skin lesions during acitretin therapy in renal transplant recipients: a double-blind, placebo-controlled study. *J Clin Oncol*. 1995;13(8):1933–1938.
13. Nijsten TE, Stern RS. Oral retinoid use reduces cutaneous squamous cell carcinoma risk in patients with psoriasis treated with psoralen-UVA: a nested cohort study. *J Am Acad Dermatol*. 2003;49(4):644–650.
14. Moon TE, Levine N, Cartmel B, et al. Effect of retinol in preventing squamous cell skin cancer in moderate-risk subjects: a randomized, double-blind, controlled trial. Southwest Skin Cancer Prevention Study Group. *Cancer Epidemiol Biomarkers Prev*. 1997;6(11):949–956.
15. Weinstock MA, Bingham SF, Lew RA, et al. Topical tretinoin therapy and all-cause mortality. *Arch Dermatol*. 2009;145(1):18–24.
16. Grau MV, Baron JA, Langholz B, et al. Effect of NSAIDs on the recurrence of nonmelanoma skin cancer. *Int J Cancer*. 2006;119(3):682–686.
17. Butler GJ, Neale R, Green AC, et al. Nonsteroidal anti-inflammatory drugs and the risk of actinic keratoses and squamous cell cancers of the skin. *J Am Acad Dermatol*. 2005;53(6):966–972.
18. Christian JB, Lapane KL, Hume AL, et al. Association of ACE inhibitors and angiotensin receptor blockers with keratinocyte cancer prevention in the randomized VATTC trial. *J Natl Cancer Inst*. 2008;100(17):1223–1232.
19. Monaco AP. The role of mTOR inhibitors in the management of posttransplant malignancy. *Transplantation*. 2009;87(2):157–163.
20. Von Hoff DD, LoRusso PM, Rudin CM, et al. Inhibition of the hedgehog pathway in advanced basal-cell carcinoma. *N Engl J Med*. 2009;361(12):1164–1172.
21. Bissonnette R. Chemo-preventative thoughts for photodynamic therapy. *Dermatol Clin*. 2007;25(1):95–100.
22. Yarosh D, Klein J, O'Connor A, et al. Effect of topically applied T4 endonuclease V in liposomes on skin cancer in xeroderma pigmentosum: a randomised study. *Lancet*. 2001;357(9260):926–929.
23. Dore DD, Lapane KL, Trivedi AN, et al. Association between statin use and risk for keratinocyte carcinoma in the Veterans Affairs Topical Tretinoin Chemoprevention Trial. *Ann Intern Med*. 2009;150(1):9–18.
24. Ming M, He YY. PTEN: new insights into its regulation and function in skin cancer. *J Invest Dermatol*. 2009;129(9):2109–2112.
25. Tang X, Kim AL, Feith DJ, et al. Ornithine decarboxylase is a target for chemoprevention of basal and squamous cell carcinomas in Ptch1+/- mice. *J Clin Invest*. 2004;113(6):867–875.
26. Einspahr JG, Stratton SP, Bowden GT, et al. Chemoprevention of human skin cancer. *Crit Rev Oncol Hematol*. 2002;41(3):269–285.
27. Katiyar SK, Roy AM, Baliga MS. Silymarin induces apoptosis primarily through a p53-dependent pathway involving Bcl-2/Bax, cytochrome c release, and caspase activation. *Mol Cancer Ther*. 2005;4(2):207–216.
28. El-Abaseri TB, Fuhrman J, Trempus C, et al. Chemoprevention of UV light-induced skin tumorigenesis by inhibition of the epidermal growth factor receptor. *Cancer Res*. 2005;65(9):3958–3965.
29. Meyskens FL, Szabo E. How should we move the field of chemopreventive agent development forward in a productive manner? *Recent Results Cancer Res*. 2005;166:113–124.
30. Demierre MF, Sondak VK. Cutaneous melanoma: pathogenesis and rationale for chemoprevention. *Crit Rev Oncol Hematol*. 2005;53(3):225–239.
31. Demierre MF, Higgins PD, Gruber SB, et al. Statins and cancer prevention. *Nat Rev Cancer*. 2005;5(12):930–942.
32. Dellavalle RP, Drake A, Graber M, et al. Statins and fibrates for preventing melanoma. *Cochrane Database Syst Rev*. 2005;(4) CD003697.
33. Farwell WR, Scranton RE, Lawler EV, et al. The association between statins and cancer incidence in a veterans population. *J Natl Cancer Inst*. 2008;100(2):134–139.
34. Koomen ER, Joosse A, Herings RMC, et al. Is statin use associated with a reduced incidence, a reduced Breslow thickness or delayed metastasis of melanoma of the skin? *Eur J Cancer*. 2007;43(17):2580–2589.
35. Harris RE, Beebe-Donk J, Namboodiri KK. Inverse association of non-steroidal anti-inflammatory drugs and malignant melanoma among women. *Oncol Rep*. 2001;8(3):655–657.
36. Ramirez CC, Ma F, Federman DG, et al. Use of cyclooxygenase inhibitors and risk of melanoma in high-risk patients. *Dermatol Surg*. 2005;31(7 Pt 1):748–752.
37. Asgari MM, Maruti SS, White E. A large cohort study of nonsteroidal anti-inflammatory drug use and melanoma incidence. *J Natl Cancer Inst*. 2008;100(13):967–971.
38. Joosse A, Koomen ER, Casparie MK, et al. Non-steroidal anti-inflammatory drugs and melanoma risk: large Dutch population-based case-control study. *J Invest Dermatol*. 2009;129(11):2620–2627.
39. Lao CD, Demierre MF, Sondak VK. Targeting events in melanoma carcinogenesis for the prevention of melanoma. *Expert Rev Anticancer Ther*. 2006;6(11):1559–1568.

**40.** Cheng AL, Hsu CH, Lin JK, et al. Phase I clinical trial of curcumin, a chemopreventive agent, in patients with high-risk or pre-malignant lesions. *Anticancer Res.* 2001;21(4B):2895–2900.

**41.** Cotter MA, Thomas J, Cassidy P, et al. N-Acetylcysteine protects melanocytes against oxidative stress/damage and delays onset of ultraviolet-induced melanoma in mice. *Clin Cancer Res.* 2007;13(19):5952–15928.

**42.** Randerson-Moor JA, Taylor JC, Elliott F, et al. Vitamin D receptor gene polymorphisms, serum 25-hydroxyvitamin D levels, and melanoma: UK case-control comparisons and a meta-analysis of published VDR data. *Eur J Cancer.* 2009;129(11):2620–2627.

**43.** Newton-Bishop JA, Beswick S, Randerson-Moor JA, et al. Serum 25-hydroxyvitamin D3 levels are associated with Breslow thickness at presentation and survival from melanoma. *J Clin Oncol.* 2009;27(32):5439–5444.

**44.** Asgari MM, Maruti SS, Kushi LH, et al. A cohort study of vitamin D intake and melanoma risk. *J Invest Dermatol.* 2009;129(7):1675–1680.

# Current Concepts in Photoprotection

*Christopher T. Burnett, Darrell Rigel, and Henry W. Lim*

## Key Points

- Photoprotection includes the complementary strategies of seeking shade when outdoors, using protective clothing, wearing a wide-brimmed hat, application of sunscreen, and wearing sunglasses.

- Protection from both UVB and UVA is important, and knowledge is also emerging regarding the cutaneous biological effects of visible light and infrared radiation.

- Avobenzone is currently the only organic ultraviolet filter available in the United States with effective protection within the UVA1 range, and photostabilized formulations of this filter are an important component of broad-spectrum sunscreen products.

- The photoprotective effect of clothing is quantified by the ultraviolet protection factor (UPF), which varies based on several factors.

## INTRODUCTION

Photoprotection broadly encompasses the various techniques used to shield the body from the harmful effects of ultraviolet radiation (UVR) produced by the sun. The ultraviolet (UV) spectrum is subdivided based on wavelength. UVC (260–290 nm) is largely filtered by the Earth's atmosphere and does not reach the surface of our planet in appreciable amounts.

Historically, attenuating UVB (290–320 nm) was the primary goal of sunscreens, as UVB is the major contributor to sunburn while also provoking DNA damage implicated in the formation of non-melanoma skin cancers.[1] UVA radiation (320–400 nm), the major spectrum responsible for tanning and photoaging, has also been shown to play a role in photoimmunosuppression and photocarcinogenesis.[2] Prompted by this knowledge, UVA protective filters have been developed in recent years, and application of a broad-spectrum sunscreen covering both the UVB and UVA ranges is currently recommended. Yet, optimal photoprotection is obtained not only by the application of sunscreen, but also by seeking shade, wearing ultraviolet (UV) protective clothing, wearing a wide-brimmed hat, and the use of sunglasses.[3] These measures, in addition to sunscreen application, are essential components of a complete photoprotective strategy.

## HISTORY

The use of topical sunscreen application dates back to the ancient Egyptians, who attempted to use olive oil as a photoprotectant.[4] The first modern use of sunscreen is credited to Veiel, who described tannin as a photoprotectant in 1887. By the 1920s tanned skin had become a popular fashion trend. As individuals spent more time outdoors in hopes of bronzing their skin, they also sought to minimize the risk of sunburn, resulting in an increased demand for sunscreens. In 1928, a product containing benzyl salicylate and benzyl cinnamate became the first commercial sunscreen.

However, sunscreen was not widely popularized until the military use of red veterinary petroleum during World War II. By the mid-1950s, several UVB filters had been developed and popularized, including para-aminobenzoic acid and salicylate derivatives. In the late 1970s, effective UVA filters were developed and combination products containing UVA filters and UVB filters allowed for broad-spectrum protection. Dibenzoylmethane derivatives were the first available long UVA filter.[4]

Sun protection factor (SPF) was adopted for use by the United States Food and Drug Administration (FDA) in 1978. In the mid-1980s, public awareness campaigns against sun exposure were developed by the American Academy of Dermatology further serving to increase public awareness of sunscreen use. In 1989 and 1992, respectively, micronized forms of titanium dioxide and zinc oxide became available.[4] The first FDA sunscreen monograph was published in 1978, with subsequent revisions in 1993 and 1999.

## SUNSCREENS

### Mechanisms

UV filters are classified into two categories: organic UV filters and inorganic UV filters. The primary difference between these categories is the mechanism of action each uses to attenuate UVR. Organic filters were previously known as chemical sunscreen filters and primarily function via a mechanism of absorption. When UVR contacts an organic filter, the molecules absorb the UVR photon, resulting in temporary excitation to a higher energy state. From this excited state, the energy may be dissipated via several reactions, including fluorescence, photoreactions, or redistribution of the energy within the molecule itself. In the latter, the energy is further attenuated by the release of heat or by collision with neighboring molecules.[5,6]

Inorganic UV filters were previously known as physical sunscreens and primarily function via reflection and scattering; two of the widely used ones are titanium dioxide and zinc oxide. Scattering occurs when photons of UVR contact submicroscopic sunscreen particles and are dispersed in various directions, thereby attenuating the incident photon energy.[6] Reflection of visible light photons from the skin surface is the reason that application of inorganic sunscreen products results in whitish discoloration of the skin. It should be noted, however, that as the particle size of inorganic filters reaches the range of nanoparticles (10–50 nm in diameter), absorption of photons occurs.[3] Therefore, a lesser amount of incident photons reaching the skin is reflected, resulting in more cosmetically acceptable final products.[7] The majority of commercially available sunscreen products contain both organic and inorganic filters.

## UV filters in sunscreen products

The United States Food and Drug Administration (FDA) views and regulates sunscreens as over-the-counter (OTC) drugs. In 1999, the FDA published the latest version of its sunscreen monograph, describing regulations for sunscreen manufacturers. The FDA identified 16 sunscreen agents which can be incorporated into commercial sunscreen products. When incorporating multiple sunscreens into a commercial product, manufacturers are required to comply with the maximum concentration assigned to each individual sunscreen, while maintaining a sun protection factor (SPF) at or above a level of two. Commonly used sunscreen agents are summarized in Table 9.1, including the 16 agents identified in the FDA monograph and others available in other parts of the world; they are further discussed below. Figure 9.1 schematizes the absorption spectra of these agents. A proposed amendment to the final monograph was released by the FDA in August 2007; it proposes to allow SPF claims to a maximum of 50, and recommended in-vitro and in-vivo testing methods for UVA protection of sunscreen products.[8] At the time of this writing, the final version of this proposed amendment has not yet been released by the FDA.

### Table 9.1 Available Sunscreen Agents

| Sunscreen | λmax (nm) | US Availability | UV Spectrum | Summary |
| --- | --- | --- | --- | --- |
| PABA | 283 | Yes | UVB | Photo/contact allergen. Stains clothes. Rarely used |
| Padimate O | 311 | Yes | UVB | Most commonly used PABA derivative |
| Octinoxate | 311 | Yes | UVB | Most common UVB filter. Photolabile. Contact allergen |
| Cinoxate | 289 | Yes | UVB | Rarely used cinnamate derivative |
| Octisalate | 307 | Yes | UVB | Weak UVB absorber |
| Homosalate | 306 | Yes | UVB | Weak UVB absorber |
| Trolamine salicylate | 260–355 | Yes | UVB | Used in hair cosmetics |
| Octocrylene | 303 | Yes | UVB | Photostabilizes avobenzone. Poor substantivity |
| Ensulizole | 310 | Yes | UVB | Used in cosmetic moisturizers |
| Parsol SLX | 312 | No | UVB | Weak UVB absorber. Large molecule (>6000 daltons) |
| Uvasorb HEB | 312 | No | UVB | Some consider as best UVB filter |
| Univil T 150 | 314 | No | UVB | Some consider as the second best UVB filter |
| Oxybenzone | 288,325 | Yes | UVA/UVB | Photolabile. Most common sunscreen photoallergen |
| Sulisobenzone | 366 | Yes | UVA/UVB | Rarely used |
| Dioxybenzone | 352 | Yes | UVA/UVB | Rarely used |
| Meradimate | 340 | Yes | UVA | Rarely used |
| Avobenzone | 357 | Yes | UVA | UVA-1 filter. Combine with others for photostability |
| Ecamsule | 345 | Yes | UVA | Photostabile. UVA absorption > benzophenones |
| Univil A Plus | 354 | No | UVA | UVA-1 filter. Photostability > avobenzone |
| Neo Helioplan AT | 334 | No | UVA | Water-soluble. Synergy with oil-phase sunscreens |
| Silatriazole | 303,344 | No | UVA/UVB | First broad-spectrum UVA/UVB photostable filter |
| Bisoctriazole | 303,344 | No | UVA/UVB | Photostable. Has inorganic and organic properties |
| Bimotrizinol | 305,360 | No | UVA/UVB | Photostable UVA/UVB filter |
| Zinc oxide | | Yes | UVA/UVB | Micronized form attenuates UVA-1 > titanium dioxide |
| Titanium dioxide | | Yes | UVA/UVB | Micronized form attenuates UVB > zinc oxide |

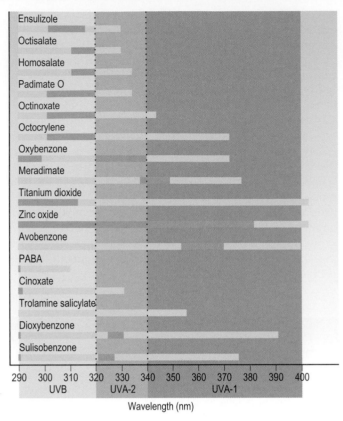

**Figure 9.1** Absorption spectra of UV filters listed in the FDA sunscreen monograph. Avobenzone is the only agent listed with an effective absorption peak within the long wavelength UVA-1 range. Modified from Diffey et al.[26]

## Organic UVB filters

### Para-aminobenzoic acid

Para-aminobenzoic acid (PABA) is an organic UV filter with a maximal absorbance within the UVB spectrum at a wavelength of 283 nm.[3] PABA is an effective UVB absorber and its high substantivity makes it durable in the face of friction and moisture.[1] However, it is now rarely used for three main reasons. First, it has the unpleasant ability to stain clothing. Second, PABA has the potential to invoke allergic contact and photoallergic dermatitis. Last, there is in-vitro evidence implicating PABA as a carcinogen, although in-vivo confirmation of this finding is lacking.[3]

### Padimate O

Another organic UV filter within the UVB spectrum is padimate O, which absorbs maximally at a wavelength of 311 nm.[3] This PABA derivative is less likely to stain clothing or result in contact hypersensitivity, but is less effective as a UV filter than its parent compound, PABA.[1] Of the PABA derivatives, padimate O is currently the most commonly used, although overall it is rarely incorporated into commercial sunscreens.

### Octinoxate

Octinoxate, a cinnamate, is the most commonly used UVB filter in the United States and has a maximum absorbance of 311 nm.[3] The agent is photolabile. Moreover, as a weak

UVB absorber, it must be combined with other UV filters in order to achieve an adequate SPF.[3] As a cinnamate, there is the potential for cross-reactivity with cocoa leaves and cinnamon-containing compounds, resulting in allergic contact dermatitis in sensitized individuals.[1] Octinoxate and other cinnamates may also contribute to a greasy sensation when applied to the skin, due to their composition of polar oils.[9] Octinoxate has the advantage of being the most widely studied sunscreen in regards to protection against photocarcinogenesis, and in general has an excellent safety profile.[10]

### Cinoxate

Another cinnamate derivative, cinoxate, absorbs maximally within the UVB range at 289 nm.[3] As a cinnamate, it shares many of the drawbacks of octinoxate. Currently, the agent is rarely used.

### Salicylates

Salicylates are commonly incorporated into sunscreen products. *Octisalate* absorbs maximally at 307 nm, *homosalate* absorbs maximally at 306 nm, and *trolamine salicylate* absorbs within a range of 260–355 nm.[1,3] Photostability and high substantivity confer advantages on the salicylates, and because of this high substantivity they are often incorporated into water-resistant products.[1] However, because of their narrow absorbance spectrum, higher concentrations are required to increase their potency as UVB absorbers.[1,3] Combining these agents with other UV filters can compensate for the lower UVB absorbance of the individual agents.[1] Trolamine salicylate is unique in that it is often used as a UV filter in hair cosmetics.[11] Combining photostable salicylates with photolabile agents such as oxybenzone or avobenzone can increase the photostability of the latter agents.[3]

### Octocrylene

Octocrylene is a UVB filter with a maximum absorbance of 303 nm.[3] Poor substantivity limits octocrylene as a sole UV filter, making it vulnerable to conditions such as friction and moisture.[1] Yet, octocrylene, because of its photostability, has been commonly used in recent years since the development of the UVA filter avobenzone. The ability to photostabilize avobenzone is the major advantage of octocrylene.[10]

### Ensulizole

The peak absorption of the UVB filter ensulizole is 310 nm with a range of 290–320 nm.[1,3] Ensulizole is water-soluble, lending to aesthetically pleasing features when applied to the skin. As such, the agent is currently popular as a component of cosmetic moisturizers.[1]

### Other UVB filters

Several UVB filters are available in Europe and other countries but are not listed in the current FDA monograph. These agents include camphor derivatives, which are the second most popular UVB filters in Europe.[12] Another agent, benxyledene malonate polysiloxane (Parsol SLX), is a large molecule at greater than 6000 daltons in size, thereby increasing safety by minimizing percutaneous absorption. However, benxyledene malonate polysiloxane only weakly absorbs UVB. Diethylhexyl butamido triazone (Uvasorb HEB) is an agent with maximum absorption at 312nm, which many consider to be the best UVB filter. Another UVB filter, ethylhexyl triazone (Univil T 150), absorbs maximally at 314nm, but is less soluble than diethylhexyl butamido triazone.[8]

## Organic UVA filters

Protection from UVB has traditionally been the focus of photoprotection and sunscreen development. This bias towards UVB is reflected in the SPF rating currently used in sunscreen assessment and labeling in the United States. SPF is defined as the ratio of the minimal erythema dose (MED) of skin following application of $2\,mg/cm^2$ of sunscreen divided by the MED of unprotected skin. Although SPF provides good assessment of a sunscreen's ability to protect against UVB, it is less indicative of the protection against UVA, which is 1000 times less erythemogenic.[5]

In recent years, the biological effects of UVA have been better elucidated. UVA reaches the Earth's surface at an intensity nearly 20-times that of UVB, penetrates window glass, penetrates more deeply into the mid dermis, and contributes to photocarcinogenesis, photoimmunosuppression, and photoaging.[13] This accumulating knowledge underscores the importance of incorporating effective UVA filters along with UVB filters in order to provide optimal broad-spectrum photoprotection. In 2007, amendments to the 1999 FDA sunscreen monograph were proposed. Among these proposals is a new standardized four-star grading system for UVA protection corresponding to low, medium, high, and highest protection based upon in-vitro and in-vivo assessments.[8]

### Benzophenones

Oxybenzone, sulisobenzone, and dioxybenzone comprise a class of UVA filters known as the benzophenones. Sulisobenzone and dioxybenzone are used rarely compared to oxybenzone, which is commonly incorporated into sunscreen products.[1] Oxybenzone has an absorption spectrum through the UVB and UVA-2 wavelengths, with two peak absorbances at 288nm and 325nm.[3] The main drawbacks of oxybenzone are photolability and its status as the most common cause of contact photoallergy among the sunscreens.[12]

### Meradimate

An overall weak UVA filter, meradimate absorbs at a peak wavelength within the UVA-2 range at 340nm. Currently, meradimate is infrequently used.[3]

### Avobenzone

Avobenzone is a UVA filter with a broad absorbance spectrum ranging between 310 and 400nm.[1] The peak absorption of avobenzone within the UVA-1 range at 357nm makes this agent a valuable contributor to broad-spectrum photoprotection.[14] In the United States, this is currently the only UV filter approved by the FDA with a peak absorbance at the UVA-1 spectrum. However, avobenzone is inherently photolabile, which in past years limited its use. Today, several agents can be combined with avobenzone to increase its photostability. These include photostable UV filters (octocrylene, salicylates and oxybenzone) and non-UV filters (diethylhexyl 2,6-naphthalate, oxynex ST, caprylyl glycol).[8] The development of photostabilized avobenzone was a major advancement

in providing adequate protection against longwave UVA. Evidence based on in-vitro studies suggests that sunscreens containing combinations of avobenzone and octocrylene currently provide the most effective UVA protection among available products in the United States.[15]

### Ecamsule

Ecamsule is the most recently introduced sunscreen agent in the United States; it is approved as an active ingredient of specific sunscreen products, with the first one reaching the US market in 2006. The absorbance spectrum for ecamsule ranges from 290 to 390nm with a peak absorption of 345nm. Unlike avobenzone, this agent is intrinsically photostable, and compared to the benzophenones, is a more efficient UVA filter.[14]

### Other UVA filters

Several UVA filters are available worldwide but are not approved for current use in the United States. One such agent, diethylamino hydroxybenzoyl hexylbenzoate (Univil A Plus), is similar to avobenzone in that it absorbs maximally at 354nm, in the UVA-1 spectrum. However, compared to avobenzone this agent has superior photostability.[16] Another filter, disodium phenyl dibenzimidazole tetrasulfonate (Neo Helipan AT), absorbs maximally within the UVA spectrum, with a peak absorption at 334nm.[16]

## Broad-spectrum UVA and UVB filters

New broad-spectrum UVA and UVB filters also exist, but are not yet available in the United States. Silatriazole (Mexoryl XL) is a broad-spectrum photostable filter with absorbance peaks in both the UVB and UVA range at 303nm and 344nm.[3] Silatriazole is the first broad-spectrum photostable filter.[5] Bisoctriazole (Tinosorb M) and bemotrizinol (Tinosorb S) are sunscreen agents currently available in many parts of the world, and are in the process of undergoing United States approval via the FDA Time and Extend Application (TEA) process. The TEA process, enacted in 2002, allows the consideration of data generated in foreign countries for the approval process.[17] Bisoctriazole (absorption peaks: 303nm and 344nm) and bemotrizinol (absorption peaks: 305nm and 360nm) are photostable agents with both UVA and UVB coverage.[8] Bisoctriazole is the first agent specifically designed to include both inorganic and organic properties.[8]

## Inorganic sunscreens

Zinc oxide and titanium dioxide are the inorganic sunscreens included in the most recent FDA monograph. These agents afford protection in the ranges of visible light, UVA and UVB, but as large molecules are cosmetically unappealing. They tend to leave a conspicuous white color when applied to the skin, may stain clothes, and can be comedogenic.[1,5] More elegant cosmetic formulations consisting of microfine particles have been developed and are now more commonly used. As the particle size of inorganic agents is decreased, a shift occurs protecting against shorter wavelengths.[14] Microfine zinc oxide attenuates most effectively in the UVA-1 spectrum within a range of 340nm to 400nm, and a peak at 380nm. Microfine titanium dioxide attenuates more effectively in the UVB and UVA-2 spectrum between 320 nm and 340 nm.[8] Zinc oxide is more cosmetically acceptable, as a lower refractive index results in a less opaque appearance.[12] Overall, these inorganic agents are considered less efficient at protecting against UVR compared to the newer organic agents.[1]

## Measuring sunscreen efficacy

The critical measurement of sunscreen efficacy should be protection from development of subsequent skin cancer, but those studies are difficult to perform. Surrogate endpoints are typically used. UVB protection is typically measured using a sun protection factor (SPF), which measures the ratio of time to sunburning with and without the use of the sunscreen being tested.[18] SPF measurements are consistent across different skin types.[19] However, SPF degrades after application by about 55% at 8 hours when the participants perform activities and by 25% when at indoor rest.[20] Sunscreens with an SPF of 30 or higher are typically recommended for adequate UVB protection.[21]

The measurement of UVA protection is less straightforward. Because the endpoint of sunburning from UVA alone at energy levels achieved in natural sunlight is difficult to attain, the in-vivo methods proposed either use artificial increased UVA intensity, increase skin sensitivity to UVA, use other endpoints besides sunburning or use in-vitro methodology. Each approach has advantages and disadvantages in measuring efficacy; all have the disadvantage of not measuring protection in an actual usage environment (Table 9.2).

The FDA has been evaluating sunscreen labeling since 1978 and is currently considering new labeling regulations to include both UVB and UVA levels. A cap on SPF of 50+ has been proposed for the labeling but higher levels of protection may be more effective in certain high UV environments.[27] UVA labeling would be derived from a combination of in-vivo and in-vitro methods. This system may be modified in response to concerns raised related to difficulty in reaching the highest level of UVA protection using currently available sunscreen agents.[28]

## Sunscreen application

In spite of continued advancement in the development of sunscreens, patient adherence and proper application are perhaps the most essential factors if sunscreens are to be effective. A given sunscreen may have a high SPF, protect against a broad spectrum of UVR, and be cosmetically elegant, but if used improperly, will not be effective. The ability of a sunscreen to filter UV is non-linear. A sunscreen with SPF 15 filters 94% of UVB, and SPF 30 filters 97%, with only marginal percent increases thereafter as the SPF increases above 30.[3] When determining the SPF, a standard application of 2 mg/cm$^2$ is used. However, in practical use, patients often apply a lesser amount, resulting in an effective SPF that may attain only 20–50% of the labeled SPF.[29] Therefore, patients should be encouraged to apply sunscreen generously and evenly. One ounce (the amount of sunscreen required to fill a shot glass) has been recommended as a helpful indicator of adequate full body coverage.[1] In anticipation of possible

| Table 9.2 Comparison of Techniques to Evaluate UVA Protection in Sunscreens | | | | |
|---|---|---|---|---|
| **Method** | **Type** | **Measure** | **Advantages** | **Disadvantages** |
| UVA from high-intensity solar simulator (PFA)[22] | In vivo | Biologic endpoint minimal erythema or tanning at 24 hours | All skin types, stable endpoint 2–24 hours | 1) Not tested at typical UVA intensity found in natural sunlight.<br>2) Larger role for UVA-2 (320–340 nm).<br>3) More powerful UVA source and longer exposures needed.<br>4) Uses human subjects |
| Skin sensitization with 8-methoxypsoralen[23] | In vivo | Subjects exposed to UVA-only component of sunlight and time to sunburning with and without sunscreen compared | In-vivo test | 1) Not tested at typical UVA intensity found in natural sunlight.<br>2) Uses human subjects |
| Immediate pigment darkening[24] | In vivo | Measures effects of 310–400 nm exposure by the development of blue-grey color that occurs and fades in minutes with and without sunscreen | Single visit, short exposure | 1) Transient endpoint.<br>2) Only works in skin types IV and V.<br>3) Uses human subjects |
| Persistent pigmented darkening[25] | In vivo | Measures dose of UVA to produce minimal persistent pigment darkening at 2–24 hours from 320 to 400 nm due to formation of epidermal melanin with and without sunscreen | Stable endpoint 2–24 hours, works for skin types II to V | 1) Only works in certain skin types.<br>2) More powerful UVA source and longer exposure needed.<br>3) Uses human subjects |
| Critical wavelength[26] | In vitro | Evaluation area under the UVA absorption spectrum curve of sunscreen agent and determining the wavelength where 90% of the area is associated with lower wavelengths. In general, higher number is better | Does not require exposure to high dose non-terrestrial UV light | 1) Water resistance cannot be measured.<br>2) Skin–sunscreen interaction not evaluated.<br>3) May not reflect photo-immunosuppression.<br>4) Higher value may have lower protection. |

under-application, it may be prudent to recommend use of sunscreen with an SPF of 30 or greater in order to maximize the effective SPF. However, a fine balance must be achieved between maximizing the effectiveness of a sunscreen and provoking non-compliance, as patients may be less likely to consistently use higher SPF sunscreens, which may feel thick or sticky.[30]

The frequent reapplication of sunscreen is another important factor to maintain the efficacy of sunscreen agents. The FDA defines a 'water-resistant' sunscreen as maintaining the SPF after 40 minutes of water immersion, and 'very water-resistant' as the ability to maintain the SPF after 80 minutes of immersion. However, using a towel to dry off the skin after water immersion can remove up to 85% of the sunscreen by friction, so reapplication after water immersion is important in spite of a sunscreen's 'waterproof' or water-resistant claims.[31] In general, sunscreen should be applied 20 minutes prior to initial sun exposure, reapplied initially 20 minutes later, and then reapplied every 2–3 hours while outside.[3]

## Protection from visible light and infrared radiation photodamage

The effects of UVR on the skin are well documented. However, until recently, the effects of radiation in the visible and infrared spectra were unknown. New and emerging data continue to elucidate the biologic effects of both visible light and infrared radiation (IR).

Visible light corresponds to wavelengths between 400 and 700 nm.[32] Visible light has been found to induce skin pigmentation and erythema, exacerbate photodermatoses, and produce reactive oxygen species with the potential for DNA damage.[32] The role visible light may play in skin cancer development is currently unknown. Current sunscreens offer little protection against visible light although antioxidants may partially protect from the damage associated with reactive oxygen species. Only inorganic, non-micronized sunscreens such as titanium dioxide and zinc oxide are able to attenuate visible light effectively, but these agents are not aesthetically elegant due to their white color.[32]

IR comprises wavelengths between 760 nm and 1 mm.[33] As the greatest component of solar radiation (54%), the skin is exposed to a substantial amount of IR.[34] Recent research suggests that IR likely contributes to photoaging, is potentially carcinogenic, and on a molecular level induces dermal matrix metalloproteinases.[33,35] Topical antioxidants, specifically those directed towards the mitochondria, may be beneficial, although more studies are needed to determine optimal use of this approach.[34]

## Sunscreens and skin cancer prevention

Multiple studies have been performed investigating the efficacy of sunscreen use in the prevention of the development of skin cancer. Sunscreen use has been demonstrated to decrease the number of existing actinic keratoses, while also decreasing the accumulation of new actinic keratoses.[36–38]

In a large, 4.5-year, randomized controlled trial performed in Australia, patients randomized to daily use of SPF 16 sunscreen developed significantly fewer squamous cell carcinomas (SCC), but without a significant effect on the development of basal cell carcinomas (BCC).[39] During an 8-year follow-up of those same study participants, SCC development was reduced by nearly 40%.[40] For BCC, the numbers trended downward (a decrease of 25%) during the extended follow-up period, but no statistical significance was seen.[40]

The relationship between sunscreen use and melanoma has been a source of controversy in the past. This controversy stemmed from the conflicting results of several case–control studies, many of which determined that sunscreen use correlated with a higher risk of melanoma, while other studies found no relationship or a decreased risk of melanoma.[41] A meta-analysis of 11 case–control studies, including over 9000 patients, found no increased risk of melanoma in relation to sunscreen use.[42] Furthermore, a quantitative review of all studies pertaining to melanoma and sunscreen use published from 1966 to 2003 also found no overall association between melanoma and sunscreen use.[43] Although the efficacy of sunscreen use in preventing melanoma remains unclear, physicians and patients can be reassured that sunscreen use does not appear to increase one's melanoma risk. Significant numbers of melanomas might be avoided by regular sunscreen use during recreational summer sun exposure, and with them appreciable financial, social and emotional costs, even for very modest estimates of the benefit of broad-spectrum sunscreens.[44] Despite the lack of evidence demonstrating the efficacy of modern sunscreens in preventing melanoma, it is argued that it would be irresponsible not to encourage their use, along with other sun protection strategies, as a means of combating the year-on-year rise in melanoma incidence.

## ADJUNCTIVE PHOTOPROTECTION

Sunscreen application should not be used as the sole defense against UVR. Rather, it should be used in conjunction with other important photoprotective measures, which include seeking shade, the use of photoprotective clothing and hats, and wearing sunglasses.

## Seeking shade

In addition to applying sunscreens and donning photoprotective clothing, using shade to minimize one's sun exposure is an important component of a complete photoprotective strategy. Complete avoidance of sunlight is an unrealistic and impractical expectation. A more attainable goal is to minimize sun exposure during peak UVB hours from 10 a.m. to 4 p.m.[3] When one's shadow is shorter than one's height, UV intensity is likely at its peak and individuals should use added caution with regard to sun exposure.[29]

When avoiding the midday sun is inescapable, as is often the case for outdoor workers, the availability and use of shade structures is recommended. In some cases, shade can attenuate UVR by 50–95%.[12] However, not all shade structures are equally effective. Studies have demonstrated that shade provided by trees often allows penetration of large amounts of UVR.[45] Trees with thicker foliage are generally thought to be more effective at attenuating sunlight. Various public shade structures may allow for the development of UV-induced erythema in relatively short time periods.[46] Moreover, even in the shade, it has been estimated that one can still be exposed to approximately 50% of UVA from sunlight.[3] Therefore, while seeking shade is an important photoprotective strategy, one should not overestimate the level of protection that it provides. Even in shaded areas, other photoprotective measures should be undertaken.

## Photoprotective clothing

The photoprotective effect of clothing is immediately evident and intuitive in both clinical and everyday experience. A clinician examining a patient with a photodermatosis such as polymorphous light eruption may note that the eruption is most evident on sun-exposed areas while sparing covered skin. Signs of chronic photodamage, including wrinkles and solar lentigines, are most pronounced on photoexposed skin, whereas skin covered by clothing may have notably less photodamage. The photoprotective ability of clothing is also immediately evident to a layperson who experiences a 'farmer's tan' with prominent pigmentation cut-offs between exposed skin and covered skin.[47] Therefore, the use of photoprotective clothing is clearly an important component of photoprotection.

The photoprotective ability of clothing is quantified and measured by the UV protection factor (UPF). The UPF is analogous to the SPF measure of sunscreens, and is similarly biased towards a measure of UVB protection given that prevention of erythema is one of the primary measurements used in its calculation.[3] Moreover, fabrics are inherently more capable of blocking UVB and less efficient at blocking UVA.[3] All clothing items are not created equal, however, and it is important for both clinicians and the public to be aware of factors that affect the UPF of a given clothing article (Fig. 9.2).

The tightness of a fabric's weave is one of the strongest determinants of UPF. Tighter weaves allow less penetration of UVR.[1] Washing clothing can shrink the gaps in the fabric fibers, thereby increasing the UPF. Wearing wet clothing increases those gaps and decreases the UPF; furthermore, the presence of water on the clothing enhances penetration of UV.[48] Tight-fitting clothing tends to be stretched, hence increasing the porosity of the fabric. Therefore, clothing that fits more loosely offers more photoprotection.[3]

The type of fabric also impacts the UPF. Polyester offers the greatest protection, followed by wool, silk and nylon, whereas cottons and rayon offer the least protection.[49] Elastic materials allow more UVR penetration when they are stretched.[3] Obviously, clothing items which cover a greater body surface area will be more protective.

Different fabric colors offer different levels of photoprotection. Darker colors absorb more UVR than lighter colors, and a given white fabric has an estimated UPF of 22 whereas a given black fabric has a UPF of 257.[48] As white has the ability to scatter and reflect light, 'off-white' or 'oatmeal' colored items may have an even lower UPF of 6, since the ability to scatter and reflect is not as great.[48] In general, the type of fabric and the tightness of its weave are greater determinants of a fabric's photoprotective ability than the color.

Chemical additives can be added to clothing to enhance its UPF. These additives include optical whitening agents that convert incident UV to visible blue light, which is reflected, hence giving the fabric a brighter appearance.[48] Similarly, bleaching of white fabrics to make them brighter can increase the UPF. UV-absorbing chemicals can also be added during laundering of clothing.[3]

A wide-brimmed hat is one specific article of clothing important in a photoprotective strategy. Human hair has a measured UPF ranging from only 5 to 17 in direct sunlight, so use of a hat to protect the scalp is beneficial.[50] The shade provided by a wide-brimmed hat (7.5 cm or greater) imparts an SPF of 7 for the nose, 3 for the cheeks, 5 for the neck, and 2 for the chin. A medium-brimmed hat (2.5–7.5 cm) provides less protection and does not impact the amount of UVR reaching the chin.[3]

Photoprotective clothing has both strengths and weaknesses compared to the use of sunscreen. Applying an article of clothing is often more convenient than applying sunscreen, especially as sunscreen needs to be reapplied in order to maintain its efficacy. Moreover, most individuals do not apply adequate amounts of sunscreen, and this drawback is clearly avoidable with application of a clothing item.[47] Yet, the use of adequate photoprotective clothing may be uncomfortably warm during hot seasons or during participation in sporting activities. These strengths and weaknesses highlight the importance of using photoprotective clothing as part of a broader photoprotection strategy.

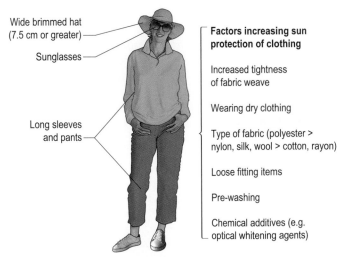

Wide brimmed hat
(7.5 cm or greater)

Sunglasses

Long sleeves
and pants

**Factors increasing sun
protection of clothing**

Increased tightness
of fabric weave

Wearing dry clothing

Type of fabric (polyester >
nylon, silk, wool > cotton, rayon)

Loose fitting items

Pre-washing

Chemical additives (e.g.
optical whitening agents)

**Figure 9.2** Ideal photoprotective clothing. The ultraviolet protection factor (UPF) indicates the efficacy of photoprotection from a clothing item and varies based on several factors listed here.

## Sunglasses

Sun exposure can also cause damaging effects to the eyes. Acute exposure to excessive amounts of UVR may result in photokeratitis, photoconjunctivitis, or even transient visual loss.[10,51] Chronic UVR exposure to the eye can invoke pterygium formation, cataracts, and squamous neoplasia of the ocular surface.[51] Although less well defined, chronic UVR exposure may also play a role in age-related macular degeneration and ocular melanoma.[51] Yet, general knowledge of these potential ill effects is lacking in the general public and current compliance in wearing sunglasses remains inadequate.[52]

Just as sunscreen application and other strategies are recommended to protect the skin from the sun's harmful effects, the use of sunglasses is recommended to protect the eyes. The sunglass standard implemented by the American National Standards Institute (ANSI) was last revised in 2001 and divides sunglasses into three categories.[53] Cosmetic sunglasses offer little protection from glare or UVR.[53] General purpose sunglasses function primarily in glare reduction but are required to minimize transmission of wavelengths below 310 nm to less than 1%.[53] The final category, special purpose sunglasses, is indicated for outdoor activities such as skiing or beach events.[53] However, in the United States, these standards are currently voluntary, so sunglass manufacturers are not required to comply with the recommendations. UV-absorbing contact lenses are also available, but given the minimal surface area covered, one should still wear sunglasses during prolonged or intense episodes of sun exposure.[54]

## Oral preparations

Polypodium leucotomos (PL) has been used for the treatment of inflammatory diseases and has shown some in-vitro and in-vivo immunomodulating properties. Twenty-one healthy volunteers (either untreated or treated with oral psoralens [8-MOP or 5-MOP]) were exposed to solar radiation for evaluation of immediate pigment darkening (IPD), minimal erythema dose (MED), minimal melanogenic dose, and minimal phototoxic dose (MPD) before and after topical or oral administration. PL was found to be photoprotective after topical application as well as oral administration. PL increased the UV dose required for IPD (P<0.01), MED (P<0.001) and MPD (P<0.001). After oral administration of PL, MED increased $2.8 \pm 0.59$ times and MPD increased $2.75 \pm 0.5$ and $6.8 \pm 1.3$ times depending upon the type of psoralen used.[55] PL may prevent UVA-induced skin photodamage possibly by preventing UVA-dependent mitochondrial DNA damage.[56] Larger studies are needed to characterize the role of PL in photoaging and skin cancer prevention.

## FUTURE OUTLOOK

The research of sunscreen products and formulation is ongoing, resulting in the development of new sunscreen technologies which may be available in the United States in the years to come. One such technology, SunSphere, consists of water-containing styrene/acrylate spheres which may be incorporated into sunscreen products to augment the SPF.[16] Once the water migrates out of the spheres, the resulting hollow beads scatter UVR at the skin surface, thereby increasing the likelihood that UVR will contact the active UV filters.[16] Another new development is the ability to encapsulate UV filters within microscopic silica glass spheres. This microencapsulation may minimize contact hypersensitivity by limiting direct skin contact with a given agent, while also allowing for the combination of previously incompatible filters by quarantining the agents to individual compartments.[16] The increasing knowledge of the effects of wavelengths beyond UV may also impact the development of future photoprotective technologies.

Newer, more effective and relevant methods of measuring sunscreen efficacy will also be developed. Biologic measures such as p53 expression,[57] chemical measures such as free radical generation,[58] and immunologic approaches that measure decreased UV-related immunosuppression during sunscreen use[59] are being evaluated. Combining all of these approaches (Integrated Protection Factor) is also being analyzed.[60]

## REFERENCES

1. Palm MD, O'Donoghue MN. Update on photoprotection. *Dermatol Ther.* 2007;20(5):360–376.
2. Scherschun L, Lim HW. Photoprotection by sunscreens. *Am J Clin Dermatol.* 2001;2(3):131–134.
3. Kullavanijaya P, Lim HW. Photoprotection. *J Am Acad Dermatol.* 2005;52(6):937–958 quiz 959–962.
4. Roelandts R. History of photoprotection. In: Lim HW, Draelos ZD, eds. *Clinical Guide to Sunscreens and Photoprotection.* New York, NY: Informa Healthcare; 2009:1–10.
5. Antoniou C, Kosmadaki M, Stratigos A, et al. Sunscreens - what's important to know. *J Eur Acad Dermatol Venereol.* 2008;22(9):1110–1118.
6. Osterwalder U, Herzog B. Chemistry and properties of organic and inorganic UV filters. In: Lim HW, Draelos ZD, eds. *Clinical Guide to Sunscreens and Photoprotection.* New York, NY: Informa Healthcare; 2009:11–38.
7. Kollias N. The absorption properties of "physical" sunscreens. *Arch Dermatol.* 1999;135(2):209–210.
8. Hexsel CL, Bangert SD, Hebert AA, et al. Current sunscreen issues: 2007 Food and Drug Administration sunscreen labelling recommendations and combination sunscreen/insect repellent products. *J Am Acad Dermatol.* 2008;59(2):316–323.
9. Tanner PR. Sunscreen product formulation. *Dermatol Clin.* 2006;24(1):53–62.
10. Nash J. Human safety and efficacy of ultraviolet filters and sunscreen products. *Dermatol Clin.* 2006;24(1):35–51.
11. González S, Fernández-Lorente M, Gilaberte-Calzada Y. The latest on skin photoprotection. *Clin Dermatol.* 2008;26(6):614–626.
12. Lautenschlager S, Wulf HC, Pittelkow MR. Photoprotection. *Lancet.* 2007;370(9586):528–537.
13. Lim HW, Naylor M, Hönigsmann H, et al. American Academy of Dermatology Consensus Conference on UVA protection of sunscreens: summary and recommendations. *J Am Acad Dermatol.* 2001;44(3):505–508.
14. Lim HW, Rigel DS. UVA: grasping a better understanding of this formidable opponent. *Skin Aging.* 2007;15(7):62.
15. Wang SQ, Stanfield JW, Osterwalder U. In vitro assessments of UVA protection by popular sunscreens available in the United States. *J Am Acad Dermatol.* 2008;59(6):934–942.
16. Tuchinda C, Lim HW, Osterwalder U, et al. Novel emerging sunscreen technologies. *Dermatol Clin.* 2006;24(1):105–117.
17. Department of Health and Human Services, Food and Drug Administration. Additional criteria and procedures for classifying over-the-counter drugs as generally recognized as safe and effective and not misbranded. *Fed Regist.* 2002;67(3060).
18. Sayre RM, Desrochers DL, Marlowe E, et al. The correlation of indoor solar simulator and natural sunlight: testing of a sunscreen preparation. *Arch Dermatol.* 1978;114(11):1649–1651.
19. Kim SM, Oh BH, Lee YW, et al. The relation between the amount of sunscreen applied and the sun protection factor in Asian skin. *J Am Acad Dermatol.* 2010;62(2):218–222.
20. Beyer DM, Faurschou A, Philipsen PA, et al. Sun protection factor persistence on human skin during a day without physical activity or ultraviolet exposure. *Photodermatol Photoimmunol Photomed.* 2010;26(1):22–27.
21. American Academy of Dermatology. Position statement on broad spectrum protection of sunscreen products. 2009. http://www.aad.org/forms/policies/Uploads/PS/PS-Broad-Spectrum%20Protection%20of%20Sunscreen%20Products%2011-16-09.pdf>. Accessed 14.03.10.
22. Cole C, VanFossen R. Measurement of sunscreen UVA protection: an unsensitized human model. *J Am Acad Dermatol.* 1992;26(2 Pt 1):178–184.
23. Lowe NJ, Dromgoole SH, Sefton J, et al. Indoor and outdoor efficacy testing of a broad-spectrum sunscreen against ultraviolet A radiation in psoralen-sensitized subjects. *J Am Acad Dermatol.* 1987;17(2 Pt 1):224–230.
24. Kaidbey KH, Barnes A. Determination of UVA protection factors by means of immediate pigment darkening in normal skin. *J Am Acad Dermatol.* 1991;25(2 Pt 1):262–266.
25. Moyal D, Wichrowski K, Tricaud C. In vivo persistent pigment darkening method: a demonstration of the reproducibility of the UVA protection factors results at several testing laboratories. *Photodermatol Photoimmunol Photomed.* 2006;22(3):124–128.

26. Diffey BL, Tanner PR, Matts PJ, et al. In vitro assessment of the broad-spectrum ultraviolet protection of sunscreen products. *J Am Acad Dermatol.* 2000;43(6):1024–1035.

27. Russak JE, Chen T, Appa Y, et al. A comparison of sunburn protection of high-sun protection factor (SPF) sunscreens: SPF 85 sunscreen is significantly more protective than SPF 50. *J Am Acad Dermatol.* 2010;62(2):348–349.

28. Dueva-Koganov OV, Rocafort C, Orofino S, et al. Addressing technical challenges associated with the FDA's proposed rules for the UVA in vitro testing procedure. *J Cosmet Sci.* 2009;60(6):587–598.

29. Eide MJ, Weinstock MA. Public health challenges in sun protection. *Dermatol Clin.* 2006;24(1):119–124.

30. Draelos ZD. Compliance and sunscreens. *Dermatol Clin.* 2006;24(1):101–104.

31. Poh Agin P. Water resistance and extended wear sunscreens. *Dermatol Clin.* 2006;24(1):75–79.

32. Mahmoud BH, Hexsel CL, Hamzavi IH, et al. Effects of visible light on the skin. *Photochem Photobiol.* 2008;84(2):450–462.

33. Schieke SM, Schroeder P, Krutmann J. Cutaneous effects of infrared radiation: from clinical observations to molecular response mechanisms. *Photodermatol Photoimmunol Photomed.* 2003;19(5):228–234.

34. Schroeder P, Calles C, Krutmann J. Prevention of infrared-A radiation mediated detrimental effects in human skin. *Skin Therapy Lett.* 2009;14(5):4–5.

35. Cho S, Shin MH, Kim YK, et al. Effects of infrared radiation and heat on human skin aging in vivo. *J Investig Dermatol Symp Proc.* 2009;14(1):15–19.

36. Darlington S, Williams G, Neale R, et al. A randomized controlled trial to assess sunscreen application and beta carotene supplementation in the prevention of solar keratoses. *Arch Dermatol.* 2003;139(4):451–455.

37. Thompson SC, Jolley D, Marks R. Reduction of solar keratoses by regular sunscreen use. *N Engl J Med.* 1993;329(16):1147–1151.

38. Naylor M, Boyd A, Smith D, et al. High sun protection factor sunscreens in the suppression of actinic neoplasia. *Arch Dermatol.* 1995;131(2):170–175.

39. Green A, Williams G, Neale R, et al. Daily sunscreen application and beta-carotene supplementation in prevention of basal-cell and squamous-cell carcinomas of the skin: a randomised controlled trial. *Lancet.* 1999;354(9180):723–729.

40. van der Pols JC, Williams GM, Pandeya N, et al. Prolonged prevention of squamous cell carcinoma of the skin by regular sunscreen use. *Cancer Epidemiol Biomarkers Prev.* 2006;15(12):2546–2548.

41. Bigby M. The sunscreen and melanoma controversy. *Arch Dermatol.* 1999;135(12):1526–1527.

42. Huncharek M, Kupelnick B. Use of topical sunscreens and the risk of malignant melanoma: a meta-analysis of 9067 patients from 11 case-control studies. *Am J Public Health.* 2002;92(7):1173–1177.

43. Dennis LK, Beane Freeman LE, VanBeek MJ. Sunscreen use and the risk for melanoma: a quantitative review. *Ann Intern Med.* 2003;139(12):966–978.

44. Diffey BL. Sunscreens as a preventative measure in melanoma: an evidence-based approach or the precautionary principle? *Br J Dermatol.* 2009;161(suppl 3):25–27.

45. Turnbull DJ, Parisi AV. Effective shade structures. *Med J Aust.* 2006;184(1):13–15.

46. Turnbull D, Parisi A. Spectral UV in public shade settings. *J Photochem Photobiol.* 2003;69(1):13–19.

47. Hatch KL, Osterwalder U. Garments as solar ultraviolet radiation screening materials. *Dermatol Clin.* 2006;24(1):85–100.

48. Gies P. Photoprotection by clothing. *Photodermatol Photoimmunol Photomed.* 2007;23(6):264–274.

49. Crews P, Kachman S, Beyer A. Influences on UVR transmission of undyed woven fabrics. *Text Chem Color.* 1999;31(6):17–26.

50. Parisi AV, Smith D, Schouten P, et al. Solar ultraviolet protection provided by human head hair. *Photochem Photobiol.* 2009;85(1):250–254.

51. Oliva MS, Taylor HAC. Ultraviolet radiation and the eye. *Int Ophthalmol Clin.* 2005;45(1):1–17.

52. Pakrou N, Casson R, Fung S, et al. South Australian adolescent ophthalmic sun protective behaviours. *Eye.* 2006;22(6):808–814.

53. Tuchinda C, Srivannaboon S, Lim HW. Photoprotection by window glass, automobile glass, and sunglasses. *J Am Acad Dermatol.* 2006;54(5):845–854.

54. Giasson C.J.O.D., Quesnel N.M.O.D., Boisjoly H. The ABCs of ultraviolet-blocking contact lenses: an ocular panacea for ozone loss? *Int Ophthalmol Clin.* 2005;45(1):117–139.

55. González S, Pathak MA, Cuevas J, et al. Topical or oral administration with an extract of Polypodium leucotomos prevents acute sunburn and psoralen-induced phototoxic reactions as well as depletion of Langerhans cells in human skin. *Photodermatol Photoimmunol Photomed.* 1997;13(1–2):50–60.

56. Villa A, Viera MH, Amini S, et al. Decrease of ultraviolet A light–induced "common deletion" in healthy volunteers after oral Polypodium leucotomos extract supplement in a randomized clinical trial. *J Am Acad Dermatol.* 2010;62(3):511–513.

57. Seité S, Moyal D, Verdier MP, et al. Accumulated p53 protein and UVA protection level of sunscreens. *Photodermatol Photoimmunol Photomed.* 2000;16(1):3–9.

58. Herrling T, Jung K, Fuchs J. Measurements of UV-generated free radicals/reactive oxygen species (ROS) in skin. *Spectrochim Acta A Mol Biomol Spectrosc.* 2006;63(4):840–845.

59. Damian DL, Barnetson RS, Halliday GM. Measurement of in vivo sunscreen immune protection factors in humans. *Photochem Photobiol.* 1999;70(6):910–915.

60. Zastrow L, Ferrero L, Herrling T, et al. Integrated sun protection factor: a new sun protection factor based on free radicals generated by UV irradiation. *Skin Pharmacol Physiol.* 2004;17(5):219–231.

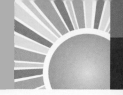

**PART 2:** Non-melanoma

# Actinic Keratoses and Other Precursors of Keratinocytic Cutaneous Malignancies

CHAPTER

# 10

*Christina L. Warner and Clay J. Cockerell*

## Key Points

- Actinic keratoses are common lesions representing an early stage in the development of invasive squamous cell carcinoma that require clinical management.

- Actinic keratoses serve as a marker of skin damage from ultraviolet light due to sun exposure.

- Bowen's disease and its variants are intraepithelial malignancies and should be removed or destroyed.

## INTRODUCTION

The recognition of risk factors, skin lesions and other conditions that predispose an individual to develop an invasive cutaneous epithelial malignancy is important as it may allow for the prevention of development of skin cancer. Patients who are predisposed to develop malignancy should be followed carefully so that cancers can be prevented or treated earlier. This chapter will focus primarily on the epidemiology, biology and classification of actinic or solar keratoses, which are the most common skin lesion associated with the development of cutaneous squamous cell carcinoma and, according to some individuals, basal cell carcinoma. Risk factors for developing cutaneous keratinocytic carcinomas, including genetic predisposition, inflammatory conditions, and environmental insults other than sun exposure, will also be discussed.

## ACTINIC KERATOSIS (SOLAR KERATOSIS)

### Definition

Actinic keratoses (AKs) are circumscribed, rough scaly lesions that develop on exposed skin surfaces and are primarily due to chronic ultraviolet irradiation that may result from sun exposure or exposure to artificial light sources such as tanning beds, ultraviolet light phototherapy, or photochemotherapy.[1,2] Similar lesions may develop following radiation from radioactive sources such as X-ray therapy. AKs were long considered in the past as premalignancies, but current thinking by most authors views these lesions as evolving squamous cell carcinoma (SCC) in situ in its earliest form.[3,4]

The term actinic keratosis (AK) was coined relatively recently. It was first used by Hermann Pinkus, and, in 1959, Becker included it in his publication on dermatological nomenclature. Historically, these lesions were recognized as a complication caused by longstanding sun exposure in seamen or farmers and were termed senile keratosis or keratosis senilis. The name was given neither because of the biology of the lesions nor because of the histopathology, but because of the rough texture that could be easily appreciated clinically. In fact, in many early textbooks, they were included in chapters with other scaly conditions often referred to as 'keratoses' such as keratodermas and keratoderma blenorrhagicum. The term solar keratosis was applied to these lesions later by Brownstein in an attempt to reflect that they are most commonly induced by sun exposure (although they can be induced by chronic exposure from artificial sources). In that the lesion is truly neoplastic, suggestions have been offered to change the name to one that more accurately reflects the acutal nature of the process rather than its clinical appearance.[3,5–8]

## Risk factors

The propensity to develop AKs is genetically influenced and those with fair skin (Fitzpatrick types I and II), blue eyes, and red or blonde hair have a markedly increased susceptibility.[8,9] Those with darker pigmentation are relatively protected, although when they become less pigmented, such as with vitiligo or albinism, AKs commonly develop. The predominant risk factor for the development of AKs is cumulative exposure to ultraviolet (UV) irradiation. Short-term, intense UV exposure also provides additional risk, although repeated long-term exposure is more important. Repeated consistent application of sunscreen has been shown to suppress the formation of AKs.[8]

Behaviors that increase cumulative UV exposure increase the risk of developing AKs, some of which include outdoor labor, leisure activities associated with sun exposure, and the use of artificial tanning beds.[2,8,9] The intensity of UV is greatest at latitudes closer to the equator and in areas of higher elevation, and therefore those who live in these areas are also at increased risk, especially if they have fair complexions. An important example of this can be seen in Australia and New Zealand, where the Caucasian population has the highest incidence of skin cancer and melanoma in the world.[10–12] More recently, ozone depletion, which permits a higher penetrance of UV irradiation to the Earth's surface, compounds this risk, even in temperate areas.[9] Finally, the increased longevity of the population also contributes to the increasing prevalence of AKs.

As noted above, cumulative lifetime UV irradiation is most important in the development of AKs and cutaneous SCC, with repeated sunburn playing a lesser role. This is thought to be the opposite of what is responsible for the development of basal cell carcinoma and melanoma, as intense intermittent exposures and severe sunburns in childhood are the most important risk factors.[13]

Immunosuppression is another independent risk factor for the development of cutaneous keratinocytic malignancies. The widespread use of immunosuppressive drugs for organ transplantation, in cancer therapy, and in the treatment of rheumatologic and other inflammatory diseases has led to a significant increase in the number of immunosuppressed patients, many of whom develop AKs and cutaneous malignancies. Often such patients have literally hundreds of lesions and cutaneous SCC is often the cause of death in these individuals. Furthermore, in immunosuppressed patients, human papillomavirus infection may be a synergistic factor in the development of AKs and SCC.[13] This relationship does not seem to hold true for immunocompetent patients, however.[14]

## Incidence and prevalence

The incidence of AK increases with age, with less than 10% of people affected in the third decade of life but 80% affected in the sixth decade.[9] Men tend to develop AKs at a younger age but the gender prevalence equalizes in the elderly population. As mentioned above, there is an inverse relationship between latitude and prevalence. For example, in Australia the prevalence of AKs in adults over 40 may be as high as 60%.[9]

## Clinical appearance

Clinically, AKs are skin-colored to reddish or yellowish brown, irregular macules or papules. They may be sharply demarcated but more commonly there is a gradual transformation from lesional to normal skin. In the elderly, multiple lesions can usually be appreciated. Although most lesions are less than 1 cm in size, sometimes large plaques may be seen (Fig. 10.1). AKs have a rough scaly texture resembling fine sandpaper and they can often be better recognized by palpation than by inspection (Fig. 10.2). Accumulation of the scale may lead to cutaneous horn formation (Fig. 10.3). Lesions develop on sun-exposed surfaces, most commonly the head and neck, and dorsal hands and forearms; however, they may occur on any area of the body that has been damaged by UV and lesions are now being recognized

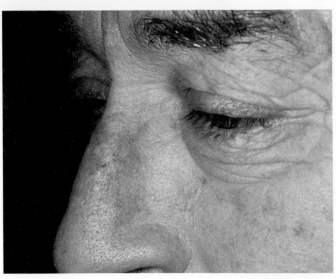

**Figure 10.2** Actinic keratosis. A scaly plaque on the bridge of the nose.

in traditionally sun-protected sites in those who frequent tanning parlors. The surrounding skin may show other evidence of sun exposure such as atrophy, pigmentary alterations and telagectasias. AKs are most often asymptomatic but patients may complain of mild irritation or pruritus.

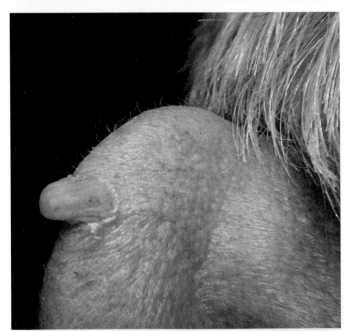

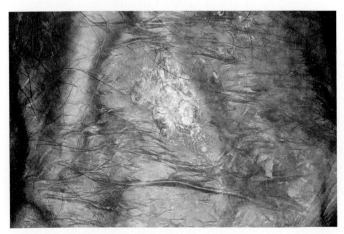

**Figure 10.1** Actinic keratosis. A large, scaly plaque on the dorsum of the hand.

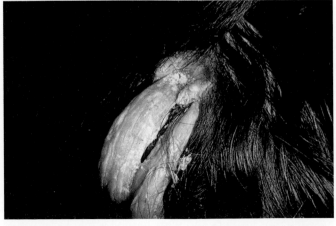

**Figure 10.3** Cutaneous horn. Biopsy of this lesion revealed an actinic keratosis.

Involvement of the lip is termed actinic chelitis. The center of the lower lip is most commonly affected and is manifest as slight thickening with scaling and crust that may be painful or associated with a burning sensation. When the entire lower lip is involved, the vermillion border becomes less distinct and small wrinkles appear perpendicular to the long axis of the lip. Solar or actinic cheilitis may evolve into SCC of the lip. These lesions have a higher risk of metastasis than SCC of glabrous skin, so it is very important to detect them as early as possible and treat them appropriately.[9] However, care should be taken to exclude verrucous candidiasis involving the lip, which can clinically mimic a squamous cell neoplasm.[15] Caution should be used whenever candidal hyphae are present in a biopsy specimen. Of course, candida may secondarily infect a carcinoma, so the patient should be closely followed and rebiopsied if the lesion persists after adequate antifungal therapy.

The development of SCC in situ in areas of actinic damage should be suspected when a thickened, sharply defined, persistent red scaly plaque, usually greater than 1 cm in diameter, is noted. When significant palpable thickening, nodules, induration, ulceration and/or bleeding develop, deeper involvement should be considered and a biopsy should be performed.

## Pathogenesis

By definition, AKs are caused by ultraviolet irradiation, especially UVB, which lies in the wavelengths between 290 and 320 nm. UVB leads to neoplastic transformation by inducing crosslinks in DNA molecules at sites of pyrimidines referred to as thymidine dimers. Mistakes of DNA enzyme-mediated repair of these crosslinks can lead to point mutations causing C to T or CC to TT transitions.[1] The importance of UV-induced DNA damage is well illustrated in patients with xeroderma pigmentosa who have inherited two defective copies of one of the DNA repair enzymes and therefore develop multiple cutaneous malignancies at an early age.

Mutations in the *p53* tumor suppressor gene, which normally halts the cell cycle to allow for DNA repair and induces cellular apoptosis in response to excessive DNA damage, are also present in AKs and SCCs. The overall incidence of *p53* mutations in AKs is greater than 50%,[8,9] and may be as high as 80% for AKs in Caucasians.[16] In SCCs, the incidence of *p53* mutations is similar but slightly higher, ranging from 69% to 90%.[16]

Some have proposed that UV-mediated inactivating mutations in *p53* are the most common 'first hit' in the development of AK, producing local immortalized clones of keratinocytes.[17] Indeed, chronically sun-exposed Caucasian skin has been shown to harbor as many as 30 to 40 *p53* clones per square centimeter.[17] Studies have shown that these clones vary in size from 60 (one stem cell unit) to 3000 and the size of these clones tends to be larger on skin that is chronically rather than intermittently sun-exposed. When skin is protected from the sun, clonal expansion is halted and clones may even regress.[17] It has been postulated that sun damage both incites immortalization of keratinocytes and then selects for *p53* clonal expansion by inducing apoptosis in adjacent normal stem cells, providing room for expansion without incurring additional mutations.[17] Despite this intriguing research, no definite 'second hit' has been identified that would allow these small immortalized clones to develop into larger clinically detectable AKs. The probability that any one of these clones will progress to an AK is very low, estimated at less than 1 in 300,000.[17]

In addition to causing DNA damage, sunlight exposure has also been shown to be immunosuppressive. Although the exact mechanisms of immunomodulation have not been elucidated, Langerhans cell numbers are decreased following sun exposure, which is a sign of local immunosuppression. UV light may play an additional role in the development of AK by inducing cutaneous immunosuppression, thereby interfering with normal immune system surveillance mechanisms that would identify and destroy abnormal cells.[8]

Finally, there are likely numerous possible genetic pathways in the development of AKs, as these lesions have a high degree of aneuploidy with loss of heterozygosity (LOH) commonly in 17p, 17q, 9p, and 9a.[8] AKs demonstrate higher rates of LOH than SCC, suggesting that the accumulation of additional genetic changes may impair clonal survival rather than promote progression.[17] It has been reported that clinically, some AKs may spontaneously regress.[8,9] While AK counts are notoriously difficult to perform and there is often significant interobserver variability, involution may occur via accumulation of additional genetic changes leading to clonal deletion or by immune rejection. Sun protection may increase the chances of an AK regressing, possibly due to improved efficacy of the immune response.

## Progression or transformation

The key genetic changes that allow transformation of AKs into invasive SCC are also not well established. Mutations in *p53* have been shown to be evenly distributed throughout this gene in AKs, but in squamous cell carcinomas *p53* mutations tend to be clustered in 'hot spots,' suggesting that certain mutations may be associated with more aggressive phenotypes.[9] Other possible associations with transformation include deletion of the 9p21 locus containing the *p16* tumor suppressor gene, activation of *ras*, and loss of an inflammatory response after invasion occurs.[1,13,17,18]

Once a clinically detectable AK has developed, the risk that an individual lesion will progress to invasive SCC is low. The majority of studies have found annual rates of transformation per lesion to be less than 0.1% per year or less than 1 in 1000.[17,19] However, as most patients have multiple lesions, over time the cumulative risk becomes more significant, and the longer a lesion remains untreated, the greater the risk. For an average patient with multiple AKs, the risk of developing an invasive SCC has been estimated to range from 10% in a 10-year period to as high as 14% in a 5-year period.[6,9,20] This risk is highest for immunocompromised patients. Although more than half of invasive SCCs on sun-damaged skin are found at sites where AK has been previously diagnosed clinically,[9] over 80–90% are found to have histopathologic evidence of associated AK.[6,9,20] Thus, some AKs associated with SCC are either too small to be clinically detected or may be overgrown by the SCC.[8]

**91**

Despite an individually low rate of transformation or progression to invasive SCC, AKs possess genetic changes that are identical to those found in SCC and are biologically considered to be intraepidermal carcinomas.[4,21,22] Their presence also serves as a sensitive indicator of excess UV exposure, thereby identifying a population at higher risk for the development not only of SCC, but also of basal cell carcinoma and melanoma. Therefore, all patients with AKs should be managed to prevent progression of individual lesions as well as to monitor for the development of other de-novo malignancies.

## Histopathology and classification schemes

Under the microscope, AKs demonstrate a broad range of histologic patterns. A number of variants have been described, including hypertrophic, atrophic, acantholytic, pigmented, lichenoid, and bowenoid.[5,8] All variants demonstrate keratinocyte atypia with disruption of normal maturation and loss of polarity, variation in cell size and shape, nuclear pleomorphism and hyperchromatism, and increased nuclear to cytoplasmic ratios. Atypical keratinocytes may also demonstrate prominent nucleoli, dyskeratosis (abnormal cornification and apoptosis of individual cells), and mitotic figures. Dermal solar elastosis, indicative of chronic actinic damage, is another characteristic feature.

The hypertrophic AK is the most common histologic variant and demonstrates parakeratosis and irregular acanthosis, sometimes interspersed with atrophic areas. Thinning or focal loss of the granular layer may be present. A common pattern of zones of parakeratosis that overlie areas of keratinocyte atypia alternating with zones of orthokeratosis that overlie an uninvolved sweat gland or hair follicle is called the 'flag sign'. Proliferation of the epidermis forming small tongues or buds is common but these are surrounded by intact basal lamina and remain contiguous to the epidermis. The atrophic variant lacks the hyperkeratosis and papillomatosis and often shows thinning of the epidermis in comparison to surrounding normal tissue. The epidermis may be only a few cell layers thick in cross-section. Acantholytic AKs demonstrate dyscohesion of keratinocytes within the epidermis, often appreciated within downward buds of keratinocytes. Pigmented AKs have increased melanin in the basal cell layer associated with slight keratinocytic atypia. Although many AKs demonstrate a slight infiltrate of lymphocytes in the superficial dermis, the lichenoid variant has features of AK with a denser band-like lymphohistiocytic infiltrate at the base of the epidermis with focal liquefactive degeneration of the basal cells resembling a benign lichenoid keratosis at low power. The bowenoid variant demonstrates keratinocytic atypia with somewhat larger-sized atypical cells and with areas that demonstrate focal full-thickness involvement of the epidermis with acanthosis, although sparing adnexal epithelium, thereby simulating SCC in situ although only in small foci.

With the exception of hyperplastic and perhaps bowenoid variants, which suggests a lesion that is evolving towards SCC, classifying actinic lesions into histologic variants does not convey significant information regarding biologic behavior. Cutaneous SCC, however, is a 'classical' neoplasm that proceeds through recognizable stages beginning in the epidermis in small foci and terminates in a lesion that involves the dermis with metastatic potential. Some authors have therefore proposed classification schemes for AKs that emphasize stages in progression towards SCC. Although it may be argued that creating a classification scheme to stratify these lesions creates artificial distinctions in a process that is really a continuum, such a schema may still be clinically useful to better predict behavior of individual lesions and allow enhanced patient management.

Goldberg et al. suggested dividing AKs into proliferative and non-proliferative lesions defined predominantly by histologic characteristics.[23] In this classification, proliferative AKs are ones that enlarge significantly over time, are often more than 1 cm in diameter, have a downward growth resembling an inverted Christmas tree, tend to involve hair follicles and sebaceous glands, and have an increased risk of progression. Berhane et al. proposed dividing lesions based on their clinical presentation into asymptomatic AKs, inflamed AKs, and SCC in situ.[18] They argued that inflamed AKs, recognized clinically as those with an erythematous halo that are tender to the touch, represent an inflammatory response to the process of transformation. They suggested that the inflammatory response would either lead to resolution of the lesion or subside allowing progression to SCC. They advocated that patients could be educated to watch for inflammation in an AK in order to detect carcinomas at their earliest stage. However, it has not been proven that all AKs that are progressing to SCC elicit an inflammatory response or that such responses will always be of sufficient severity and duration to be clinically noticeable.[8] A final problem with this classification scheme is its lack of correlation with histopathologic patterns.

Cockerell et al.[3,5-8] have proposed a three-tiered classification scheme termed keratinocytic intraepidermal neoplasia (KIN) which is similar to that used in grading cervical intraepithelial neoplasia (CIN). KIN I is defined as keratinocyte atypia confined to the bottom third of the epithelium with the basal and suprabasal cells showing some nuclear enlargement and hyperchromasia. Nuclei maintain their round or oval shape but show variation in size, mild nuclear outline irregularities, and small nucleoli. There is usually no overlying hyperkeratosis or parakeratosis. These subtle changes are best appreciated by comparing the abnormal nuclei to adjacent normal epidermis or to the uninvolved adnexal epithelium. KIN II is defined as atypia involving the lower two-thirds of the epidermis and the majority of clinically diagnosed AKs would fall into this category. Abnormal keratinocytes display more obvious nuclear enlargement, membrane irregularities, hyperchromasia, and prominent nucleoli. Increased numbers of mitotic figures are present. Alternating parakeratosis and orthokeratosis is common overlying adjacent zones of atypia and zones of more normal epidermis, respectively. Cockerell et al. further divided this second stage into KIN IIa, where the process lacks significant acanthosis and spares adnexal structures, and KIN IIb, where the atypical keratinocytes have involved adnexa, show significant acanthosis or budding of keratinocytes into the superficial papillary dermis, or demonstrate areas of acantholysis. KIN III represents carcinoma in situ with full-thickness atypia involving the epidermis and adnexal structures. This scheme has been shown to have a high degree of interobserver agreement and could allow for a considerable simplification in terminology. Although a uniform classification scheme could enhance communication between clinicians and pathologists, potentially improving patient care, the KIN nomenclature has not yet been generally adopted.

## Treatment and prevention

Treatment of AKs, though medically necessary, should be conservative. Counseling regarding the relationship of AK to excess sun exposure should be emphasized during office visits. Patients should be informed that the rate of AK development might be slowed with the use of photoprotection.

Options for therapy of AKs include chemotherapeutic agents, surgical procedures, and light-based treatments. Biopsy may be indicated if a lesion has not responded to more conservative therapy, if the dermatologic surgeon is concerned that a lesion may truly represent SCC, or if it is deemed that the cosmetic result warrants the procedure.

Cryosurgery with liquid nitrogen is the procedure performed most commonly by practicing dermatologists (Chapter 42). It is effective for most AKs but can produce dyspigmentation, especially in darker-skinned patients. The procedure is somewhat painful and results in a blister which generally heals within 5–7 days. Multiple lesions may be treated in an office visit but follow-up is indicated to ensure eradication. Another not widely utilized technique is to apply liquid nitrogen over a large area to peel the skin and treat subclinical lesions. Similarly, a chemodestructive peel using tri- or bichloracetic acid to individual lesions or a large area is effective but also is not commonly utilized.

When there is clinical suspicion that the lesion might be SCC, a common treatment is sharp curettage followed by electrodesiccation (Chapter 41). This also allows the physician to obtain biopsy material. Tissue removed can be submitted for histopathologic analysis. Although this form of treatment results in a cure in 99% of lesions, it may leave scarring at the site.

Photodynamic therapy (Chapter 45) may produce less dyspigmentation than cryotherapy. A photosensitizer, aminolevulinic acid (ALA) or methyl-aminolevulinic acid (m-ALA), is applied to the area to be treated. After approximately 12 hours incubation, the area is exposed to a specific frequency of visible light. The patient develops inflammation and over the next 7–10 days the area heals and the AKs are destroyed.

Topical chemotherapy (Chapter 43) was developed to be both a therapy and a preventative agent. Immune response modifiers have been shown by multiple studies to have efficacy in AK therapy.[24–26] Originally developed for treatment of genital warts, imiquimod has been used as a topical therapy. It is typically applied two times per week for up to 16 weeks. Salasche et al.[26] have demonstrated the effectiveness of imiquimod use in 4-week on and off cycles. As with 5-fluorouracil, imiquimod causes diffuse inflammation at both clinical and subclinical sites. These inflammations are a positive signal of therapy effectiveness. More recent studies have shown lower strengths (3.75%) of imiquimod used in cycle therapy (2 weeks on, 2 weeks off, 2 weeks on) to have better efficacy with lower levels of inflamatory response.[26a] Finally, Grimaitre et al.[27] demonstrated effectiveness of colchicine in a small group of patients, and other molecules are currently being developed as topical preparations.

Topical 5-fluorouracil is available as a cream or lotion in varying concentrations from 1% to 5%. In addition, a newer 'microsponge' system has been approved by the FDA.[28] The medication often is applied daily to affected areas for 4–6 weeks, which causes both clinical and subclinical lesions to become red and irritated. The irritation can be intense and become exudative. Some patients are unable to maintain a normal social life because of their appearance (Fig. 10.4). Although the recommended length of treatment is between 4 and 6 weeks, many patients tolerate less than 3 weeks, which limits efficacy. Application of topical corticosteroids may diminish the inflammatory reaction, although some experts state that the inflammation is required for the medication to be effective.

Topical retinoids have shown efficacy in treating mild AKs, and have even been advocated for the reversal of sun damage.[29–31] However, application must be continuous for many months and long-term efficacy needs further investigation. Furthermore, irritation, erythema and dryness are side effects. Oral retinoids have been used to suppress keratinocytic neoplasia in organ transplant recipients.[31] Topical diclofenac, a non-steroidal anti-inflammatory drug, is also approved for treatment of AKs.[32] Daily application over 3–6 months results in a statistically significant reduction in AKs. The drug is less irritating than 5-fluorouracil but must be used for longer and is generally considered to be less effective (Table 10.1).

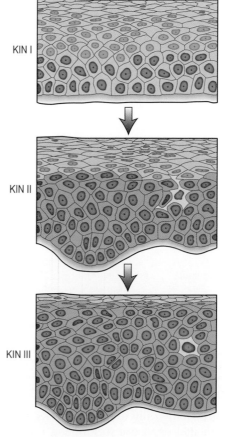

Histological features of keratinocytic intraepidermal neoplasia

KIN I

KIN II

KIN III

**Figure 10.4** Diagrammatic representation of histological features of KIN.

Table 10.1 Therapies and Therapeutic Options for Actinic Keratoses

| Approach | 100% Clearance Rate | Median Lesion Reduction % | Advantages | Disadvantages |
|---|---|---|---|---|
| *Topical chemotherapies* | | | *Treat multiple lesions at once, and also treat clinically inapparent lesions* | *Long-term regimen, difficulties with patient compliance* |
| 5% 5-fluorouracil | 80%[33] | 86%[33] | Effective, less costly, minimal scarring | Potent irritant that some patients can't tolerate, may cause severe inflammatory reactions, healing can take 1–2 months, may mask deeper skin cancers |
| Diclofenac | 40%[34]–50%[32] | 64%[35] | Well tolerated with minimal to moderate irritation, no scarring | Prolonged treatment time required |
| Imiquimod | 50%[36] | 87%[37] | Induces patient's own immune system, may produce immunologic memory, no scarring | Sometimes induces brisk inflammation with poor patient compliance, can cause systemic flu-like symptoms, myalgia, headache |
| Topical retinoids | 55% (3% ointment)[38] | 30.3%[38] | Mild to moderate irritation, can serve as adjunctive treatment | Treatment lengthy, not sufficiently efficacious to generally use as monotherapy |
| Ingenol mebutate | 40%[39] | 75–100%[39] | 1 or 2 applications needed | Can have very brisk inflammatory response that occasionally leads to scarring |
| *Destructive therapies* | | | *Fewer problems with patient compliance* | |
| Cryosurgery | 67%[40]–75%[38] | 88%[41] | Rapid procedure, few side effects, heals with minimal scarring, well tolerated, high patient compliance | Painful, can heal with some scarring, hypo- or hyperpigmentation, difficult to treat numerous lesions |
| Photodynamic therapy | 69%–91%[38] | 78%[41] | Useful to treat numerous AKs, or to treat areas of poor healing such as legs, good cosmetic results | Two-step process, severe stinging and burning during treatment, costly equipment, problems with reimbursement |
| Shave excision or curettage (and electrodesiccation) | High | High | Allows for pathologic diagnosis, good choice for hypertrophic or thick lesions, as well as ones that do not respond to initial therapy | Scarring, delayed healing in sites with poor circulation |
| Peels, dermabrasion, laser resurfacing | High | High | Treat multiple lesions at once | Healing can take weeks, may leave scarring or hypo- or hyperpigmentation |
| *Combination therapies* | | | *Potential higher efficacy* | |
| Imiquimod and cryosurgery | Insufficient data | Insufficient data | Cryosurgery during imiquimod treatment may potentiate the development of anti-tumor immune response[42] | Treatment lengthy, may cause systemic symptoms |
| Diclofenac and cryosurgery | 64%[43] | 88%[43] | Well tolerated | Treatment lengthy |
| PDT and imiquimod | Insufficient data | 90%[44] | Treat multiple lesions, good cosmetic response | Treatment lengthy |

## OTHER LESIONS ASSOCIATED WITH KERATINOCYTIC MALIGNANCIES

### Radiation, arsenical and tar keratoses

Skin lesions histologically identical to AKs can be induced by environmental exposure to ionizing radiation, arsenic and tar. Exposure to ionzing radiation can induce a number of different harmful disorders of the skin, including radio-dermatitis, radiation-induced keratoses, and frank malignancy, especially SCC. Radiation exposure may be incurred medically for diagnosis as well as for treatment of malignancies both internal and cutaneous. Less commonly, it may be used for the treatment of benign skin conditions. Therapy of benign dermatoses with low doses of radiation using superficial X-ray or Grenz ray is generally safe but should be reserved for recalcitrant dermatoses only and administered in limited doses. In the 1950s the most common uses for X-ray therapy for cutaneous disease were for acne, hirsutism, and refractory tinea capitis. The development of radiation-induced malignancy is directly related to the dose administered. The latency between therapy and development of neoplasia may be as short as a few years but is usually more than 10 years. Careful long-term follow-up is necessary.

Long-term arsenic exposure characteristically produces large numbers of small hyperkeratotic lesions on acral skin, especially the palms and soles (Fig. 10.5). Epidemiological studies in humans also suggest that it is related to the development not only of keratoses but also of SCC and superficial basal cell carcinoma.[45] SCC with the potential for metastasis can arise from arsenical keratoses with a low risk for metatasis. Arsenic exposure was more common in the past when adequate precautions were not taken to protect workers. Arsenic trioxide administered in a product known as Fowler's solution was also historically used as a treatment of disorders such as psoriasis and asthmatic bronchitis. Arsenic is also a contaminant in drinking water in some areas of the world. Treatment of patients with arsenical keratoses can be difficult as hundreds of lesions may be present.

Keratosis and cancer of the skin that develop following chronic exposure to tar, pitch, coal, soot and/or mineral oil products were among the first recognized occupational-related diseases. This association led to early understanding of chemical carcinogenesis. Tar keratoses are uncommon today in the United States with the safeguards that have been instituted for those who may come in contact with tar and pitch containing products, such as roofers and road workers. Clinically, lesions are similar in appearance to AK and arsenical keratoses, being elevated crusty, keratotic papules that occur on skin that has been exposed to tar. Treatment of these lesions is also similar.

## PUVA keratoses

Keratoses related to psoralen–ultraviolet A (PUVA) therapy, used primarily to treat psoriasis, appear clinically similar to AKs, presenting as warty hyperkeratotic and scaly papules measuring from several millimeters up to 1 cm in diameter. Histologically, the lesions demonstrate acanthosis, papillomatosis, hyperkeratosis, and focal parakeratosis. Not all lesions demonstrate significant nuclear atypia and when nuclear atypia is present, it is usually relatively minimal. PUVA-induced keratoses may not possess the same risk of evolution to SCC as do conventional AKs although they do serve as a marker of an increased risk for the development of cutaneous non-melanoma skin cancer. The incidence of the development of SCC in patients who have undergone long-term PUVA therapy has been demonstrated to be signicantly increased.[46]

## Scars, chronic inflammation, and chronic infection

Scars that result from cutaneous injuries or from chronic inflammation of the skin may predispose an individual to develop cutaneous malignancy, in particular SCC.[47] The recognition that SCC may develop within a burn scar is credited to Marjolin and is termed Marjolin's ulcer. It has since become recognized that SCC may develop in scars that develop as a consequence of a number of other injuries, including frostbite, electrical burns, chronic sinuses or fistulas, chronic osteomyelitis, chronic stasis dermatitis, prurigo nodularis and following a variety of cutaneous infections.

SCCs that develop in areas of chronic inflammation and ulceration are thought to have a somewhat more aggressive biologic behavior with rates of metastasis reported from 18% to 40%, while metastasis rates for squamous cell carcinomas developing in burn scars have been reported as high as 60%.[48-50] This may be a generalization, however, as in a study of SCC of the skin, Headington and Callen observed two histopathologic variants of SCC arising in scars: an aggressive, invasive anaplastic lesion and a lesion with histologic features similar to verrucous carcinoma.[51] Patients with the former frequently experienced an aggressive course and had metastases at the time of diagnosis. In contrast, those with a verrucous carcinoma pattern rarely had metastasis and were cured with local excisional surgery. Thus, it is obviously important to biopsy any non-healing chronically inflamed skin lesion to identify malignancy and its histologic pattern to prevent sequelae.

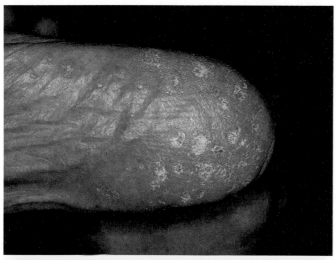

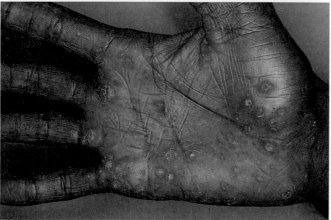

**Figure 10.5** Multiple volar keratoses are representative of arsenical keratoses.

## Human papillomavirus-associated lesions

Epidermodysplasia verruciformis (EV) is a rare genetically inherited skin condition associated with an inability to mount an effective immune response to certain strains of the human papillomavirus.[14] Many different subtypes have been associated with EV, including 5, 8, 9, 12, 14, 15, 17, 19, 25, 36, 38, 47 and 50. Two loci, EV1 and EV2 on chromosomes 17 and 2 respectively, have so far been identified as being associated with the condition.[14] Affected individuals develop numerous flat warty lesions that are histologically similar to verrucae planae. Infected keratinocytes show pronounced viral changes with perinuclear halos, prominent eosinophilic inclusions, and a bluish-grey cytoplasm on hematoxylin and eosin staining. About one-half of EV patients will develop a cutaneous malignancy in the fourth or fifth decade.

Verrucous carcinoma, fist described by Ackerman in 1948, is a low-grade variant of SCC that is commonly seen in the upper respiratory and digestive tracts, in the anogenital region, and on palmoplantar skin.[14] Oroaerodigestive lesions, also called oral florid papillomatosis or giant mucocutaneous papillomatosis, have been associated with low-risk HPV types 6 and 11 and high-risk HPV types 16 and 18. The development of these lesions is also associated with the use of chewing tobacco or snuff. Anogenital verrucous carcinoma, classically called giant condyloma of Buschke–Lowenstein, has been more commonly associated with low-risk rather than high-risk HPV types. It characteristically has a deceptively benign histologic appearance with minimal nuclear atypia. The epidermis is markedly acanthotic with bulbous epidermal retia that extend deep into the dermis and deeper structures. There is usually a prominent granular layer with hyperkeratosis and often parakeratosis. Some lesions demonstrate viral cytopathic effect. Although verrucous carcinoma usually does not metastasize, it can be very locally aggressive, resulting in considerable tissue destruction, and may recur repeatedly if not treated appropriately.

Bowenoid papulosis (BP) represents a clinical variant of SCC in situ in the genital region caused by oncogenic subtypes of HPV. Various types of high-risk HPV have been identified, including 16, 18, 31–35 as well as a few others.[14] Patients are usually young adults in their third through fifth decades and present with multiple reddish brown to violaceous papules, macules or plaques that may be confluent. Affected females have an increased incidence of associated cervical dysplasia. Histologically, lesions have an architectural appearance similar to that of a condyloma acuminatum but with acanthosis and a proliferation of atypical keratinocytes in the epidermis with close crowding of nuclei demonstrating disordered maturation. Multinucleate and necrotic keratinocytes are common, and atypical mitoses are often present. Although infection with oncogenic HPV likely plays the major role in the development of these lesions, an ineffective host immune response may be contributory as some patients have been shown to have cutaneous anergy and decreased populations of T helper cells. Furthermore, the incidence of BP is greater in HIV-infected patients. Although BP lesions may sometimes regress, they do have a 2.6% chance of evolving into invasive SCC.[14]

Most cutaneous SCC is not associated with HPV in the immunocompetent population even if patients are infected with an oncogenic strain of HPV. However, HPV infection in immunocompromised individuals likely plays at least some role in the development of SCC as their risk of developing SCC is 64–250 times greater than that of the normal population.[14] Significantly higher levels of HPV DNA have been recovered from SCC arising in immunocompromised and transplant patients as compared with those in normal individuals.[14] Cutaneous SCC is a major complication of long-term immunosuppression, and in those who undergo successful long-term organ transplantation, SCC is the most common cause of death. Therefore, all individuals who are immunocompromised for long periods should be closely monitored and treated aggressively.

## CUTANEOUS SQUAMOUS CELL CARCINOMA IN SITU AND ITS VARIANTS

Bowen's disease is defined by many as a distinct clinical variant of SCC in situ. It presents as a slightly scaly and crusted, discrete erythematous plaque with a sharp but often irregular or undulating border (Figs 10.6 and 10.7). The surface characteristics vary and include hyperkeratosis, fissures, dyspigmentation, erosions, and/or ulcerations. It is most common in fair-skinned older individuals on

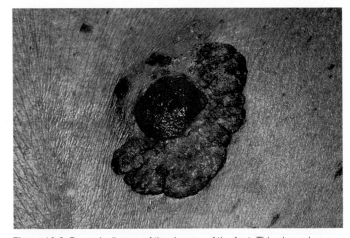

Figure 10.6 Bowen's disease of the dorsum of the foot. This plaque has a scaly surface with an undulating border.

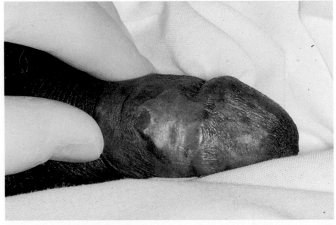

Figure 10.7 Erythroplasia of Queyrat.

sun-exposed areas, although it may occur in darker-skinned patients where it is often found on protected skin. The lesion usually grows in a slow but progressive manner with up to an 8% risk of involving the dermis if left untreated.[52] Previously some authors argued that Bowen's disease was a marker for internal malignancy but repeated studies have failed to demonstrate this association.[53] Histopathologic examination demonstrates acanthosis with atypical keratinocytes present within the entire epithelium involving adnexal structures and with parakeratosis overlying. There is usually prominent cytologic atypia with some individual cell dyskeratosis and increased mitoses.

Erythroplasia of Queyrat is a clinical variant of SCC in situ of the genital area. It is most commonly found on the glans penis in uncircumcised men and presents as a sharply circumscribed bright red shiny plaque. The histologic changes are the same as those seen in Bowen's disease although the dermal inflammatory infiltrate is often rich in plasma cells.

The choices of therapy for these in-situ carcinomas include surgical excision, electrodesiccation and curettage, cryotherapy with liquid nitrogen, local irradiation, topical chemotherapy with imiquimod or 5-fluorouracil, laser surgery, and microscopically controlled surgery. These lesions should be treated to resolution because if left untreated they may involve deeper structures with a possibility for metastasis.

## FUTURE OUTLOOK

The prevalence of AKs will likely increase as the population continues to live longer and as drugs and therapies that are chemotherapeutic agents or immunosuppressive agents become even more widely used in the management of patients with inflammatory diseases, organ transplantation, or cancer. In patients with immunosuppression, whether organic or iatrogenic, there is a greater risk of development of SCC that may be aggressive, so early identification and treatment will become increasingly important. Such patients need to be evaluated and treated prior to undergoing immunosuppression in efforts to decrease the morbidity that they will inevitably face. Furtheremore, efforts at education regarding the dangers of excessive sun exposure must be continued and development of methods to provide passive protection will likely help to reduce future AKs.

## REFERENCES

1. Hussein M. Ultraviolet radiation and skin cancer: molecular mechanisms. *J Cutan Pathol.* 2005;32:191–205.
2. Cox NJ. Actinic keratosis induced by a sunbed. *BMJ.* 1994;308:977–978.
3. Cockerell CJ, Wharton JR. New histopathological classification of actinic keratosis (incipient intraepidermal squamous cell carcinoma). *J Drugs Dermatol.* 2005;4:462–467.
4. Ackerman AB. Solar keratosis is squamous cell carcinoma. *Arch Dermatol.* 2003;139:1216–1217.
5. Cockerell CJ. Histopathology of incipient intraepidermal squamous cell carcinoma. *J Am Acad Dermatol.* 2000;42:11–17.
6. Yantsos VA, Conrad N, Zabawski E, et al. Incipient intraepidermal cutaneous squamous cell carcinoma: a proposal for reclassifying and grading solar (actinic) keratoses. *Semin Cutan Med Surg.* 1999;18:3–14.
7. Wendy F, Cockerell CJ. The actinic (solar) keratosis: a 21st-century perspective. *Arch Dermatol.* 2003;139:66–70.
8. Anwar J, Wrone D, Kimyai-Asadi A, et al. The development of actinic keratoses into invasive squamous cell carcinoma: evidence and evolving classification schemes. *Clin Dermatol.* 2004;22:189–196.
9. Schwartz R, Bridges T, Butani A, et al. Actinic keratosis: an occupational and environmental disorder. *J Eur Acad Dermatol Venereol.* 2008;22:606–615.
10. Green A, Beardmore G, Hart V, et al. Skin cancer in a Queensland population. *J Am Acad Dermatol.* 1988;19:1045–1052.
11. Marks R, Ponsford M, Selwood T, et al. Non-melanotic skin cancer and solar keratoses in Victoria. *Med J Aust.* 1983;2:618–622.
12. Siskind V, Aitkin J, Green A, et al. Sun exposure and interaction with family history in risk of melanoma in Queensland, Australia. *Int J Cancer.* 2002;97:90–95.
13. Pons M, Quintanilla M. Molecular biology of malignant melanoma and other cutaneous tumors. *Clin Transl Oncol.* 2006;8:466–474.
14. Dubina M, Goldenberg G. Viral-associated nonmelanoma skin cancers: a review. *Am J Dermatopathol.* 2009;31:561–573.
15. Terai H, Shimahara M. Cheilitis as a variation of Candida-associated lesions. *Oral Dis.* 2006;12:349–352.
16. Park WS, Lee HK, Lee JY, et al. p53 mutations in solar keratoses. *Hum Pathol.* 1996;27:1180–1184.
17. Takata M, Saida T. Early cancers of the skin: clinical, histopathological, and molecular characteristics. *Int J Clin Oncol.* 2005;10:391–397.
18. Berhane T, Halliday GM, Cooke B, et al. Inflammation is associated with progression of actinic keratoses to squamous cell carcinoma in humans. *Br J Dermatol.* 2002;146:810–815.
19. Quaedvlieg P, Tirsi E, Thissen M, et al. Actinic keratosis: how to differentiate the good from the bad ones? *Eur J Dermatol.* 2006;16:335–339.
20. Moon TE, Levine N, Carmel B, et al. Effect of retinol in preventing squamous cell cancer in moderate-risk subjects. *Cancer Epidemiol Biomarkers Prev.* 1997;6:949–956.
21. Jonason AS, Kunala S, Price GJ, et al. Frequent clones of p53-mutated keratinocytes in normal human skin. *Proc Natl Acad Sci U S A.* 1996;93:14025–14029.
22. Cockerell CJ. Pathology and pathobiology of the actinic (solar) keratosis. *Br J Dermatol.* 2003;149:34–36.
23. Goldberg LH, Joseph AK, Tschen JA. Proliferative actinic keratosis. *Int J Dermatol.* 1994;33:341–345.
24. Walker JK, Koenig C. Is imiquimod effective and safe for actinic keratosis? *J Fam Pract.* 2003;52:184–185.
25. Stockfleth E, Meyer T, Benninghoff B, et al. A randomized, double-blind, vehicle-controlled study to assess 5% imiquimod cream for the treatment of multiple actinic keratoses. *Arch Dermatol.* 2002;138:1498–1502.
26. Salasche SJ, Levine N, Morrison L. Cycle therapy of actinic keratoses of the face and scalp with 5% topical imiquimod cream: an open-label trial. *J Am Acad Dermatol.* 2002;47:571–577.
26a. Swanson et al. *J Am Acad Dermatol.* 2009.
27. Grimaitre M, Etienne A, Fathi M, et al. Topical colchicine therapy for actinic keratoses. *Dermatology.* 2000;200:346–348.
28. Jorizzo J, Stewart D, Bucko A, et al. Randomized trial evaluating a new 0.5% fluorouracil formulation demonstrates efficacy after 1-, 2-, or 4-week treatment in patients with actinic keratosis. *Cutis.* 2002;70:335–339.
29. Baranco VP, Olson RL, Everett MA. Response of actinic keratosis to topical vitamin A acid. *Cutis.* 1980;6:681.
30. Weiss JS, Ellis CN, Headington JT, et al. Topical tretinoin improves photoaged skin. A double-blind vehicle-controlled study. *JAMA.* 1988;259:527–532.
31. De Graaf YG, Euvrard S, Bouwes Bavinck JN. Systemic and topical retinoids in the management of skin cancer in organ transplant recipients. *Dermatol Surg.* 2004;30:656–661.
32. Wolf Jr JE, Taylor JR, Tschen E, et al. Topical 3.0% diclofenac in 2.5% hyaluronan gel in the treatment of actinic keratoses. *Int J Dermatol.* 2001;40:709–713.
33. Askew DA, Mickan SM, Soyer HP, et al. Effectiveness of 5-fluorouracil treatment for actinic keratosis – a systematic review of randomized controlled trials. *Int J Dermatol.* 2009;48:453–463.
34. Pirard D, Vereecken P, Mélot C, et al. Three percent diclofenac in 2.5% hyaluronan gel in the treatment of actinic keratoses: a meta-analysis of the recent studies. *Arch Dermatol Res.* 2005;297:185–189.
35. Rivers JK, Arlette J, Shear N, et al. Topical treatment of actinic keratoses with 3.0% diclofenac. *Br J Dermatol.* 2002;146:94–100.
36. Hadley G, Derry S, Moore RA. Imiquimod for actinic keratosis: systematic review and meta-analysis. *J Invest Dermatol.* 2006;126:1251–1255.
37. Korman N, Moy R, Ling M, et al. Dosing with 5% imiquimod cream 3 times per week for the treatment of actinic keratosis. *Arch Dermatol.* 2005;141:467–473.
38. de Berker D, McGregor JM, Hughes BR. Guidelines for the management of actinic keratoses. *Br J Dermatol.* 2007;156:222–230.
39. Anderson L, Schmieder GJ, Werschler WP, et al. Randomized, double-blind, double-dummy, vehicle-controlled study of ingenol mebutate gel 0.025% and 0.05% for actinic keratosis. *J Am Acad Dermatol.* 2009;60(6):934–943.

40. Thai K, Fergin P, Freeman M, et al. A prospective study of the use of cryosurgery for the treatment of actinic keratoses. *Int J Dermatol.* 2004;43:687–692.

41. Kaufmann R, Spelman L, Weightman W, et al. Multicentre intraindividual randomized trial of topical methyl aminolaevulinate–photodynamic therapy vs. cryotherapy for multiple actinic keratoses on the extremities. *Br J Dermatol.* 2008;158:994–999.

42. Bassukas ID, Gaitanis G. Combination of cryosurgery and topical imiquimod: does timing matter for successful immunocryosurgery? *Cryobiology.* 2009;59(1):116–117.

43. Berlin JM, Rigel DS. Diclofenac sodium 3% gel in the treatment of actinic keratoses post cryosurgery. *J Drugs Dermatol.* 2008;7:669–673.

44. Shaffelburg M. Treatment of actinic keratoses with sequential use of photodynamic therapy; and imiquimod 5% cream. *J Drugs Dermatol.* 2009;8(1):35–39.

45. Graham JH, Helwig EB. Cutaneous precancerous conditions in man. *NCI Monogr.* 1963;10:323.

46. Stern RS, Lunder EJ. Risk of squamous cell carcinoma and methoxsalen (psoralen) and UV-A radiation (PUVA). *Arch Dermatol.* 1998;134:1582–1585.

47. Kaplan RP. Cancer complicating chronic ulcerative and scarring mucocutaneous disorders. *Adv Dermatol.* 1987;2:19.

48. Johnson TM, Rowe DE, Nelson BR, et al. Squamous cell carcinoma of the skin (excluding lip and oral mucosa). *J Am Acad Dermatol.* 1992;26:467–484.

49. McGrath JA, Schofield OM, Mayou BJ, et al. Epidermolysis bullosa complicated by squamous cell carcinoma: report of 10 cases. *J Cutan Pathol.* 1992;19:116–123.

50. Aron NK, Tajuri S. Postburn scar carcinoma. *Burns.* 1989;15:121–124.

51. Callen JP, Headington J. Bowen's and non-Bowen's squamous intraepithelial neoplasia of the skin. Relationship to Internal malignancy. *Arch Dermatol.* 1980;116:422–426.

52. Kao GF. Carcinoma arising in Bowen's disease. *Arch Dermatol.* 1986;122:1124–1126.

53. Arbesman H, Ransohoff DF. Is Bowen's disease a predictor for the development of internal malignancy? *JAMA.* 1987;257:516–518.

# Basal Cell Carcinoma

*Clay J. Cockerell, Kien T. Tran, John Carucci, Emily Tierney, Pearon Lang, John C. Maize Sr., and Darrell S. Rigel*

## Key Points

- Basal cell carcinoma (BCC) is the most common malignancy occurring in humans, appearing most often as a translucent papule with rolled borders and telangiectasias.

- Although most lesions are related to excess ultraviolet exposure, BCC is multifactorial in origin.

- Clinical–pathological correlation is critical when planning the treatment of a BCC.

- Many modalities exist for removal of BCC, with Mohs micrographic surgery offering the highest cure rates for aggressive-growth BCC, recurrent BCC, and BCCs in cosmetically sensitive or high-risk anatomic sites.

- Discovery of a molecular defect in the hedgehog pathway led to development of a hedgehog inhibitor currently in clinical trials for treatment of advanced BCC.

## INTRODUCTION

Basal cell carcinoma (BCC) is a skin cancer derived from non-keratinizing cells that form the basal layer of the epidermis. Tumor size can vary from a few millimeters to several centimeters in diameter. BCC tends to invade locally if left untreated, which can result in compromised function and cosmesis secondary to massive tissue loss. BCC is the most common of all cancers diagnosed in the United States with over 2,000,000 cases diagnosed annually.[1] Although BCCs rarely metastasize and thus rarely cause death, they can result in significant morbidity. This is especially true if they are not correctly diagnosed and managed in a proper and timely manner.

## HISTORY

BCC was first described in 1824 by Jacob.[2] Later, Krompecher suggested that it arose from the basal cells of the epidermis.[3] Subsequently, a number of other theories were put forth as regards the site of origin of this tumor, including the hair follicle and other appendageal structures. The association of the patched gene (*PTCH*) with hereditary nevoid basal cell carcinoma syndrome (Gorlin syndrome) was vital to understanding the pathogenesis of BCCs.[4-7]

## EPIDEMIOLOGY

BCC is the most common cancer occurring in man and accounts for approximately 75% of all non-melanoma skin cancers (NMSCs) along with approximately 25% of all cancers diagnosed in the United States.[8] The estimated lifetime risk of BCC in the white population is 33–39% for men and 23–28% for women.

Although once thought to be a disease of the elderly, BCC is becoming increasingly common in younger patients. Christenson et al. noted a disproportionate increase in BCC in women under 40.[9] BCC characteristically develops on sun-exposed skin of lighter-skinned individuals, with approximately 30% occurring on the nose. Risk factors for BCC have been well characterized and include ultraviolet light (UVL) exposure, male sex, light hair and eye color, northern European ancestry, and inability to tan.[8] Tanning-bed users are at increased risk for developing BCC.[10] Bower et al. recently reported that individuals with BCC had a threefold increased risk for melanoma, but no increased risk for any other type of cancer.[11] BCCs tend to show a typical body distribution: 70% on the head (most frequently on face),[12] 25% on the trunk,[13] and 5% on the penis,[14] vulva,[15] or perianal skin.

## PATHOGENESIS

The causes of BCC are summarized in Table 11.1.[16-29] The key etiologic agent responsible for development of BCC is exposure to ultraviolet light (UVL), particularly the ultraviolet B (UVB) spectrum (290 to 320 nm) that induces mutations in tumor suppressor genes.[30,31] Some have reported that intermittent, brief exposures may place patients at higher risk than occupational exposure.[32] Ramani and Bennett reported a significant increased incidence of BCCs in World War II servicemen stationed in the Pacific theater as compared to those stationed in Europe.[33] This suggests that several months or years of intense exposure to UVL may have deleterious long-term effects. Other factors that appear to be involved in the pathogenesis include mutations in regulatory genes,[5] exposure to ionizing radiation,[34] and iatrogenic immune suppression after solid organ transplant.[35]

Several heritable conditions predispose to BCC. These include the nevoid basal cell carcinoma syndrome (NBCCS) (Fig. 11.1),[36] Bazex syndrome,[37] and Rombo syndrome.[38] Patients with NBCCS may develop hundreds of BCCs and may exhibit a broad nasal root, frontal bossing, borderline intelligence, jaw cysts, palmar pits, and multiple skeletal abnormalities. NBCCS occurs due to mutations in the tumor suppressor *PTCH* gene located on chromosome arm 9q.[39,40] Bazex syndrome is transmitted in an X-linked dominant fashion.[37] In this syndrome, patients present with multiple BCCs, follicular atrophoderma, dilated follicular ostia

## Table 11.1 BCC Causes and Associations

| Causes | Associations |
|---|---|
| Sun exposure | Primarily UVB, 290–320 nm |
| Gene mutations | *p53* gene mutations[16–18] |
| Exposure to artificial UV light | Tanning booths, UV light therapy,[19] PUVA[20] |
| Ionizing radiation exposure | Radiation therapy[21,22] |
| Arsenic exposure | Fowler's solution of potassium; contaminated water source has been the most common source of arsenic ingestion[22] |
| Immunosuppression | Transplant recipients[23] |
| Xeroderma pigmentosum | Inability to repair UV-induced DNA damage[24] |
| Nevoid basal cell carcinoma syndrome | *PTCH* gene mutation. Medulloblastomas, meningioma, fetal rhabdomyoma, and ameloblastoma also can occur[25,26] |
| Bazex syndrome | Atrophoderma ('ice pick' marks, especially on dorsal hands), multiple basal cell carcinomas, and local anhidrosis (decreased or absent sweating)[27] |
| Personal and family history of previous non-melanoma skin cancer (NMSC) | The risk of developing new NMSC is 35% at 3 years and 50% at 5 years after an initial skin cancer diagnosis[28] |
| Skin type | Skin types I and II are especially susceptible, as are patients with albinism[29] |

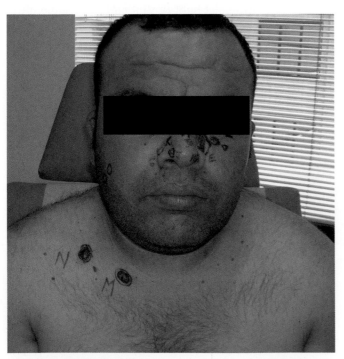

**Figure 11.1** Patient with basal cell nevus syndrome with multiple BCCs present. Note the frontal bossing.

with ice-pick scars, hypotrichosis, and hypohidrosis. In contrast, Rombo syndrome is transmitted in an autosomal dominant fashion.[38] Patients present with vermiculate atrophoderma, milia, hypertrichosis, trichoepitheliomas, BCCs, and peripheral vasodilation.

UVL-induced epidermal DNA damage is thought to be the primary carcinogenic event occurring in the development of BCC. Xeroderma pigmentosum (XP) is characterized by the development of NMSC at an early age secondary to an ability to repair UVL-induced DNA damage.[41] Using XP as a model, investigators have sought to determine if an inability to repair UVL-induced DNA damage might also explain the genesis of skin cancer in non-XP patients. However, due to the conflicting results of current studies, one cannot conclude at this time that an inability to repair damaged DNA explains the development of all BCC. Cumulative lifetime UV exposure appears to increase the probability of developing BCC. However, recent studies also suggest that, like melanoma, intermittent intense sun exposure early in life may also be a risk factor.[42] The development and distribution of squamous cell carcinoma (SCC) may more accurately reflect cumulative sun damage than does that of BCC, as a significant percentage of BCCs occur on non-sun-exposed skin.[43]

UVL from sources besides sunlight, including tanning beds[44] and UVL used for therapeutic purposes (PUVA),[20] may contribute to the development of BCC. UVL may mediate its carcinogenic effect not only by damaging epithelial DNA but also by creating an immune tolerant state in the skin.[45] In addition, UVL may bring about the development of BCC through mutations in tumor suppressor gene *p53* and other genes.[46] Mutations in *p53* are thought to prevent the death of cells damaged by UVL, which would allow the propagation of these abnormal cell(s).[46] As with basal cell nevus syndrome, the patched gene may play a pathogenesis role in patients with sporadic BCCs.[5]

Other environmental factors beyond UVL may lead to the development of BCC. The risk for developing BCCs within sites previously treated with radiation for management of cancers is well established.[47,48] Ionizing radiation given for benign conditions (e.g. tinea capitis, hirsutism, acne) in doses as low as 450 rads, has been associated with BCC formation.[49] The latency for tumor development is usually long and evidence of radiation damage need not be present.

Arsenic exposure, especially to inorganic arsenic, has been associated with the development of multiple NMSC including BCC.[50] Lesions most commonly occur on the trunk. Sources of arsenic exposure include well water, pesticides (e.g. Paris green), medications (Fowler's solution, herbal remedies) and industry (mining, smelting, sheep dippings to control lice and blowfly infestation).

BCC may arise in a nevus sebaceous.[51] Nevus sebaceous commonly presents as a flesh-colored to yellow plaque on the scalp at birth. The lifetime risk for development of BCC in these lesions varies between 5% and 20%.

The role of the immune system in the pathogenesis of skin cancer is not completely understood. Immunosuppressed patients with lymphoma or leukemia,[52] and organ transplant recipients,[35] have a marked increase in the incidence of SCC, but only a slight increase in the incidence of BCC.

Bastiaens et al. found that transplant recipients developed more BCCs on the trunk and arms than did non-immunosuppressed patients (~10-fold).[23] Patients with HIV develop BCCs at the same rate as immunocompetent individuals, based on similar risk factors.[53] BCC may subvert immune response through several mechanisms. Kaporis et al. showed that BCC is associated with immunosuppressive regulatory T cells.[54] Nickoloff and colleagues demonstrated that UVL-induced BCCs express Fas ligand (CD95L).[55] They further showed that these cells were associated with CD95-bearing cytotoxic T cells undergoing apoptosis. Thus, the presence of regulatory T cells may serve to attenuate anti-tumor immunity at the T-cell level while CD95L[+] BCCs may send a 'death signal' to any surviving functional cytotoxic T cells in the tumor microenvironment.

Mutations in the gene encoding the *p53* tumor suppressor have been found in more than half of sporadic BCCs. The inactivating mutations usually bear evidence of UV induction, bearing CC $\Rightarrow$ TT and C $\Rightarrow$ T substitutions produced by the photoproducts of adjacent pyrimidines. The pathways through which hedgehog signaling induces tumorigenesis remain unclear. Patched1 may have cell cycle gatekeeper functions (see Chapter 2).

## BIOLOGICAL BEHAVIOR

### Local invasion

The greatest danger of BCC results from local invasion. In general, BCC is a slow-growing tumor that invades locally rather than metastasizes. The rate of doubling is estimated to be between 6 months and 1 year. If left untreated, the tumor will progress to invade subcutaneous tissue, muscle, and even bone. Anatomic fusion planes appear to provide a low resistance path for tumor progression. Tumors along the nasofacial or retroauricular sulcus may be extensive. In one case, a patient documented the progression of his own tumor with photographs over a 27-year period.[56] The lesion, which encompassed an entire side of the face, including the maxillary sinus, apparently doubled over a 10-year period and grew rapidly in the 2 years prior to presentation. This scenario tends to occur in the context of physical or psychiatric disability that interferes with judgment or access to healthcare. In another case, a 35 cm BCC on the back of a 65-year-old man recurred after wide local excision and XRT, resulting in spinal cord compression.[57] Lethal extension to the central nervous system from aggressive scalp BCC has been reported.[58]

### Perineural invasion

Perineural invasion is uncommon in BCC and occurs most often in histologically aggressive or recurrent lesions.[59] Perineural invasion is more likely to be encountered with recurrent tumors located in the preauricular and malar areas. Ratner et al. reported an incidence of 3.8% in their series.[60] Leibovitch et al.[61] reported perineural spread in >50% of periocular BCCs eventuating in orbital invasion. Perineural spread may present with pain, paresthesias, weakness, or paralysis. The presence of focal neurologic symptoms at the site of a previously treated skin cancer should raise concern about nerve involvement. When perineural invasion is detected, every effort should be made to clear the tumor, preferably by Mohs surgery. Patients with gross perineural invasion manifested by neurologic symptoms would benefit from preoperative MRI to assess extent of tumor spread. Classic examples might include brow paralysis due to involvement of the temporal branch of the facial nerve or midface paresthesias secondary to involvement of the trigeminal nerve.

## Metastasis

Metastasis of BCC occurs only rarely, with rates varying from 0.0028% to 0.55%.[62-64] Involvement of lymph nodes and lungs were most common. von Domarus et al. reported five cases of metastatic BCC in which perineural or intravascular invasion had been noted in three of the five cases.[65] Squamous differentiation was not observed in the primary tumors in the cases they presented, but was noted in two of five cases of metastatic cancer. Overall, squamous differentiation was present in 15% of the primary or metastatic tumors from the 170 cases reviewed. Aggressive histologic characteristics including morpheaform characteristics, squamous differentiation and perineural invasion have been identified as risk factors for metastasis.

## CLINICAL PRESENTATION OF BCC

Basal cell carcinoma may look only slightly different than normal skin. Classically, BCC appears as a pearly papule with colors ranging from white to flesh-colored and in cases of pigmented BCC, brown (Figs 11.2 and 11.3). In some cases the skin may be just slightly raised or even flat. BCCs may have one or more visible and irregular blood vessels, an ulcerative area in the center that often is pigmented, and black-blue or brown areas. Large BCCs may have oozing or crusted areas.

Patients commonly report the following:

- a skin lesion that bleeds easily
- a lesion that does not heal
- oozing or crusting spots in a lesion
- appearance of a scar-like lesion without having injured the area
- irregular blood vessels in or around the lesion
- a lesion with a central depression.

Consider BCC in any patient with a non-healing lesion of 3–4 weeks on sun-exposed skin, especially if there is central depression (Fig. 11.2). These tumors may take many months or years to reach even 1 cm in diameter.

Patients often have a history of chronic sun exposure that may be recreational sun exposure (sunbathing, outdoor sports, fishing, boating) or occupational sun exposure (lifeguard, farming, construction). Occasionally, patients have a history of exposure to ionizing radiation, including X-ray therapy for acne, which was commonly used until 1950. Finally, patients can have a history of arsenic intake from well water.

Clinical appearance of BCC varies by type:

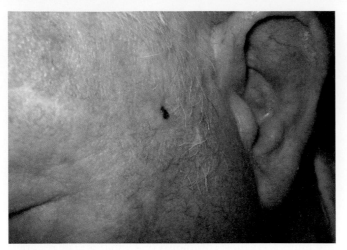

Figure 11.2 Basal cell cancer presenting as a non-healing ulcer.

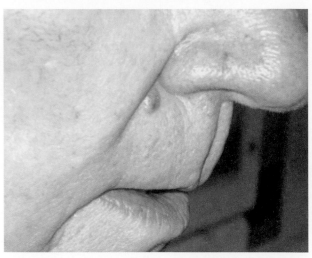

Figure 11.3 Nodular basal cell carcinoma demonstrating classic rolled borders with telangiectasias. (Courtesy of Brook Brouha, MD.)

## Nodular BCC (noduloulcerative, 'rodent ulcer')

Nodular BCC accounts for half of all BCCs and is characterized by nodules of large, basophilic cells and stromal retraction (Fig. 11.3).[66] As it enlarges, it frequently ulcerates centrally, leaving a raised, pearly border with telangiectasias, which aids in making the diagnosis (noduloulcerative BCC) (Fig. 11.4). Melanin pigment may be present in variable amounts, so one may observe a few flecks of brown pigment or the lesion may be black or blue-black and may be confused with a melanocytic lesion (Fig. 11.5). When left alone, these tumors may reach a large size and extend deeply, destroying an eyelid, nose, or ear. Thus the term 'rodent ulcer' originated because of the resemblance to tissue gnawed by a rat. In large lesions, tissue destruction and ulceration may dominate the picture such that the inexperienced clinician does not recognize the true nature of the ulcer. Careful examination, however, will often reveal at the edge of the ulcer an elevated translucent telangiectatic border.

## Superficial (multicentric) BCC

Superficial BCC (sBCC) is more frequently found on the trunk and extremities but can also be seen on the head and neck.[23] Typically, the sBCC lesion is flat and pink or red (Fig. 11.6). A slight amount of scale may be present and there may be a thready translucent elevated border. Areas of spontaneous regression characterized by atrophy and hypopigmentation may be present. The diameter of the lesion varies from a few millimeters to several centimeters. The lesion may be confused with a benign inflammatory condition such as nummular dermatitis and psoriasis. Variable amounts of pigment can be present, leading to confusion with a melanocytic lesion. Initially, the growth pattern is primarily horizontal. With the passage of time, these tumors can become deeply invasive with induration, ulceration, and nodule formation. Extensive subclinical lateral spread accounts for the significant recurrence rate of these tumors after routine excision. Budding of tumor islands off the hair follicles

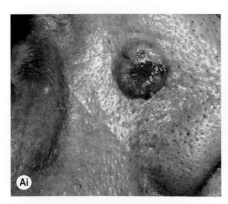
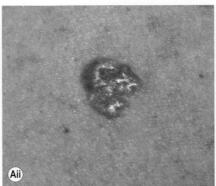
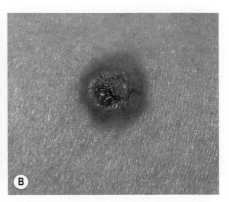

Figure 11.4 A) Nodulocystic basal cell carcinomas demonstrating classic rolled borders with telangiectasias. B) Nodular basal cell carcinoma with central ulceration, a common clinical finding. (Courtesy of Darrel Rigel, MD.)

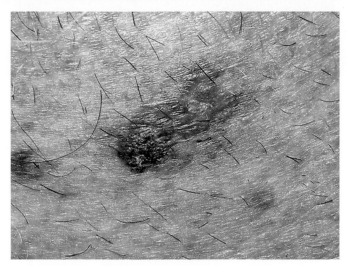

**Figure 11.5** Pigmented basal cell carcinoma.

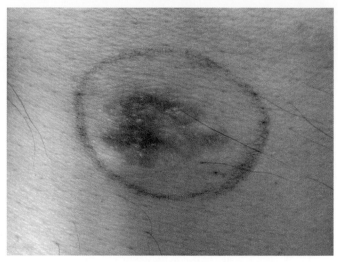

**Figure 11.7** Morpheic basal cell carcinoma. Note the white to pink plaque with telangiectasia. (Courtesy of Brook Brouha, MD.)

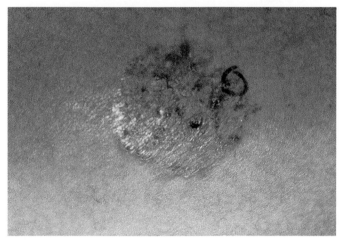

**Figure 11.6** Superficial basal cell carcinoma.

can explain a recurrence after curettage and electrodesiccation or topical therapy.

## Morpheaform BCC

The name for this variant of BCC is derived from its resemblance to a plaque of morphea (localized scleroderma). Typically, the lesion is indurated and ivory in color, and there may be overlying telangiectasia (Fig. 11.7). Although the lesion has been likened to morphea, usually it is not difficult to distinguish between the two. Occasionally, however, metastatic carcinoma may be misdiagnosed clinically and histologically as a morpheaform BCC. The morpheaform BCC is noted for its subclinical spread and high recurrence rate after treatment.[67]

## Cystic BCC

Cystic degeneration in a BCC often is not clinically obvious and thus the lesion may appear to be a typical nodular BCC.[8] However, in instances in which there are histologically marked cystic changes, the BCC clinically may have a clear or blue-gray cystic appearance and exude a clear fluid if

punctured or cut. If such a lesion is in the periorbital area, it may be confused with a hidrocystoma.

## BCC with squamous metaplasia (basosquamous or metatypical carcinoma)

BCC with squamous metaplasia (basosquamous carcinoma) is primarily a histologic variant of BCC and there are usually no clinical features that allow one to make the diagnosis preoperatively. Basosquamous carcinoma may be much more aggressive and destructive in its behavior, more likely to metastasize and more likely to recur after treatment.[68] Recurrent BCCs have been observed to undergo squamatization contributing to more aggressive behavior. It has been estimated that basosquamous carcinoma constitutes 1–2.5% of all NMSC. The incidence of metastases with this variant of BCC has been estimated to be as high as 9.7%.[68]

## BCC with an aggressive (infiltrative or micronodular) growth pattern

BCCs of this type are notorious for their aggressive and destructive behavior, subclinical spread, and high recurrence rate. It is therefore important to recognize these clinicopathologic variants. Up to 20% of all primary BCCs fall into this category. Clinically, these lesions are flat or only slightly elevated plaques. They are ill-defined in contrast to the purely nodular BCC. If there is a significant sclerosing stromal component (so-called sclerosing BCC), they may present as a firm plaque and demonstrate some of the clinical features of a morphea-like BCC.

## Premalignant fibroepithelioma of Pinkus

This is a rare variant of BCC which has unique histologic features. In most instances, the lesion is situated on the lower back but it can occur elsewhere. The typical lesion is a smooth, slightly red, moderately firm nodule that may be pedunculated. Clinically, the lesion resembles a fibroma.

## Pigmented BCC

This is an uncommon variant of BCC that has brown-black macules in some or all areas, often making it difficult to differentiate from melanoma (Fig. 11.5). Typically, some areas of these tumors do not retain pigment; pearly, raised borders with telangiectasias that are typical of a nodular BCC can be observed. This aids clinically in differentiating this tumor from a melanoma.

## Basal cell nevus syndrome (Gorlin syndrome)

BCC is also a feature of basal cell nevus syndrome (i.e. Gorlin syndrome), an autosomal dominant inherited condition (see Chapter 33).[4] The lesions in these patients cannot be distinguished histologically from ordinary BCCs. The gene responsible for this syndrome is located on chromosome arm 9q, and chromosome abnormalities develop in some patients.[69] The number of BCCs in patients with this syndrome may total from one to hundreds (Fig. 11.8A–C). Multiple BCCs begin to appear after puberty on the face, trunk, and extremities. In many cases, the tumors are highly invasive and

involve areas of the face, especially around the eyes and nose (Fig. 11.9). Other features associated with Gorlin syndrome include the following:

- mental retardation
- frontal bossing
- congenital agenesis of the corpus callosum and medulloblastoma
- odontogenic jaw cysts
- bifid ribs and pectus excavatum
- absent or undescended testes
- mesenteric lymphatic cysts
- palmar and plantar pits (Fig. 11.8B,C)
- ectopic calcification (particularly of the falx cerebri)
- ocular and skeletal abnormalities (e.g. hypertelorism, shortening of the fourth and fifth metacarpals).

## HISTOLOGY

Typically, BCCs are undifferentiated histologically, but some may show a degree of differentiation toward epithelial structures or adnexa. These neoplasms arise from the

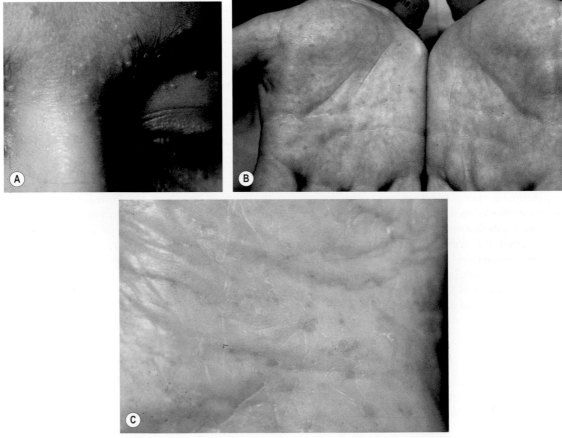

**Figure 11.8** A patient with basal cell nevus syndrome with: **A)** multiple BCCs on the face; and **B,C)** palmar and plantar pits.

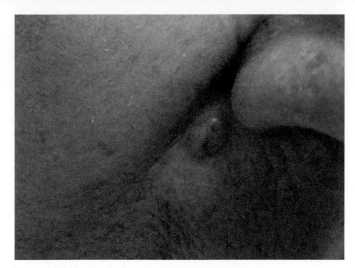

**Figure 11.9** Basal cell carcinoma near the alar crease.

pluripotential germinative cells of the skin that reside in the basal layer of the epidermis or the epithelial structures of adnexa. BCCs have many different clinical and histologic appearances as may be expected in so common a neoplasm. The two major factors that influence the histologic appearance of BCCs are the potential of its cells to differentiate and proliferate and the stromal response evoked by the epithelial component. Differentiation of neoplastic basal cells, just as of normal germinative basal cells in embryonic epidermis, may be toward follicular, sebaceous, eccrine or apocrine structures, although incompletely in neoplasia. The stroma may be mucinous, edematous or scirrhous.

BCCs have three well-recognized growth patterns: (1) nodular, (2) superficial, and (3) morpheic. The superficial and morpheic types each have a characteristic histopathologic picture that varies little from lesion to lesion. Nodular BCCs, however, may show many different histopathologic variants. The major ones have been classified as solid (primordial), keratotic (pilar), cystic and adenoid types. The adamantinoid and granular types are much rarer.[8]

Many nodular BCCs show secondary changes or unusual features. Some such changes are common and may have prognostic importance. A common finding is squamous differentiation. Some authors regard this as a metaplastic change that may correlate with a more aggressive biologic behavior.[68] Another common change is sclerosis of the stroma, which is usually found in recurrent lesions (especially in the deep portion) and renders them difficult to treat.[70]

Locally aggressive BCCs have been described that histologically show a diffuse, infiltrative pattern in the primary lesion that differs from the usually expansile nature of the nodular BCC.[71,72] This type of BCC is poorly circumscribed; the epithelial nests are widely separated from each other, show little palisading of the peripheral basal cells and often have a spiky shape. The well-developed stromal–parenchymal interaction that characterizes the usual nodular BCC is lacking. Some of these lesions have a central tumor nodule with infiltrative margins but others have no central nodular mass.

## Classification

BCCs have also traditionally been histologically classified according to their degree and mode of differentiation, e.g. solid (primordial), adenoid, keratotic, pigmented and so forth. However, there is an accumulating body of evidence suggesting that the growth pattern of the neoplasm is more relevant than the degree of differentiation from the perspective of providing the clinician with information that may be helpful in planning the optimal therapeutic procedure.[71]

## Circumscribed BCC

The typical and most common BCC is the nodular or noduloulcerative type, which is a dome-shaped lesion. It is composed of irregularly sized and shaped islands of basaloid cells. Characteristically, the islands are relatively large and are aggregated in a cohesive cluster bound together by a fibrovascular stroma. The tumor margins are convex and the neoplasm grows in an expansile fashion. This tendency of the neoplasm to cohesiveness and expansile growth accounts for the circumscription of the tumor at the deep and lateral margins. The fact that the great majority of BCCs have a circumscribed growth pattern mainly accounts for their high cure rate. This type of BCC is usually symmetric and the margins can usually be easily determined clinically by inspection and palpation. Such lesions can be adequately treated by removal with a narrow margin of normal skin.[73]

## Solid BCC

The solid BCC is composed primarily of large aggregates of basaloid cells with no evidence of differentiation toward any adnexal structure (Fig. 11.10). The cells are relatively uniform in size and have large nuclei with inapparent nucleoli and scant cytoplasm. The cell borders are not crisply defined as are those of SCC and it is often difficult to see intercellular bridges. Desmosomes are present, however, as has been readily demonstrated by electron microscopy and immunohistochemical studies and they can be visualized by light microscopy in about 60% of cases.[74] The cells at

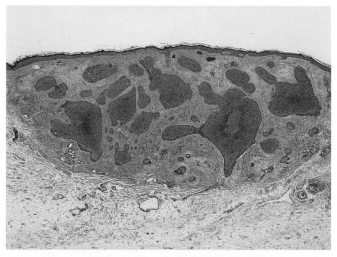

**Figure 11.10** Solid basal cell carcinoma. Note the symmetry and circumscription of the tumor. It was composed predominantly of large islands of uniform cells. (H&E; original magnification ×25.)

the periphery of the islands tend to align in a parallel array with the base of the cell contacting the basement membrane and the apex pointing inward toward the center of the island. This picket fence-like arrangement is referred to as palisading (Fig. 11.11). Mitotic figures are usually not found and, when present, usually appear normal. The large islands of basal cells often show central necrosis. This leads to the formation of lacunae, which contain amorphous debris and degenerated cells.

The islands of basaloid epithelial cells comprise the tumor parenchyma. They are embedded in a fibrovascular stroma that consists of plump fibroblasts in a meshwork of fine collagen fibers and abundant ground substance. The stroma serves a sustentacular role. The stroma often contains abundant mucin, especially adjacent to the islands of epithelial cells (Fig. 11.12). Because of the high content of glycosaminoglycans in the stroma which are removed during routine tissue processing, the stroma often pulls away from the palisaded row of basal cells at the edges of the islands, thereby producing artefactual clefts. These clefts are found so regularly in paraffin-embedded specimens that they have taken on diagnostic importance. Inflammation is not usually prominent in tumors that are not ulcerated. There often is a sparse to moderate infiltrate of mononuclear cells in the stroma with little or no exocytosis in the islands of basal cells. However, if the lesion becomes ulcerated, the inflammatory infiltrate becomes more pronounced and can be dense. Plasma cells are commonly found in the stroma of lesions from the face and scalp.

## BCC with squamous metaplasia (basosquamous or metatypical carcinoma)

Some BCCs show regions with cellular features resembling SCC (Figs 11.13 and 11.14). This type of BCC is composed of cells that are both basaloid and squamoid in appearance while retaining the typical organization of basal cell carcinoma. The presence of the stroma serves to distinguish BCC with squamous differentiation from SCC that does not evoke a stromal proliferation. There usually are some islands of basaloid tumor cells and others in which basal cells merge into a region composed of atypical squamoid cells. Some

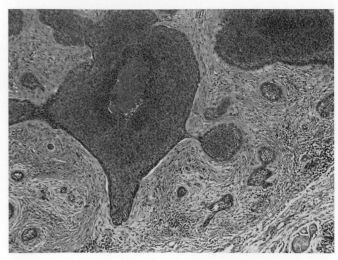

Figure 11.11 Prominent palisading of the outermost row of basal cells. Clear zone adjacent to the palisaded cells is due to loss of mucin from this area during tissue processing. (H&E; original magnification ×200.)

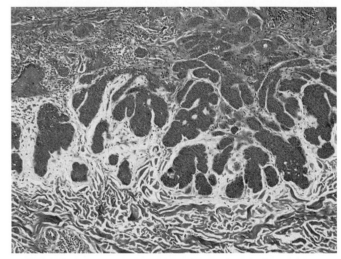

Figure 11.12 Basal cell carcinoma with myxoid stroma. (H&E; original magnification ×100.)

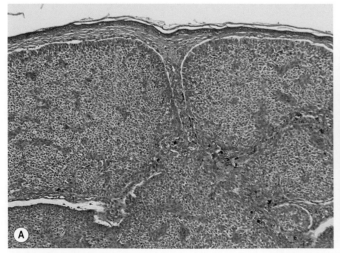

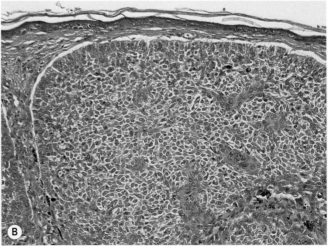

Figure 11.13 A) Basal cell carcinoma with squamous metaplasia. This neoplasm has the usual organization of solid basal cell carcinoma. (H&E; original magnification ×40.) B) At higher magnification, it can be seen that many of the cells have abundant cytoplasm, are angulated rather than round, and show intercellular bridges. (H&E; original magnification ×100.)

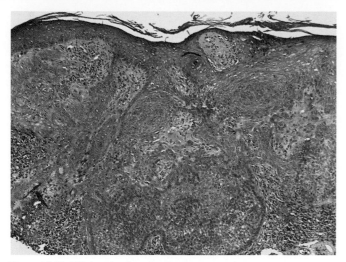

**Figure 11.14** This basal cell carcinoma shows prominent squamous differentiation in the superficial portion of the tumor. The deeper portion shows more typically basaloid cells and prominent peripheral palisading. (H&E; original magnification ×100.)

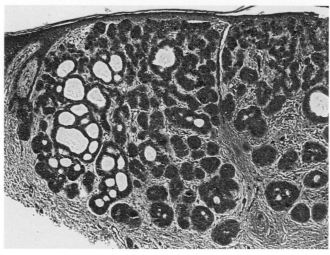

**Figure 11.15** Adenoid basal cell carcinoma. The tumor islands are composed of basaloid epithelial cells surrounded by myxoid stroma. The arrangement of basaloid cells around the stroma focally resembles tubular structures. (H&E; original magnification ×40.)

authors consider squamous metaplasia in BCC to be a sign of differentiation, whereas others correlate this finding with the potential for more aggressive biologic behavior.[68,75]

Some solid BCCs demonstrate abortive differentiation. These neoplasms have abundant mucin in the intercellular spaces and the basal cells become stellate in shape. Cystic degeneration may occur in the center of some islands. There is a distinct palisade of the peripheral row of basal cells that maintain their normal morphology. This type of BCC may represent differentiation toward follicular sheath. Granular BCC is a rare variant of solid BCC in which several of the basal cell lobules are replaced by cells which have eccentric nuclei and cytoplasmic granules identical to the cells of granular cell tumor. Some BCCs may show foci of differentiation toward sebaceous cells. If sebaceous differentiation is prominent, the neoplasm may be classified as a sebaceous epithelioma.[76] These lesions must be distinguished from clear cell BCC, in which the tumor cells have abundant cytoplasmic accumulations of glycogen.

## Adenoid BCC

This type of BCC is characterized by interweaving cords and varying-sized islands of basal cells, which are surrounded by a mucinous stroma (Fig. 11.15). The entrapment of the mucinous stroma between anastomosing strands of cells and within cell islands produces the appearance of gland-like or tubular structures. Adenoid BCCs showing cystic change have been called adenocystic BCC. This term should probably be avoided as it may cause confusion with a different entity, adenoid cystic carcinoma.[8]

## Cystic BCC

Microcysts are commonly found in islands of basal cells in solid BCCs. These are the result of necrosis of cells in the central portion of the islands. Some BCCs show a unique histologic picture that merits the designation 'cystic'.[74] These uncommon tumors consist of one or a few exceptionally large islands of basal cells in which there is a large central

lacuna containing amorphous debris and partially degenerated acantholytic epithelial cells (Fig. 11.16).

## Cornifying (keratotic) BCC

Rarely, BCCs demonstrate the capacity to cornify, usually in the center of the basaloid islands (Fig. 11.17). The keratin may be ortho- and/or parakeratotic. These lesions can be distinguished from trichoepithelioma by the absence of abortive hair papilla formation in them, the unusual presence of stromal retraction around the islands of basaloid cells present, and predominance of the epithelial component over the stromal component.

## Follicular BCC (infundibulocystic BCC)

Follicular BCC is a peculiar variant that occurs on the face.[77] These lesions characteristically are small and are composed of aggregates of basaloid cells containing microcysts (Figs 11.18 and 11.19). The microcysts have delicately laminated orthokeratotic material in them and often show squamoid metaplasia around the cysts. Some of the basaloid islands may rarely resemble hair follicles in telogen. They share features in common with trichoepithelioma, but they can be distinguished in several ways. In follicular BCC (in contrast to trichoepithelioma) the aggregates of cells frequently are in continuity with the epidermis, the stroma comprises the minority rather than the majority of the tumor, there are no foreign body reactions to keratin, and structures reminiscent of hair papillae are lacking.

## Fibroepithelioma of Pinkus

This type of BCC is composed of lace-like fronds of basaloid cells that anastomose in an edematous-appearing fibrous stroma (Fig. 11.20). The strands of basaloid cells emanate from the basal layer of the epidermis. Often there are more typical islands of basaloid cells with peripheral palisading.

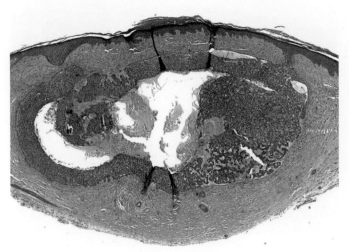

Figure 11.16 Cystic basal cell carcinoma. The bulk of this neoplasm is composed of an exceptionally large island of basal cells which shows central cystic degeneration. (H&E; original magnification ×80.)

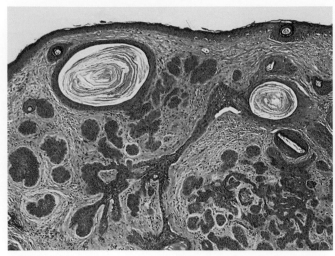

Figure 11.18 Basal cell carcinoma with follicular differentiation. This tumor is characteristically small, symmetric, well-circumscribed and superficial. Many of the aggregates of basaloid cells resemble telogen follicles. Microcysts are present (H&E; original magnification ×40.)

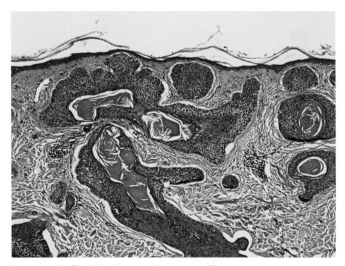

Figure 11.17 Cornifying basal cell carcinoma. There are central cystic structures containing masses of orthokeratin and a granular zone adjacent to the keratin. The structures resemble aberrant follicular units. (H&E; original magnification ×40.)

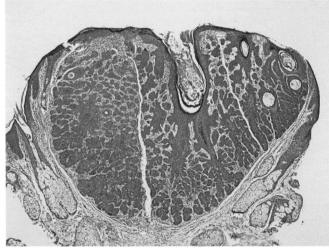

Figure 11.19 Basal cell carcinoma with follicular differentiation. This lesion shows occasional small horn cysts and fissures in the stroma. (H&E; original magnification ×80.)

## Pigmented BCC

Melanin pigmentation may occur in all types of BCC with the possible exception of the morphea type. However, most pigmented BCCs are of the solid type (Fig. 11.21). In pigmented BCCs, melanocytes are interspersed among the basal cells and variable amounts of melanin are present within the cytoplasm of the neoplastic basal cells.[78] There are also numerous macrophages with melanin pigment in the stroma.

## BCC with diffuse growth pattern

As opposed to the common nodular BCC which presents clinically as a dome-shaped lesion with fairly well-defined borders, lesions of the diffuse growth variant tend to be plaque-like or flat, spread horizontally in the skin and have poorly defined margins. These lesions tend to have a higher recurrence rate because they extend insidiously beyond the clinically visible or palpable border. Therefore, it is often difficult for the clinician to accurately gauge how much normal-appearing tissue around the tumor must be sacrificed in order to achieve total removal.

## Superficial BCC

Histologically, these tumors show horizontally arranged lobules of atypical basal cells in the papillary dermis that have broad-based connections with the epidermis (Fig. 11.22). All islands of basal cells contact the epidermis. Therefore, there is no downward extension into the middle or deep dermis but rather only superficial centrifugal growth is typically seen. The lobules of basal cells show palisading of the peripheral basal cells as do other types of BCC. A thin fibrovascular stroma, often with a host response of lymphocytes and histiocytes, underlies the tumor nests.

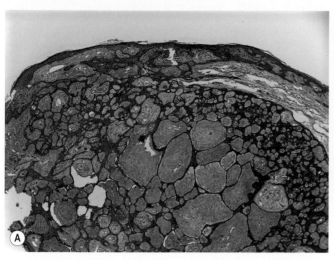
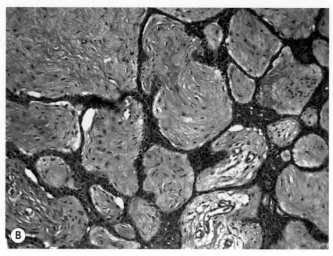

**Figure 11.20** Fibroepithelioma. The bulk of this neoplasm is composed of the myxoid stroma. The epithelial component is made up mainly of anastomosing cords of basal cells. There is a fairly large aggregate of basal cells in the upper right corner beneath the epidermis. (H&E; original magnification ×40 and ×100.)

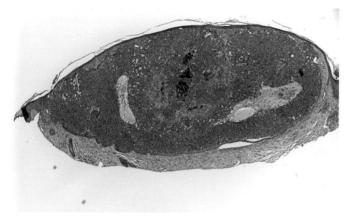

**Figure 11.21** Pigmented basal cell carcinoma. This solid tumor shows many macrophages in the stroma and in the area of cystic necrosis that contain melanin pigment. (H&E; original magnification ×40).

## Morpheic BCC

Morpheic BCCs are notoriously difficult to treat because of their insidious centrifugal extensions, which make it difficult to determine margins by clinical inspection or palpation. Salasche and Ammonette found morphologic extensions averaging approximately 7mm in these lesions.[79] The dense fibrous stroma, which comprises the majority of the tumor volume, precludes treatment by curettage.

Morpheic BCCs often show no connection with the epidermis and the epithelial structures of adnexa are completely effaced. There are often cords, strands and small nests of basaloid cells enmeshed in a dense stroma of thickened collagen bundles (Figs 11.23 and 11.24). Mucin is scant to absent, so there often is no evidence of retraction of the stroma from the epithelial cells. Because the nests and cords of cells are so thin, there is no palisading of the basal cells except in some of the small islands that may be present in some tumors. These strands and cords of cells most often are arranged parallel to the surface or at an acute angle to it.

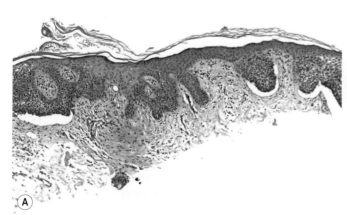
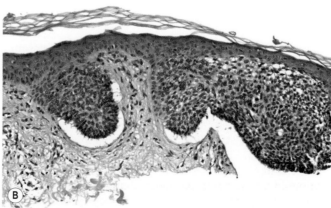

**Figure 11.22** Superficial basal cell carcinoma. The periphery of the lesion is at the left. The 'shoulder' of the tumor is composed of horizontally oriented nests of basal cells that are connected to the epidermis. The stroma encases these islands. Evidence exists of regression in the central portion of the lesion, where there is fibrosis in the upper dermis and a dense host response of mononuclear cells. (H&E; original magnification ×40 and ×100.)

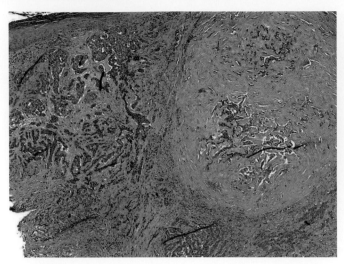

**Figure 11.23** Morpheic basal cell carcinoma. The epithelial component is made up of small angulated nests, cords and strands of basal cells. These are surrounded by a dense collagenous stroma. Inflammation is characteristically sparse or absent and palisading is not present. There is usually no connection of the tumor islands with the epidermis, although this lesion does have some epidermal connection. (H&E; original magnification ×40.)

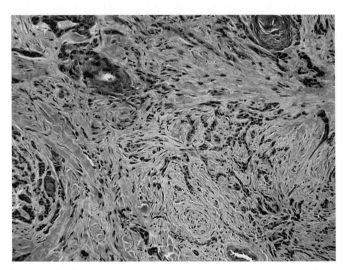

**Figure 11.24** This morpheic basal cell carcinoma shows only strands of hyperchromatic basal cells in the abundant fibrotic stroma. It resembles metastatic scirrhous carcinoma of the breast. There is a focus of calcification at the far left. (H&E; original magnification ×80.)

Morpheic BCCs must be distinguished histologically from syringoma, desmoplastic trichoepithelioma and metastatic adenocarcinoma. Syringoma has as its hallmark small tubular epithelial structures embedded in a sclerotic stroma. However, in some sections (especially in those taken near the periphery of the lesion), the lumina may not be evident and one sees only strands of epithelial cells in a dense collagenous stroma. Simply cutting and examining more sections will differentiate these lesions because the lumina will be found and morpheic BCCs never demonstrate lumina in the epithelial strands. Desmoplastic trichoepithelioma (Fig. 11.25) can also usually be distinguished from morpheic BCC through the presence in these tumors of microcysts containing keratin, which are not found in morpheic BCCs.[80]

Most problematic is distinguishing metastatic adenocarcinoma (especially breast carcinoma which may induce a scirrhous tissue reaction) from morpheic BCC. Careful examination of the tissue sections may reveal foci of glandular differentiation in metastatic adenocarcinoma or mucin droplets in the cytoplasm may be detectable with a mucicarmine stain. Furthermore, some metastatic adenocarcinomas will show the presence of carcinoembryonic antigen on staining by the immunoperoxidase method whereas BCCs do not.

### Infiltrating BCC

This term has been used to denote a peculiar type of BCC that, untreated, may pursue a particularly aggressive course of local tissue destruction.[72] These lesions lack a central cohesive mass of basal cell islands as seen in nodular BCC. Instead, they consist of elongated islands and cords of atypical basal cells that are widely separated spatially. The nests of tumor cells are often angulated and may be oriented almost perpendicular to the surface (Fig. 11.26). Palisading may be present but often is not well developed. The stroma may be mucinous, edematous or fibrotic. The dispersion of the tumor islands produces a poorly marginated flattish or plaque-like lesion. These tumors expand peripherally as do morpheic-type BCCs but typically show simultaneous deep extension to underlying prominences of soft tissue whereas morpheic BCC usually remains confined to the reticular dermis.

### Micronodular BCC

Micronodular BCC shares with infiltrating BCC the propensity for dispersion of the nests of epithelial cells. These neoplasms are made of small, round aggregates of basal cells rather than large aggregates as seen in solid BCCs.[66] Palisading is often well developed. The islands approximate the size of hair bulbs. These lesions, too, usually are poorly defined and flat with indistinct borders and have the capacity to invade deeply. A unique aspect is the fact that the nests of cells at the deep aspect of the lesion often seem to be lying free in the tissue without surrounding stroma (Fig. 11.27). This may indicate that these clones have acquired an autonomous nature unlike ordinary solid BCCs, in which the epithelial component is intimately dependent upon the connective tissue stroma for its propagation.

It is not uncommon to see BCCs that have a mixture of growth patterns in varying combinations. For example, some lesions may have a micronodular component admixed with a solid component or a micronodular component with an infiltrative one. The presence of an infiltrative and/or micronodulary component along with a solid central or eccentric nodule indicates the potential for more aggressive local growth than in solid, purely nodular BCCs.[81]

### Eccrine and apocrine epithelioma

Just as some BCCs may show follicular or sebaceous differentiation, others may show eccrine or apocrine features, although this presentation is much less common.[82,83] Depending upon the individual lesion, eccrine epitheliomas may show a combination of fairly typical islands of BCCs, small cystic islands or syringoma-like areas in varying proportions within a scirrhous stroma. Eccrine epitheliomas, which have been

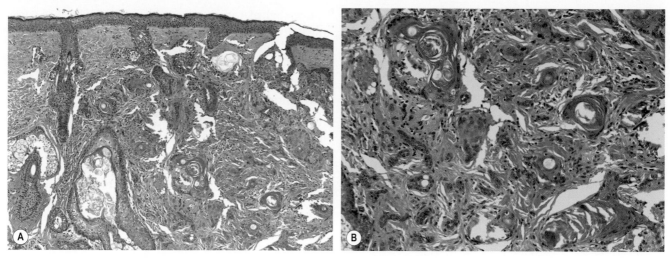

**Figure 11.25** Desmoplastic trichoepithelioma. Note the horn cysts and an abortive follicle. Horn cysts and follicular differentiation are not found in morpheic basal cell carcinomas. (H&E; original magnification ×40 and ×100).

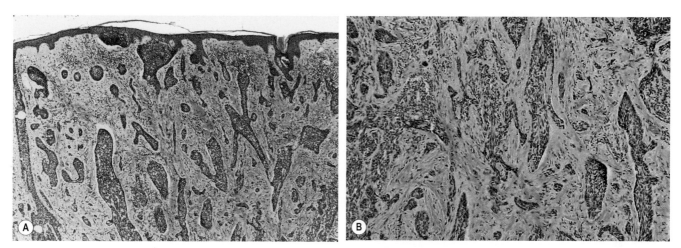

**Figure 11.26 A)** Infiltrating basal cell carcinoma. There is no central mass of basaloid cells. The epithelial component is composed of irregularly shaped islands and strands of basaloid cells dispersed in the stroma. The tumor is a plaque with a flat surface. Note extensions into the subcutaneous fat. (H&E; original magnification ×40.) **B)** The cellular aggregates have poorly developed palisading. (H&E; original magnification ×80.)

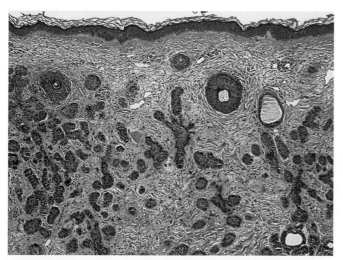

**Figure 11.27** Micronodular basal cell carcinoma. Instead of large islands of basal cells, this variant is made up of small aggregates of cells. Palisading is often apparent around the periphery of the small nests, but stromal retraction is not usually present. (H&E; original magnification ×80.)

found most commonly in the scalp, tend to recur as do other BCCs with a diffuse growth pattern. Apocrine epithelioma is rare: only one case has been reported.

## Basaloid hyperplasia in dermatofibroma

There seems to be a stimulus for epidermal proliferation elaborated by the stromal cells in the dermis of dermatofibromas. Almost all dermatofibromas show epidermal hyperplasia with orthohyperkeratosis and peculiar elongation of the rete ridges, giving them a 'boot of Italy' appearance. Some dermatofibromas also show induction of hair germs from the base of the epidermis (Fig. 11.28). These buds of hyperplastic basal cells show peripheral palisading, are surrounded by a cellular myxoid stroma and resemble the basaloid lobules of superficial BCC. The small size and rounded contour of these buds are clues to their benign nature. Furthermore, usually only one or a few such buds are present in the lesion. In rare instances, however, true BCC evolves from the epidermis of dermatofibroma (Fig. 11.29).

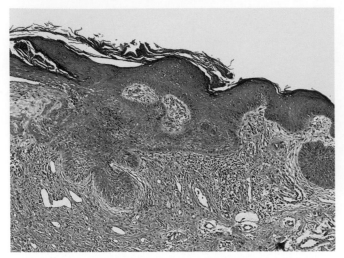

Figure 11.28 Dermatofibroma with induction of follicular germs. There are aggregates of basaloid cells emanating from the base of the epidermis; these show the organization of primitive follicles. (H&E; original magnification ×80.)

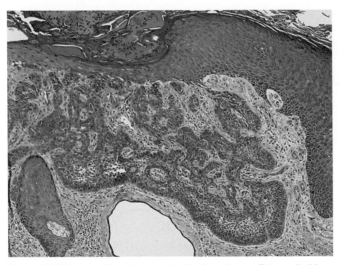

Figure 11.29 Basal cell carcinoma originating in a dermatofibroma. In this lesion, the islands of basal cells are not showing any evidence of follicular differentiation, the islands are multifocal and the epidermis is ulcerated. (H&E; original magnification ×80.)

## Evolutionary histologic changes

Necrosis is common in islands of neoplastic basal cells. Sometimes entire islands of cells become necrotic. A sequela of necrosis is dystrophic calcification. Calcium is commonly found in small aggregates in BCCs. On occasion, these calcium deposits serve as the nidus for metaplastic bone formation.

Partial regression may also occur in BCCs. Some investigators have noted regression in 20% of lesions.[84] Regression is characterized by a zone of fibrosis within the tumor. This is the result of the host immune response and of apoptosis. Areas of active regression show a dense mononuclear cell infiltrate around the lobules of basal cells. These contain many necrotic cells that can be identified by their pyknotic nuclei and eosinophilic cytoplasm.

Another finding associated with cell death in BCCs is the deposition of amyloid in the stroma.[85] It has been demonstrated that the amyloid in macular and lichen amyloidosis is the result of death of epidermal cells with the conversion of tonofilaments to amyloid fibrils. A similar phenomenon probably accounts for the common finding of amyloid globules in BCCs.

## Perineural and perifollicular extensions of BCC

Neoplasms often show a propensity to follow the paths of least resistance in their local growth. In the skin, nerves (see Fig. 11.33C) and hair follicles (Fig. 11.30) offer potential pathways along which BCC may extend beyond the main tumor body. Because these tumor extensions are not bulky, they are imperceptible to the physician during surgery and may be left behind to serve as a nidus for recurrence. Perifollicular extension is especially common on the scalp where there are terminal follicles that are deeply rooted in the subcutaneous tissue. An excision that does not extend deeply enough may result in tumor being buried in the base of the wound even though the main portion of the tumor has been adequately excised. It is important for the pathologist to scan the histologic sections for evidence of perineural and perifollicular extensions of BCC.

## Ultrastructural features of BCC

By electron microscopy, undifferentiated BCCs are composed of two cell types. The major cell type has a large nucleus, sparse mitochondria and granular endoplasmic reticulum, abundant tonofilaments and prominent desmosomes. The second, less common cell type has dark granular cytoplasm and an irregular nucleus. The dark appearance of the cytoplasm results from a large number of free RNA particles. The morphologic features of undifferentiated BCC cells, therefore, are similar to normal epidermal basal and squamous cells. Pilar and eccrine differentiation may occur in some tumors. Some authors have found evidence of neuroendocrine differentiation in rare examples of BCC.[86]

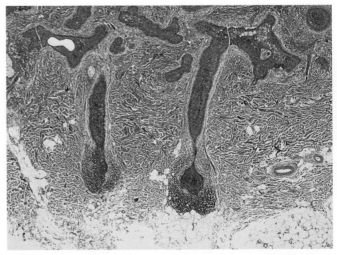

Figure 11.30 In this neoplasm, the atypical basal cells have extended downward in the tracts of follicular units. (H&E; original magnification ×80.)

## IMMUNOHISTOCHEMICAL FEATURES

AE 1 is a monoclonal antikeratin antibody that has specificity for normal epidermal basal cells. BCCs show weak homogeneous staining with AE 1 by the peroxidase-antiperoxidase method.[87] Moll et al. used monoclonal antibodies to desmoplakins to study various tumors for desmosome expression by immunofluorescence microscopy and demonstrated that desmosomes in BCC are detectable by this technique.[88]

Stanley et al.[89] also used immunofluorescence to study the components of the basement membrane around the tumor aggregates in BCC. Laminin, type IV collagen and bullous pemphigoid antigen are definite protein components of normal epidermal basement membrane. Antibodies to laminin and to type IV collagen were found to react with the basement membrane around all tumor aggregates. Bullous pemphigoid antigen, which is produced by normal epidermal basal cells, was not detected strongly or continuously around the islands of neoplastic basal cells, indicating that there is a selective defect of bullous pemphigoid antigen in the basement membrane of BCC. Alpha-smooth muscle actin has been documented in 66% of micronodular, 62% of morpheic and 0% of nodular BCCs.[90] The presence of actin may be a marker for aggressive invasion in micronodular tumors. Expression of stromolysin 3, a member of the metalloproteinase family, is increased in deeply invasive BCC and morpheic BCC compared to the global rate of expression in BCC and may facilitate invasion.[91] The monoclonal antibody Ber-EP4 is an epithelial marker that targets a partially formalin resistant epitope on two glycoproteins of unknown function. It shows promise in distinguishing BCC from SCC[92-95] and microcystic adnexal carcinoma.[96]

## TREATMENT

There are relatively few double-blind randomized controlled trials that address treatment of BCC. The National Comprehensive Cancer Network (NCCN) convenes a panel of clinician experts. This panel periodically updates practice guidelines based on continual review of published clinical evidence and vast anecdotal personal experience. The most current guidelines may be found in the NCCN Guidelines & Clinical Resources section under the 'Basal and Squamous Cell Skin Cancers' link at http://www.nccn.org/professionals/physician_gls/f_guidelines.asp

NCCN makes complete cure of the BCC the primary goal of management. Without tumor elimination, the following secondary goals, though desirable, are ultimately compromised: 1) preservation of normal tissue, 2) preservation of function, and 3) optimal cosmetic result. Robins and Albom showed a high recurrence rate for BCCs in young women, presumably because the secondary goal of cosmesis had taken precedence over the primary goal of definitive treatment.[97]

Though indolent in nature, a repeatedly undertreated BCC can ultimately lead to the loss of an eye or nose. If the physician managing a patient with a BCC decides to forego the primary goal of complete destruction and employ palliative therapy, informed consent should be obtained.

Ideally, all BCCs should be biopsied, allowing selection of the most appropriate treatment (see Chapter 40). When clinical diagnosis is certain, or a biopsy is not feasible, the clinician may treat empirically. However, a specimen from the treatment should be submitted for pathologic examination and, if necessary, the patient can be further treated.

When the clinical diagnosis of BCC, the extent, or the histologic subtype is not certain, a biopsy should be performed before treatment. This information allows selection of the most appropriate therapeutic course. Post-treatment biopsies may be helpful when margins were not evaluated during therapy, for example, with blind modalities such as cryosurgery, radiation, or topical therapy. Curettings submitted for pathologic evaluation may confirm the diagnosis of BCC but rarely allow a determination of histologic pattern or depth. A shave, punch, or incisional biopsy will provide a better diagnostic specimen. Even a shave may miss an aggressive growth pattern or a deeply buried recurrent BCC since the tumor may be below the epidermis or papillary dermis.

Management of BCC is related to the biologic behavior of the tumor. Although a comprehensive review of each treatment approach is provided elsewhere in this text, a description of their application to BCC is provided below.

## Treatment algorithm

Selection of appropriate treatment depends on whether the particular BCC has even a single risk factor for recurrence. The following nine items comprise the complete NCCN list of risk factors:

- diameter greater than 20 mm on trunk and extremities
- diameter greater than 10 mm on cheeks, forehead, scalp, or neck
- diameter greater than 6 mm on genitalia, hands, feet, or face excepting cheeks and forehead
- poorly defined borders
- recurrence
- immunosuppression
- area of prior radiation therapy
- any sign of morpheaform, sclerosing, mixed infiltrative, or micronodular histologic features
- perineural involvement.

If the BCC has none of these risk factors, treatment generally starts with standard excision or curettage and electrodesiccation in non-hair-bearing skin. If the BCC possesses even a single risk factor, treatment typically begins with Mohs surgery but occasionally excision is employed if the only risk factor is a diameter greater than 20 mm on the trunk and extremities. However, each BCC is a unique situation and treatment using a variety of therapeutic techniques is tailored to yield the optimal outcome. Table 11.2 shows the subtypes of BCC and their recommended treatment.

## Curettage and electrodesiccation

Curettage and electrodesiccation (CE) is the most commonly employed technique for BCC management (see Chapter 41). Cure rates up to 98% have been reported in the literature when used for appropriate lesions.[98] Some authors advocate that CE should be performed for a fixed number of cycles,[99] while others[98] feel the procedure should be repeated until a healthy base is encountered.

Table 11.2  Subtypes of Basal Cell Carcinoma (BCC) and their Recommended Treatment

| Type of BCC | Treatment Options |
|---|---|
| Nodular ≤2 cm (trunk, extremities) | Excision<br>Curettage and electrodesiccation (lesions should not be deeply invasive)<br>Cryosurgery ± curettage<br>Radiation*<br>Note: for lesions >2 cm, Mohs surgery is preferred |
| Nodular <1 cm (cheeks, forehead, scalp or neck) | Excision<br>Curettage and electrodesiccation (lesions should not be deeply invasive)<br>Cryosurgery ± curettage (skilful clinicians only)<br>Radiation*<br>Note: for lesions >1 cm, Mohs surgery is preferred |
| Nodular <0.6 cm (face except cheeks or forehead, genitalia, hands or feet) | Excision Mohs surgery†<br>Cryosurgery ± curettage (skilful clinicians only – may want pre- and post-treatment biopsies)<br>Radiation (may want pre- and post-treatment biopsies)*<br>Note: for lesions >0.6 cm, Mohs surgery is preferred |
| Superficial (multicentric) | Shave excision with curettage ± electrodesiccation<br>Curettage and electrodesiccation<br>5% Imiquimod<br>5-Fluorouracil (may need to use with curettage or occlusion)<br>Photodynamic therapy<br>Cryosurgery<br>Excision<br>Mohs surgery (if recurrent or large, e.g. >2cm)<br>Radiation (extremely superficial X-ray required; not a usual or preferred method)* |
| Morpheaform | Mohs surgery†<br>Excision (if Mohs surgery not available) |
| Aggressive growth pattern | Mohs surgery†<br>Excision (if Mohs surgery not available)<br>Radiation (may require pre- and post-treatment biopsies)* |
| 'Field fire' | Mohs surgery (allow wound to heal on its own if possible)†<br>Excision<br>Note: cryosurgery or radiation is not ideal; especially if possibly recurrent BCC |
| Metatypical | Mohs surgery†<br>Excision (if Mohs surgery not available)<br>Radiation (may need pre- and post-treatment biopsies)* |
| Recurrent | Mohs surgery†<br>Excision (if Mohs surgery not available) |
| Neurotropic | Mohs surgery†<br>Excision (if Mohs surgery not available)<br>Some of these patients may require postoperative radiation |
| Incompletely excised | Re-excise in conventional manner or by Mohs surgery |
| Unresectable and advanced disease | Cisplatin + doxorubicin + radiation |
| Metastases to regional nodes | Surgical removal of the nodes; may need to combine with radiation |
| Systemic metastases | Cisplatin + doxorubicin; may use with radiation when necessary |

*Should not be used in younger patients.

†Preferred treatment.

Both technique and lesion selection are crucial. The curette is ineffective when the BCC: 1) is enmeshed in a sclerotic stroma and/or has an aggressive histologic growth pattern (i.e. recurrent BCC, morpheaform BCC, sclerosing BCC, micronodular BCC); 2) buds off or is concealed between pilosebaceous units (e.g. nose, scalp); 3) is deeply invasive (e.g. perineural, deep dermis, subcutaneous fat, perichondrium, periosteum); or 4) cannot be immobilized (e.g. lips, eyelids).

CE should be used with caution in areas at high risk for recurrence, i.e. embryonic fusion planes, scalp, ear, lips, eyelids, nose and temples. The curette may track into the resulting hole, rendering curettage unreliable.[100,101] If curettage does not yield a firm base, the tumor may be extensive. The margin control achieved by Mohs surgery or even conventional excision in such cases provides critical information.

CE appears best suited for well-defined exophytic, nodular BCCs under 1cm located in areas at a lower risk for recurrence. The size limitation does not apply to sBCCs. CE is quick and particularly useful in a patient with multiple lesions. However, the technique is subtle and high cure rates require experience. It can cause hypopigmentation and hypertrophic scarring (especially in young adults and on the trunk and extremities) which generally improves with time[99] and can be treated with corticosteroids. CE done near a free margin (e.g. eyelids, lip) can result in notching and ectropion. The lack of margin evaluation inherent in CE may leave deep foci of BCC capable of prolonged undetected growth.[102]

To improve cosmetic results, some investigators have omitted electrodesiccation. This appears to minimize hypertrophic scarring but not hypopigmentation.[103] The cure rate appears to be only slightly compromised.[104]

## Surgical excision

Excision offers the potential of histologic margin control, rapid healing and optimal cosmetic result (Chapter 46). Potentially, it can be used for all types of BCCs in all locations. However, it is time-consuming, sacrifices normal tissue and requires much more skill and training than does CE. It is less suitable for numerous lesions and reconstruction may be required to prevent or correct resultant cosmetic and functional defects.[105] The histologic control it offers in treating recurrent BCC,[106] morpheaform BCC,[79,107] BCCs with an aggressive histology,[108,109] sBCC,[71] and BCC in high-risk areas[105,110] is inferior to that achieved by Mohs surgery. Thus, recurrence rates are higher for these subtypes.

Excision of large sBCCs, often located on the trunk and extremities, may require grafting and often results in sacrifice of healthy tissue and an unsightly spreading scar.[101] A similar cosmetic result may be achieved by CE or cryosurgery.

Margins for excision of BCCs range from 3–5mm for small primary BCCs to 1.5–3.0cm for recurrent BCCs.[66] Sexton et al. found more marginal involvement when excising aggressive growth pattern BCCs.[66] Wolf and Zitelli[73] found 4-mm margins sufficient to eradicate 98% of 'well-defined' non-morpheaform BCCs up to 2cm in diameter. In lesions greater than 2cm in diameter, they found subclinical spread to be so variable that concrete margin recommendations could not be made. Given these data, for morpheaform BCCs, recurrent BCCs, BCCs greater than 2cm in size, and BCCs with aggressive histologic patterns, margins of 1cm or greater may be necessary.

An excision to the level of fat is generally adequate for small primary BCCs. However, large, longstanding BCCs, recurrent BCCs, and those in high-risk areas may penetrate more deeply.

Though excisional surgery complications include scarring, hypopigmentation, infection and cosmetic deformity, cosmetic results improve with time and scar revision is possible.[111]

### Mohs micrographic surgery

The complete histologic margin evaluation unique to Mohs surgery allows for maximum tissue preservation during the complete eradication of nearly any BCC (Chapter 47).[112]

It is the treatment of choice for any of the high-risk BCCs as defined at the beginning of this section, including the following: large invasive BCCs; those with morpheaform or aggressive histologic features; those in high-risk areas; those which are recurrent;[112] those which exhibit perineural spread;[113] those which are ill-defined; those which have been incompletely excised; as well as those in areas where tissue preservation is important (Fig. 11.31).

In addition to the disadvantages and complications associated with any excision, Mohs surgery can be time-consuming and tedious. The added training, equipment and personnel limit its availability in some regions. However, when appropriately utilized for BCC, Mohs surgery is cost-effective[114] since: 1) an office setting, not an operating room, is generally utilized; 2) the Mohs surgeon is also the pathologist; and 3) with the high cure rate, expensive recurrences are rare.

Though there are no monoclonal antibodies specific to BCC, Mohs surgeons use certain staining patterns to distinguish tumor cells from epithelial and adenexal structures. These antibodies seem particularly useful in finding subtle tumor cells amongst dense inflammation, as seen in patients with CLL, or finding tumor around nerves, as seen with aggressive subtypes.[115-120]

In patients with basal cell nevus syndrome burdened with numerous lesions, clearing lateral margins may create an impractically large Mohs defect. In such circumstances, one may choose to settle for clearing only deep margins and consider using less invasive modalities (ie. imiquimod) to manage the epidermal component.

## Radiation therapy

Radiation therapy has the advantages of sparing normal tissue, eliminating the need for reconstructive surgery and providing an alternative to a surgical procedure (see Chapter 52). However, great care in patient selection is required as there are several potential pitfalls. It is often employed for BCCs of the nose, ear and periocular area because it may decrease collateral damage to delicate

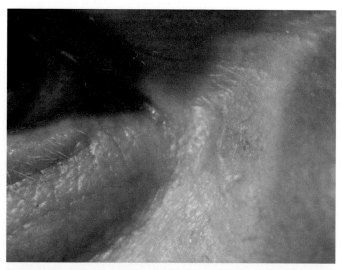

**Figure 11.31** Periocular location of this basal cell carcinoma is an indication for Mohs surgery. (Courtesy of Brook Brouha, MD.)

structures such as the lacrimal collecting system.[121] It also is an additional option for poor surgical candidates.[122] There is a significant failure rate for high-risk areas and for recurrent, large, and/or aggressive subtype BCCs. Moreover, there is the inconvenience and expense of multiple treatments. Lastly, in contrast to the invasive therapies, the cosmetic result of radiation deteriorates with time. Radiation therapy can work as palliation, debulking an otherwise inoperable BCC.[123] Radiation may also be used adjunctively when recurrence is a concern.

Radiation therapy should be avoided in younger patients[124] in the treatment of morpheaform BCCs because of poor cosmetic outcomes,[125] and in patients with basal cell nevus syndrome because of the possibility of stimulating additional BCCs.[126] However, with optimal lesion and patient selection, radiation therapy can result in 5-year cure rates of 90–95%.[122,125,127–129] Unfortunately, there is a decrease in cure rate in larger lesions[110,123] and at certain sites such as the nose.[110] Also, radiation therapy can miss deep tumor. The resulting undetected growth, particularly in the periocular area, can result in disastrous loss of function.

Although certain small BCCs can be effectively managed by a single radiation session, fractionation of the dose over time is better tolerated by normal tissue and leads to a better cosmetic result. Unfortunately, the appearance of an irradiated area deteriorates with time and, depending on the locations, will be characterized by atrophy, telangiectasia and/or hypopigmentation.[122,125] Other complications of radiation therapy include comedones and chronic radiation dermatitis.[127] Scalp lesions generally are avoided because of resultant alopecia.[125]

The 27% failure rate noted when irradiating recurrent BCCs illustrates that high cure rates seen with certain primary BCCs are not universally applicable.[122] These recurrent lesions, as well as certain large or aggressive subtype primary BCCs, may be ill-defined and/or have substantial subclinical extension. To compensate for subclinical spread, wider margins are included in the radiation field. In recurrent or high-risk primary BCCs, delineation of the tumor through pretreatment biopsies may be advisable.[122] Under certain circumstances, post-treatment biopsies may also be appropriate.

The healing process after irradiation may require weeks to months, especially on the trunk and extremities.[122] Erythema then often oozing and crusting result. These symptoms may be accompanied by itching, burning and crawling sensations. Subsequently, the area ulcerates and slowly heals. Massive necrosis signifies a large tumor and biopsies should be performed if this was not anticipated.

## Cryosurgery

When using cryosurgery to treat a BCC, a cryoprobe with a liquid nitrogen spray unit is necessary (see Chapter 42). Discs or cotton-tipped swabs dipped in liquid nitrogen are typically not sufficient for treating any BCC.

An adequate tumor kill requires a double freeze–thaw cycle with a tissue temperature of −50°C.[130] Electrical impedance of the tissue may be the most useful variable to follow.[130] Tumors overlying cartilage or bone may be frozen until the tissue becomes fixed to the underlying structure,

signifying sufficient depth.[131] In sBCC, a single freeze may be adequate for cure. As with other modalities, treatment of a margin of 'clinically normal' skin may compensate for subclinical involvement.[130,132]

Though opinion varies, great care should be exercised if cryosurgery is chosen to treat BCCs with aggressive histologic features, recurrent BCCs, morpheaform BCCs, metatypical BCCs and BCCs located in high-risk areas.[130,132–136] Sclerosing BCCs may respond poorly to cryosurgery because of their ill-defined nature and because the sclerotic tissue may be insulating.[134] Preoperative biopsies may help determine extent of the tumor. Post-treatment biopsies may discover buried foci of residual tumor, an important concern with this modality. For this reason, cryosurgery should not be performed on the scalp. Similarly, cryosurgery on lower legs results in slow healing, poor cosmetic results and an increased infection risk.[134]

Cure rates as high as 97% have been achieved for nodular BCCs less than 1cm in size,[133] and in primary BCCs 2cm or less in size have been reported to be as high as 97–98%.[131,137] Cure rates drop for BCCs greater than 2cm and for recurrent BCCs, morpheaform BCCs, sBCCs, BCCs with an aggressive histologic growth pattern, and BCCs in high-risk areas.[131,133,135,137] Cryosurgery may also be used for palliation.[131] Aggressive treatment of BCCs overlying superficial nerves (e.g. ulnar area, finger) may result in neuralgia and neuropathy that may persist up to 2 years but usually resolves.[136] Excepting sBBC, tumors greater than 3cm are poor candidates for cryosurgery.[136]

A lasting depression may follow, particularly on the tip of the nose, forehead, back, chest and ear. Cryosurgery near the vermilion of the upper lip or the cartilage of the ear may result in notching. Hypertrophic scars, when present, are generally visible by 6 weeks.

In summary, cryosurgery is tissue-sparing and is especially useful in patients in poor health, taking anticoagulants and/or with pacemakers. Used properly, it produces high cure rates for small nodular BCCs. However, it is a blind treatment modality and should be used with great caution for high-risk lesions. Cosmetically, the results compare to those achieved with CE.

## Lasers

Superficial BCC can be treated by the carbon dioxide ($CO_2$) laser in a defocused vaporizing mode combined after curettage. High cure rates, minimal discomfort, rapid healing and usually excellent cosmesis have been reported, though follow-up in some cases has been limited.[138–140] However, because of hypertrophic scars in 5% of patients and common hypopigmentation, this indication appears to offer no advantage over CE.

The $CO_2$ laser used in focused or incisional mode can excise BCCs much like a scalpel. Unlike electrosurgery, the $CO_2$ laser does not compromise histologic examination of the specimen. The $CO_2$ laser may be useful in patients on anticoagulants or with pacemakers as it seals blood and lymph vessels. It may also decrease wound infections as it sterilizes as it cuts and can also remove involved cartilage or bone.[141]

## Photodynamic therapy

Photodynamic therapy (PDT) can be used for BCC treatment (Chapter 45).[142,143] The tumor concentrates the photosensitizing agent relative to surrounding skin. A light source, shone on the skin, activates the photosensitizer, causing necrosis of the tumor.

The reduced penetration associated with topical application usually limits utility to thin lesions. Response rates of 92% for sBCC and 71% for nodular BCC have been reported at 6 months,[144] but in other studies recurrence is significant (11–44%).[145,146] PDT has also been succesfully used to treat BCCs in patients with Gorlin syndrome.[147]

## Topical chemotherapy

### Immune response modifiers

Imiquimod cream acts through Toll-like receptor 7 to produce interferon-alpha, tumor necrosis factor-alpha and other cytokines (Chapter 44). It primarily targets antigen-presenting cells such as monocytes, dendritic cells and epidermal Langerhans cells.[148,149]

The initial studies treating primary nodular and superficial BCCs were encouraging.[150] Three-month studies show a better response rate for sBCCs than for nodular BCCs (81% average vs 76%).[151-156] Imiquimod also shows promise as an adjunct in the management of large sBCCs[157] and multiple sBCCs.[158,159]

### Other agents

Topical 5-fluorouracil (5-FU), because of its variable penetration, should be used at a concentration of at least 5%, and then only for treating sBCC.[160] 5-FU is not effective in eradicating invasive BCC or BCC with follicular involvement.[161] When used on deeper tumors, 5-FU may treat the surface but a residual hidden component may grow extensively before discovery.[162]

Topical 5% 5-FU is applied twice daily to sBCC for no less than 6 weeks. Three months may be necessary. Approximately 3% of patients, usually those with multiple lesions, may become allergic to 5-FU.[163] Because topical 5-FU can conceal deep foci of BCC, requires prolonged treatment, and can be painful, it should be reserved as a last resort. However, 5-FU may have prophylactic value in patients who develop multiple BCCs, e.g. basal cell nevus syndrome.[160]

Ingenol-3-angelate (Ing3A), extracted from *Euphorbia peplus*, is currently in clinical trials for eradicating BCC by topical application. Early studies suggest that efficacy appears to be dose-related.[164] Ing3A induced acute neutrophilic inflammation on mouse skin and caused subcutaneous hemorrhage and vascular damage. Both Ing3A and phorbol 12-myristate 13-acetate (PMA) activated extracellular signal-regulated kinase 1/2 (ERK1/2) in epidermis, but Ing3A also activated ERK1/2 in skin dermal fibroblasts and endothelial cells. Study results suggest that P-glycoprotein-mediated absorptive transport, dermal penetration, and vascular damage contribute to the anticancer activity of Ing3A in vivo.[165]

## Systemic retinoids

Etretinate, isotretinoin and acitretin may be used in the management of BCCs in patients with Gorlin syndrome.[166] Doses of 4.5 mg/kg per day of isotretinoin and 1 mg/kg per day of etretinate are necessary to bring about what is sometimes only partial regression of BCCs.[166] Even the necessary chronic use of 1.5 mg/kg per day of isotretinoin as a preventive measure is not tolerated in some patients, and unfortunately once these agents are discontinued, relapse may occur.

## Systemic chemotherapy

Chemotherapy has been used to manage both metastatic BCC and uncontrolled local disease. Disseminated metastatic BCC, with few exceptions, has a usual survival period of 10 to 20 months.[167] If metastases are confined to the nodes, surgery or surgery plus radiation therapy may be successful.[168] For disseminated metastases, systemic chemotherapy alone or with radiation therapy is indicated. Cisplatin appears to be more effective than bleomycin, cyclophosphamide, 5-FU and vinblastine and has been associated with long-term survival. For unresectable BCCs, cisplatin and doxorubicin alone or with radiation are reasonably well tolerated and yield prolonged disease control.[169]

GDC-0449, an orally active small molecule that targets the hedgehog pathway, appears to have anti-tumor activity in locally advanced or metastatic BCC.[170] Hedgehog signaling is activated in a variety of solid tumors and hematologic malignancies by point mutations in hedgehog pathway members or autocrine or paracrine ligand secretion. Several hedgehog inhibitors were developed to block hedgehog pathway activity at the level of the activating receptor, smoothened. GDC-0449 is a systemic smoothened inhibitor entering clinical trials. It was successfully tested in a phase I clinical trial, showing objective response in several BCCs.[171]

## Interferon

For patients with BCC in whom surgical intervention is not optimal, local treatment with interferon alfa-2b is an alternative.[172] Regimens of 5 million IU three times per week for 4 to 8 weeks are typically used. The most frequent adverse events were transient, mild-to-moderate flu-like symptoms in 95% of patients and asymptomatic leukopenia or neutropenia in 25%.[173] Also noted are fever, malaise, rheumatic complaints, altered psyche, chills, transient leukopenia, and injection site pain and itching. Cure rates are approximately 80%.[174]

## Combination therapy

Varous combinations of therapies have also been used to enhance BCC cure rates. Imiquimod has been used with CE and with curettage alone, with cure rates approaching 100%.[175,176] Photodynamic therapy has also been augmented by systemic retinoids to reduce BCC recurrence rates.[177] In sBCCs or 'thin' BCCs, curettage followed by 25% topical 5-FU under occlusion for 3 weeks, appears to be more effective than occluded topical 5-FU alone, demonstrating a 94% 5-year cure rate.[163]

Cryosurgery may also be combined with curettage. With larger tumors, an initial debulk followed by cryosurgery of the base may aid in the removal of tumor and help to delineate subclinical extensions.[137] Preoperative imiquimod or topical 5-FU may also help demonstrate the extent of the BCC.[136,178]

## Other factors in BCC management

### Age and cosmetic results

Most elderly individuals tolerate both the local anesthesia and the removal of even large BCCs. Consequently, all but the most infirm are typically good surgical candidates. However, elderly individuals scar less and are often less concerned about appearances, making many of them excellent candidates for CE or cryosurgery. Younger individuals, on the other hand, are more prone to hypertrophic scarring and generally desire the more subtle scar of an excision. Radiation therapy is usually reserved for older individuals, because of long-term sequelae involving cosmesis, carcinogenic effect (albeit small), and late radiation necrosis.

### Number of lesions

Situations exist where excision of innumerable BCCs in a patient may be neither the most practical nor the best treatment. For example, excising multiple sBCCs will be time-consuming and require the sacrifice of extensive healthy tissue for what may eventually become spreading scars. In such a circumstance, topical chemotherapy, cryosurgery or CE might yield satisfactory therapeutic and cosmetic results.

### Lesion size

The size of the lesion may direct therapy. For example, topical chemotherapy, CE or cryosurgery to manage a 5cm sBCC on the back might produce a better cosmetic result than excision and grafting. However, with large, invasive BCCs, excision or Mohs surgery is generally the treatment of choice, although radiation therapy at times may be preferable (Fig. 11.32).

## Distinctness of the tumor borders

Well-demarcated, exophytic BCC is usually circumscribed on histology and generally cured by CE, cryosurgery, radiation therapy or excision. However, ill-defined, flat or plaque-like BCC often demonstrates aggressive growth patterns best managed by Mohs surgery.

## Primary versus recurrent BCC

Numerous studies employing different techniques have shown that there is a dramatic decline in cure rate for recurrent as opposed to primary BCC.[137] Recurrent tumors are ill-defined, embedded in a sclerotic matrix and often demonstrate extensive subclinical spread.[106,107] Mohs surgery, with its exact histologic control, offers patients with recurrent lesions the highest likelihood of cure (Fig. 11.33).[106,112,179–181]

## Anatomic location

The treatment of BCC may be complicated by anatomic considerations in the following areas: lips, eyelids, scalp, distal nose and lower leg (Fig. 11.31). To perform effective curettage, tissue immobilization is paramount. This is difficult on the lips or eyelids and a chalazion clamp may aid in stabilizing the tissue.[182] The scalp and distal nose are rich in pilosebaceous units that can shield BCCs from the curette. Also, the deep dermis of the distal nose is so dense that tumor islands are not entirely removed by curettage,[182] and the scalp is so vascular that an adequate freeze is difficult and recurrences are common.[131] Cryosurgery on the leg generally results in prolonged healing time, increased infection risk, and poor cosmetic results.[131] Even on the trunk, scar spreading after an excision may result in inferior cosmesis compared to other methods. Radiation therapy should generally be reserved for BCCs on the head and neck, as poor cosmetic outcomes arise from treatments on the trunk and extremities.[122]

## Variants requiring special approaches

### 'Field fire' BCC

This variant of BCC may reside in a previously irradiated field or may represent a multifocal recurrent BCC. Clinically, it may be difficult to determine margins; therefore, Mohs surgery is

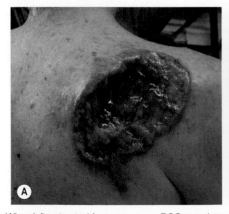
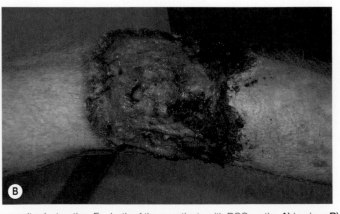

**Figure 11.32** When left untreated for many years, BCCs can become quite destructive. For both of these patients with BCC on the **A)** back or **B)** arm, a multidisciplinary approach was utilized, including imaging studies for metastatic spread and radiation oncology. **(A,** courtesy of John O'Brian, MD.)

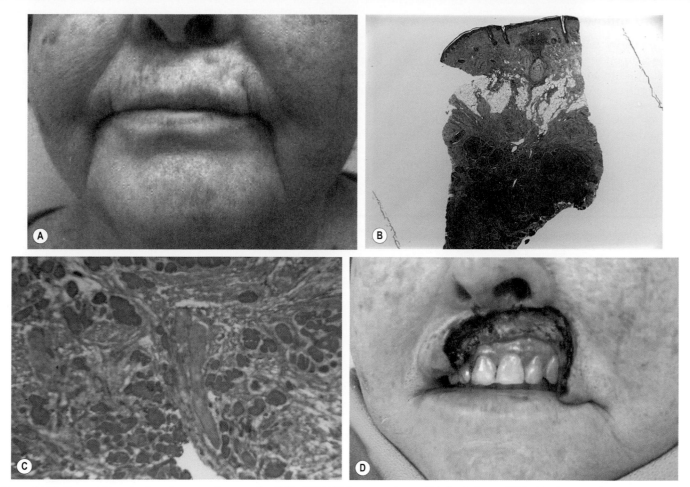

**Figure 11.33** Recurrent basal cell carcinoma on the upper lip. **A)** The BCC initially appeared as an ill-defined plaque. **B)** The histology revealed a deep-seated tumor with a prior scar overlying it. **C)** The fourth layer of Mohs revealed perineural involvement. (Frozen section; original magnification ×40.) **D)** After five stages of Mohs surgery, the recurrent BCC was cleared and the wound was repaired. (**A** and **B** courtesy of the University of Texas Southwestern Mohs Surgery Unit.)

the treatment of choice. The surgeon should avoid closures with dog-ear excisions or flaps which may conceal tumor or introduce tumor cells into a wound. If there is a known history of radiation to a limited region, it may be best to excise the entire area to prevent further tumor development.

## Incompletely excised BCC

Based on certain studies,[183] some clinicians elect to simply follow patients when pathologic examination of excised BCCs shows positive margin involvement. In the cited studies, only one-third of the presumably incompletely excised BCCs recurred and in cases where the area was immediately re-excised, residual tumor was found in only 50% of the specimens.[184]

The most likely explanation is that those tumors were entirely excised, albeit with cells at the margin.[183] This would explain why no residual tumor was found in many of the specimens. Other possibilities are that an inflammatory response eliminated residual tumor[185] or that residual tumor was devitalized by the procedure.[183] The lack of residual tumor in re-excision specimens may also be explained by the residual amount being minimal

and evading detection in the 'incomplete' histopathologic examination.

Other studies have shown that incompletely excised BCCs recur as often as 86% of the time.[185,186] Dellon et al.[185] have shown that incompletely excised BCCs with aggressive growth patterns are more likely to recur than those with nodular growth and have postulated the necessity of immediate re-excision only for BCCs with aggressive histology. However, any recurrent BCC can behave aggressively, so it has been recommended that every incompletely excised BCC be re-excised.[186-188] In addition, whenever a major reconstruction is planned, it is important to know that the BCC be completely excised before the defect is reconstructed.

## Perineural BCC

Mohs surgery allows the precise tracing of a perineural BCC. This may even entail multidisciplinary input. Hanke et al.[189] have recommended the removal of an additional layer after free margins have been obtained to search for non-contiguous tumor, but this approach is not universally accepted. Once the tumor has spread into the cranium, surgery is usually no longer feasible and radiation therapy can then be considered.

## Patient follow-up

The regularity with which BCC patients need to be seen depends upon the number, the frequency, and the severity of the BCCs treated and how much background sun damage is present. Although recurrent BCC tends to present within 5 years, some may recur later.[190] In addition, these patients often develop additional primary BCCs. Between 20% and 33% of patients develop a new BCC within a year of having been treated for the initial BCC and by the fifth year, up to 45% will develop an additional BCC.[191,192]

## FUTURE OUTLOOK

As the most common cancer in man, the need for better diagnostic and therapeutic approaches will continue to be critical. Targeted gene therapy and the use of immune response modifiers are among the active areas of research in BCC. The use of topical endonuclease which decreases numbers of BCCs in patients with xeroderma pigmentosum may have promise.[193] Multiphoton laser scanning microscopy is being investigated as a non-invasive diagnostic method.[194] Finally, inflammatory response pathways and their inhibitors may have a role in lifetime basal cell risk.[195]

Given the magnitude of the BCC problem, the development of new diagnostic and therapeutic modalities will continue to be of the utmost importance.

## REFERENCES

1. Rogers HW, Weinstock MA, Harris AR, et al. Incidence estimate of nonmelanoma skin cancer in the United States, 2006. *Arch Dermatol.* 2010;146(3):283–287.

2. Jacob A. Observations respecting an ulcer of peculiar character, which attacks the eyelids and other parts of the face. *Dublin Hospital Reports.* 1824;(4):232–239.

3. Krompecker E. Der Basalzellenkrebs. Jena: Fischer; 1903.

4. Gorlin RJ, Goltz RW. Multiple nevoid basal-cell epithelioma, jaw cysts and bifid rib. A syndrome. *N Engl J Med.* 1960;262:908–912.

5. Gailani MR, Stahle-Backdahl M, Leffell DJ, et al. The role of the human homologue of Drosophila patched in sporadic basal cell carcinomas. *Nat Genet.* 1996;14(1):78–81.

6. Hahn H, Wicking C, Zaphiropoulous PG, et al. Mutations of the human homolog of Drosophila patched in the nevoid basal cell carcinoma syndrome. *Cell.* 1996;85(6):841–851.

7. Johnson RL, Rothman AL, Xie J, et al. Human homolog of patched, a candidate gene for the basal cell nevus syndrome. *Science.* 1996;272(5268):1668–1671.

8. Crowson AN. Basal cell carcinoma: biology, morphology and clinical implications. *Mod Pathol.* 2006;19(suppl 2):S127–S147.

9. Christenson LJ, Borrowman TA, Vachon CM, et al. Incidence of basal cell and squamous cell carcinomas in a population younger than 40 years. *JAMA.* 2005;294(6):681–690.

10. Karagas MR, Stannard VA, Mott LA, et al. Use of tanning devices and risk of basal cell and squamous cell skin cancers. *J Natl Cancer Inst.* 2002;94(3):224–226.

11. Bower CP, Lear JT, Bygrave S, et al. Basal cell carcinoma and risk of subsequent malignancies: a cancer registry-based study in southwest England. *J Am Acad Dermatol.* 2000;42(6):988–991.

12. Erba P, Farhadi J, Wettstein R, et al. Morphoeic basal cell carcinoma of the face. *Scand J Plast Reconstr Surg Hand Surg.* 2007;41(4):184–188.

13. Fresini A, Rossiello L, Severino BU, et al. Giant basal cell carcinoma. *Skinmed.* 2007;6(4):204–205.

14. Shindel AW, Mann MW, et al. Mohs micrographic surgery for penile cancer: management and long-term followup. *J Urol.* 2007;178(5):1980–1985.

15. Mulvany NJ, Allen DG. Differentiated intraepithelial neoplasia of the vulva. *Int J Gynecol Pathol.* 2008;27(1):125–135.

16. Fabricius EM, Kruse-Boitschenko U, Khoury R, et al. Localization of telomerase hTERT protein in frozen sections of basal cell carcinomas (BCC) and tumor margin tissues. *Int J Oncol.* 2009;35(6):1377–1394.

17. Nan H, Qureshi AA, Hunter DJ, et al. A functional SNP in the MDM2 promoter, pigmentary phenotypes, and risk of skin cancer. *Cancer Causes Control.* 2009;20(2):171–179.

18. Rodust PM, Stockfleth E, Ulrich C, et al. UV-induced squamous cell carcinoma–a role for antiapoptotic signalling pathways. *Br J Dermatol.* 2009;161(suppl 3):107–115.

19. Situm M, Buljan M, Bulat V, et al. The role of UV radiation in the development of basal cell carcinoma. *Coll Antropol.* 2008;32(suppl 2):167–170.

20. Stern RS. Putting iatrogenic risk in perspective: basal cell cancer in PUVA patients and Australians. *J Invest Dermatol.* 2009;129(9):2315–2316.

21. Cognetta AB, Green WH, Marks MM, et al. Basal cell carcinoma and World War II-era cathode ray oscilloscope exposure. *J Am Acad Dermatol.* 2005;52(2 suppl 1):1–7.

22. Suarez B, Lopez-Abente G, et al. Occupation and skin cancer: the results of the HELIOS-I multicenter case-control study. *BMC Public Health.* 2007;7:180.

23. Bastiaens MT, Hoefnagel JJ, Bruijn JA, et al. Differences in age, site distribution, and sex between nodular and superficial basal cell carcinoma indicate different types of tumors. *J Invest Dermatol.* 1998;110(6):880–884.

24. Applebaum KM, Karagas MR, Hunter DJ, et al. Polymorphisms in nucleotide excision repair genes, arsenic exposure, and non-melanoma skin cancer in New Hampshire. *Environ Health Perspect.* 2007;115(8):1231–1236.

25. Garcia de Marcos JA, Dean-Ferrer A, Arroyo Rodriguez S, et al. Basal cell nevus syndrome: clinical and genetic diagnosis. *Oral Maxillofac Surg.* 2009;13(4):225–230.

26. Takahashi C, Kanazawa N, Yoshikawa Y, et al. Germline PTCH1 mutations in Japanese basal cell nevus syndrome patients. *J Hum Genet.* 2009;54(7):403–408.

27. Alcalay J, Ben-Amitai D, Alkalay R. Idiopathic basal cell carcinoma in children. *J Drugs Dermatol.* 2008;7(5):479–481.

28. Ramachandran S, Rajaratnam R, Smith AG, et al. Patients with both basal and squamous cell carcinomas are at a lower risk of further basal cell carcinomas than patients with only a basal cell carcinoma. *J Am Acad Dermatol.* 2009;61(2):247–251.

29. Asuquo ME, Ngim O, Ebughe G, et al. Skin cancers amongst four Nigerian albinos. *Int J Dermatol.* 2009;48(6):636–638.

30. Gailani MR, Leffell DJ, Ziegler A, et al. Relationship between sunlight exposure and a key genetic alteration in basal cell carcinoma. *J Natl Cancer Inst.* 1996;88(6):349–354.

31. van Dam RM, Huang Z, Rimm EB, et al. Risk factors for basal cell carcinoma of the skin in men: results from the health professionals follow-up study. *Am J Epidemiol.* 1999;150(5):459–468.

32. Naldi L, DiLandro A, D'Avanzo B, et al. Host-related and environmental risk factors for cutaneous basal cell carcinoma: evidence from an Italian case-control study. *J Am Acad Dermatol.* 2000; 42(3):446–452.

33. Ramani ML, Bennett RG. High prevalence of skin cancer in World War II servicemen stationed in the Pacific theater. *J Am Acad Dermatol.* 1993;28(5 Pt 1):733–737.

34. Karagas MR, McDonald JA, Greenberg ER, et al. Risk of basal cell and squamous cell skin cancers after ionizing radiation therapy. For The Skin Cancer Prevention Study Group. *J Natl Cancer Inst.* 1996;88(24):1848–1853.

35. Berg D, Otley CC. Skin cancer in organ transplant recipients: epidemiology, pathogenesis, and management. *J Am Acad Dermatol.* 2002;47(1):1–17 quiz 18-20.

36. Gorlin RJ. Nevoid basal cell carcinoma syndrome. *Dermatol Clin.* 1995;13(1):113–125.

37. Goeteyn M, Geerts ML, Kint A, et al. The Bazex-Dupre-Christol syndrome. *Arch Dermatol.* 1994;130(3):337–342.

38. Ashinoff R, Jacobson M, Belsito DV. Rombo syndrome: a second case report and review. *J Am Acad Dermatol.* 1993;28(6):1011–1014.

39. Bale AE, Gailani MR, Leffell DJ. Nevoid basal cell carcinoma syndrome. *J Invest Dermatol.* 1994;103(5 suppl):126S–130S.

40. Bale AE, Gailani MR, Leffell DJ. The Gorlin syndrome gene: a tumor suppressor active in basal cell carcinogenesis and embryonic development. *Proc Assoc Am Physicians.* 1995;107(2):253–257.

41. Cleaver JE, Lam ET, Revet I. Disorders of nucleotide excision repair: the genetic and molecular basis of heterogeneity. *Nat Rev Genet.* 2009;10(11):756–768.

42. Gallagher RP, Lee TK. Adverse effects of ultraviolet radiation: a brief review. *Prog Biophys Mol Biol.* 2006;92(1):119–131.

43. Gallagher RP, Hill GB, Bajdik CD, et al. Sunlight exposure, pigmentary factors, and risk of nonmelanocytic skin cancer. I. Basal cell carcinoma. *Arch Dermatol.* 1995;131(2):157–163.

44. Westerdahl J, Ingvar C, Masback A, et al. Risk of cutaneous malignant melanoma in relation to use of sunbeds: further evidence for UV-A carcinogenicity. *Br J Cancer.* 2000;82(9):1593–1599.

45. Wang L, Toda M, Saito K, et al. Post-immune UV irradiation induces Tr1-like regulatory T cells that suppress humoral immune responses. *Int Immunol.* 2008;20(1):57–70.

46. Brash DE, Ziegler A, Jonanson AS, et al. Sunlight and sunburn in human skin cancer: p53, apoptosis, and tumor promotion. *J Investig Dermatol Symp Proc*. 1996;1(2):136–142.

47. Krasin MJ, Hoth KA, Hua C, et al. Incidence and correlates of radiation dermatitis in children and adolescents receiving radiation therapy for the treatment of paediatric sarcomas. *Clin Oncol (R Coll Radiol)*. 2009;21(10):781–785.

48. Schwartz JL, Kopecky KJ, Mathes RW, et al. Basal cell skin cancer after total-body irradiation and hematopoietic cell transplantation. *Radiat Res*. 2009;171(2):155–163.

49. Karagas MR, Nelson HH, Zens MS, et al. Squamous cell and basal cell carcinoma of the skin in relation to radiation therapy and potential modification of risk by sun exposure. *Epidemiology*. 2007;18(6):776–784.

50. Cabrera HN, Gomez ML. Skin cancer induced by arsenic in the water. *J Cutan Med Surg*. 2003;7(2):106–111.

51. Rosen H, Schmidt B, Lam HP, et al. Management of nevus sebaceus and the risk of basal cell carcinoma: an 18-year review. *Pediatr Dermatol*. 2009;26(6):676–681.

52. Ramsay HM, Fryer A, Strange RC, et al. Multiple basal cell carcinomas in a patient with acute myeloid leukaemia and chronic lymphocytic leukaemia. *Clin Exp Dermatol*. 1999;24(4):281–282.

53. Lobo DV, Chu P, Grekin RC, et al. Nonmelanoma skin cancers and infection with the human immunodeficiency virus. *Arch Dermatol*. 1992;128(5):623–627.

54. Kaporis HG, Guttman-Yassky E, Lowes MA, et al. Human basal cell carcinoma is associated with Foxp3+ T cells in a Th2 dominant microenvironment. *J Invest Dermatol*. 2007;127(10):2391–2398.

55. Gutierrez-Steil C, Wrone-Smith T, Sun X, et al. Sunlight-induced basal cell carcinoma tumor cells and ultraviolet-B-irradiated psoriatic plaques express Fas ligand (CD95L). *J Clin Invest*. 1998;101(1):33–39.

56. Sherman JE, Talmor M. Slow progression and sequential documentation of a giant basal cell carcinoma of the face. *Surgery*. 2001;130:90–92.

57. Fogarty GB, Ainslie J. Recurrent basal cell carcinoma causing spinal cord compression. *ANZ J Surg*. 2001;71:129–131.

58. Kovarik CL, Stewart D, Barnard JJ. Lethal basal cell carcinoma secondary to cerebral invasion. *J Am Acad Dermatol*. 2005;52:149–151.

59. Niazi ZB, Lamberty BG. Perineural infiltration in basal cell carcinomas. *Br J Plast Surg*. 1993;46:156–157.

60. Ratner D, Lowe L, Johnson TM, et al. Perineural spread of basal cell carcinomas treated with Mohs micrographic surgery. *Cancer*. 2000;88:1605–1613.

61. Leibovitch I, McNab A, Sullivan T, et al. Orbital invasion by periocular basal cell carcinoma. *Ophthalmology*. 2005;112:717–723.

62. Mikhail GR, Nims LP, Kelly Jr AP, et al. Metastatic basal cell carcinoma: review, pathogenesis, and report of two cases. *Arch Dermatol*. 1977;113:1261–1269.

63. Safai B, Good RA. Basal cell carcinoma with metastasis. Review of literature. *Arch Pathol Lab Med*. 1977;101:327–331.

64. Ting PT, Kasper R, Arlette JP. Metastatic basal cell carcinoma: report of two cases and literature review. *J Cutan Med Surg*. 2005;9:10–15.

65. von Domarus H, Stevens PJ. Metastatic basal cell carcinoma. Report of five cases and review of 170 cases in the literature. *J Am Acad Dermatol*. 1984;10:1043–1060.

66. Sexton M, Jones DB, Maloney ME. Histologic pattern analysis of basal cell carcinoma. Study of a series of 1039 consecutive neoplasms. *J Am Acad Dermatol*. 1990;23(6 Pt 1):1118–1126.

67. Bart RS, Kopf AW, Gladstein AH. Treatment of morphea-type basal cell carcinomas with radiation therapy. *Arch Dermatol*. 1977;113(6):783–786.

68. Garcia C, Poletti E, Crowson AN. Basosquamous carcinoma. *J Am Acad Dermatol*. 2009;60(1):137–143.

69. Gailani MR, Bale AE. Developmental genes and cancer: role of patched in basal cell carcinoma of the skin. *J Natl Cancer Inst*. 1997;89(15):1103–1109.

70. Freeman RG, Duncan C. Recurrent skin cancer. *Arch Dermatol*. 1973;107(3):395–399.

71. Sloane JP. The value of typing basal cell carcinomas in predicting recurrence after surgical excision. *Br J Dermatol*. 1977;96(2):127–132.

72. Jacobs GH, Rippey JJ, Altini M. Prediction of aggressive behavior in basal cell carcinoma. *Cancer*. 1982;49(3):533–537.

73. Wolf DJ, Zitelli JA. Surgical margins for basal cell carcinoma. *Arch Dermatol*. 1987;123(3):340–344.

74. Reidbord HE, Wechsler HL, Fisher ER. Ultrastructural study of basal cell carcinoma and its variants with comments on histogenesis. *Arch Dermatol*. 1971;104(2):132–140.

75. Ting PT, Kasper R, Arlette JP. Metastatic basal cell carcinoma: report of two cases and literature review. *J Cutan Med Surg*. 2005;9(1):10–15.

76. Barr RJ, Graham JH. Granular cell basal cell carcinoma. A distinct histopathologic entity. *Arch Dermatol*. 1979;115(9):1064–1067.

77. Walsh N, Ackerman AB. Infundibulocystic basal cell carcinoma: a newly described variant. *Mod Pathol*. 1990;3(5):599–608.

78. McGibbon DH. Malignant epidermal tumours. *J Cutan Pathol*. 1985;12(3–4):224–238.

79. Salasche SJ, Amonette RA. Morpheaform basal-cell epitheliomas. A study of subclinical extensions in a series of 51 cases. *J Dermatol Surg Oncol*. 1981;7(5):387–394.

80. Takei Y, Fukushiro S, Ackerman AB. Criteria for histologic differentiation of desmoplastic trichoepithelioma (sclerosing epithelial hamartoma) from morphea-like basal-cell carcinoma. *Am J Dermatopathol*. 1985;7(3):207–221.

81. Hendrix Jr JD, Parlette HL. Micronodular basal cell carcinoma. A deceptive histologic subtype with frequent clinically undetected tumor extension. *Arch Dermatol*. 1996;132(3):295–298.

82. Sanchez NP, Winkelmann RK. Basal cell tumor with eccrine differentiation (eccrine epithelioma). *J Am Acad Dermatol*. 1982;6(4 Pt 1):514–518.

83. Sakamoto F, Ito M, Sato S, et al. Basal cell tumor with apocrine differentiation: apocrine epithelioma. *J Am Acad Dermatol*. 1985;13(2 Pt 2):355–363.

84. Curson C, Weedon D. Spontaneous regression in basal cell carcinomas. *J Cutan Pathol*. 1979;6(5):432–437.

85. Weedon D, Shand E. Amyloid in basal cell carcinomas. *Br J Dermatol*. 1979;101(2):141–146.

86. Dardi LE, Memoli VA, Gould VE. Neuroendocrine differentiation in basal cell carcinomas. *J Cutan Pathol*. 1981;8(5):335–341.

87. Kariniemi AL, Holthofer H, Vartio T, et al. Cellular differentiation of basal cell carcinoma studied with fluorescent lectins and cytokeratin antibodies. *J Cutan Pathol*. 1984;11(6):541–548.

88. Moll R, Cowin P, Kapprell HP, et al. Desmosomal proteins: new markers for identification and classification of tumors. *Lab Invest*. 1986;54(1):4–25.

89. Stanley JR, Beckwith JB, Fuller RP, et al. A specific antigenic defect of the basement membrane is found in basal cell carcinomas but not in other epidermal tumors. *Cancer*. 1982;50:1486.

90. Christian MM, Moy RL, Wagner RL, et al. A correlation of alpha-smooth muscle actin and invasion in micronodular basal cell carcinoma. *Dermatol Surg*. 2001;17:441–445.

91. Cribier B, Noacco G, Peltre B, et al. Expression of stromolysin 3 in basal cell carcinomas. *Eur J Dermatol*. 2001;11:530–533.

92. Tellechea O, Reis JP, Domingues JC, et al. Monoclonal antibody Ber EP4 distinguishes basal-cell carcinoma from squamous-cell carcinoma of the skin. *Am J Dermatopathol*. 1993;15(5):452–455.

93. Jones MS, Helm KF, Maloney ME. The immunohistochemical characteristics of the basosquamous cell carcinoma. *Dermatol Surg*. 1997;23(3):181–184.

94. Beer TW, Shepherd P, Theaker JM. Ber EP4 and epithelial membrane antigen aid distinction of basal cell, squamous cell and basosquamous carcinomas of the skin. *Histopathology*. 2000;37(3):218–223.

95. Rossen K, Thomsen HK. Ber-EP4 immunoreactivity depends on the germ layer origin and maturity of the squamous epithelium. *Histopathology*. 2001;39(4):386–389.

96. Krahl D, Sellheyer K. Monoclonal antibody Ber-EP4 reliably discriminates between microcystic adnexal carcinoma and basal cell carcinoma. *J Cutan Pathol*. 2007;34(10):782–787.

97. Robins P, Albom MJ. Recurrent basal cell carcinoma in young women. *J Dermatol Surg*. 1975;1:49–51.

98. Spiller WF, Spiller RF. Treatment of basal cell epithelioma by curettage and electrodesiccation. *J Am Acad Dermatol*. 1984;11:808–814.

99. Kopf W, Bart RS, Schrager D, et al. Curettage-electrodesiccation treatment of basal cell carcinomas. *Arch Dermatol*. 1977;113:439–443.

100. Freeman RG, Duncan WC. Recurrent skin cancer. *Arch Dermatol*. 1973;107:395–399.

101. Popkin GL, Bart RS. Excision versus curettage and electrodesiccation as dermatologic office procedures for the treatment of basal cell carcinomas. *J Dermatol Surg*. 1975;1:33–35.

102. Grande DJ, Whitaker DC, Koranda FC. Subdermal basal-cell carcinoma. *J Dermatol Surg Oncol*. 1982;8:779–781.

103. McDaniel WE. Therapy for basal cell epitheliomas by curettage only. Further study. *Arch Dermatol*. 1983;119:901–903.

104. Barlow JO, Zalla M, Kyle A, et al. Treatment of basal cell carcinoma with curettage alone. *J Am Acad Dermatol*. 2006;54:1039–1045.

105. Bart RS, Schrager D, Kopf AW, et al. Scalpel excision of basal cell carcinomas. *Arch Dermatol*. 1978;14:739–742.

106. Menn H, Robins P, Kopf AW, et al. The recurrent basal cell epithelioma. A study of 100 cases of recurrent re-treated basal cell epitheliomas. *Arch Dermatol*. 1971;103:628–631.

107. Burg G, Hirsch RD, Konz B, et al. Histographic surgery: accuracy of visual assessment of the margins of basal-cell epithelioma. *J Dermatol Surg*. 1975;1:21–24.

108. Thackray AC. Histological classification of rodent ulcers and its bearing on their prognosis. *Br J Cancer*. 1951;5:213.

109. Dellon AL. Histologic study of recurrent basal cell carcinoma. *Plast Reconstr Surg*. 1985;75:853–859.

110. Dubin N, Kopf AW. Multivariate risk score for recurrent cutaneous basal cell carcinomas. *Arch Dermatol*. 1983;119:373–377.

111. MacFarlane AW, Curley RK, Graham RM. Recurrence rates of basal cell carcinomas according to site, methods of removal, histological type and adequacy of excision. *Br J Dermatol*. 1986;115(suppl):23.

112. Drake LA. Guidelines of cure for Mohs micrographic surgery. *J Am Acad Dermatol*. 1995;33:271.

113. Lever WF, Schaumburg-Lever G. *Histopathology of the Skin*. 6th ed. Philadelphia: Lippincott; 1983:562–575.

114. Cook J, Zitelli J. Mohs micrographic surgery: a cost analysis. *J Am Acad Dermatol*. 1995;39:698–703.

115. Morhenn VB, Roth S, Roth R. Use of monoclonal antibody (VM-2) plus the immunogold-silver technique to stain basal cell carcinoma cells. *J Am Acad Dermatol*. 1987;17:765–769.

116. Smeets NW, Stavast-Kooy AJ, Krekels GA, et al. Adjuvant cytokeratin staining in Mohs micrographic surgery for basal cell carcinoma. *Dermatol Surg*. 2003;29:375–377.

117. Kist D, Perkins W, Christ S, et al. Antihuman epithelial antigen (Ber-EP4) helps define basal cell carcinoma masked by inflammation. *Dermatol Surg*. 1997;23:1067–1070.

118. Krunic AL, Garrod DR, Viehman GE, et al. The use of antidesmoglein stains in Mohs micrographic surgery. A potential aid for the differentiation of basal cell carcinoma from horizontal sections of the hair follicle and folliculocentric basaloid proliferation. *Dermatol Surg*. 1997;23:463–468.

119. Ramnavain ND, Walker NP, Markey AC. Basal cell carcinoma: rapid techniques using cytokeratin markers to assist treatment by micrographic (Mohs) surgery. *Br J Biomed Sci*. 1995;52:184–187.

120. Jimenez FJ, Grchnik JM, Buchanan MD, et al. Immunohistochemical techniques in Mohs micrographic surgery: their potential use in the detection of neoplastic cells masked by inflammation. *J Am Acad Dermatol*. 1995;32:89–94.

121. Leshin B, Yeatts P, Anscher M, et al. Management of periocular basal cell carcinoma: Mohs micrographic surgery versus radiotherapy. *Surv Ophthalmol*. 1993;38:193–212.

122. Gladstein AH, Kopf AW, Bart RS. Radiotherapy of cutaneous malignancies. In: Goldschmidt H, ed. *Physical Modalities in Dermatologic Therapy. Radiotherapy, Electrosurgery, Phototherapy, Cryosurgery*. New York, NY: Springer-Verlag; 1978:95.

123. Hunter RD. Skin. In: Easson EC, Pointon RCS, eds. *The Radiotherapy of Malignant Disease*. New York, NY: Springer-Verlag; 1985:135.

124. Thissen MR, Neumann MH, Schouten LJ. A systematic review of treatment modalities for primary basal cell carcinomas. *Arch Dermatol*. 1999;135:1177–1183.

125. Brady LW, Binnick SA, Fitzpatrick PJ. Skin cancer. In: Perez CA, Brady LW, eds. *Principles and Practice of Radiation Oncology*. Philadelphia, PA: Lippincott; 1987:377.

126. Gorlin RJ. Nevoid basal cell carcinoma syndrome. *Medicine*. 1987;66:98–113.

127. Braun-Falco O, Lukacs S, Goldschmidt H. *Dermatologic Radiotherapy*. New York, NY: Springer; 1976:69.

128. Chahbazian CM, Brown GS. Radiation therapy for carcinoma of the skin of the face and neck. Special considerations. *JAMA*. 1980;244:1135–1137.

129. Chahbazian CM, Brown GS. Skin cancer. In: Gilbert HA, ed. *Modern Radiation Oncology: Classic Literature and Current Management*. Philadelphia, PA: Harper & Row; 1984:158.

130. Zacarian SA. Cryogenics: the cryolesion and the pathogenesis of cryonecrosis. In: Zacarian SA, ed. *Cryosurgery for Skin Cancer and Cutaneous Disorders*. St Louis, MO: Mosby; 1985:1.

131. Zacarian SA. Cryosurgery for cancer of the skin. In: Zacarian SA, ed. *Cryosurgery for Skin Cancer and Cutaneous Disorders*. St Louis: Mosby; 1985:96.

132. Kuflik EG. Cryosurgery for cutaneous malignancy; an update. *Dermatol Surg*. 1997;23:1081–1087.

133. Fraunfelder FT. Cryosurgery of eyelid, conjunctival and intraocular tumors. In: Zacarian SA, ed. *Cryosurgery for Skin Cancer and Cutaneous Disorders*. St Louis, MO: Mosby; 1985:259.

134. Gage AA. Cryosurgery of advanced tumors of the head and neck. In: Zacarian SA, ed. *Cryosurgery for Skin Cancer and Cutaneous Disorders*. St Louis, MO: Mosby; 1985:163.

135. Kuflik EG. Cryosurgery for carcinoma of the eyelids. A 12-year experience. *J Dermatol Surg Oncol*. 1985;11:243–246.

136. Zacarian SA. Complications, indications and contraindications in cryosurgery. In: Zacarian SA, ed. *Cryosurgery for Skin Cancer and Cutaneous Disorders*. St Louis, MO: Mosby; 1985:283.

137. Spiller WF, Spiller RF. Cryosurgery and adjuvant surgical techniques for cutaneous carcinomas. In: Zacarian SA, ed. *Cryosurgery for Skin Cancer and Cutaneous Disorders*. St Louis, MO: Mosby; 1985:187.

138. Wheeland RG, Bailin PL, Ratz JL, et al. Carbon dioxide laser vaporization and curettage in the treatment of large or multiple superficial basal cell carcinomas. *J Dermatol Surg Oncol*. 1987;13:119–125.

139. Humphreys TR, Malhotra R, Scharf MJ, et al. Treatment of superficial basal cell carcinoma and squamous cell carcinoma in situ with a high-energy pulsed carbon dioxide laser. *Arch Dermatol*. 1998;134:1247–1252.

140. Horlock N, Grobbelaar AO, Gault DT. Can the carbon dioxide laser completely ablate basal cell carcinomas? A histological study. *Br J Plast Surg*. 2000;53:286–293.

141. Bailin PL, Ratz JL, Lutz-Nagey L. CO2 laser modification of Mohs surgery. *J Dermatol Surg Oncol*. 1981;7:621–623.

142. Szeimies RM. Methyl aminolevulinate-photodynamic therapy for basal cell carcinoma. *Dermatol Clin*. 2007;25(1):89–94.

143. Choudhary S, Nouri K, Elsaie ML. Photodynamic therapy in dermatology: a review. *Lasers Med Sci*. 2009;24(6):971–980.

144. Zeitouni NC, Shieh S, Oseroff AR. Laser and photodynamic therapy in the management of cutaneous malignancies. In: Ellerin B, ed. *Clinics in Dermatology*. New York, NY: Elsevier; 2001:328–339.

145. Basset-Sequin N, Ibbotson S, Emestam L, et al. *Photodynamic therapy using methylaminolevalinate is as efficacious as cryotherapy in primary superficial basal cell carcinoma but with better cosmetic outcome*. San Francisco: American Academy of Dermatology Annual Meeting; 2003.

146. Fink-Puches R, Soyer HP, Hofer A, et al. Longterm follow-up and histological changes of superficial non melanoma skin cancers treated with topical aminolevulinic acid photodynamic therapy. *Arch Dermatol*. 1998;134:821–826.

147. Schweiger ES, Kwasniak L, Tonkovic-Capin V. A patient with nevoid basal cell carcinoma syndrome treated successfully with photodynamic therapy: case report and review of the literature. *J Drugs Dermatol*. 2010;9(2):167–168.

148. Stanley MA. Mechanism of action of imiquimod. *Pap Rep*. 1999;10:23–29.

149. Hemmi H, Kaisho T, Takeuchi O, et al. Small antiviral compounds activate immune cells via the TUR 7 MYD88-dependent signaling pathway. *Nat Immunol*. 2002;3:196–200.

150. Beatner KR, Geisse JK, Helman D, et al. Therapeutic response of basal cell carcinoma to the immune response modifier imiquimod 5% cream. *J Am Acad Dermatol*. 1999;41:1002–1007.

151. Gollnick H, Barona CG, Frank RG, et al. Recurrence rate of superficial basal cell carcinoma following treatment with imiquimod 5% cream: conclusion of a 5-year long-term follow-up study in Europe. *Eur J Dermatol*. 2008;18(6):677–682.

152. Shumack S, Robinson J, Kossard S, et al. Efficacy of topical 5% imiquimod cream for the treatment of nodular basal cell carcinoma: comparison of dosing regimens. *Arch Dermatol*. 2002;138(9):1165–1171.

153. Geisse JK, Rich P, Pandya A, et al. Imiquimod 5% cream for the treatment of superficial basal cell carcinoma: a double-blind, randomized, vehicle-controlled study. *J Am Acad Dermatol*. 2002;47(3):390–398.

154. Schulze HJ, Cribier B, Requena L, et al. Imiquimod 5% cream for the treatment of superficial basal cell carcinoma: results from a randomized vehicle-controlled phase III study in Europe. *Br J Dermatol*. 2005;152(5):939–947.

155. Geisse J, Caro I, Lindholm J, et al. Imiquimod 5% cream for the treatment of superficial basal cell carcinoma: results from two phase III, randomized, vehicle-controlled studies. *J Am Acad Dermatol*. 2004;50(5):722–733.

156. Elliot Love W, Bernhard JD, Bordeaux JS. Topical imiquimod or fluorouracil therapy for basal and squamous cell carcinoma; a systematic review. *Arch Dermatol*. 2009;145(12):1431–1438.

157. Chen TM, Rosen T, Orengo I. Treatment of a large superficial basal cell carcinoma with 5% imiquimod: a case report and review of the literature. *Dermatol Surg*. 2002;28:344–346.

158. Micali G, de Pasquale R, Caltabiano R. Topical imiquimod treatment of superficial and nodular basal cell carcinomas in patients affected by basal cell nevus syndrome: a preliminary report. *J Dermatol Treat*. 2002;3:123–127.

159. Drehs MM, Cook-Bolden F, Tanzi EL. Successful treatment of multiple superficial basal cell carcinomas with topical imiquimod: case report and review of the literature. *Dermatol Surg*. 2002;28:427–429.

160. Klein E, Stoll HL, Miller E, et al. The effects of 5-fluorouracil (5-FU) ointment in the treatment of neoplastic dermatoses. *Dermatologica*. 1970;140(suppl):21–33.

161. Reymann F. A follow-up study of treatment of basal cell carcinoma with 5-fluorouracil ointment. *Dermatologica*. 1972;144:205–208.

162. Mohs FE, Jones DL, Bloom RF. Tendency of fluorouracil to conceal deep foci of invasive basal cell carcinoma. *Arch Dermatol*. 1978;114:1021–1022.

163. Epstein E. Fluorouracil paste treatment of the basal cell carcinoma. *Arch Dermatol*. 1985;121:207–213.

164. Siller G, Rosen R, Freeman M, et al. PEP005 (ingenol mebutate) gel for the topical treatment of superficial basal cell carcinoma: results of a randomized phase IIa trial. *Australas J Dermatol*. 2010;51(2):99–105.

165. Li L, Shukla S, Lee A, et al. The skin cancer chemotherapeutic agent ingenol-3-angelate (PEP005) is a substrate for the epidermal multidrug transporter (ABCB1) and targets tumor vasculature. *Cancer Res*. 2010;70(11):4509–4519.

166. Peck GL. Topical tretinoin in actinic keratoses and basal cell carcinoma. *J Am Acad Dermatol*. 1986;15:829–835.

167. Farmer ER, Helwig EB. Metastatic basal cell carcinoma: a clinicopathologic study of 17 cases. *Cancer*. 1980;46:748–757.

168. Wieman TJ, Shiveley EH, Woodcock TM. Responsiveness of metastatic basal cell carcinoma to chemotherapy. A case report. *Cancer*. 1983;52:1583–1585.

169. Robinson JK. Use of a combination of chemotherapy and radiation therapy in the management of advanced basal cell carcinoma of the head and neck. *J Am Acad Dermatol*. 1987;17:770.

170. Von Hoff DD, LoRusso PM, Rudin CM, et al. Inhibition of the hedgehog pathway in advanced basal-cell carcinoma. *N Engl J Med*. 2009;361(12):1164–1172.

171. Dierks C. GDC-0449 – targeting the hedgehog signaling pathway. *Recent Results Cancer Res*. 2010;184:235–238.

172. Cornell RC, Greenway HT, Tucker SB, et al. Intralesional interferon therapy for basal cell carcinoma. *J Am Acad Dermatol*. 1990;23(4 Pt 1):694–700.

173. Fernández-Vozmediano JM, Armario-Hita JC. Treatment of basal cell carcinoma of the nasal pyramid with intralesional interferon alfa-2b. *J Drugs Dermatol*. 2010;9(4):381–384.

174. Vine JE. Skin cancer update. Treatment alternatives for basal cell and squamous cell carcinoma. *N J Med*. 2001;98:35–37.

175. Rigel DS, Torres AM, Ely H. Imiquimod 5% cream following curettage without electrodesiccation for basal cell carcinoma: preliminary report. *J Drugs Dermatol*. 2008;7(1 suppl 1):s15–s16.

176. Spencer JM. Pilot study of imiquimod 5% cream as adjunctive therapy to curettage and electrodesiccation for nodular basal cell carcinoma. *Dermatol Surg*. 2006;32(1):63–69.

177. Lin MH, Lee JY, Ou CY, et al. Sequential systemic retinoid and photodynamic therapy for multiple keratotic pigmented nodular basal cell carcinomas on the scalp. *J Dermatol*. 2009;36(9):518–521.

178. Macpherson N, Lamrock E, Watt G. Effect of inflammation on positive margins of basal cell carcinomas. *Australas J Dermatol*. 2010;51(2):95–98.

179. Mohs FE. Carcinoma of the skin. A summary of therapeutic results. In: *Chemosurgery: Microscopically Controlled Surgery for Skin Cancer*. Springfield, IL: Charles C Thomas; 1978:153.

180. Robins P. Chemosurgery: my 15 years of experience. *J Dermatol Surg Oncol*. 1981;7:779–789.

181. Tromovitch TA, Stegman SJ. Microscopic-controlled excision of cutaneous tumors. Chemosurgery fresh tissue technique. *Cancer*. 1978;41:653–658.

182. Salasche SJ. Curettage and electrodesiccation in the treatment of mid facial basal cell epithelioma. *J Am Acad Dermatol*. 1983;8:496–503.

183. Gooding CA, White G, Yatsuhashi M. Significance of marginal extension in excised basal cell carcinoma. *N Engl J Med*. 1965;273:923.

184. Sarma DP, Griffing CC, Weilbaecher TG. Observations on the inadequately excised basal cell carcinomas. *J Surg Oncol*. 1984;25:79–80.

185. Dellon AL, DeSilva S, Connolly M, et al. Prediction of recurrence in incompletely excised basal cell carcinoma. *Plast Reconstr Surg*. 1985;75:860–871.

186. Shanoff LB, Spira M, Hardy SA. Basal cell carcinoma. A statistical approach to rational management. *Plast Reconstr Surg*. 1967;39:619–624.

187. Koplin L, Zarem HA. Recurrent basal cell carcinoma: review concerning the incidence, behavior and management of recurrent basal cell carcinoma with emphasis on the incompletely excised lesion. *Plast Reconstr Surg*. 1980;65:656–664.

188. Robinson JK. What are adequate treatment and follow-up care for nonmelanoma cutaneous cancer? *Arch Dermatol*. 1987;123:331–333.

189. Hanke CW, Wolf RL, Hochman SA, et al. Perineural spread of basal cell carcinoma. *J Dermatol Surg Oncol*. 1983;9:742–747.

190. Grover RW. Basal cell carcinoma. *Arch Dermatol*. 1973;107:138.

191. Robinson JK. Risk of developing another basal cell carcinoma. A 5-year prospective study. *Cancer*. 1987;60:118–120.

192. Marghoob A, Kopf AW, Bart RS, et al. Risk of another basal cell carcinoma developing after treatment of a basal cell carcinoma. *J Am Acad Dermatol*. 1993;28:22–28.

193. Yarosh D, Klein J, O'Connor A, et al. Effect of topically applied T4 endonuclease V in liposomes in skin cancer in xeroderma pigmentosum: a randomized study. *Lancet*. 2001;357:926–929.

194. Paoli J, Smedh M, Ericson MB. Multiphoton laser scanning microscopy – a novel diagnostic method for superficial skin cancers. *Semin Cutan Med Surg*. 2009;28(3):190–195.

195. Vogel U, Christensen J, Wallin H, et al. Polymorphisms in COX-2, NSAID use and risk of basal cell carcinoma in a prospective study of Danes. *Mutat Res*. 2007;617(1–2):138–146.

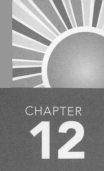
# 12   Squamous Cell Carcinoma

*Sanjay Bhambri, Scott Dinehart, and Avani Bhambri*

---

## Key Points

- The incidence of squamous cell carcinoma (SCC) is rising and thought to occur secondary to numerous factors including increasing UV exposure, prevalence of human papillomavirus, and immunosuppression.

- Awareness of the varied clinical and histologic presentations of SCC is essential for appropriate workup and management.

- Several limitations exist in the current AJCC staging system for SCC. Proposed changes to the staging classification system consist of including tumor size, presence of perineural invasion, tumor depth, and number and size of nodal metastasis, as these features impart important prognostic information.

- Treatment selection is dependent on numerous factors including associated clinical and histologic features as well as therapeutic morbidity, patient cost, convenience, and preference.

- Primary prevention of SCC is aimed at encouraging the limiting of UV exposure, advocating the use of regular sunscreen and sun protective clothing, and recommending regular skin examinations.

---

## INTRODUCTION AND HISTORY

Cutaneous squamous cell carcinoma (SCC) is a malignancy arising from epithelial keratinocytes.[1] It is the second most common skin malignancy after basal cell carcinoma in Caucasians and its incidence has been rapidly increasing. Excessive ultraviolet exposure represents the most important risk factor in the development of SCC as it most commonly occurs on sun-exposed skin. SCC displays a spectrum of clinical and histologic features. If detected and treated early, it has a 95% cure rate. However, SCC can also be aggressive with potential for local destruction as well as metastasis. Many new medical and surgical treatments are continuing to be examined so that the morbidity and mortality associated with this disease can be curtailed.

## EPIDEMIOLOGY

Non-melanoma skin cancer (NMSC) comprises one-third of all cancers in the United States and the incidence is 18–20 times higher than that of melanoma. NMSC has an annual incidence of over 600,000 cases, of which approximately 500,000 are basal cell carcinomas (BCCs) and 100,000 to 150,000 are SCCs.[2] Since common BCCs and SCCs are not reported to SEER (Surveillance, Epidemiology and End Results), few resources are available that accurately document incidence rates. Weinstock calculated the NMSC (SCC+BCC) incidence to be as high as 900,000 to 1,200,000 with a 7%–11% lifetime risk of developing SCC.[3,4] The incidence of SCC in men is significantly higher than in women, with a ratio as high as 3:1 and an annual incidence rate of 81–136 per 100,000 in men and 26–59 per 100,000 in women.[5,6] The difference in gender predilection may be accounted for by lesser protective clothing and higher overall lifetime accumulation of ultraviolet (UV) exposure among men. SCC predominantly affects fair-skinned individuals, usually over the age of 40.[7]

There has been an increase in incidence rates of all skin cancers over the past several decades. A study revealed the incidence of SCC from 1976 to 1989 to be 39 per 100,000 in women and 63 per 100,000 in men. From 1990 to 1992, the incidence rate of SCC increased to 100 per 100,000 for women and 191 per 100,000 for men in the United States.[7,8] Incidence rates of SCC vary worldwide, with incidence rates doubling every 8–10 degree decline in geographic latitude.[9] Given its fair-skinned population and increased sun exposure, Australia has the highest worldwide incidence rate of SCC. Queensland, Australia has an SCC incidence rate of 1332 per 100,000 for men and 755 per 100,000 for women.[10]

Although BCCs outnumber SCCs, SCCs have a greater tendency to recur and metastasize. The 3-year cumulative risk of developing a subsequent SCC given a prior history of SCC is 18%, whereas the risk of developing an SCC after a prior history of BCC is 6%.[11] Cutaneous SCC causes the majority of deaths among NMSC and results in approximately 2500 deaths per year in the United States.[9] SCC occurs most commonly in individuals with fair skin and has a higher predilection for occurring on sun-exposed skin of the head and neck (see Chapter 5).[12]

The rising incidence of SCC is thought to occur secondary to numerous factors, including increased UV exposure, ozone depletion, changes in lifestyle including changes in activities and clothing, increased prevalence of human papillomavirus (HPV), ionizing radiation, genetics, and immunosuppression.[13] Additionally, increased awareness of skin cancer may be leading to higher incidence rates but also reduction in diagnostic delay.[14]

In addition to skin type, cumulative sun exposure, and geographic latitude, chronic immunosuppression is another important risk factor for the development of SCC. Chronic immunosuppression – whether caused by disease such as leukemia/lymphoma or HIV/AIDS, or iatrogenically induced in patients with autoimmune disease or in organ transplant recipients – has become increasingly important in impacting the rising rates of NMSC, particularly SCC. Solid organ transplant recipients, including kidney, heart, lung, and pancreatic patients, represent a population particularly at risk for the development of SCC. Interestingly, this population has a higher incidence of SCCs compared to BCCs, with a ratio of 4:1, in contrast to a ratio of 1:4 in the general population.[15] With the advent of improved immunosuppressive medications and regimens, overall survival and organ transplant rejection have decreased; however, the rate of skin cancer development in this population has increased. The mean time to develop SCC after transplantation is 8 years.[15] Organ transplant patients may have an increased risk of skin cancer development secondary to the presence of foreign graft antigens as well as immunosuppression.[16] The incidence of SCC in renal transplant patients is 18 to 36 times that of the general population.[17,18] The incidence of SCC is highest in heart transplant patients compared to kidney and liver transplant patients, with one study reporting a threefold higher incidence of SCC occurring among heart transplant patients compared to kidney patients.[19] An Australian study showed that among heart transplant patients surviving beyond 4 years post transplant, skin cancer was related to the cause of death in 27% of cases. An increase of 34% in incidence rate occurred between the fifth and tenth years after transplantation. The overall higher risk of skin cancer among heart transplant patients may be related to the higher doses of immunosuppression.[20–22] Additionally, the type of immunosuppression adopted after transplant has an impact on development of SCC. A study by Ingvar et al. supported a strong association between the development of cutaneous SCC with azathioprine but not with ciclosporin.[23] The International Transplant Skin Cancer Collaborative (ITSCC) has presented guidelines for the management of SCC in organ transplant recipients. Initial screening of transplant patients should include past history of sunburns, skin cancer and HPV infection, as well as assessment of type and duration of immunosuppression, and skin type. In instances of rapid development of SCC, ITSCC guidelines recommend decreasing the dose of immunosuppression. More research studies are needed to effectively characterize how immune responses affect the development of SCC.[24,25]

## PATHOGENESIS

The pathogenesis of SCC is multifactorial, with both environmental and genetic factors influencing its development. Cumulative sun exposure is believed to be the most important factor contributing to the development of SCC, as evidenced by the majority of SCCs occurring on sun-exposed skin.[26] UVB (290–320 nm) is more carcinogenic in SCC development than is UVA (320–400 nm).[27] The role of UV radiation in promoting development of SCC is manifold and is related to its ability to act as a tumor initiator and promoter. UVB causes the formation of thymidine dimers and subsequently induces DNA point mutations which promote the development of SCC. The majority of UVB-induced damage to DNA is repaired; however, mismatching of DNA base pairs can occur, resulting in mutations. Patients with xeroderma pigmentosa have defective excision repair mechanisms of thymidine dimer base pairs and therefore display greater photosensitivity and higher incidence of SCC development. UV radiation produces mutations in the *p53* tumor suppressor gene and promotes the development of SCC.[28] Mutations in the *p53* tumor suppressor gene subsequently result in the clonal expansion of abnormal keratinocytes.

UVA also plays a role, although lesser than UVB, in the development of SCC. Studies suggest that UVA helps to expand tumor cells via activation of the signal transduction molecule protein C kinase.[29] UVA also has a role in immunosuppression via modulation of the IL-10 pathway activation of suppressor T cells.[30] Impaired immunity against early clonal expansion of abnormal keratinocytes leads to the progression of carcinoma. Patients who receive long-term treatment with psoralen plus UVA (PUVA) are also at higher risk for the development of SCC.[31]

A variety of exposures and conditions lead to an increased risk of SCC (Table 12.1). Scars and chronic dermatoses also predispose to SCC development. Marjolin's ulcers are SCCs developing within areas of chronic scarring

### Table 12.1 Exposures and Conditions that Lead to an Increased Risk Of SCC[5]

| Scarring Processes or Sites of Chronic Inflammation or Infection | Exposures | Associated Primary Dermatoses (Often Scarring or Photosensitivity) |
| --- | --- | --- |
| Chronic osteomyelitis sinus<br>Burn scar<br>Vaccination scar<br>Chronic venous ulcer<br>Pilonidal cyst<br>Branchial cleft cyst<br>Chromoblastomycosis<br>Hyalohyphomycosis<br>Lymphogranuloma venereum<br>Granuloma inguinale<br>Lupus vulgaris<br>Acrodermatitis chronica atrophicans<br>Plantar ulcers of leprosy | Arsenic<br>Polycyclic aromatic hydrocarbons<br>Immunosuppression<br>X-ray therapy<br>PUVA | Dystrophic epidermolysis bullosa<br>Epidermodysplasia verruciformis<br>Xeroderma pigmentosum<br>Oculocutaneous albinism<br>Porokeratosis of Mibelli<br>Linear porokeratosis<br>Disseminated superficial actinic porokeratosis<br>Porokeratosis palmaris et plantaris disseminatum<br>Discoid lupus erythematosus<br>Lichen planus<br>Lichen sclerosus et atrophicus<br>Dissecting perifolliculitis of the scalp<br>Acne conglobata<br>Hidradenitis suppurativa<br>Mutilating keratoderma<br>Necrobiosis lipoidica diabeticorum<br>Nevus sebaceous |

(see below). SCCs also develop with greater frequency in areas of chronic trauma and inflammation, such as that caused by radiation therapy. Additionally, several chemical compounds, including arsenic, polycyclic aromatic hydrocarbons, and insecticides, can predispose to the development of SCC.

Finally, human papillomavirus (HPV) has been implicated in the development of SCC. HPV viral proteins E6 and E7 have been shown to inhibit the tumor suppressor gene *p53*. There is also evidence that HPV may act in p53-independent pathways to prevent apoptosis. HPV has been estimated to be involved in the pathogenesis of up to 90% of NMSCs in immunocompromised individuals and up to 50% of NMSCs in immunocompetent individuals (see Chapter 19).[24]

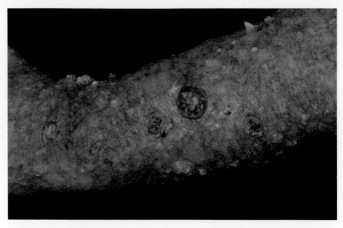

**Figure 12.1** Multiple AKs and SCC on the forearm

## CLINICAL FEATURES

SCC presents in a spectrum of clinical appearance which includes many subtypes and widely varying clinical behaviors. The variety of morphologies depends on the location, background pigmentation, and clinical setting. On a continuum, primary morphologies range from ill-defined rough pink patches to well-circumscribed hyperkeratotic plaques. Typically, SCCs arising in sun-exposed, actinically damaged skin are most commonly found on the head, neck, and upper extremities, and, in women, the lower extremities are often involved. Fewer SCCs occur on sun-covered locations such as the genitalia, buttocks, and feet, suggesting a role for factors apart from actinic damage in the development of SCCs.

Actinic keratoses (AKs) represent proliferations of atypical keratinocytes confined to the epidermis, which are induced by UV exposure in sunlight (see Chapter 10). Although AKs have traditionally been thought of as representing precancerous or premalignant lesions, the view that these lesions exist on a continuum with SCC in situ and SCC is becoming more widely accepted. There is even more disagreement over the rate of transformation of AK to invasive carcinoma, mostly arising because it is difficult to accurately assess this transformation in the controlled study environment. One study has proposed that the likelihood of an invasive SCC evolving from a given AK ranges from 0.075% to 0.096% per lesion per year. Thus, for a person with 7.7 AKs, the average number for an affected person, invasive SCC would develop at a rate of 10.2% over 10 years if left untreated. Others have proposed higher estimates, with the rate of transformation to invasive SCC being 13–20% over a 10-year period.[32–35]

AKs represent one of the most commonly encountered lesions in clinical dermatology practice. They occur most frequently on sun-exposed skin of the face, neck, scalp of bald individuals, extremities, and upper trunk. Clinically they appear as rough, scaly, red-brown papules and plaques. Variants of AKs include hypertrophic, pigmented, lichenoid, and atrophic types. Hypertrophic AKs are thickened hyperkeratotic lesions that may be difficult to distinguish from early SCC. Early AKs may only display slight erythema with minimal scale. Advanced lesions typically are more hyperkeratotic, erythematous, and can occasionally be painful. Lesions range in size from a few millimeters to several centimeters in diameter and can be clinically similar to early SCCs (Fig. 12.1). Since AKs generally develop secondary to increased cumulative sun exposure over years, older individuals develop lesions with greater frequency, with the number of lesions increasing with age. Fair-skinned individuals are more susceptible to developing AKs than patients with darker skin types. Patients who are immunosuppressed as well as those with certain genetic abnormalities, including albinism and xeroderma pigmentosum, are more susceptible to development of AKs. Actinic keratoses as well as disseminated superficial actinic porokeratosis and porokeratosis of Mibelli may demonstrate malignant potential for the development of SCC, especially when associated with pain. Although up to 25% of AKs may regress spontaneously with sun protective measures, treatment is generally indicated for those lesions that are thick or symptomatic, and for those occurring in immunosuppressed individuals.[36]

Squamous cell carcinoma in situ, also known as Bowen's disease, represents an intraepidermal malignancy which generally appears as a scaly enlarging plaque on sun-exposed skin, usually arising in elderly individuals (Fig. 12.2). Lesions may arise from pre-exisiting actinic keratoses or de novo. In addition to chronic actinic damage, other risk factors for Bowen's disease include fair skin, radiation and arsenic exposure, immunosuppression, and human papillomavirus infection. The rate of transformation of Bowen's disease to invasive SCC has been estimated to be 3–8%, and the metastatic potential following development of invasive carcinoma is 3–5%.[37–40] If left untreated, Bowen's disease may progress and become invasive, especially on the genitalia. Bowen's disease on sun-exposed skin is more common and less aggressive compared to that on sun-protected areas. Lesions of Bowen's disease may at times be difficult to clinically distinguish from AK, tinea, psoriasis, nummular eczema, and superficial BCC. Erythroplasia of Queyrat represents SCC in situ presenting on the mucous membranes of the glans penis, vulva, and oral mucosa. Factors related to its development are thought to include trauma, poor hygiene, irritation, friction, syphilis, and other inflammatory conditions. Important to include in the differential with Bowen's disease and erythroplasia of Queyrat is bowenoid papulosis. Whether this condition represents true SCC in situ versus a benign

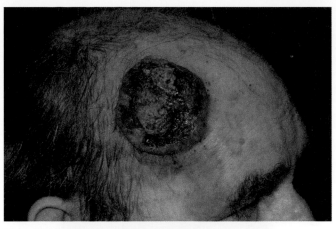

Figure 12.4 Large ulcerated SCC on the head.

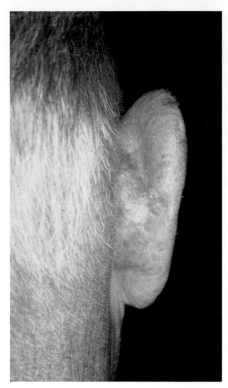

Figure 12.2 Bowen's disease.

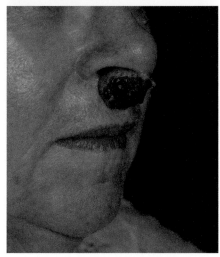

Figure 12.5 SCC nodule.

condition is a matter of debate. Lesions of bowenoid papulosis, which present as multiple small brown papules usually on the penile shaft, rarely become invasive. Bowen's disease occurring secondary to arsenic exposure clinically resembles classic Bowen's disease but tends to arise on sun-protected areas of the trunk. Other clinical findings associated with arsenic-induced Bowen's disease include palmoplantar keratoses and guttate hypopigmentation. When associated with arsenic exposure, Bowen's disease may occur with internal malignancies.

The characteristic clinical presentation for invasive SCC is a raised, firm, erythematous keratotic papule or nodule with more substance than a typical AK (Fig. 12.3). Lesions classically arise in sun-exposed regions, often on a background of actinically damaged skin (Figs 12.4 and 12.5). Rapid growth, induration, and erosions in an AK or porokeratosis, especially when associated with pain, are often harbingers of SCC transformation. SCCs are most

often keratotic; however, they can present as nodular lesions without significant epidermal change. SCC may vary in size from a few millimeters to several centimeters if left untreated. Large SCCs often present with erosion, ulceration, and can be painful if deeply invasive (Fig. 12.6). Paresthesias, dysesthesias, or motor nerve paresis may reflect underlying perineural spread but is generally a late manifestation. Larger lesions are not uncommonly associated with metastasis, and therefore it is important

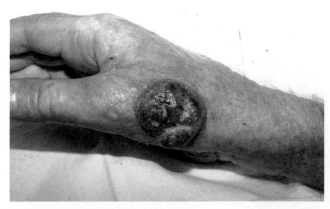

Figure 12.3 Large SCC nodule on the hand.

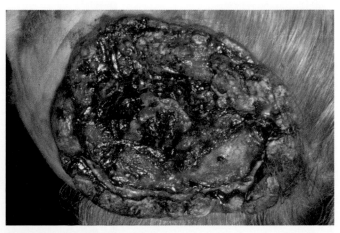

Figure 12.6 Ulcerated SCC plaque.

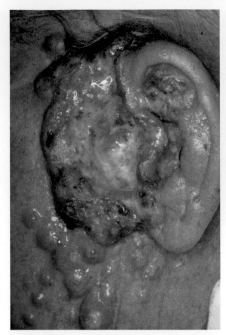

**Figure 12.7** SCC nodules with metastasis.

to evaluate local lymph nodes during clinical examination (Fig. 12.7). The rate of growth of SCCs is variable; however, rapidly growing tumors tend to have more aggressive features including deeper invasion and poor differentiation.

Rapidly growing SCCs in certain locations are more high risk, including those found on the ear and lip (Fig. 12.8). One explanation for this observation could be a lack of a protective fat buffer layer in these locations, whereby the lymphatics of underlying perichondrium and muscle could facilitate metastasis. SCC involving the lip may metastasize at a rate of 10–14%, and that of the ear at a rate of 11%.[41] A low threshold should be maintained in identifying and treating these lesions. SCC of the lip is primarily limited to the lower lip. The precursor lesion for SCC of the lip is actinic cheilitis, where the vermillion border loses its definition and becomes dry, keratotic, atrophic, and irregularly hypopigmented. New erythema, induration, erosion, or elevation in previously stable actinic cheilitis may signal transformation to SCC. Intraoral SCCs are even more aggressive than lip lesions and metastasis rates range from 20% to 70%.[42] Intraoral SCC commonly presents on the anterior floor of the mouth, anterior tongue, and buccal vestibule. The precursor lesion for intraoral SCC is leukoplakia. Risk factors include tobacco chewing and smoking, Betel nut chewing, alcohol, human papillomavirus infections, erosive lichen planus, Plummer–Vinson syndrome, and dyskeratosis congenita.

SCC involving the anogenital region is also considered high risk and may have developed in the setting of human papillomavirus. Irritation, pruritus, pain, erythema, erosion, and bleeding are common signs and symptoms associated with anogenital SCC. Maceration, lack of scale, induration, and ulceration rather than hyperkeratotic exophytic lesions are common. Vulvar and scrotal lesions may develop secondary to chronic occupational exposure to aromatic hydrocarbons found in mineral oil, pitch, and tar. Penile lesions of the glans are typically associated with lack of circumcision, poor hygiene, and chronic inflammation from processes such as lichen sclerosus (Fig. 12.9). Vulvar lesions have a metastasis rate of 13% and those involving the penis have a local recurrence rate of 40%.

The diagnosis of periungal SCC (Fig. 12.10) is often delayed as it is often verrucous in appearance and commonly misdiagnosed as periungal verruca vulgaris. Lesions may also mimic paronychia, with swelling, erythema, and pain, and cause onychodystrophy. Chronic paronychia unresponsive to repeated treatment with antibiotics and antifungals should be biopsied to evaluate for possible malignancy. Periungal SCCs may have high local recurrence rates but they display low metastatic potential at a rate of less than 2%.

**Figure 12.8 A)** SCC ear. **B)** SCC posterior ear.

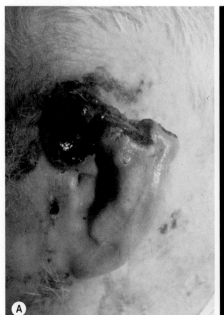
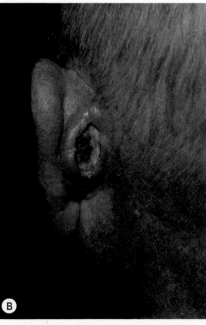

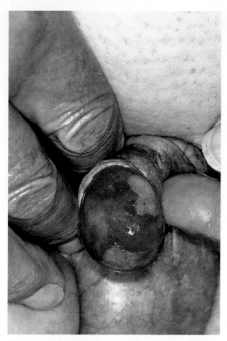

Figure 12.9 SCC on glans penis.

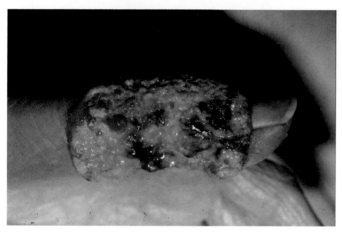

Figure 12.10 Periungal SCC.

Marjolin's ulcer is an eponym for SCC that develops in injured or chronically damaged skin affected by chronic dermatoses and wounds, including skin affected by long-standing ulcers, sinus tracts, osteomyelitis, radiation dermatitis, and vaccination scars (Fig. 12.11). Tumors arising at these sites may demonstrate a high rate of metastasis and they are particularly aggressive early on. Tenderness, pruritus, and irritation may be associated symptoms. There should be a low threshold for biopsy in any ulcer that has changed in size or symptoms. Certain inflammatory conditions are associated with a higher risk of SCC development, including discoid lupus erythematosus, lichen sclerosus, lichen planus, and dystrophic epidermolysis bullosa. It is unclear why these conditions predispose to higher rates of SCC development. There is a long latency period of 20–30 years before SCC develops in these settings. Skin damaged by radiation has the shortest latency period to malignancy.

SCC is less common in darker skin types than in fair-skinned individuals, but similarly affects elderly patients and is most often found on the face and extremities.

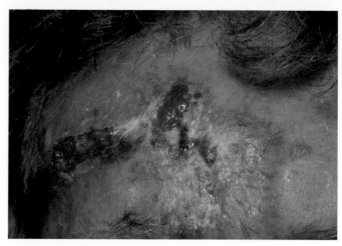

Figure 12.11 Marjolin's ulcer.

SCCs are more common than basal cell carcinomas in this population and frequently develop in sites of previous injury and scarring. Tumors in covered locations are also more common in darker-skinned individuals than in Caucasians.

Verrucous carcinoma is considered a low-grade subtype of SCC. Although it rarely metastasizes, it can become deeply invasive. Clinically it appears as a verrucous plaque that can have a 'cauliflower-like' growth. Verrucous carcinoma is referred to by different names depending on location. Buschke–Löwenstein tumor is found in the anogenital region (Fig. 12.12), Ackerman tumor is found on the oral mucosa, and epithelioma cuniculatum is found on the feet (Fig. 12.13). Risk factors for the development of verrucous carcinoma include human papillomavirus types 6 and 11, chronic inflammatory processes, chronic trauma, and chemical carcinogens including tobacco and Betel nuts. Aggressive anaplastic transformation has been reported in verrucous carcinomas treated with radiation therapy.[43]

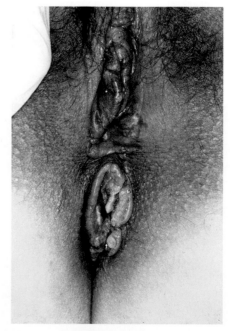

Figure 12.12 Verrucous carcinoma: Buschke–Löwenstein tumor.

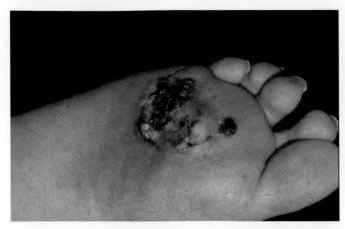

**Figure 12.13** Verrucous carcinoma.

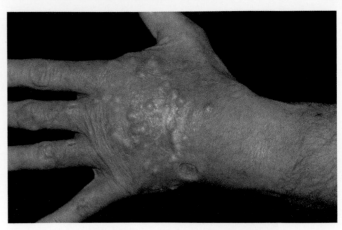

**Figure 12.15** Multiple keratoacanthomas.

Keratoacanthoma (KA) is a variant of SCC and is characterized by a rapid growth phase followed by spontaneous regression or involution.[44] Controversy exists over the clinical nature of KAs, whether they represent a benign cutaneous tumor or a well-differentiated squamous cell carcinoma. Clinically, a well-circumscribed papule or nodule rapidly enlarges over several weeks, stabilizes in growth, followed by spontaneous regression over several weeks to years with residual tissue scarring. Lesions generally range between 1 cm and 3 cm in size and typically occur on sun-exposed skin (Fig. 12.14). Although most KAs spontaneously regress, some KAs have been reported to have aggressive clinical behavior leading to metastasis.[45] Several variants of KA exist; however, solitary KA is the most common. Keratoacanthoma centrifugum marginatum is a variant characterized by large size and slow healing with scarring. Multiple KAs can be seen in several syndromes, including Ferguson–Smith, Grzybowski, and Muir–Torre (Fig. 12.15). Ferguson–Smith syndrome, an autosomal dominant condition, is characterized by multiple KAs appearing in sun-exposed areas which usually spontaneously regress. The Grzybowski variant, in contrast, is marked by the appearance of hundreds to thousands of smaller-sized lesions. Muir–Torre syndrome is characterized by the presence of multiple keratoacanthomas, sebaceous tumors, and visceral cancers, most commonly involving the colon.

## PATIENT EVALUATION, DIAGNOSIS, AND DIFFERENTIAL DIAGNOSIS

Clinical suspicion of SCC can be confirmed with histologic evaluation. Various biopsy techniques can be employed, including shave, punch, incision, and excision, to evaluate for the presence of SCC. Regardless of the type of technique employed, all biopsy samples should include an adequate sampling of the base of the lesion, including the dermis, so that the pathologist is able to effectively assess for possible invasion. Adequate measurement of depth of invasion will allow the clinician to effectively determine subsequent therapy options.

The differential diagnosis of cutaneous SCC most commonly includes hypertrophic actinic keratosis, verruca vulgaris, and inflamed or irritated seborrheic keratosis. SCC lesions involving the mucosa, however, can mimic and be difficult to distinguish from inflammatory processes. A high level of suspicion should be maintained for lesions involving mucosa as these tumors can be more aggressive.

Patient history should include a comprehensive review of any potential risk factors, including prior treatment, radiation exposure, scars, immunosuppression, rapid growth, and symptoms including pain or paresthesia. A comprehensive skin examination is essential when assessing for the presence of skin cancer. SCC can be present in both sun-exposed and covered areas, therefore careful examination of covered areas should be pursued (Figs 12.16 and 12.17). Additionally, mucosal surfaces should be examined as lesions involving the mucosa can be more aggressive. Palpation of lesions can be helpful since many AKs often are not readily apparent but can be felt. Palpation of perilesional skin and regional soft tissue should be performed to assess for adherence, induration, pain, and in-transit metastasis (Figs 12.18 and 12.19).

Since cutaneous SCC has the potential to metastasize, physical examination of regional lymph nodes is essential, especially for lesions that are invasive, recurrent, or high risk. Even for unilateral tumors, bilateral palpation of lymph nodes should be done, as contralateral spread can occur. Radiologic examination may be helpful for evaluation of aggressive high-risk SCCs or for the presence of clinically palpable nodes. Computerized axial tomography examination can allow for identification of lymph nodes which may not be clinically palpable as well as bony

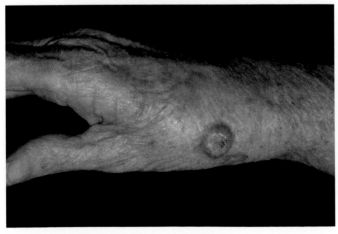

**Figure 12.14** Keratoacanthoma.

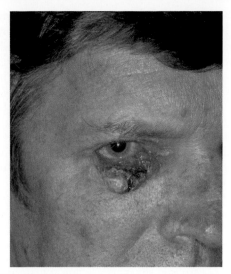

**Figure 12.16** Periocular SCC.

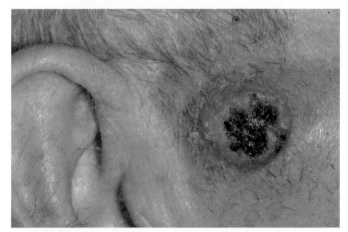

**Figure 12.17** Preauricular SCC.

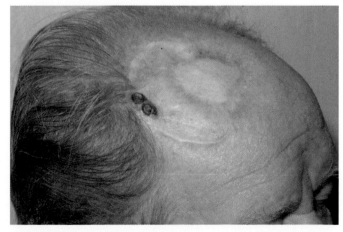

**Figure 12.18** Recurrent SCC on the scalp.

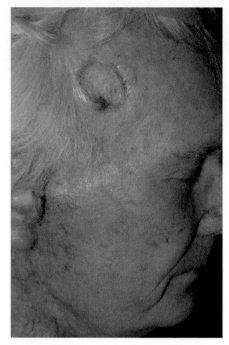

**Figure 12.19** Recurrent SCC.

considerable debate since its benefit in predicting recurrence and improving outcome is unclear.[47]

Patients with SCC traditionally have been staged according to the American Joint Commission on Cancer (AJCC) criteria, which stages patients according to primary tumor size, regional lymph node status, and the presence of distant metastasis. However, AJCC criteria fails to include certain histologic variables, including tumor differentiation, the presence of perineural involvement, and depth of tumor invasion. Since many important prognostic factors have been neglected from the AJCC criteria, the current staging system may need to be revised. A 2006 study proposed that metastatic SCC involvement of parotid and cervical lymph nodes imparts important prognostic implications. In a follow-up multicenter study involving six institutions, three from the United States and three from Australia, 322 patients with metastatic cutaneous SCC were restaged according to a newly proposed system which separated parotid involvement from cervical involvement. Survival was worse for patients with advanced parotid disease compared to those with early parotid disease (69% vs 82%). Neck node involvement when occurring with parotid disease imparted worse survival than parotid disease alone (61% vs 79%).[48] Proposed changes for the TNM classification system consist of including stratified tumor size, presence of perineural invasion, tumor thickness, and number and size of nodal metastasis. The inclusion of these factors in the staging of cutaneous SCC may more accurately reflect the prognosis and natural history of the disease.[49]

## PATHOLOGY

The biologic behavior of SCC is influenced by the histologic type, tumor size, depth, level of differentiation, and the presence of perineural invasion, all of which should be assessed when examining a biopsy sample. In addition

invasion. Ultrasound and fine needle aspiration of clinically positive lymph nodes may also be useful. Magnetic resonance imaging (MRI) allows for examination of soft tissue and perineural involvement. Positive emission tomography (PET) scanning is useful when evaluating an unknown primary, assessing treatment response, and determining persistent or recurrent disease.[46] The use of sentinel lymph node biopsy for evaluation of metastatic SCC is still under

to the mentioned histologic criteria, a patient's immune response also influences behavior of SCC.

Invasive SCC consists of a proliferation of atypical keratinocytes arising from the epidermis with extension to the dermis and deeper structures. Atypical keratinocytes may exhibit glassy eosinophilic cytoplasm, hyperchromatic nuclei, prominent nucleoli, atypical mitoses, as well as disorganized architecture (Fig. 12.20). Detached islands of squamous epithelial cells are present in the dermis. Keratinization may occur extracellularly as horn pearls or be seen within individual cells. Except for poorly differentiated SCCs, the presence of desmosomal attachments and keratin production may help to identify the lesion's keratinocyte origin. In SCC in situ, atypical keratinocytes span the entire thickness of the epidermis (Fig. 12.21). There is hyperkeratosis, parakeratosis, and acanthosis, although occasionally the epidermis can be atrophic. Atypical keratinocytes often demonstrate a loss of polarity with abnormal maturation. Distinction between hypertrophic AK and SCC in situ may be subtle. Extensive involvement of adnexal structures as well as diffuse confluent parakeratosis help favor a diagnosis of SCC in situ. Nuclear pleomorphism and the presence of mitoses are also more numerous in SCC in situ compared to AK. If left untreated, SCC in situ may progress to invasive SCC.[9]

Pseudoepitheliomatous hyperplasia (PEH) may clinically and histologically simulate SCC. PEH is a benign well-differentiated proliferation of epidermis that tends to arise in the setting of chronic inflammation caused by wounds, ulcers, or primary dermatoses, and also can occur overlying certain benign tumors. Histologically, features favoring PEH include well-differentiated, vertically oriented proliferation into the dermis with lack of atypical mitotic figures, nuclear pleomorphism, and individual cell keratinization. Dermal edema and an inflammatory infiltrate may be present. Many cases of PEH are difficult to distinguish from SCC and therefore deeper sections or repeat biopsies are often needed for definitive distinction.

Histologic grading of SCC was initially proposed by Broder. The Broder system grades SCC from I to IV based on the degree of cellular differentiation. In grade I tumors, 75% of cells are differentiated, compared to grades II, III, and IV where 50–75%, 25–50%, and less than 25% of cells are differentiated, respectively.[50] Although this system provided defined guidelines for grading of SCC, it has not been widely accepted, and most pathologists classify lesions as well, moderately, or poorly differentiated (Figs 12.22 and 12.23). Broder believed that the grade of SCC directly correlated with malignant potential. Although grading of SCC certainly has a definite role in predicting biologic behavior, it is not the sole predictive factor. Most metastatic SCCs are well differentiated due to the greater overall numbers of well-differentiated tumors. However, a greater

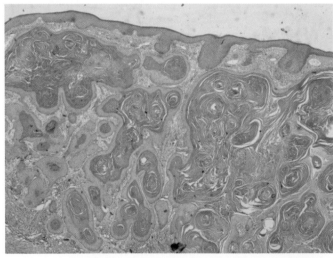

**Figure 12.20** Invasive SCC.

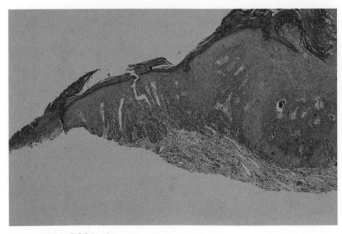

**Figure 12.21** SCC in situ.

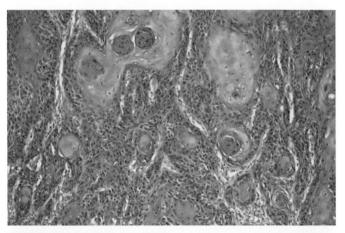

**Figure 12.22** Well-differentiated SCC.

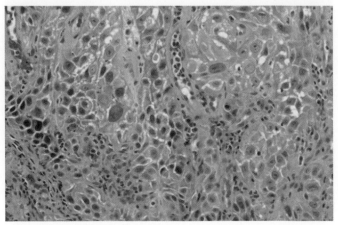

**Figure 12.23** Poorly differentiated SCC.

percentage of poorly differentiated SCCs metastasize compared with their well-differentiated counterparts, 17% versus 0.6%, respectively.[51]

Several histologic variants of SCC have been characterized. Adenoid or acantholytic SCC displays a pseudoglandular acantholytic appearance which is the result of dyskeratosis and acantholysis. Lesions commonly appear as eroded nodules on sun-exposed skin of the head, neck, and upper extremities. The rate of metastasis can range from 3% to as high as 19%.[52]

Adenosquamous carcinoma, also known as mucoepidermoid carcinoma, is a rare variant of SCC displaying both squamous and glandular differentiation (Fig. 12.24). Squamous differentiation, primarily located superficially, shows positive immunohistochemical staining for cytokeratin. Glandular differentiation, located in the deeper dermis and subcutis, displays positive immunohistochemical staining for carcinoembryonic antigen. In contrast to acantholytic SCC which is pseudoglandular in appearance, adenosquamous carcinoma contains glandular mucin-secreting epithelium. Lesions are typically located centrofacially and present in the elderly. Tumors tend to be aggressive with higher tendency towards perineural invasion and metastasis.[53]

Verrucous carcinoma is a low-grade, well-differentiated variant of SCC and is commonly found on the skin, oral cavity, genitalia, and feet (Fig. 12.25). A deep biopsy sample is needed to effectively provide diagnosis, since superficially the tumor simulates a verruca vulgaris with hyperkeratosis, parakeratosis, papillomatosis, and acanthosis. The tumor is large with rete ridges extending into the dermis and a pushing border. Proliferating keratinocytes with minimal cytologic atypia can also be seen. The presence of proliferating cell nuclear antigen (PCNA) at the borders may be helpful in distinguishing verrucous carcinoma from other types of SCC which stain more diffusely with PCNA.[54] Although rarely prone to metastasis, verrucous carcinoma tends to be slow growing with tendency for local invasion and recurrence if incompletely removed.[5]

The histologic diagnosis of keratoacanthoma is based largely on the architecture of the lesion, however it can be difficult to differentiate KA from SCC. Most clinicians consider KA to be a form of SCC, and more pathologists recently have been diagnosing this lesion as squamous cell carcinoma, keratoacanthoma type. KAs typically have a

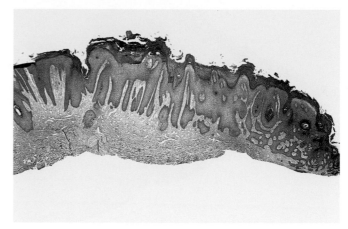

**Figure 12.25** Verrucous carcinoma.

well-circumscribed volcano or crateriform architecture with a central core filled with cornified material and surrounded by well-differentiated keratinocytes with glassy eosinophilic cytoplasm (Fig. 12.26). There is minimal cytologic atypia and mitoses. An associated mixed inflammatory infiltrate consisting of lymphocytes, eosinophils, and neutrophils may be present in the underlying dermis. Immunohistochemical analysis may assist in differentiating KA from SCC. The presence of PCNA-positive cells predominantly in the periphery of squamous nests in KA can be contrasted with the diffuse staining pattern of PCNA seen in SCC.[44]

Spindle cell SCC is a rare variant of SCC. Clinically, lesions resemble ulcerated, eroded, and often exophytic tumors, commonly appearing on the sun-exposed skin of elderly patients. Histologically, the tumor is composed of atypical, poorly differentiated spindle cells with large nuclei, scant cytoplasm, numerous mitoses, and cellular pleomorphism (Figs 12.27 and 12.28). Evidence of keratinization may or may not be present. Tumor borders are poorly defined with tumor infiltration occurring as either strands or individual cells extending to the deep dermis and subcutaneous fat. Histologically, it may be difficult to differentiate from other spindle cell neoplasms, and generally, immunohistochemical study has to be pursued for definitive diagnosis. Spindle cell SCC generally maintains expression of cytokeratin. Other entities to be considered in the differential diagnosis of spindle cell SCC include

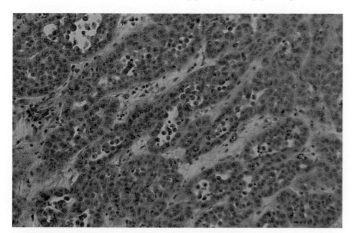

**Figure 12.24** Adenosquamous or acantholytic SCC.

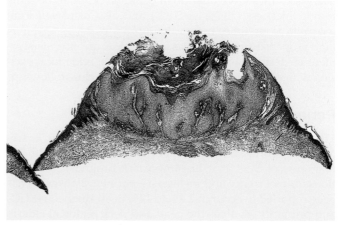

**Figure 12.26** Keratoacanthoma.

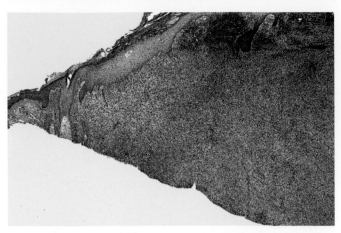

Figure 12.27 Spindle cell SCC.

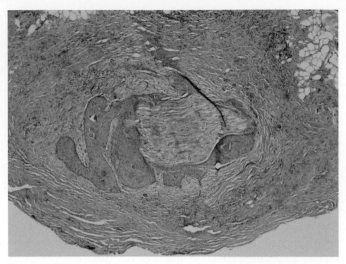

Figure 12.29 Perineural invasion.

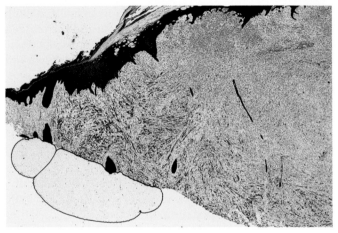

Figure 12.28 Spindle cell SCC (cytokeratin stain).

may mask the presence of perineural invasion. Therefore, careful pathologic review is mandatory in these instances. Most patients with a diagnosis of SCC with perineural invasion are asymptomatic and pain or tenderness may signal deeper extension of disease. Both sensory nerves and larger cranial nerves can be involved, with facial nerves and the second division of the trigeminal nerve being the most commonly involved.[9] If left untreated, perineural involvement can lead to facial paralysis and diplopia. Perineural invasion is typically associated with poor prognosis, with a local recurrence rate of 47%, a 35% rate of metastasis to regional lymph nodes, and a 15% distant metastasis rate.[57]

## Tumor depth

SCC tumor depth is believed to have important prognostic implications affecting recurrence and metastasis. Despite the importance that tumor depth is believed to impart, the measurement and reporting of SCC tumor thickness is often overlooked. As in melanoma, the reporting of SCC tumor depth may allow the clinician to optimize his ability to correlate treatment options with prognosis and survival. In addition to the patient's immune status, tumor location, tumor size, tumor grade, and presence of perineural invasion, tumor thickness is an important factor to consider when assessing the risk of metastasis. The histologic features and rate of metastasis were assessed in 673 cases of SCC. Tumors with a depth of less than 2 mm, which comprised half of all cases, did not metastasize. Tumors with a thickness between 2 mm and 6 mm metastasized at a rate of 4.5%, and those with a depth of greater than 6 mm had a metastatic rate of 15%. Similarly, only one tumor with invasion involving the entire dermis metastasized; however, tumors invading the subcutaneous fat had a metastatic rate of 4.1%, and those involving the underlying muscle, cartilage, or bone had a metastatic rate of 12.5%. Based on these results, Khanna and colleagues provided correlation between tumor thickness and overall risk for metastasis. Tumors with a thickness of less than 2 mm should be regarded as low risk, those with a thickness between 2 mm and 6 mm are intermediate risk, and those with a thickness greater than 6 mm are considered high risk.[59] In the

atypical fibroxanthoma which expresses vimentin, leiomyosarcoma which expresses desmin, and melanoma which typically expresses S-100 and Melan-A. Given its poor differentiation, this variant is thought to be relatively aggressive with poor prognosis.[55]

Desmoplastic SCCs commonly appear on the sun-exposed skin of the head and neck. Histologic features include a trabecular growth pattern, desmoplastic stromal reaction, and frequent perineural invasion. Desmoplastic SCC tends to have a worse prognosis than conventional SCC. In a study by Breuninger et al.,[56] desmoplastic SCCs were found to metastasize six times more often than common SCCs of the same tumor thickness (22.7% vs 3.8%) and also displayed local recurrences ten times more often (27.3% vs 2.6%). Given its high propensity for metastasis and local recurrence, management of desmoplastic SCC should include wide local excision with examination of lymph nodes, and close follow-up.

## Perineural invasion

The presence of perineural invasion (Fig. 12.29) is frequently reported in biopsy reports in conjunction with the diagnosis of SCC as it has important prognostic implications for recurrence and metastasis. Perineural invasion has been reported to occur in 2.4% to 14% of all cutaneous SCCs and primarily involves the head and neck region of elderly individuals.[57,58] The presence of perineural inflammation

author's (SD) own experience, examination of a series of 22 patients with metastatic cutaneous SCC revealed an average primary tumor thickness of 6.6 mm.[60] Measurement of invasive SCC tumor thickness should be another important component – as are tumor differentiation[61] and the presence of perineural invasion – in the diagnostic reporting of SCC, since it confers important information for prognosis and survival.

## Metastasis

Metastasis from SCC is not uncommon, and, as noted, high-risk SCCs have a higher rate of metastasis.[58] A study examining 365 cases of cutaneous SCC treated by Mohs surgery showed an overall 7.4% metastatic rate, with tumors arising on the lip, temple, and dorsum of the hand having a higher rate.[62] In the author's experience, more than 90% of tumors metastasize within the first 2 years after Mohs surgery and therefore close follow-up is extremely important. Recurrent disease is often present at the time of lymph node involvement and distant visceral spread is rare without local or regional disease. Additionally, overall 5-year survival after regional metastasis is only 25%.[61,63] More recently, the overall metastatic rate for SCC was calculated as 2.3% to 5.2%, dependent on whether follow-up was less than or greater than 5 years, respectively. The risk of metastasis and recurrence was based on several clinical and histologic features (Table 12.2) including anatomic location, size, treatment history, immune status, degree of histologic differentiation, depth of invasion, and the presence of perineural invasion. In general, SCCs located on sun-exposed areas have lower risk for metastasis, except for those located on the ear and lip. Patients with primary tumors have a rate of metastasis of 5.2% compared to 30.3% for recurrent tumors. Additionally, chronically immunosuppressed individuals are at higher risk for developing metastasis. Histologic features also carry important prognostic value, as poorly differentiated tumors and those with greater depth of invasion predict worse metastatic potential. The presence of perineural invasion portends a significantly worse prognosis and is associated with a metastatic rate of 47.3%.[64] Cutaneous SCC metastasis may occur through many routes, including lymphatic, perineural, hematogenous, and along fascial planes. Brodland and Zitelli proposed that metastasis involves detachment of the primary tumor, invasion and circulation through vascular or lymphatic vessels, with subsequent invasion into a recipient tissue.[65] Local metastasis tends to occur in the primary regional lymphatic system, with the parotid and cervical nodes being most common, given that most cutaneous SCCs occur on the head and neck (Figs 12.30 and 12.31). Distant metastasis most commonly spreads to the lungs, liver, brain, skin, or bone.[9]

## TREATMENT

Clinical guidelines for the management of SCC are available from the American Academy of Dermatology (www.aad.org) and the National Comprehensive Cancer network (www.nccn.org). Many modalities are available in the treatment of patients with SCC. As noted by Motley et al., several factors should influence the choice of treatment; these include the ability to locally remove the tumor, the possibility of in-transit metastasis, and the possibility of the presence of lymph node metastasis.[66] The majority of patients presenting with SCC have low-risk localized disease. However, when determining treatment options, it is important to ascertain which lesions are high risk and therefore may have higher potential for recurrence and/or metastasis.

### Table 12.2 Risk of Recurrence and Metastasis from Clinical and Histologic Features[63]

| Clinical Features | Recurrence (%) | Metastasis (%) |
|---|---|---|
| **Anatomic location** | | |
| Sun-exposed skin | 7.9 | 5.2 |
| Scarred areas in sun-protected skin | Not available | 37.9 |
| Lip | 10.5 | 13.7 |
| Ear | 18.7 | 11.0 |
| **Size (diameter)** | | |
| <2 cm | 7.4 | 9.1 |
| >2 cm | 15.2 | 30.3 |
| **Treatment history** | | |
| Primary | 7.9 | 5.2 |
| Recurrent | 23.3 | 30.3 |
| **Immune status** | | |
| Immunosuppressed | 13.4 | 8 |
| **Histologic Features** | | |
| **Differentiation** | | |
| Well-differentiated | 13.6 | 9.2 |
| Poorly differentiated | 28.6 | 32.8 |
| **Depth of invasion** | | |
| <4 mm (Clark level <IV) | 5.3 | 6.7 |
| >4 mm (Clark level ≥IV) | 17.2 | 45.7 |
| **Nerve involvement** | | |
| Perineural invasion | 47.2 | 47.3 |

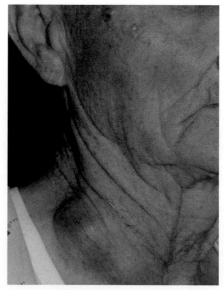

**Figure 12.30** Large metastatic nodule.

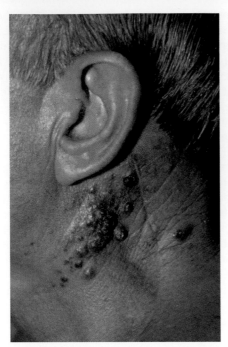

**Figure 12.31** Metastatic SCC.

Treatment selection is dependent on numerous factors but priority should be maintained to arrive at oncologic cure. Success of treatment can therefore be determined by the rate of recurrence and/or metastasis. In addition to assessing the associated clinical and histologic features, including tumor size and depth, location, grade of differentiation, symptoms, and immune status, other variables which should be considered when selecting treatment include therapeutic morbidity as well as patient cost, convenience, and preference. Treatment options can be categorized based on whether they permit or preclude histologic evaluation of margins. Destructive methods prevent histologic margin control and include cryotherapy, electrodesiccation and curettage, chemotherapy, and radiotherapy. Surgical options, including standard excision and Mohs micrographic surgery, allow for adequate histologic margin evaluation.

Cryotherapy has been used effectively in the treatment of AKs and SCCs for several decades with successful results (see Chapter 42). Typically, small, low-risk, minimally invasive SCCs with well-defined borders can be treated with cryotherapy. Large, invasive, recurrent, or high-risk SCCs should be treated with alternative methods since cryotherapy does not provide for adequate assessment of margin control. The cryogen most commonly used is liquid nitrogen (−196°C). The lesion is rapidly frozen to a temperature of −40 degrees to −60 degrees. The freezing time varies depending on the clinician, but typically lasts for at least 60 seconds. The lesion is allowed to thaw and then freezing is repeated. Generally, normal skin around the lesion is also treated to allow for better chance of cure. Several reports of disease-free survival have been published in the literature, however no controlled trials have been performed. Kuflik and Gage reported a 5-year cure rate of 96.1% in a group of 52 patients.[67] In an older study, Zacarian reported a 97% disease-free survival rate in 203 treated SCC lesions with follow-up ranging from less than 3 months to greater than 10 years.[68] Cryotherapy is generally well tolerated and patients may experience transient burning, blistering, erythema, and edema. Risks of alopecia, scarring, and post-inflammatory pigmentation should be discussed with the patient. A potential drawback to the use of cryotherapy is the development of recurrence which may be difficult to assess secondary to scar formation.

Electrodesiccation and curettage (ED&C) is a well-tolerated, minimally invasive treatment that has been used effectively in the treatment of in-situ and minimally invasive SCCs (see Chapter 41). ED&C should be avoided in invasive SCC with follicular extension, given a higher risk for recurrence. The main disadvantage to this treatment option is the lack of histologic margin control that can be achieved. Given the usual hypopigmented sclerotic scar that results from this procedure, ED&C is generally reserved for treating lesions on the trunk and extremities. Additionally, this technique should be used with caution and careful monitoring in those patients with pacemakers and defibrillators. Reported cure rates with ED&C have ranged from 96% to 99% in the treatment of in-situ and minimally invasive SCCs measuring less than 2 cm in diameter.[69-71] Honeycutt and Jansen reported a 99% cure rate following treatment of 281 SCCs in a 4-year follow-up period.[69] In another study, Whelan and colleagues treated 26 SCCs and reported a disease-free survival of 100% in a 2- to 9-year follow-up period.[72] Since ED&C is a technique-dependent treatment option, cure rates are largely dependent upon the practitioner's level of experience.

Radiation therapy (RT) can be used as primary and adjuvant therapy in the management of SCC (see Chapter 52). RT is used as a primary treatment modality in patients where cosmetic and/or functional outcome outweighs that which can be obtained with surgery. It is a beneficial treatment option in patients with unresectable tumors and also in instances where the patient is a poor surgical candidate. Adjuvant RT can be used in the treatment of metastatic disease as well as high-risk SCCs, particularly those with perineural invasion and positive surgical margins. In addition to helping to reduce the risk of local recurrence, RT has a palliative role in patients with advanced disease.[73-75] RT has a higher recurrence rate compared to several other treatment modalities. A study by Rowe and colleagues reported a local recurrence rate of 10% after 5 years or more in 160 patients receiving RT for primary SCC[64]. Surgery with adjuvant RT is currently used in the treatment of patients with regional nodal metastasis. RT generally entails three to five treatments per week for 4 to 8 weeks. Common side effects of RT include inflammation, erythema, tenderness, fibrosis, atrophy, and telangiectasia. Additionally, RT, unlike other treatment modalities, carries the risk of promoting SCC development after a repeated number of treatments.

Non-surgical treatments including topical chemotherapy and immune response modifiers are also frequently used in the management of AKs and superficial SCCs (see Chapter 43). Topical 5-fluorouracil (5-FU) interferes with DNA synthesis, therefore causing disruption in growth of malignant cells. 5-FU has been used in the treatment of AKs and non-invasive SCCs. Imiquimod 5% cream is a topical immune response modifier that stimulates the production of interferon-alpha and several cytokines, including tumor necrosis factor-alpha (TNF-α) and interleukins (IL) 1, 6, 8, and 12. It has shown efficacy in the treatment of SCC in situ. In one study, imiquimod applied to SCC in situ lesions produced a 93% positive treatment response with no residual tumor present in 6-week post-treatment biopsy specimens.[76] 5-FU and imiquimod provide a convenient and non-invasive alternative for the management of AKs and SCC in situ, however they are not recommended for the treatment of invasive SCC.[77]

Photodynamic therapy (PDT) has been used increasingly in the management of widespread AKs (see Chapter 45). PDT involves administering a photosensitive chemical compound with subsequent activation with a light source. Upon absorbing light, the photosensitive compound releases oxygen species cable of causing direct cellular damage and local inflammation. Precancerous and malignant cells selectively uptake the photosensitizer compared with normal skin.[78] Although currently used in the management of AKs, the efficacy of PDT use in management of Bowen's disease is still being investigated. Several studies have shown higher recurrence rates with PDT compared to other treatment modalities in the treatment of SCC in situ.[79–81] Further studies are needed to evaluate the role of PDT in the management of SCC.

Standard surgical excision represents one of the most common treatment modalities for the management of invasive SCC (see Chapter 46). It represents the treatment of choice for most cutaneous SCCs, since it allows for adequate histologic margin evaluation. Varied recommendations relating to margin width have been presented and debated in the literature; however, in 1992, Brodland and Zitelli presented a pivotal study.[65] Tumors were excised with progressive 1 mm margins and subsequently examined with Mohs micrographic surgery. The authors reported a 95% clearance of low-risk tumors (less than 2 cm, well differentiated, without involvement of subcutaneous tissue, located on trunk or extremities) with 4 mm margins, and 6 mm for high-risk tumors (greater than 2 cm, invasive to subcutaneous tissue, located on the face or anogenital region) (Fig. 12.32). The 5-year cure rate for primary SCC with standard excision is 92% and for recurrent SCC is 77%.[64]

Mohs micrographic surgery (MMS) is the standard of care for high-risk SCCs, including those located on the face, large tumors, and recurrent tumors (see Chapter 47). Benefits of MMS include tissue sparing, margin control, and high cure rate. MMS allows for determination of continuous tumor spread (Fig. 12.33) but does not identify discontinuous tumor such as in-transit metastasis. In 1992, Rowe and colleagues presented a review of all studies published since 1940 on the prognosis of SCC of the skin, ear, and lip. MMS had lower recurrence rates compared to other treatments, including surgical excision, ED&C, and RT: 3.1% versus 10.9% for primary SCC of the skin and lip; 5.3% versus 18.7% for SCC of the ear; 10% versus 23.3% for locally recurrent SCC; 0% versus 47% for SCC with perineural invasion; 25.2% versus 41.7% for SCC greater than 2 cm in diameter; 32.6% versus 53.6%

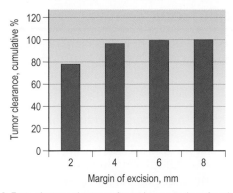

Figure 12.32 Rate of tumor clearance for various margins of excision.[65]

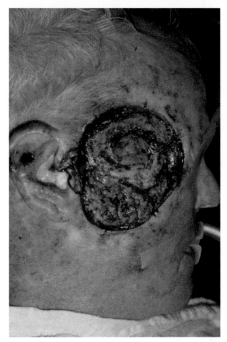

Figure 12.33 Post Mohs surgery defect.

for poorly differentiated SCC.[64] MMS should be considered over other treatment modalities in the treatment of high-risk SCCs.

## PREVENTION

Primary prevention of SCC is aimed at promoting patient education and increased awareness. Photoprotection is strongly encouraged by advocating the use of regular sunscreen and sun protective clothing, along with limiting UV exposure. Prevention strategies have also focused on early detection of skin cancer. Regular skin self-examination and physician visits are recommended. Early detection strategies for NMSC have focused not only on informing patients of the early signs of skin cancer, but also on educating clinicians, not just dermatologists, on early recognition and diagnosis. Chemopreventive agents currently being evaluated for the treatment and prevention of NMSC include retinoids, difluoromethylornithine, T4 endonuclease V, polyphenolic antioxidants such as epigallocatechin gallate found in green tea and grape seed extract, silymarin, isoflavone genistein, NSAIDs, curcumin, lycopene, vitamin E, beta-carotene, and selenium.[82]

## FUTURE OUTLOOK

Several new advances in the understanding of pathogenesis and management of SCC are currently underway. Recently, the association between diet and skin cancer development has garnered much attention. Ibiebele and colleagues studied the association between dietary patterns and development of NMSC. The authors concluded that a dietary pattern characterized by high meat and fat intake increases the risk of SCC development, particularly in persons with a history of skin cancer.[83] Additional studies are needed to further characterize this association. The role of human papillomavirus (HPV) in cutaneous, as well as mucous membrane, SCCs is being further characterized.

Determining which tumors are high risk as well as those most likely to metastasize will influence guidelines for clinical management. Current AJCC staging is inadequate in fully characterizing the risk of invasive SCC. Specifically, the role of tumor depth, desmoplasia, and degree of immunosuppression should be incorporated in the assessment of tumor risk as these features clearly influence tumor behavior.[84]

## REFERENCES

1. Rapini RP. *Practical Dermatopathology*, first ed. Philadelphia: Mosby; 2005:244–246.
2. Diepgen TL, Mahler V. The epidemiology of skin cancer. *Br J Dermatol.* 2002;146(suppl 61):1–6.
3. Weinstock MA. Epidemiologic investigation of nonmelanoma skin cancer and mortality: the Rhode Island Follow-Back Study. *J Invest Dermatol.* 1994;102:6S–9S.
4. Weinstock MA. Epidemiology of nonmelanoma skin cancer: clinical issues, definitions and classification. *J Invest Dermatol.* 1994;102:4S–5S.
5. Goldman GD. Squamous cell cancer: a practical approach. *Semin Cutan Med Surg.* 1998;17:80–95.
6. Miller D, Weinstock MA. Nonmelanoma skin cancer in the United States: incidence. *J Am Acad Dermatol.* 1994;30:774–778.
7. Gray DJ, Suman VJ, Su WP, et al. Trends in the population-based incidence of squamous cell carcinoma of the skin first diagnosed between 1984 and 1992. *Arch Dermatol.* 1997;133:735–740.
8. Chuang T-Y, Popescu NA, Su WP, et al. Squamous cell carcinoma: a population-based incidence study in Rochester, Minn. *Arch Dermatol.* 1990;126(2):185–188.
9. Johnson T, Rowe DE, Nelson BR, et al. Squamous carcinoma of the skin (excluding lip and oral mucosa). *J Am Acad Dermatol.* 1992;26:467–484.
10. Buettner PG, Raasch BA. Incidence rates of skin cancer in Townsville, Australia. *Int J Cancer.* 1998;78:587–593.
11. Marcil I, Stern RS. Risk of developing a subsequent nonmelanoma skin cancer in patients with a history of nonmelanoma skin cancer: a critical review of the literature and meta-analysis. *Arch Dermatol.* 2000;136:1524–1530.
12. Karjalainen S, Salo H, Teppo L. Basal cell and squamous cell carcinoma of the skin in Finland: site distribution and patient survival. *Int J Dermatol.* 1989;28:445–450.
13. Leiter U, Garbe C. Epidemiology of melanoma and nonmelanoma skin cancer – the role of sunlight. *Adv Exp Med Biol.* 2008;624:89–103.
14. Chow CW, Tabrizi SN, Tiedemann K, et al. Squamous cell carcinomas in children and young adults: a new wave of a very rare tumor? *J Pediatr Surg.* 2007;42:2035–2039.
15. Ramsay HM, Fryer AA, Reece S, et al. Clinical risk factors associated with nonmelanoma skin cancer in renal transplant recipients. *Am J Kidney Dis.* 2000;36(1):167–176.
16. Maddox JS, Soltani K. Risk of nonmelanoma skin cancer with azathioprine use. *Inflamm Bowel Dis.* 2008;14(10):1425–1431.
17. Gupta AK, Cardella CJ, Haberman HF. Cutaneous malignant neoplasms in patients with renal transplants. *Arch Dermatol.* 1986;122:1288–1293.
18. Hoxtell EO, Mandel JS, Murray SS, et al. Incidence of skin carcinoma after renal transplantation. *Arch Dermatol.* 1977;113:436–438.
19. Jensen P, Hansen S, Moller B, et al. Skin cancer in kidney and heart transplant recipients and different long-term immunosuppressive therapy regimens. *J Am Acad Dermatol.* 1999;40:177–186.
20. Ulrich C, Schmook T, Sachse M, et al. Comparative epidemiology and pathogenic factors for nonmelanoma skin cancer in organ transplant patients. *Dermatol Surg.* 2004;30:622–627.

21. Ong CS, Keogh AM, Kossard S, et al. Skin cancer in Australian heart transplant recipients. *J Am Acad Dermatol.* 1999;40:27–34.
22. Euvrard S, Kanitakis J, Pouteil-Noble C, et al. Comparative epidemiological study of premalignant and malignant epithelial cutaneous lesions developing after kidney and heart transplantation. *J Am Acad Dermatol.* 1995;33:222–229.
23. Ingvar A, Smedby KE, Lindelof B, et al. Immunosuppressive treatment after solid organ transplantation and risk of post-transplant cutaneous squamous cell carcinoma. *Nephrol Dial Transplant.* 2010;25:2764–2771.
24. Garcia-Zuazaga J, Olbricht SM. Cutaneous squamous cell carcinoma. *Adv Dermatol.* 2008;24:33–57.
25. Stasko T, Brown MD, Carucci JA, et al. International transplant-skin cancer collaborative; European skin care in organ transplant patients network. Guidelines for the management of squamous cell carcinoma in organ transplant recipients. *Dermatol Surg.* 2004;30(4 Pt 2):642–650.
26. Kricker A, Armstong BK, English DR. Sun exposure and nonmelanocytic skin cancer. *Cancer Causes Control.* 1994;5:367–392.
27. Kwa RE, Campana K, Moy RL. Biology of cutaneous squamous cell carcinoma. *J Am Acad Dermatol.* 1992;26(1):1–26.
28. Ziegler A, Jonason AS, Lefell DJ. Sunburn and p53 in the onset of skin cancer. *Nature.* 1994;372:773–776.
29. Matsui MS, DeLeo VA. Longwave radiation and promotion of skin cancer. *Cancer Cell.* 1991;3(1):8–12.
30. Nghiem DX, Kazimi N, Mitchell DL, et al. Mechanisms underlying the suppression of established immune responses by ultraviolet radiation. *J Invest Dermatol.* 2002;119:600–608.
31. Studniberg HM, Weller P. PUVA, UVB, psoriasis, and nonmelanoma skin cancer. *J Am Acad Dermatol.* 1993;29:1013–1022.
32. Fu W, Cockerell CJ. The actinic (solar) keratosis. *Arch Dermatol.* 2009;139:66–70.
33. Marks R, Rennie G, Selwood TS. Malignant transformation of solar keratoses to squamous cell carcinoma. *Lancet.* 1988;1:795–797.
34. Dodson JM, DeSpain J, Hewett JE, et al. Malignant transformation of actinic keratosis and the controversy over treatment: a patient-oriented perspective. *Arch Dermatol.* 1991;127:1029–1031.
35. Montgomery H, Dorffel J. Verruca senilis und keratoma senile. *Arch Dermatol Syphilol.* 1939;39:387–408.
36. Marks R, Foley P, Goodman G, et al. Spontaneous remission of solar keratoses: the case for conservative management. *Br J Dermatol.* 1986;115:649–655.
37. Hansen JP, Drake AL, Walling HW. Bowen's disease: a four-year retrospective review of epidemiology and treatment at a university center. *Dermatol Surg.* 2008;34:878–883.
38. Cox NH, Eedy DJ, Morton CA. Guidelines for management of Bowen's disease: 2006 update. *Br J Dermatol.* 2007;156:11–21.
39. Jacobs DM, Sandles LG, Leboit PE. Sebaceous carcinoma arising from Bowen's disease of the vulva. *Arch Dermatol.* 1986;122:1191–1193.
40. Kao GF. Carcinoma arising in Bowen's disease. *Arch Dermatol.* 1986;122:1124–1126.
41. Rudolph R, Zelac DE. Squamous cell carcinoma of the skin. *Plast Reconstr Surg.* 2004;114(6):82e–94e.
42. Neville BW, Day TA. Oral cancer and precancerous lesions. *CA Cancer J Clin.* 2002;52:195–215.
43. Perez CA, Kraus FT, Evans JC, et al. Anaplastic transformation in verrucous carcinoma of the oral cavity after radiation therapy. *Radiology.* 1996;86:108–115.
44. Phillips P, Helm KF. Proliferating cell nuclear antigen distribution in keratoacanthoma and squamous cell carcinoma. *J Cutan Pathol.* 1993;20:424–428.
45. Hodak E, Jones RE, Ackerman AB. Solitary keratoacanthoma is a squamous cell carcinoma: three examples with metastasis. *Am J Dermatopathol.* 1993;15:332–342.
46. Hyde NC, Prvulovich E, Newman L, et al. A new approach to pre-treatment assessment of N0 neck in oral squamous cell carcinoma: the role of sentinel node biopsy and positron emission tomography. *Oral Oncol.* 2003;39:350–360.
47. Weisberg NK, Bertagnolli MM, Becker DS. Combined sentinel lymphadenectomy and Mohs micrographic surgery for high-risk cutaneous squamous cell carcinoma. *J Am Acad Dermatol.* 2000;43:483–488.
48. Andruchow JL, Veness MJ, Morgan GJ, et al. Implications for clinical staging of metastatic cutaneous squamous carcinoma of the head and neck based on a multicenter study of treatment outcomes. *Cancer.* 2006;106:1078–1083.
49. Dinehart SM, Peterson S. Evaluation of the American Joint Committee on Cancer staging system for cutaneous squamous cell carcinoma and proposal of a new staging system. *Dermatol Surg.* 2005;31:1379–1384.
50. Broders AC. Practical points on the microscopic grading of carcinoma. *N Y State J Med.* 1932;32:667.
51. Breuninger H, Black B, Rassner G. Microstaging of squamous cell carcinomas. *Am J Clin Pathol.* 1990;94:624–627.
52. Nappi O, Pettinato G, Wick MR. Adenoid (acantholytic) squamous cell carcinoma of the skin. *J Cutan Pathol.* 1989;16:114–121.

53. Banks ER, Cooper PH. Adenosquamous carcinoma of the skin: a report of 10 cases. *J Cutan Pathol*. 1991;18:227–234.

54. Noel JC, Heenen M, Peny MO, et al. Proliferating nuclear antigen distribution in verrucous carcinoma of the skin. *Br J Dermatol*. 1995;133:868–873.

55. Kane CL, Keehn CA, Smithberger E, et al. Histopathology of cutaneous squamous cell carcinoma and its variants. *Semin Cutan Med Surg*. 2004;23(1):54–61.

56. Breuninger H, Schaumberg-Lever G, Holzschuh J, et al. Desmoplastic squamous cell carcinoma of skin and vermilion surface: a highly malignant subtype of skin cancer. *Cancer*. 1997;79:915–919.

57. Bernstein SC, Lim KK, Brodland DG, et al. The many faces of squamous cell carcinoma. *Dermatol Surg*. 1996;22:243–254.

58. Goepfert H, Dichtel WJ, Medina JE, et al. Perineural invasion in squamous cell carcinoma of the head and neck. *Am J Surg*. 1984;148:542–547.

59. Khanna M, Fortier-Riberdy G, Smoller B, et al. Reporting tumor thickness for cutaneous squamous cell carcinoma. *J Cutan Pathol*. 2002;29:321–323.

60. Dinehart SM, Nelson-Adesokan P, Cockerell C, et al. Metastatic cutaneous squamous cell carcinoma derived from actinic keratosis. *Cancer*. 1997;79(5):920–923.

61. Jensen V, Prasad A, Smith A, et al. Prognostic criteria for squamous cell cancer of the skin. *J Surg Res*. 2010;159(1):509–516.

62. Dinehart SM, Pollack SV. Metastases from squamous cell carcinoma of the skin and lip. *J Am Acad Dermatol*. 1989;21:241–248.

63. Epstein E. Malignant sun-induced squamous cell carcinoma of the skin. *J Dermatol Surg Oncol*. 1983;9:505–506.

64. Rowe DE, Carroll RJ, Day CL. Prognostic factors for local recurrence, metastasis, and survival rates in squamous cell carcinoma of the skin, ear, and lip. *J Am Acad Dermatol*. 1992;26:976–990.

65. Brodland DG, Zitelli JA. Mechanisms of metastasis. *J Am Acad Dermatol*. 1992;27(1):1–8.

66. Motley R, Kersey P, Lawrence C. Multiprofessional guidelines for the management of the patient with primary cutaneous squamous cell carcinoma. *Br J Dermatol*. 2002;146(1):18–25.

67. Kuflik EG, Gage AA. The five-year cure rate achieved by cryosurgery for skin cancer. *J Am Acad Dermatol*. 1991;24:1002–1004.

68. Zacarian SA. Cryosurgery of cutaneous carcinomas. An 18-year study of 3,022 patients with 4,228 carcinomas. *J Am Acad Dermatol*. 1983;9:947–956.

69. Freeman RG, Knox JM, Heaton CL. The treatment of skin cancer: a statistical study of 1,341 skin tumors comparing results obtained with irradiation, surgery, and curettage followed by electrodesiccation. *Cancer*. 1964;17:535–538.

70. Honeycutt WM, Jansen GT. Treatment of squamous cell carcinoma of the skin. *Arch Dermatol*. 1973;108:670–672.

71. Williamson GS, Jackson R. Treatment of squamous cell carcinoma of the skin by electrodesiccation and curettage. *Can Med Assoc J*. 1964;90:408–413.

72. Whelan CS, Deckers PJ. Electrocoagulation for skin cancer: an old oncologic tool revisited. *Cancer*. 1981;47:2280–2287.

73. Veness MJ. The important role of radiotherapy in patients with non-melanoma skin cancer and other cutaneous entities. *J Med Imaging Radiat Oncol*. 2008;52:278–286.

74. Jambusaria-Pahlajani A, Miller CJ, Quon H, et al. Surgical monotherapy versus surgery plus adjuvant radiotherapy in high-risk cutaneous squamous cell carcinoma: a systematic review of outcomes. *Dermatol Surg*. 2009;35:574–585.

75. Han A, Ratner D. What is the role of adjuvant radiotherapy in the treatment of cutaneous squamous cell carcinoma with perineural invasion. *Cancer*. 2007;109:1053–1059.

76. Mackenzie-Wood A, Kossard S, de Launey J, et al. Imiquimod 5% cream in the treatment of Bowen's disease. *J Am Acad Dermatol*. 2001;44:462–470.

77. Del Rosso JQ. The treatment of viral infections and nonmelanoma skin cancers. *Cutis*. 2007;79(suppl 4):29–35.

78. Fien SM, Oseroff AR. Photodynamic therapy for non-melanoma skin cancer. *J Natl Compr Canc Netw*. 2007;5(5):531–540.

79. Tierney E, Barker A, Ahdout J, et al. Photodynamic therapy for the treatment of cutaneous neoplasia, inflammatory disorders, and photaging. *Dermatol Surg*. 2009;35:725–746.

80. Salim A, Leman JA, McColl JH, et al. Randomized comparison of photodynamic therapy with topical 5-fluorouracil in Bowen's disease. *Br J Drematol*. 2003;148:539–543.

81. Morton C, Horn M, Lehman J, et al. A 24-month update of placebo controlled European study comparing MAL-PDT with cryosurgery and 5-fluorouracil in patient's with Bowen's disease. *J Eur Acad Dermatol Venerol*. 2005;19(suppl 2):237–238.

82. Wright TI, Spencer JM, Flowers FP. Chemoprevention of nonmelanoma skin cancer. *J Am Acad Dermatol*. 2006;54(6):933–946.

83. Ibiebele TI, van der Pols JC, Hughes MC, et al. Dietary pattern in association with squamous cell carcinoma of the skin: a prospective study. *Am J Clin Nutr*. 2007;85(5):1401–1408.

84. Bergstrom KG. Rethinking squamous cell carcinoma: which are high risk, which could benefit from lymph node dissection, what's coming up in the future? *J Drugs Dermatol*. 2008;7(9):903–906.

# Adnexal Carcinomas of the Skin

*Sarah N. Walsh and Daniel J. Santa Cruz*

## Key Points

- Adnexal carcinomas are rare and often misdiagnosed both clinically and histologically.
- Lesions can develop de novo or in conjunction with a pre-existing benign adenoma.
- Recognition and separation of these lesions into distinct entities is important, given the therapeutic and prognostic implications.
- Complete excision with clear margins, including by Mohs micrographic surgery, is the primary treatment of choice.

## INTRODUCTION

Adnexal carcinomas are rare and troublesome neoplasms, which are often lumped together as a single entity. However, well-defined distinct lesions do exist and should be separated out, given the therapeutic and prognostic implications, as tumors with a propensity for local invasion and destruction only versus those that frequently metastasize can then be identified. Biopsy is necessary for diagnostic purposes and complete excision with clear margins is the primary mode of treatment. Chemotherapy and/or radiation have been used for lesions that follow a more aggressive course. Continued follow-up is necessary, especially for those tumors which pose a definite threat for metastasis.

## EPIDEMIOLOGY

Adnexal carcinomas are rare (US age-adjusted incidence of 0.5/100,000 per year), with the incidence rate among men being statistically significantly higher than among women (0.6 vs 0.4; male to female incidence ratio 1.5; $P < 0.001$). Hispanic whites (incidence 0.4/100,000 per year), blacks (0.3), and Asian/Pacific Islanders (0.2) all had significantly lower rates than non-Hispanic whites (0.6) ($P < 0.001$). Incidence rates rose 100-times with age, from 0.037 for age 20 to 29 years to 3.8 for those 80 years or older. From 1978–1982 to 2002–2005, the rates increased 150%, from 0.2 to 0.5; the apocrine–eccrine carcinoma incidence increased from 0.1 to 0.3 (170%) and the sebaceous carcinoma increased from 0.06 to 0.2 (217%). Five-year US survival rates overall were 99% for localized versus 43% for distant disease.[1]

## CARCINOMAS OF THE ECCRINE AND APOCRINE GLANDS

### Microcystic adnexal carcinoma

Microcystic adnexal carcinoma (MAC) was first described by Goldstein, Barr, and Santa Cruz in 1982.[2] Lesions typically are located on the face, with preference for the upper lip. There is a female predilection, with lesions most commonly developing in adults in their mid-sixties.

Lesions present as an ill-defined indurated firm plaque or discrete nodule. The epidermal surface is smooth or crusted and yellowish to flesh-colored. The neoplasm grows slowly, from 1 to 17 years on average.

Microscopic examination shows small keratinous cysts admixed with solid strands, some with lumens, of small basaloid cells within the superficial portion of the lesion (Fig. 13.1). Within the mid portion, there is a predominance of basaloid strands and cords, which decrease in size with increasing depth into the dermis. In the deep portions, the basaloid strands diminish to clusters of only two or three cells. The overall architecture is of a deeply infiltrative lesion which lacks cytological pleomorphism (Fig. 13.2). Mitoses are rare but perineural invasion is common (Fig. 13.3).

Several conditions enter into the differential diagnosis. The most likely lesion for MAC to be confused with is desmoplastic trichoepithelioma. The MAC cells resemble those of syringomas and poromas, while the ones from trichoepitheliomas resemble those of basal cell carcinomas with more angulated cell cords. Both lesions may deeply penetrate the dermis, but the characteristic perineural invasion of MAC is not seen in desmoplastic trichoepithelioma. Syringoma, particularly the plaque-type variant, and infiltrative basal cell carcinoma may also pose diagnostic problems. Syringomas tend to be more superficially located and usually occur periorbitally, while basal cell carcinomas have retraction artifact and an epidermal connection.

Treatment options include standard surgical excision, Mohs micrographic surgery (MMS), irradiation, chemotherapy, and observation.[3] While MACs are typically thought to be locally aggressive with a propensity for recurrence, there have been several reported cases with hematogenous, lymphatic, and/or perineural spread with both regional and distant metastases, resulting in at least one death.[3,4]

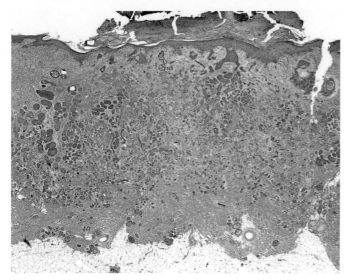

Figure 13.1 Microcystic adnexal carcinoma at low power, showing the solid nests of basaloid cells in the upper portions, which progressively diminish to strands and cords in the deeper portions of the lesion.

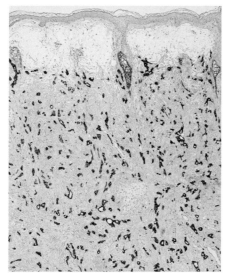

Figure 13.2 Immunohistochemical staining with CK7 best highlights the deeply infiltrative architecture of MACs.

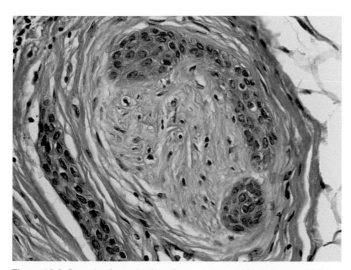

Figure 13.3 Strands of neoplastic cells are present within a nerve, which is a common finding in MACs.

## Adenoid cystic carcinoma

True adenoid cystic carcinoma of the skin is a very rare lesion which was first described by Boggio in 1975.[5] This neoplasm most commonly occurs on the scalp and typically affects middle-aged to elderly females. Lesions arise as an asymptomatic crusted verrucous plaque or deep-seated nodule.

The solid to cystic dermal nests of adenoid cystic carcinoma have no connection to the overlying epidermis, have a swiss-cheese, cribriform, or sieve-like appearance, and are composed of small, basophilic cells with scant cytoplasm (Fig. 13.4). An important diagnostic clue is the extensive perineural invasion (Fig. 13.5).

Histologically, adenoid cystic carcinoma poses a difficult differential with the so-called 'adenoid cystic' variant of basal cell carcinoma. The epidermal origin of basal cell carcinoma is helpful, as is the prominent perineural invasion common in adenoid cystic carcinoma. Primary salivary gland adenoid cystic carcinoma can, rarely, directly invade or metastasize to the skin and should be considered in the differential diagnosis.

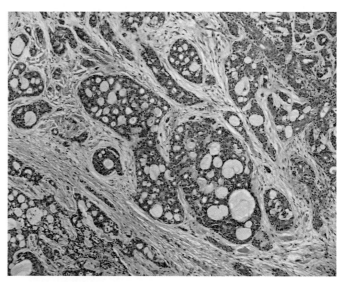

Figure 13.4 The classic cribriform nests of adenoid cystic carcinoma.

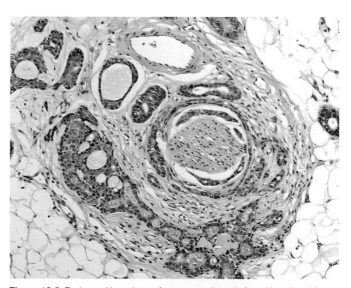

Figure 13.5 Perineural invasion, a feature consistently found in adenoid cystic carcinomas.

Adenoid cystic carcinomas have an indolent but progressive course with a high rate of local recurrence.[6] However, recurrence rates have been lowest when Mohs technique is used.[7] Metastases have been reported in the lungs and pleura and in lymph nodes.[8] Close long-term follow-up is necessary.

## Mucinous carcinoma

Mucinous carcinoma is one of the most common adnexal carcinomas of the skin. The lesion was originally described by Lennox et al. in 1952.[9] The tumor presents as a painless slow-growing solitary nodule that is usually flesh colored, and has a soft, spongy consistency. These tumors often can be transilluminated.

The large majority of lesions are located on the head and neck, with a predilection for the eyelids. Lesions occur in twice as many females as males and typically present between the ages of 31 to 89.[10]

Grossly, mucinous carcinomas have a lobulated, mucoid, glistening appearance. Histologically, they are composed of cords, tubules, and lobules of epithelial cells, floating in large pools of slightly basophilic mucin, separated by thin fibrovascular septa (Fig. 13.6). The neoplastic epithelial cells have bland cytological features with monomorphous round nuclei (Fig. 13.7).

The most important differential diagnosis is metastatic mucinous carcinoma, particularly originating from the breast or gastrointestinal tract. Cutaneous metastasis of breast carcinoma typically occurs in the chest, breast, and axilla, whereas primary cutaneous mucinous carcinoma is predominantly located on the head and neck.[10] Morphologically, primary gastrointestinal carcinomas metastatic to skin have cytological pleomorphism and dirty necrosis, which are not seen in primary cutaneous mucinous carcinomas. In addition, the presence of sulfomucins is highly distinctive of carcinomas of gastrointestinal origin, while sialomucins are generally seen in primary cutaneous mucinous carcinoma.

Treatment includes wide local excision with clear margins.[11] Success has been reported with MMS. Cutaneous mucinous carcinoma usually has an indolent course.

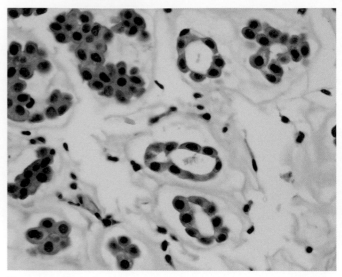

**Figure 13.7** The lack of cellular pleomorphism in mucinous carcinoma can be appreciated at high power.

Recurrence typically occurs in the first few years. While this tumor generally has a low metastatic potential, regional and distant metastases have been reported.[12]

## Porocarcinoma

Malignant poroma was described by Pinkus and Mehregan in 1963.[13] Porocarcinoma has been reported in association with either hidroacanthoma simplex or poroma.[14,15] There is a slight female predominance with a wide age range. The most common location is the lower extremities. Clinically, the lesion presents as a nodule, usually ulcerative, or an infiltrative plaque showing verrucous features.

Porocarcinomas have lobular downgrowths emanating from the epidermis composed of small cells with vesicular nuclei and scant cytoplasm, which are sharply demarcated from the surrounding epidermal keratinocytes (Fig. 13.8). While the neoplastic cells generally have monomorphous nuclei (Fig. 13.9), those located near sites of dermal invasion

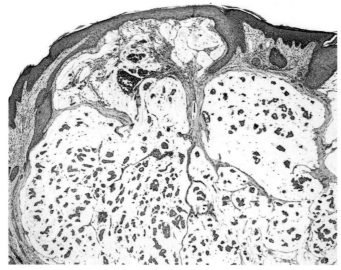

**Figure 13.6** A low-power view of mucinous carcinoma showing large pools of mucin separated by thin fibrous septa containing collections of epithelial cells.

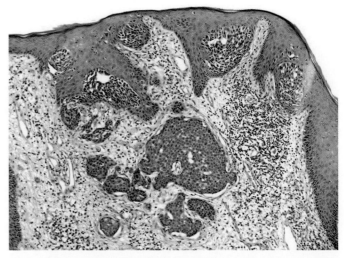

**Figure 13.8** The nests and lobules of poroid cells in porocarcinoma, including intraepidermal collections, are easily distinguished from the surrounding keratinocytes, even at low magnification.

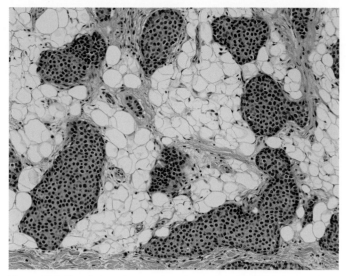

Figure 13.9 Despite invasion into the subcutaneous adipose tissue, porocarcinoma often has deceptively bland cytological features.

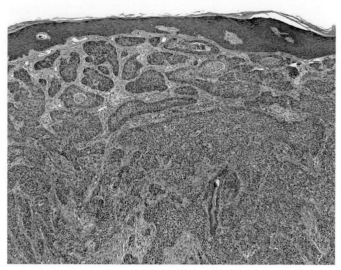

Figure 13.10 At low power, acrospirocarcinoma shows irregular infiltrating nests of cells with clear to lightly eosinophilic cytoplasm.

may have a greater degree of cytological pleomorphism and display cytoplasmic vacuolization with formation of intracellular lumens.

The intraepidermal phase of porocarcinoma must be distinguished from hidroacanthoma simplex, squamous cell carcinoma in situ, and extramammary Paget's disease. In the invasive phase, the most difficult differential diagnosis is with non-keratinizing squamous cell carcinomas arising in Bowen's disease and metastatic carcinoma.

Wide local excision has been the primary treatment for porocarcinoma. Approximately 20% of porocarcinomas recur locally, 20% metastasize to regional lymph nodes, and 12% metastasize to distant sites.[14]

## Acrospirocarcinoma

Most malignant acrospiromas arise de novo, although some are associated with a pre-existent acrospiroma. These lesions have a predilection for the face and extremities. There is a slight female predominance and patients are typically above 50 years old.[16] Lesions usually appear as a large, ulcerated mass or nodule or an infiltrative plaque.

Microscopically, tumors are centered in the dermis and are composed of solid sheets, nests, or lobules of polygonal cells with pale to clear cytoplasm and distinct cell borders (Fig. 13.10). An important clue to the diagnosis is intra- or intercellular lumen formation (Fig. 13.11). Areas with mitoses and pronounced nuclear pleomorphism are present.

The main differential is with acrospiroma, which can be difficult since benign lesions may display mild nuclear pleomorphism and increased mitotic activity. These changes, however, are usually focal. Metastatic carcinomas could be considered, but evidence of ductal differentiation along with immunohistochemical staining will assist in resolving this dilemma.

Primary treatment includes wide local excision with or without sentinel lymph node biopsy or lymph node dissection.[17] Tumors have a high rate of local recurrence and a propensity for metastasizing to regional lymph nodes and distant sites, including lungs, bones, brain, and liver.[17–20]

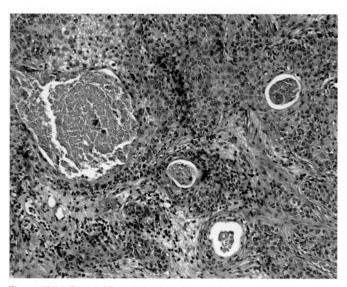

Figure 13.11 Ductal differentiation is an important diagnostic clue in acrospirocarcinoma.

## Malignant mixed tumor

Malignant mixed tumors of the skin (malignant chondroid syringomas) are very rare, and malignant areas can be seen in conjunction with benign areas. The average patient age is 48.3 years, with females outnumbering males.[21] Tumors occur mainly on the extremities and have a slow rate of growth. They often present as cystic structures with a mucoid consistency. Infiltrative growth is common, therefore these tumors do not enucleate out like the benign counterpart.

Histologically, malignant mixed tumors have strands and cords of epithelial cells scattered among mesenchymal elements (Fig. 13.12). Most neoplasms present with variable degrees of cellular pleomorphism, mitoses, and areas of poorly differentiated epithelial structures.

The main differential diagnostic problem is with benign mixed tumors. Criteria for malignancy have been proposed by Harrist et al.[22] Soft tissue tumors, such as extraskeletal myxoid chondrosarcoma, may also have nests and cords of cells with a distinctive epithelioid appearance; however,

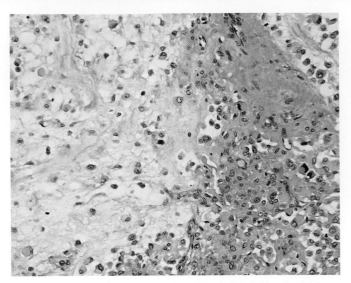

Figure 13.12 Both mesenchymal (on the left) and epithelial (on the right) components of malignant mixed tumor are seen.

immunohistochemistry can aid in distinguishing between the two.

Complete excision with wide margins is the treatment of choice. Chemotherapy and radiation therapy have not been effective.[21] Local recurrence is common and satellite lesions around the main tumor are also frequently seen.[21] Nodal metastases and distant metastases, most commonly to the lungs, bones, and brain, have been reported.[21]

## Spiradenocarcinoma

Malignant changes within a benign longstanding spiradenoma were first described by Dabska in 1972.[23] Tumors most commonly occur on the trunk, extremities, or head and neck. There has been no reported sex predilection, and most patients present in the sixth decade of life.[24] The usual history is that of a longstanding nodule that has recently grown rapidly.

The histological diagnosis depends mainly on identifying a portion of benign spiradenoma. While areas with lumen formation can be found (Fig. 13.13), the malignant

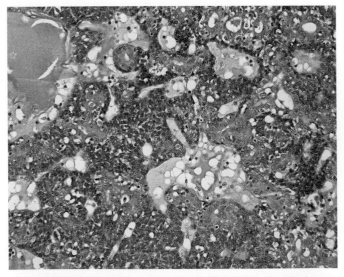

Figure 13.13 The architecture, including ductal differentiation, of a spiradenoma is retained, but the cells are overlapping and have pleomorphic nuclei.

portion can show solid sheets of non-keratinizing basaloid cells, as well as areas with squamous and adenocarcinomatous features. Vascular invasion has been noted.

In the absence of an identifiable spiradenoma, these carcinomas can be difficult to classify due to their relatively undifferentiated nature. On the hands and feet, aggressive digital papillary adenocarcinoma may be considered. However, spiradenocarcinoma should be suspected in any high-grade cutaneous carcinoma arising in a longstanding, deep-seated nodule.

Complete surgical excision with 1 cm margins and depth to the fascia or MMS are both acceptable.[24] Adjunctive therapy with tamoxifen has been given in those cases with positivity for estrogen receptors.[25] Metastases develop in up to 57% of patients, most commonly to the regional lymph nodes, lungs, brain, liver, skin, spinal cord, and parotid gland.[24]

## Cylindrocarcinoma

Malignant cylindroma is a rare tumor, which was first described by Wiedemann in 1929.[26] Malignant change within a pre-existing cylindroma is more common in patients with multiple lesions, particularly in those with Brooke–Spiegler syndrome.[27] Patient age ranges from 50 to 96 years and women are slightly more affected than men.[27] Tumors typically occur on the scalp. Clinical signs suspicious for malignant changes within a pre-existing cylindroma include rapid growth, tenderness, ulceration, discoloration, and bleeding.[28]

The tumors have dermal nests and cords of basaloid cells with marked cellular pleomorphism and focal necrosis. An associated benign cylindroma component is nearly always identified. It is debatable if a diagnosis of malignant cylindroma can be made in the absence of the benign counterpart.

Similar to spiradenocarcinoma, the malignant components of cylindroma lack sufficient differentiating features, and identification of a benign cylindroma component is necessary, making for a limited differential diagnosis.

Complete surgical excision is the primary treatment. Radiotherapy has been used for inoperable tumors and in those patients with metastatic disease.[27] Malignant cylindromas have an aggressive course, with a tendency for local destruction, recurrence, and frequent metastases. Death from disease is common.

## Apocrine adenocarcinoma

Approximately 75 cases to date of apocrine adenocarcinoma have been reported in the English literature.[29] Lesions are typically solitary and arise in the axillary or anogenital regions. Patient age ranges from 18 to 81 years.[29] There is no gender predilection, and lesion duration is frequently less than 1 year.[18]

Patients may experience some discomfort but usually no pain. Tumor size typically ranges from 1.5 to 8 cm.[30] The most common clinical impression is basal cell carcinoma.[29]

Microscopically, tumors are intradermal and are composed of cells with abundant eosinophilic finely granular cytoplasm that have tubular, tubulopapillary, or solid patterns (Fig. 13.14). Decapitation secretion is usually present.

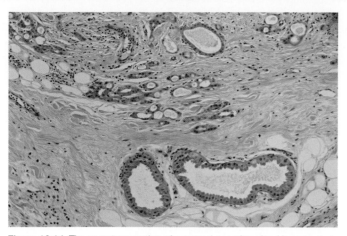

**Figure 13.14** The secretory portion of a normal apocrine gland is present at the bottom of the field, in contrast to the irregular eosinophilic tubules above of apocrine adenocarcinoma.

Additional features include an infiltrative margin, necrosis, and lymphovascular invasion.

Distinguishing between an apocrine adenoma and an apocrine adenocarcinoma can be difficult. A combination of histological features, including degree of cellular pleomorphism, hyperchromasia, mitotic activity, and the presence of stromal invasion, has been suggested to separate adenocarcinomas from adenomas.[30] It is also difficult, if not impossible, to differentiate primary cutaneous apocrine adenocarcinoma from metastatic breast carcinoma, with clinical history and correlation with other laboratory and radiological data being the best method at this time.

Complete local excision remains the current treatment. In general, local recurrence and regional lymph node metastasis are relatively frequent.[29] However, widespread metastatic dissemination and death from disease are much less common.[29]

There is also a variant of apocrine carcinoma, described by Requena et al in 1998, named primary cutaneous cribriform carcinoma, which microscopically is composed of interconnected aggregates of pleomorphic cells that form cribriform spaces of variable size and shape, and thus far follows an indolent course (Fig. 13.15).[31]

## Aggressive digital papillary adenocarcinoma

This neoplasm was first reported by Helwig in 1984.[32] It has a preference for the upper-extremity digits and typically affects older males.[33,34] Clinically, aggressive digital papillary adenocarcinoma (ADPA) presents as a solitary firm gray-tan rubbery nodule. The average tumor size has been reported as 1.7 cm.[34]

Histologically, lesions are well-circumscribed dermal nodules with papillary, cystic, and solid areas composed of basaloid cells with pleomorphic nuclei and scant cytoplasm arranged as compact glands and papillary projections (Fig. 13.16). Abundant mitoses are present (Fig. 13.17).

It is very difficult, if not impossible, to differentiate those tumors that are locally aggressive from those that may metastasize, therefore the distinction between the so-called adenomas and adenocarcinomas is probably futile.[33] We interpret all these lesions as adenocarcinomas.

Complete local surgical excision, including by MMS, has been utilized, although amputation is usually required.[34]

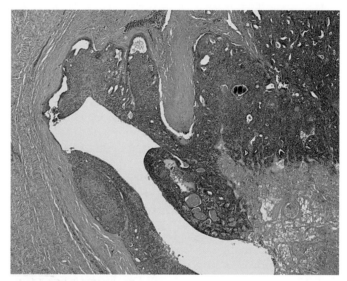

**Figure 13.16** At low power, aggressive digital papillary adenocarcinoma shows cystic and solid areas of compact glands with a large area of necrosis.

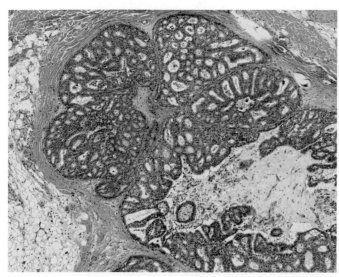

**Figure 13.15** Cribriform apocrine carcinoma has lobules of pleomorphic cells forming cribriform spaces of variable size and shape.

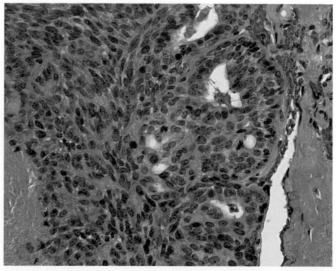

**Figure 13.17** Cellular pleomorphism and numerous mitoses are seen at high magnification of aggressive digital papillary adenocarcinoma.

Aggressive digital papillary adenocarcinomas have a high rate of recurrence and metastatic potential, with the lungs being the most common site of metastasis.[33]

## Syringocystadenocarcinoma papilliferum

While cases describing a malignant syringocystadenoma papilliferum had been written about as far back as 1911, it was not until 1980 that the first well-documented cases were reported.[35,36] The mean patient age at detection is 65.9 years. Tumors are described as exophytic verrucous plaques or nodules, typically less than 4 cm, and usually present on the scalp.[36]

On microscopic examination, syringocystadenocarcinoma papilliferum is composed of cystic to papillary epidermal invaginations, with the upper portions of the lesion showing keratinizing squamous epithelium and the lower portions being covered by two-cell layered epithelium (Fig. 13.18). There is nuclear overlap and pleomorphism, numerous mitoses, and necrosis (Fig. 13.19). Surrounding clusters of plasma cells are consistently identified.

The main histological differential diagnosis includes papillary adenocarcinoma or apocrine adenocarcinoma. Tumor location is helpful, as papillary carcinoma occurs on the digits (aggressive digital papillary adenocarcinoma) and apocrine adenocarcinoma is typically seen in the axilla. The identification of an associated syringocystadenoma papilliferum is the most reliable histological feature.

Treatment is complete surgical excision, including by MMS. Metastatic spread to regional lymph nodes is exceedingly rare.[37] Death from disease has not been documented.

## CARCINOMAS OF THE HAIR FOLLICLE

### Tricholemmomal carcinoma

Tricholemmomal carcinoma (also called tricholemmal carcinoma) is the malignant counterpart to tricholemmoma. Males are more commonly affected than females, with a mean patient age of 71 years.[38] Lesions typically occur

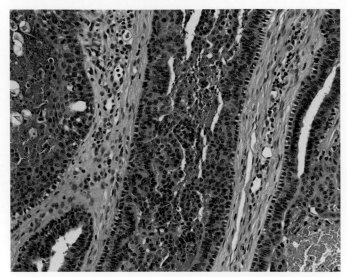

Figure 13.19 A double layer of columnar and cuboidal epithelium characteristic of syringocystadenoma papilliferum is retained at one edge, while the central portion shows features of carcinoma with the nuclear overlapping, pleomorphism, and necrosis.

on the head and neck and extremities.[38] Tumors present as slow-growing papules or nodules that are commonly misdiagnosed clinically as basal cell carcinoma.

Histological sections show lobules with wide epidermal connections invading the dermis with pushing borders. Evidence of tricholemmal differentiation is seen (Fig. 13.20). Frequently, there is nuclear enlargement, prominent nucleoli, and a high mitotic index.

These tumors may be confused with other malignant skin tumors with clear cell changes, including clear cell squamous cell carcinoma and clear cell malignant acrospiromas (acrospirocarcinoma, porocarcinoma). Immunohistochemical evidence of tricholemmal differentiation can help in resolving these dilemmas.

Despite their seemingly malignant cytological appearance, these lesions uncommonly have deep invasion, local recurrence, or metastasis.[38,39] Thus, conservative

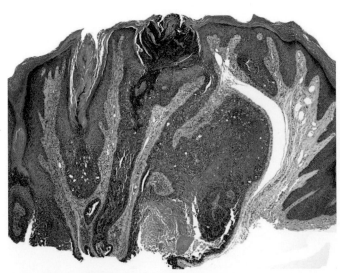

Figure 13.18 • The architecture of syringocystadenocarcinoma papilliferum is best appreciated at low power, which highlights the endophytic invaginations of epithelium extending down from the epidermis into the dermis.

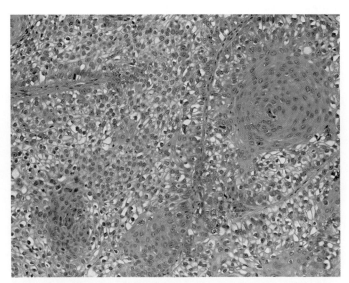

Figure 13.20 The distinguishing feature of tricholemmomal carcinoma is highlighted, with the neoplastic clear cells that are characteristic of outer root sheath differentiation.

surgical excision with clear margins appears to be the treatment of choice. Mohs surgical technique has also been used.

## Proliferating tricholemmal cystic carcinoma

In 1976, Headington suggested the malignant variant of proliferating tricholemmal tumor be termed 'malignant proliferating tricholemmal tumor' in order to separate it from tricholemmal (or tricholemmomal) carcinoma, which is the malignant form of tricholemmoma.[40] While some authors believe these lesions should be regarded as a high-risk subtype of squamous cell carcinoma, we think proliferating tricholemmal cystic carcinomas are distinct follicular neoplasms with differentiation towards the tricholemmal sheath at the isthmus.[41] The separation is important given the increased rates of recurrence and metastasis in proliferating tricholemmal cystic carcinomas as compared to conventional cutaneous squamous cell carcinomas.[42]

Proliferating tricholemmal cystic carcinomas (or malignant proliferating tricholemmal tumors) most commonly occur on sun-exposed areas of elderly females, with a predilection for the scalp. Patients often give a history of a subcutaneous mass present for decades, which has gradually or rapidly increased in size. Clinically, tumors appear as a firm painless nodule, with overlying alopecia and/or ulceration, and are most often confused with a squamous cell carcinoma.

Variably sized dermal lobules with solid and cystic areas and a jagged outline are seen microscopically (Fig. 13.21). The cells have abundant eosinophilic cytoplasm with nuclear pleomorphism and numerous mitoses. The distinguishing feature is the tricholemmal cornification within the tumor (Fig. 13.22).

The main differential is with a proliferating tricholemmal tumor. This can be difficult as proliferating tricholemmal tumors can have some cytological and architectural pleomorphism. Clinical and histological criteria

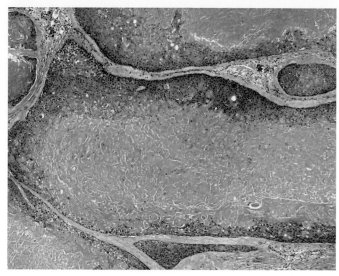

**Figure 13.22** A high-power image highlighting the tricholemmal cornification of proliferating tricholemmal cystic carcinoma.

for separating the two have been proposed.[42,43] Squamous cell carcinomas also enter into the differential, but these lack the tricholemmal cornification characteristic of proliferating tricholemmal cystic carcinomas.

Treatment includes local excision with wide margins or MMS.[43] Lymph node dissection, radiation, and chemotherapy have also been used with variable to limited success.[43] Lesions have a high rate of metastasis, including to regional lymph nodes, lungs, mediastinum, liver, and fibromuscular tissue.[44]

## Matrical carcinoma

The terms matrical carcinoma, pilomatrix carcinoma, and calcifying epitheliocarcinoma of Malherbe were first proposed in 1980, although an 'aggressive' pilomatricoma that required amputation after multiple local recurrences was reported in 1927.[45,46] Unlike their benign counterparts, malignant pilomatricomas typically occur in adult males, with a mean age of 46.3 years.[47] Lesions are predominantly located on the head and neck. Clinically, tumors present as a slowly growing, firm, non-tender solitary nodule that is clinically mistaken for a pilomatricoma, keratinous cyst, or basal cell carcinoma.[47]

Histological examination shows dermal lobules, strands, and serpiginous cords of basaloid cells with nuclear pleomorphism and numerous mitoses (Fig. 13.23). Squamous eddies and keratin pearls are present in the lobules; ghost cells and necrosis en masse are common (Fig. 13.24).

The main differential diagnoses are proliferating pilomatricoma and basal cell carcinoma with matrical differentiation. While proliferating pilomatricoma can have cytological pleomorphism and mitoses, there is architectural symmetry and circumscription and the sex distribution is different. Even though some basal cell carcinomas can have matrical differentiation, the other histological features typical of basal cell carcinoma, such as peripheral palisading and retraction artifact, are present.

Recurrence rates of greater than 50% have been reported with simple excision, therefore a wide excision with 0.5 to 1.0 cm margins is recommended.[47] Success

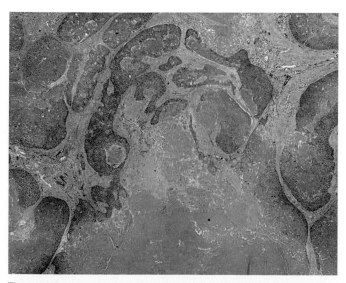

**Figure 13.21** Large irregular infiltrating cystic lobules of proliferating tricholemmal cystic carcinoma with central dense keratin showing tricholemmal cornification.

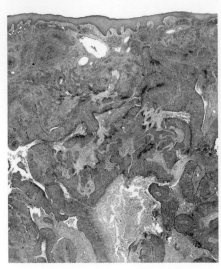

Figure 13.23 Scanning magnification of matrical carcinoma shows islands, strands, and serpiginous cords of basophilic cells with central eosinophilic necrosis.

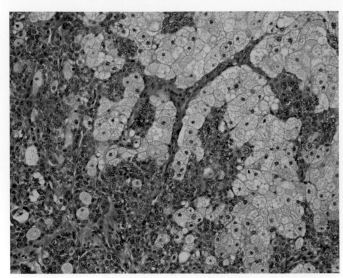

Figure 13.25 Typical features of sebaceous carcinoma are seen, including a predominance of basaloid cells with nuclear overlap and pleomorphism along with the bubbly cells of sebaceous differentiation.

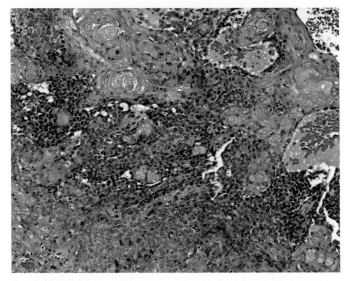

Figure 13.24 High-power microscopy of matrical carcinoma demonstrates the basaloid cells with nuclear pleomorphism, as well as numerous keratin pearls and focal shadow cells.

with MMS has also been reported. Metastases are common and mainly occur in the lungs and lymph nodes.[47] Radiation may be used when complete surgical excision is not possible.[47]

## CARCINOMAS OF THE SEBACEOUS GLANDS

### Sebaceous carcinoma

In 1942, Woolhander and Becker reported a diagnosis of a true adenoma of sebaceous gland origin and considered the possibility that the lesion may represent an early carcinoma.[48] However, in 1943, examples of sebaceous adenoma and sebaceous carcinoma were presented.[49] Some believe that lesions once called sebaceous adenoma should now be classified as sebaceous carcinoma.

Sebaceous carcinomas are slightly more common in men and have a strong predilection for elderly Caucasians.[50]

Most lesions occur on the head and neck, with more than 50% of these being on the eyelid. Lesions usually present as a slow-growing firm subcutaneous nodule, sometimes with overlying ulceration. Because there is not a specific clinical appearance, diagnosis can be delayed by 1 to 2.9 years.[50] There is a well-known association of sebaceous carcinoma with Muir–Torre Syndrome (MTS), with the incidence being 66–100%.[51]

Histologically, sebaceous carcinoma is a dermal neoplasm with an asymmetrical architecture that is focally infiltrative, and is composed of lobules of basaloid cells with pleomorphic nuclei, abundant mitoses, and foci of necrosis. Sebaceous differentiation within the basaloid lobules can be focal or diffuse (Fig. 13.25).

The main differential diagnosis is with carcinomas showing clear cell changes, including basal cell carcinoma and non-cornifying squamous cell carcinoma, and metastases, such as renal cell carcinoma. However, the sebocytes of sebaceous carcinoma have a distinct clear cell appearance, with numerous small round vacuoles within the cytoplasm and a central scalloped nucleus.

Sebaceous carcinoma is primarily treated by standard excision with wide margins or MMS. Both ocular and extraocular sebaceous carcinomas can spread to regional lymph nodes and metastasize to distant sites, resulting in death from metastatic disease. Given the association with Muir–Torre syndrome, diagnosis of a sebaceous neoplasm outside of the head and neck in a patient under 50 years old mandates an additional workup, with immunohistochemical staining for MLH-1, MSH-2, and MSH-6 being the initial screening test.[51] Microsatellite instability analysis can subsequently be performed if warranted.

## FUTURE OUTLOOK

While conventional complete surgical excision is the primary treatment for adnexal carcinomas, Mohs micrographic surgery has emerged as an excellent modality in many cases. Chemotherapy or radiation has been used as adjuvant therapy in those neoplasms that follow a more aggressive course. Close clinical follow-up is necessary to monitor for tumor persistence, recurrence, or metastasis. Knowledge of these lesions and information about prognosis will continue to accumulate as this rare and difficult class of malignancies is better recognized and reported.

## REFERENCES

1. Blake PW, Bradford PT, Devesa SS, et al. Cutaneous appendageal carcinoma incidence and survival pattern in the United States: a population-based study. *Arch Dermatol*. 2010;146(6):625–632.

2. Goldstein DJ, Barr RJ, Santa Cruz DJ. Microcystic adnexal carcinoma: a distinct clinicopathologic entity. *Cancer*. 1982;50(3):566–572.

3. Wetter R, Goldstein GD. Microcystic adnexal carcinoma: a diagnostic and therapeutic challenge. *Dermatol Ther*. 2008;21(6):452–458.

4. Snow S, Madjar DD, Hardy S, et al. Microcystic adnexal carcinoma: report of 13 cases and review of the literature. *Dermatol Surg*. 2001;27(4):401–408.

5. Boggio R. Adenoid cystic carcinoma of scalp. *Arch Dermatol*. 1975;111(6):793–794.

6. Barnes J, Garcia C. Primary cutaneous adenoid cystic carcinoma: a case report and review of the literature. *Cutis*. 2008;81(3):243–246.

7. Lang Jr PG, Metcalf JS, Maize JC. Recurrent adenoid cystic carcinoma of the skin managed by microscopically controlled surgery (Mohs surgery). *J Dermatol Surg Oncol*. 1986;12(4):395–398.

8. Pappo O, Gez E, Craciun I, et al. Growth rate analysis of lung metastases appearing 18 years after resection of cutaneous adenoid cystic carcinoma. Case report and review of the literature. *Arch Pathol Lab Med*. 1992;116(1):76–79.

9. Lennox B, Pearse AG, Richards HG. Mucin-secreting tumours of the skin with special reference to the so-called mixed-salivary tumour of the skin and its relation to hidradenoma. *J Pathol Bacteriol*. 1952;64(4):865–880.

10. Kazakov DV, Suster S, LeBoit PE, et al. Mucinous carcinoma of the skin, primary, and secondary: a clinicopathologic study of 63 cases with emphasis on the morphologic spectrum of primary cutaneous forms: homologies with mucinous lesions in the breast. *Am J Surg Pathol*. 2005;29(6):764–782.

11. Santa Cruz DJ, Meyers JH, Gnepp DR, et al. Primary mucinous carcinoma of the skin. *Br J Dermatol*. 1978;98(6):645–653.

12. Snow SN, Reizner GT. Mucinous eccrine carcinoma of the eyelid. *Cancer*. 1992;70(8):2099–2104.

13. Pinkus H, Mehregan AH. Epidermotropic eccrine carcinoma. A case combining features of eccrine poroma and Paget's dermatosis. *Arch Dermatol*. 1963;88:597–606.

14. Robson A, Greene J, Ansari N, et al. Eccrine porocarcinoma (malignant eccrine poroma): a clinicopathologic study of 69 cases. *Am J Surg Pathol*. 2001;25(6):710–720.

15. Ishida M, Hotta M, Kushima R, Okabe H. A case of porocarcinoma arising in pigmented hidroacanthoma simplex with multiple lymph node, liver and bone metastases. *J Cutan Pathol*. 2011;38(2):227–231.

16. Requena L, Kutzner H, Hurt MA, et al. Malignant tumors with apocrine and eccrine differentiation. In: LeBoit PE, Gunter B, Weedon D, et al., eds. *World Health Organization Classification of Tumors. Pathology & Genetics. Skin Tumours*. Lyon, France: IARC Press; 131, 2006:134–135.

17. Nash JW, Barrett TL, Kies M, et al. Metastatic hidradenocarcinoma with demonstration of Her-2/neu gene amplification by fluorescence in situ hybridization: potential treatment implications. *J Cutan Pathol*. 2007;34(1):49–54.

18. Stout AP, Cooley SG. Carcinoma of sweat glands. *Cancer*. 1951;4(3):531–536.

19. Hernández-Pérez E, Cestoni-Parducci R. Nodular hidradenoma and hidradenocarcinoma. A 10-year review. *J Am Acad Dermatol*. 1985;12 (1 Pt 1):15–20.

20. Keasbey LE, Hadley GG. Clear-cell hidradenoma. Report of three cases with widespread metastases. *Cancer*. 1954;7(5):934–952.

21. Takahashi H, Ishiko A, Kobayashi M, et al. Malignant chondroid syringoma with bone invasion: a case report and review of the literature. *Am J Dermatopathol*. 2004;26(5):403–406.

22. Harrist TJ, Aretz TH, Mihm Jr MC, et al. Cutaneous malignant mixed tumor. *Arch Dermatol*. 1981;117:719–724.

23. Dabska M. Malignant transformation of eccrine spiradenoma. *Pol Med J*. 1972;11:388–396.

24. Hantash BM, Chan JL, Egbert BM, et al. De novo malignant eccrine spiradenoma: a case report and review of the literature. *Dermatol Surg*. 2006;32:1189–1198.

25. Sridhar KS, Benedetto P, Otrakji CL, et al. Response to eccrine spiradenocarcinoma to tamoxifen. *Cancer*. 1989;64:366–370.

26. Wiedemann A. Weitere Beitrage zur Kenntnis der sogenannten Zylindrome der Kopfhaut. *Arch Dermatol*. 1929;159:180–187.

27. Durani BK, Kurzen H, Jaeckel A, et al. Malignant transformation of multiple dermal cylindromas. *Br J Dermatol*. 2001;145(4):653–656.

28. Gerretsen AL, van der Putte SC, Deenstra W, et al. Cutaneous cylindroma with malignant transformation. *Cancer*. 1993;72(5):1618–1623.

29. Robson A, Lazar AJ, Ben Nagi J, et al. Primary cutaneous apocrine carcinoma: a clinico-pathologic analysis of 24 cases. *Am J Surg Pathol*. 2008;32(5):682–690.

30. Warkel RL, Helwig EB. Apocrine gland adenoma and adenocarcinoma of the axilla. *Arch Dermatol*. 1978;114(2):198–203.

31. Requena L, Kiryu H, Ackerman AB. Cribriform carcinoma. In: Requena L, Kiryu H, Ackerman AB, eds. *Neoplasms with Apocrine Differentiation*. Philadelphia: Lippincott-Raven, Ardor Scribendi; 1998:879–905.

32. Helwig EB. Eccrine acrospiroma. *J Cutan Pathol*. 1984;11(5):415–420.

33. Kao GF, Helwig EB, Graham JH. Aggressive digital papillary adenoma and adenocarcinoma. A clinicopathological study of 57 patients, with histochemical, immunopathological, and ultrastructural observations. *J Cutan Pathol*. 1987;14(3):129–146.

34. Frey J, Shimek C, Woodmansee C, et al. Aggressive digital papillary adenocarcinoma: a report of two diseases and review of the literature. *J Am Acad Dermatol*. 2009;60(2):331–339.

35. Hedinger E. Zur Frage des plasmocytomes(Granulationsplasmocytom in Kombination mit einem krebsig umgewandelten Schweissdrusenadenom des behaarten Kopfes). *Frankfurt Ztschr Path*. 1911;7:343–350.

36. Dissanayake RVP, Salm R. Sweat gland carcinomas: prognosis related to histological type. *Histopathology*. 1980;4:445–466.

37. Numata M, Hosoe S, Itoh N, et al. Syringadenocarcinoma papilliferum. *J Cutan Pathol*. 1985;12:3–7.

38. Allee JE, Cotsarelis G, Solky B, et al. Multiple recurrent trichilemmal carcinoma with perineural invasion and cytokeratin 17 positivity. *Dermatol Surg*. 2003;29(8):886–889.

39. Billingsley EM, Fedok F, Maloney ME. Trichilemmal carcinoma. *J Am Acad Dermatol*. 1997;36(1):107–109.

40. Headington JT. Tumors of the hair follicle. A review. *Am J Pathol*. 1976;85(2):479–514.

41. Cassarino DS, Derienzo DP, Barr RJ. Cutaneous squamous cell carcinoma: a comprehensive clinicopathologic classification—part two. *J Cutan Pathol*. 2006;33(4):261–279.

42. Kini JR, Kini H. Fine-needle aspiration cytology in the diagnosis of malignant proliferating trichilemmal tumor: report of a case and review of the literature. *Diagn Cytopathol*. 2009;37(10):744–747.

43. Satyaprakash AK, Sheehan DJ, Sangüeza OP. Proliferating trichilemmal tumors: a review of the literature. *Dermatol Surg*. 2007;33(9):1102–1108.

44. Noto G, Pravatà G, Aricò M. Proliferating tricholemmal cyst should always be considered as a low-grade carcinoma. *Dermatology*. 1997;194(4):374–375.

45. Weedon D, Bell J, Mayze J. Matrical carcinoma of the skin. *J Cutan Pathol*. 1980;7(1):39–42.

46. Lopansri S, Mihm MC. Pilomatrix carcinoma or calcifying epitheliocarcinoma of Malherbe: a case report and review of literature. *Cancer*. 1980;45(9):2368–2373.

47. Hardisson D, Linares MD, Cuevas-Santos J, et al. Pilomatrix carcinoma: a clinicopathologic study of six cases and review of the literature. *Am J Dermatopathol*. 2001;23(5):394–401.

48. Woolhander HW, Becker SW. Adenoma of sebaceous glands (adenoma sebaceum) with consideration of keratotic adenoma sebaceum and true adenoma of sebaceous glands. *Arch Derm Syph*. 1942;45:734–756.

49. Warren S, Warvi WN. Tumor of sebaceous glands. *Am J Pathol*. 1943;19:441–459.

50. Dasgupta T, Wilson LD, Yu JB. A retrospective review of 1349 cases of sebaceous carcinoma. *Cancer*. 2009;115(1):158–165.

51. Abbas O, Mahalingam M. Cutaneous sebaceous neoplasms as markers of Muir-Torre syndrome: a diagnostic algorithm. *J Cutan Pathol*. 2009;36(6):613–619.

# Paget's Disease

*Gagik Oganesyan, S. Brian Jiang, and Dirk M. Elston*

---

## Key Points

- Mammary Paget's disease (MPD) is almost always associated with underlying breast carcinoma. If an underlying mass is palpated, the patient should be referred for a fine needle biopsy of the mass or an excisional biopsy.

- The immunostaining pattern of MPD and extramammary Paget's disease (EMPD) show substantial overlap, but EMPD is more likely to stain positively for gross cystic disease fluid protein 15 and less likely to stain for the human milk-fat-globule membrane protein MFGM-gp 155.

- Expression of histo-blood group A type 1/2, and type 3 antigens by tumor cells of EMPD may correlate with a greater risk of invasive carcinoma.

- CK20 staining in EMPD suggests underlying carcinoma of the colon.

- Recent evidence suggests that EMPD tumor cells grow in a contiguous fashion, and that long finger-like projections may account for the high incidence of local recurrence.

- Mohs micrographic surgery (MMS) is a valuable technique for the removal of tumors with irregular growth patterns, and has proved useful as a tissue-sparing form of surgical therapy for EMPD. Immunostains can improve the sensitivity of margin control with MMS.

---

## INTRODUCTION

The term Paget's disease incorporates two unrelated groups of disorders. The first is Paget's disease of the bone, also known as osteitis deformans. The second comprise malignant neoplasms affecting the skin. When occurring on the breast or nipple, the condition is referred to as mammary Paget's disease (MPD). It is called extramammary Paget's disease (EMPD) if it occurs anywhere else. Both may be associated with underlying malignancies. An underlying malignancy is almost always present in MPD (Table 14.1).

## MAMMARY PAGET'S DISEASE

### History

The initial clinical description of the disease was provided by a French physician, Alfred Velpeau, in his book entitled *A Treatise on the Diseases of the Breast and Mammary Region*, published in 1856. He described the condition as an unusual irritation of the nipple resembling eczema or psoriasis,

where 'the nipple looked like a raspberry or strawberry'. However, Velpeau classified this condition as a benign eczematous process and provided no clear etiology for the disease. It was the British physician Sir James Paget who described the association of the condition with an underlying malignancy, and his name is now associated with the disease. In his report, which was published in 1874 in St. Bartholomew's Hospital Reports in London, Paget gave a similar clinical description to that of Velpeau, but he noted that in every case there was an underlying carcinoma identified within 2 years. In all the patients described by Paget, the skin eruption preceded the malignancy, and Paget concluded that the malignancy was likely a secondary event due to chronic irritation of the underlying structures. It was not until 1881 that George Thin described the pathology of the lesions and was first to state that the observed skin condition was a neoplastic process secondary to an underlying ductal carcinoma.

## Epidemiology

Paget's disease of the breast is a relatively rare condition, and it accounts for roughly 0.6–3.2% of all the breast carcinomas. The median age of onset is 54–57 years, with a male to female ratio of 1:50–200. In 82–100% of patients, MPD is associated with an underlying breast malignancy. Of these malignancies, 74–90% are either invasive or in-situ ductal adenocarcinomas, 18% are unspecified adenocarcinomas, and 1% are lobular carcinomas.[1] Survival rates vary, but with recent advances in diagnostic and surgical techniques, the 5-year survival rate is estimated to be 88–93% for invasive disease and 98–100% for non-invasive disease. The 5-year disease-free survival rate is approximately 75% in both groups.[2]

## Pathogenesis and etiology

While the majority of cases of MPD represent extensions of underlying breast adenocarcinoma, rarely, cases can be limited to the epidermis and are referred to as primary MPD. Some cases of primary MPD may arise from Toker cells, while other apparent cases of primary MPD may simply represent tissue sampling error. Toker cells, first described by Cyril Toker, are large intraepidermal cells with ample pale cytoplasm. They are usually found in the basal layer of normal nipple epidermis at the openings of the lactiferous ducts, and appear to give rise to clear cell papulosis as well as EMPD. Some regard clear cell papulosis as the benign counterpart of EMPD and primary MPD.

## Table 14.1 Mammary vs Extramammary Paget's Disease

|  | Mammary Paget's Disease | Extramammary Paget's Disease |
|---|---|---|
| Epidemiology | 0.6–3.2% of all breast carcinomas<br>Median age of onset 54–57 years<br>Male to female ratio 1:50–200 | 14% of all Paget's disease<br>Median age of onset 72–75 years<br>Male to female ratio 1:1.2 |
| Anatomic locations | Breast | Vulva, perineal region, scrotum, axillae |
| Pathology | Large cells with pale cytoplasm within the epidermis, usually appear to 'crush' the basal epidermal layer<br>Common markers: EMA, CEA, CK7<br>Specific markers*: Her2/Neu, ER | Large cells with pale cytoplasm within the epidermis, usually appear to 'crush' the basal epidermal layer<br>Common markers: EMA, CEA, CK7*<br>Specific markers*: GCDFP-15, CK20[†]<br>Histo-blood group A type 1, 2, 3 antigens[‡] |
| Prognosis | 5-year survival rate of 88–93% for invasive and 98–100% for non-invasive disease | 5-year-survival rate of 85% for minimally invasive and as low as 25% for deeply invasive disease |
| Therapy | Treatment based on the standards for the underlying breast malignancy, usually breast-conserving surgery + XRT+ SNLB | Local excision preferably by Mohs surgery for isolated lesions<br>Otherwise, treatment based on the standards for the underlying malignancy and the depth of invasion |

*Positive only in certain percentage of cases.

[†]Usually positive when EMPD is associated with underlying colorectal carcinoma or transitional cell carcinoma of the bladder.

[‡]May correlate with greater risk of invasive disease in EMPD.

## Clinical features

MPD typically presents as a chronic unilateral erythematous scaly plaque on the nipple or the areola (Figs 14.1 and 14.2). Ulceration, edema, bloody discharge, and nipple inversion are also common clinical presentations. Many of the patients suffer from significant pain and abnormal sensation around the area. In 15–30% of patients, there is an underlying palpable breast mass, and 32–77% of the patients will have an abnormal suspicious mammogram.[2] Uncommonly, MPD may present as a pigmented lesion that could be confused clinically with malignant melanoma.

## Patient evaluation, diagnosis and differential diagnosis

The differential diagnosis of MPD includes allergic contact dermatitis, dermatophytosis, psoriasis, erosive adenomatosis of the nipple, melanoma, and Bowen's disease. A positive potassium hydroxide (KOH) preparation confirms the

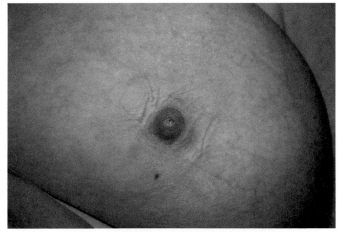

Figure 14.2 Mammary Paget's disease. Subtle erythema of nipple.

diagnosis of dermatophytosis. The presence of extramammary lesions favors a diagnosis of psoriasis, and an acute onset of pruritic skin lesions suggests an episode of allergic contact dermatitis. Whenever MPD is suspected, a careful physical examination of the breast and lymph nodes is warranted. A skin biopsy should be performed to confirm the diagnosis. If an underlying mass is palpated, the patient should be referred for a fine needle biopsy of the mass or an excisional biopsy. If no mass is palpated, the patient should be referred for mammography. Up to 77% of patients with MPD have positive mammography results, but a negative result does not rule out the possibility of underlying carcinoma. Upon final diagnosis of MPD, the patient should be referred to specialists in medical, surgical and radiation oncology for definitive treatment.

## Pathology

The histologic appearance of Paget's disease is typically diagnostic. Large cells with ample pale-staining cytoplasm and large cytologically atypical nuclei are noted within the

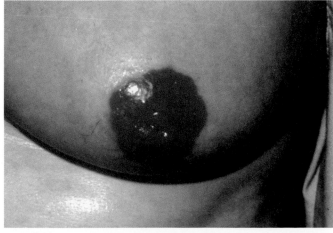

Figure 14.1 Mammary Paget's disease. Bright red erythema of nipple and areola.

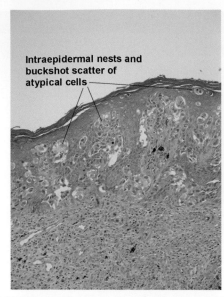

Intraepidermal nests and
buckshot scatter of
atypical cells

**Figure 14.3** Histologic section of mammary Paget's disease (H&E stain ×100).

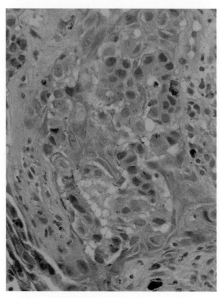

**Figure 14.4** Histologic section of mammary Paget's disease. Nests of malignant cells may form glandular structures. Cells demonstrate atypia and a high nuclear to cytoplasmic ratio (H&E stain × 400).

epidermis. The cells may be distributed singly, aggregated in nests close to the basal layer, or may appear to replace the entire epidermis (Figs 14.3 and 14.4). A flattened or 'crushed' basal layer is often noted below the tumor cells. The overlying epidermis may demonstrate para- or orthokeratosis or may be eroded. Underlying ductal carcinoma in situ (DCIS) or invasive disease may be present. Typically, Paget's cells stain positively for low molecular weight cytokeratins 8 and 18, cytokeratin 7 (CK7), carcinoembryonic antigen (CEA), epithelial membrane antigen (EMA), and high molecular weight glycoprotein mucin-1 (MUC1). The cells also stain positively for Her2/Neu receptor, estrogen receptor, and progesterone receptor in 88%, 30%, and 40% of the cases respectively.[2]

Other clear cell changes of the nipple epidermis may mimic MPD histologically. Glycogenated epidermal cells may appear large and pale, but typically demonstrate a rim of cytoplasm at the periphery of the cell. Clear cell papulosis and Toker cell hyperplasia are distinguished

by a lack of cytologic atypia.[3] Another distinguishing feature is that benign Toker cells typically stain negatively or weakly for CEA and Her2/Neu, while both benign Toker cells and MPD will stain for EMA, low molecular weight keratins and CK7.[4] Other conditions that need to be distinguished from MPD include pagetoid dyskeratosis of the nipple epidermis, malignant melanoma, and Bowen's disease. Pagetoid dyskeratosis and Bowen's disease will stain positively for high molecular weight cytokeratin and negatively for CK7, EMA, CEA and Her2/Neu. Melanoma will stain positive for S100, HMB-45 and Melan-A, and negative for the other above-mentioned antigens. It should be noted that pigmented Paget's disease may be heavily colonized by melanocytes and immunohistochemical staining of dendritic processes with melanocytic markers has resulted in an incorrect diagnosis of melanoma.[5]

## Treatment

Traditionally, the primary therapy recommended for MPD has been mastectomy with axillary lymph node dissection. More recently, the combination of breast-conserving therapy followed by radiotherapy and sentinel lymph node biopsy (SLNB) has been shown to be a safe alternative for the treatment of breast cancer and may be effective for MPD.[6–8]

### EXTRAMAMMARY PAGET'S DISEASE

Extramammary Paget's disease (EMPD) is an uncommon epidermal malignant neoplasm that is clinically and histologically similar to MPD. However, EMPD, as its name implies, occurs outside of the breast, usually on apocrine gland-bearing skin, including the skin of the vulva, scrotum, perineal region, and axillae. Unlike MPD, EMPD is more commonly limited to the skin without an associated underlying malignancy.

## History

In 1888, Radcliffe Cocker, a well-known British dermatologist, reported a male patient with a clinical presentation similar to that of Paget's disease of the nipple, but occurring on the scrotum. Initially, the lesion presented as a well-defined plaque resembling eczema, but progressed to become nodular with ulcerations. Histologically, the tumor was similar to Paget's disease of the nipple. Shortly thereafter, perianal and vulvar EMPD were reported in 1893 and 1901 respectively.

## Epidemiology

EMPD is estimated to have an incidence of 0.11 in 100,000 people, and it comprises about 14% of all cases of Paget's disease. The mean age at diagnosis is 72–75 years.[9] Previous reports have estimated the male to female ratio at about 1:3.2, but more recent larger studies estimate the ratio to be much closer to 1:1.2 in Caucasians. Interestingly, it appears that in Asian populations the male to female ratio is reversed to about 3:1, likely due to genetic variations. Familial cases of EMPD have also been described, further highlighting the importance of genetic influence on this disease. About 11–45% of patients will have associated visceral malignancies, which include breast, colorectal, genitourinary, and hepatocellular carcinoma. When EMPD is located in the perianal area, there is a higher incidence of co-existing internal malignancies. The level of invasion is of great prognostic importance, with deeper tumors presenting a greater risk of metastasis. The overall 5-year survival for invasive EMPD is estimated to be 72%. Minimally invasive disease has a 5-year survival rate of 85%, whereas deeply invasive disease has a survival rate of 25%.

## Pathogenesis and etiology

There are two main categories of EMPD: primary and secondary. The pathogenesis of primary EMPD is controversial. Some suggest that Paget's cells in primary EMPD may originate from the intraepidermal portions of apocrine or eccrine ducts, which is supported by the fact that most cases of EMPD occur on apocrine-bearing skin. In a recent study, 23 EMPD cases were analyzed by extensive immunohistochemical staining, and all were consistent with the hypothesis that these cells may have a sweat gland origin.[10] Others have suggested that primary EMPD may arise from Toker cells.[11] Mammary-like ducts along the milk line, and pluripotential stem cells that follow the distribution of the milk line have also been suggested as sources for primary EMPD. Secondary EMPD arises either by direct extension or via epidermotropic metastasis from an underlying malignancy, most commonly rectal carcinoma. Urogenital carcinoma, prostate carcinoma, and primary cutaneous adnexal carcinomas are other sources for secondary EMPD.

Nuclear overexpression of both *p53* and *p73* protein is common in EMPD and their expression in tumor cells is significantly higher than in normal skin.[12] Both proteins have been implicated in tumor progression. Specificity protein 1 (*Sp1*), a sequence-specific DNA-binding protein, activates a broad spectrum of mammalian genes, including the gene for vascular endothelial growth factor (VEGF). A study of 35 EMPD specimens, including invasive and metastatic tumors, showed strong nuclear positive staining for *Sp1* together with strong cytoplasmic positive staining for VEGF. Expression levels were significantly higher than those in normal skin, suggesting that overexpression of *Sp1* and VEGF may also play a pivotal role in the tumorigenesis.[13]

Expression of adhesion molecules has been shown to be important in both growth and metastasis of many cancers, including EMPD. E-cadherin, plakoglobin and beta-catenin have all been shown to play important roles in cell adhesion. A study of 63 cases of Paget's disease of the vulva (including eight with invasive disease) and 23 cases of Paget's disease of the breast showed that 66% (41/54) of the cases of in-situ Paget's disease of the vulva expressed E-cadherin in >50% of Paget cells, compared with only 28% (2/7) of the cases of Paget's disease of the vulva associated with invasive disease (p = 0.039). The same investigators found that 25% (14/55) of cases of intraepidermal Paget's disease of the vulva showed expression of plakoglobin protein in >50% of Paget cells, compared with 12% (1/8) of cases of Paget's disease of the vulva with invasive disease. Beta-catenin expression was not significantly different between invasive and non-invasive disease. There

were no significant differences in expression for Paget's disease of the breast. The results suggest that E-cadherin and plakoglobin expression may have a role to play a role in the pathogenesis and progression of Paget's disease of the vulva, while there is no evidence that they play a role in mammary Paget's disease.[14]

## Clinical features

The clinical appearance of EMPD is very similar to that of MPD. It most often presents as an erythematous scaly plaque, but crusting, maceration and/or ulceration are common. Common sites of occurrence include the vulva, perineal region, scrotum, and axillae (Figs 14.5–14.7). EMPD has also been reported in sites that do not contain apocrine glands, such as the lower extremities and head and neck region. Most lesions are chronic and they may be pruritic or painful. EMPD may also present with hair loss (alopecia neoplastica), although the background skin is rarely completely normal in appearance.

## Patient evaluation, diagnosis and differential diagnosis

As with MPD, EMPD can resemble other inflammatory and neoplastic conditions. Given that EMPD commonly presents in anogenital, inguinal and axillary areas, common

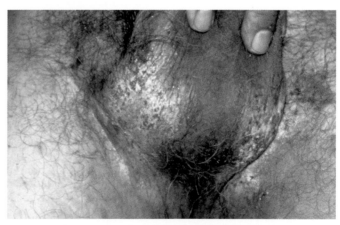

**Figure 14.5** Extramammary Paget's disease. Fissuring and maceration could be misinterpreted as eczematous dermatitis or benign familial pemphigus (Hailey–Hailey disease).

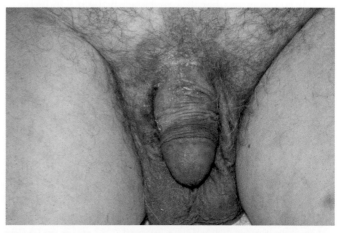

**Figure 14.6** Extramammary Paget's disease. Erythematous scaly patches.

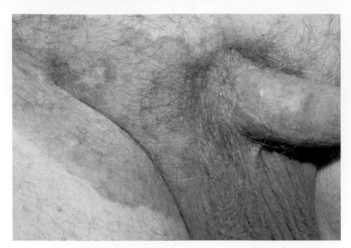

**Figure 14.7** Extramammary Paget's disease. Erythema and scale with a slightly raised border.

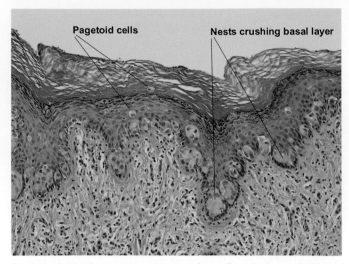

**Figure 14.8** Histologic section of extramammary Paget's disease (H&E stain × 40).

misdiagnoses include fungal infections, psoriasis, lichen sclerosus et atrophicans, hidradenitis, and Bowen's disease. As many of the lesions may be colonized with yeast, a positive KOH or culture does not exclude the possibility of EMPD. There should be a very low threshold for performing a skin biopsy in lesions recalcitrant to treatments with antifungals or topical steroids. Further testing may include endoscopy, especially in perianal or periurethral sites. For women, a pelvic ultrasound may be indicated. Metastatic EMPD arises in patients with dermal invasion, and lymphovascular involvement visible in histologic sections is correlated with a higher risk of metastatic disease. Imaging studies, including $^{18}$F-fluorodeoxyglucose positron emission tomography (PET)–computed tomography (CT) scans. can be used to detect distant metastases. Serum CEA levels can be used to monitor for recurrence in those with metastatic disease.

## Pathology

Histologically, EMPD appears almost identical to MPD. Hematoxylin and eosin (H&E) staining will show large cells with ample pale amphophilic cytoplasm and atypical nuclei within the epidermis. They can be scattered throughout the epidermis individually, form clusters resembling glandular structures, or, in some instances, appear to replace the entire epidermis (Figs 14.8–4.10). As with MPD, nests often appear to crush the basal layer beneath them. Underlying invasive carcinoma may be present. The underlying carcinoma may be the result of invasion from the malignant population of cells in the epidermis, or the epidermotropic component may arise from an underlying carcinoma. Extragenital lesions may be associated with primary carcinoma arising in a pre-existing apocrine adenoma or other pre-existing adnexal tumor.[15] The immunostaining pattern is similar to that for MPD, but the cells of EMPD are more likely to stain positively for gross cystic disease fluid protein 15 (GCDFP-15). They are much less likely than cells of MPD to stain for the human milk-fat-globule membrane protein MFGM-gp 155. Additionally, EMPD that is associated with underlying colorectal cancers will stain for CK20 (often coexpressing CK7 and CK20) and will commonly fail to stain for GCFPD-15. CK20- and CK7-positive EMPD

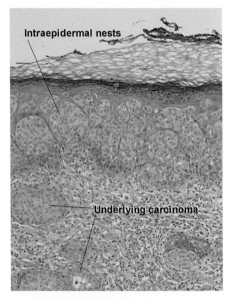

**Figure 14.9** Histologic section of extramammary Paget's disease (H&E stain × 100).

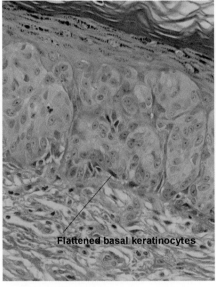

**Figure 14.10** Histologic section of extramammary Paget's disease (H&E stain × 200).

has also been linked to other visceral malignancies, including transitional cell carcinoma of the bladder. Expression of histo-blood group A type 1/2, and type 3 antigens by tumor cells may correlate with a greater risk of invasive carcinoma, although additional studies are needed to bear out this observation.[16]

EMPD should be differentiated histologically from melanoma and Bowen's disease. Melanoma will stain for S100 and HMB-45, while Bowen's disease will be positive for high molecular weight keratins and *p63*. Primary EMPD stains negative for *p63*, while EMPD secondary to urethral carcinoma can stain positive.[17]

## Treatment

The treatment of EMPD depends largely on whether the lesion is a primary, or is secondary to an underlying carcinoma. For secondary EMPD, treatment must be directed toward the underlying tumor in addition to local control of the disease. While surgery has been the mainstay therapy for primary EMPD, the overall recurrence rate of EMPD treated with traditional wide surgical excision is estimated to be about 20–44%. The invasive component has higher recurrence rates compared to in-situ disease, providing metastasis does not occur. That is to say, it is typically the in-situ component that proves most difficult to control. Mohs micrographic surgery (MMS) has emerged as a tissue-sparing surgical therapy for EMPD. Its main advantage is that it allows maximal tissue conservation, while providing 100% margin evaluation during the surgery. Recent studies have demonstrated that the recurrence rate of EMPD in patients treated with MMS is significantly lower than in those treated with traditional surgical techniques.[18] Immunostaining has proved helpful in the evaluation of margins during MMS, and may further diminish the rate of recurrence.[19]

Use of MMS is predicated upon contiguous growth of tumor cells. Traditionally, extramammary Paget's disease was thought to be multifocal in origin, and this was thought to contribute to the high rate of recurrences after wide local excision. However, a recent report using information from scouting biopsies as well as the Mohs map which created a two-dimensional reconstruction of the tumor, refuted this concept. The study demonstrated two contiguous, thin, long, projections that extended from the main body of the tumor. In various planes of section, this would have given the appearance of a multifocal tumor. Conventional tumor sectioning techniques could easily have led to the incorrect conclusion that the initial margins were free of tumor. The study suggested that extramammary Paget's disease demonstrates contiguous tumor growth with a highly irregular pattern of finger-like projections beyond the bulk of the tumor, and that it is this irregular pattern of growth that may account for the high rate of recurrence. MMS using CK7 immunostaining was helpful in identifying and removing foci of Paget's cells that extended beyond the main body of the tumor.[20] Taken together, the emerging body of evidence suggests that MMS should be considered as a first-line surgical treatment option for primary EMPD. Although the surgical defects are often quite large, good functional results and quality of life can be achieved after resection and repair of large perianal defects.[21]

5-Fluorouracil- or docetaxel-based chemotherapy has demonstrated some efficacy in patients with metastatic disease. Systemic chemotherapeutic agents have also been used in selected cases of EMPD without spread. Several regimens have been used, including mitomycin C or carboplatin in combination with 5-fluorouracil, and low-dose mitomycin C, cisplatin and etoposide. Systemic chemotherapy should be used as an adjuvant or in patients who have contraindications to surgery or radiotherapy. Other therapeutic options include topical 5-fluorouracil and photodynamic therapy (PDT).[22] When used alone, responses with these modalities are often incomplete and partial surgical excision may be necessary. Ionophoresis has been used to improve topical drug delivery, but the results have not been spectacular. With any 'blind' treatment modality, the risk of long-term recurrence is high, and patients must be monitored for any sign of recurrence. PDT with 5-aminolevulinic acid/protoporphyrin IX (PpIX)-mediated fluorescence has been used to help visualize the clinical margins of the lesion, and could theoretically help to decrease recurrence rates. Some evidence suggests that PDT can improve the response to $CO_2$ laser therapy, and combined modalities deserve further study.[23] Further study is needed to determine whether fluorescent examination can detect narrow finger-like extensions of the tumor.

Topical imiquimod therapy appears promising for patients with contraindications to other forms of treatment, or as an adjunct to more limited surgery in order to preserve sexual function.[24-26] Activation of the serine/threonine kinase, protein kinase B (AKT) is frequently detected in EMPD and promotes cell proliferation by interacting with the mammalian target of rapamycin (mTOR).[27] Further study is needed before rapamycin becomes part of the standard armamentarium for treatment of this disease.

Radioisotope navigation, which is standard in the identification of sentinel nodes in melanoma patients, is problematic in extramammary Paget's disease because of overlapping radioactivity from the primary tumor. Fluorescence navigation with indocyanine green and a handheld gamma probe has shown promise in this setting, as it is less prone to background uptake.[28]

Radiotherapy has been used for some patients who are poor surgical candidates.[29] Radiosensitization with a hydrogen peroxide solution-soaked gauze has been used for a variety of unresectable tumors.[30] Experimentally, hydrogen peroxide has been shown to be a strong radiosensitizer for a highly radioresistant osteosarcoma cell line designated HS-Os-1. This observation led to a clinical trial of radiosensitization therapy for a variety of tumor types. After exposure to hydrogen peroxide, the patients are treated with radiation therapy by means of a high-energy electron beam from a linear accelerator. The total dose given is in the range of 48 Gy, in fractions of 4 Gy. Radiation is delivered three times per week. Prior to each radiation treatment, the lesion is covered with gauze soaked in hydrogen peroxide solution and the lesion is then gently massaged to facilitate penetration of the solution. Radiosensitization may relate to blockade of anti-oxidative enzymes, including peroxidases. This modality deserves further study for patients with extensive disease.

## FUTURE OUTLOOK

Combination therapy may improve patient morbidity and mortality from MPD and EMPD. Studies are needed to evaluate the efficacy of combining radiotherapy with tissue-conserving surgical techniques such as MMS in the treatment of large or poorly defined lesions of primary EMPD. Combining modalities such as surgery, topical drug delivery, radiosensitization and photodynamic therapy may improve the future outlook for patients with this disorder.

## ACKNOWLEDGEMENT

Images contributed by Dr. Elston were produced while the author was a full-time federal employee. They are in the public domain.

## REFERENCES

1. Dalberg K, Hellborg H, Warnberg F. Paget's disease of the nipple in a population based cohort. *Breast Cancer Res Treat*. 2008;111(2):313–319.
2. Caliskan M, Gatti G, Sosnovskikh I, et al. Paget's disease of the breast: the experience of the European Institute of Oncology and review of the literature. *Breast Cancer Res Treat*. 2008;112(3):513–521.
3. Nofech-Mozes S, Hanna W. Toker cells revisited. *Breast J*. 2009;15(4):394–398.
4. Garijo MF, Val D, Val-Bernal JF. An overview of the pale and clear cells of the nipple epidermis. *Histol Histopathol*. 2009;24(3):367–376.
5. Petersson F, Ivan D, Kazakov DV, et al. Pigmented Paget disease—a diagnostic pitfall mimicking melanoma. *Am J Dermatopathol*. 2009;31(3):223–226.
6. Bijker N, Rutgers EJ, Duchateau L, et al. Breast-conserving therapy for Paget disease of the nipple: a prospective European Organization for Research and Treatment of Cancer study of 61 patients. *Cancer*. 2001;91(3):472–477.
7. Goodwin A, Parker S, Ghersi D, et al. Post-operative radiotherapy for ductal carcinoma in situ of the breast. *Cochrane Database Syst Rev*. 2009;(3) CD000563.
8. Buchholz TA. Radiation therapy for early-stage breast cancer after breast-conserving surgery. *N Engl J Med*. 2009;360(1):63–70.
9. Hatta N, Yamada M, Hirano T, et al. Extramammary Paget's disease: treatment, prognostic factors and outcome in 76 patients. *Br J Dermatol*. 2008;158(2):313–318.
10. Liegl B, Leibl S, Gogg-Kamerer M, et al. Mammary and extramammary Paget's disease: an immunohistochemical study of 83 cases. *Histopathology*. 2007;50(4):439–447.
11. Fernandez-Flores A. Toker-cell pathology as a unifying concept. *Histopathology*. 2008;52(7):889–891.
12. Chen S, Moroi Y, Urabe K, et al. Differential expression of two new members of the p53 family, p63 and p73, in extramammary Paget's disease. *Clin Exp Dermatol*. 2008;33(5):634–640.
13. Chen SY, Takeuchi S, Moroi Y, et al. Concordant over-expression of transcription factor Sp1 and vascular endothelial growth factor in extramammary Paget's disease. *Int J Dermatol*. 2008;47(6):562–566.
14. Ellis PE, Cano SD, Fear M, et al. Reduced E-cadherin expression correlates with disease progression in Paget's disease of the vulva but not Paget's disease of the breast. *Mod Pathol*. 2008;21(10):1192–1199.
15. Miyamoto T, Adachi K, Fujishima M. Axillary apocrine carcinoma with Paget's disease and apocrine naevus. *Clin Exp Dermatol*. 2009;34(5):e110–e113.
16. Tanaka A, Kimura A, Yamamoto Y, et al. Expression of histo-blood group A type 1, 2 and 3 antigens in normal skin and extramammary Paget's disease. *Acta Histochem Cytochem*. 2008;41(6):165–171.
17. Yanai H, Takahashi N, Omori M, et al. Immunohistochemistry of p63 in primary and secondary vulvar Paget's disease. *Pathol Int*. 2008;58(10):648–651.
18. Lee KY, Roh MR, Chung WG, et al. Comparison of Mohs micrographic surgery and wide excision for extramammary Paget's disease: Korean experience. *Dermatol Surg*. 2009;35(1):34–40.
19. Stranahan D, Cherpelis BS, Glass LF, et al. Immunohistochemical stains in Mohs surgery: a review. *Dermatol Surg*. 2009;35(7):1023–1034.
20. Hendi A, Perdikis G, Snow JL. Unifocality of extramammary Paget disease. *J Am Acad Dermatol*. 2008;59(5):811–813.
21. Conklin A, Hassan I, Chua HK, et al. Long-term functional and quality of life outcomes of patients after repair of large perianal skin defects for Paget's and Bowen's disease. *J Gastrointest Surg*. 2009;13(5):951–955.
22. Wang XL, Wang HW, Guo MX, et al. Treatment of skin cancer and pre-cancer using ALA-PDT—a single hospital experience. *Photodiagnosis Photodyn Ther*. 2008;5(2):127–133.
23. Fukui T, Watanabe D, Tamada Y, et al. Photodynamic therapy following carbon dioxide laser enhances efficacy in the treatment of extramammary Paget's disease. *Acta Derm Venereol*. 2009;89(2):150–154.
24. Badgwell C, Rosen T. Treatment of limited extent extramammary Paget's disease with 5 percent imiquimod cream. *Dermatol Online J*. 2006;12(1):22.
25. Challenor R, Hughes G, Fitton AR. Multidisciplinary treatment of vulval extramammary Paget's disease to maintain sexual function: an imiquimod success story. *J Obstet Gynaecol*. 2009;29(3):252–254.
26. Hatch KD, Davis JR. Complete resolution of Paget disease of the vulva with imiquimod cream. *J Low Genit Tract Dis*. 2008;12(2):90–94.
27. Chen S, Nakahara T, Uchi H, et al. Immunohistochemical analysis of the mammalian target of rapamycin signalling pathway in extramammary Paget's disease. *Br J Dermatol*. 2009;161(2):357–363.
28. Tsujino Y, Mizumoto K, Matsuzaka Y, et al. Fluorescence navigation with indocyanine green for detecting sentinel nodes in extramammary Paget's disease and squamous cell carcinoma. *J Dermatol*. 2009;36(2):90–94.
29. Kim TH, Chang IH, Kim TH, et al. Extramammary Paget's disease of scrotum treated with radiotherapy. *Urology*. 2009;74(2):474 e1–3.
30. Ogawa Y, Ue H, Tsuzuki K, et al. New radiosensitization treatment (KORTUC I) using hydrogen peroxide solution-soaked gauze bolus for unresectable and superficially exposed neoplasms. *Oncol Rep*. 2008;19(6):1389–1394.

# Sarcomas of the Skin

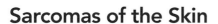

*Tawnya L. Bowles, Merrick I. Ross, and Alexander J. Lazar*

## Key Points

- Sarcomas of the skin comprise numerous rare entities that commonly present as nodules or plaques.
- Cutaneous sarcomas exhibit differentiation toward a variety of mesenchymal lineages.
- Dermatofibrosarcoma protuberans, atypical fibroxanthoma, and cutaneous leiomyosarcoma are the most common types.
- Diagnosis is aided by key immunohistochemical, cytogenetic, and molecular diagnostic studies.
- Complete surgical extirpation is the mainstay of therapy.
- Radiotherapy is used as adjuvant therapy in select patients; chemotherapy plays a limited role.

## INTRODUCTION

Sarcomas of the skin are a heterogeneous group of non-epithelial primary skin neoplasms. These rare tumors are composed of neoplastic spindle, round, or epithelioid cells that exhibit mesenchymal differentiation. Cutaneous sarcomas are histologically classified according to the mature cell type they resemble, including smooth muscle cells, adipocytes, vascular endothelial cells, skeletal muscle cells, fibroblasts, chondrocytes, osteocytes, and Schwann cells, among other cell types (Table 15.1). Cutaneous sarcomas have a different biologic behavior than their subfascial counterparts, and are generally associated with a better prognosis. While cutaneous sarcomas represent a large group of pathologically diverse tumors, there are common themes in the clinical presentation, diagnosis, and treatment. In addition to a general discussion on the management of cutaneous sarcomas, this chapter includes clinicopathologic descriptions of several of the more common subtypes, including dermatofibrosarcoma protuberans (DFSP), atypical fibroxanthoma (AFX), and superficial leiomyosarcoma (SLMS). Other rare tumor types receive more limited discussion. Some sarcomas arsing within the subcutis are also included in this chapter. While these sarcomas are not technically skin sarcomas, they present as superficial tumors that can involve the overlying skin and often exhibit a biologic behavior that should be distinguished from their subfascial counterparts. Kaposi sarcoma, a tumor of vascular origin associated with human herpesvirus-8 infection, is discussed separately in Chapter 16. Additional vascular neoplasms, such as angiosarcoma and epithelioid hemangiomaendothelioma, are discussed in Chapter 18.

## HISTORY

Modern concepts of cutaneous sarcomas emerged gradually from small case series and have further evolved with the development of special techniques such as electron microscopy, immunohistochemistry, cytogenetics, and molecular biology. In 1924, Darier and Ferrand recognized the high local recurrence rate of the tumor now known as DFSP. AFX, first described by Helwig in 1961, shows some histologic features of undifferentiated pleomorphic sarcoma/malignant fibrous histiocytoma, but is pathogenically distinct and has a much better clinical outcome.[1] While generally characterized by a benign course, case reports later described the metastatic potential of AFX.[2] SLMS was originally described in 1958 by Stout and Hill.[3] While subcutaneous and visceral leiomyosarcoma are known for their metastatic potential, cutaneous leiomyosarcomas have a much lower rate of metastatic potential and are, therefore, considered a separate entity.[4]

## EPIDEMIOLOGY

Sarcomas of the skin are rare. Melanoma, carcinomas, and benign mesenchymal skin tumors are much more commonly found than cutaneous sarcomas.[5] Because of their rarity, national cancer registries do not typically report cutaneous sarcomas as a separate category.

Cutaneous sarcomas are variously categorized as 'non-melanoma skin cancer', 'sarcoma', or 'miscellaneous tumors'. When categorized as 'non-melanoma skin cancer', the relatively uncommon primary cutaneous sarcomas are overshadowed even by relatively unusual cutaneous carcinomas such as Merkel cell carcinoma. Similarly, the more common subfascial sarcomas represent the majority of cases categorized as 'sarcomas'. Histologic information for the more common cutaneous sarcomas is available through the Surveillance, Epidemiology, and End Results (SEER) Program of the National Cancer Institute. A SEER review of more than 12,000 patients with cutaneous sarcoma[6] published in 2008 included more than 8500 cases of Kaposi sarcoma. Of the approximately 3500 remaining cutaneous sarcomas, DFSP was the most common type, with an incidence of 4.5 per 1 million persons, followed by cutaneous undifferentiated pleomorphic sarcoma/malignant fibrous histiocytoma (UPS/MFH) (1.5 per 1 million persons), SLMS (0.6 per 1 million persons) and cutaneous angiosarcoma (0.4 per 1 million persons). These four diagnostic categories accounted for approximately 95% of reported cases after

## Table 15.1 Sarcomas Found in or Close to the Skin

| Histologic Type | |
|---|---|
| Adipocytic | Liposarcoma<br>　Well differentiated (atypical lipomatous tumor)<br>　Dedifferentiated<br>　Myxoid and round cell<br>　Pleomorphic |
| Fibroblastic/<br>myofibroblastic | Dermatofibrosarcoma protuberans<br>Desmoid fibromatosis<br>Atypical fibroxanthoma (AFX)<br>Acral myxoinflammatory fibroblastic sarcoma<br>Infantile or congenital fibrosarcoma<br>Low-grade fibromyxoid sarcoma<br>Undifferentiated pleomorphic sarcoma/ malignant fibrous histiocytoma (UPS/MFH) |
| Smooth or skeletal muscle | Superficial leiomyosarcoma (SLMS)<br>Myoepithelial carcinoma<br>Rhabdomyosarcoma<br>　Alveolar<br>　Embryonal |
| Vascular origin* | Kaposi sarcoma†<br>Angiosarcoma (vasoformative and epithelioid)<br>Epithelioid hemangioendothelioma<br>Atypical vascular lesions |
| Uncertain differentiation | Pleomorphic hyalinizing angioectatic tumor<br>Clear cell sarcoma (melanoma of soft parts)<br>Epithelioid sarcoma<br>Ewing sarcoma<br>Synovial sarcoma |
| Other | Sarcoma metastatic to skin<br>(e.g. leiomyosarcoma to scalp) |

*Discussed in Chapter 18.

†Discussed in Chapter 16.

This list is not comprehensive for all sarcomas, but includes sarcomas described as occurring as primary lesions in the skin or subcutis or extending to involve these.

excluding Kaposi sarcoma. Gender distributions indicated that most cutaneous sarcomas other than DFSP were more common in men, and, overall, blacks had a higher incidence of most sarcomas than did whites or Asians.

Of note, the histologic classification of MFH has evolved over time. AFX was originally described as a superficial variant of MFH. Currently most soft tissue pathologists conceptualize AFX and UPS/MFH as separate entities, as discussed further below. AFX is not reportable for SEER databases.

## PATHOGENESIS AND ETIOLOGY

Cutaneous sarcomas typically arise spontaneously without a clear etiology. Ultraviolet (UV) radiation has been associated with development of AFX,[7] and therapeutic irradiation predisposes to DFSP. Cutaneous trauma, in the form of burns, venous stasis ulcers, insect bites, and even tattoos, has been anecdotally associated with SLMS.[3]

Genetic alterations in cutaneous sarcomas have been characterized. Two broad genetic classes of sarcomas are recognized. The first group has simple cytogenetic features as assessed by a traditional karyotype and is associated with a characteristic chromosomal translocation that is usually balanced or a characteristic gene mutation. The second group has complex cytogenetic features and lack known characteristic mutations; aberrations in the telomerase pathway are common. These distinctions hold true for deep, subfascial sarcomas, but there is less cytogenetic information on cutaneous tumors since they are not commonly analyzed in this fashion. Nonetheless, tumors such as DFSP represent the first class with a characteristic translocation between chromosomes 17 and 22 that results in overexpression from the platelet-derived growth factor-β gene ($PDGF\beta$).[8]

Another example is clear cell sarcoma, which can be differentiated from melanoma by identification of a reciprocal translocation between chromosomes 12 and 22 that results in fusion of the Ewing sarcoma region 1 gene ($EWSR1$) and activating transcription factor 1 ($ATF1$) genes.[9] Translocations and mutations characteristic of particular tumor types are listed in Table 15.2.

Other examples of molecular derangements driving tumorigenesis include amplification of the 1213~15 locus involving the $MDM2$ gene and others in well-differentiated liposarcoma, and point mutations in $CTNNB1$, the gene encoding β-catenin, in desmoid tumors. These two tumors are usually subfascial and large, but can involve the skin from time to time and are mentioned more for illustration of possible molecular mechanisms.

$p53$ is mutated with loss of function in sarcomas and many other tumors, usually during tumor progression. Its importance in this process is underscored by the many varieties of tumors encountered in Li–Fraumeni syndrome, where one non-functional copy of this gene is inherited with subsequent somatic loss of heterozygosity associated with the tumors encountered in these patients. Characteristic $p53$ mutations have also been associated with UV radiation and the development of AFX tumors, as discussed in detail in the AFX section below.

## GENERAL PRINCIPLES OF NATURAL HISTORY AND DIAGNOSIS

### Natural history

Cutaneous sarcomas typically have a good prognosis, with some propensity for local recurrence but limited metastatic potential, with several exceptions. Epithelioid sarcoma is particularly aggressive, even when superficial. Patients can rapidly develop regional lymph node involvement and distant bony or pulmonary metastases, often within 1 year of the initial diagnosis. In addition, clear cell sarcoma (melanoma of soft parts) resembles malignant melanoma in the propensity to involve lymph nodes prior to giving rise to distant metastases. Very unlike most other sarcomas, these two metastasize early to lymph nodes while most sarcomas bypass lymphoid tissue and involve lung or other distant organ sites as the initial site of metastasis via a hematogenous route. However, as noted above, more superficially located sarcomas tend to be less associated with metastatic behavior, possibly due to their superficial location, but perhaps also because they tend to be of smaller size. The specific histologic types seen in the skin, such as DFSP, are also generally less likely to metastasize.

**Table 15.2 Genetic Alterations of Sarcomas that May Present in the Skin**

| Histologic Type | Genetic Alteration | Involved Gene(s) |
|---|---|---|
| Alveolar rhabdomyosarcoma | t(2;13)(q35;q14)<br>t(1;13)(p36;q14), double minutes<br>t(2;2)(q35;p23)<br>t(X;2)(q35;q13) | PAX3-FOXO1A fusion<br>PAX7-FOXO1A fusion<br>PAX3-NCOA1<br>PAX3-AFX |
| Alveolar soft part sarcoma | t(X;17)(p11;q25) | TFE3-ASPSCR1 fusion |
| Angiomatoid fibrous histiocytoma | t(12;16)(q13;p11)<br>t(12;22)(q13;q12)<br>t(2;22)(q33;q12) | FUS-ATF1 fusion<br>EWSR1-ATF1 fusion<br>EWSR1-CREB1 fusion |
| Atypical fibroxanthoma | C to T transitions<br>C to G transversions | P53 |
| Clear cell sarcoma (melanoma of soft parts) | t(12;22)(q13;q12)<br>t(2;22)(q34;q12) | EWSR1-ATF1 fusion<br>EWSR1-CREB1 fusion |
| Dermatofibrosarcoma protuberans | t(17;22)(q22;q13)<br>Ring form of chromosomes 17 and 22 | COL1A1-PDGFβ fusion<br>COL1A1-PDGFβ fusion |
| Desmoid fibromatosis | Point mutations in β-catenin gene | CTNNB1 |
| Desmoplastic small round cell tumor | t(11;22)(p13;q12) | EWSR1-WT1 fusion |
| Endometrial stromal sarcoma | t(7;17)(p15;q21)<br>t(6;7)(p21;7p15)<br>t(6;10)(p21;p11) | JAZF1-JJAZ1 fusion<br>JAZF1-PHF1 fusion<br>EPC1-PHF1 fusion |
| Epithelioid sarcoma | Loss of heterozygosity (22q11) | INI1 loss |
| Ewing sarcoma/PNET | t(11;22)(q24;q12)<br>t(21;22)(q12;q12)<br>t(2;22)(q33;q12)<br>t(7;22)(p22;q12)<br>t(17;22)(q12;q12)<br>inv(22)(q12q12)<br>t(16;21)(p11;q22) | EWSR1-FLI1 fusion<br>EWSR1-ERG fusion<br>EWSR1-FEV fusion<br>EWSR1-ETV1 fusion<br>EWSR1-E1AF fusion<br>EWSR1-ZSG<br>FUS-ERG |
| Extraskeletal myxoid chondrosarcoma | t(9;22)(q22;q12)<br>t(9;17)(q22;q11)<br>t(9;15)(q22;q21)<br>t(3;9)(q11;q22) | EWSR1-NR4A3 fusion<br>TAF2N-NR4A3 fusion<br>TCF12-NR4A3 fusion<br>TFG-NR4A3 fusion |
| Infantile fibrosarcoma | t(12;15)(p13;q26) | ETV6-NTRK3 fusion |
| Inflammatory myofibroblastic tumor | t(1;2)(q22;p23)<br>t(2;19)(p23;p13)<br>t(2;17)(p23;q23)<br>t(2;2)(p23;q13) | TPM3-ALK<br>TPM4-ALK<br>CLTC-ALK<br>RANB2-ALK |
| Low-grade fibromyxoid sarcoma | t(7;16)(q33;p11)<br>t(11;16)(p11;p11) | FUS-CREB3L2 fusion<br>FUS-CREB3L1 fusion |
| Myxoid/round cell liposarcoma | t(12;16)(q13;p11)<br>t(12;22)(q13;q12) | FUS-DDIT3 fusion<br>EWSR1-DDIT3 fusion |
| Synovial sarcoma | t(X;18)(p11;q11)<br>t(X;18)(p11;q11) | Predominantly SS18-SSX1 fusion<br>SS18-SSX1, SSX2 or SSX4 fusion |
| Well-differentiated liposarcoma | Amplification of 12q13~15 locus | MDM2, CDK4 and others |

## Biopsy technique

Biopsy is absolutely necessary to establish a new diagnosis of cutaneous sarcoma. A representative specimen should be obtained. Evaluation of a small biopsy specimen may be non-diagnostic or indeterminate. Punch or elliptic excisional biopsies are commonly employed. A high clinical suspicion should prompt re-biopsy if pathologic findings are discordant with the clinical impression. If an incisional biopsy is planned, the orientation of the incision should be carefully planned so as to be easily encompassed by the subsequent therapeutic excision.

## Histopathologic diagnosis

In order to differentiate among the various cutaneous sarcomas, a thorough knowledge of the classic histopathologic features and common variant patterns is essential.

**159**

Supportive immunohistochemical (IHC) studies are essential in the great majority of cases, because the differential diagnosis often includes biologically diverse tumors of epithelial, melanocytic, and lymphoid differentiation. Almost no IHC marker is entirely sensitive or specific. It is essential to interpret the results of a well-chosen panel of markers in the context of all available clinical and histopathologic data. Molecular testing, when applicable, can be extremely helpful in the settings of uncommon clinical scenarios or unusual histologic features (see Table 15.2 for listing).

Concerning hypercellularity can be seen in reactive conditions such as nodular fasciitis, perhaps the most common benign soft tissue tumor misdiagnosed as sarcoma. Nodular fasciitis is associated with sudden rapid onset, usually good circumscription, histologic similarity to cells in tissue culture, and variably fibrous or myxoid stroma. Nodular lesions of verruga peruana, the cutaneous manifestation of *Bartonella bacilliformis* infection, are proliferations of hypercellular epithelioid and spindle cells that sometimes resemble Kaposi sarcoma, leiomyosarcoma, fibrosarcoma, or spindle cell melanoma. Consideration of an infectious rather than a neoplastic etiology is based on the clinical presentation of miliary or nodular angiomatous lesions in a patient from endemic regions of Peru, Ecuador, or Colombia. Of note, the mere presence of histologically "sarcomatous" elements in a tumor does not necessarily point to a diagnosis of sarcoma. Such elements can occur focally in primary cutaneous malignancies such as melanoma, squamous cell carcinoma, basal cell carcinoma, Merkel cell carcinoma, and various adnexal carcinomas. In addition, sarcoma in the skin is occasionally metastatic from deeper primary tumors, most commonly from leiomyosarcoma of the uterus or to a lesser degree from other sites with additional histologies. Usually these are late events in disease progression and thus clinical history will help establish the diagnosis.

## Electron microscopy

Although IHC studies now provide much information regarding cellular differentiation, this was formerly the domain of electron microscopy. Electron microscopy remains a useful modality in selected cases. For example, electron microscopy can sometimes provide clues as to the differentiation of very poorly differentiated neoplasms that have lost expected IHC markers. However, currently this technique is only very rarely employed in most centers.

## Other advanced techniques: cytogenetics, in-situ hybridization, and RT-PCR

A number of subfascial sarcomas are associated with characteristic cytogenetic abnormalities that are readily identified on G-banded karyotypes prepared from short-term cell cultures (Table 15.2). This requires procurement of fresh tissue with prompt transport to a specialized cytogenetics laboratory. Cytogenetic evaluation can be employed with larger cutaneous sarcomas when a portion of the tumor can be spared and devoted to establishing a short-term cell culture. In smaller cutaneous tumors, there may not be sufficient neoplastic tissue for such studies.

When fresh tissue is not available, fluorescence in-situ hybridization (FISH) techniques can be employed on archival paraffin-embedded tissue to search for specific locus re-arrangements, such as those involving the *EWSR1* locus at 22q12 in Ewing family tumors, clear cell sarcoma, and other deep sarcomas.

Reverse transcription polymerase chain reaction (RT-PCR) can also be used to demonstrate a specific fusion transcript such as the *EWSR1–ATF1* resulting from the balanced translocation t(12;22)(q13;q2) in clear cell sarcoma. This technique can be used for fresh, frozen and archival formalin-fixed material as well, though the success yield drops considerably in archival cases older than 5 years. In comparison, since FISH relies on DNA as the analyte rather than RNA for RT-PCR, the former technique is often more robust in older or less well-preserved tissues.

## CLINICOPATHOLOGIC FEATURES OF SPECIFIC TYPES OF CUTANEOUS SARCOMAS

## Dermatofibrosarcoma protuberans

### Clinical features

DFSP is a low-grade sarcoma, apparently showing fibroblastic differentiation, that presents as a nodular, cutaneous mass on the trunk or extremities that is slow-growing and rarely metastasizes unless it shows fibrosarcomatous ("higher grade") differentiation. The head and neck is a less common site. Over time, the tumor takes on a characteristic protuberant appearance that may have one or more nodules (Fig. 15.1). Tumors may be flesh-colored or show a pink or violet-red coloration. DFSP typically affects adults in middle to later life, but has also been described in infants and children. Men and women are affected equally. Unusual presentations include the depressed indurated plaque of non-protuberant ('atrophic') DFSP and pedunculated lesions that closely simulate neurofibromas or fibroepithelial polyps. While regional and distant metastases are uncommon, local recurrence rates for DFSP in various reports range from 0% to 60%. The high propensity for

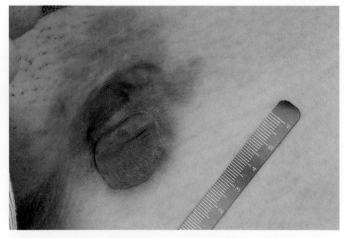

Figure 15.1 Dermatofibrosarcoma protuberans (DFSP) involving the groin of a young adult. (Image courtesy of Raphael Pollock MD/PhD, Department of Surgical Oncology, and Medical Graphics and Photography at M. D. Anderson Cancer Center, Houston, TX.)

local recurrence may be related to tumor growth into the subcutaneous tissue through finger-like extensions, which may preclude complete resection.

## Pathologic and radiologic diagnosis

Clinical suspicion is confirmed by biopsy. On histologic examination, classic DFSP is composed of relatively small, uniform spindle cells arranged at least focally in a distinctly storiform or whorled pattern (Fig. 15.2). Mitotic activity is usually low. DFSP tumors are diffusely positive for CD34 on IHC staining. This can help distinguish DFSP from dermatofibromas, which generally lack significant CD34 expression. Some find factor XIIIa helpful, as it is expressed by most dermatofibromas but is absent in DFSP. DFSP tumors are also negative for S100 protein, smooth muscle actin, desmin, keratins, and epithelial membrane antigen. A minority of tumors have areas of fibrosarcomatous differentiation (DFSP-FS). DFSP-FS is usually seen in larger tumors and seems to represent an aggressive form of tumor progression as its presence is associated with higher rates of local recurrence and acquisition of metastatic potential.[10] A pediatric form of DFSP with identical genetics is termed giant cell fibroblastoma and is characterized by the presence of multinucleate giant cells and angiectoid spaces. The spindle cell component is usually less cellular with a more fibrotic appearance; CD34 reactivity is retained. Hybrid lesions with classic DFSP are noted. Other histologic variants of DFSP include a myxoid variant, which can complicate recognition on small biopsy. While usually not necessary for diagnosis, both FISH and RT-PCR methods are available to detect evidence of the marker or ring chromosomes containing a translocation t(17;22)(q22;q13) which brings the *PDGF-β* gene encoding the ligand platelet-derived growth factor-β under the control of the strong constitutive promotor COL1A1 encoding collagen type 1a1. This combination ultimately leads to intense overexpression of wild-type PDGF-β protein after proteolytic processing and the presence of this factor appears to drive the pathogenesis of this neoplasm (Fig. 15.3).

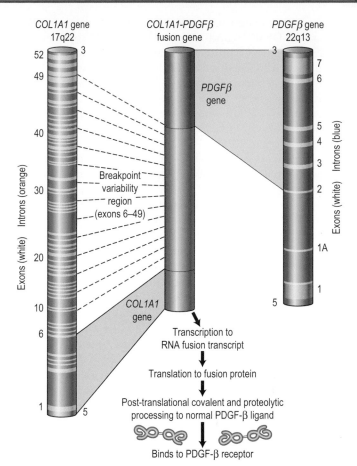

**Figure 15.3** Molecular pathogenesis of DFSP. A translocation between chromosomes 17 and 22 results in the creation of a fusion gene consisting of *COL1A1* and *PDGFβ*. The strong *COL1A1* promoter replaces the self-inhibitory *PDGFβ* promoter, causing upregulated transcription of the RNA fusion transcript. This is translated into a fusion protein that is proteolytically processed to produce normal PDGF-β which is secreted in an unregulated fashion. PDGF-β acts as a growth factor that stimulates tumor growth, but its interaction with PDGF receptors can be blocked by tyrosine kinase receptors with therapeutic efficacy in cases not amenable to surgical extirpation.

Radiographic imaging is not necessary in all cases but computed tomography (CT) or magnetic resonance imaging (MRI) may be useful in defining the subcutaneous extent of large or recurrent DFSP tumors, particularly in anatomically sensitive areas. DFSP demonstrates similar signal attenuation to that of skeletal muscle on CT and non-specifically prolonged T1 and T2 relaxation times on MRI.

## Treatment

The primary treatment of DFSP is surgical. The options for resection include traditional wide local excision, typically with 2–3 cm margins around the gross tumor and including the subcutaneous tissue and investing fascia, or Mohs micrographic surgery (MMS). The size and location of the tumor will dictate the most appropriate technique of resection. The presence of infiltrative tentacle-like extensions of tumor can make achieving a negative-margin resection difficult. Ensuring histologically negative margins while conserving tissue is critical, especially in aesthetically or functionally sensitive areas such as the face or distal extremities. Traditional wide local excision

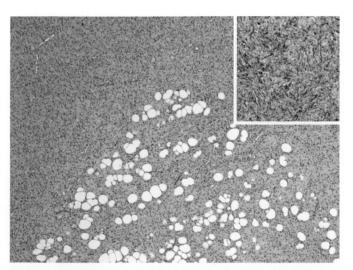

**Figure 15.2** DFSP is composed of spindle cells arranged in a storiform pattern that often infiltrate around individual adipose cells, as seen on H&E stain. Strong and diffuse reactivity for CD34 on immunohistochemistry is characteristic (inset).

has been associated with a local recurrence rate of 4–17% for classic DFSP[10,11] and 52% for DFSP-FS.[10] Proponents of MMS emphasize the tissue-sparing advantage of MMS in cosmetically sensitive areas. Studies of MMS for DFSP show a local recurrence rate of 0–6%.[12] However, these studies of MMS for DFSP are limited by lack of long-term follow-up and small sample size, and may preferentially include patients with smaller tumors and more limited disease.

Radiation therapy has been used as adjuvant treatment following surgical resection.[13] Postoperative radiation therapy should be considered for large tumors at high risk for local recurrence, in the setting of close or positive margins where further resection is not possible due to functional or cosmetic limitations, and for recurrent DFSP. Patients with DFSP who were deemed inoperable due to poor health status or unresectability of tumor have occasionally been treated successfully with radiation therapy as the only modality.[14]

While chemotherapy has traditionally played a minimal role in the treatment of DFSP, the discovery that DFSP tumors overexpress (PDGFβ) has opened the door for targeted therapy.[15] As discussed above, a chromsomal translocation [t(17:22)] drives overexpresssion of PDGFβ (Fig. 15.3). The fusion product, which retains growth factor activity, is overexpressed.[8] Imatinib mesylate, a protein tyrosine kinase inhibitor that inhibits PDGFRβ and other targets, has shown activity against localized and metastatic DFSP containing t(17:22).[15-17] Imatinib mesylate is approved by the Food and Drug Administration for the treatment of unresectable, recurrent, and metastatic DFSP. Clinical trials of imatinib mesylate as neoadjuvant treatment of DFSP are ongoing.

## Atypical fibroxanthoma

### Clinical features

Atypical fibroxanthoma (AFX) is a low-grade dermal neoplasm that commonly occurs as an ulcerated nodule on sun-damaged skin in the head and neck region of elderly individuals (Fig. 15.4).[1] It is rare outside of this clinical context. Men are affected more often than women.[18] Patients often have a history of other skin cancers, such as basal and squamous cell carcinoma, and the clinical appearance of AFX may resemble these more common skin cancers. The local recurrence rate for AFX is low (2–9%) and metastases are very uncommon.[2,19,20] AFX is histologically similar to other spindle cell neoplasms such as cutaneous malignant fibrous histiocytoma (MFH), and the pathologic distinction between the two has been controversial. Previous reports on the incidence of MFH most likely included tumors that are now recognized as AFX.[6]

AFX tumors typically form in skin exposed to UV radiation. The mechanism by which UV radiation can promote AFX tumor formation may be explained by specific mutations in the tumor suppressor gene *p53*. AFX tumors have been shown to harbor *p53* gene mutations, consisting of C to T transitions or C to G transversions, which are characteristic of UV-induced mutagenesis.[7] AFX has also been reported in immunosuppressed transplant-recipient patients.

### Pathologic diagnosis

Classic AFX is composed of haphazardly arranged, pleomorphic spindle and giant cells, often with a high mitotic rate and many abnormal mitotic figures (Fig. 15.5). Strictly defined, AFX should be confined to the dermis and has virtually no metastatic potential. Lesions histologically identical to AFX which involve the subcutis gain an increased likelihood of local recurrence and acquire some limited metastatic potential. In recognition of this, these tumors are termed unclassified dermal sarcoma by some, but as this tumor does not clearly share pathogenic features of undifferentiated pleomorphic sarcoma/malignant fibrous histiocytoma (UPS/MFH), it is no longer considered within this spectrum by many authorities. Regardless of this shift in nomenclature and conceptualization, the important issue is that AFX is defined by confinement to the dermis and basically lacks metastatic potential, while AFX-like tumors involving the subcutis acquire some metastatic potential and warrant closer follow-up.

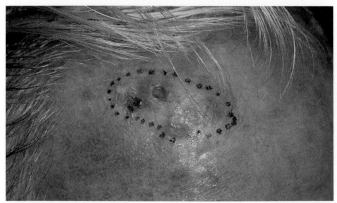

**Figure 15.4** Atypical fibroxanthoma on the forehead of an elderly male patient. Clinically, this tumor was a group of papules merging to a plaque involving sun-damaged skin. (Image courtesy of Val Thomas MD, Department of Dermatology, M. D. Anderson Cancer Center, Houston, TX.)

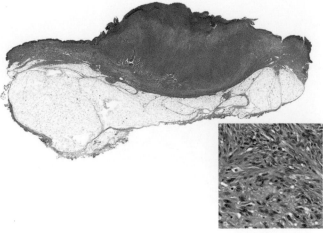

**Figure 15.5** An H&E low-power view of this atypical fibroxanthoma shows a papular to nodular lesion with extensive ulceration. At higher power, the lesion is composed of pleomorphic spindle cells (inset).

On immunohistochemical analysis, AFX is a diagnosis of exclusion. The most important exclusion is melanoma, but spindle cell squamous cell carcinoma and leiomyosarcoma can also be included in the differential diagnosis. AFX tumors are negative for S100 protein, cytokeratins, and desmin, differentiating it from melanoma, squamous cell carcinoma, and leiomyosarcoma, respectively. Numerous reports have suggested stains to be specific for AFX and differentiate it from other potential mimics, but none of these have proper specificity.

## Treatment

Surgical excision is the primary treatment for AFX. Wide local excision with 2 cm margins of normal tissue with resection down to and including the investing fascia is generally recommended. MMS has also been advocated for AFX tumor resection, particularly when tissue conservation is of primary concern. As with DFSP, these studies are limited by small sample size and short length of follow-up, but advocates suggest the local recurrence rate in MMS is equivalent to or lower than that for traditional wide local excision.

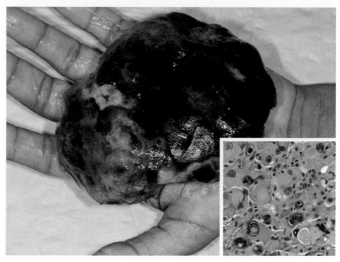

**Figure 15.6** A dramatic presentation of undifferentiated pleomorphic sarcoma/malignant fibrous histiocytoma (UPS/MFH) involving the palmar hand of an adult patient. Extreme nuclear pleomorphism can be encountered (H&E, inset). (Clinical image courtesy of Raphael Pollock MD/PhD, Department of Surgical Oncology, and Medical Graphics and Photography, M. D. Anderson Cancer Center, Houston, TX.)

## Undifferentiated pleomorphic sarcoma/ malignant fibrous histiocytoma

### Clinical features

Undifferentiated pleomorphic sarcoma (UPS) is the term recommended in the 2002 World Health Organization (WHO) classification for the tumor known historically as malignant fibrous histiocytoma (MFH). UPS is a pleomorphic spindle cell neoplasm and the subfascial form was previously regarded as the most common soft tissue sarcoma in adults. The morphologic pattern historically considered to be MFH is now known to be shared by a variety of poorly differentiated sarcomas that can be classified into separate categories using modern methodologies such as immunohistochemistry and molecular diagnostics.[21] UPS/MFH is currently considered a diagnosis of exclusion and accounts for no more than 5% of adult soft tissue sarcomas. In addition, AFX, as discussed above, is a distinct pathologic diagnosis that may have previously been considered as superficial MFH.

UPS/MFH most commonly arise from subfascial soft tissues; less than 10% are primarily in the subcutaneous tissue.[22] While the overlying skin may be involved, these tumors rarely arise in the skin, but are included as part of this discussion because of their superficial presentation and different biologic behavior than the more common subfacial type. On examination, subcutaneous UPS/ MFH most commonly presents as a subcutaneous mass or ulcerated nodule on the extremity of elderly adults (Fig. 15.6). While the pathogenesis of UPS/MFS is not fully understood, tumors have been reported in scar tissue from surgical sites and sometimes in burn scars. Cases have also been reported in immunosuppressed patients with HIV or after organ transplantation.

UPS/MFH is regarded as an aggressive sarcoma with significant metastatic potential, although the subfascial tumors have a greater propensity for metastases than subcutaneous tumors.[22] A metastatic rate of 17% was reported for subcutaneous MFH, compared to 29% for subfascial MFH, in one series. Local recurrence ranges from 17% to 40% with standard wide local excision.[22]

### Pathologic diagnosis

UPS/MFH is a diagnosis of exclusion. MFH-like tumors are a heterogeneous group that have in common cytologic and nuclear pleomorphism, spindle cells, and histiocyte-like cells characterized by foamy cytoplasm (Fig. 15.7). A solid mass composed of spindle and pleomorphic cells is characteristic. A superfical form has been described where tumor involves primarily fibrous septa and is highly infiltrative. This form may have an increased propensity for local recurrence.

UPS/MFH has no specific immunohistochemical profile and this is thus a diagnosis of exclusion. Important exclusions include spindle cell carcinoma, melanoma, and leiomyosarcoma.

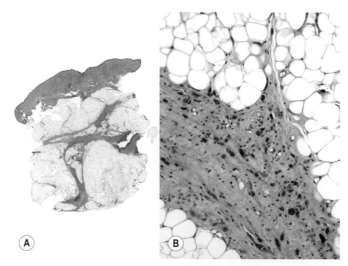

**Figure 15.7** The superficial form of undifferentiated pleomorphic sarcoma/malignant fibrous histiocytoma (UPS/MFH) can show extensive involvement of fibrous septa that can complicate local excision (H&E stain, **A**). A higher power image shows that the widened septa are colonized by pleomorphic tumor cells (**B**).

## Treatment

Surgical resection by wide local excision is the mainstay of treatment for this neoplasm. Some have advocated MMS for subcutaneous UPS/MFH, citing reduced local recurrence, but many of these tumors are large and better handled by a traditional surgical approach. Postoperative radiation therapy may be used to reduce local recurrence.[23] Patients require diligent surveillance for development of recurrent or metastatic disease.

## Acral myxoinflammatory fibroblastic sarcoma

### Clinical features

Acral myxoinflammatory fibroblastic sarcoma (AMFS) is a rare, low-grade neoplasm that most commonly presents as a painless nodule of the distal extremities in a middle-aged patient.[24] The tumor is poorly circumscribed and, due to its common location and appearance, can be mistaken for ganglion cyst, tenosynovitis, or giant cell tumor of the tendon sheath. Local recurrence is common, with a reported incidence up to 67%.[24] Metastases are uncommon but reported.[24]

### Pathologic and radiographic diagnosis

On histopathologic review, AMFS is characterized by a predominant inflammatory infiltrate with a complex mix of epithelioid, spindle, and Reed–Sternberg-like cells in a fibrosclerotic/myxoid stroma. The tumor may be confined to the dermis or extend into the subcutaneous tissue. Prominent nuclear atypia, other than the Reed–Sternberg-like cells, is uncommon, and mitotic figures are infrequent.[25] Tumors are variably immunoreactive to CD68 and CD34, and rarely reactive to smooth muscle actin. Important negative markers include CD30, leukocyte common antigen, and T- and B-cell markers to exclude hematopoietic malignancies.[21]

Radiographic imaging is sometimes utilized to determine the subcutaneous extent of the tumor. On MRI, AMFS resemble benign cysts with a low intensity on T1-weighted images and a high intensity on T2-weighted images. MRI is, therefore, unlikely to discriminate between benign entities and AMFS.

### Treatment

Resection by wide local excision with histologically negative margins is recommended. While adjuvant radiotherapy and chemotherapy have been anecdotally reported,[24] long-term results in a large sample of patients are lacking and the low risk of metastatic behavior should be taken into account.

## Superficial leiomyosarcoma

### Clinical features

Superficial leiomyosarcoma (SLMS) is a malignant neoplasm showing smooth muscle differentiation that originates in the dermis and appears as a small (typically less than 3 cm), firm, tender nodule with a predilection for the extremities and scalp. Tumors may also arise on the trunk.

The clinical appearance is often nondescript and prone to misdiagnosis as a benign tumor such as an epidermoid cyst. SLMS are more common in men than women and typically occur in the sixth decade of life. SLMS are very rare malignancies, with a reported incidence of 0.6 per 1,000,000 persons.[6] Compared to the more common visceral leiomyosarcomas, SLMS that are confined to the dermis have a better prognosis and rarely, if ever, metastasize.[4,26] Like other cutaneous sarcomas, SLMS can recur locally, at a rate of 14–40%.[4] SLMS that arise from within or show extensive growth into the subcutis resemble soft tissue leiomyosarcomas in biologic behavior and result in metastases in 30–40% of patients.[4]

### Diagnosis

SLMS is characterized pathologically as dermal lesions with variable subcutaneous extensions. Bundles of elongated, spindle-shaped cells are observed. Two growth patterns have been described: nodular and diffuse.[5] The nodular pattern is characterized by a cellular background with nuclear atypia and frequent mitotic figures. The diffuse pattern is less cellular and mitotic figures are rare.

On IHC evaluation, SLMS tumors stain positively for smooth muscle actin (SMA) and desmin. The latter stain is the most specific for smooth muscle differentiation as SMA is noted in multiple spindle cell proliferations. An important pitfall is that SLMS can express cytokeratins. S100 protein is generally negative.

### Treatment

Surgical resection is the primary treatment for SLMS. Due to the rarity of the tumor, the minimum resection margin is not known, but general recommendations are for resection with a 2–3 cm margin around the gross tumor with deep resection including the subcutaneous tissue and investing fascia. MMS has also been used, with favorable recurrence rates noted, although sample sizes in the available studies have been small.[27] No role has been established for the use of radiation therapy or chemotherapy in SLMS.

## Clear cell sarcoma of soft tissue (melanoma of soft parts)

### Clinical features

Clear cell sarcoma of soft tissue (CCS), also known as malignant melanoma of soft parts, is a sarcoma with melanocytic differentiation that typically presents in young adults as a small to mid-sized (<6 cm), slow-growing extremity mass, with 40% of tumors located on the foot or ankle (Fig. 15.8).[21,28] Tumors are often associated with tendons or aponeuroses but can extend into the subcutaneous tissue and lower dermis. CCS can rarely involve the viscera, retroperitoneum, and bone.

CCS has morphologic similarities to malignant melanoma, but has distinct genetic features (Fig. 15.9). Cytogenetic analysis of CCS has demonstrated a characteristic reciprocal chromosomal translocation [t(12;22)(q13;q12)][9] that results in fusion of the Ewing sarcoma region 1 (EWSR1) gene with activating transcription factor 1 (ATF1).[29] A less common translocation, [t(2;22)(q34;q12)],

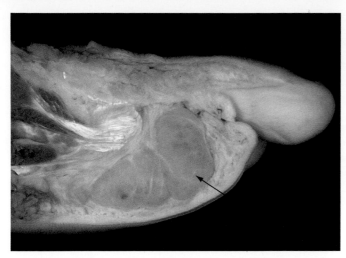

**Figure 15.8** Clear cell sarcoma characteristically involves the deep fascial planes, as in this sagittal section of the foot from an amputation, but these tumors can be more superficial on rare occasion. (Image courtesy of Heinz-Herbert Homann MD, University of Ruhr, Bochum, Germany.)

results in fusion of *EWSR1* to the ATF1 homolog cyclic adenosine monophosphate responsive element binding protein 1 (*CREB1*).[30]

Local recurrence rates for CCS range from 14% to 23%[31] and lymph node metastases occur in 12% to 43% of patients.[31-33] Distant metastases have been documented in 13% of patients identified through the SEER database.[32] Due to the propensity of CCS to metastasize to lymph nodes and distant sites, the 5-year overall survival rates range from 40% to 68%. Blazer et al.[32] found that disease stage, truncal tumor site, and non-Caucasian ethnicity were predictors of decreased disease-specific survival in patients with CCS.

## Pathologic diagnosis

CCS is composed of nests of spindle-shaped or polygonal cells with eosinophilic or clear cytoplasm delineated by fibrous septa. The mitotic rate is low and the nuclei have a prominent nucleolus. Tumors show strong staining for S100 protein, HMB45, and other melanocytic antigens. On specific histochemical staining, melanin pigment can sometimes be visualized.

## Treatment

Surgical resection by wide local excision is the primary treatment. Evaluation of regional lymph node basins and consideration for lymphadenectomy is advocated, due to the propensity of CCS to metastasize to lymph nodes. While sentinel lymph node biopsy is commonly used in malignant melanoma, its role in CCS has yet to be defined. Chemotherapy treatments, most commonly platinum-based regimens, have been used but show limited benefit.[33] Targeted therapies based on MET expression induced by the characteristic fusion protein are currently being evaluated.

## Pleomorphic hylanizing angiectatic tumor

### Clinical features

Pleomorphic hylanizing angiectatic tumor (PHAT) is a low-grade, slow-growing tumor of uncertain differentiation that typically arises in the subcutaneous tissue on the lower extremities of adults.[21] Tumors have also been noted on the arms, buttocks, and chest wall. Men and women are affected equally. PHAT tends to recur locally (>50% incidence) but no metastases have been reported.

PHAT was recognized by Smith et al. in 1996 and several case reports and small series of patients have since been reported.[34,35] Prior to 1996, tumors were often misdiagnosed as schwannoma or low-grade MFH. In addition, PHAT, considered a benign tumor, can be confused with myxofibrosarcoma, a common malignant sarcoma with metastatic potential.

### Pathologic diagnosis

PHAT is a pleomorphic tumor characterized by thin-walled dilated vessels and significant perivascular hyalinization. Significant atypia is present but mitotic figures are rare. A variable inflammatory component is also noted. The degree of atypia may resemble MFH, but PHAT can be differentiated by intranuclear cytoplasmic inclusions, the scarcity of mitotic figures, and variable reactivity to CD34.[34] The ectatic vessels of PHAT resemble those identified in schwannomas, but PHAT lacks encapsulation and is negative for S100 protein on IHC.

### Treatment

Surgical resection by wide local excision is recommended. No role for radiotherapy or chemotherapy has been established.

## OTHER SARCOMAS IN THE SKIN

A variety of other sarcomas can present primarily in the skin or superficial subcutis, including Ewing sarcoma (Fig. 15.10), alveolar rhabdomyosarcoma, and atypical lipomatous tumor/well-differentiated liposarcoma, to name a few. When such cases are encountered, it is best to apply multiple diagnostic modalities – including molecular diagnostic testing, if relevant – to confirm the diagnosis, since they are rare.

Metastases can occur from subfascial sarcomas to the skin. In a subset of cases, skin can be the initial metastatic event, but this is rare. More often, skin metastases are a late event in sarcoma progression and herald a very poor prognosis. In our experience, sarcoma skin metastases are seen in fewer than 1 in 400 patients, with subfascial leiomyosarcoma being the most common source, accounting for approximately 40% of sarcoma metastases to the skin. The head and neck region, specifically the scalp, is the most frequent site of skin metastasis. Since the scalp is a common site of primary dermal SLMS, the possibility of metastasis should be considered. However, careful clinical correlation will most often solve this problem.

## SURVEILLANCE

In patients with a history of cutaneous sarcoma, surveillance to detect local recurrence or metastases is recommended. In general, most experts recommend close follow-up in the first 5 years after diagnosis and treatment. Surveillance primarily consists of a thorough physical examination, including a head-to-toe skin examination with a low threshold for

**Figure 15.9** Detection of gene rearrangements and fusion transcripts in clear cell sarcoma. The *ATF1/EWSR1* fusion gene is formed by a reciprocal translocation involving chromosomes 12 and 22 **(A).** Fluorescence in-situ hybridization (FISH) probes to the centromeric (red) and telomeric (green) DNA flanking region of the *EWSR1* locus can be used to detect this event. The spectral overlap of the two probes produces a yellow signal when juxtaposed. With *EWSR1* rearrangement, separate nuclear signals are discerned. In panel **B,** the pattern of fluorescent signals is illustrated for a cell lacking a translocation (left) and with a rearrangement of the *EWSR1* locus (right). There is a diagram (circle) followed by an actual DAPI-stained nucleus (square). PCR amplification of reverse-transcribed tumor RNA can be used to detect a specific fusion transcript. A type 1 fusion is shown on gel electrophoresis with confirmation by Sanger sequencing **(C).** Molecular diagnostic techniques can be very helpful in unusual cases. Abbreviations: der, derivative chromosome; M, size marking standards.

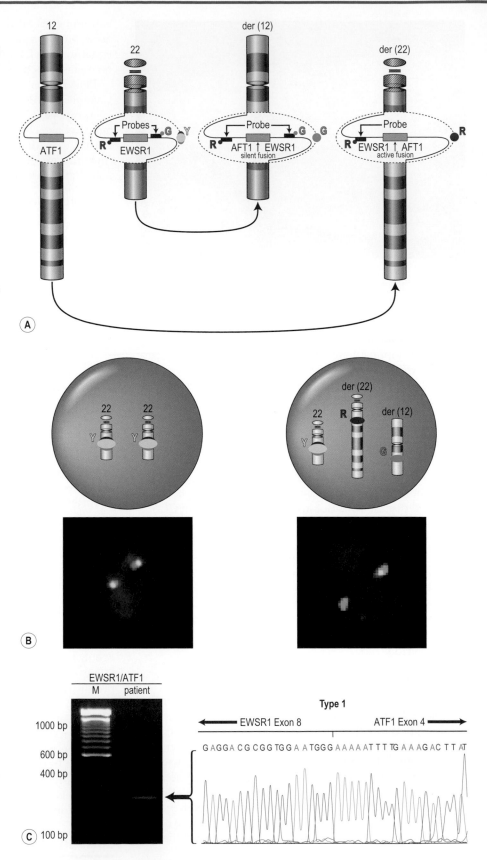

biopsy of suspicious lesions. This is often supplemented by radiography of pulmonary fields or other areas, based on the degree of risk of the intial lesion and the natural history of the particular diagnosis. Other than epithelioid sarcoma, most of the superficial sarcomas have limited metastatic potential, as discussed above. In the case of the primarily subfascial sarcomas that present superficially on rare occasion, these appear to be usually less aggressive than their deep conterparts but there are generally not large series to support a specific approach. The management of these complex cases is probably best performed in large referral centers with extensive multidisciplinary expertise.

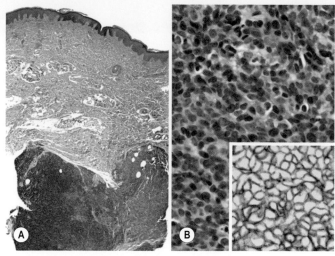

**Figure 15.10** Rare case of primary cutaneous Ewing sarcoma involving the dermis (H&E, **A**). Higher power reveals a small round blue cell neoplasm (H&E, **B**), with characteristic membrane accentuation of CD99 reactivity seen on immunohistochemistry (**B,** inset).

## FUTURE OUTLOOK

Much of what is known about cutaneous sarcomas is based on case reports and relatively small series. More accurate epidemiological data regarding the incidence and mortality of this category of skin cancer will require greater attention from regional and national cancer registries. A more complete understanding of the natural behavior and a more rigorous assessment of different treatment approaches would probably benefit from cooperative multicenter studies. This would be especially helpful in characterizing the rarest entities.

The advent of modern biological therapies, such as imatinib mesylate, holds out the promise of pharmacological agents targeted at specific molecules expressed by tumor cells, and eventually such agents could prove to be useful adjuncts or even primary therapies for these tumors. In the meantime, complete surgical excision will likely remain the mainstay of therapy for the foreseeable future.

## ACKNOWLEDGEMENT

David R. Guillén and Clay J Cockerell are thanked for their work on the previous version of this chapter.

## REFERENCES

1. Helwig EB. Atypical fibroxanthoma. In: Tumor Seminar Proceedings of 18th Annual Tumor Seminar of San Antonio Society of Pathologists, 1961. *Tex J Med.* 1963;59:664–667.
2. Dahl I. Atypical fibroxanthoma of the skin. A clinico-pathological study of 57 cases. *Acta Pathol Microbiol Scand A.* 1976;84(2):183–197.
3. Stout AP, Hill WT. Leiomyosarcoma of the superficial soft tissues. *Cancer.* 1958;11(4):844–854.
4. Fields JP, Helwig EB. Leiomyosarcoma of the skin and subcutaneous tissue. *Cancer.* 1981;47(1):156–169.
5. Leboit PE. *Pathology and Genetics of Skin Tumours.* Lyon: IARC Press; 2006.
6. Rouhani P, Fletcher CD, Devesa SS, et al. Cutaneous soft tissue sarcoma incidence patterns in the U.S.: an analysis of 12,114 cases. *Cancer.* 2008;113(3):616–627.
7. Dei Tos AP, Maestro R, Doglioni C, et al. Ultraviolet-induced p53 mutations in atypical fibroxanthoma. *Am J Pathol.* 1994;145(1):11–17.
8. Simon MP, Pedeutour F, Sirvent N, et al. Deregulation of the platelet-derived growth factor B-chain gene via fusion with collagen gene COL1A1 in dermatofibrosarcoma protuberans and giant-cell fibroblastoma. *Nat Genet.* 1997;15(1):95–98.
9. Peulvâe P, Michot C, Vannier JP, et al. Clear cell sarcoma with t(12;22) (q13-14;q12). *Gene Chromosome Canc.* 1991;3(5):400–402.
10. Bowne WB, Antonescu CR, Leung DH, et al. Dermatofibrosarcoma protuberans: a clinicopathologic analysis of patients treated and followed at a single institution. *Cancer.* 2000;88(12):2711–2720.
11. Fiore M, Miceli R, Mussi C, et al. Dermatofibrosarcoma protuberans treated at a single institution: a surgical disease with a high cure rate. *J Clin Oncol.* 2005;23(30):7669–7675.
12. Snow SN, Gordon EM, Larson PO, et al. Dermatofibrosarcoma protuberans: a report on 29 patients treated by Mohs micrographic surgery with long-term follow-up and review of the literature. *Cancer.* 2004;101(1):28–38.
13. Ballo MT, Zagars GK, Pisters P, et al. The role of radiation therapy in the management of dermatofibrosarcoma protuberans. *Int J Radiat Oncol.* 1998;40(4):823–827.
14. Suit H, Spiro I, Mankin HJ, et al. Radiation in management of patients with dermatofibrosarcoma protuberans. *J Clin Oncol.* 1996;14(8):2365–2369.
15. Sjèoblom T, Shimizu A, O'Brien KP, et al. Growth inhibition of dermatofibrosarcoma protuberans tumors by the platelet-derived growth factor receptor antagonist STI571 through induction of apoptosis. *Cancer Res.* 2001;61(15):5778–5783.
16. McArthur GA, Demetri GD, van Oosterom A, et al. Molecular and clinical analysis of locally advanced dermatofibrosarcoma protuberans treated with imatinib: Imatinib Target Exploration Consortium Study B2225. *J Clin Oncol.* 2005;23(4):866–873.
17. Rubin BP, Schuetze SM, Eary JF, et al. Molecular targeting of platelet-derived growth factor B by imatinib mesylate in a patient with metastatic dermatofibrosarcoma protuberans. *J Clin Oncol.* 2002;20(17):3586–3591.
18. Mirza B, Weedon D. Atypical fibroxanthoma: a clinicopathological study of 89 cases. *Australas J Dermatol.* 2005;46(4):235–238.
19. Fretzin DF, Helwig EB. Atypical fibroxanthoma of the skin. A clinicopathologic study of 140 cases. *Cancer.* 1973;31(6):1541–1552.
20. Ang GC, Roenigk RK, Otley CC, et al. More than 2 decades of treating atypical fibroxanthoma at Mayo Clinic: what have we learned from 91 patients? *Dermatol Surg.* 2009;35(5):765–772.
21. Fletcher CDM, Unni KK, Mertens F. *Pathology and Genetics of Tumours of Soft Tissue and Bone.* Lyon: IARC Press; 2002.
22. Weiss SW, Enzinger FM. Malignant fibrous histiocytoma: an analysis of 200 cases. *Cancer.* 1978;41(6):2250–2266.
23. Le Doussal V, Coindre JM, Leroux A, et al. Prognostic factors for patients with localized primary malignant fibrous histiocytoma: a multicenter study of 216 patients with multivariate analysis. *Cancer.* 1996;77(9):1823–1830.
24. Meis-Kindblom JM, Kindblom LG. Acral myxoinflammatory fibroblastic sarcoma: a low-grade tumor of the hands and feet. *Am J Surg Pathol.* 1998;22(8):911–924.
25. Fetsch JF, Laskin WB, Miettinen M. Superficial acral fibromyxoma: a clinicopathologic and immunohistochemical analysis of 37 cases of a distinctive soft tissue tumor with a predilection for the fingers and toes. *Hum Pathol.* 2001;32(7):704–714.
26. Svarvar C, Bohling T, Berlin O, et al. Clinical course of nonvisceral soft tissue leiomyosarcoma in 225 patients from the Scandinavian Sarcoma Group. *Cancer.* 2007;109(2):282–291.
27. Huether MJ, Zitelli JA, Brodland DG. Mohs micrographic surgery for the treatment of spindle cell tumors of the skin. *J Am Acad Dermatol.* 2001;44(4):656–659.
28. Enzinger FM. Clear-cell sarcoma of tendons and aponeuroses. An analysis of 21 cases. *Cancer.* 1965;18:1163–1174.
29. Fujimura Y, Ohno T, Siddique H, et al. The EWS-ATF-1 gene involved in malignant melanoma of soft parts with t(12;22) chromosome translocation, encodes a constitutive transcriptional activator. *Oncogene.* 1996;12(1):159–167.
30. Antonescu CR, Nafa K, Segal NH, et al. EWS-CREB1: a recurrent variant fusion in clear cell sarcoma – association with gastrointestinal location and absence of melanocytic differentiation. *Clin Cancer Res.* 2006;12(18):5356–5362.
31. Lucas DR, Nascimento AG, Sim FH. Clear cell sarcoma of soft tissues. Mayo Clinic experience with 35 cases. *Am J Surg Pathol.* 1992;16(12):1197–1204.
32. Blazer 3rd DG, Lazar AJ, Xing Y, et al. Clinical outcomes of molecularly confirmed clear cell sarcoma from a single institution and in comparison with data from the Surveillance, Epidemiology, and End Results registry. *Cancer.* 2009;115(13):2971–2979.
33. Finley JW, Hanypsiak B, McGrath B, et al. Clear cell sarcoma: the Roswell Park experience. *J Surg Oncol.* 2001;77(1):16–20.
34. Smith ME, Fisher C, Weiss SW. Pleomorphic hyalinizing angiectatic tumor of soft parts. A low-grade neoplasm resembling neurilemoma. *Am J Surg Pathol.* 1996;20(1):21–29.
35. Folpe AL, Weiss SW. Pleomorphic hyalinizing angiectatic tumor: analysis of 41 cases supporting evolution from a distinctive precursor lesion. *Am J Surg Pathol.* 2004;28(11):1417–1425.

# Kaposi's Sarcoma

*Miguel Sanchez*

## Key Points

- Kaposi's sarcoma is a multicentric, mostly oligoclonic neoplastic proliferation of endothelial cells that have been infected and transformed by human herpesvirus-8.

- Four epidemiologic types of Kaposi's sarcoma are recognized: classic (typically found sporadically in elderly persons of Mediterranean descent), epidemic (AIDS-related), endemic (occurring in Africa), and iatrogenic (immunosuppression-associated, transplant-associated).

- While there are numerous clinical variants, the typical lesions are well-demarcated, smooth purple macules, plaques and nodules that histologically show slit-like vascular channels and spindle-shaped tumor cells.

- Clinical course varies from the development of few, indolent-growing cutaneous lesions to aggressive, life-threatening dissemination of tumors affecting skin, lymph nodes and systemic organs.

- Treatment may be localized or systemic depending on the type, extent, complications, rate of progression, and organ invasion.

## INTRODUCTION

Kaposi's sarcoma (KS) is a reactive, multifocal, multicentric, angiogenic neoplastic proliferation that is thought to originate from endothelial cells that are infected with the human herpesvirus-8 (HHV-8), also known as KS-associated herpesvirus (KSHV). Most cases present with lesions on the skin and/or mucous membranes, but, as the course progresses, tumors may also arise in the lymph nodes and visceral organs.

## HISTORY

In 1872, Moritz Kaposi reported an 'idiopathic multiple pigmented sarcoma of the skin' which became known as 'classic' Kaposi sarcoma. In the 1950s, a more aggressive 'endemic' form of the malignancy, with a prevalence in equatorial and southern Africa as high as 200 times that of the classic type, was described in English language journals.[1] An 'iatrogenic' KS variant was distinguished in the 1970s in transplant patients receiving immunosuppressive

therapy. However, KS remained a relatively uncommon disease until 1981, when a virulent and disseminated 'epidemic' type associated with life-threatening opportunistic infections was described in men who have sex with men (MSM) and blood transfusion recipients.[2]

## PATHOGENESIS

In 1994, DNA sequences of a new human gammaherpesvirus (HHV-8) were identified in KS tissue examined by representational difference analysis.[3] Since then, the virus has been detected in more than 90% of KS tumors and all four main types.[4] The virus is recovered most often and in higher titers in saliva, suggesting that intimate sexual or asexual oral contact increases the risk of transmission. Less effective transmission occurs via blood and semen. Annually, only 0.03% of men and 0.015% of women over 50 years of age who are infected with HHV-8 develop classic KS.[5] In contrast, the 10-year probability of developing KS for persons co-infected with HHV-8 and HIV is nearly 50%.[6] Molecular diagnostic techniques comparing viral HHV-8 DNA of the tumors have demonstrated that at least 80% of the tumors arise independently from multiple cells.[7]

Much remains to be learned about the mechanisms by which HHV-8 and co-factors, such as HIV, trigger KS lesions. HIV infection potentiates oncogenesis and increases the risk of developing KS lesions by up to a factor of 10,000.[8] The viral–host interaction is complex and appears to involve HHV-8 infection of the cells with growth factors secreted by the spindle cells, mononuclear and endothelial cells. It is postulated that HHV-8 transforms a lymphatic or vascular endothelial cell or its precursor into a spindle cell, and then helps to sustain its unregulated proliferation by interacting with the multifunctional proangiogenic HIV-1 transcriptional transactivator (TAT) protein, inhibiting apoptosis, accelerating tumorigenesis in part by activating nuclear factor-kappa B, and stimulating angiogenesis by upregulating various angiogenic cytokines and growth factors, including vascular endothelial growth factor (VEGF). A number of cytokines stimulate KS spindle cell growth in vitro and possibly in vivo.[8]

## CLINICAL FINDINGS

Typically, KS lesions progress from well-demarcated, non-blanching, reddish to dark purple, oval or circular, ecchymotic-like macules or patches to firm, indurated

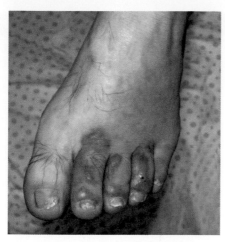

Figure 16.1 Characteristic purple papules and plaques on the toes of a man with KS.

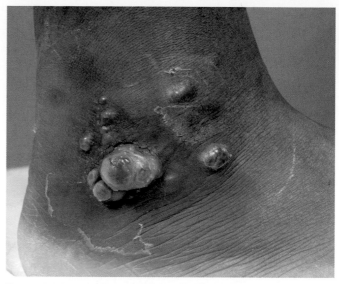

Figure 16.3 Exophytic, pyogenic granuloma-like KS resembles bacillary angiomatosis.

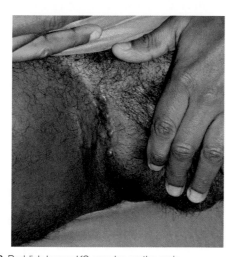

Figure 16.2 Reddish brown KS papules on the groin.

papules, plaques or nodules that enlarge to measure several centimeters in length (Fig. 16.1). These lesions may coalesce to form larger infiltrated plaques that cover large areas. In dark-skinned persons, the lesions are often brown (Fig. 16.2). Less frequently, the initial lesions are plaques or subcutaneous nodules, or exophytic papules may be the initial disease manifestation (Fig. 16.3). Several clinical and histological KS variants have been described (Table 16.1).[9]

## CLINICAL VARIANTS

### Classic KS

This type of KS characteristically develops in middle-aged or elderly men living in or descending from the Mediterranean basin and Eastern or Southern Europe.[10,11] While the highest incidences have been found in Sardinia (29.2 per million in men and 19.6 per million in women) and Sicily (30.1 per million in men and 5.4 per million in women), cases of classic KS have been reported from every continent except Antarctica.[12] The male-to-female gender ratio is approximately 3:1, although ratios as high as 15:1 have been calculated in some populations. Less than 8% of cases present before the age of 50 and cases in adolescents and young adults are rare.[11]

| Table 16.1 Morphologic Variants of Kaposi's Sarcoma |
| --- |
| **Anaplastic:** Rare histologic phenotype with marked cytologic atypia, numerous mitoses, a propensity for acral locations, and a high degree of aggressiveness and local invasion. |
| **Bullous:** Tense blister(s) within KS tumor plaques that histologically show subepidermal or intraepidermal edema. |
| **Ecchymotic:** Bluish or purplish bruise-like KS lesion characterized by vast extravasation of red blood cells. |
| **Exophytic:** Well-demarcated, smooth-surfaced, red papules and nodules above the surface of the skin. |
| **Intravascular:** Rare type in which spindle cell proliferation is limited to intravenous areas. |
| **Lymphangiomatous:** Invasion of lymphatics by tumors producing cutaneous lymphedema. This variant typically occurs in the lower extremities and results in gross swelling with cobblestoning violaceous papules, nodules and occasionally bullae that may ulcerate. |
| **Hyperkeratotic:** Verrucous indurated plaques associated with chronic lymphedema, with markedly thickened stratum corneum, verruciform epidermal acanthosis, and often fibrosis in the upper dermis. |
| **Keloidal:** Firm, thick, rubbery nodules which histologically show dense, hyalinized collagen, usually seen in African-Americans. |
| **Lymphangiectactic:** Pseudoblister-like nodules with large, dilated ectatic lymphatic vessels. |
| **Lymphadenopathic:** Enlarged palpable lymph nodes from KS invasion. |
| **Lymphangioma-like:** Also known as lymphangiomatous or cavernous KS, this rare type is characterized by a proliferation of wide, irregular anastomosing channels lined by a monolayer of plump sarcoma cells separating the collagen bundles. The spaces contain frothy, pale eosinophilic fluid rather than erythrocytes. A pseudo-bullous appearance, considered a clinical hallmark of this type, occurs in about half of the cases. |
| **Micronodular:** Minute, unencapsulated nodules of proliferating spindle cells in the reticular dermis. |
| **Pyogenic granuloma-like:** An exophytic KS variant consisting of bright red, friable polypoid papules or nodules which may bleed, erode, ulcerate or crust. These lesions are often misdiagnosed clinically as bacillary angiomatosis. |
| **Telangiectatic:** Lesion studded with numerous telangiectasias on their surface. An uncommon variant is a well-demarcated patch of spider telangiectasias that eventually becomes a solid purple plaque. |

An elevated risk of classic KS, independent of HHV-8 infection, has been reported in patients with low absolute lymphocytes, including low CD4+ and CD8+ T cells.[13] Other reported risk factors include exposure to southern Italian volcanic soil, living in areas contaminated with arthropods, chronic leg edema, diabetes mellitus, and reduced numbers of B cells. In men, multivariate analysis has demonstrated an elevated KS risk with the use of topical corticosteroids, infrequent bathing, and a history of asthma or of allergy. Recent studies have indicated that classic KS is promoted by interleukin-13 (IL-13) and haplotypes of the IL-8 receptor-beta genes. Notably, the risk of developing KS may be decreased by cigarette smoking in men – by approximately 20% for each 10 pack-years reported, sevenfold with more than 40 pack-years, and 80% overall in current smokers.[12]

Characteristic violaceous, purple or brown macules or patches evolve into papules, plaques, or deep-seated indurated nodules. The tumors gradually grow horizontally and vertically, coalescing into larger plaques or nodules and occasionally become hyperkeratotic. Although lesions may develop over any other part of the body, especially the upper legs, face, and trunk, the most frequently involved location is the lower extremities, commonly the ankles and soles (Fig. 16.4). The lesions typically present on a single extremity but in time the distribution often becomes bilateral and multifocal.

The course of classic KS is usually chronic, indolent and protracted, and only rarely acute, rapidly progressive, or characterized by rapidly enlarging tumors after periods of relative quiescence. Over 2 years, only 34% of 39 untreated asymptomatic patients remained progression-free. However, most cases survive 10 to 15 years after diagnosis, dying of unrelated causes.[11] In one study, only 2% of 438 patients with classic KS died of disseminated disease after 4.8 years, although 14% died of second malignancies and 22% died of other unrelated medical conditions.[11] In a smaller series, only one of 41 patients died from KS after 10 years of observation.[14]

The most common complications are edema, ulceration and bleeding. The tumors are disfiguring and those on the soles or oral cavity become especially painful. Lymphatic obstruction eventuates in gross lymphedema. Tumor ulceration increases the risk of cellulitis and sepsis. Oral mucosal lesions are rare,[10] but lymph node and gastrointestinal lesions

## Table 16.2 Clinical Staging for Classic Kaposi Sarcoma

| Stage 1 | (maculonodular)*: Small macules and papules are confined to lower extremities |
|---------|------------------------------------------------------------------------------|
| Stage 2 | (infiltrative)*: Plaques, sometimes associated with nodules, present mainly on the lower extremities |
| Stage 3 | (florid)†: Widespread plaques and nodules, many ulcerated, predominantly localized on the lower extremities |
| Stage 4 | (disseminated)†: Tumors on various areas of the body beyond the extremities |

\* Slow rate of progression, fewer complications, low incidence of visceral involvement.
† More rapid progression, greater risk of systemic involvement, and significant functional impairment.

occur more commonly than previously appreciated.[15,16] In one report, tumors were found endoscopically in the gastrointestinal tract (all on the stomach, 27% on the esophagus and 11% on the duodenum) in 82% of classic-KS patients,[15] and in another study 23% had regional lymph node involvement.[16] Intestinal involvement may produce nausea, vomiting, abdominal cramps, weight loss, and anemia from chronic bleeding. Based on lesion distribution and disease progression a classification system for staging classic KS has been proposed (Table 16.2).[17]

Up to a third of classic KS cases develop a second primary malignancy, often non-Hodgkin lymphoma.[18] There are conflicting data on the risk of other malignancies, either before or following a diagnosis of classic KS. Although some studies have reported an association, particularly with non-Hodgkin lymphoma and other lymphohematopoietic malignancies, larger, population-based studies have failed to document higher rates of these or other types of cancer.[11] On the other hand, a population-based study from Israel found higher rates of KS in individuals, especially immigrants from the Soviet Union and Poland, previously diagnosed with lymphoma, leukemia and breast cancer.[11] It remains to be determined whether cancer-induced immunosuppression predisposes persons from HHV-8 endemic areas to develop classic KS. Treatment is palliative and administered to halt disease progression, decrease edema, and enhance function. Unfortunately, there are few prospective, well-designed classic-KS trials to assist the clinician to select a best practice approach. Localized radiotherapy to individual tumors is particularly valuable in the elderly, whose shorter life expectancy precludes the probability of severe chronic radiation dermatitis. Other therapies, including cryotherapy, intralesional vinblastine and laser or surgical destruction for localized cutaneous disease, and chemotherapy or interferon for symptomatic progressive skin or systemic disease, have been effectively used.

## Epidemic (AIDS-related) KS

The development of epidemic KS tumors represents recognizable stigmata that publicly reveal the person's HIV status and are considered by many patients to be the most dreaded complication of HIV infection. Tumors may arise on any body region, including the face, hands, anogenital area and mucous membranes (see Chapter 19). On the trunk, the lesions often follow Langer's cleavage lines (Fig. 16.5). Oral

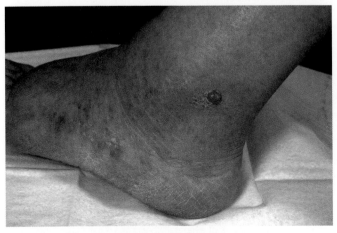

**Figure 16.4** Classic KS involving the ankle and foot.

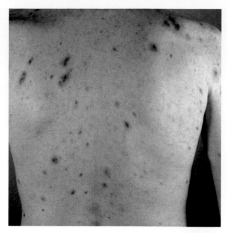

**Figure 16.5** Epidemic KS plaques along the Langer's lines on the back.

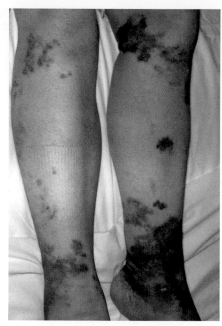

**Figure 16.7** Disseminated KS in a profoundly immunocompromised HIV-infected man.

lesions develop in a third of cases and may be the presenting site in about 15%, with the hard palate being the most commonly involved oral cavity area followed by the soft palate, gingiva, uvula, pharynx, and tongue (Fig. 16.6). While mucocutaneous lesions are usually the presenting manifestation, lymphatic and visceral tumors may precede those on the skin. Lymph node involvement is frequent but only detected on autopsy in many cases.

Untreated HIV-infected persons with KS usually die of other opportunistic infections. However, death may be caused by complications from internal organ involvement, including respiratory failure, gut perforation, cardiac tamponade, and brain metastasis. The course of pulmonary KS may be slowly progressive or aggressive, especially in profoundly immunocompromised persons, requiring prompt treatment. Pulmonary tumors present with bronchospasm, cough, dyspnea and/or hemoptysis. The gastrointestinal tract (stomach, colon) is the most commonly involved organ (40% at initial presentation, 80% at autopsy) but the lesions are frequently asymptomatic and may not influence prognosis. Other organs (heart, adrenal glands, urethra, bone, brain) are rarely involved. Low CD4 counts and elevated HIV-1 viral loads are independently poor prognostic factors for the development of epidemic KS (Fig. 16.7).

Previous to the introduction of antiretroviral therapy, as many as 40% of HIV-infected men who have sex with men (MSM) developed KS, in contrast to 3% of heterosexual injection drug users, 3% of transfusion recipients, 3% of women or children, and 1% of hemophiliacs.[19] With the introduction of highly active antiretroviral therapy, the KS incidence in the HIV French Hospital Database decreased from 32 cases/1000 person-years in 1993 to 3 cases/1000 person-years after 1999.[20] Among HIV-infected women, the incidence of KS is 15-fold lower than in HIV-infected men, but the disease is often more aggressive, with higher rates of lymph node and visceral involvement and poorer survival than in men, even after adjustment for CD4 lymphocyte counts. The development of classic KS is associated with high HHV-8 lytic and latent antibody titers.[11]

Since KS is a multicentric disease, conventional cancer staging has been a challenge and not found to be clinically valuable. No system has been universally accepted for clinical staging, but the AIDS Clinical Trials Group classification, which is based on immune status, extent of tumor involvement, and presence of systemic illnesses, is used for clinical studies of AIDS-associated KS and has been associated with survival (Table 16.3).[21]

## Non-epidemic gay-related KS in MSM

KS develops at a higher rate than in the general population in MSM without evidence of HIV infection or immunodeficiency. The lesions most commonly appear on the extremities or genitalia, but in contrast to the epidemic type, the extent of disease is limited and the prognosis is good. Patients are younger than those with the classic variant. However, these patients may have a higher risk of developing lymphoproliferative neoplasms (Castleman disease, follicular lymphoma and Burkitt lymphoma).[20]

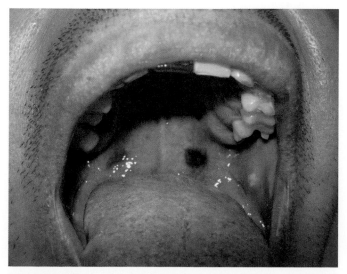

**Figure 16.6** Bluish-red tumors on the palate of a man with AIDS-associated KS.

| Table 16.3 The AIDS Clinical Trials Group Classification |
| --- |
| **T (tumor) status** |
| $T_0$ (good risk): Localized tumor confined to skin and/or lymph nodes and/or minimal non-nodular oral disease limited to the palate<br>$T_1$ (poor risk): Widespread KS tumors and presence of one of the following:<br>• Disease-induced edema<br>• Extensive oral KS: nodular or extrapalatal<br>• Visceral lesions in organs other than lymph nodes |
| **I (immune system) status** |
| $I_0$ (good risk): CD4 cell count is ≥ 200 (or 150 or 100) cells per μL<br>$I_1$ (poor risk): CD4 cell count ≤ 200 cells per μL |
| **S (systemic illness) status** |
| $S_0$ (good risk): No systemic illness, no history of opportunistic infections (OI) or thrush, Karnofsky performance status score ≥70 and absence of the following B symptoms:<br>• Unexplained fever<br>• Night sweats<br>• More than 10% involuntary weight loss<br>• Diarrhea persisting more than 2 weeks<br>$S_1$ (poor risk): OI or thrush, presence of B symptoms and/or Karnofsky performance status score ≤70 |

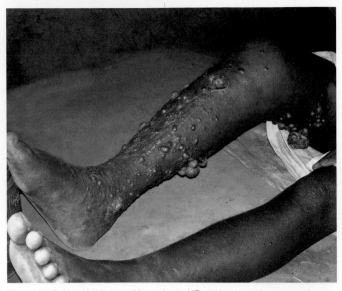

**Figure 16.8** Lymphadenopathic endemic KS with gross edema, woody induration, and exophytic and subcutaneous tumors in an African man. (Courtesy of Jason Prystowsky, M.D.)

## Endemic KS

Prior to the HIV epidemic, Taylor et al. distinguished four clinical manifestations of KS in Africans: a benign disease resembling classic KS; a prepubertal lymphadenopathic form that predominantly affects boys; an aggressive and destructive type affecting skin and bone in the extremities; and a disseminated, systemic kind that was fatal within 3 years in nearly all cases.[22] The first two types are the most common.

In the past two decades, the prevalence of endemic KS has increased, especially in Malawi, Swaziland, Uganda, Zambia and Zimbabwe.[23] Males are affected about 15 times more often than females, except in the lymphadenopathic type, which is only three times more prevalent in males (Fig. 16.8). This type constitutes 12% of all endemic KS cases but 42% of childhood cases.[23]

## Post-transplant (iatrogenic) KS

This clinical variant occurs nearly exclusively in post-transplant patients but has also been reported during treatment with high-dose corticosteroids or immunosuppressants for conditions such as asthma, pemphigus, or connective tissue disease.[24] The incidence in renal transplant recipients may be as high as 3.5% in regions endemic for KS versus 0.4% in Western Europe and the United States. In 10% of cases, KS develops only in extracutaneous visceral organs. Men are affected 3.3 times more frequently than women. Most cases have Mediterranean, Middle Eastern, Jewish, Caribbean or African ancestry. The average time to develop KS is 16 months after transplantation. Depending on the degree of immunosuppression, the course can be aggressive and fulminant but tumor regression may follow discontinuation of immunosuppressants or change to sirolimus.[25]

## DIFFERENTIAL DIAGNOSIS

Depending on the type of lesion, KS can resemble numerous skin lesions, most of which are vascular in nature (Table 16.4).

## EVALUATION

### Laboratory diagnosis

In classic KS, a physical examination, routine laboratory tests, and confirmatory histological examination of tissue from a punch or a deep shave biopsy usually suffice, except in cases with clinically suspected systemic disease, in which imaging, endoscopy or fiberoptic bronchoscopy may be indicated.

### Histopathology

*Patches* of KS histologically demonstrate irregular, somewhat jagged, thin-walled, slit-like vascular spaces that are lined by a single layer of flattened endothelial cells and may contain erythrocytes. These channels surround pre-existing blood vessels and cutaneous appendages in the upper dermis and may seem to dissect collagen bundles. The dermis is sparsely studded with a superficial infiltrate of lymphocytes, plasma cells and often hemosiderin-laden macrophages, as well as variable erythrocyte extravasation. The presence of a pre-existing blood vessel protruding into an abnormal vascular space has been termed the 'promontory sign'.

*Plaques* of KS show many dissecting erythrocyte-filled vascular channels surrounded by whorls of spindle-shaped cells (Figs 16.9 and 16.10). A dense dermal mononuclear infiltrate may extend to the adipose tissue. Intra- and extracellular hyaline globules probably represent 'effete' erythrocytes. There is no significant nuclear or cytological pleomorphism and mitotic figures are sparse. Cross-section of a spindled endothelial cell may show an erythrocyte present within a clear paranuclear vacuole in its cytoplasm, a finding called 'autolumination'.

## Table 16.4 Differential Diagnosis

**Vascular lesions**

Acroangiodermatitis of Malli (Pseudo-Kaposi sarcoma)
Angiokeratoma
Angioma serpiginosum
Arteriovenous hemangioma
Arteriovenous malformations
Blue rubber bleb syndrome
Cherry angioma
Cobb syndrome
Epithelioid hemangioma (angiolymphoid hyperplasia with eosinophilia)
Eruptive pseudoangiomatosis
Glomeruloid hemangioma
Infantile hemangioma
Kaposiform hemangioendothelioma
Lobular capillary hemangioma (pyogenic granuloma)
Lymphangioma circumscriptum
Microvenular hemangioma
Pigmented purpuric dermatitis
Purpura
Pyogenic granuloma
Retiform hemangioendothelioma
Targetoid hemosiderotic hemangioma
Tufted angioma
Verrucous hemangioma

**Infections**

Bacillary angiomatosis
*M. marinum* infection
Sporotrichosis

**Systemic**

Systemic amyloidosis
Verruga peruana

**Malignant neoplasms**

Angiosarcoma
Leukemia cutis
Metastatic carcinoma cutis (especially renal)

**Other histologic considerations**

Intravascular papillary endothelial hyperplasia (Masson's tumor)
Intravenous pyogenic granuloma
Intravascular fasciitis
Papillary intralymphatic angioendothelioma (Dabska tumor)
Intravascular myopericytoma

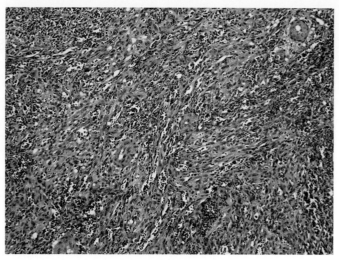

**Figure 16.10** Higher magnification shows the vascular slit-like channels interspersed between neoplastic spindle-shaped cells that form large fascicles and phagocytose erythrocytes.

*Nodules* of KS contain numerous erythrocyte-filled, slit-like channels interspersed between neoplastic spindle-shaped endothelial cells that form large fascicles. More dilated vascular channels, typical of a cavernous hemangioma, may be seen at the periphery of the lesion. The lining cells of the vascular structures stain immunohistochemically with endothelial cell markers such as factor VIII-related antigen, human leukocyte antigen DR (HLA-DR), von Willebrand factor, and monoclonal antibodies EN4 and PAL E. The spindle cells are positive for CD34 and often CD31 as well. Formalin-fixed and frozen tissues can be stained with monoclonal antibodies to HHV-8 latency-associated nuclear antigen (LANA), a highly sensitive and specific marker that has not been found to be expressed in other vascular tumors.[26]

### Serology

Detection of HHV-8 in peripheral blood by PCR supports the diagnosis of KS. However, not all KS patients are HHV-8 viremic. The presence of LANA in serum is strongly correlated with the risk of developing KS in immunocompromised individuals.[26] About 85% of patients in whom HHV-8 DNA has been found in their KS lesions have HHV-8 serum antibodies, usually in high titers, demonstrable by the direct immunofluorescence assay (IFA).[3]

### Systemic organ evaluation

Due to the poor prognosis associated with pulmonary KS, evaluation with chest radiographs is warranted in all patients except those with classic cutaneous KS without respiratory symptoms. Radiographic findings are not specific and usually show diffuse bilateral infiltration of the lungs, with irregular nodules of varying sizes located more commonly in the lower lobes. Other findings include hilar or mediastinal lymphadenopathy and pericardial or pleural effusions which may be sanguinous. Fiberoptic bronchoscopy visualizes endobronchial lesions but biopsy is not routinely performed due to the high risks of bleeding and perforation.

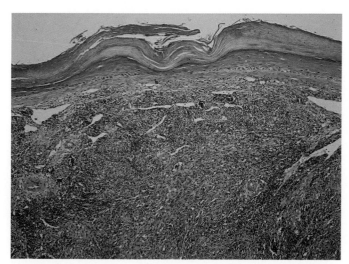

**Figure 16.9** Histopathologic examination of a KS plaque shows dermal whorls of haphazardly arranged atypical spindle-shaped cells and irregular channels filled with red blood cells. (Courtesy of Shane Mehan M.D.)

Esophagogastroduodenoscopy or colonoscopy is reserved for symptomatic patients. However, biopsies may not be revealing since the tumors frequently are localized below the mucosa.

## TREATMENT

### Systemic therapy

The objectives of treatment are case-specific but center on achieving clinical remission, prolonging life, improving disfigurement and quality of life, reducing the size and progression of tumors, and preventing or palliating complications, such as edema.

### Classic KS

Observation and conservative care is acceptable in asymptomatic patients. Individual lesions may regress spontaneously even as new lesions appear. Compression, foot orthotics, and wound care should be considered when appropriate. Since early localized lesions are exquisitely radiosensitive, radiation therapy is a reasonable choice, especially for older patients. Other local treatments also do not alter the disease course but can shrink or eradicate individual lesions. Considerations for systemic treatment include development of more than 10 new lesions per month, symptomatic lung disease, and disabling lymphedema.[11]

### Epidemic KS

The standard initial treatment is the administration of antiretroviral therapy (ART) regimens that effectively reduce HIV and HHV-8 viral loads and increase CD4 T-cell counts. Highly active antiretroviral therapy (HAART) has been reported to decrease the risk of developing KS by 66% within 15 months.[27] Clinical trials with HAART have reported resolution of KS in 44–74% and reduction in the risk of death by 81%,[28] but in many of these trials, chemotherapy was also administered to some patients.[29,30] In most cases that develop KS while on HAART, the lesions are smaller, less extensive, and more likely to remit spontaneously.[30]

In a group of HAART-treated KS patients, only 25% required systemic antitumor therapy within 5 years.[30] In one study, the overall 5-year survival rates for patients with nodular, patch, and plaque episodic KS on ART were 79%, 91%, and 92% (total 89%), respectively.[30] Survival rates were deemed lower in patients with nodular KS because of their higher prevalence of T1 staging.[30] Indeed, unfavorable responses to HAART are associated with T1 tumor stage, CD4 cell count below 200 cells/μL, positive HHV-8 DNA and absence of antibodies against HHV-8 lytic antigens at the time of diagnosis.[31] Although HIV protease inhibitors have been reported to inhibit angiogenesis independently of their effects on HIV, NNRTI-based HAART appears to be as effective as regimens with protease inhibitors in preventing development of lesions, inducing remission and prolonging time to treatment failure.[32]

The survival rate of patients with pulmonary KS improved from only 10% to 53% after initiation of HAART.[33] However, KS can develop or persist in some HAART-treated patients despite effective HIV control and high CD4 counts.[34,35] A good prognosis was reported in KS patients with CD4 counts above 300 cells/mm$^3$ and undetectable HIV viral loads, with only 22% having newly diagnosed, persistent or progressive KS.[30] Even those who required systemic therapy for KS had lower risks of death than patients with lower CD4 counts.[30]

Individual patches and thin plaques may respond to topical therapies. Small flat macules and patches have the best response. *Chemotherapy* is required for KS patients with extensive (>25) cutaneous lesions, rapid skin progression that is unresponsive to local therapy, symptomatic organ involvement, edema that is extensive or interferes with function, or persistent KS-associated immune reconstitution inflammatory syndrome (KS-IRIS) that fails to resolve with continued antiretroviral therapy.

In up to 7% of HIV-infected patients, initiation of ART elicits an IRIS response that leads to enlargement of lesions and an eruption of new tumors that can be fulminant and lethal.[36] Possible but not well-established risk factors for KS-IRIS are KS-associated edema, higher CD4 counts than in KS patients without IRIS, and combined treatment with both protease inhibitor and non-nucleosides.[36]

### Post-transplant KS

Dose reduction or withdrawal of immunosuppressants, especially calcineurin inhibitors, is the first-line treatment. Substitution of ciclosporin with the mTor inhibitor sirolimus, which directly affects the mTOR pathway that is upregulated by KSHV and which has both antitumor and immunosuppressive effects, induced remission of KS tumors in 15 kidney-transplant recipients.[25,37]

### Endemic KS

Treatment is challenging and usually palliative, since availability of immunotherapy and access to chemotherapy and radiotherapy is very limited in many African countries.

### Topical therapy

*Topical therapy* should be considered for patients with small lesions and limited disease, especially to improve disfigurement, to reduce disease-related anxiety, and to decrease the size of individual KS patches, papules or plaques.

*Alitretinoin (9-cis-retinoic acid) gel* is FDA-approved for the treatment of AIDS-associated KS. Complete or partial responses after application to lesions two to four times daily for 12 weeks were achieved in 35% of patients also treated with HAART.[38] Macules, small patches and thin papules are most likely to show favorable responses. Irritation-associated symptoms are common during treatment and post-inflammatory hyperpigmentation is induced in dark-skinned patients.

*Vinblastine* can be injected intralesionally into the involved dermis, usually starting at 0.1 mg/mL and 0.1 mg/0.5 cm$^2$ and increasing every 1–2 weeks up to 0.3 mg/mL until the desired effect is obtained. In one study, intralesional injections of 0.2 mg/mL resulted in over 50% regression of intraoral tumors with a mean response duration of 3.52 months, in 74% of cases.[39] Some clinicians simultaneously treat lesions with intralesional vinblastine to destroy the deeper areas and cryotherapy for the more superficial dermal involvement of the tumor. The injections are painful and frequently cause erythema, erosion, ulceration and crusting. This treatment can effectively eradicate small, localized lesions but is disappointing in infiltrated plaques or nodules.

*Cryotherapy with liquid nitrogen* at −196°C sprayed from a cryogun or applied with a cotton swab to the tumor destroys individual lesions. Depending on the depth of the lesion, spray freezing times ranging from 10 to 40 seconds are needed to destroy the lesion. This amount of freezing causes blistering, and ulceration. An 80% complete lesional response was reported with treatments consisting of two freeze–thaw cycles,[40] but recurrences were common. Macules and small patches may be successfully eradicated, leaving hypopigmented scars. Cryotherapy destroys the surface of plaques or nodules, imparting an appearance of remission, though the tumor usually remains in the deeper dermis and invariably grows back in time. While nodules and plaques may be completely destroyed with prolonged freezing, the long healing time of the ensuing ulcers and remaining scars make treatment of medium to large lesions impractical.

## Radiotherapy

*Radiotherapy* is an option as palliative treatment and in the elderly, whose life expectancies may mitigate concerns about the development of chronic radiation dermatitis.

KS is exquisitely sensitive to ionizing radiation and responses occur in 80–90% treated cases. Treatments may be administered either as low-voltage (100 kv) photons or electron beam radiotherapy. Radiotherapy may eradicate even large and widespread localized lesions indefinitely, including those in acral areas, palliate extensive symptomatic disease and improve lymphedema. This treatment may be more effective in new than in longstanding lesions. After administration of 8.0 Gy (given in one fraction in about half the cases), 11% and 63% of patients with epidemic KS had complete and partial responses, respectively, whereas 29% of African-endemic KS had complete responses and another 29% had partial responses.[41] Even better results were obtained with a higher dose of 21 Gy administered in 3.5 Gy fractions three times a week. This regimen achieved a 91% overall and 80% complete lesional responses.[42]

*Electron beam therapy* is reserved for superficial lesions and usually administered once weekly in 4 Gy fractions. Because recurrence may be common in adjacent, untreated areas, radiation oncologists may prefer extended-field radiotherapy to effect a higher cure rate. In a large retrospective case series of 643 patients with epidemic KS treated with extended-field irradiation using 4 MeV electron beam and/or localized field irradiation of 45–100 kV X-rays, an objective response was observed in 92% of patients (CR: 66%; PR: 26%; no response: 8%).[43] Development of severe radiation-induced mucositis limits radiotherapy as a treatment for oral lesions. Localized hyperpigmentation, desquamation, and ulceration are more common in epidemic KS lesions.

## Other therapies

*Recombinant interferon-alpha* has antiviral, antiproliferative and immunologic activities. In clinical studies, this therapy has improved KS in 30–40% of cases with CD4 cell counts higher than 150 cells/μL, and predominantly indolent KS lesions limited to the skin. Responses are often slow over months of treatment.[44,45] Early studies used very high doses but subsequent trials of recombinant alpha-2b interferon in combination with antiretrovirals reported benefit with less toxicity in doses as low as 1 million IU subcutaneously daily.[45] Side effects, especially flu-like symptoms and neutropenia, limit dose escalation. In such cases, a change to less myelosuppressive antiretroviral agents or treatment with granulocyte–macrophage colony-stimulating factor (GM-CSF) should be considered. Recombinant interferon-alpha-2b in doses of 5 million units can be administered safely to patients on HAART.[46] Case reports have suggested that combined with antiretroviral therapy, pegylated interferon-alpha-2b, which has greater resistance to proteolytic breakdown and increased biological half-life, is more effective due to its superior viral suppression.[47]

*Interleukin-12*, which has angiogenic inhibitory activity, achieved a 71% response rate among 24 evaluable patients at doses of 300 ng/kg or greater.[48] In patients on HAART IL-12 at a dose of 300 ng/kg subcutaneously twice weekly combined with six 3-week cycles of 20 mg/m² of pegylated liposomal doxorubicin and then followed by a maintenance IL-12 dose of 500 ng/kg twice weekly for up to 3 years in patients on HAART yielded an 83% major response rate (CR: 25%). Furthermore, 56% of patients with residual lesions after the end of chemotherapy had a new major response during maintenance interleukin therapy.[49]

*Chemotherapy* with cytotoxic agents administered singly (etoposide, bleomycin, vincristine) or as part of regimens (doxorubicin–bleomycin–vincristine or vinblastine–bleomycin) have been reported to induce response rates between 21% and 80% with median duration of response from 1 to 9 months. Due to a lack of standardization of criteria used to stage patients and to evaluate response to treatment in these studies, it is not always feasible to compare response rates.[44] The addition of HAART significantly improves responses and outcomes.

The liposomal anthracyclines are considered the initial chemotherapeutic agents of choice in most cases. Pegylated liposomal doxorubicin (PLD) administered as a slow 30–60-minute infusion of 20 mg/m² every 3 weeks, relieves symptoms in up to half of patients even without the addition of antiretroviral drugs.[50] Objective response rates are better, faster and safer than regimens containing either doxorubicin, or bleomycin, or vincristine. In a small but carefully conducted randomized study of patients with moderate to severe KS, a complete or partial remission was achieved after 48 weeks in 76% of the group treated with PLD and HAART, but only in 20% of the control cohort on HAART alone.[51] Notably, 10 patients in the control group required rescue chemotherapy. At a median follow-up of 29 months, although 30% of PLD-treated patients had died, only 3% expired from KS progression.[51] While patients may develop neutropenia, anemia or acute transient reactions to the infusion, the risk of alopecia, nausea or vomiting, and cardiotoxicity are markedly reduced compared to regimens containing non-liposomal doxorubicin.

In a randomized, double-blind study, clinical benefit and tumor responses were observed in 80% and 55%, respectively, of KS cases treated with pegylated liposomal doxorubicin ($20 \, mg/m^2$) and 63% and 32%, respectively, of those treated with liposomal daunorubicin ($40 \, mg/m^2$). The clinical benefit was maintained for a median of 63 days after treatment with doxorubicin and 55 days after treatment with daunorubicin.[52] Better responses may be obtained with a higher ($60 \, mg/m^2$) dose of daunorubicin. In general, patient response to PLD requires fewer treatment cycles and thus is more cost-effective. More cycles of liposomal anthracyclines are needed in HAART-treated patients.

Recurrent or resistant KS may respond to *paclitaxel* or *docetaxel*. Not only do these taxanes inhibit mitosis by preventing depolymerization of microtubules but they also suppress angiogenesis. Approximately 56% of patients treated with four cycles of paclitaxel experienced responses that lasted an average of 9 months and improved quality of life. Even better major response rates have been achieved at higher doses, even in patients with pulmonary KS and those who failed anthracyclines. Similar response rates have been obtained with docetaxel, which also prevented disease progression in another third of treated patients.[53] Premedication with a corticosteroid such as dexamethasone, at a dose of 20 mg given orally at 12 and 6 hours before infusion of paclitaxel. This diminishes the risk of a hypersensitivity reaction. Interaction with other drugs that are metabolized by cytochrome P450 enzymes should be considered. Neutropenia and thrombocytopenia are common without co-administration of hematopoietic growth factors.

*Thalidomide*, an oral immunomodulator that inhibits angiogenesis induced by basic fibroblast growth factor, has induced KS regression in 34–47% of AIDS-KS cases in small clinical trials but the required dose may be high and about a third of patients develop neuropathy.[44,45]

*Indinavir*, a protease inhibitor, at a dose of 800 mg twice daily for 12 months, resulted in one complete remission, two partial regressions, five disease improvements, and eight disease stabilizations among 26 patients with classic KS. Patients with early KS lesions less than 3 months had especially favorable outcomes, while those with late disease had higher non-response and relapse rates.[54]

*Imiquimod cream* under occlusion with a polyurethane dressing for at least 24 weeks produced two complete and three partial clinical responses and decreased induration in another six cases, but did not prevent progression in the other six patients in an uncontrolled series of both HIV-associated and classic KS.[55] Treatment was well tolerated with only irritation.

*Photodynamic therapy* involving application of an ointment containing 20% delta-aminolevulinic acid occluded with a transparent dressing for 6 hours followed by irradiation with a 600–730 nm red light with 90 to $250 \, mW/cm^2$ (exposure time varies between 6 and 20 minutes for a total dose of 100 to $150 \, J/cm^2$) may be cosmetically valuable in superficial lesions.[56] In one study, complete and partial palliative responses were achieved respectively in 32.5% and 63.3% of cases treated with exposure to

## Table 16.5 Non-Chemotherapy KS Treatments

| |
|---|
| Alitretinoin gel (PR: 35–37%) |
| Cryotherapy (partial tumor response: up to 80%) |
| Interferon alpha, subcutaneous, with antiretroviral agent(s), 1 million units (CR: 40%) or 10 million units daily (CR: 55%) |
| Intralesional vinblastine (clinical response: 60–90%) |
| Photodynamic treatment (CR: 32.5%; PR: 63%) |
| Radiotherapy (up to 80% complete lesional response depending on dose) |
| Surgery (variable) |
| Thalidomide, 200–1000 mg (median 600 mg daily) (PR: 47%) |

CR, complete response; PR, partial response.

$100–400 \, J/cm^2$ of 630 nm light 2 hours after an oral dose of $1.0 \, mg/kg$ of Photofrin.[57] Median duration of response for complete responders was 26 weeks and for partial responders was 8 weeks.

*Surgical excision* is impractical except possibly as treatment of localized small tumors when patients prefer a scar to the appearance of the lesions or as palliative therapy of painful lesions. Recurrences are high unless the tumors are excised with wide margins and there have been no studies comparing Mohs micrographic surgery to conventional excisional surgery.

*Laser therapy* with the pulsed dye (535 nm) laser may lighten or eradicate the surface of tumors but in most patients recurrence is noted within 12 weeks.[58] Ablative lasers ($CO_2$, erbium) offer an advantage of controlled bleeding over surgery but are avoided due to concerns about viral vaporization and high recurrence rates (Table 16.5).

## FUTURE OUTLOOK

Future significant advancements in this disease will most likely occur in the area of therapeutics. *Bevacizumab*, a promising humanized monoclonal anti-VEGF antibody, is being trialed in combination with PLD. *Incyclinide (Metastat)*, a chemically modified, highly anti-inflammatory tetracycline which inhibits production and activity of MMP-2, induced a response rate of 40% at an oral dose of $50 \, mg/day$.[59] *Imatinib*, an oral tyrosinase kinase inhibitor, targets c-kit and platelet-derived growth factor receptor signaling and produced partial clinical regression in half of patients in a small pilot study.[60] Multikinase inhibitors, such as sorafenib and sunitinib, which have anti-angiogenic activity and target the 'mTOR' signaling pathway, may be valuable in other types of KS in addition to the post-transplant form.

The outcome of retrospective studies evaluating the effect of ganciclovir or foscarnet on subsequent KS development has been variable. In a pilot study, all seven patients treated with cidofovir continued to have progression of KS.[61] Other potential future treatments that need to be evaluated include bortezomib, a proteasome inhibitor; calcipotriene, a vitamin D analog; histone deacetylase inhibitors that reverse herpesvirus latency and induce apoptosis of infected cells; and Cdk inhibitors, which inhibit VEGF production and HHV-8 replication.[6]

# ACKNOWLEDGEMENT

Susan E. Krown, M.D., Attending Physician and Member, Memorial Sloan-Kettering Cancer Center, Professor of Medicine, Weill Cornell Medical College, and Member, Melanoma and Sarcoma Service, Memorial Sloan-Kettering Cancer Center, reviewed, provided guidance and assisted with the preparation of this article.

# REFERENCES

1. Matondo P. Clinical classification of African Kaposi's sarcoma: time for reappraisal. *Int J Dermatol*. 1995;34:166–167.
2. Friedman-Kien AE. Disseminated Kaposi's sarcoma syndrome in young homosexual men. *J Am Acad Dermatol*. 1981;5:468–471.
3. Chang Y, Cesarman E, Pessin MS, et al. Identification of new herpesvirus-like DNA sequences in AIDS-associated Kaposi's sarcoma. *Science*. 1996;266:1865–1869.
4. Rizza G, Andreoni M, Dorrucci M, et al. Human herpesvirus 8 seropositivity and risk of Kaposi's sarcoma and other acquired immunodeficiency syndrome-related diseases. *J Natl Cancer Inst*. 1999;91(17):1440–1441.
5. Vitale F, Briffa DV, Whitby D, et al. Kaposi's sarcoma herpes virus and Kaposi's sarcoma in the elderly populations of 3 Mediterranean islands. *Int J Cancer*. 2001;91(4):588–591.
6. Martin JN, Ganem DE, Osmond DH, et al. Sexual transmission and the natural history of human herpesvirus 8 infection. *N Engl J Med*. 1998;338:948–954.
7. Duprez R, Lacoste V, Brière J, et al. Evidence for a multiclonal origin of multicentric advanced lesions of Kaposi sarcoma. *J Natl Cancer Inst*. 2007;99(14):1086–1094.
8. Escalon MP, Hagemeister FB. AIDS-related malignancies. In: Kantarjian HM, Wolff RA, Koller CA, eds. *MD Anderson Manual of Medical Oncology*. New York: McGraw-Hill; 2006:903–910.
9. Grayson W, Pantanowitz L. Histological variants of cutaneous Kaposi's sarcoma. *Diagn Pathol*. 2008;3:31.
10. Iscovich J, Boffetta P, Franceschi S, et al. Classic Kaposi sarcoma: epidemiology and risk factors. *Cancer*. 2000;88(3):500–517.
11. Krown SE, Singh JC. *Classic Kaposi's sarcoma: epidemiology, risk factors, pathology, and molecular pathogenesis*. Up to Date; Version 17.3, www.uptodate.com; 2009.
12. Anderson LA, Lauria C, Romano N, et al. Risk factors for classical Kaposi sarcoma in a population-based case-control study in Sicily. *Cancer Epidemiol Biomarkers Prev*. 2008;17(12):3435–3443.
13. Brown EE, Whitby D, Vitale F, et al. Virologic, hematologic, and immunologic risk factors for classic Kaposi's sarcoma. *Cancer*. 2006;107(9):2282–2290.
14. Azzarelli A, Mazzaferro V, Quagliuolo V, et al. Kaposi's sarcoma: malignant tumor or proliferative disorder? *Eur J Cancer Clin Oncol*. 1988;24(6):973–978.
15. Kolios G, Kaloterakis A, Filiotou A, et al. Gastroscopic findings in Mediterranean Kaposi's sarcoma (non-AIDS). *Gastrointest Endosc*. 1995;42(4):336–339.
16. Stratigos JD, Potouridou I, Katoulis AC, et al. Classic Kaposi's sarcoma in Greece: a clinico-epidemiological profile. *Int J Dermatol*. 2008;36(10):735–740.
17. Brambilla L, Boneschi V, Taglioni M, et al. Staging of classic Kaposi's sarcoma: a useful tool for therapeutic choices. *Eur J Dermatol*. 2003;13:83.
18. Hiatt KM, Nelson AM, Lichy JH, et al. Classic Kaposi sarcoma in the United States over the last two decades: a clinicopathologic and molecular study of 438 non-HIV-related Kaposi sarcoma patients with comparison to HIV-related Kaposi sarcoma. *Mod Pathol*. 2008;21(5):572–582.
19. Grabar S, Abraham B, Mahamat A, et al. Differential impact of combination antiretroviral therapy in preventing Kaposi's sarcoma with and without visceral involvement. *J Clin Oncol*. 2006;24(21):3408–3414.
20. Lanternier FA, Lebbe CF, Schartz NC, et al. Kaposi's sarcoma in HIV-negative men having sex with men. *AIDS*. 2008;22(10):1163–1168.
21. Krown SE, Testa MA, Huang J. AIDS-related Kaposi's sarcoma: prospective validation of the AIDS Clinical Trials Group staging classification. AIDS Clinical Trials Group Oncology Committee. *J Clin Oncol*. 1997;15(9):3085–3092.
22. Taylor JF, Templeton AC, Vogel CL, et al. Kaposi's sarcoma in Uganda: a clinico-pathological study. *Int J Cancer*. 1971;8:122–135.
23. de-Thé G, Bestetti G, van Beveren M, et al. Prevalence of human herpesvirus 8 infection before the acquired immunodeficiency disease syndrome-related epidemic of Kaposi's sarcoma in East Africa. *J Natl Cancer Inst*. 1999;91(21):1888–1889.
24. Louthrenoo W, Kasitanon N, Mahanuphab P, et al. Kaposi's sarcoma in rheumatic diseases. *Semin Arthritis Rheum*. 2003;32(5):326–333.
25. Stallone G, Schena A, Infante B, et al. Sirolimus for Kaposi's sarcoma in renal-transplant recipients. *N Engl J Med*. 2005;352(13):1317–1323.
26. Hammock L, Reisenauer A, Wang W, et al. Latency-associated nuclear antigen expression and human herpesvirus-8 polymerase chain reaction in the evaluation of Kaposi sarcoma and other vascular tumors in HIV-positive patients. *Mod Pathol*. 2005;18:463–468.
27. Ledergerber B, Egger M, Erard V, et al. AIDS-related opportunistic illnesses occurring after initiation of potent antiretroviral therapy: the Swiss HIV Cohort Study. *JAMA*. 1999;282(23):2220–2226.
28. Tam HK, Zhang ZF, Jacobson LP, et al. Effect of HAART on survival among HIV-infected men with Kaposi sarcoma or non-Hodgkin lymphoma. *Int J Cancer*. 2002;98:916–922.
29. Nguyen HQ, Magaret AS, Kitahata MM, et al. Persistent Kaposi sarcoma in the era of highly active antiretroviral therapy: characterizing the predictors of clinical response. *AIDS*. 2008;22:937–945.
30. Mani D, Neil N, Israel R, et al. A retrospective analysis of AIDS-associated Kaposi's sarcoma in patients with undetectable HIV viral loads and CD4 counts greater than 300 cells/mm³. *J Int Assoc Physicians AIDS Care*. 2009;8(5):279–285.
31. El Amari EB, Toutous-Trellu L, Gayet-Ageron A, et al. Predicting the evolution of Kaposi sarcoma, in the highly active antiretroviral therapy era. *AIDS*. 2008;22(9):1019–1028.
32. Portsmouth S, Stebbing J, Gill J, et al. A comparison of regimens based on nonnucleoside reverse transcriptase inhibitors or protease inhibitors in preventing Kaposi's sarcoma. *AIDS*. 2003;17:17–22.
33. Holkova B, Takeshita K, Cheng DM, et al. Effect of highly active antiretroviral therapy on survival in patients with AIDS-associated pulmonary Kaposi's sarcoma treated with chemotherapy. *J Clin Oncol*. 2001;19(18):3848–3851.
34. Maurer T, Ponte M, Leslie K. HIV-associated Kaposi's sarcoma with a high CD4 count and a low viral load [letter]. *N Engl J Med*. 2007;57:1352–1353.
35. Krown SE, Lee JY, Dittmer DP, for the AIDS Malignancy Consortium. More on HIV-associated Kaposi's sarcoma [letter]. *N Engl J Med*. 2008;358:535–536.
36. Bower M, Nelson M, Young AM, et al. Immune reconstitution inflammatory syndrome associated with Kaposi's sarcoma. *J Clin Oncol*. 2005;23(22):5224–5228.
37. Monaco AP. The role of mTOR inhibitors in the management of post-transplant malignancy. *Transplantation*. 2009;87(2):157–163.
38. Bodsworth NJ, Bloch M, Bower M, et al. Phase III vehicle-controlled, multi-centered study of topical alitretinoin gel 0.1-percent in cutaneous AIDS-related Kaposi's sarcoma. *Am J Clin Dermatol*. 2001;2(2):77–87.
39. Boudreaux A, Smith L, Cosby C, et al. Intralesional vinblastine for cutaneous Kaposi's sarcoma associated with acquired immunodeficiency syndrome. A clinical trial to evaluate efficacy and discomfort associated with injection. *J Am Acad Dermatol*. 1993;28(1):61–65.
40. Tappero JW, Burger TG, Kaplan LD, et al. Cryotherapy for cutaneous Kaposi's sarcoma associated with acquired immunodeficiency syndrome (AIDS). *J Acquir Immune Defic Syndr*. 1991;4(9):839–846.
41. Kigula-Mugambe JB, Kavuma A. Epidemic and endemic Kaposi's sarcoma: a comparison of outcomes and survival after radiotherapy. *Radiotherapy Oncol*. 2005;76:59–62.
42. Gressen EL, Rosenstock JG, Xie Y, et al. Palliative treatment of epidemic Kaposi's sarcoma of the feet. *Am J Clin Oncol*. 1999;22(3):286–290.
43. Kirova YM, Belembaogo E, Frikha H, et al. Radiotherapy in the management of epidemic Kaposi's sarcoma: a retrospective study of 643 cases. *Radiother Oncol*. 1998;46:19–22.
44. Vanni T, Sprinz E, Machado MW, et al. Systemic treatment of AIDS-related Kaposi's sarcoma: current status and perspectives. *Cancer Treat Rev*. 2006;32(6):445–455.
45. Krown SE. Management of Kaposi sarcoma: the role of interferon and thalidomide. *Curr Opin Oncol*. 2001;13:374–381.
46. Krown SE, Lee JY, Lin L, et al. Interferon-alpha 2b with protease inhibitor-based antiretroviral therapy in patients with AIDS-associated Kaposi sarcoma: an AIDS malignancy consortium phase I trial. *J Acquir Immune Defic Syndr*. 2006;41(2):149–153.
47. Van der Ende M, Mulder JW, van den Berge M, et al. Complete clinical and virological remission of refractory HIV-related Kaposi's sarcoma with pegylated interferon alpha. *AIDS*. 2007;21(12):1661–1662.
48. Yarchoan R, Pluda JM, Wyvill KM, et al. Treatment of AIDS-related Kaposi's sarcoma with interleukin-12: rationale and preliminary evidence of clinical activity. *Crit Rev Immunol*. 2007;27(5):401–414.
49. Little RF, Aleman K, Kumar P, et al. Phase 2 study of pegylated liposomal doxorubicin in combination with interleukin-12 for AIDS-related Kaposi sarcoma. *Blood*. 2007;110(13):4165–4171.
50. Krown SE, Northfelt DW, Osoba J, et al. Use of liposomal anthracyclines in Kaposi's sarcoma. *Semin Oncol*. 2004;31(suppl 13):36–52.
51. Martín-Carbonero L, Palacios R, Valenica E, et al. Long-term prognosis of HIV-infected patients with Kaposi sarcoma treated with pegylated liposomal doxorubicin. *Clin Infect Dis*. 2008;47(3):410–417.

52. Cooley T, Henry D, Tonda M, et al. A randomized, double-blind study of pegylated liposomal doxorubicin for the treatment of AIDS-related Kaposi's sarcoma. *Oncologist*. 2007;12:114–123.

53. Lim ST, Tupule A, Espina BM, et al. Weekly docetaxel is safe and effective in the treatment of advanced-stage acquired immunodeficiency syndrome-related Kaposi sarcoma. *Cancer*. 2005;103:417–421.

54. Monini P, Sgadari C, Grosso MG, et al. Clinical course of classic Kaposi's sarcoma in HIV-negative patients treated with the HIV protease inhibitor indinavir. *AIDS*. 2009;23(4):534–538.

55. Celestin-Schartz NE, Chevret S, Paz C, et al. Imiquimod 5-percent cream for treatment of HIV-negative Kaposi's sarcoma skin lesions: a phase I to II, open-label trial in 17 patients. *J Am Acad Dermatol*. 2008;58(4):585–591.

56. Park MY, Kim YC. Classic Kaposi sarcoma treated with intralesional 5-aminolevulinic acid injection photodynamic therapy. *Arch Dermatol*. 2009;145(10):1200–1202.

57. Bernstein ZP, Wilson BD, Oseroff AR, et al. Photofrin, photodynamic therapy for treatment of AIDS-related cutaneous Kaposi's sarcoma. *AIDS*. 1999;113(13):1697–1704.

58. Tappero JW, Grekin RC, Zanelli GA, et al. Pulsed-dye laser therapy for cutaneous Kaposi's sarcoma associated with acquired immunodeficiency syndrome. *J Am Acad Dermatol*. 1992;27:526–530.

59. Aldenhoven M, Barlo NP, Sanders CJ. Therapeutic strategies for epidemic Kaposi's sarcoma. *Int J STD AIDS*. 2006;17(9):571–578.

60. Dittmer DP, Krown SE. Targeted therapy for Kaposi's sarcoma and Kaposi's sarcoma-associated herpesvirus. *Curr Opin Oncol*. 2007;19(5):452–457.

61. Little RF, Merced- Galindez F, Staskus K, et al. A pilot study of cidofovir in patients with Kaposi sarcoma. *J Infect Dis*. 2003;187:149–153.

# Merkel Cell Carcinoma

## CHAPTER 17

*Jayasri G. Iyer, Renee Thibodeau, and Paul Nghiem*

---

## Key Points

- Merkel cell carcinoma (MCC) is an uncommon neuroendocrine skin cancer with a 5-year disease-associated mortality of 46%.
- The reported incidence of MCC has tripled in the past 20 years and there are approximately 1500 new cases each year in the US.
- Risk factors include age over 50 years, profound immune suppression, UV exposure, and fair skin.
- Unfortunately, despite its lack of tenderness, MCC is often thought to be an inflamed/ruptured cyst, leading to delayed diagnosis.
- Management is distinct from other skin cancers in that microscopic node evaluation and adjuvant radiation therapy are often indicated.
- The Merkel cell polyomavirus was discovered in 2008. DNA from this virus is present in approximately 80% of MCC tumors.

## INTRODUCTION

Merkel cell carcinoma (MCC) is an uncommon but often lethal neuroendocrine skin cancer. Its incidence of ~1500 cases per year in the US is similar to that of cutaneous T-cell lymphoma and dermatofibrosarcoma protuberans. MCC is the second most common cause of non-melanoma skin cancer death, after squamous cell carcinoma. MCC has a higher 5-year relative mortality (46%) than malignant melanoma (15%). MCC presenting without clinical evidence of nodal disease has a 32% chance of microscopic nodal involvement. MCC management has been challenging due to lack of prospective clinical studies, and a paucity of centers with expertise or interest in this rare disease.

## HISTORY

Prior to 1972, when the cancer we now call 'MCC' was properly identified, it was referred to as 'undifferentiated carcinoma of the skin'. In 1972, Toker referred to it as 'trabecular carcinoma of the skin' in recognition of one of its characteristic histologic patterns. In 1978, Tang and Toker used electron microscopy to reveal intracytoplasmic dense-core neurosecretory granules in MCC that are similar to those seen in neuroendocrine cells. In 1980, DeWolf-Peeters named it Merkel cell carcinoma because of the neuroendocrine features shared between this cancer and the normal Merkel cell present in the epidermis (Fig. 17.1).

The introduction of specific immunostains in the 1990s decreased the frequent mischaracterization of MCC as lymphoma, metastatic carcinoma, or melanoma.

## EPIDEMIOLOGY

Prior to the 1980s, the diagnosis of Merkel cell carcinoma was only rarely made. With the introduction of the cytokeratin 20 (CK20) antibody in the early 1990s, the diagnosis of MCC could be made more readily and its reported incidence increased significantly. MCC predominantly affects fair-skinned individuals over the age of 70. Only 5% of cases occur in patients under the age of 50. MCC tends to affect men more than women.[1] The reported incidence of MCC in the US is currently approximately 1500 cases per year[2] and has more than tripled in the past 20 years[3] due to: 1) improved diagnosis as described above, 2) increased numbers of immune-suppressed patients (HIV, solid organ transplant recipients, chronic lymphocytic leukemia), and 3) an increase in the number of older individuals with prior extensive sun exposure. MCC incidence is likely to continue to grow in the US as these at-risk populations increase. Although the incidence of MCC is currently about 30 times less than that of melanoma, MCC has a higher 5-year disease-associated mortality of 46%[4] as compared to 12.5% among all those diagnosed with invasive melanoma.[5]

## PATHOGENESIS AND ETIOLOGY

### UV exposure

Several lines of evidence suggest that UV exposure is an important risk factor for MCC. This cancer occurs almost exclusively in fair-skinned individuals, with 94–98% of US cases occurring in Caucasians. MCC arises more often on sun-exposed sites such as the head, neck and dorsal arm. The incidence of MCC is greater in geographic locations with higher UV indices.[1] Patients who received numerous treatments of methoxsalen plus UVA for psoriasis had an approximately 100-fold increased incidence for MCC.[6] In spite of these strong links with UV, not all cases arise on sun-exposed skin. Approximately 15% of MCC cases occur in sun-protected areas such as the buttocks, genitals, or hair-covered scalp.

### Profound immune suppression

The risk of MCC is markedly elevated in patients with advanced HIV/AIDS (13-fold),[7] solid organ transplant recipients on chronic immunosuppressive medications

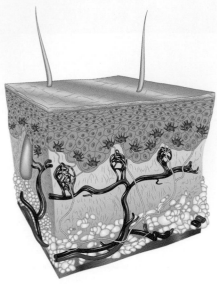

Figure 17.1 Normal Merkel cells in the skin. In this schematic, normal Merkel cells are indicated as red cells connected to nerves (yellow). Merkel cells are located in the basal layer of the epidermis and are required for light touch sensation in the skin.

(10-fold),[8] and patients with chronic lymphocytic leukemia (30- to 50-fold)[9] These links suggest an important role for T-cell immune surveillance in preventing the development of clinically apparent MCC.

## Merkel cell polyomavirus

Because of the strong links between immune suppression and MCC, several groups searched for an associated pathogen. In 2008, a novel human polyomavirus was found to be present in ~80% of MCC tumors and was named the Merkel cell polyomavirus (MCPyV).[10] Several lines of evidence suggest a probable role for MCPyV in this cancer: 1) MCPyV DNA is integrated into the genome of many MCC tumors, a hallmark of oncogenic viruses. 2) Viral sequences can be detected in the majority of MCCs but only rarely in normal skin or other skin tumors. 3) MCC patients are more likely than age-matched controls to have antibodies to the Merkel cell polyomavirus capsid protein[11] (88% for MCC patients versus 53% for the general population).[12] 4) Proteins derived from MCPyV that are likely to have a role in oncogenesis are persistently expressed in many MCC tumors.[13] 5) Certain portions of a critical oncoprotein (large T antigen) that are likely to be detrimental to the cancer (via promoting excessive DNA replication at the site of viral integration) are often deleted in the integrated/truncated viral sequences. These mutations are suggestive of a strong selection for the cancer-promoting functions of MCPyV.

Despite this overwhelming evidence linking this new polyomavirus to MCC, it is also clear that viral infection is not sufficient to cause this cancer. Seroprevalence studies indicate that a majority of the general population are exposed to this virus in childhood, yet MCC remains a rare cancer that typically arises after age 50. It also appears that MCPyV is not necessary because no viral DNA can be detected in approximately 20–30% of MCC tumors. These tumors may have either developed without any involvement of MCPyV,

or the virus may have only been important for tumor initiation and then subsequently lost.

## Collision tumors

MCC sometimes develops in the setting of other skin malignancies such as squamous cell carcinoma or Bowen's disease. This is particularly relevant since it has recently been established that Merkel cells are derived from an epidermal (not neural crest) origin and thus epidermal premalignant progenitor cells could theoretically differentiate in a squamous or neuroendocrine pattern.

## CLINICAL FEATURES

MCC typically presents as a rapidly growing, firm, asymptomatic, red, pink, purple, or skin-colored nodule[9] (Fig. 17.2). MCC most commonly occurs on sun-exposed areas, particularly the head and neck; however, in approximately one in six patients, it presents on a sun-protected site. Nodal or visceral presentation of MCC in the absence of a discernable primary lesion occurs in approximately 15% of cases.[9] Most primary MCCs (56%) were thought to be some type of benign lesion at the time of biopsy (cyst/acneiform lesion was the single most common pre-biopsy diagnosis). Clinical features commonly associated with lesions that turn out to be Merkel cell carcinoma can be summarized with the letters AEIOU: Asymptomatic, Expanding rapidly, Immune suppressed, Older than 50 years, and UV-exposed fair skin. Among patients presenting with a primary cutaneous MCC, 89% had three or more of these five features.[9]

## PATIENT EVALUATION, DIAGNOSIS, AND DIFFERENTIAL DIAGNOSIS

The clinical presentation of MCC may be non-specific and its differential diagnosis includes a spectrum of benign and malignant diseases including cyst, acneiform lesion, cutaneous lymphoma, melanoma, non-melanoma skin cancer, and cutaneous metastasis of carcinoma. The diagnosis of MCC is of necessity made only upon detailed histologic evaluation including an appropriate panel of immunostains.

## Staging and prognosis

As for other cancers, the stage at presentation of MCC is a key determinant of prognosis as well as of recommended treatment. MCC with no apparent nodal involvement on clinical examination has a 32% chance of microscopic lymph node involvement.[14] Hence, sentinel lymph node biopsy (SLNB) is an important procedure to determine microscopic involvement of nodes and accurately establish the stage of disease at diagnosis. This also helps to determine the need for nodal basin therapy. Importantly, SLNB should be performed prior to wide excision as local lymphatics are disturbed by surgery, making the test less reliable following wide excision. The 5-year relative survival rate for MCC patients who were pathologically determined to be node-negative was 76% as compared to 59% for patients whose nodes were determined to be negative by clinical examination only (p<0.0001).[4]

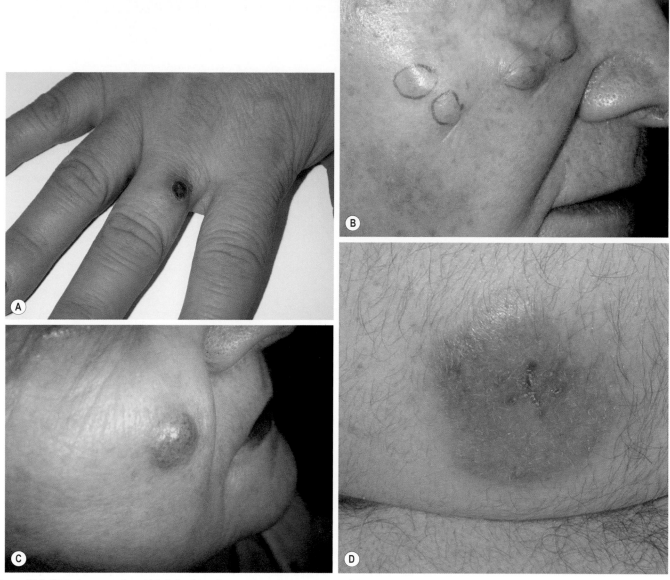

**Figure 17.2** Clinical presentation of Merkel cell carcinoma. Examples of primary MCC tumors: **A)** middle finger; **B)** orbital region of the face with satellite nodules seen inferolaterally; **C)** cheek (photo courtesy of Barry Paul, MD); **D)** buttock. Although MCC lesions often resemble a rapidly growing red/purple inflamed cyst, the lack of tenderness (88% are non-tender) can be an important clue that a biopsy should be carried out for such a lesion (especially on the sun-exposed skin of an elderly or immune-suppressed person).

## The new staging system

A new consensus staging system for MCC has been adopted for worldwide use as of 2010.[4] This four-tiered system (Table 17.1) is the first MCC-specific staging system created by the American Joint Committee on Cancer (AJCC). Two key features of this new staging system are the inclusion of the *method* of nodal examination used to determine node negativity for 'local-only' disease (microscopic or clinical-only node examination) and the *extent* of nodal involvement (microscopic-only disease or clinically evident nodal disease). Both of these factors were found to be highly significant in the cohort of 5823 MCC patients used to derive the new system. Table 17.1 includes survival data (relative to age- and sex-matched controls) for each sub-stage of the new AJCC staging system.

## Radiologic imaging studies

MCC not only has a high propensity for invading local and regional nodal basins, but also exhibits a significant tendency for distant spread. Imaging studies (CT/PET) are therefore critical for staging patients who present with higher-risk disease (large primary tumor or known nodal involvement). However, for patients with a small primary lesion and microscopically negative nodal involvement, scans may not be indicated or may be obtained primarily as a baseline study. Imaging studies often miss microscopic nodal disease that would be detected by sentinel lymph node biopsy.[14] Therefore, imaging should not be viewed as a substitute for microscopic nodal evaluation. Imaging studies may reveal a benign lesion that is undistinguishable from a malignant one unless biopsied. This may lead to

## Table 17.1 Merkel cell carcinoma staging system

| Stage | Stage Grouping | Stage Description | 1-Year Relative Survival | 3-Year Relative Survival | 5-Year Relative Survival |
|---|---|---|---|---|---|
| Stage 0: | 0 | Tumor in situ | ----* | ----* | ----* |
| Stage I: Local, tumor diameter ≤2 cm | IA | Nodes microscopically negative and not clinically detectable | 100 | 86 | 79 |
| | IB | Nodes not clinically detectable (no pathologic eval of nodes done) | 90 | 70 | 60 |
| Stage II: Local, tumor diameter >2 cm | IIA | Nodes microscopically negative and not clinically detectable | 90 | 64 | 58 |
| | IIB | Nodes not clinically detectable (no pathologic eval of nodes done) | 81 | 58 | 49 |
| | IIC | Primary tumor invading bone/muscle/fascia/cartilage | 72 | 55 | 47 |
| Stage III: Regional nodal disease | IIIA | Micrometastasis† | 76 | 50 | 42 |
| | IIIB | Macrometastasis‡ (clinically detectable node or intransit metastases§) | 70 | 34 | 26 |
| Stage IV: Distant metastatic disease | IV | Distant Metastatic Disease | 44 | 20 | 18 |

This table summarizes the first-ever American Joint Committee on Cancer staging system specific for Merkel cell carcinoma. It was adopted for worldwide use in 2010.

*No data are available for in-situ MCC tumors, but survival is expected to be excellent.

†Micrometastases are diagnosed after sentinel or elective lymphadenectomy.

‡Macrometastases are defined as clinically detectable nodal metastases confirmed pathologically by biopsy or therapeutic lymphadenectomy.

§In-transit metastasis is a tumor distinct from the primary lesion and located either 1) between the primary lesion and the draining regional lymph nodes or 2) distal to the primary lesion.

unnecessary invasive procedures, worry and complications that are not warranted when the prior probability of metastatic disease is very low.

## New MCC-specific diagnostic codes

Seven new MCC-specific International Classification of Diseases (ICD) diagnostic codes were adopted for use in late 2009[15] (Table 17.2). Prior to 2009, MCC was classified as 'malignant carcinoma of the skin' (ICD code 173.x) along with numerous other less aggressive carcinomas (such as basal cell carcinoma) that rarely require imaging studies or hospitalization. Introduction of these specific codes will facilitate MCC patients in obtaining appropriate insurance approval for treatment and help clinicians and researchers track MCC-associated costs.

## PATHOLOGY

### Histology

MCC often presents as a dermal proliferation of undifferentiated small to intermediate sized, round to oval shaped, blue cells extending into subcutaneous fat, fascia and muscle, arranged in sheets and trabeculae. The histologic differential diagnosis for MCC is broad and immunohistochemical stains play a key role in differentiating this tumor from lymphoma, melanoma or other metastatic carcinoma. Involvement of epidermal and adnexal structures by MCC is uncommon. The overlying epidermis is

## Table 17.2 Diagnostic Codes for Merkel Cell Carcinoma*

| ICD Code | Disease |
|---|---|
| 209.31 | Merkel cell carcinoma of the face |
| 209.32 | Merkel cell carcinoma of the scalp and neck |
| 209.33 | Merkel cell carcinoma of the upper limb |
| 209.34 | Merkel cell carcinoma of the lower limb |
| 209.35 | Merkel cell carcinoma of the trunk |
| 209.36 | Merkel cell carcinoma of other sites including buttocks and genitals |
| 209.37 | Secondary Merkel cell carcinoma (presenting in nodal or visceral sites without known primary) |
| V10.91 | Personal history of malignant neuroendocrine tumor (should be used when seeing a patient more than 5 years after an MCC tumor was last treated) |

*Eight International Classification of Diseases (ICD) codes were assigned to Merkel cell carcinoma in late 2009.

only rarely ulcerated. Nuclei are round and hyperchromatic with evenly dispersed ('salt and pepper') chromatin and inconspicuous nucleoli. Cytoplasm is scant in tumor cells. Frequent findings include mitotic figures, fragmented nuclei, areas of necrosis, characteristic crush artifact, and lymphocytic infiltrates. Lymphovascular invasion is often seen in the primary lesion and has been linked with outcome.[16] Pathology reports may not include comment on this parameter. Because it can be important in determining management, a simple request to pathology to comment on this finding may be indicated.

## Immunohistochemistry

MCC cells typically express cytokeratin 20 (CK20) with a characteristic 'perinuclear dot' staining pattern (Fig. 17.3). Tumor cells are variably positive for neuroendocrine markers, such as neuron-specific enolase, chromogranin A, and synaptophysin. Tumor cells are typically negative for TTF-1, S100 and leukocyte common antigen, facilitating differentiation from several other small blue round cell tumors (Table 17.3). In addition, MCPyV oncoproteins (T antigens) that are persistently expressed in many MCC tumors[13] can be stained using a monoclonal antibody specific for the large T antigen of MCPyV (Fig. 17.4).

## TREATMENT

Treatment depends on the stage of presentation and may involve surgical management, radiation therapy and chemotherapy. The National Comprehensive Cancer Network

(NCCN) publishes a multidisciplinary treatment guideline for MCC that is updated annually (http://www.nccn.org). This algorithm and other updated treatment information are available at www.merkelcell.org/usefulinfo/index.php.

**Table 17.3 Immunohistochemical Stains for the Differential Diagnosis of MCC\***

| Stain | MCC | Small Cell Lung Cancer | Lymphoma | Melanoma |
|---|---|---|---|---|
| CK20 | + perinuclear dot-like pattern | – | – | – |
| CK7 | – | + | | – |
| TTF-1 | – | + | | – |
| LCA | – | – | + | – |
| S100 | – | | | + |

\*The table indicates stains commonly used to differentiate between small cell lung cancer, lymphoma and melanoma. It should be noted that not all MCC tumors follow the classical CK20-positive/CK7-negative expression pattern.

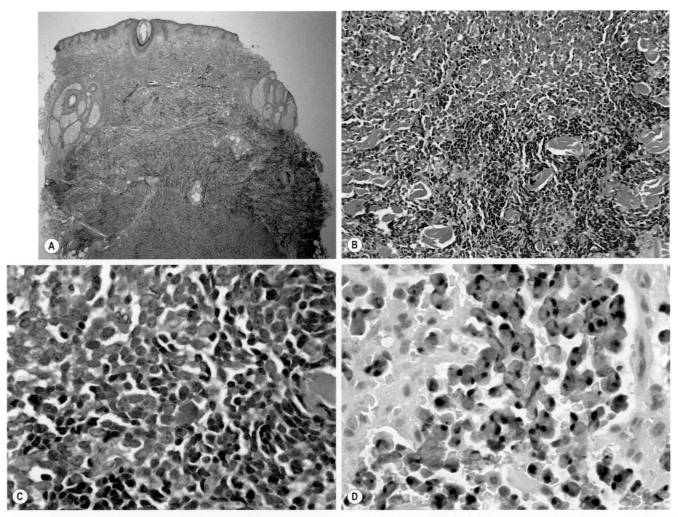

**Figure 17.3** Merkel cell carcinoma histology. **A)** As in this case, MCC tumors often appear distinct from the overlying epidermis. **B)** Small round cells with scant cytoplasm invade and disrupt collagen bundles. **C)** Hyperchromatic nuclei with evenly dispersed ('salt and pepper') chromatin. **D)** Cytokeratin-20 immunostain demonstrates expression in a classic perinuclear dot-like pattern.

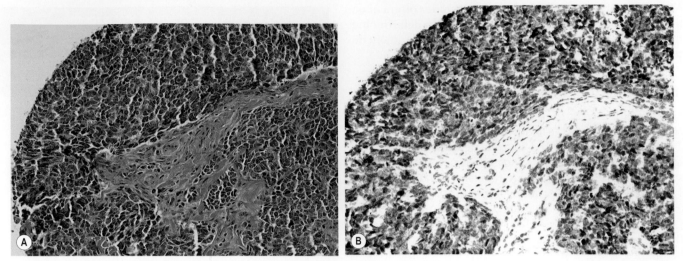

**Figure 17.4** Large T antigen expression in MCC tumors. An antibody directed against a unique portion of the Merkel cell polyomavirus large T antigen demonstrates expression of this oncoprotein in MCC tumor cells of one of our cases but not adjacent stroma (**A,** H&E; **B,** anti-MCPyV T antigen antibody, CM2B4, gift of P Moore and Y Chang). Previously published studies have demonstrated persistent expression of this oncoprotein in approximately half of MCC tumors.[13]

## Surgery

Surgical excision of the tumor with microscopically negative margins is typically a key aspect of managing primary Merkel cell carcinoma. The addition of postoperative radiation to the primary site has been associated with decreased local recurrence rates.[17] Emerging data from several groups,[18] including our own, suggest that there exists a subset of low-risk MCC patients who do not require adjuvant radiation (primary tumor ≤1 cm, negative sentinel lymph node biopsy, no chronic immune suppression, no lymphovascular invasion in the primary tumor, confidently negative microscopic margins after excision). If radiation will be delivered subsequently, aggressive surgery (amputation, or very wide margins requiring skin grafts) is typically not indicated, as this increases morbidity and delays the initiation of radiation therapy. For microscopic node-positive MCC, either completion lymph node dissection (CLND) or radiation therapy can offer excellent regional control rates.[19] Combining both CLND and radiation therapy does not appear to offer additional benefit for patients with microscopic-only nodal disease but may be indicated for clinically apparent nodal disease.

## Radiation therapy

MCC is an unusually radiation-sensitive tumor. Inclusion of postoperative radiation has been associated with lower locoregional recurrence of MCC as compared with surgical excision alone.[17] In patients for whom surgical excision is not feasible, radiation monotherapy may be a reasonable option[20] (Fig. 17.5).

## Chemotherapy

Most local and regional Merkel cell carcinomas can be effectively managed with a combination of surgery and radiation therapy. Adjuvant chemotherapy has not been demonstrated to improve survival and is infrequently used. For MCC that is not amenable to surgery or radiation, chemotherapy is often initially effective in controlling this tumor. However, unfortunately, MCC typically recurs with multi-drug resistance. The most commonly used regimen for MCC is the typical small cell lung cancer/neuroendocrine regimen: a combination of etoposide with either carboplatin or cisplatin.

## Follow-up

Because of its high recurrence rate during the first 3 years after diagnosis, patients should typically be seen every 3–6 months during this period. Visits should include a comprehensive skin and lymph node examination along with detailed review of systems. For patients who have not had any recurrence for 3–4 years after diagnosis, the risk of subsequently developing recurrent disease is approximately 90% less than at the time of their initial presentation.[18]

### FUTURE OUTLOOK

MCC has a high mortality rate even for the best prognostic group (stage Ia, 21% disease-associated 5-year mortality). Therefore, traditional anatomical staging alone is not sufficient for an accurate prognosis. Development of novel biomarkers that complement stage is likely to aid in prognostic accuracy as well as improving therapeutic decision-making.

A particularly exciting area for MCC is immunotherapy. Because of the persistent expression of Merkel cell polyomavirus proteins that are likely involved in oncogenesis, development of therapeutic vaccination, locally targeted immunostimulation, or MCPyV-targeted cellular therapy may hold promise in treating this cancer.

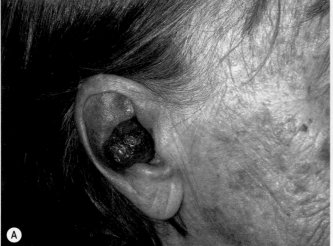

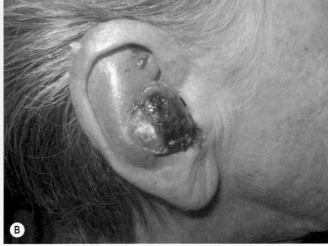

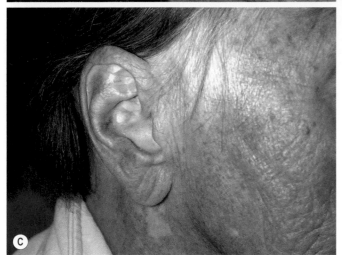

**Figure 17.5** Merkel cell carcinoma is typically very radiation-sensitive. **A)** An 87-year-old woman presented with an MCC of the right ear. She refused surgical excision and underwent radiation monotherapy. **B)** Necrosis of the lesion 3 weeks after beginning radiation therapy. **C)** Complete resolution of the MCC tumor several months after radiation therapy. She remained disease-free for approximately 24 months and died of an unrelated cause.

## REFERENCES

1. Agelli M, Clegg LX. Epidemiology of primary Merkel cell carcinoma in the United States. *J Am Acad Dermatol.* 2003;49:832–841.
2. Lemos B, Nghiem P. Merkel cell carcinoma: more deaths but still no pathway to blame. *J Invest Dermatol.* 2007;127:2100–2103.
3. Hodgson NC. Merkel cell carcinoma: changing incidence trends. *J Surg Oncol.* 2005;89:1–4.
4. Lemos BD, Storer BE, Iyer JG, et al. *Development of the first American Joint Committee on Cancer staging system for Merkel cell carcinoma based on prognostic factors analysis of 5,823 National Cancer Data Base cases.* doi:10.1016/j.jaad.2010.02.056.
5. American Cancer Society. *Cancer Facts & Figures 2009.* Atlanta: American Cancer Society; 2009.
6. Lunder EJ, Stern RS. Merkel-cell carcinomas in patients treated with methoxsalen and ultraviolet A radiation. *N Engl J Med.* 1998;339:1247–1248.
7. Engels EA, Frisch M, Goedert JJ, et al. Merkel cell carcinoma and HIV infection. *Lancet.* 2002;359:497–498.
8. Penn I, First MR. Merkel's cell carcinoma in organ recipients. report of 41 cases. *Transplantation.* 1999;68:1717–1721.
9. Heath ML, Jaimes N, Lemos B, et al. Clinical characteristics of Merkel cell carcinoma at diagnosis in 195 patients: the AEIOU features. *J Am Acad Dermatol.* 2008;58:375–381.
10. Feng H, Shuda M, Chang Y, et al. Clonal integration of a polyomavirus in human Merkel cell carcinoma. *Science.* 2008;319:1096–1100.
11. Tolstov YL, Pastrana DV, Feng H, et al. Human Merkel cell polyomavirus infection II. MCV is a common human infection that can be detected by conformational capsid epitope immunoassays. *Int J Cancer.* 2009;125:1250–1256.
12. Carter JJ, Paulson KG, Wipf GC, et al. Association of Merkel cell polyomavirus-specific antibodies with Merkel cell carcinoma. *J Natl Cancer Inst.* 2009;101:1510–1522.
13. Shuda M, Arora R, Kwun HJ, et al. Human Merkel cell polyomavirus infection I. MCV T antigen expression in Merkel cell carcinoma, lymphoid tissues and lymphoid tumors. *Int J Cancer.* 2009;125:1243–1249.
14. Gupta SG, Wang LC, Penas PF, et al. Sentinel lymph node biopsy for evaluation and treatment of patients with Merkel cell carcinoma: the Dana-Farber experience and meta-analysis of the literature. *Arch Dermatol.* 2006;142:685–690.
15. Iyer JG, Koba S, Nghiem P. Toward better management of Merkel cell carcinoma using a consensus staging system, new diagnostic codes and a recently discovered virus. *Actas Dermosifiliogr.* 2009;100(suppl 2):49–54.
16. Andea AA, Coit DG, Amin B, et al. Merkel cell carcinoma: histologic features and prognosis. *Cancer.* 2008;113:2549–2558.
17. Lewis KG, Weinstock MA, Weaver AL, et al. Adjuvant local irradiation for Merkel cell carcinoma. *Arch Dermatol.* 2006;142:693–700.
18. Allen PJ, Bowne WB, Jaques DP, et al. Merkel cell carcinoma: prognosis and treatment of patients from a single institution. *J Clin Oncol.* 2005;23:2300–2309.
19. Fang CL, Lemos BD, Douglas J, et al. Radiation monotherapy as regional treatment for node-positive Merkel cell carcinoma. *Cancer.* 2010;116:1783–1790.
20. Mortier L, Mirabel X, Fournier C, et al. Radiotherapy alone for primary Merkel cell carcinoma. *Arch Dermatol.* 2003;139:1587–1590.

# Malignant Neoplasms: Vascular Differentiation

*Omar P. Sangueza and Luis C. Requena*

## Key Points

- Clinical presentation is frequently a red- to purple-colored macule, plaque or nodule.

- Helpful diagnostic clues include sharp circumscription versus infiltrative edges of the neoplasm, size and multicentricity, as well as site of involvement, age, and other associated disease states such as immunosuppression, but biopsy is required to confirm diagnosis.

- Conservative excision is effective for benign lesions but other extensive treatment modalities may be needed for malignancies.

- High metastatic and mortality rates for vascular malignancies.

## INTRODUCTION

Angiosarcomas (AS) are rare, aggressive and malignant neoplasms. These lesions can be classified as low-grade and high-grade neoplasms. Low-grade AS include: endovascular papillary angioendothelioma (Dabska's tumor), retiform hemangioendothelioma, epithelioid hemangioendothelioma and composite hemangioendothelioma. Endovascular papillary angioendothelioma and retiform hemangioendotheliomas are probably the same entity. These lesions are locally aggressive and seldom metastasize. High-grade AS include: AS of the face and scalp of the elderly, AS associated with lymphedema, and radiation-induced AS.[1]

## HISTORY

In 1903, Mallory introduced the term hemangioendothelioma to describe a vascular tumor that infiltrated surrounding tissue, recurred locally, and may metastasize distally.[2] In 1943, Arthur Purdy Stout used the term hemangioendothelioma to describe vascular neoplasms with malignant behavior.[3] Angiosarcoma of the scalp and face of the elderly was first described by Caro and Stubenranch in 1945,[4] but it was Wilson Jones in 1964 who first provided detailed information about the clinical and histopathologic aspects of this variant of cutaneous angiosarcoma.[5] In 1948, Stewart and Treves reported six cases of angiosarcoma in postmastectomy lymphedema.[6] In 1982, Weiss and Enzinger proposed the terms hemangioendothelioma and epithelioid angiosarcoma.[7] In 1969, Maria Dabska reported an unusual neoplasm in six children who ranged in age from 4 months to 15 years.[8] She denominated this neoplasm endovascular papillary angioendothelioma. The term retiform hemangioendothelioma was coined by Calonje et al.[9] Finally, Nayler et al. introduced the term composite hemangioendothelioma in 2000.[10]

## EPIDEMIOLOGY

Angiosarcomas are an exceedingly rare type of vascular sarcoma. Approximately one-third of the reported cases occur in the skin. Approximately 50% of angiosarcomas occur in the head and neck. The African-American population and those individuals younger than 50 years of age are rarely affected. Of all the sarcomas affecting the head and neck, 10% are angiosarcomas.[11]

High-grade angiosarcomas have a poor prognosis, they are highly aggressive and are often multicentric. These neoplasms have high recurrence and mortality rates. They tend to metastasize quite readily because of their intrinsic biologic properties. The 5-year survival rate is around 20%.[12,13] Between 20% and 30% of AS metastasize to regional lymph nodes, which is higher than for most sarcomas.[11]

Angiosarcomas can affect any location of the body, but they have a predilection for skin and superficial soft tissue and are usually found on the head and neck of elderly people. The peak age of incidence for AS is around the seventh decade, with a range of 18 to 91 years.[14] The median age ranges from 60 to 71 years, and the male:female distribution is roughly equal.[15] However, for head and neck angiosarcomas, the male:female ratio is almost 2:1, and the median age is 71 years.[16,17]

## PATHOGENESIS AND ETIOLOGY

Vascular endothelial growth factor (VEGF) is involved in the regulation of endothelial cell proliferation, angiogenesis, and vascular permeability. VEGF-D is a member of the VEGF family of glycoproteins and has been found to be upregulated in the tumor cells of some malignancies. A study compared the serum VEGF-D levels in 11 patients with cutaneous angiosarcoma of the face and scalp and 18 healthy controls and found that serum VEGF-D levels were significantly elevated in angiosarcoma patients compared with the controls.[17]

Chronic lymphedema is a predisposing factor, but only 10% of AS are associated with this condition. There are also several case reports of angiosarcoma developing near defunctionalized arteriovenous fistulas in patients with renal transplants.[18] Sun exposure and trauma have also been proposed as risk factors in the development of AS, although no definitive evidence for these associations have been demonstrated.[19] Radiation is an important factor in the development of AS from the head and neck as well as the breast.[20]

## LOW-GRADE ANGIOSARCOMAS

### Retiform hemangioendothelioma and endovascular papillary angioendothelioma (Dabska's tumor)

Endovascular papillary angioendothelioma (EPE) and retiform hemangioendothelioma (RH) are low-grade angiosarcomas. EPE mainly affects children and young adults, while RH has been reported in patients within an age range of 9 to 78 years.[21,22] Clinically, EPE presents as enlarging cutaneous lesions that occur either as a diffuse swelling or as an intradermal tumor. Affected sites include the head, neck and extremities. RH preferentially affects the lower and upper limbs, although isolated lesions have been reported on the scalp, trunk and penis. Their etiology is unknown. One case of RH has been described in a setting of chronic lymphedema and another following radiation treatment.[23]

However, the majority of cases arise spontaneously with no known precipitating event.

Histopathologically, EPE is composed of irregular, interconnecting, vascular channels lined by atypical, endothelial cells. A very characteristic histopathological feature is the presence of papillary plugs of atypical endothelial cells that project into the lumina of the vessels (Fig. 18.1). The endothelial cells are round to polyhedral with atypical hyperchromatic and eccentrically placed nuclei, always in the luminal border of the cell. The cytoplasm of some hobnail endothelial cells contains vacuoles as an expression of primitive lumen formation. Mitotic figures may be seen. Some of the endothelial papillae possess a central sclerotic core of connective tissue. In some vessels, intraluminal lymphocytes are intermingled with endothelial cells.

RH, histopathologically, consists of elongated arborizing blood vessels involving the dermis in a pattern reminiscent of the normal rete testis architecture. These arborizing blood vessels are lined by monomorphic hobnail endothelial cells. In some areas, this pattern is obscured by the presence of a dense inflammatory infiltrate of mature lymphocytes (Fig. 18.2). However, in addition to the retiform pattern, more solid areas containing epithelioid or spindle cells with cytological atypia can also be identified. In many cases the same type of papillary projections which are the

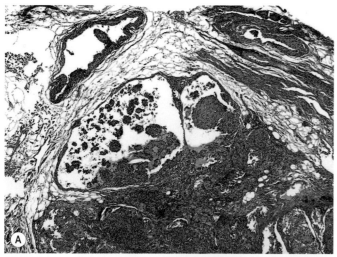

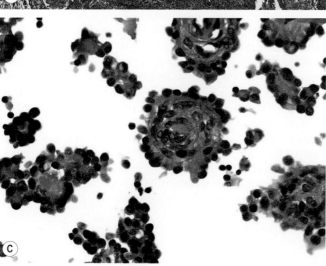

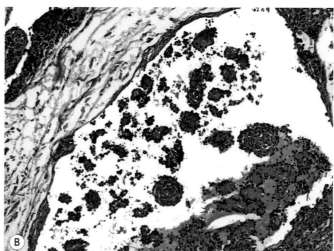

Figure 18.1 Endovascular papillary angioendothelioma (Dabska's tumor).

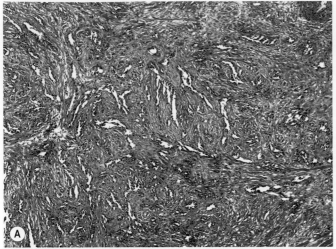

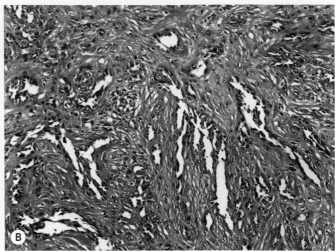

Figure 18.2  Retiform hemangioendothelioma.

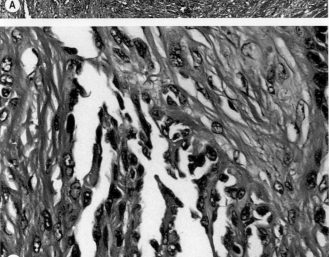

hallmark of Dabska's tumor can be identified in RH. By the same token, typical cases of EPE can present focally a retiform pattern. Immunohistochemically, neoplastic endothelial cells of RH express CD31 and CD34, but not D2-40 and VEGFR-3, which support a blood rather than lymphatic endothelial cell differentiation.[24]

These lesions also have similar clinical behavior with a high tendency to local recurrence but a low metastatic rate. To date, there is only one reported case of RH with lymph node metastasis.[25]

The differential diagnosis is mainly with high-grade angiosarcomas. EPE/RH and angiosarcoma are infiltrative. However, EPE/RH differs from angiosarcoma by lacking cytologic atypia and high mitotic rates. Furthermore, EPE/RH frequently recurs but rarely metastasizes, unlike angiosarcoma. The treatment for both neoplasms consists of surgical excision.

## Composite hemangioendothelioma

Composite cutaneous hemangioendothelioma is the most recently described tumor within the spectrum of hemangioendotheliomas. It is characterized by a mixture of histologic patterns including epithelioid hemangioendothelioma, retiform hemangioendothelioma, and spindle cell hemangioma.[10] So far, all the cases reported have involved adult patients, with a median age of 39.5 years. The lesions arose predominantly on the hands and feet, presenting mostly as solitary, slow-growing nodular tumors, which are usually present for several years before diagnosis.

Composite hemangioendothelioma consists of an admixture of different components that vary from lesion to lesion (Fig. 18.3). There is also variation in the proportion of each of the components; as well as the manner in which each component is distributed throughout the lesion. In most cases, the predominant histopathologic components are those of epithelioid and retiform hemangioendothelioma, but areas with spindle cells are also identified in some neoplasms. Angiosarcoma-like areas are at least focally present in most cases. One of the reported neoplasms was associated with an arteriovenous malformation and another was associated with a superficial lymphatic malformation.

Immunohistochemically, lesions of composite hemangioendothelioma stain positive with the endothelial markers CD31 and CD34,[10] but they also express podoplanin, Lyve-1 and Prox-1, which support an endothelial lymphatic line of differentiation.[26] Smooth muscle actin stain is usually confined to the stroma and the walls of the nonneoplastic vessels.

Composite hemangioendothelioma should not be confused with polymorphous hemangioendothelioma, which is an extremely rare vascular neoplasm mainly occurring

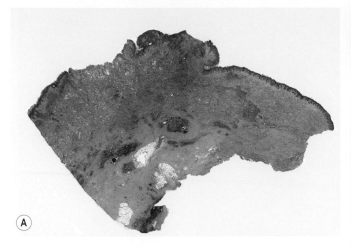

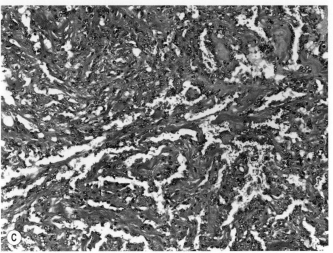

**Figure 18.3** Composite cutaneous hemangioendothelioma.

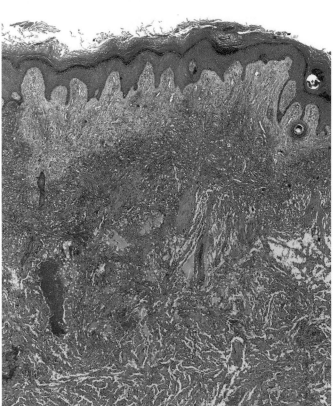

in lymph nodes, although it has been also reported in soft tissue.[27] Histopathologically, polymorphous hemangioendothelioma is characterized by a combination of solid, primitive vascular and angiomatous patterns, with relatively uniform cytologic features. In other words, polymorphous hemangioendothelioma refers to lesions showing a combination of solid and angiomatous components, whereas the term composite hemangioendothelioma describes lesions combining different types of hemangioendotheliomas in the same lesion.

The treatment of choice is surgical excision.[10] Metastatic disease, when present, is usually confined to the regional lymph nodes and histopathologic study of the involved lymph nodes demonstrates that the epithelioid component of the neoplasm is responsible for the metastases.[26] No

tumor-related deaths due to composite hemangioendothelioma have been reported so far.

## INTERMEDIATE GRADE ANGIOSARCOMAS (EPITHELIOID HEMANGIOENDOTHELIOMA)

Epithelioid hemangioendothelioma is a malignant neoplasm which has a better prognosis than conventional angiosarcoma of the soft tissues, but is able to metastasize and should be regarded as a fully malignant, rather than borderline, vascular neoplasm.

Clinically, this neoplasm appears as a solitary, slightly painful, soft tissue tumor,[28] although similar lesions have also been reported in the skin[29,30] and oral cavity.[31] In some cases the lesions consist of ulcerated nodules.[32] Epithelioid

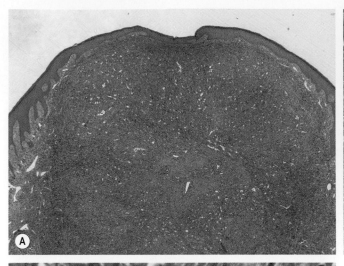

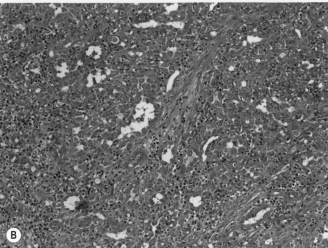

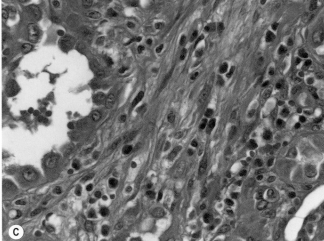

**Figure 18.4** Epithelioid hemangioendothelioma.

hemangioendothelioma is most commonly located on the extremities, but it can affect other anatomical sites, including the head, trunk and mucosae. Cutaneous lesions may be associated with subsequent bone, lymph node, and pulmonary lesions.

Histopathologically, epithelioid hemangioendothelioma presents as a dermal nodule composed of cords, strands and nests of plump epithelioid cells embedded in a fibromyxoid or sclerotic stroma. Many of the neoplastic cells contain vacuoles in their cytoplasm as a sign of primitive vascular differentiation (Fig. 18.4). Slight cellular pleomorphism and occasional mitotic figures may be seen. Rarely, large distinct vascular channels are mainly present in the central areas of the neoplasm. Occasionally, the stroma may show foci of osseous metaplasia.[33]

In many cases epithelioid hemangioendotheliomas are difficult to differentiate from metastatic adenocarcinomas, which contain mucin vacuoles within the neoplastic cells. A helpful feature that allows this distinction is the presence of erythrocytes in the vacuoles of epithelioid hemangioendothelioma.[34] Immunohistochemistry is also useful in this differential diagnosis. The neoplastic cells of epithelioid hemangioendothelioma express immunoreactivity for the vascular markers CD31 and CD34,[34] but they may also stain with cytokeratins[35], alpha-smooth muscle actin, and FLI-1.[34,35] Other neoplasms that need to be considered in the differential diagnosis include cutaneous epithelioid angiomatous nodule

(CEAN) and the epithelioid form of angiosarcoma involving the skin and superficial soft tissues. CEAN is a peculiar and recently recognized vascular proliferation.[36–38] Clinically these lesions affect different areas of the body and histologically are characterized by a well-circumscribed, mainly unilobular, solid proliferation of endothelial cells with prominent epithelioid features. The cytoplasm is abundant and eosinophilic, and many of the neoplastic cells contain prominent vacuoles. Inflammatory infiltrates are variable. All the cases reported thus far have followed a benign course. Epithelioid angiosarcoma is composed of solid sheets of neoplastic cells, many of them atypical, with abundant mitotic figures and with necrosis occurring in both individual cells and large areas of the neoplasm (necrosis en masse). Occasional tumors may demonstrate t(1;3)(p36.3;q25)(G).[39]

Treatment of superficial forms of epithelioid hemangioendothelioma includes wide local excision without adjuvant radiotherapy or chemotherapy and clinical evaluation of the regional lymph nodes, since this is the most common metastatic site. Metastases occur more frequently in the histopathologically malignant forms. In one study, fewer than half of the patients who developed metastases died of their disease, because most of the metastases occur in regional lymph nodes and excision of these structures is curative, or at least provides long-term disease-free survival.[40] However, follow-up of a recent series of 30 patients with epithelioid hemangioendothelioma of the skin and soft tissues demonstrated systemic metastases in 21% of the cases (lung, lymph node most common) and 17% of the patients died because of the tumor.[34] The follow-up of another recent series of 49 cases of epithelioid hemangioendothelioma involving the skin and soft tissues demonstrated that increased mitotic activity and size of the neoplasm were the two features more directly associated with decreased survival, whereas tumor site, cytologic atypia, the presence of necrosis, and tumor spindling were not significant.[40]

## HIGH-GRADE ANGIOSARCOMAS

This group of malignant neoplasms includes cutaneous angiosarcoma of the face and scalp, angiosarcomas secondary to chronic lymphedema, and angiosarcomas of the breast secondary to radiation. Despite their clinical differences, all angiosarcomas share common histological features.

Cutaneous angiosarcoma of the face and scalp predominantly affects white elderly patients and is usually located on the scalp and upper forehead. The clinical presentation of angiosarcomas varies from ill-defined bruise-like lesions simulating hematoma to facial edema; especially of the eyelids with minimal erythema.[41,42] More advanced lesions may present as indurate plaques or nodules that may ulcerate. In some instances, there are satellite lesions in the vicinity. Some cases are multifocal, which makes it difficult to determine clinically the extension of the lesion.[43] The neoplasm spreads gradually and centrifugally in a relatively short period of time, and in advanced cases, large parts of the scalp, face, and neck become affected. Atypical presentations of angiosarcoma of the face and scalp include superinfected angiosarcoma simulating an inflammatory process,[44] angiosarcoma resembling rosacea,[45] and an angiosarcoma presenting with edema in the periorbital region.

There are around 300 cases of Stewart–Treves syndrome reported worldwide. Angiosarcomas associated with chronic lymphedema appear as purplish, bruise-like areas or violaceous nodules superimposed on the browny non-pitting edema of the affected limb.[46] After the appearance of the lesions, there is a rapid increase in their number and size and they may undergo ulceration. Advanced cases spread distally to the hands and proximally to the chest wall. The clinical appearance and the histological behavior of angiosarcomas in lymphedematous extremities unassociated with mastectomy are essentially identical to those of postmastectomy angiosarcoma.

The clinical appearance of postirradiation cutaneous angiosarcoma varies from case to case. The different clinical presentations of this type of angiosarcoma often produces delays in the diagnosis. Diffuse infiltrative plaques, papulonodules, and ulcerated lesions have been described. All lesions occur in the area of irradiation or its immediate vicinity, and because most of the cases appear following radiation for breast and genitourinary malignant tumors, the chest wall and the lower abdominal wall are the sites most frequently involved by postirradiation angiosarcomas. Most of these patients have no evidence of lymphedema, suggesting that radiation is the most important etiologic factor.

Histopathologically, angiosarcomas usually extend far beyond the clinically visible boundaries of the lesion.[3] There is a considerable amount of morphological variation from lesion to lesion, and within different areas of the same tumor. Well-differentiated angiosarcomas appear as irregular, dilated, vascular channels lined with flattened endothelial cells with an innocuous appearance, which may lead them to be confused with a hemangioma or lymphangioma. However, careful observation of these lesions reveals the presence of irregular vascular channels dissecting through the dermis. These channels tend to communicate with each other, forming an anastomosing network. Furthermore, some of the endothelial cells appear as large, hyperchromatic, and pleomorphic, protruding within the vascular lumina, forming small papillations. In less differentiated angiosarcomas, there are solid proliferations of polygonal or spindle-shaped pleomorphic endothelial cells, with prominent mitotic activity and poorly formed vascular spaces (Fig. 18.5). This sometimes makes it difficult to distinguish them from carcinoma, melanoma or a high-grade fibrosarcoma. Of considerable value for the diagnosis of these cases is the presence of cytoplasmic vacuoles within the neoplastic cells.[3] Patchy lymphoid infiltrates are also a common finding in angiosarcomas of the face and scalp. In rare instances, dense nodular infiltrates of lymphocytes with germinal center formation may be seen scattered throughout the lesion, and at first glance the neoplasm may be misinterpreted as a cutaneous lymphoma or pseudolymphoma.[47] The number of erythrocytes present within the vascular spaces varies from a few to none in the poorly differentiated areas. Pre-existing adnexal, neural and vascular structures of the dermis are frequently involved and destroyed by the tumor. Uncommon cytologic variants of cutaneous angiosarcoma of the face and scalp include granular cell angiosarcoma[48,49] and angiosarcoma with foamy cells.[50] In some angiosarcomas, numerous single necrotic neoplastic cells are scattered throughout the neoplastic aggregations of endothelial cells, giving the lesions a starry-sky appearance.[51]

Immunohistochemically, angiosarcomas are usually positive for the endothelial markers CD34[52] and CD31,[53,54] although not all angiosarcomas express this latter marker.[54] More recent immunohistochemical studies have shown that angiosarcomas express vascular endothelial growth factor receptor-3 (VEGFR-3)[55-58] and podoplanin,[59] suggesting a lymphatic differentiation. Overexpression of basic fibroblastic growth factor,[60] angiopoietin-2 and Tie-1 and Tie-2 receptors of endothelium,[61] and Ets-1 proto-oncogene and metalloproteinase genes such as collagenase-1 (MMP-1) have been correlated with the growth and progression of angiosarcoma.

The prognosis of cutaneous angiosarcoma is poor. In the largest series reported to date, Holden et al.[62] found that only 12% of patients survived five or more years, with approximately half of the patients dying within 15 months of the debut of the tumor. Maddox and Evans[63] documented similar findings in a series of 17 patients. These authors also noted an increase in survival in patients with lesions less than 5 cm in diameter and in tumors with a prominent lymphocytic infiltrate. There was no prognostic correlation with the sex, location of the lesion, histologic differentiation or mitotic activity. When the lesions metastasize, the cervical lymph nodes are the earliest involved sites, but widespread dissemination to lung, liver, spleen, and the skeleton appear shortly thereafter. The ideal therapy is wide surgical excision of the lesion, followed by radiotherapy,[64,65] but this cannot be readily accomplished

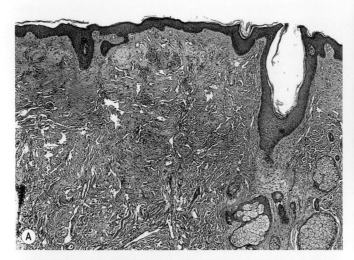

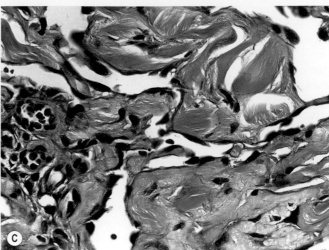

Figure 18.5 Cutaneous angiosarcoma.

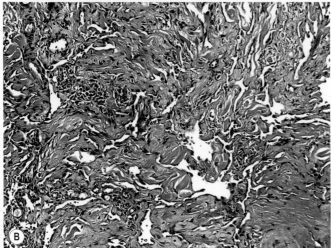

with angiosarcomas of the face and scalp, because they frequently extend beyond the clinically apparent margins of the lesion. Preoperative assessment of the tumor margins by biopsies of the periphery of the lesion with the use of immunohistochemical markers including CD31, CD34, podoplanin and the proliferation marker Ki-67 are helpful in delineating the extension of the tumor and to plan adequate treatment. Despite the overall poor prognosis, seven patients with cutaneous angiosarcoma of the face and scalp treated with wide-field electron-beam therapy have shown apparent eradication of cutaneous lesions and prolonged survival, although pulmonary metastases developed 10 years later in two of these patients. Adjuvant systemic chemotherapy with liposome-encapsulated doxorubicin,[66,67] interferon alfa-2a and 13-cis-retinoic acid,[68] paclitaxel,[69] or intralesional interferon alfa-2b and interleukin-2[70] has been used in patients with angiosarcoma of the scalp and face with variable results.

## GLOMANGIOSARCOMAS

Malignant glomus tumors (also known as glomangiosarcomas) are rare neoplasms, and some authors even doubt that such lesions exist, the most controversial issue being the recognition and acceptance of those in which no benign component is present. In addition to the soft tissue, malignant glomus tumors have been reported in a variety of sites, including skin, bone, bladder, central nervous system, lung, and gastrointestinal tract.[71-74]

The lesions of glomangiosarcoma are larger and more deeply located than conventional glomus tumors. They are predominantly located on the extremities, appearing as subcutaneous masses and have occurred equally in men and women. While most malignant glomus tumors do not metastasize, there are several reports of patient death as a consequence of widespread disease.[71,75,76]

Microscopically, malignant glomus tumor consists of sarcomatous areas intermingled with areas of benign glomus tumor. When present, identification of foci of typical glomus tumor is the most important clue to the histopathologic diagnosis of glomangiosarcoma. The malignant areas are poorly circumscribed, infiltrative, and composed of fascicles of spindle cells or aggregations of round glomoid cells with nuclear pleomorphism, frequent mitotic figures, and foci of necrosis en masse. In some neoplasms, there is a peculiar arrangement of the neoplastic cells, with small round glomus cells at the periphery and spindled cells centrally[71] (Fig. 18.6). A diagnosis of glomangiosarcoma should be not misconstrued in cases of longstanding glomus tumors, which contain glomus cells with large hyperchromatic nuclei, probably a result of degenerative changes similar to those seen in ancient schwannoma. Some authors

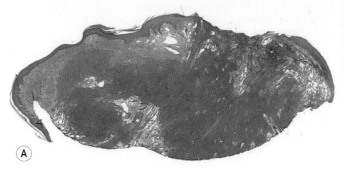

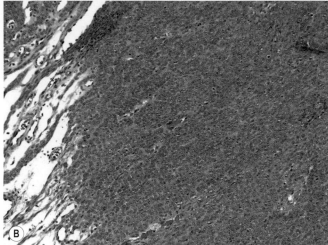

**Figure 18.6** Glomangiosarcoma.

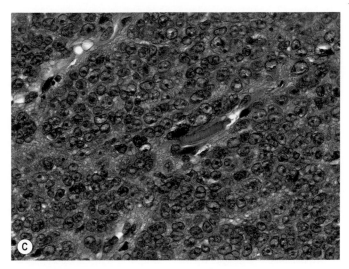

have proposed the name symplastic glomus tumor for these benign glomus tumors with nuclear atypia.[71]

In the absence of a benign glomus tumor component, the diagnosis of glomangiosarcoma nearly always necessitates the use of immunohistochemistry. Malignant glomus tumors have demonstrated immunoreactivity for vimentin, collagen type IV, muscle-specific actin, and smooth muscle actin, whereas neuron-specific enolase, desmin, Leu-7, CD34, and S-100 positivities are detected focally in only some cases.[71,77,78] Some neoplastic cells express caldesmon and calponin as well.[71] Factor VIII-related antigen is negative in neoplastic cells.[79] In one example of glomangiosarcoma arising in a benign glomus tumor, immunohistochemical studies demonstrated that bcl-2, an inhibitor of apoptosis, was strongly expressed in the glomangiosarcoma areas with only weak staining in the benign areas. The proliferation index of glomangiosarcoma was almost 10-fold higher than that of the benign glomus tumor. Numerous nuclei of glomangiosarcoma were intensely positive for the tumor suppressor protein p53.[80] Ultrastructural studies demonstrated that neoplastic cells of glomangiosarcoma showed prominent nucleoli, poorly developed organelles, and some bundles of tonofilaments.[76,77] Micropinocytotic vesicles have been also identified in some cases.[77]

Criteria for malignancy and classification of atypical glomus neoplasms were proposed,[71] categorizing problematic lesions as either 'symplastic', 'of uncertain malignant potential', or 'malignant'. Tumors with a deep location and size >2 cm or atypical mitoses or moderate to high nuclear grade with >5 mitoses/50 HPF were considered 'malignant'. Those that had a high nuclear grade but lacked other malignant features were termed 'symplastic'. The designation 'of uncertain malignant potential' was given to tumors that did not fulfill the criteria for 'malignant' or 'symplastic' but had a high mitotic rate and a superficial location or a large size only or were deeply located.

## FUTURE OUTLOOK

Vascular sarcomas remain a challenge to manage given the multiple variants and rarity of this tumor and the related lack of large studies. Complete removal by surgical excision will continue to be essential in an attempt to avoid local recurrence and metastasis.

## REFERENCES

**1.** Sangueza OP, Requena L. *Pathology of Vascular Skin Lesions*. Totowa, NJ: Human Press; 2003:236–274.
**2.** Mallory FB. The results of the application of special histological methods to the study of tumors. *J Exp Med*. 1908;10:575–593.
**3.** Purdy Stout A. Hemangio-endothelioma: a tumor of blood vessels featuring vascular endothelial cells. *Ann Surg*. 1943;118:445–464.
**4.** Caro MR, Stubenrauch Jr CH. Hemangioendothelioma of the skin. *Arch Dermatol Syph*. 1945;51:295–304.

5. Wilson Jones E. Malignant angioendothelioma of the skin. *Br J Dermatol.* 1964;76:21–39.

6. Stewart FW, Treves N. Lymphangiosarcoma in postmastectomy lymphedema. *Cancer.* 1948;1:64–81.

7. Weiss SW, Enziner FM. Epithelioid hemangioendothelioma: a vascular tumor often mistaken for a carcinoma. *Cancer.* 1982;50:970–981.

8. Dabska M. Malignant endovascular papillary angioendothelioma of the skin in childhood. Clinicopathologic study of 6 cases. *Cancer.* 1969;24:503–510.

9. Calonje E, Fletcher CD, Wilson-Jones E, et al. Retiform hemangioendothelioma. A distinctive form of low-grade angiosarcoma delineated in a series of 15 cases. *Am J Surg Pathol.* 1994;18:115–125.

10. Nayler SJ, Rubin BP, Calonje E, et al. Composite hemangioendothelioma: a complex, low-grade vascular lesion mimicking angiosarcoma. *Am J Surg Pathol.* 2000;24:352–361.

11. Aust MR, Olsen KD, Lewis JE, et al. Angiosarcomas of the head and neck: clinical and pathologic characteristics. *Ann Otol Rhinol Laryngol.* 1997;106:943–951.

12. Weedon D. Pathology of the skin. In: *Systemic Pathology.* vol. 9. London: Churchill Livingstone; 1992:1026.

13. Freedman AN. Angiosarcoma of the scalp: case report and literature review. *Can J Surg.* 1987;30:197–198.

14. Mark RJ, Tran LM, Sercarz J, et al. Angiosarcoma of the head and neck. The UCLA experience 1955 through 1990. *Arch Otolaryngol Head Neck Surg.* 1993;119:973–978.

15. Koch M, Nielsen GP, Yoon SS. Malignant tumors of blood vessels: angiosarcomas, hemangioendotheliomas, and hemangiopericytomas. *J Surg Oncol.* 2008;97:321–329.

16. Fury MG, Antonescu CR, Van Zee KJ, et al. A 14-year retrospective review of angiosarcoma: clinical characteristics, prognostic factors, and treatment outcomes with surgery and chemotherapy. *Cancer J.* 2005;11:241–247.

17. Mendenhall WM, Mendenhall CM, Werning JW, et al. Cutaneous angiosarcoma. *Am J Clin Oncol.* 2006;29:524–528.

18. Wehrli BM, Janzen DL, Shokeir O, et al. Epithelioid angiosarcoma arising in a surgically constructed arteriovenous fistula: a rare complication of chronic immunosuppression in the setting of renal transplantation. *Am J Surg Pathol.* 1998;22:1154–1159.

19. Lydiatt WM, Shaha AR, Shah JR. Angiosarcoma of the head and neck. *Am J Surg.* 1994;168:451–454.

20. Sasaki R, Soejima T, Kishi K, et al. Angiosarcoma treated with radiotherapy: impact of tumor type and size on outcome. *Int J Radiat Oncol Biol Phys.* 2002;52:1032–1040.

21. Manivel JC, Wick MR, Swanson PE, et al. Endovascular papillary angioendothelioma of childhood: a vascular lesion possibly characterized by 'high' endothelial cell differentiation. *Hum Pathol.* 1986;17:1240–1244.

22. Duke D, Dvorak AM, Harris TJ, et al. Multiple retiform hemangioendotheliomas. A low-grade angiosarcoma. *Am J Dermatopathol.* 1996;18:606–610.

23. Fukunaga M, Endo Y, Masui F, et al. Retiform haemangioendothelioma. *Virchows Arch.* 1996;428:301–304.

24. Parsons A, Sheehan DJ, Sangueza OP. Retiform hemangioendotheliomas usually do not express D2-40 and VEGFR-3. *Am J Dermatopathol.* 2008;30:31–33.

25. Bhutoria B, Konar A, Chakrabarti S, et al. Retiform hemangioendothelioma with lymph node metastasis: a rare entity. *Indian J Dermatol Venereol Leprol.* 2009;75:60–62.

26. Requena L, Díaz Recuero JL, Manzarbeitia F, et al. Cutaneous composite hemangioendothelioma with satellitosis and lymph node metastases. *J Cutan Pathol.* 2008;35:225–230.

27. Nascimento AG, Keeney GL, Sciot R, et al. Polymorphous hemangioendothelioma. A report of two cases, one affecting extranodal soft tissues and review of the literature. *Am J Surg Pathol.* 1997;21:1083–1089.

28. Weiss SW, Ishak KG, Dial DH, et al. Epithelioid hemangioendothelioma and related lesions. *Semin Diagn Pathol.* 1986;3:259–287.

29. Ellis GL, Kratochvill FJ. Epithelioid hemangioendothelioma of the head and neck: a clinicopathologic report of twelve cases. *Oral Surg Oral Med Oral Pathol.* 1986;61:61–68.

30. Tyring S, Guest P, Lee P, et al. Epithelioid hemangioendothelioma of the skin and femur. *J Am Acad Dermatol.* 1989;20:362–366.

31. Orsini G, Fioroni M, Rubini C, et al. Epithelioid hemangioendothelioma of the oral cavity: report of case. *J Oral Maxillofac Surg.* 2001;59:334–337.

32. Grezard P, Balme B, Ceruse P, et al. Ulcerated cutaneous epithelioid hemangioendothelioma. *Eur J Dermatol.* 1999;9:487–490.

33. Kiryu H, Hashimoto H, Hori Y. Ossifying epithelioid hemangioendothelioma. *J Cutan Pathol.* 1996;23:558–561.

34. Mentzel T, Beham A, Calonje E, et al. Epithelioid hemangioendothelioma of skin and soft tissues: clinicopathologic and immunohistochemical study of 30 cases. *Am J Surg Pathol.* 1997;21:363–374.

35. Gray MH, Rosenberg AE, Dicersin GR, et al. Cytokeratin expression in epithelioid vascular neoplasms. *Hum Pathol.* 1990;21:212–217.

36. Clarke LE, Lee R, Militello G, et al. Cutaneous epithelioid hemangioendothelioma. *J Cutan Pathol.* 2008;35:236–240.

37. Brenn T, Fletcher CDM. Cutaneous epithelioid angiomatous nodule: a distinct lesion in the morphologic spectrum of epithelioid vascular tumors. *Am J Dermatopathol.* 2004;26(1):14–21.

38. Sangüeza OP, Walsh SN, Sheehan DJ, et al. Cutaneous epithelioid angiomatous nodule: a case series and proposed classification. *Am J Dermatopathol.* 2008;30(1):16–20.

39. Mendlick MR, Nelson M, Pickering D, et al. Translocation t(1;3)(p36.3;q25) is a nonrandom aberration in epithelioid hemangioendothelioma. *Am J Surg Pathol.* 2001;25(5):684–687.

40. Deyrup AT, Tighiouart M, Montag AG, et al. Epithelioid hemangioendothelioma of soft tissue: a proposal for risk stratification based on 49 cases. *Am J Surg Pathol.* 2008;32:924–927.

41. Holden CA, Spittle MF, Wilson Jones E. Angiosarcoma of the face and scalp, prognosis and treatment. *Cancer.* 1987;59:1046–1057.

42. Tay YK, Ong BH. Cutaneous angiosarcoma presenting as recurrent angio-oedema of the face. *Br J Dermatol.* 2000;143:1346–1348.

43. Kacker A, Antonescu CR, Shaha AR. Multifocal angiosarcoma of the scalp: a case report and review of the literature. *Ear Nose Throat J.* 1999;78:302–305.

44. Diaz-Cascajo C, de la Vega M, Rey-López A. Superinfected cutaneous angiosarcoma: a highly malignant neoplasm simulating an inflammatory process. *J Cutan Pathol.* 1997;24:56–60.

45. Mentzel T, Kutzner H, Wollina U. Cutaneous angiosarcoma of the face: clinicopathologic and immunohistochemical study of a case resembling rosacea clinically. *J Am Acad Dermatol.* 1998;38:837–840.

46. Bisceglia M, Attino V, D'Addeta C, et al. Le sindrome di Stewart e Treves in fase precoce: presentazione di due casi e revisione della letteratura. *Pathologica.* 1996;88:483–490.

47. Requena L, Santonja C, Stutz N, et al. Pseudolymphomatous cutaneous angiosarcoma: a rare variant of cutaneous angiosarcoma readily mistaken for cutaneous lymphoma. *Am J Dermatopatol.* 2007;29:342–350.

48. McWilliam LJ, Harris M. Granular cell angiosarcoma of the skin: histology, electron microscopy and immunohistochemistry of a newly recognized tumor. *Histopathology.* 1985;9:1205–1216.

49. Hitchcock MG, Hurt MA, Santa Cruz DJ. Cutaneous granular cell angiosarcoma. *J Cutan Pathol.* 1994;21:256–262.

50. Ackerman AB, Guo Y, Vitale P, et al. *Clues to Diagnosis in Dermatopathology III.* Chicago: ASCP Press; 1993:357–360.

51. Smith KJ, Lupton GP, Skelton HG. Cutaneous angiosarcomas with a starry-sky pattern. *Arch Pathol Lab Med.* 1997;121:980–984.

52. Orchard GE, Zelger B, Jones EW, et al. An immunohistochemical assessment of 19 cases of cutaneous angiosarcoma. *Histopathology.* 1996;28:235–240.

53. Yonezawa S, Marayuma I, Tanaka S, et al. Thrombomodulin as a marker for vascular tumors: comparative study with factor VIII and Ulex europaeus I lectin. *Am J Clin Pathol.* 1987;88:405–411.

54. DeYoung BR, Wick MR, Fitzgibbon JF, et al. CD31: an immunospecific marker for endothelial differentiation in human neoplasms. *Appl Immunohistochem.* 1993;1:97–103.

55. Poblet E, Gonzalez Palacios F, Jimenez FJ. Different immunoreactivity of endothelial markers in well and poorly differentiated areas of angiosarcomas. *Virchows Arch.* 1996;428:217–221.

56. Hashimoto M, Ohsawa A, Onhnishi A, et al. Expression of vascular endothelial growth factor and its receptor mRNA in angiosarcoma. *Lab Invest.* 1995;73:859–863.

57. Brown LF, Tognazzi K, Dvorak HF, et al. Strong expression of kinase insert domain-containing receptor, a vascular permeability factor/vascular endothelial growth factor receptor in AIDS-associated Kaposi's sarcoma and cutaneous angiosarcoma. *Am J Pathol.* 1996;148:1065–1074.

58. Folpe AL, Veikkola T, Valtola R, et al. Vascular endothelial growth factor receptor-3 (VEGFR-3): a marker of vascular tumors with presumed lymphatic differentiation, including Kaposi's sarcoma, kaposiform and Dabska-type hemangioendotheliomas, and a subset of angiosarcomas. *Mod Pathol.* 2000;13:180–185.

59. Breiteneder-Geleff S, Soleiman A, Kowalski H, et al. Angiosarcomas express mixed endothelial phenotypes of blood and lymphatic capillaries. Podoplanin as a specific marker for lymphatic endothelium. *Am J Pathol.* 1999;154:385–394.

60. Yamamoto T, Umeda T, Yokozeki H, et al. Expression of basic fibroblast growth factor and its receptor in angiosarcoma. *J Am Acad Dermatol.* 1999;41:127–129.

61. Brown LF, Dezube BJ, Tognazzi K, et al. Expression of Tie1, Tie2, and angiopoietins 1, 2, and 4 in Kaposi's and cutaneous angiosarcoma. *Am J Pathol.* 2000;156:2179–2183.

62. Holden CA, Spittle MF, Wilson Jones E. Angiosarcoma of the face and scalp, prognosis and treatment. *Cancer.* 1987;59:1046–1057.

63. Maddox JC, Evans HL. Angiosarcoma of skin and soft tissue. A study of forty-four cases. *Cancer.* 1981;48:1907–1921.

64. Mark RJ, Poen JC, Tran LM, et al. Angiosarcoma: a report of 67 patients and a review of the literature. *Cancer.* 1996;77:2400–2406.

65. Brand CU, Yawalkar N, von Briel C, et al. Combined surgical and X-ray treatment for angiosarcoma of the scalp: report of a case with a favourable outcome. *Br J Dermatol.* 1996;134:763–765.

66. Jackel A, Deichmann M, Waldmann V, et al. Regression of metastatic angiosarcoma of the skin after systemic treatment with liposome-encapsulated doxorubicin and interferon alpha. *Br J Dermatol.* 1999;140:1187–1188.

67. Wollina U, Fuller J, Graefe T, et al. Angiosarcoma of the scalp: treatment with liposomal doxorubicin and radiotherapy. *J Cancer Res Clin Oncol.* 2001;127:396–399.

68. Spieth K, Gille J, Kaufmann R. Therapeutic efficacy of interferon alfa-2a and 13-cis-retinoic acid in recurrent angiosarcoma of the head. *Arch Dermatol.* 1999;135:1035–1037.

69. Fata F, O'Reilly E, Ilson D, et al. Paclitaxel in the treatment of patients with angiosarcoma of the scalp of face. *Cancer.* 1999;15:2034–2037.

70. Ulrich L, Krause M, Brachmann A, et al. Successful treatment of angiosarcoma of the scalp by intralesional cytokine therapy and surface irradiation. *J Eur Acad Dermatol Venereol.* 2000;14:412–415.

71. Folpe AL, Fanburg-Smith JC, Mietinen M, et al. Atypical and malignant glomus tumors. Analysis of 52 cases, with a proposal for the reclassification of glomus tumors. *Am J Surg Pathol.* 2001;25:1–12.

72. Hiruta N, Kameda N, Tokudome T, et al. Malignant glomus tumor: a case report and review of the literature. *Am J Surg Pathol.* 1997;21:1096–1103.

73. Wetherington RW, Lyle WG, Sangueza OP. Malignant glomus tumor of the thumb: a case report. *J Hand Surg [Am].* 1997;22:1098–1102.

74. López Rios F, Rodriguez Peralto JL, Castaño E, et al. Glomangiosarcoma of the lower limb: a case report with a literature review. *J Cutan Pathol.* 1997;24:571–574.

75. Brathwaite CD, Poppiti Jr RJ. Malignant glomus tumor. A case report of widespread metastases in a patient with multiple glomus body hamartomas. *Am J Surg Pathol.* 1996;20:233–238.

76. Watanabe K, Sugino T, Kusakabe T, et al. Glomangiosarcoma of the hip: report of a highly aggressive tumour with widespread distant metastases. *Br J Dermatol.* 1998;139:1097–1101.

77. Khoury T, Balos L, McGrath B, et al. Malignant glomus tumor: a case report and review of literature, focusing on its clinicopathologic features and immunohistochemical profile. *Am J Dermatopathol.* 2005;27:428–431.

78. Aiba M, Hirayama A, Kuramochi S. Glomangiosarcoma in a glomus tumor. An immunohistochemical and ultrastructural study. *Cancer.* 1988;61:1467–1471.

79. Gould EW, Manivel JC, Albores-Saavedra J, et al. Locally infiltrative glomus tumors and glomangiosarcomas. A clinical, ultrastructural, and immunohistochemical study. *Cancer.* 1990;65:310–318.

80. Hegyi L, Cormack GC, Grant JW. Histochemical investigation into the molecular mechanisms of malignant transformation in a benign glomus tumour. *J Clin Pathol.* 1998;51:872–874.

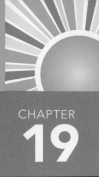

# Cutaneous Neoplastic Disorders Related to HPV and HIV Infection

*Kien T. Tran, Jane M. Grant-Kels, and Clay J. Cockerell*

## Key Points

- Epidermodysplasia verruciformis (EV) is a genetic lifelong disease associated with specific human papillomaviruses (HPV) and multiple skin cancers. Immunosuppressed patients have an increased risk of developing EV lesions.

- Bowenoid papulosis presents as wart-like papules usually affecting the genitals of young sexually active adults. HPV genotype is detected in most lesions of bowenoid papulosis with HPV-16 being the most commonly identified.

- Progression of bowenoid papulosis to invasive squamous cell carcinoma is relatively uncommon but may occur, especially in immunocompromised hosts.

- Verrucous carcinoma is a locally aggressive low-grade malignancy with minimal atypia and is often associated with HPV infection. The lesions rarely metastasize but are associated with local morbidity.

- Cutaneous neoplasms are common in HIV-infected patients. As these individuals are now living longer as a consequence of administration of HAART, these are becoming a more important ongoing problem in management.

## INTRODUCTION

As we gain increasing knowledge into the pathophysiology of cutaneous malignant neoplasms, it becomes increasingly evident that many are driven by virally mediated mechanisms. These processes, especially in HPV-induced condyloma near the anogenital region, can lead to squamous cell carcinoma (SCC). Human papillomavirus is a small double-stranded DNA virus that is phylogenetically divided into five genera, the most relevant in the skin being the alpha and gamma papillomavirus.[1] Most alpha HPVs infect the mucosal environment surrounding the anogenital region along with the adjacent skin and include types 6 and 11, found in 90% of genital warts. The beta papillomavirus genus refers to the group related to epidermodysplasia verruciformis, with types 5 and 8 related to skin cancer. The viral genome of HPV encodes proteins E6 and E7 that modulate cellular regulatory proteins. E6 binds to and enhances the ubiquitination and degradation of the global tumor suppressor *p53*. E7 inactivates the retinoblastoma tumor suppressor gene, which is responsible for halting progression through the cell cycle.

HIV infection and the concomitant immunodeficiency lends itself to increased rates of cutaneous neoplasm. Some are specific to HIV patients, such as Kaposi sarcoma. Others are related to the prolonged immunodeficiency from the infection. Since the introduction of highly active antiretroviral therapy (HAART), the lifespan for HIV-infected patients has expanded, resulting in many patients suffering from common cutaneous malignancies that are endemic to the normal population, albeit at a higher rate.

## NEOPLASTIC DISORDERS IN HPV-INFECTED PATIENTS

## Epidermodysplasia verruciformis

### Introduction

Epidermodysplasia verruciformis (EV) serves as a unique model for the study of HPV-mediated oncogenesis. EV is a rare, mainly autosomal recessive, virally mediated genetic disease associated with mutations in the *EVER1* and *EVER2* genes (band 17q25).[2] The disease is characterized by pityriasis versicolor-like macular and planar verruca-like lesions over sun-exposed areas that develop early in life and transform into squamous cell carcinoma later in adulthood. Although patients are infected with multiple beta-HPV types, only a select few (HPV-5 and HPV-8 mainly) are associated with the development of cutaneous malignancies. In addition, immunosuppressed patients are at increased risk of developing EV lesions that resolve with improvement of the immune status. As such, the genodermatosis and its associated genes lend a unique perspective on inherent anti-HPV pathways and virally mediated skin oncogenesis.

### History

EV was first described as a genodermatosis by Lewandowsky and Lutz in 1922 and as a model of viral cutaneous oncogenesis in 1972.[3] The oncogenic EVHPV types were discovered in 1978.[4] Genetic analysis of the 17q25.3 region led to the discovery of the *EVER1* and *EVER 2* genes.[5]

### Epidemiology

The disease is rare in the general population. The largest series to date involves fewer than 200 patients, mainly in Eastern Europe and Latin America.

### Pathogenesis and etiology

A large proportion of patients are born to consanguineous parents, with the proportion approaching one-third. The mode of inheritance for the vast majority is autosomal recessive. An X-linked recessive mode of inheritance has also been reported.[6] The classically associated *EVER1* and *EVER2* genes, also termed *TMC6* and *TMC8*, encode TMC (transmembrane channel-like) proteins that localize to the endoplasmic reticulum with features of integral membrane proteins. The exact function in prevention of persistent infections has not yet been revealed. EV is associated commonly with specific benign and malignant strains of beta HPVs that share nucleotide homology. Of about 20 characterized EVHPVs, high-risk HPV-5 and HPV-8 are predominantly associated with malignant lesions.

The pathogenesis of EV has not clearly been elucidated. It has been hypothesized that the *EVER* genes play a role in immune response to the infection or control of the infection within keratinocytes. A cell-mediated immunity defect relating to inhibition of natural cytotoxicity and T lymphocyte proliferation to HPV infection has been shown. The exact role that HPV plays in the development of cutaneous carcinoma is also unclear. Some have suggested that EVHPV infection is a cofactor in the pathogenesis of skin carcinoma, with cancers occuring more commonly in sun-exposed areas and higher viral loads discovered in actinic keratosis than in squamous cell carcinoma for EV patients.

## Clinical features

The first cutaneous lesions appear at the age of 5–8 years, usually as flat plane warts localized mainly on the face and hands, spreading progressively all over the body. Somewhat later, red plaques, located usually on the neck and trunk, appear (Fig. 19.1). Skin changes are polymorphous. There can also be brown, red and achromic plaques and pityriasis versicolor-like lesions (Fig. 19.2). The plane wart-like lesions can display a Koebner phenomenon. Malignant transformation occurs in about half of the cases and usually in the third decade. The preferential localization of neoplasms is the forehead and temporal areas, with premalignant lesions resembling actinic keratosis. The rate of progression depends on the viral type of EVHPVs and the extent of sun exposure (Fig. 19.3).[7] Cancers – although persistent – are usually only locally destructive with low metastatic potential. The disease is characterized by a lifelong persistence of cutaneous disease, usually with no involvement of internal

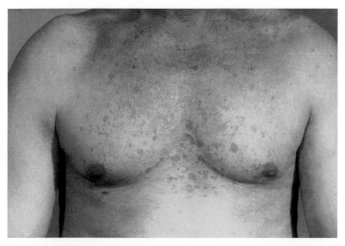

**Figure 19.1** Widespread red plaques on the trunk induced by several EVHPVs, mainly EVHPV5.

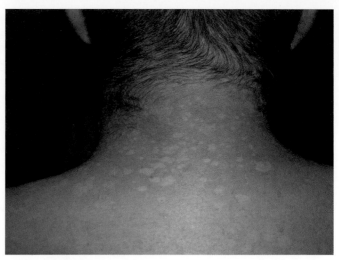

**Figure 19.2** Pityriasis versicolor-like lesions, widespread on the trunk, found to be induced by several EVHPVs.

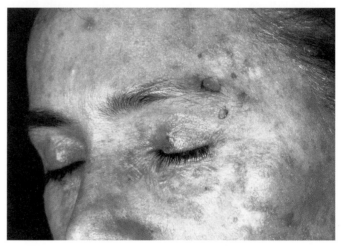

**Figure 19.3** Wart-like lesions on the face, some larger, deeper, covered with crusts (early carcinoma in situ).

organs, mucous membranes or lymph nodes. The overall prognosis is good.

## Patient evaluation, diagnosis and differential diagnosis

The diagnosis of EV is based on clinicopathological correlation along with virological findings. EV-like lesions can be found incidentally in normal skin and in immunosuppressed patients and histological findings by themselves do not constitute a diagnosis. In the correct clinical setting and with physical findings, the diagnosis can be confirmed by skin biopsy. This demonstrates highly characteristic cytopathic effects of bluish-purple color to ballooned keratinocytes in the epidermis (Fig. 19.4A). Characterization of mutations of specific genes *EVER1* and *EVER2* provides confirmation of the diagnosis. As the strain of EVHPVs causing the condition cannot be elucidated by histology alone, PCR analysis of paraffin-embedded tissue can confirm the presence of an oncogenic or non-oncogenic strain. Southern blot analysis is highly specific for HPV typing (Fig. 19.4B). The clinical differential diagnoses include tinea versicolor, planar warts, and widespread macular

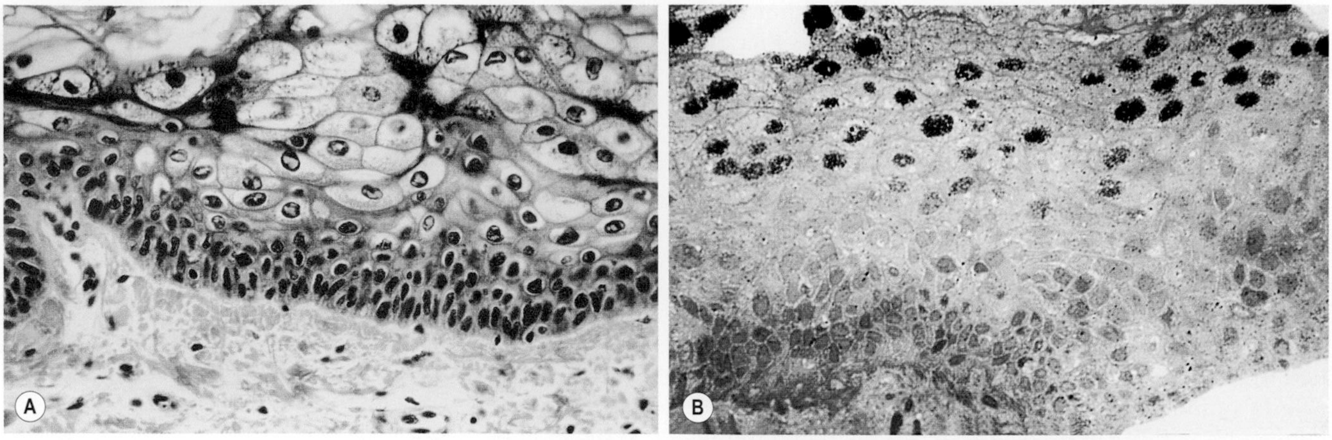

**Figure 19.4 A)** Characteristic cytopathic effect of EVHPV-induced lesion. Clarified dysplastic cells, starting suprabasally, with small pyknotic nuclei, replacing almost the entire epidermis. **B)** Molecular hybridization in situ showing abundant EVHPV5 DNA in the clarified cells. (Courtesy of Scott Boswell, MD.)

seborrheic keratoses. The extent of the disease, clinical history, prevalence in sun-exposed portions of the body, and early appearance of the disease in cases with genetic predisposition are clues to diagnosis.

## Pathology

The classic histological presentation of EV on low-power histological evaluation is that of a planar wart-like papule with hyperkeratosis, hypergranulosis and acanthosis. The keratinocytes possess a blue-gray pallor with perinuclear halos and keratohyaline granules. They are arranged in columns or nests, with the pallor being most conspicuous in the superficial granular layer. Premalignant lesions appear clinically and histologically similar to actinic keratosis with atypical keratinocytes in the epidermis as well as in adnexal epithelium. As the lesions progress to frank carcinoma, the keratinocytes lose typical EV findings and appear more as traditional SCC in situ and invasive SCC (Fig. 19.5).

## Treatment

No therapy for EV secondary to a genetic defect is definitive. Treatment includes preventive modalities, especially sun protection and avoidance. For patients with EV secondary to immunosuppression (Fig. 19.6), reconstitution of the immune system is key, although complete resolution of EV lesions is unlikely. Various modalities have been employed in case reports and case series for treatment of malignant lesions. including surgery, systemic retinoids, interferon-alpha, imiquimod, cimetidine, 5-fluorouracil, and photodynamic therapy. Cidofovir has been shown to be unsuccessful in one case report. For neoplasms in a localized region, auto-transplantation from uninvolved skin has been reported with some success. Radiotherapy should be avoided.

## Bowenoid papulosis

### Introduction

There is no other condition that better exemplifies the need for clinicopathological correlation than bowenoid papulosis (BP). BP lesions are banal in clinical appearance

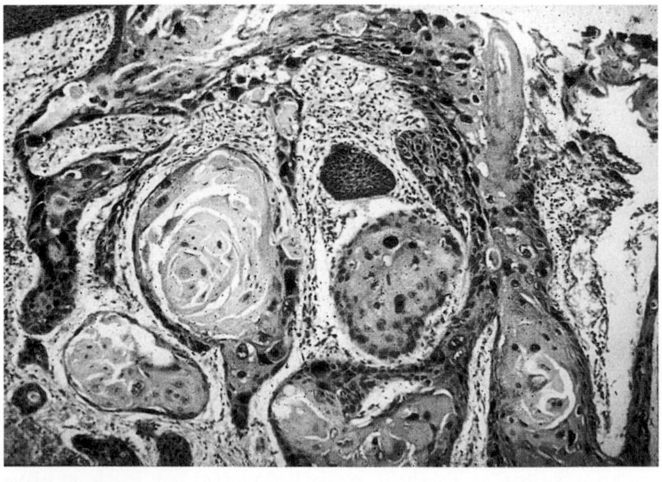

**Figure 19.5** Carcinoma Bowen's type with numerous dyskeratotic and pleomorphic cells in and around hair follicles, which are partly filled with keratotic masses.

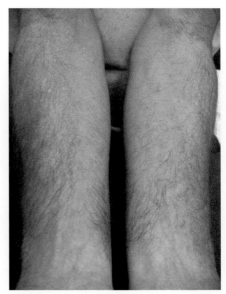

**Figure 19.6** Acquired EV in a patient with HIV infection. (Image courtesy of Yale Dermatology Residency Collection.)

although the biopsy of these lesions appears malignant. The true biologic potential of BP lesions lies somewhere in the middle and depends on the immune status of the patient. Only when the clinical lesion and pathologic findings are closely correlated is one able to make an accurate diagnosis and institute proper therapy.

## History

The term bowenoid papulosis was first presented in the literature by Kopf and Bart in 1977.[8] Wade, Kopf and Ackerman further delineated the entity in additional publications in 1978[9] and 1979. Other authors reported similar descriptions of wart-like papules with the histology of squamous cell carcinoma in situ during the 1970s.

## Epidemiology

Bowenoid papulosis most commonly affects young sexually active adults, although rare cases in younger patients due to sexual abuse or incidental contact have been reported. No racial predilection has been observed, although Wade et al. noted that the 11 patients in their initial series were Caucasian.[9] Often patients with BP have a history of prior infectious or inflammatory genital dermatoses, including condylomata acuminata, herpes simplex virus, psoriasis, lichen planus and lichen sclerosus. HPV genotypes are usually identified in lesions of BP. Immunosuppression and advancing age are thought to be risk factors for progression of BP to invasive squamous cell carcinoma.[10]

## Pathogenesis and etiology

The link between HPV and BP has been established via electron microscopic evidence of viral particles within lesions with immunoperoxidase and immunofluorescence microscopy confirmation, and by DNA hybridization. HPV genotype is detected in most lesions of BP, with HPV-16 being most commonly identified, although HPV types 6b, 18, 31–35, 39, 42, 48, 51–55 and 67 have also been detected.[11,12] Types 16, 18 and 33 are the most highly oncogenic, with HPV-16 and HPV-18 closely linked to cervical carcinoma.

## Clinical features

Bowenoid papulosis is characterized by flat papules that vary in color from pink to violaceous to reddish brown or deeply pigmented. The surface of the papules may be velvety, scaly or smooth. The number of papules ranges from several to many and they may coalesce to form plaques. Bowenoid papulosis may affect the shaft, glans, foreskin, inguinal fold, or perianal region in males and the vulva, perineum, and perianal region in females (Figs 19.7–19.9). It can also involve extragenital regions. Patients often present with BP of many months' to years' duration. Even in patients with longstanding lesions, progression to invasive squamous cell carcinoma is relatively uncommon. Bowenoid papulosis and invasive squamous

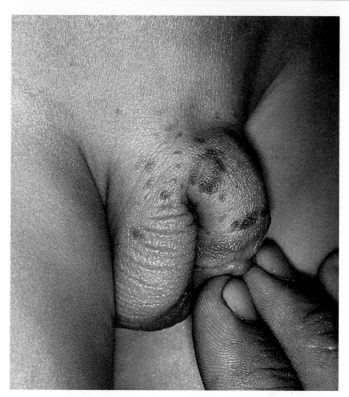

**Figure 19.7** Multiple papules of bowenoid papulosis of the penile shaft and scrotum. (Image courtesy of Yale Dermatology Residency Collection.)

cell carcinoma have rarely been reported to occur concomitantly. When immunosuppression is reversed, BP may spontaneously remit.

## Patient evaluation, diagnosis and differential diagnosis

The diagnosis of BP is established on the basis of clinicopathological correlation. Application of white vinegar (5% acetic acid) can highlight lesions that are difficult to visualize, and following its application, lesions appear white, known as acetowhite lesions. All patients should be followed for the development of invasive carcinoma or for development of anal intraepithelial neoplasia (AIN) if perianal involvement is seen. Females affected with BP should be evaluated for cervical HPV infection and CIN. Sexual partners of patients with BP should also be evaluated. HPV typing is an optional study and is not routinely performed. The presence of more highly oncogenic genotypes may identify individuals who should have more frequent monitoring. The clinical differential diagnosis of BP includes condylomata acuminata, flat warts, seborrheic keratosis, epidermal nevus, granuloma annulare, melanocytic nevus, lichen planus and psoriasis (Table 19.1). These can usually be readily distinguished histologically.

## Pathology

From scanning magnification the lesions of BP have architectural features of condylomata acuminata (Fig. 19.10A,B).

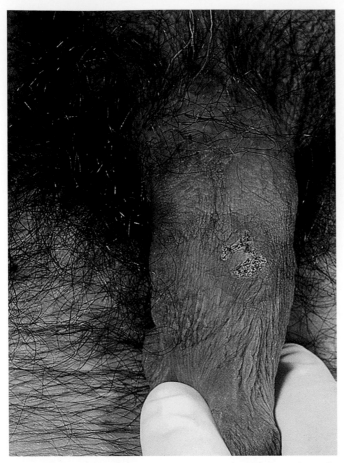

Figure 19.8 Multiple pigmented papules of bowenoid papulosis on the penile shaft. (Image courtesy of Yale Dermatology Residency Collection.)

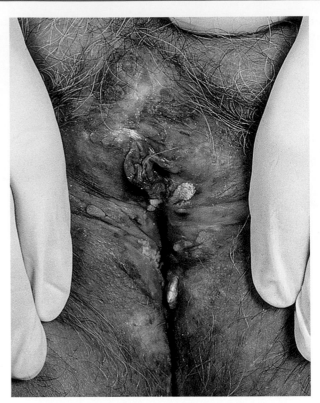

Figure 19.9 Multiple papules of bowenoid papulosis affecting the vulva. (Image courtesy of New York University Department of Dermatology.)

## Table 19.1 Clinical Differential Diagnosis: Diagnosis Made by Biopsy

| | Clinical Criteria | Histologic Criteria |
|---|---|---|
| Condylomata acuminatum | Verrucous papules | Papillated epidermal hyperplasia, parakeratosis, mitotic figures, vacuolated epithelial cells, arborization, no atypia, dilated tortuous capillaries |
| Flat warts | Flat smooth papules | Acanthosis, hyperkeratosis, vacuolization of epithelial cells, no atypia |
| Seborrheic keratosis | Stuck on, brownish keratotic papules and plaques with plugging | Papillated acanthosis with hyperkeratosis and horn (pseudo)cysts |
| Epidermal nevus | Linearly arranged keratotic papules | Papillated acanthosis with hyperkeratosis |
| Granuloma annulare | Pale pink papules annularly arranged | Palisaded granulomas with mucin |
| Melanocytic nevus | Tan to brown papule | Nests of melanocytic nevus cells |
| Lichen planus | Flat-topped violaceous papules with Wickham's striae | Hyperkeratosis, acanthosis, wedge-shaped hypergranulosis, vacuolar alteration, band-like infiltrate |
| Psoriasis | Red papules and plaques with silvery scale | Psoriasiform epidermal hyperplasia, hyperkeratosis layered with neutrophils and mounds of parakeratosis, dilated tortuous capillaries |
| Pearly penile papule | Small skin-colored papule | Fibrosis, stellate fibroblasts, and increased number of dilated vascular spaces |

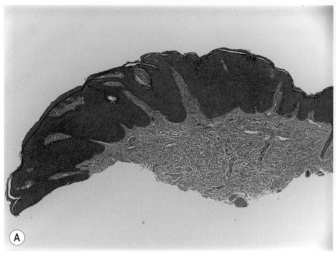

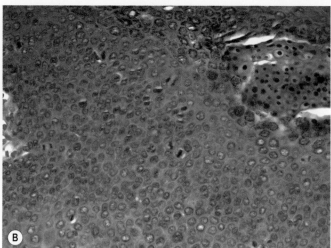

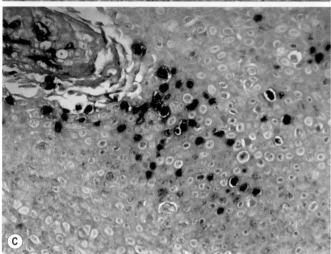

**Figure 19.10 A)** Papillated epithelial hyperplasia with a suggestion of arborization of peripheral rete (×25; H&E). **B)** High-power view of epithelium demonstrating disarray, dyskeratosis, and mitotic figures (×400). **C)** In-situ hybridization revealing infection by HPV-16.

The epidermis is papillated and hyperplastic with focal hypergranulosis, arborization of the peripheral rete ridges, and dilated tortuous papillary blood vessels. On occasion, one can discern focal vacuolization of the granular cell zone. At all levels of the epidermis there are atypical keratinocytes in disarray demonstrating large, hyperchromatic and pleomorphic nuclei with eosinophilic cytoplasm, as well as crowding of the epithelial nuclei. Dyskeratotic keratinocytes, typical and atypical mitotic figures, multinucleated keratinocytes, and hyperkeratosis with focal or confluent parakeratosis are prominent features. A superficial perivascular and often band-like lymphohistiocytic infiltrate is usually identified in the underlying dermis. The degree of cytologic atypia varies from lesion to lesion. In-situ hybridization can help determine the oncogenic type infecting the cells (Fig. 19.10C).

The histopathologic differential diagnosis includes Bowen's disease (Table 19.2). Lesions of Bowen's disease are usually broader and demonstrate confluent rather than focal parakeratosis. They generally show more prominent cytologic atypia with numerous atypical mitotic figures and multinucleated keratinocytes. Bowen's disease does not usually demonstrate hypergranulosis, dilated and tortuous papillary blood vessels, or papillated epidermal hyperplasia. Another diagnostic entity that should be considered is that of a condyloma acuminatum that has been treated chemically with podophyllin resin. Podophyllin

| Table 19.2 Pathologic Differential Diagnosis: Diagnosis Made by Clinical Pathologic Correlation | | |
|---|---|---|
| | **Clinical Criteria** | **Histologic Criteria** |
| Bowen's disease | Red, scaling and/or crusting patch | Confluent parakeratosis, acanthosis, full-thickness epidermal atypia with mitoses |
| Recently treated condyloma | History of condyloma recently treated with podophyllin resin | Condyloma with necrotic keratinocytes and bizarre mitotic figures |
| Bowenoid papulosis | Small red-brown papules, usually multiple in number, occasionally verrucoid | Focal parakeratosis, acanthosis, and papillomatosis, full-thickness epidermal atypia with mitoses |

resin application results in necrotic keratinocytes and bizarre mitotic figures, especially within the first 72 hours after application.[13] It has been reported that after 2 weeks, these changes are no longer present.

## Treatment

The biologic potential of BP directly impacts treatment. Although there have been reports of spontaneous regression, regression is most commonly noted when an immunosuppressive state is reversed. There are numerous reports of BP progressing to invasive squamous cell carcinoma, especially in immunocompromised hosts, so the condition should not be regarded lightly. Ablation rather than observation is usually chosen not only to remove malignant potential but also to reduce the threat of transmission. Condom use along with other barriers during sexual encounters is mandatory.

Bowenoid papulosis may be treated by a variety of surgical and medical modalities. Porter et al. recommend circumcision to eliminate a major risk factor for invasive carcinoma and HPV infection.[14] These authors also contend that circumcision allows for more effective follow-up and treatment. Partial or total vulvectomy may be performed in women with extensive disease and who are immunocompromised, but is rarely necessary. Local ablative options include shave removal, curettage, electrosurgery, cryotherapy, and laser destruction using Nd:Yag or $CO_2$ lasers. Topical therapeutic measures include application of trichloroacetic acid, 5-fluorouracil, cidofovir, interferon, and imiquimod.[15,16] One effective regimen has been the application of cidofovir 0.4% cream twice daily for 5 days, repeated every 15 days, for three cycles. In HIV-positive patients, surgical and topical therapy is generally ineffective until HAART is initiated.[14]

## Verrucous carcinoma

### Introduction

Verrucous carcinoma represents a unique variant of a low-grade squamous cell carcinoma associated with HPV infection. The lesion histologically has features similar to a verruca and is not significantly atypical. Clinically, however, it does not behave like a verruca. Verrucous carcinomas are locally aggressive and have high rates of recurrence.

### History

Verrucous carcinoma was originally described as a unique variant of a well-differentiated squamous carcinoma in 1948.[17] Over the years, the term has been expanded to include lesions in the larynx, genitalia, skin, esophagus, and even bladder.

### Epidemiology

The incidence of verrucous carcinoma is unknown, although it is likely higher than reported.

### Pathogenesis and etiology

The pathogenesis of the lesion is unknown but a viral etiology is strongly implicated. HPV types 1, 2, 11, 16 and 18 have been implicated via in-situ hybridization and types 6 and 11 are found in Buschke–Löwenstein tumors.[18–22] Other etiologies include chronic inflammation, inflammatory diseases such as erosive lichen planus, and chronic exposure to tobacco, alcohol or dipped snuff, especially in the oral mucosa. Oral verrucous carcinoma is associated more often with male immunocompromised patients.[23] Anal and penile lesions are also associated with HPV infection, although other etiologies have been postulated, including chronic infection, phimosis, poor hygiene, and trauma.[24]

## Clinical features

Early lesions of verrucous carcinoma are clinically indistinguishable from verruca. The oral cavity is the most common site of involvement. Incipient lesions appear as white patches on an erythematous base. Later, they develop into exophytic soft white warty tumors that extend over large portions of the oral mucosa. The tumor may ulcerate and extend locally into underlying tissues and bone. Most lesions do not metastasize to lymph nodes. Epithelioma cuniculatum, which refers to palmoplantar verrucous carcinoma, is found primarily on the soles but can involve the wrists, fingers and nail bed (Fig. 19.11). It presents as a hyperkeratotic warty lesion with keratin-filled sinuses. Epithelioma cuniculatum is slow growing, locally invasive and may result in bony destruction. The Buschke–Löwenstein variant is similar in appearance and develops as an exophytic tumor of the anogenital region that may ulcerate and develop sinuses. It arises at the site of a verruca. Recurrence rate for these lesions may be as high as 70%.[25]

## Patient evaluation, diagnosis and differential diagnosis

The diagnosis of verrucous carcinoma requires clinicopathological confirmation. The classic scenario is that of a locally aggressive and recurrent neoplasm with a surprisingly benign histological appearance. A skin biopsy is a prerequisite for diagnosis and the biopsy must be taken in a fashion that allows for assessment of the depth of the extension of the lesion. After a diagnosis is established, physical palpation and imaging studies such as CT scans, MRI or X-ray should be performed to examine if there is bony and/or soft tissue involvement. The differential diagnosis includes common verruca, keratoacanthoma, squamous cell carcinoma, pseudoepitheliomatous hyperplasia, and even verrucous psoriasis.

## Pathology

Verrucous carcinoma on scanning examination is an exoendophytic tumor that resembles a verruca with the exophytic portion demonstrating hyperkeratosis and parakeratosis and the endophytic component showing well-differentiated squamous epithelium with minimal atypia (Fig. 19.12A). The lesion extends into deep tissues,

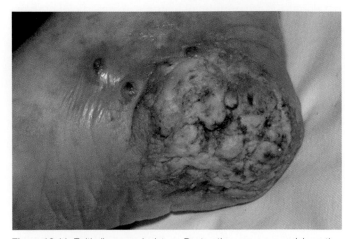

**Figure 19.11** Epithelioma cuniculatum. Destructive verrucous nodule on the heel of a patient.

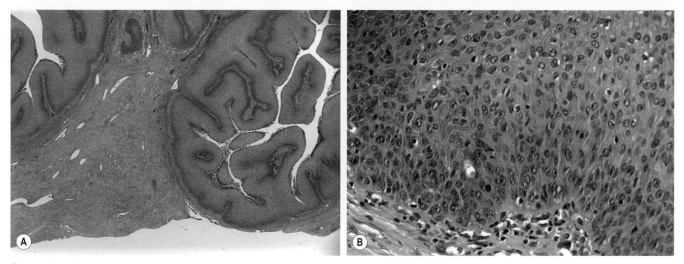

**Figure 19.12 A)** Scanning view of a verrucous carcinoma that appears like a verrucous nodule with a marked endophytic component (×20). **B)** Although clinically invasive, marked atypia is not seen in verrucous carcinoma (×400).

including even tendons, muscle and bone. Unlike routine squamous cell carcinoma, the lesion does not demonstrate striking keratinocytic atypia or mitoses (Fig. 19.12B). In contrast, verrucae and keratoacanthoma do not extend deeply into the tissue.

## Treatment

Surgical excision is the primary treatment for verrucous carcinoma. Although conventional surgery can be curative, Mohs surgery is advantageous as it allows for examination of all margins and is tissue sparing.[26,27] Other forms of therapy include cryosurgery, radiotherapy, or curettage and electrodesiccation. Carbon dioxide laser, imiquimod, photodynamic therapy, and local or systemic chemotherapy have also been attempted with variable success.[28,29] As the lesion has a high recurrence rate, vigilant follow-up is required.

## VACCINATION FOR HPV

The final FDA approval of two vaccines (Gardasil and Cervarix) against oncogenic types of human papillomavirus represents a major scientific development. The two vaccines are the first that target oncogenic viruses and if successful can potentially decrease the occurrence of the second most common cancer among women worldwide and the most common sexually transmitted disease in the world. Gardasil represents a quadrivalent vaccine containing virus-like particles made from the L1 capsid protein plus an adjuvant of types 6, 11, 16 and 18.[30] In randomized, double-blind, placebo-controlled trials, the vaccine was determined to decrease the incidence of CIN, cervical cancer, anogenital warts, and persistent viral infection of HPV types 6, 11, 16 and 18 by approximately 90% over a 3-year period.[30,31] Gardasil is indicated in girls and women aged 9 through 26 years and in boys and men aged 9 through 26 years. The most common side effect was headache, followed by fever, nausea, dizziness, and injection site pain. However, a disproportionate number of syncope and venous thromboembolic events was noted in one study.[32] Cervarix represents a bivalent vaccine to HPV genotypes 16 and 18 and utilizes a new adjuvant, 3-deacetylated

monophosphoyl lipid A with aluminum hydroxide, which has been shown to produce higher antibody titers.[33] Both vaccines have been demonstrated to provide cross-protection to other HPV subtypes, namely HPV-31 for the quadrivalent vaccine and HPV-31 and HPV-45 for the bivalent vaccine. Both vaccines are Pregnancy Class B. The safety and effectiveness of the vaccines have not been established in the very young, elderly, or immunocompromised patients. Epidemiological modeling suggests that herd immunity through vaccination of both boys and girls will result in a pronounced decrease in the prevalence of the disease.

## NEOPLASTIC DISORDERS IN HIV-INFECTED PATIENTS

Cutaneous neoplasms are common problems in individuals infected with the human immunodeficiency virus (HIV). Lesions can arise in both immunocompromised and immunocompetent patients.

### Kaposi sarcoma

Kaposi sarcoma (KS) is a vascular neoplastic disorder that prior to the onset of the AIDS pandemic was observed only in a very small select subset of individuals (see Chapter 16). It was the most frequent neoplastic disorder to develop in patients with AIDS prior to the advent of HAART. The disease is seen primarily in HIV-positive homosexual men and its onset, severity, and progression are not related to the degree of immunosuppression. In general, however, more extensive disease is seen in patients with CD4+ cell counts below 200 cells/mm³. HHV-8 is strongly associated, infecting both vascular and lymphatic endothelial cells. Clinically, KS skin lesions may be pink, red, brown or purple macules, patches or plaques (Fig. 19.13). Purpuric nodules may also develop (Figs 19.14 and 19.15). Early lesions are commonly mistaken for purpura or nevi. About one-third to one-half of patients have lesions on the lower extremity, similar to that seen in the classic form.[34] Lesions commonly develop on other sites, including the mucous membranes, the trunk and the scalp. Internal organ involvement is common and, as a general rule, one internal lesion develops for every

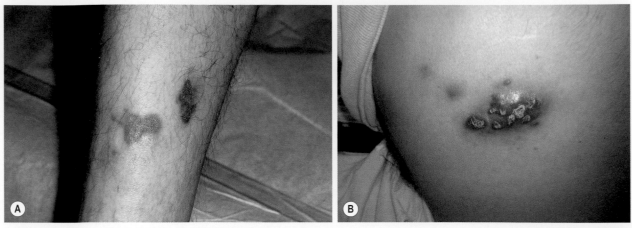

**Figure 19.13** Plaque-stage Kaposi sarcoma. Note the purplish plaques present on the lower extremity **(A)** and on the abdomen **(B).** These lesions have been found to be caused by human herpesvirus type 8.

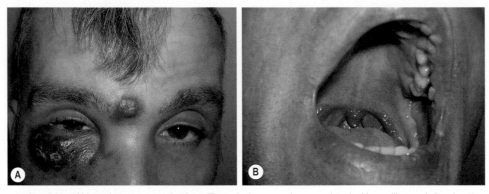

**Figure 19.14 A)** Plaques and nodules of Kaposi sarcoma on the face. These lesions may be associated with swelling and discoloration, as is evident in this case. **B)** Kaposi sarcoma is also frequently found on the oral mucosa.

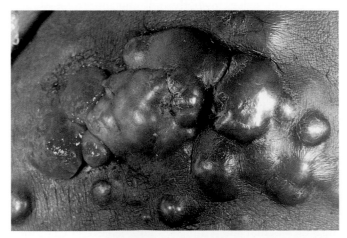

**Figure 19.15** Multiple erosive nodules of Kaposi sarcoma. When present in multiplicity, these may be debilitating and deforming.

of HIV-related KS should be made with caution in women and children from the United States as the neoplasm occurs only rarely in these patient populations.

HIV-related KS will generally resolve with antiretroviral therapy. Local destructive measures are generally effective for isolated or sporadic lesions if treatment is desired. Liquid nitrogen cryotherapy is usually the first therapeutic option for superficial lesions along with laser surgery, topical alitretinoin gel, and photodynamic therapy. Radiation treatment and electron beam therapy may be used in selected cases of multifocal but localized disease. Radiotherapy is quite effective for painful lesions of the palms and soles. Other modalities have some evidence of efficacy, including intralesional injections of vinblastine sulfate, interferon alfa-2b, systemic therapy with interferon and liposomally encapsulated doxorubicin and daunorubicin.[35]

## Cutaneous epithelial neoplasms in HIV patients

HIV patients have an increased incidence of epithelial neoplams, most commonly involving oral, cervical and anorectal sites. Women with AIDS have a twofold increased

five skin lesions.[33] Involvement of the gastrointestinal tract may be dangerous if it causes blockage or hemorrhage. When tumors involve the lymphatics, marked edema may develop. No specific laboratory findings are seen. Diagnosis is based on clinicopathological correlation. The diagnosis

risk for the development of cervical cancer as compared to the general population, and American AIDS patients have a greater than 40-fold increased risk for the development of anal cancer.[36] Bowenoid papulosis as well as cloacogenic carcinoma are also increased in incidence in these patients. Although basal cell carcinomas and squamous cell carcinomas have been suggested over the years to be increased in incidence in HIV patients, a more recent retrospective study spanning two decades failed to show an association between these cancers and the immune status of HIV patients, CD4 count, or receipt of HAART. Cutaneous non-AIDS-defining cancers such as BCC, SCC and melanoma were associated with traditional risk factors such as aging and skin color.[37] As to whether future research will support the findings of this group remains to be seen.

## Lymphoreticular malignancies

Lymphoreticular malignancies of both B- and T-cell lineage may develop, especially in those with CD4+ counts <200 cells/mm³. The majority of these involve lymph nodes and the reticuloendothelial system. The skin may be involved either primarily or secondarily at a higher rate than in traditional lymphomas at initial presentation. Unlike in the general population, non-Hodgkin lymphoma and B-cell lymphomas are seen most commonly (Fig. 19.16). Approximately half of all the non-Hodgkin lymphomas are associated with EBV infection. Children afflicted with HIV infection have a higher incidence of mucosa-associated lymphoid tissue (MALT) lymphomas involving the salivary tissue, pulmonary, and gastric mucosa.[38] Pink to purplish papules or nodules are typical for patients afflicted with cutaneous non-Hodgkin lymphoma. Any site may be involved.

Cutaneous Hodgkin disease is extremely rare and usually a consequence of direct extension from underlying nodal disease. HIV-related cutaneous T-cell lymphoma may have a clinical appearance similar to mycosis fungoides and can manifest as widespread plaques that may progress to erythroderma.[11] HTLV-1-associated lymphoma may also resemble mycosis fungoides although it can also appear like a viral exanthem. The routine diagnosis of this neoplasm is based on the characteristic clinical appearance taken in the context of histopathologic features. In many

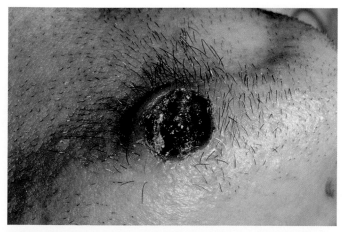

**Figure 19.16** Cutaneous B-cell lymphoma. Patients who have infection are prone to develop lymphoreticular malignancies, some of which may affect the skin, as in this case.

cases, gene rearrangement studies, immunophenotyping, flow cytometric immunologic analysis and the use of DNA probes are necessary to subtype the neoplasm. Treatment consists of the standard therapy for systemic lymphoma.

## FUTURE OUTLOOK

As scientific knowledge progresses, addtional cutaneous cancers will be identified that have a direct or indirect relationship with HPV or HIV infection. Research into the mechanisms by which these viruses mediate cutaneous oncogenesis will result in new treatments for the resulting ailments. Vaccination against the oncogenic HPV viruses is a testament to continued advances in the treatment of these oncogenic infections and the hope that this form of tumorigenesis can be circumvented.[39]

## REFERENCES

1. de Villiers EM, Fauquet C, Broker TR, et al. Classification of papillomaviruses. *Virology*. 2004;324(1):17–27.
2. Ramoz N, Rueda LA, Bouadjar B, et al. Mutations in two adjacent novel genes are associated with epidermodysplasia verruciformis. *Nat Genet*. 2002;32(4):579–581.
3. Lewandowsky F, Lutz W. Fall einer bisher nicht beschriebenen Hauterkrankung (Epidermodysplasia verruciformis). *Arch Derm Syph (Berlin)*. 1922;141:193–203.
4. Orth G, Jablonska S, Favre M, et al. Characterization of two types of human papillomaviruses in lesions of epidermodysplasia verruciformis. *Proc Natl Acad Sci USA*. 1978;75(3):1537–1541.
5. Ramoz N, Rueda LA, Bouadjar B, et al. A susceptibility locus for epidermodysplasia verruciformis, an abnormal predisposition to infection with the oncogenic human papillomavirus type 5, maps to chromosome 17qter in a region containing a psoriasis locus. *J Invest Dermatol*. 1999;112(3):259–263.
6. Androphy EJ, Dvoretzky I, Lowy DR. X-linked inheritance of epidermodysplasia verruciformis. Genetic and virologic studies of a kindred. *Arch Dermatol*. 1985;121(7):864–868.
7. Termorshuizen F, Feltkamp MC, Struijk L, et al. Sunlight exposure and (sero)prevalence of epidermodysplasia verruciformis-associated human papillomavirus. *J Invest Dermatol*. 2004;122(6):1456–1462.
8. Kopf AW, Bart RS. Tumor conference No. 11: multiple bowenoid papules of the penis: a new entity? *J Dermatol Surg Oncol*. 1977;3(3):265–269.
9. Wade TR, Kopf AW, Ackerman AB. Bowenoid papulosis of the penis. *Cancer*. 1978;42(4):1890–1903.
10. Obalek S, Jablonska S, Beaudenon S, et al. Bowenoid papulosis of the male and female genitalia: risk of cervical neoplasia. *J Am Acad Dermatol*. 1986;14(3):433–444.
11. Parker SC, Fenton DA, McGibbon DH. Homme rouge and the acquired immunodeficiency syndrome. *N Engl J Med*. 1989;321(13):906–907.
12. Yoneta A, Yamashita T, Jin HY, et al. Development of squamous cell carcinoma by two high-risk human papillomaviruses (HPVs), a novel HPV-67 and HPV-31 from bowenoid papulosis. *Br J Dermatol*. 2000;143(3):604–608.
13. Wade TR, Ackerman AB. The effects of resin of podophyllin on condyloma acuminatum. *Am J Dermatopathol*. 1984;6(2):109–122.
14. Porter WM, Francis N, Hawkins D, et al. Penile intraepithelial neoplasia: clinical spectrum and treatment of 35 cases. *Br J Dermatol*. 2002;147(6):1159–1165.
15. Snoeck R, Van Laethem Y, De Clercq E, et al. Treatment of a bowenoid papulosis of the penis with local applications of cidofovir in a patient with acquired immunodeficiency syndrome. *Arch Intern Med*. 2001;161(19):2382–2384.
16. Descamps V, Duval X, Grossin M, et al. Topical cidofovir for bowenoid papulosis in an HIV-infected patient. *Br J Dermatol*. 2001;144(3):642–643.
17. Ackerman LV. Verrucous carcinoma of the oral cavity. *Surgery*. 1948;23(4):670–678.
18. Noel JC, Peny MO, Goldschmidt D, et al. Human papillomavirus type 1 DNA in verrucous carcinoma of the leg. *J Am Acad Dermatol*. 1993;29(6):1036–1038.
19. Boshart M, zur Hausen H. Human papillomaviruses in Buschke-Lowenstein tumors: physical state of the DNA and identification of a tandem duplication in the noncoding region of a human papillomavirus 6 subtype. *J Virol*. 1986;58(3):963–966.
20. Noel JC, Peny MO, Detremmerie O, et al. Demonstration of human papillomavirus type 2 in a verrucous carcinoma of the foot. *Dermatology*. 1993;187(1):58–61.

21. Garven TC, Thelmo WL, Victor J, et al. Verrucous carcinoma of the leg positive for human papillomavirus DNA 11 and 18: a case report. *Hum Pathol*. 1991;22(11):1170–1173.

22. Schell BJ, Rosen T, Rady P, et al. Verrucous carcinoma of the foot associated with human papillomavirus type 16. *J Am Acad Dermatol*. 2001;45(1):49–55.

23. Walvekar RR, Chaukar DA, Deshpande MS, et al. Verrucous carcinoma of the oral cavity: A clinical and pathological study of 101 cases. *Oral Oncol*. 2009;45(1):47–51.

24. Yeager JK, Findlay RF, McAleer IM. Penile verrucous carcinoma. *Arch Dermatol*. 1990;126(9):1208–1210.

25. Chu QD, Vezeridis MP, Libbey NP, et al. Giant condyloma acuminatum (Buschke-Lowenstein tumor) of the anorectal and perianal regions. Analysis of 42 cases. *Dis Colon Rectum*. 1994;37(9):950–957.

26. Padilla RS, Bailin PL, Howard WR, et al. Verrucous carcinoma of the skin and its management by Mohs' surgery. *Plast Reconstr Surg*. 1984;73(3):442–447.

27. Alkalay R, Alcalay J, Shiri J. Plantar verrucous carcinoma treated with Mohs micrographic surgery: a case report and literature review. *J Drugs Dermatol*. 2006;5(1):68–73.

28. Nikkels AF, Thirion L, Quatresooz P, et al. Photodynamic therapy for cutaneous verrucous carcinoma. *J Am Acad Dermatol*. 2007;57(3):516–519.

29. Heinzerling LM, Kempf W, Kamarashev J, et al. Treatment of verrucous carcinoma with imiquimod and CO2 laser ablation. *Dermatology*. 2003;207(1):119–122.

30. Villa LL, Costa RL, Petta CA, et al. Prophylactic quadrivalent human papillomavirus (types 6, 11, 16, and 18) L1 virus-like particle vaccine in young women: a randomised double-blind placebo-controlled multicentre phase II efficacy trial. *Lancet Oncol*. 2005;6(5):271–278.

31. Villa LL, Costa RL, Petta CA, et al. High sustained efficacy of a prophylactic quadrivalent human papillomavirus types 6/11/16/18 L1 virus-like particle vaccine through 5 years of follow-up. *Br J Cancer*. 2006;95(11):1459–1466.

32. Slade BA, Leidel L, Vellozzi C, et al. Postlicensure safety surveillance for quadrivalent human papillomavirus recombinant vaccine. *JAMA*. 2009;302(7):750–757.

33. Bonanni P, Boccalini S, Bechini A. Efficacy, duration of immunity and cross protection after HPV vaccination: a review of the evidence. *Vaccine*. 2009;27(suppl 1):A46–A53.

34. Krigel RL, Friedman-Kien AE. Epidemic Kaposi's sarcoma. *Semin Oncol*. 1990;17(3):350–360.

35. Dittmer DP, Krown SE. Targeted therapy for Kaposi's sarcoma and Kaposi's sarcoma-associated herpesvirus. *Curr Opin Oncol*. 2007;19(5):452–457.

36. Fowler MG, Melnick SL, Mathieson BJ. Women and HIV. Epidemiology and global overview. *Obstet Gynecol Clin North Am*. 1997;24(4):705–729.

37. Crum-Cianflone N, Hullsiek KH, Satter E, et al. Cutaneous malignancies among HIV-infected persons. *Arch Intern Med*. 2009;169(12):1130–1138.

38. Mueller BU. HIV-associated malignancies in children. *AIDS Patient Care STDS*. 1999;13(9):527–533.

39. Dunne EF, Datta SD, Markowitz LE. A review of prophylactic human papillomavirus vaccines: recommendations and monitoring in the US. *Cancer*. 2008;113(suppl 10):2995–3003.

# Pseudolymphomas of the Skin

*Lorenzo Cerroni and Helmut Kerl*

## Key Points

- Cutaneous pseudolymphomas are benign inflammatory skin diseases that mimic malignant lymphomas either clinically, histopathologically, or both.
- Cutaneous pseudolymphomas should be classified precisely according to specific clinicopathologic entities.
- Integration of clinical, histopathologic, immunophenotypic and molecular genetic features is crucial for the diagnosis of cutaneous pseudolymphomas.
- Some non-lymphoid malignant neoplasms may simulate histopathologically the picture of a cutaneous lymphoma.

## INTRODUCTION

Pseudolymphomas of the skin are benign lymphocytic proliferations that simulate cutaneous malignant lymphomas clinically and/or histopathologically.[1] The term pseudolymphoma does not refer to any particular disease but rather to a heterogeneous group of inflammatory conditions and benign 'tumors' of diverse causes. For proper treatment, it is important to identify specific entities. In addition to benign inflammatory skin disorders, some non-lymphoid malignant neoplasms may simulate histopathologically the picture of a cutaneous lymphoma.

## HISTORY AND CLASSIFICATION

Cutaneous pseudolymphomas have been known for a long time.[2,3] In recent years, many inflammatory skin diseases have been added to the group of the cutaneous pseudolymphomas, mainly because of the presence of histopathologic features similar to those observed in malignant lymphomas of the skin.[1] Table 20.1 shows a modern clinicopathologic classification of conditions that are currently viewed as cutaneous pseudolymphomas.

## EPIDEMIOLOGY

There are no exact data concerning the incidence, prevalence, and geographic distribution of cutaneous pseudolymphomas. Cutaneous pseudolymphomas induced by the spirochetal microorganism *Borrelia burgdorferi* (i.e. *Borrelia lymphocytoma*) commonly arise in regions with endemic *Borrelia burgdorferi* infection.

## PATIENT EVALUATION, DIAGNOSIS AND DIFFERENTIAL DIAGNOSIS

The clinical manifestations of cutaneous pseudolymphomas are variable, depending on the specific entity: some resemble mycosis fungoides and present with patches and/or plaques, others resemble subcutaneous lymphoma and present with panniculitic lesions, still others resemble cutaneous B-cell lymphomas and present with papules, nodules and/or tumors. Cutaneous pseudolymphomas may also show the features of generalized erythroderma.

Histologic diagnosis of cutaneous pseudolymphomas depends upon two main considerations: (1) the architectural pattern of the infiltrate, which can be studied only in adequate biopsy specimens, and (2) the cellular composition of those infiltrates, which frequently shows a mixed character.[1,4-6] Histologic features should be integrated by phenotypic and gene rearrangement data that can be obtained on routinely fixed, paraffin-embedded sections of tissue. New, standardized methods of analysis of T-cell receptor (TCR) and immunoglobulin genes have been introduced recently.[7] In this context, it should be reminded that, although monoclonality of B lymphocytes in B-cell pseudolymphomas is infrequent, rare cases of otherwise typical *Borrelia burgdorferi*-associated lymphocytoma cutis with monoclonal rearrangement of the immunoglobulin heavy chain genes have been observed. Beside genuine monoclonality, 'pseudoclonality' is not infrequent in cutaneous pseudolymphomas.[8]

## SPECIFIC CLINICOPATHOLOGIC ENTITIES

### Actinic reticuloid

Actinic reticuloid is a severe persistent photodermatitis that usually affects older men, characterized by extreme photosensitivity to a broad spectrum of UV radiation and by clinicopathologic similarities to mycosis fungoides (see Chapter 21).[9,10] The patients present in the early stages with erythemas on the face and neck and on dorsa of the hands. As the eruption progresses, it becomes lichenified and reddish-purple (Fig. 20.1). The patient's face may have a leonine appearance with deep furrowing of markedly thickened skin. Diffuse alopecia can also be seen. The course may be characterized by recurrent erythroderma, and circulating Sézary cells may be found in the peripheral blood of patients with actinic reticuloid. Pruritus is generally severe and intractable. The disease is chronic and shows no tendency to spontaneous remission.[11]

## Table 20.1 Classification of Cutaneous Pseudolymphomas

| Clinicopathological Entity | Simulated Malignant Lymphoma |
| --- | --- |
| Actinic reticuloid | Mycosis fungoides/Sézary syndrome |
| Lymphomatoid contact dermatitis | |
| Solitary T-cell pseudolymphoma (superficial type) | |
| Lichenoid ('lymphomatoid') keratosis | |
| Lichenoid pigmented purpuric dermatitis (including lichen aureus) | |
| Lichen sclerosus et atrophicus | |
| Vitiligo (inflammatory stages) | |
| Annular lichenoid dermatitis of youth (exact nosology yet unclear) | |
| CD8+ cutaneous infiltrates in HIV-infected patients | |
| Lymphomatoid drug reaction, T-cell type | |
| Pseudolymphomas in tattoos, T-cell type | |
| Pseudolymphomas at sites of vaccination, T-cell type | |
| Mycosis fungoides-like infiltrates in regressing malignant epithelial and melanocytic tumors | |
| Pseudolymphomas in herpes simplex or herpes zoster infections | Cytotoxic NK/T-cell lymphomas *or* Lymphomatoid papulosis/cutaneous anaplastic large cell lymphoma |
| PLEVA, including the febrile ulcero-necrotic variant | |
| Atypical lymphoid infiltrates (CD30) associated with: orf, milker's nodule, molluscum contagiosum and other infectious disorders | Lymphomatoid papulosis/cutaneous anaplastic large cell lymphoma |
| Persistent arthropod bite reactions (including nodular scabies) | |
| Drug eruptions with clusters of CD30+ lymphocytes | |
| Lupus panniculitis | Subcutaneous 'panniculitis-like' T-cell lymphoma |
| Lymphocytoma cutis | Follicle center lymphoma Marginal zone B-cell lymphoma Diffuse large B-cell lymphoma |
| Lymphomatoid drug reaction, B-cell type | Follicle center lymphoma |
| Pseudolymphoma after vaccination, B-cell type | |
| Pseudolymphoma in tattoos, B-cell type | Marginal zone B-cell lymphoma |
| Morphea, inflammatory stage | |
| Syphilis (secondary) | |
| 'Acral pseudolymphomatous angiokeratoma' (small papular pseudolymphoma) | |
| Inflammatory pseudotumor (plasma cell granuloma) Cutaneous plasmacytosis | Marginal zone B-cell lymphoma, plasmacytic variant |
| Lymphocytic infiltration of the skin (Jessner-Kanof) | Cutaneous manifestations of B-cell chronic lymphocytic leukemia |
| Cutaneous extramedullary hematopoiesis | Cutaneous manifestations of myeloid leukemia |
| Reactive angioendotheliomatosis/Intravascular histiocytosis | Intravascular diffuse large cell lymphoma |
| Benign intravascular proliferation of lymphoid blasts | |

Histologic examination reveals dense, band-like or patchy, mixed-cell infiltrates of lymphocytes, histiocytes, plasma cells and eosinophils, as well as some atypical mononuclear cells with hyperchromatic lobulated nuclei in the upper part of the dermis (Fig. 20.2).[1] The papillary dermis is usually thickened; stellate and multinucleated fibroblasts are present. Lymphocytes can be found in the hyperplastic epidermis. A histopathologic feature useful in distinction from mycosis fungoides is the presence of lichen simplex chronicus superimposed upon an inflammatory process.

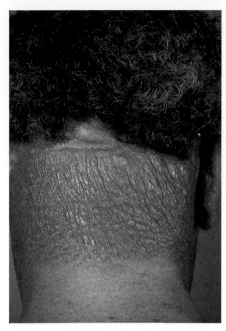

Figure 20.1 Actinic reticuloid. Thickened and furrowed skin on the neck.

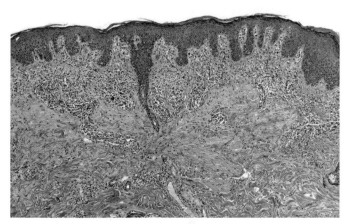

Figure 20.2 Actinic reticuloid. Histology reveals psoriasiform epidermal hyperplasia and a patchy band-like inflammatory infiltrate resembling mycosis fungoides.

On phototesting, patients with chronic actinic dermatitis were found to be sensitive to UVB, UVA, and, in most instances, to visible light. Fluorescent light is said to lead sometimes to exacerbation of the disease. The minimal erythema dose is lower than normal. Some investigators believe that progression to malignant lymphoma can occasionally occur, although this remains controversial.

Treatment of chronic actinic dermatitis is difficult and numerous therapeutic approaches have been proposed. Photoprotection is most important. Any relevant associated contact or photocontact allergens have to be identified and avoided. Some patients have been reported to respond to corticosteroids, photochemotherapy with PUVA, alpha-interferon, or to a combination treatment with azathioprine, hydroxychloroquine and prednisone. Ciclosporin A (sometimes combined with bath-PUVA) and topical tacrolimus ointment (especially for facial lesions) appear also to be effective.

## Lymphomatoid contact dermatitis

Clinically, lymphomatoid contact dermatitis is characterized by pruritic erythematous plaques (Fig. 20.3).[12] The clinical picture and histologic features are highly suggestive of mycosis fungoides. The lesions grow progressively, and exfoliative erythroderma can be observed. Lymphomatoid contact dermatitis typically undergoes phases of exacerbation and remission. Although the disease has been reported to evolve into true malignant lymphoma, it is more likely that such patients had malignant lymphoma from the outset.

Histologically, lymphomatoid contact dermatitis resembles mycosis fungoides ('spongiotic simulator of cutaneous T cell lymphoma') (Fig. 20.4).[1] The differentiation from mycosis fungoides is usually done on the basis of changes within the epidermis. In lymphomatoid contact dermatitis, there are only a few lymphocytes in the epidermis in the context of more pronounced spongiosis. Small collections of CD1a+ Langerhans' cells may also be observed ('pseudo-Pautrier' microabscesses).

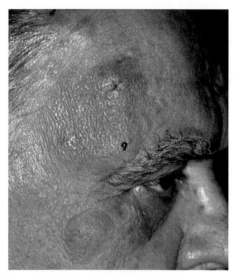

Figure 20.3 Lymphomatoid contact dermatitis. Eczematous papules and plaques on the cheek and forehead.

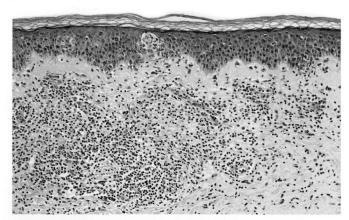

Figure 20.4 Lymphomatoid contact dermatitis. Dense band-like infiltrate in the superficial dermis. Note the small intraepidermal collection of cells representing a 'Pautrier's microabscess'-like cluster of Langerhans cells and lymphocytes.

**209**

Patch tests to a variety of common antigens can give a positive reaction. For the management of patients, a thorough search for antigens is necessary in order to interrupt the process. When contact with the responsible allergen(s) is avoided, the lesions heal in a relatively short time.

## Lymphomatoid drug reactions

A large number of drugs may induce atypical lymphoid infiltrates in the skin that simulate malignant lymphoma (Fig. 20.5A,B).[13,14] Table 20.2 lists the most common drugs implicated in the onset of cutaneous pseudolymphomas. The external use of etheric plant oils may also cause lymphoproliferative reactions that mimic malignant lymphomas, clinically and histologically.

Histologically, pseudolymphomatous drug eruptions are characterized by dense band-like or nodular and diffuse infiltrates of sometimes atypical lymphocytes revealing T- (mycosis fungoides-like) or B-cell (follicle center lymphoma-like or marginal zone lymphoma-like) patterns (Fig. 20.6A,B). Eosinophils may or may not be present.

Lymphomatoid drug reactions regress when the drug is withdrawn. One single case of progression into mycosis fungoides has been documented.

## CD30+ (T-cell) pseudolymphomas

The presence of CD30+ large blasts simulating the picture of a CD30+ cutaneous lymphoproliferative disorder has been observed in the skin in several reactive conditions, including arthropod reactions, scabies, and drug eruptions among many others.[15] This type of pseudolymphoma is related often to infectious disorders, particularly to viral infections (orf, milker's nodule, molluscum contagiosum, herpes simplex, herpes zoster, and others) (Fig. 20.7A–C).[16]

Besides the presence of large, atypical CD30+ cells, histology reveals the typical changes of the specific underlying disorder. Moreover, in these reactive conditions, CD30+ lymphocytes are present in small numbers scattered throughout the infiltrate and are usually not arranged in clusters or sheets as observed in lymphomatoid papulosis or anaplastic large cell lymphoma. However, in given cases, differentiation may be very difficult or even impossible on histologic and immunohistochemical grounds alone. Unlike the situation in lymphomatoid papulosis and anaplastic large cell lymphoma, gene rearrangement studies in CD30+ pseudolymphomas reveal the presence of a polyclonal population of T lymphocytes.

## Persistent nodular arthropod bite reactions

The most typical example of this group of lymphomatoid infiltrates is nodular scabies. Clinically, elevated, round or oval, bright red to brownish red papules and nodules occur, most frequently on the genitalia, elbows and in the axillae (Fig. 20.8). The lesions are found in about 7% of patients with scabies. The nodules are very pruritic and may persist for many months or even years.

The mite and its parts are seldom identified in long-standing papules or nodules of scabies. The clinical differential diagnosis includes prurigo nodularis and malignant lymphoma.

Histologically, dense, superficial and deep, perivascular, predominantly lymphohistiocytic, infiltrates with plasma cells and varying numbers of eosinophils are seen (Fig. 20.9A,B). Eosinophils are also scattered among collagen bundles. The epidermis may be slightly spongiotic, hyperplastic and hyperkeratotic. Large, activated (atypical-looking) lymphocytes are a frequent finding.

Immunohistologic investigations reveal T lymphocytes as the predominant cells of nodular scabies. In some cases,

**Figure 20.5** Lymphomatoid drug reactions.
**A)** Disseminated, lichenoid papules and plaques simulating a cutaneous T-cell lymphoma.
**B)** Generalized papules and small nodules on the back simulating cutaneous B-cell lymphoma.

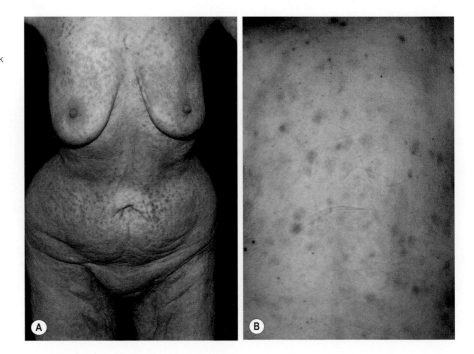

## Table 20.2 Important Drugs Involved in Cutaneous Pseudolymphomas

| Category | Drug |
| --- | --- |
| Anticonvulsant | Carbamazepine<br>Clonazepam<br>Lamotrigine<br>Phenytoin |
| Antidepressant | Amitriptyline<br>Desipramine<br>Doxepin<br>Fluoxetine<br>Lithium |
| Antipsychotic | Chlorpromazine<br>Perphenazine<br>Thioridazine |
| Anxiolytic tranquilizer | Alprazolam<br>Lorazepam |
| Uricosuric | Allopurinol |
| Diuretic | Furosemide<br>Hydrochlorothiazide |
| Beta-adrenergic blocker | Atenolol |
| Antihypertensive | Clonidine<br>Losartan |
| Calcium channel blocker | Diltiazem |
| Cephalosporic antibiotic | Cefixime |
| Macrolide antibiotic | Clarithromycin |
| Urinary tract antibiotic | Nitrofurantoin |
| Sulfonamide | Sulfasalazine |
| Antibacterial | Co-trimoxazole<br>Sulfamethoxazole |
| H2-receptor antihistamine | Cimetidine<br>Nizatidine<br>Ranitidine |
| H1-receptor antihistamine | Terfenadine |
| Antineoplastic, anti-inflammatory | Methotrexate |
| Immunosuppressant | Ciclosporin |
| Antiarthritic | Gold/gold compounds |
| Antihyperlipidemic | Gemfibrozil |

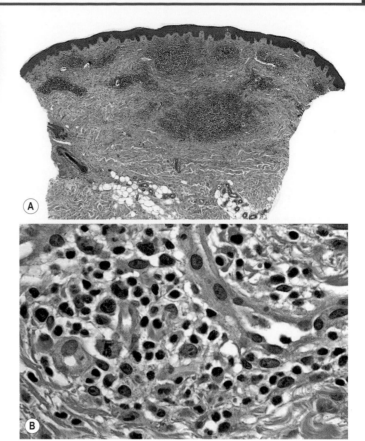

**Figure 20.6** Lymphomatoid drug reaction. **A)** Dense nodular dermal infiltrates of lymphocytes and histiocytes. **B)** Note large atypical cells.

positivity of large lymphoid cells for the CD30 antigen may simulate the immunophenotypic pattern of lymphomatoid papulosis. Occasionally, a B-cell pattern analogous to lymphocytoma cutis can be recognized in persistent nodular arthropod bite reactions.

Antiscabietic therapy is usually ineffective. Intralesional injection of corticosteroids in larger nodules may be helpful. Spontaneous resolution in time is the rule.

## Lymphocytoma cutis

Lymphocytoma cutis is a pseudolymphoma with a B-cell pattern, which can be caused by various stimuli, including insect bites, drugs, vaccinations, acupuncture, wearing of gold pierced earrings, medicinal leech therapy, and tattoos.[1,17] One of the most common associations is found with the spirochete *Borrelia burgdorferi*.[18] It should be remembered that *Borrelia* infection has been convincingly linked to some cases of cutaneous B-cell lymphoma as well, thus detection of *Borrelia* DNA is not equivalent to a diagnosis of benignancy.

There are numerous clinical presentations of lymphocytoma cutis.[1] Frequently, a firm solitary nodule or tumor can be observed. However, lesions may be clustered in a region or, rarely, may be scattered widely. Scaling and ulceration are absent. Involvement of special body sites (earlobe, nipple, scrotum) is almost pathognomonic of *Borrelia burgdorferi*-associated lymphocytoma cutis (Fig. 20.10A,B).[18] The *Borrelia burgdorferi*-associated type of lymphocytoma cutis often occurs in children.

Histologic examination shows dense, nodular, mixed-cell infiltrates, often with formation of lymphoid follicles (Fig. 20.11A,B). Although the infiltrates are frequently 'top-heavy', in lymphocytoma cutis there may be dense diffuse lymphoid infiltrates simulating the histopathologic picture of a B-cell lymphoma.

Differentiation of lymphocytoma cutis from malignant lymphoma may be extremely difficult or even impossible on histologic grounds alone. Reactive lymphoid follicles are frequently found in both lymphocytoma cutis and marginal zone B-cell lymphoma. Complete histopathologic, immunophenotypic (Fig. 20.12) and molecular analyses

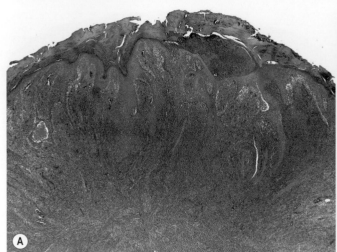

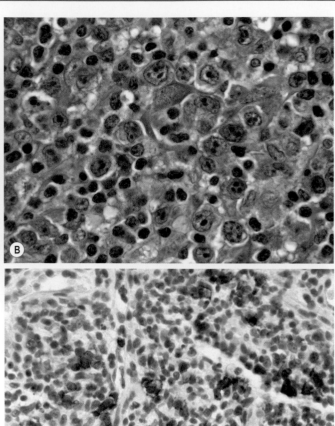

**Figure 20.7** Milker's nodule. **A)** Epidermal hyperplasia and dense lymphohistiocytic infiltrate. **B)** Note large atypical cells and **C)** positivity for CD30.

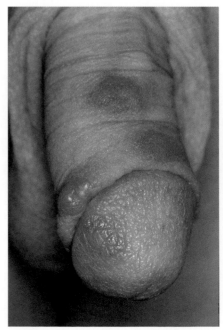

**Figure 20.8** Nodular lesions of scabies on genital skin.

are crucial in distinguishing lesions of lymphocytoma cutis from those of cutaneous B-cell lymphomas.[5,19]

Lymphocytoma cutis may resolve spontaneously in several months or years. Small nodules can be removed by surgical excision, and local injection of corticosteroids or interferon-α may result in regression. Patients with lesions of lymphocytoma cutis and detection in serum of immunoglobulins specific for *Borrelia burgdorferi* or detection on tissue sections of *Borrelia* DNA by polymerase chain reaction can be treated with antibiotics (*Borrelia*-induced lymphocytoma is usually treated with a 3-week course of minocycline or with intravenous administration of ceftriaxone). Resolution may be slow after the end of antibiotic treatment.

## Other pseudolymphomas

Several other inflammatory disorders may mimic the clinical and/or histopathologic picture of cutaneous lymphoma.

Lichenoid (lymphomatoid) keratosis (Fig. 20.13A,B), lichenoid pigmented purpuric dermatitis (including lichen aureus) (Fig. 20.14A,B) and lichen sclerosus on genital skin can also be added to the list of cutaneous T-cell pseudolymphomas.[20] The histopathological features, with dense

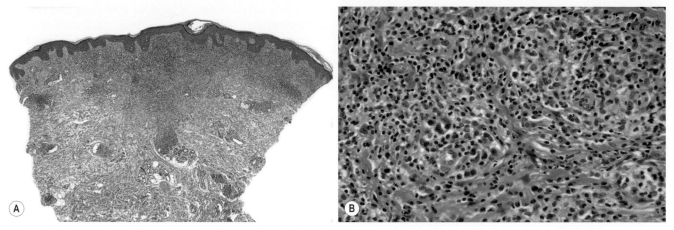

**Figure 20.9** Nodular scabies. **A)** Dense lymphoid infiltrates with a 'top-heavy' arrangement. Note a cuniculus within the horny layer. **B)** The inflammatory infiltrate is composed of lymphocytes, histiocytes, plasma cells and eosinophils.

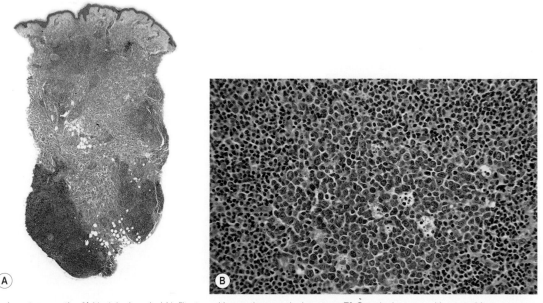

**Figure 20.10** *Borrelia*-induced lymphocytoma cutis. **A)** Involvement of the ear. **B)** Typical manifestation on the nipple.

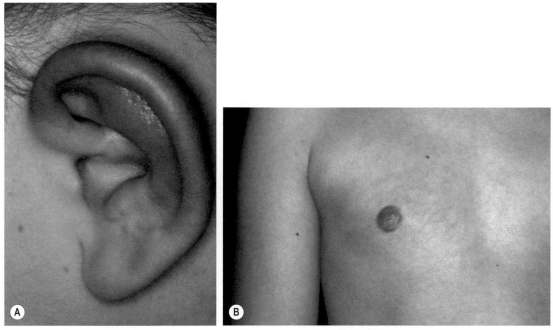

**Figure 20.11** Lymphocytoma cutis. **A)** Nodular lymphoid infiltrates with reactive germinal centers. **B)** Germinal center with centroblasts, centrocytes and 'tingible body'-macrophages. This case, located on the nipple, was due to infection with *Borrelia burgdorferi*.

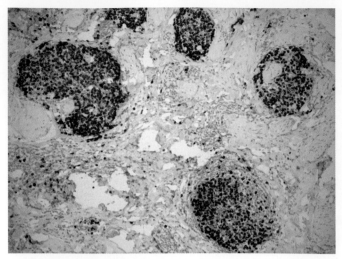

**Figure 20.12** Lymphocytoma cutis. Staining for proliferating cells (MIB-1/Ki67) reveals high proliferation within reactive germinal centers.

band-like inflammatory lymphoid infiltrates and often epidermotropism of lymphocytes, may be indistinguishable from those of mycosis fungoides. Moreover, T-lymphocyte clonality can be sometimes found in these diseases. Accurate clinicopathological correlation is crucial to establish a correct diagnosis.

Reactions to tattoos (Fig. 20.15A,B) may sometimes reveal lymphoid follicular structures or a mycosis fungoides-like pattern. The presence of pigment suggests the correct diagnosis; however, one well-documented case of cutaneous lymphoma arising in a tattoo has been reported and follow-up should be performed very carefully.

Lupus profundus (lupus panniculitis) may mimic lesions of subcutaneous panniculitis-like T-cell lymphoma both clinically and histologically.[21] Lupus panniculitis reveals clinically subcutaneous plaques and indurations, mostly located on the extremities. Antinuclear antibodies and other markers of systemic lupus erythematosus may be absent. Histology shows a lobular panniculitis, often with

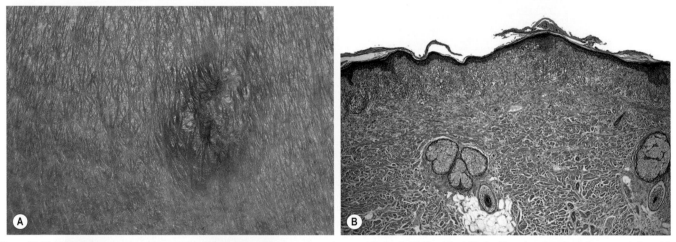

**Figure 20.13** Lichenoid (lymphomatoid) keratosis. **A)** Solitary, small erythematous plaque on the trunk. **B)** Band-like infiltrate of lymphocytes simulating mycosis fungoides.

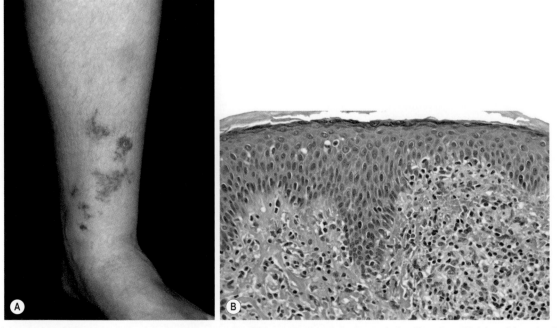

**Figure 20.14** Lichen aureus. **A)** Red-orange macules located on one leg. **B)** Lymphocytes and extravasated erythrocytes with intraepidermal cells simulating a mycosis fungoides.

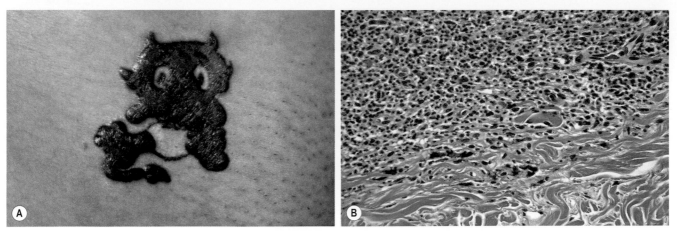

**Figure 20.15** Pseudolymphoma within a tattoo. **A)** Reddish plaques within a tattoo. **B)** Dense lymphoid infiltrates with large cells; note pigment at the base of the infiltrate.

concomitant presence of broadened, fibrotic septa. A useful feature for differentiation of subcutaneous panniculitis-like T-cell lymphoma from lupus panniculitis is the presence in the former of so-called 'rimming' of fat cells by pleomorphic, atypical CD8+ T lymphocytes that are positive for proliferation markers.[22] In contrast to subcutaneous panniculitis-like T-cell lymphoma, B cells, plasma cells and germinal centers are commonly a prominent feature in lupus panniculitis. Moreover, the dermoepidermal junction may show features of lupus erythematosus (interface dermatitis). Analysis of T-cell receptor gene rearrangement reveals polyclonal populations of T and B lymphocytes in lupus panniculitis, in contrast to subcutaneous panniculitis-like T-cell lymphoma, where monoclonality of T lymphocytes is found as a rule. It should be underlined that a precise distinction between lupus panniculitis and panniculitis-like T-cell lymphoma cannot be made in every case, and that cases with overlapping clinicopathologic features of lupus panniculitis and subcutaneous T-cell lymphoma recently have been described, thus suggesting that a relationship between the two entities may exist.[23,24]

Localized scleroderma/morphea (inflammatory stage) and secondary syphilis may simulate cutaneous lymphomas, especially marginal zone B-cell lymphoma, histopathologically. A polyclonal pattern of immunoglobulin light chain expression favors a diagnosis of an inflammatory process. Besides serologic tests for syphilis, presence of *Treponema pallidum* can be demonstrated on routinely processed material by immunohistochemistry.

Acral pseudolymphomatous angiokeratoma is characterized by unilateral clustered red-violaceous papules and small nodules, usually located on the hands and feet of children.[25,26] Histopathologic investigations reveal a dense nodular lymphoid infiltrate with occasional plasma cells and eosinophils. The term angiokeratoma is misleading, and based on the distinctive clinicopathologic features, the designation 'small papular pseudolymphoma' has been suggested for this benign lymphoproliferative disease.

Annular lichenoid dermatitis of youth is a term recently coined for a peculiar disease in children, characterized by annular erythematous patches that clinically resemble inflammatory morphea, but present histopathologically with band-like infiltrates of T lymphocytes suggestive of mycosis fungoides (Fig. 20.16).[27] The T lymphocytes are polyclonal, and follow-up data suggest that this condition is not related to mycosis fungoides.

Recently, a benign proliferation of blasts simulating the histopathologic picture of an intravascular lymphoma has been described in the skin after trauma.[28] Neoplastic cells have a T-helper phenotype. In contrast to intravascular lymphoma, in the reactive condition, lymphoid blasts are located within the lymphatic rather than the blood vessels. Similar findings have been described rarely in other organs as well.

Differentiation of so-called 'idiopathic solitary T-cell pseudolymphoma' from primary cutaneous small–medium pleomorphic T-cell lymphoma is almost impossible on clinicopathologic grounds, and the term 'solitary small-to medium-sized pleomorphic T-cell nodule of undetermined significance' has been proposed.[29] Patients present with solitary lesions located in the vast majority of cases on the head and neck area, characterized histopathologically by dense infiltrates of pleomorphic T-helper lymphocytes admixed with variable numbers of B cells (Fig. 20.17A,B). Follow-up seems to be invariably benign.

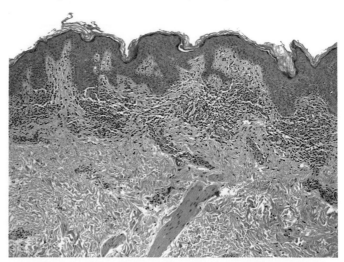

**Figure 20.16** Annular lichenoid dermatitis of youth. Band-like lymphocytic infiltrate simulating a mycosis fungoides.

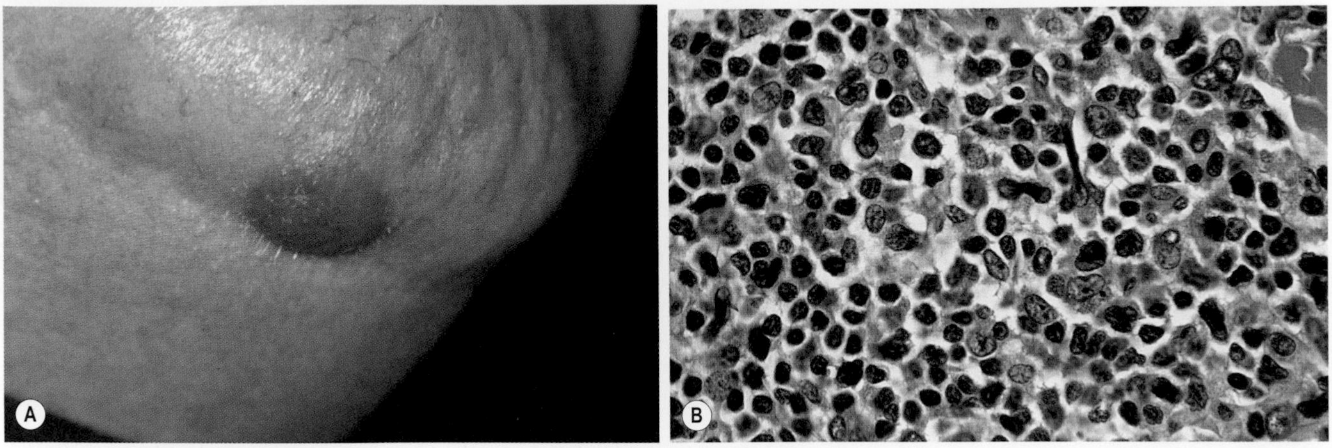

**Figure 20.17** Solitary small to medium-sized pleomorphic T-cell nodule of undetermined significance. **A)** Solitary nodule on the chin. **B)** Dense infiltrate of small- to medium-sized pleomorphic lymphocytes.

Finally, besides inflammatory skin disorders, some malignant cutaneous neoplasms may present with histopathologic features that mimic those of a cutaneous lymphoma. Lymphoepithelial-like carcinoma is a typical example, as the prominent reactive lymphoid infiltrates may mask the dermal clusters of neoplastic epithelial cells. Dense, pseudolymphomatous infiltrates may be observed rarely also in cases of cutaneous angiosarcoma,[30] representing a source of diagnostic pitfall. Complete phenotypic analyses are crucial in order to establish the correct diagnosis.

## FUTURE OUTLOOK

Pseudolymphoma of the skin is a convenient term for a group of disorders that are characterized by the same problem, namely, similarity to malignant lymphomas. In order to better allow for tailored treatment, these entities should be classified precisely according to specific categories. A synthesis of clinical, histopathologic, immunophenotypic and gene rearrangement studies will be necessary for precise classification, and for differentiation from malignant lymphomas. Improvement in genetic investigations may provide for more precise and reliable tools for differentiation of benign from malignant lymphoid infiltrates of the skin.

## REFERENCES

1. Cerroni L, Gatter K, Kerl H. *Skin Lymphoma – The Illustrated Guide*. 3rd ed. Oxford: Wiley-Blackwell; 2009.
2. Caro WA, Helwig EB. Cutaneous lymphoid hyperplasia. *Cancer*. 1969;24:487–502.
3. Clark WH, Mihm MC, Reed RJ, et al. The lymphocytic infiltrates of the skin. *Hum Pathol*. 1974;5:25–43.
4. Nihal M, Mikkola D, Horvath N, et al. Cutaneous lymphoid hyperplasia: a lymphoproliferative continuum with lymphomatous potential. *Hum Pathol*. 2003;34:617–622.
5. Leinweber B, Colli C, Chott A, et al. Differential diagnosis of cutaneous infiltrates of B lymphocytes with follicular growth pattern. *Am J Dermatopathol*. 2004;26:4–13.
6. Reddy K, Bhawan J. Histologic mimickers of mycosis fungoides: a review. *J Cutan Pathol*. 2007;34:519–525.
7. van Dongen JJM, Langerak AW, Brüggemann M, et al. Design and standardization of PCR primers and protocols for detection of clonal immunoglobulin and T-cell receptor gene recombinations in suspect lymphoproliferations: Report of the BIOMED-2 Concerted Action BMH4-CT98-3936. *Leukemia*. 2003;17:2257–2317.
8. Böer A, Tirumalae R, Bresch M, et al. Pseudoclonality in cutaneous pseudolymphomas: a pitfall in interpretation of rearrangement studies. *Br J Dermatol*. 2008;159:394–402.

9. Ive FA, Magnus IA, Warin RP, et al. Actinic reticuloid: a chronic dermatosis associated with severe photosensitivity and the histological resemblance to lymphoma. *Br J Dermatol*. 1969;81:469–485.
10. Norris PG, Hawk JLM. Chronic actinic dermatitis: a unifying concept. *Arch Dermatol*. 1990;126:376–378.
11. Dawe RS, Crombie IK, Ferguson J. The natural history of chronic actinic dermatitis. *Arch Dermatol*. 2000;136:1215–1220.
12. Gomez Orbaneja J, Iglesias Diez L, Sanchez Lozano JL, et al. Lymphomatoid contact dermatitis. *Contact Dermatitis*. 1976;2:139–143.
13. Magro CM, Crowson AN, Kovatich AJ, et al. Drug-induced reversible lymphoid dyscrasia: a clonal lymphomatoid dermatitis of memory and activated T cells. *Hum Pathol*. 2003;34:119–129.
14. Ploysangam T, Breneman DL, Mutasim DF. Cutaneous pseudolymphomas. *J Am Acad Dermatol*. 1998;38:877–905.
15. Werner B, Massone C, Kerl H, et al. Large CD30-positive cells in benign, atypical lymphoid infiltrates of the skin. *J Cutan Pathol*. 2008;35:1100–1107.
16. Leinweber B, Kerl H, Cerroni L. Histopathologic features of cutaneous herpes virus infections (herpes simplex, herpes varicella/zoster). A broad spectrum of presentations with common pseudolymphomatous aspects. *Am J Surg Pathol*. 2006;30:50–58.
17. Cerroni L, Borroni RG, Massone C, et al. Cutaneous B-cell pseudolymphoma at the site of vaccination. *Am J Dermatopathol*. 2007;29:538–542.
18. Colli C, Leinweber B, Müllegger R, et al. Borrelia burgdorferi-associated lymphocytoma cutis: clinicopathologic, immunophenotypic, and molecular study of 106 cases. *J Cutan Pathol*. 2004;31:232–240.
19. Cerroni L, Arzberger E, Pütz B, et al. Primary cutaneous follicle center cell lymphoma with follicular growth pattern. *Blood*. 2000;95:3922–3928.
20. Fink-Puches R, Wolf P, Kerl H, et al. Lichen aureus. Clinicopathologic features, natural history, and relationship to mycosis fungoides. *Arch Dermatol*. 2008;144:1169–1173.
21. Massone C, Kodama K, Salmhofer W, et al. Lupus erythematosus panniculitis (lupus profundus): clinical, histopathological, and molecular analysis of nine cases. *J Cutan Pathol*. 2005;32:396–404.
22. Lozzi GP, Massone C, Citarella L, et al. Rimming of adipocytes by neoplastic lymphocytes. A histopathologic feature not restricted to subcutaneous T-cell lymphoma. *Am J Dermatopathol*. 2006;28:9–12.
23. Magro CM, Schaefer JT, Morrison C, et al. Atypical lymphocytic lobular panniculitis: a clonal subcutaneous T-cell dyscrasia. *J Cutan Pathol*. 2008;35:947–954.
24. Pincus L, LeBoit PE, McCalmont TH, et al. Subcutaneous panniculitis-like T-cell lymphoma with overlapping clinicopathologic features of lupus erythematosus: coexistence of 2 entities? *Am J Dermatopathol*. 2009;31:520–526.
25. Kaddu S, Cerroni L, Pilatti A, et al. Acral pseudolymphomatous angiokeratoma. *Am J Dermatopathol*. 1994;16:130–133.
26. Okuyama R, Masu T, Mizuashi M, et al. Pseudolymphomatous angiokeratoma: report of three cases and an immunohistological study. *Clin Exp Dermatol*. 2009;34:161–165.
27. Cesinaro AM, Sighinolfi P, Greco A, et al. Annular lichenoid dermatitis of youth… and beyond: a series of 6 cases. *Am J Dermatopathol*. 2009;31:263–267.
28. Baum CL, Stone MS, Liu V. Atypical intravascular CD30+ T-cell proliferation following trauma in a healthy 17-year-old male: first reported case of a potential diagnostic pitfall and literature review. *J Cutan Pathol*. 2009;36:350–354.
29. Beltraminelli H, Leinweber B, Kerl H, et al. Primary cutaneous CD4+ small-/medium-sized pleomorphic T-cell lymphoma: a cutaneous nodular proliferation of pleomorphic T lymphocytes of undetermined significance? A study of 136 cases. *Am J Dermatopathol*. 2009;31:317–322.
30. Requena L, Santonja C, Stutz N, et al. Pseudolymphomatous cutaneous angiosarcoma: a rare variant of cutaneous angiosarcoma readily mistaken for cutaneous lymphoma. *Am J Dermatopathol*. 2007;29:342–350.

# Cutaneous T-cell Lymphoma: Mycosis Fungoides and Sézary Syndrome

*Brittany A. Zwischenberger, Amit G. Pandya, and Joan Guitart*

## Key Points

- Cutaneous T-cell lymphoma (CTCL) is a malignant neoplasia of T cells with homing features in the skin.
- Mycosis fungoides and Sézary syndrome are the most common variants of CTCL.
- Mycosis fungoides is often a slow-growing, indolent epidermotropic malignancy, while Sézary syndrome progresses rapidly.
- The clinical presentations of mycosis fungoides are protean including patches, plaques, tumors and erythroderma.
- Sézary syndrome is characterized by erythroderma, lymphadenopathy, and malignant T cells in the peripheral circulation.
- Prognosis and treatment of CTCL is dependent on stage of disease.

## INTRODUCTION

Cutaneous T-cell lymphoma (CTCL) is a group of non-Hodgkin lymphomas with primary cutaneous manifestation but can also involve the blood, lymph nodes, and visceral organs. Mycosis fungoides (MF) is the most common variant and accounts for 54–72% of all cases of CTCL.[1,2] Sézary syndrome (SS) represents 2.5% of all cases of CTCL and is an aggressive, leukemic variant of CTCL.[1] MF and SS are considered different presentations of the same disease and, therefore, are referred to as MF/SS and included in a single staging system.[3] However, recently published studies using gene expression analysis revealed a different expression profile for MF and SS.[4]

MF/SS is characterized by a predominance of memory helper T cells (CD4+/CD45R0+) with loss of mature T-cell antigens.[3] Clinically, MF presents with lesions limited to the skin and follows an indolent course over several years; SS presents with generalized erythroderma, lymphadenopathy and blood involvement. Other cutaneous lymphomas, in order of decreasing frequency, include primary cutaneous peripheral T-cell lymphoma, CD30+ lymphoproliferative disorders (lymphomatoid papulosis and anaplastic large T-cell lymphoma), subcutaneous panniculitic T-cell lymphoma, NK/T-cell lymphoma, angioimmunoblastic T-cell lymphoma, and adult T-cell leukemia/lymphoma (HTLV-1+).[2] Since MF and SS are the most common type of CTCL, they will be the focus of this chapter.

## HISTORY

Mycosis fungoides was first described by Alibert in 1806 through a case series of patients with mushroom-like cutaneous lesions.[5] Sézary later described a patient with erythroderma, leukocytosis, and lymphadenopathy in 1936.

## EPIDEMIOLOGY

MF/SS is rare, with an annual incidence of 6.4 per million patient-years in the United States from 1973 to 2002.[1] MF is substantially more common in blacks than whites (incidence rate ratio 1.6) and even less common in Asians (incidence rate ratio of 0.6 compared to whites). Conversely, SS occurs more commonly in whites than blacks.[1] The onset of disease increases in incidence with age (median age at diagnosis, 57–61 years).[1,6–8] However, MF/SS has been described in patients of all ages.[9] Epidemiologic data accumulated between 1973 and 2002 appeared to show an increased incidence of MF/SS.[1] CTCL incidence positively correlates with high physician density, high density of medical specialists, high median family income, and high percentage of adults with a bachelor's degree or higher.[1] These data indicate that the true incidence of CTCL is likely underrepresented with current epidemiological data.

## PATHOGENESIS AND ETIOLOGY

The etiology of the proliferation of malignant T cells in MF/SS is unknown, but has been attributed to chronic antigenic stimulation and possibly viral infections. The physiologic role of memory CD4+ helper T cells improves our understanding of the pathogenesis of MF/SS. Memory CD4+ helper T cells are part of the response to skin injury; activated antigen presenting cells (APCs) recruit memory T cells to the affected site. Memory T cells contain skin homing signals (cutaneous lymphocyte antigen [CLA] and CC-chemokine receptor 4 [CCR4]). Increased CLA and CCR4 expression is found in malignant T cells of mycosis fungoides.[10] Also, patients with CTCL demonstrate memory T cells in the dermis and blood even in the absence of visible lesions.[11] The degree of cell marker expression reflects severity of disease. As disease severity increases, cell marker expression of CCR4 and CXCR3/4 decreases, causing malignant cells to spread beyond the confines of the skin.[12] MF/SS, therefore, may arise from deregulation of normal skin immune surveillance.[11]

Epidermal Langerhans cells may lead to continuous antigenic stimulation of T cells eventually leading to CTCL.[13]

The skin-associated microbes *Staphylococcus aureus* and *Chlamydia* species may offer such a persistent stimulation through the production of superantigens.[14–16] Viral etiologies are also suggested, including human T-cell lymphotrophic virus (HTLV-1), cytomegalovirus (CMV), and Epstein-Barr virus (EBV), but a causal role is questionable.[17–21] Finally, CTCL has been associated with several HLA-class 2 alleles: DQB1*03 in MF/SS, HLA-DR5 in MF, and DQB1*0502 in SS.[22] Besides the persistent activation of T cells in the early stages of CTCL, defects in apoptotic pathways have been documented in numerous studies.[23,24] Regardless of the precipitant, the persistence of T cells in the skin leads to chronic inflammation with a predominance of a Th2 cytokine profile (IL-4, IL-5, IL-10).

Chromosomal abnormalities have also been described in biopsies from patients with MF/SS indicating a dominant clonal population. These defects are usually detected in more advanced stages. Chromosomal alterations in MF and SS were identified with comparative genomic hybridization (CGH) analysis, fluorescent in-situ hybridization (FISH), and allelotyping, and demonstrated similar patterns of chromosomal imbalances in MF and SS.[25] The shared gains and losses of copy numbers were present in 12–38% of cases. However, improved techniques investigating changes in DNA copy number in MF and SS demonstrate differences between the two.[4] Gains occur more frequently than losses in tumor-stage MF, with the long arm of chromosome 7 most commonly involved in gains (59% of samples showed gains on 7q36, which rarely occurs in SS). MF chromosomal alterations also frequently involve gains on chromosome 1 and losses on chromosomes 5 and 9. In contrast, malignant T cells in SS demonstrate a different pattern: gain of 17q23–25 (80%), gain of 8q24 (75%), and loss of 17p13 (75%).[4] The different chromosomal aberrations suggest that MF and SS each have a unique pathogenesis.

## CLINICAL FEATURES

MF/SS often has an indolent course, causing a delay in diagnosis as long as 7 years. Since skin biopsies can be non-specific early in the course of the disease, multiple, sequential biopsies are often needed before the diagnosis is confirmed. Patients are often treated with topical steroids for a presumptive diagnosis of eczema, atopic dermatitis, psoriasis or other dermatoses before a diagnosis of MF/SS is finally made. According to the WHO–EORTC (World Health Organization–European Organization for Research and Treatment of Cancer) classification, there are three variants of MF: folliculotropic MF (FMF), pagetoid reticulosis, and granulomatous slack skin.[26]

The cutaneous lesions of MF are asymmetrical, well demarcated but not as sharply demarcated as psoriasis, variable in size, and often progress from patches to plaques and, occasionally, tumors. The extent of skin involvement varies widely, but patients often present with multiple lesions located in different anatomic sites. Importantly, lesions can be irregular in size as they undergo progression and spontaneous regression. Classically, the breasts, buttocks, and intertriginous regions are involved, creating a 'bathing suit' distribution, but MF can also involve other sun-protected areas, such as the flanks, inner thighs,

inner arms, and periaxillary areas. In general, the patches are several centimeters in diameter, well circumscribed, circular, oval or annular, and pink to red in appearance (Fig. 21.1). Plaques are similar in appearance but have overlying fine scale (Fig. 21.2). Longstanding lesions are often atrophic, resulting in a 'cigarette paper' wrinkled appearance. MF palmaris et plantaris (MFPP) is a rare variant that includes hyperkeratotic patches and plaques of the palms and soles.[27]

Tumor-stage CTCL presents as dome-shaped nodules >1 cm in diameter, often with ulceration and pain (Fig. 21.3). The distribution of tumor lesions is random without a specific pattern related to sun exposure. It is important to recognize and document all lesions due to prognostic and treatment implications.[3] Poikiloderma is fairly specific to MF/SS, which helps rule out other variants of CTCL and benign dermatoses (Fig. 21.4).[28]

FMF preferentially involves the head, neck and upper torso (Fig. 21.5). The majority (68%) of patients report severe pruritus.[29] Alopecia is characteristic of FMF, reported in 65%

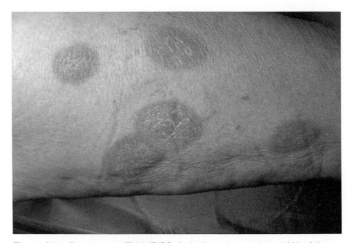

**Figure 21.1** Patch-stage (T1) MF/SS: limited patch covering <10% of the body surface area.

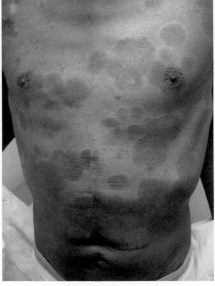

**Figure 21.2** T2 patch/plaque-stage MF: multiple hyperpigmented plaques on patient's trunk covering ≥10% of the body surface area.

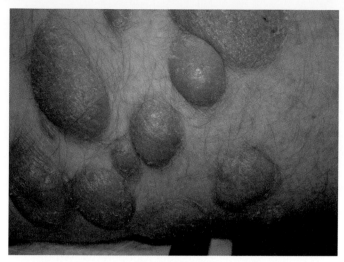

Figure 21.3 T3 tumor-stage MF: multiple tumors on thigh.

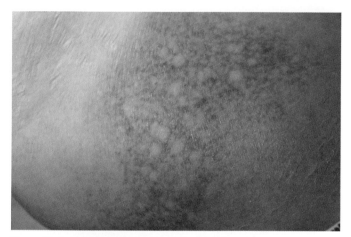

Figure 21.4 Poikiloderma associated with MF.

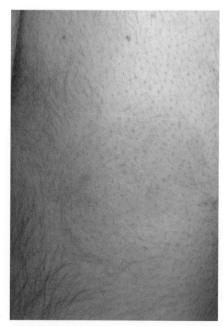

Figure 21.5 Folliculotropic MF: erythematous plaque with alopecia on extremity.

of patients, and typically is seen on the scalp, eyebrows, eyelashes, beard area and body.[29] Plaques may coalesce at the eyebrow and forehead, resulting in leonine facies. Finally, patients commonly develop acneiform lesions. In general, the patches/plaques are poorly defined with prominent follicular papules and excoriations.[29] Importantly, prognosis is similar to classical tumor-stage MF; 5-year survival is 80%.[26] However, survival rates tend to drop drastically between 10 and 15 years after diagnosis.[29]

Pagetoid reticulosis and granulomatous slack skin have an excellent prognosis, with 100% 5-year survival.[26] Patients with pagetoid reticulosis tend to be young and present with a single or, less commonly, multiple, psoriasiform, verrucous or hyperkeratotic patch or plaque on an extremity. Granulomatous slack skin, an extremely rare subtype, is characterized by large indurated plaques that progress to erythematosus nodules and loss of skin elasticity with resulting exaggerated folds of lax skin in existing skin folds.

Erythrodermic MF presents with diffuse erythema and may include palms and soles (Fig. 21.6). Sézary syndrome is characterized as generalized erythroderma affecting over 80% of the body surface area, edema, and fine scale (Fig. 21.7). The erythroderma is light pink to violaceous and individual lesions are usually not seen. Palmoplantar keratoderma with

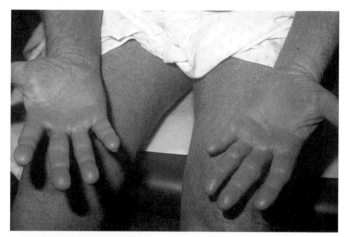

Figure 21.6 T4 erythrodermic MF: diffuse erythroderma, including hyperkeratosis of palms and soles.

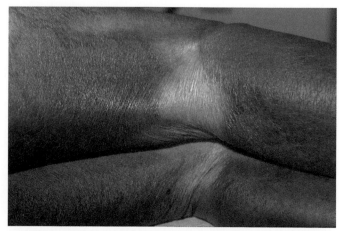

Figure 21.7 Sézary syndrome: erythroderma covering ≥ 80% of the body surface area.

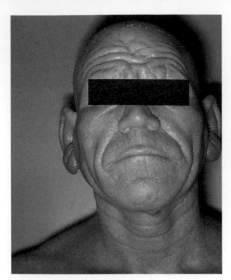

**Figure 21.8** Sézary syndrome with 'lion facies'.

hyperkeratosis and fissuring is a common manifestation of SS. Alopecia and ectropion are often observed in these patients. Extracutaneous manifestations of MF/SS include involvement of the peripheral blood, lymphoid nodes, liver, spleen, lungs, and central nervous system.

Patients with skin of color often have pigmentary changes associated with hyper-/hypopigmentation MF/SS.[30] Furthermore, pruritus may lead to secondary changes, such as lichenification and post-inflammatory hyperpigmentation. The erythroderma of SS may present on flexural surfaces as linear bands that alternate with uninvolved areas to form a 'deck chair sign' or 'folded luggage' pattern.[30] Exaggeration of normal skin folds, or a 'lion-like' facies, may develop secondary to skin infiltration, particularly of dermal adnexal structures (Fig. 21.8).

Patients with CTCL have an increased incidence of second malignancies (standardized incidence ratio [SIR] = 1.79),[31] including non-cutaneous lymphomas, lung, colon, urinary, melanoma, and biliary cancer, with no single cancer prevailing. Importantly, most patients will develop the second cancer within 25 months of CTCL diagnosis and risk decreases with time.

## DIAGNOSIS, STAGING AND PATHOLOGY

The diagnosis of MF/SS is predominantly based on history, physical examination and the histopathologic findings of a skin biopsy. Staging is based on the results of these examinations, as well as blood, lymph node and occasionally other tissue evaluations (Table 21.1). A firm diagnosis of MF/SS is often made after other diagnoses are excluded. The International Society for Cutaneous Lymphomas (ISCL) has proposed an algorithm for the diagnosis of early MF which has not yet been validated but may be useful in making a diagnosis (Table 21.2).[3]

The ISCL/EORTC revised the staging of mycosis fungoides and Sézary syndrome using the TNMB system into stages 1–4 (Table 21.3).[3] In order to accurately stage a patient with MF/SS, a thorough staging evaluation should be performed (Table 21.4). This includes history and physical examination with particular attention to morphology and extent of disease (T classification), lymphadenopathy, hepatosplenomegaly, laboratory tests (CBC, LFT, LDH), chest X-ray, and PCR or Southern blot for T-cell receptor gene rearrangement of peripheral blood or skin biopsies. If the patient is stage IIB or higher or demonstrates elevated LDH or rapidly progressive disease, then a CT scan or PET/CT scan of chest/abdomen/pelvis is appropriate.[32] If the patient has large palpable nodes of more than 1.5–2 cm in greatest dimension, lymph nodes should be biopsied. Finally, a bone marrow biopsy is not necessary unless there are significant cytopenias or other hematological complications.[33]

The majority of patients present with early MF (T1 or T2 disease).[8] The earlier classification system published in 1979 by the Mycosis Fungoides Cooperative Group was based on the TNMB system and organized into a staging system based on disease extent and survival.[34] Of note, the B (blood) classification was not included in staging. The early classification system was recently revised to reflect the advancing knowledge of the characteristics and prognosis of MF/SS, which are distinctly different from other CTCL variants.[3] The revised classification by the ISCL/EORTC maintains the earlier TNMB classification system (Table 21.1).[3]

The revised T classification has more specific descriptions of the skin lesions that reflect induration and size. The revised N (node) classification is based on excisional biopsies of clinically palpable lymph nodes only (≥1.5 cm) and, therefore, does not require unsolicited biopsies of clinically normal lymph nodes for staging purposes (Table 21.5). Additionally, palpable nodes should be examined with an imaging study to confirm appropriateness of biopsy and identify the largest peripheral node. The preference of biopsy sites, in descending order, is cervical, axillary, and inguinal. Biopsies are examined for histology, immunohistochemistry, flow cytometry, and/or molecular genetic or cytogenetic analysis. If lymph node biopsies demonstrate atypia, specifically disruption of the nodal architecture according to the NCI/VA system or Dutch system, then Southern blot or PCR analysis may be performed to detect clonality. Lymph node (LN) staging is based on the number of atypical lymphocytes and disruption of nodal architecture.

The revised M (metastasis) classification requires pathology to confirm visceral involvement. Also, the organ of metastases should be noted. The presence of lymphoma cells in the peripheral blood is now identified as an independent adverse prognostic indicator.[8] Likewise, the revised B (blood) classification uses clonal expansion of *TCR* gene rearrangement (Southern blot or PCR clonal analysis) to identify malignant cells in the peripheral blood. B2 disease is defined as those patients with a high tumor burden of Sézary cells, ≥1000/µL, in peripheral blood. If patients have B2 involvement or unexplained hematologic abnormalities, a bone marrow biopsy is recommended. Flow cytometric analysis of T-cell receptor-Vβ expression may help characterize blood involvement in the future by identifying clonality, quantifying tumor burden, and following response

**Table 21.1 ISCL/EORTC Revision to the Classification of Mycosis Fungoides and Sézary Syndrome**

| TNMB Stages | | |
|---|---|---|
| Tumor (skin) | T1 | Limited patches, papules, and/or plaques covering <10% of the skin surface. May further stratify into T1a (patch only) vs T1b (plaque ± patch) |
| | T2 | Patches, papules or plaques covering ≥10% of the skin surface. May further stratify into T2a (patch only) vs T2b (plaque ± patch) |
| | T3 | One or more tumors (≥1 cm diameter) |
| Nodes | T4 | Confluence of erythema covering ≥80% body surface area |
| | N0 | No clinically abnormal peripheral lymph nodes; biopsy not required |
| | N1 | Clinically abnormal peripheral lymph nodes; histopathology Dutch grade 1 or NCI LN 0–2 |
| | a | Clone negative* |
| | b | Clone positive* |
| | N2 | Clinically abnormal peripheral lymph nodes; histopathology Dutch grade 2 or NCI LN 3 |
| | a | Clone negative* |
| | b | Clone positive* |
| | N3 | Clinically abnormal peripheral lymph nodes; histopathology Dutch grade 3–4 or NCI LN 4; clone positive or negative |
| | Nx | Clinically abnormal peripheral lymph nodes; no histologic confirmation |
| Visceral | M0 | No visceral organ involvement |
| | M1 | Visceral involvement (must have pathology confirmation[†] and organ involved should be specified) |
| Blood | B0 | Absence of significant blood involvement: ≤5% of peripheral blood lymphocytes are atypical (Sézary) cells[‡] |
| | a | Clone negative* |
| | b | Clone positive* |
| | B1 | Low blood tumor burden: >5% of peripheral blood lymphocytes are atypical (Sézary) cells but does not meet the criteria of B2 |
| | a | Clone negative* |
| | b | Clone positive* |
| | B2 | High blood tumor burden: ≥1000/μL Sézary cells[‡] with positive clones |

* A T-cell clone is defined by PCR or Souther blot analysis of the T-cell receptor gene.

†For viscera, spleen and liver may be diagnosed by imaging criteria.

‡If Sézary cells are not able to be used to determine tumor burden for B2, then one of the following modified ISCL criteria along with a positive clonal rearrangement of the TCR may be used instead: 1. Expanded CD4+ or CD3+ cells with CD4/CD8 ratio of 10 or more, 2. Expanded CD4+ cells with abnormal immunophenotype including loss of CD7 or CD26.

(Adapted from Olsen et al.[3])

to therapy,[35] with a specificity of 100%. Presently, this approach is considered a research tool, as it is expensive and not practical since a large panel of antibodies is used for the test.

The characteristic clinical features include persistent and/or progressive patches and/or plaques in non-sun-exposed areas, of variable sizes and shapes, and poikiloderma. Biopsies should sample the oldest and newest lesions after topical treatments have been discontinued for at least 2 to 4 weeks.[28] Several histologic features have been identified as sensitive and specific markers of early MF in order to differentiate it from benign dermatoses. The most consistent finding is medium- to large-sized (7–9 μm in diameter) convoluted (cerebriform) mononuclear cells, also known as 'Sézary cells' (Fig. 21.9). Most of the atypical lymphocytes are located in the epidermis (epidermotropism), typically at the basal layer (Fig. 21.10). As expected, epidermotropism is more prominent in plaques than patches.[26] Cells organized linearly or in small clusters (Pautrier's microabscesses) in the epidermis carry sensitivity and specificity of 100% and 92.3%, respectively.[3,36] The more clinically advanced tumor stage is associated with migration of atypical cells into the dermis (Fig. 21.11). Clusters of malignant T cells in the dermis is 91.7% sensitive

### Table 21.2 Algorithm for the Diagnosis of Early Mycosis Fungoides*

| Criteria | | Scoring System |
|---|---|---|
| Clinical:<br>  – Basic<br>  – Additional | Persistent and/or progressive patches/thin plaques<br><br>1. Non-sun-exposed location<br>2. Size/shape variation<br>3. Poikiloderma | 2 points = basic criteria PLUS two additional criteria<br>1 point = basic criteria PLUS one additional criterion |
| Histopathologic:<br>  – Basic<br><br>  – Additional | Superficial lymphoid infiltrate<br><br>1. Epidermotropism without spongiosis<br>2. Lymphoid atypia[†] | 2 points = basic criteria and two additional criteria<br>1 point = basic criteria and one additional criterion |
| Molecular biological: | Clonal TCR gene rearrangement | 1 point = clonality |
| Immunopathologic: | 1. <50% CD2+, CD3+, and/or CD5+ T cells<br>2. <10% CD7+ T cells<br>3. Epidermal/dermal discordance of CD2, CD3, CD5, or CD7[‡] | 1 point = one or more criteria |

TCR, T-cell receptor.

*A total of 4 points is required for the diagnosis of mycosis fungoides based on any combination of points from the clinical, histopathologic, molecular biological, and immunopathologic criteria.

[†]Lymphoid atypia is defined as cells with enlarged hyperchromatic nuclei and irregular or cerebriform nuclear contours.

[‡]T-cell antigen deficiency confined to the epidermis.

(Adapted from Pimpinelli et al.[28])

### Table 21.3 ISCL/EORTC Revision to the Staging of Mycosis Fungoides and Sézary Syndrome

| | T | N | M | B |
|---|---|---|---|---|
| IA | 1 | 0 | 0 | 0, 1 |
| IB | 2 | 0 | 0 | 0, 1 |
| II | 1, 2 | 1, 2 | 0 | 0, 1 |
| IIB | 3 | 0–2 | 0 | 0, 1 |
| III | 4 | 0–2 | 0 | 0, 1 |
| IIIA | 4 | 0–2 | 0 | 0 |
| IIIB | 4 | 0–2 | 0 | 1 |
| IVA1 | 1–4 | 0–2 | 0 | 2 |
| IVA2 | 1–4 | 3 | 0 | 0–2 |
| IVB | 1–4 | 0–3 | 1 | 0–2 |

TNMB definitions in Table 21.1 (Adapted from Olsen et al.[3])

and 100% specific; a band-like infiltrate may also be seen in the upper dermis.

Ancillary techniques serve a valuable role in detection of early MF/SS and following response to treatment. A dominant clonal T-cell receptor gene rearrangement is often found in MF/SS specimens. PCR of frozen tissue can demonstrate a dominant clonal T-cell population based on T-cell receptor gene rearrangement.[28] Newer, more sensitive PCR techniques, such as PCR with denaturing gradient gel electrophoresis/temperature gradient gel electrophoresis/single-stranded conformational polymorphism analysis, are preferred because they improve clonal detection to a lower threshold of 1%.[28] The newest and most reliable method of T-cell clonality in the skin is capillaroscopy with Gene Scan.[37] This method allows for a precise definition of the clone by using standard BIOMED probes. Immunopathologically, there is a loss of pan-T-cell markers. The phenotype of classical MF is CD3+, CD4+, CD45RO+, and CD8−. Although not part of the diagnostic criteria, cells express CD4 and CD45RO indicating derivation from the memory T-cell population. Again, the degree of cell marker expression reflects severity of disease.[12] Pan-T-cell antigens include CD2, CD3 and CD5. Early MF may show a deficiency of T cells expressing CD2, CD3 and/or CD5 (<50%) and particularly CD7 (<10%). There may also be discordance in the expression of CD2, CD3, CD5 and CD7 in the epidermis compared to the dermis.

Folliculotropic MF pathology demonstrates folliculotropic infiltrates with atypical lymphocytes which are CD3+, CD4+, CD8− (Figs 21.12 and 21.13).[29] Five patterns are described as characteristic of FMF by Gerami and Guitart:[38] (1) basaloid folliculolymphoid hyperplasia with folliculotropism; (2) granulomatous dermatitis closely associated with destructive process of the follicular unit with evidence of folliculotropism; (3) eosinophilic folliculitis-like presentation with folliculotropism; (4) formation of dilated follicular cysts with folliculo-tropism; (5) the prototypical follicular mycosis fungoides with intact follicles with folliculotropism with or without follicular mucinosis. Specimens usually demonstrate epidermal sparing (74%) and follicular mucinosis is seen in

**Table 21.4 Recommended Evaluation/Initial Staging of the Patient with Mycosis Fungoides/Sézary Syndrome**

| | Instructions | Comments |
|---|---|---|
| Complete physical examination | 1. Identify type(s) of skin lesions | – If only patch/plaque disease or erythroderma, then estimate percentage of body surface area involved, note ulceration<br>– If tumors present, determine total number of lesions, aggregate volume, largest size lesions, and regions of body involved |
| | 2. Identify palpable lymph nodes, especially those ≥1.5 cm in largest diameter or firm, irregular, clustered, or fixed | |
| | 3. Identify organomegaly | |
| Skin biopsy | 1. Immunophenotyping to include at least the following markers: CD2, CD3, CD4, CD5, CD7, CD8, and a B-cell marker (CD20). Add CD30 if differential diagnosis includes lymphomatoid papulosis, anaplastic lymphoma, or large-cell transformation | – If only one biopsy taken, choose most indurated area |
| | 2. Evaluation for clonality of TCR gene rearrangement | |
| Blood tests | 1. CBC with manual differential, liver function tests, LDH, comprehensive chemistries | |
| | 2. TCR gene rearrangement and relatedness to any clone in skin | |
| | 3. Analysis for abnormal lymphocytes by either Sézary cell count with determination absolute number of Sézary cells and/or flow cytometry (including CD4+/CD7– or CD4+/CD26–) | |
| Radiologic tests | 1. Chest X-ray or ultrasound of the peripheral nodal groups to corroborate absence of adenopathy | – If patient with T1N0B0 stage disease who is otherwise healthy and without complaints directed to a specific organ system<br>– Selected patients with T2N0B0 disease with limited skin involvement |
| | 2. CT scan of chest, abdomen, and pelvis alone ± FDG-PET scan to evaluate potential lymphadenopathy, visceral involvement, or abnormal laboratory tests. MRI may substitute for CT scan | All other patients |
| Lymph node biopsy | 1. Excisional biopsy if node is either ≥1.5 cm in diameter and/or is firm, irregular, clustered, or fixed | |
| | 2. Site of biopsy: largest lymph node draining an involved area of the skin | – If FDG-PET scan data are available, the node with highest standardized uptake value (SUV)<br>– If multiple nodes are enlarged and otherwise equal in size or consistency, the order of preference is cervical, axillary, and inguinal areas |
| | 3. Analysis: pathologic assessment by light microscopy, flow cytometry, and TCR gene rearrangement | |

(Adapted from Olsen et al.[3])

about half of patients (51%).[29,38] A combination of patterns can be found in a single patient and/or a single biopsy specimen.

Follicular mucinosis is the accumulation of mucin around the outer root sheaths of hair follicles. It is not a reliable indicator of FMF because it can be present in benign dermatoses. Patients with benign or idiopathic follicular mucinosis (IFM) are more likely to be younger (mean age 39 years) and present with a single lesion; while lymphoma-associated follicular mucinosis (LAFM) usually presents in older patients (mean age 54 years) and with multiple lesions.[39] Histologically, the two conditions may be impossible to distinguish. Epidermal involvement is often absent in LAFM and, in general, cytological atypia is not prominent.

In contrast, histology of pagetoid reticulosis shows markedly atypical intermediate to large cells located primarily in the epidermis and arranged singly (pagetoid pattern) or in nests.[26] Immunohistochemical analysis of atypical T cells reveals they are often CD8+ and less often CD4+ or null phenotype and occasionally with CD30 expression. Pathology of granulomatous slack skin shows a granulomatous infiltrate of neoplastic T cells and loss of elastic tissue. The phenotype is consistently CD3+, CD4+, CD8–, similar to FMF.

SS was previously defined by the presence of generalized erythroderma, lymphadenopathy, and other systemic manifestations, with ≥5% Sézary cells in the peripheral blood.[40] However, reactive T cells resembling

## Table 21.5 Histopathologic Staging of Lymph Nodes in Mycosis Fungoides and Sézary Syndrome

| Updated ISCL/EORTC Classification | Dutch System | NCI-VA Classification[85] |
|---|---|---|
| N1 | Grade 1: dermatopathic lymphadenopathy (DL) | LN0: no atypical lymphocytes |
| | | LN1: occasional and isolated atypical lymphocytes (not arranged in clusters) |
| | | LN2: many atypical lymphocytes or in 3–6 cell clusters |
| N2 | Grade 2: DL; early involvement by MF (presence of cerebriform nuclei >7.5 μm) | LN3: aggregates of atypical lymphocytes; nodal architecture preserved |
| N3 | Grade 3: partial effacement of LN architecture; many atypical cerebriform mononuclear cells (CMCs) | LN4: partial/complete effacement of nodal architecture by atypical lymphocytes or frankly neoplastic cells |
| | Grade 4: complete effacement | |

(Adapted from Olsen et al.[3])

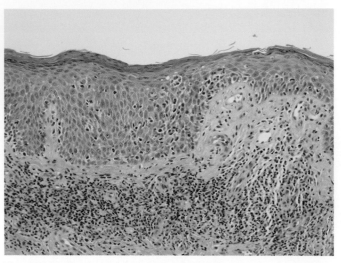

**Figure 21.10** Histology of patch/plaque-stage MF with a superficial dermal infiltrate and multiple atypical cells in epidermis.

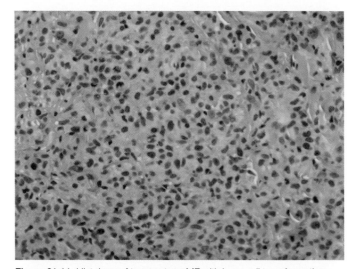

**Figure 21.11** Histology of tumor-stage MF with large cell transformation.

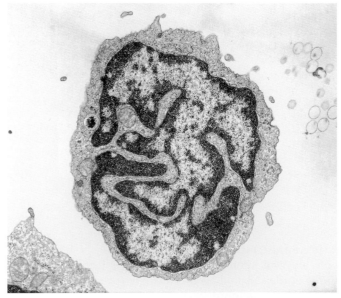

**Figure 21.9** Sézary cell. This electron micrograph of the Sézary cell shows the convoluted nuclei, also known as 'cerebriform'. (Image courtesy of Dr. Dorothea Zucker-Franklin, New York University Medical Center.)

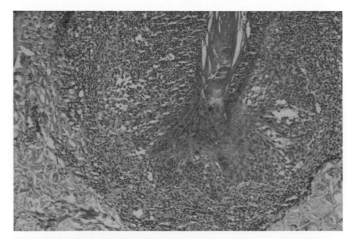

**Figure 21.12** Folliculotropic MF: histology, transverse section showing folliculotropism with multiple atypical lymphocytes.

Sézary cells are often identified, especially in patients with extensive inflammatory dermatosis or erythroderma and rarely in healthy individuals.[41] Recent revisions in classification emphasize cell markers by flow cytometry for diagnosis.[3]

Patients with SS who present without a previous diagnosis of MF are considered to have primary SS and demonstrate unique histologic and immunologic cell markers compared to secondary SS.[42] The majority (71%) of skin biopsies from patients with primary SS demonstrate a

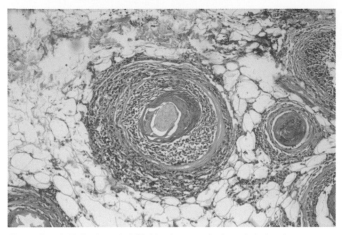

**Figure 21.13** Folliculotropic MF: histology, vertical section showing folliculotropism with multiple atypical lymphocytes.

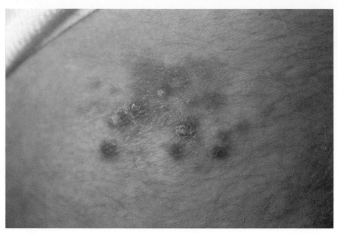

**Figure 21.15** Lymphomatoid papulosis (LyP).

perivascular dermal lymphoid infiltrate. The CD7 cell marker is often decreased in skin and blood samples. Epidermotropism of atypical lymphocytes, a feature of classic MF, is present in a minority of biopsies (39%). Both primary and secondary SS may show peripheral eosinophilia. Flow cytometry of peripheral blood in patients with SS usually detects a population of aberrant cells with CD3+, CD4+, CD7−, CD26− phenotype.

MF is often diagnosed after treatment for more common diseases has failed. Early MF can be similar in presentation to large plaque parapsoriasis, chronic eczema, poikiloderma atrophicans vasculare, drug eruptions, psoriasis, lichen planus, pityriasis lichenoides, and other dermatoses. The differential diagnosis in skin of color includes lichen planus pigmentosus inversus, inflammatory vitiligo, progressive macular hypomelanosis, digitate dermatosis, pityriasis lichenoides chronica, actinic reticuloid, and sarcoidosis.[30]

CTCL variants are also in the differential diagnosis of MF/SS, including lymphomatoid papulosis, subcutaneous panniculitis-like T-cell lymphoma, and adult T-cell leukemia/lymphoma (ATLL). Like MF, the variants follow indolent courses (except for ATLL). Lymphomatoid papulosis (LyP) is a CTCL variant under the subtype of primary cutaneous CD30+ lymphoproliferative disorders, which also includes primary cutaneous anaplastic large cell lymphoma (C-ALCL) (Fig. 21.14). LyP is characterized by recurrent eruption of papules and nodules that resolve spontane-

ously with hemorrhagic necrotic features on biopsy, often leaving hyperpigmentation and pox-like scars (Fig. 21.15). LyP and C-ALCL represent a spectrum of the same disease, in which LyP follows an indolent course with 100% survival at 5 years.[26] Importantly, patients with LyP have a 10–20% risk for developing a second malignant cutaneous lymphoma, most commonly MF, C-ALCL, or Hodgkin lymphoma. Lesions of C-ALCL do not spontaneously regress but are associated with a 95% 5-year survival.

Subcutaneous panniculitis-like T-cell lymphoma (SPTL) is characterized by atypical cells in the subcutaneous tissue, especially the lower extremities, and a relative sparing of the dermis and epidermis.[26] SPTL is associated with an 82% 5-year survival rate. An important complication is hemophagocytic syndrome, which carries a poor prognosis, particularly in women.

Adult T-cell leukemia/lymphoma is associated with human T-cell leukemia virus 1 (HTLV-1); likewise, it is found most commonly in areas where HTLV-1 is endemic, such as Japan and the Caribbean. The disease is usually disseminated and atypical cells in the periphery have 'floral' or 'clover leaf' nuclei. Cutaneous lesions are present in about 50% of patients and are usually nodules and tumors, with papules and plaques being less common.[26] The phenotype of malignant cells in ATLL corresponds to T regulatory cells with high CD25 and FOX-P3 expression.[43] Extracutaneous manifestations include hypercalcemia, bone lesions, lymphadenopathy, splenomegaly, pulmonary infiltrates, and opportunistic infections. Unlike other CTCL variants, ATLL has a poor prognosis with most patients with acute phase disease surviving 2 weeks to 1 year.

## PROGNOSIS

Patients with MF/SS have a decreased overall survival compared with age-, sex-, and race-matched controls. Exceptions include patients with T1 or stage IA disease, who have survival similar to the normal population.[8,44] More advanced disease is associated with increased likelihood of disease progression and worsened survival; however, even patients with stage 1B and 2A disease had a relatively good prognosis, with only 21% of patients advancing to higher stages.[8] Independent predictors of survival include age at presentation (increased age associated with worse prognosis),

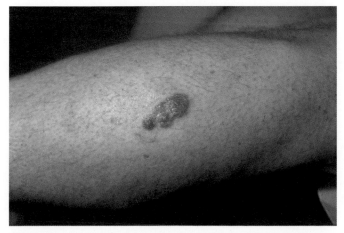

**Figure 21.14** Nodule of primary cutaneous CD30+ T-cell lymphoma on leg.

T classification, and presence or absence of extracutaneous (stage IV) disease.

Published estimates of survival must be interpreted with caution as the classification system was recently updated. In 2003, patients with MF had a relative risk for death of 2.4 when compared to the general population.[8] Specifically, the relative risk for death was 2.2 in stage IB/IIA, 3.9 in stage IIB/III, and 12.8 in stage IV. Patients with T2, T3 and T4 disease had a median survival of 12.1, 3.3, and 4.0 years, respectively. Patients with erythrodermic CTCL, which includes primary and secondary SS, advanced age and elevated lactate dehydrogenase (LDH) demonstrated the strongest association with a poor prognosis.[45] Other significant predictors of poor prognosis were white blood cell count ≥20,000 and treatment with systemic steroids.

## TREATMENT

While the goal of treating malignancies is complete remission and eradication of malignant clone, patients with MF/SS rarely achieve this endpoint. Nevertheless, early-stage disease can be controlled with skin-directed therapies, achieving prolonged remissions. Patients with advanced or recalcitrant disease often require the addition of systemic therapies. A list of treatments is outlined in Table 21.6.

## Topical therapy

Like for psoriasis and eczema, MF/SS treatment should include skin protection and moisturizers, as patients often have significant xerosis and erythema. Several skin-directed therapies can be used for MF/SS, including topical

### Table 21.6 List of Treatments Ordered from Least Toxic to Most Toxic

| | Treatment | Comments |
|---|---|---|
| Topical: | Corticosteroids | High-potency, class I, for patch disease |
| | Antibiotics | In cases of erythrodermic patients with *S. aureus* colonization |
| | Bexarotene gel 1% | Only topical with FDA approval for MF |
| | Phototherapy: PUVA BB UVB NB UVB UVA-1 308-xenon chloride laser | SE: erythema, pigmentation (especially BB UVB) PUVA is more effective for thicker lesions than UVB |
| | Total skin electron beam (TSEB) | SE: *acute* – erythema, dry desquamation; *chronic* – permanent alopecia (dose-dependent); *other* – radiation-induced secondary cutaneous malignancies, loss of fingernails and toenails, telangiectasias, pigmentation, pruritus, anhidrosis |
| | Mechlorethamine (nitrogen mustard) | SE: aqueous form associated with contact dermatitis, ointment and gel forms less irritating |
| | Carmustine (BCNU) | SE: bone marrow suppression is rare |
| Systemic: | IFN-alpha (monotherapy or combined with PUVA) | SE: fever, fatigue, decreased white count, anemia, hepatitis |
| | Bexarotene (oral) | Retinoid Response dose-dependent and limited by SE SE: hypertriglyceridemia, central hypothyroidism |
| | Extracorporeal photopheresis (ECP) | Usually well tolerated |
| | Methotrexate (MTX) | Particularly helpful for lymphomatoid papulosis |
| | Denileukin diftitox (IV) | SE: vascular leak syndrome (temporize with pretreatment hydration, corticosteroids) |
| | Vorinostat | HDAC inhibitor |
| | Alemtuzumab | SE: opportunistic infection, neutropenia, cardiotoxicity |
| | Gemcitabine | SE: myelosuppression |
| | Doxorubicin (pegylated, liposomal) | Avoids cardiotoxicity and nephrotoxicity of conventional doxorubicin |
| | Stem cell transplant | Allogeneic versus autologous Combine allogeneic with low-dose non-myeloablative chemotherapy for graft-versus-tumor effect SE: GVHD and death (allogeneic) |

SE, side effect; BB UVB, broadband ultraviolet B light; NB UVB, narrowband UVB; IV, intravenous; GVHD, graft-versus-host disease.

corticosteroids, topical retinoid (bexarotene gel), topical nitrogen mustard, topical carmustine (BCNU), psoralen and ultraviolet A light (PUVA), ultraviolet B light (UVB) and total skin electron beam therapy (TSEB). Considering the delayed diagnosis of MF/SS, lesions are frequently treated with topical corticosteroids before clinical confirmation of MF/SS. However, topical corticosteroids, particularly high-potency class I formulations, may be effective in patients with patch-stage disease.[7] Side effects include reversible depression of cortisol levels (13%).

MF/SS may respond to antibiotics, particularly in patients with erythroderma and *S. aureus* colonization on the skin and nares.[16] Eradication of colonization with antibiotics for 4–8 weeks in erythrodermic patients is associated with clinical improvement in 58%.

The only topical therapy with FDA approval for MF is 1% bexarotene gel, a topical retinoid. Bexarotene produces a 76% response rate when used to treat CTCL.[46] However, the complete response rate is low and a common side effect is severe skin irritation.

Topical mechlorethamine (nitrogen mustard) is used as an aqueous solution, gel or ointment, and must be compounded. In patients with clinical stage I–III, overall response rate is reported to be 83% and complete response 50%.[47] Complete response rates are greater in earlier stages of disease. Up to 40% of patients receiving the aqueous form develop contact dermatitis (irritant or hypersensitivity), and mechlorethamine is occasionally associated with squamous cell carcinoma when patients have been previously treated with phototherapy. With a recent increase in the price of mustargen, this option is not cost-effective and rarely selected presently. The ointment form is less frequently associated with contact hypersensitivity while still giving similar efficacy.[47,48] Hypersensitivity can be tempered with desensitization. Topical carmustine (BCNU) uncommonly causes contact hypersensitivity and is useful for patients unable to tolerate mechlorethamine; however, carmustine can cause bone marrow suppression (30%).[49]

Phototherapy for MF/SS includes PUVA, broadband (BB) UVB (290–320nm), narrowband (NB) UVB (311–313nm), and UVA-1.[50] A higher complete response is achieved when phototherapy is given to patients with early MF/SS (Fig. 21.16). Phototherapy is usually administered three times per week. Overall complete response to PUVA is 65% in stage IA, IB, and IIA.[51] BB UVB achieves a complete response in 89% and 44% of stage IA and IB MF cases, respectively. NB UVB is predominantly effective in early patch disease and less effective in thin plaque MF.[50,52,53] The majority of patients demonstrate complete response after 20–37 treatments. The effectiveness of NB UVB in patch lesions is similar to that of PUVA but it induces less erythema and pigmentation than BB UVB.[54,55] Patients with plaques and follicular MF benefit more from PUVA. The complete response, partial response, and failure rates of NB UVB are reported as 68%, 26%, and 5%, respectively, when used to treat early-stage MF, and the time to relapse is comparable to that with PUVA. When compared to BB UVB, NB UVB has greater complete response rates in more advanced disease (78% vs 44% in stage IB MF treated with NB and BB, respectively) and a lower relapse rate.[56] Maintenance NB UVB is recommended for 18 months to prevent relapse after complete response.[53] UVA-1 has deeper penetration of the skin, but the therapeutic effects of UVA-1 in MF/SS are not well known. The 308-nm xenon chloride laser is also effective in stage 1A or 1B CTCL that is refractory to topical steroids.[57] Of note, patients with skin of color are more difficult to treat with phototherapy due to increased photoprotection.[30]

MF/SS is extremely radiosensitive. Local and total skin electron beam therapy (TSEB) has been used for several decades and is particularly effective in the treatment of thick plaques and advanced disease. The rate of complete response with TSEB is better in early disease but it is frequently reserved for more advanced disease.[58] TSEB is more effective than topical mechlorethamine in late disease in the absence of systemic involvement, including those with

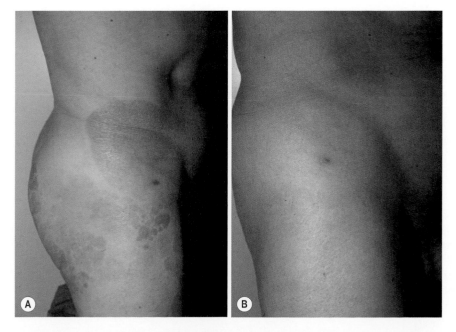

**Figure 21.16** Plaque-stage MF before **(A)** and after **(B)** treatment with PUVA.

lymphadenopathy.[59] Patients who have a complete response to treatment experience a longer freedom from relapse when given adjuvant mechlorethamine.[60] Erythrodermic MF/SS responds to TSEB with a 3-year disease-free survival of 49%, which increases to 81% when TSEB is combined with extracorporeal photopheresis (ECP).[61] The most common acute complications are erythema and dry desquamation. Most patients experience some degree of permanent alopecia but severity is dose dependent. Other side effects include radiation-induced secondary cutaneous malignancies, loss of fingernails and toenails, telangiectasia, pigmentation, pruritus, and anhidrosis.

## Systemic therapy

Traditional systemic therapies for MF/SS include interferon (IFN)-alpha and retinoids (acitretin and isotretinoin). Response (complete or partial) to IFN-alpha as monotherapy is 87.5%, 77.5%, and 25% in stage I, II, and III–IV, respectively, and is most likely in the first 6 months.[62] Regardless of stage of disease, relapse is common (57%). A randomized controlled trial compared the efficacy of IFN-alpha plus acitretin to IFN-alpha plus PUVA. Patients included in the study were diagnosed with stage I/II disease and complete response rates were significantly better for PUVA/IFN-alpha (70%) than for IFN-alpha/acitretin (38%).[63] Side effects of IFN-alpha include fever, fatigue, decreased white count, anemia, and hepatitis.

Oral bexarotene (Targretin), an RXR retinoid analog, is appropriate for patients with relapsed or refractory CTCL, including the erythrodermic subtype. Sixty-six patients with stage I–IV MF/SS were treated with bexarotene and 33% demonstrated a response by 8 weeks (only two patients had complete response).[64] The response is dose dependent and limited by the side effects, especially hypertriglyceridemia. Patients receiving bexarotene must be monitored for the dose-related side effects of hypertriglyceridemia, hyperlipidemia, and hypothyroidism.

Extracorporeal photopheresis (ECP) is a unique mode of therapy that exposes peripheral mononuclear cells to 8-MOP and then UVA irradiation after they have been collected from the patient. Blood is removed from the patient, and separated by centrifugation into cellular and plasma components. The peripheral mononuclear cells are exposed to 8-MOP and UVA radiation, then reinfused.[65] ECP allows the use of irradiation towards the malignant lymphocytes without the risks of skin exposure. ECP is usually reserved for severe, erythrodermic MF/SS with blood involvement.[61,66,67] More specifically, patients expected to experience the best response to ECP have the following characteristics: erythrodermic skin stage (especially primary erythroderma), WBC counts less than 25,000/mm³, disease of short duration, normal percentage of CD8 cells (>15% of total lymphocytes), immunocompetence, absence of bulky lymph nodes or overt visceral disease, the presence of circulating CD4⁺/CD7⁻ lymphocytes <6000/mm³, a CD4⁺/CD8⁺ ratio of <10 in skin and blood, and the presence of circulating Sézary cells.[67] As a monotherapy, ECP demonstrates a 72% overall response rate and a 25% complete response rate.[68] Disease responsiveness improves when ECP is combined with biological modifiers, such as IFN-gamma and retinoids.[69]

Intravenous denileukin diftitox (Ontak), a high-affinity IL-2 receptor fusion protein, and vorinostat, a histone deacetylase (HDAC)-inhibitor, are FDA-approved biologic agents for treatment of CTCL. Denileukin diftitox, composed of IL-2 plus diphtheria toxin, is effective in advanced stages of MF/SS and has a 30% response rate.[70] The IL-2 binds with the IL-2 receptor on malignant cells, becomes internalized, and inhibits protein synthesis due to the toxin.[71] Twenty-five percent of patients experience vascular leak syndrome, which can be life-threatening and is defined as the simultaneous occurrence of two or more of the following: hypotension, edema, and hypoalbuminemia.[70] This side effect can be temporized with pretreatment hydration and corticosteroids.

The HDAC inhibitor (HDAC-I) vorinostat is the most recent advancement in MF/SS treatment and is appropriate in patients who have failed prior therapies.[72] HDAC-I permits normal DNA transcription by blocking HDAC enzymes, which are often overexpressed in cancer cells and facilitate the silencing of normal gene transcription by causing chromatin to compact.[72,73] Results of clinical studies in patients with advanced disease showed a response in over 30% of cases and 30% of patients experiencing pruritus relief.[74] Many other HDAC-Is are becoming available, including romidepsin.

The immunotherapeutic agent alemtuzumab is a humanized recombinant IgG monoclonal antibody that targets the CD52 cell surface glycoprotein on the surface of T cells, normal and malignant; therefore, patients are at risk of opportunistic infection, neutropenia, and cardiotoxicity. Alemtuzumab (30 mg per infusion, three times per week for 12 weeks) has a partial response rate of 38% when used to treat patients with stage IIB–IVB MF/SS but a similar percentage of patients experience progressive disease.[75] Patients tend to relapse within 4 months. Median disease-free survival is 6 months.[76] Alemtuzumab is particularly useful to treat erythrodermic MF and SS. The majority (84%) of patients respond (partial or complete) when administered the standard regimen.[76] This drug provides rapid symptom relief in most patients with severe pruritus associated with erythroderma.

## Other therapy

Management of advanced-stage or refractory CTCL is challenging, as MF and SS are relatively chemoresistant conditions. TSEB combined with parenteral chemotherapy (cyclophosphamide, doxorubicin, etoposide, and vincristine), for example, leads to a higher rate of complete response compared with TSEB only, but does not improve disease-free or overall survival.[58] Other single-agent regimens that produce clinical responses in advanced MF/SS are methotrexate (high dose, 25–50 mg/week) and gemcitabine.[77,78] Gemcitabine provides an overall response rate of 68%, with 8% complete response.[79] Gemcitabine is generally well tolerated, with myelosuppression as the most significant side effect. Pegylated and liposomal doxorubicin is also highly effective, with a response rate of over 80% and without the cardiotoxicity or nephrotoxicity of conventional doxorubicin.[80,81]

Refractory, progressive MF/SS can be treated with stem cell transplant (SCT). A meta-analysis of allogeneic versus autologous hematopoietic stem cell transplant in patients with MF/SS suggests that allogeneic SCT leads to significantly increased survival and, importantly, a significantly greater event-free survival compared to autologous SCT.[82] Overall survival rates at 1 and 5 years are 85% and 80%, respectively, for patients receiving allogeneic SCT, and 68% and 23%, respectively, for patients receiving autologous SCT. Graft-versus-host disease (GVHD) occurs in the majority of patients (90%) receiving allogeneic SCT, but death is rare. GVHD does not occur in those receiving autologous SCT. The new approach to allogeneic SCT is with low nonmyeloablative chemotherapy conditioning relying on the graft to clear the malignancy. It has been shown that the main benefit of this treatment modality is the graft-versus-tumor effect.[83]

## Integrated therapeutic approach

Based on the literature and clinical experience, the following recommendations can be made:

Patients with stage IA, chronic, or slowly growing disease can be managed initially with potent topical steroids, nitrogen mustard, bexarotene gel, or NB UVB. Patients with extensive skin involvement (IB, IIA) will benefit from total skin-directed therapy like NB UVB (thin lesions) or PUVA (thick lesions and FMF). In general, add low-dose retinoids, especially when using PUVA therapy. This combination expedites the treatment course and may provide a photo-chemopreventive effect.[84] Resistant cases should be treated with oral bexarotene, PUVA plus IFN, PUVA plus oral bexarotene, or total skin electron beam radiation plus nitrogen mustard. Rapidly progressive or advanced disease should be initially approached with single-agent chemotherapy, denileukin diftitox, multi-agent chemotherapy, photopheresis, or bone marrow transplantation.

## FUTURE OUTLOOK

Although much progress has been made in the diagnosis and treatment of CTCL, there needs to be a better overall knowledge of this disease. Future epidemiologic and laboratory studies will help to understand the etiology of the disease. Quality-of-life and economic impact studies are needed to determine the overall effect of CTCL on patients. Diagnosis of early disease and variants is still difficult in many cases and should be further refined with validation of diagnostic protocols. As therapies for CTCL are associated with significant side effects and cost, larger randomized, controlled trials and meta-analyses will be needed to determine the best treatment options for early, moderate, and advanced disease.

## REFERENCES

1. Criscione VD, Weinstock MA. Incidence of cutaneous T-cell lymphoma in the United States, 1973-2002. *Arch Dermatol*. 2007;143(7):854–859.
2. Bradford PT, Devesa SS, Anderson WF, et al. Cutaneous lymphoma incidence patterns in the United States: a population-based study of 3884 cases. *Blood*. 2009;113:5064–5073.
3. Olsen E, Vonderheid E, Pimpinelli N, et al. Revisions to the staging and classification of mycosis fungoides and Sézary syndrome: a proposal of the International Society for Cutaneous Lymphomas (ISCL) and the cutaneous lymphoma task force of the European Organization of Research and Treatment of Cancer (EORTC). *Blood*. 2007;110:1713–1722.
4. Van Doorn R, can Kester MS, Dijkman R, et al. Oncogenomic analysis of mycosis fungoides reveals major differences with Sézary syndrome. *Blood*. 2009;113:127–136.
5. Alibert JLM. *Tableau de plan fongoide: Description des maladies de la peau observe a l'hopital St. Louis et exposition des meilleures methodes suivies pour leur traitement*. Paris, France: Barior l'Aine et Files; 1806.
6. Van Doorn R, van Hasele CW, van Voorst PC, et al. Mycosis fungoides: disease evolution and prognosis of 309 Dutch patients. *Arch Dermatol*. 2000;136:504–510.
7. Zackheim HS, Amin S, Kashani-Sabet M, et al. Prognosis in cutaneous T-cell lymphoma by skin stage: long-term survival in 489 patients. *J Am Acad Dermatol*. 1999;40:418–425.
8. Kim YH, Liu HL, Mraz-Gernhard S, et al. Long-term outcome of 525 patients with mycosis fungoides and Sézary syndrome: clinical prognostic factors and risk for disease progression. *Arch Dermatol*. 2003;139:857–866.
9. Tuyp E, Burgoyne A, Aitchison T, et al. A case-control study of possible causative factors in mycosis fungoides. *Arch Dermatol*. 1987;123:196–200.
10. Kamarashev J, Burg G, Kempf W, et al. Comparative analysis of histological and immunohistological features in mycosis fungoides and Sézary syndrome. *J Cutan Pathol*. 1998;25:407–412.
11. Kim EJ, Hess S, Richardson SK, et al. Immunopathogenesis and therapy of cutaneous T cell lymphoma. *J Clin Invest*. 2005;115(4):798–812.
12. Kallinich T, Muche JM, Qin S. Chemokine receptor expression on neoplastic and reactive T cells in the skin at different stages of mycosis fungoides. *J Invest Dermatol*. 2003;121(5):1045–1052.
13. Berger CL, Hanlon D, Kanada D, et al. The growth of cutaneous T-cell lymphoma is stimulated by immature dendritic cells. *Blood*. 2002;99(8):2929–2939.
14. Jackow CM, Cather JC, Hearne V, et al. Association of erythrodermic cutaneous T-cell lymphoma, superantigen-positive *Staphylococcus aureus*, and oligoclonal T-cell receptor V beta gene expression. *Blood*. 1997;89:32–40.
15. Abrams JT, Balin BJ, Vonderheid EC. Association between Sézary T cell-activating factor, *Chlamydia pneumoniae*, and cutaneous T cell lymphoma. *Ann N Y Acad Sci*. 2001;941:69–85.
16. Talpur R, Bassett R, Duvic M. Prevalence and treatment of Staphylococcus aureus colonization in patients with mycosis fungoides and Sézary syndrome. *Br J Dermatol*. 2008;159(1):105–112.
17. Zucker-Franklin D, Pancake BA. The role of human T-cell lymphocytic viruses (HTLV-I and II) in cutaneous T-cell lymphomas. *Semin Dermatol*. 1994;13:160–165.
18. Wood GS, Salvekar A, Schaffer J, et al. Evidence against a role for human T-cell lymphotrophic virus type I (HTLV-1) in the pathogenesis of American cutaneous T-cell lymphoma. *J Invest Dermatol*. 1996;107:301–317.
19. Bazarbachi A, Soriano V, Pawson R, et al. Mycosis fungoides and Sézary syndrome are not associated with HTLV-I infection: an international study. *Br J Haematol*. 1997;98:927–933.
20. Herne KL, Talpur R, Breuer-McHam J, et al. Cytomegalovirus seropositivity is significantly associated with mycosis fungoides and Sézary syndrome. *Blood*. 2003;101:2132–2136.
21. Chang YT, Liu HN, Chen CL, et al. Detection of Epstein-Barr virus and HTLV-1 in T-cell lymphomas of skin in Taiwan. *Am J Dermatopathol*. 1998;20:250–254.
22. Jackow CM, McHam JB, Friss A, et al. HLA-DR5 and DQB1*03 class II alleles are associated with cutaneous T-cell lymphoma. *J Invest Dermatol*. 1996;107(3):373–376.
23. Zoi-Toli O, Vermeer MH, De Vries E, et al. Expression of Fas and Fas-ligand in primary cutaneous T-cell lymphoma (CTCL): association between lack of Fas expression and aggressive types of CTCL. *Br J Dermatol*. 2000;143(2):313–319.
24. Dereure O, Portales P, Clot J, et al. Decreased expression of Fas (APO-1/CD95) on peripheral blood CD4+ T lymphocytes in cutaneous T-cell lymphomas. *Br J Dermatol*. 2000;143(6):1205–1210.
25. Mao X, Lillingto D, Scarisbrick JJ, et al. Molecular cytogenetic analysis of cutaneous T-cell lymphomas: identification of common genetic alterations in Sézary syndrome and mycosis fungoides. *Br J Dermatol*. 2002;147:464–475.
26. Willemze R, Jaffe ES, Burg G, et al. WHO-EORTC classification for cutaneous lymphomas. *Blood*. 2005;105:3768–3785.
27. Kim ST, Jeon YS, Sim HJ, et al. Clinicopathologic features and T-cell receptor gene rearrangement findings of mycosis fungoides palmaris et plantaris. *J Am Acad Dermatol*. 2006;54(3):466–471.
28. Pimpinelli N, Olsen EA, Santucci M, et al. Defining early mycosis fungoides. *J Am Acad Dermatol*. 2005;53:1053–1063.
29. Gerami P, Rosen S, Kuzel T, et al. Folliculotropic mycosis fungoides: an aggressive variant of cutaneous T-cell lymphoma. *Arch Dermatol*. 2008;144(6):738–746.
30. Hinds GA, Heald P. Cutaneous T-cell lymphoma in skin of color. *J Am Acad Dermatol*. 2009;60:359–375.
31. Brownell I, Etzel CJ, Yang DJ, et al. Increased malignancy risk in the cutaneous T-cell lymphoma patient population. *Clin Lymphoma Myeloma*. 2008;8(2):100–105.
32. Tsai EY, Taur A, Espinosa L, et al. Staging accuracy in mycosis fungoides and Sézary syndrome using integrated positron

emission tomography and computed tomography. *Arch Dermatol.* 2006;142(5):577–584.

33. Beylot-Barry M, Parrens M, Delaunay M, et al. Is bone marrow biopsy necessary in patients with mycosis fungoides and Sézary syndrome? A histological and molecular study at diagnosis and during follow-up. *Br J Dermatol.* 2005;152(6):1378–1379.

34. Bunn PA, Lamberg SI. Report of the committee on staging and classification of cutaneous T-cell lymphomas. *Cancer Treat Rep.* 1979;63:725–728.

35. Feng B, Jorgensen JL, Jones D, et al. Flow cytometric detection of peripheral blood involvement by mycosis fungoides and Sézary syndrome using T-cell receptor Vβ chain antibodies and its application in blood staging. *Mod Pathol.* 2010;23(2):284–295.

36. Santucci M, Biggeri A, Feller AC, et al. Efficacy of histologic criteria for diagnosing early mycosis fungoides: an EORTC cutaneous lymphoma study group investigation. *Am J Surg Pathol.* 2000;24:40–50.

37. Shaheen D, Elkader AA, Marouf S, et al. Molecular immunoglobulin/T-cell receptor clonality diagnosis by gene scan in lymphoproliferative disorder. *Hematology.* 2006;11(2):77–86.

38. Gerami R, Guitart J. The spectrum of histopathologic and immunohistochemical findings in folliculotropic mycosis fungoides. *Am J Surg Pathol.* 2007;31(9):1430–1438.

39. Rongioletti F, De Lucchi S, Meyes D, et al. Follicular mucinosis: a clinicopathologic, histochemical, immunohistochemical and molecular study comparing the primary benign form and the mycosis fungoides-associated follicular mucinosis. *J Cutan Pathol.* 2009;37(1):15–19.

40. Hwang ST, Janik JE, Jaffe ES, et al. Mycosis fungoides and Sézary syndrome. *Lancet.* 2008;371:945–957.

41. Meijer C. J. L. M., van Leeuwen A. W. F. M., van der Loo EM, et al. Cerebriform (Sézary like) mononuclear cells in healthy individuals: a morphologically distinct population of T cells: relationship with mycosis fungoides and Sézary Syndrome. *Virchows Arch.* 1977;25:95–104.

42. Diwan AH, Prieto VG, Herling M, et al. Primary Sézary syndrome commonly shows low-grade cytologic atypia and an absence of epidermotropism. *Am J Clin Pathol.* 2005;123:510–515.

43. Walsh PT, Benoit BM, Wysocka M, et al. A role for regulatory T cells in cutaneous T-cell lymphoma; induction of a CD4+ CD25+ Foxp3+ T-cell phenotype associated with HTLV-1 infection. *J Invest Dermatol.* 2006;126(3):690–692.

44. Kim YH, Jensen RA, Watanabe GL, et al. Clinical stage IA (limited patch and plaque) mycosis fungoides. *Arch Dermatol.* 1996;132:1309–1313.

45. Vidulich KA, Talpur R, Bassett RL, et al. Overall survival in erythrodermic cutaneous T-cell lymphoma: an analysis of prognostic factors in a cohort of patients with erythrodermic cutaneous T-cell lymphoma. *Int J Dermatol.* 2009;48:243–252.

46. Breneman D, Duvic M, Kuzel T, et al. Phase 1 and 2 trial of bexarotene gel for skin-directed treatment of patients with cutaneous T-cell lymphoma. *Arch Dermatol.* 2002;60:5165–5170.

47. Kim YH, Martinez G, Varghese A, et al. Topical nitrogen mustard in the management of mycosis fungoides: an update of the Stanford experience. *Arch Dermatol.* 2003;139(2):165–173.

48. Whittaker SJ, Foss FM. Efficacy and tolerability of currently available therapies for the mycosis fungoides and Sézary syndrome variants of cutaneous T-cell lymphoma. *Cancer Treat Rev.* 2007;33:146–160.

49. Zackheim HS, Epstein EH, Crain WR. Topical carmustine (BCNU) for cutaneous T cell lymphoma: a 15-year experience in 143 patients. *J Am Acad Dermatol.* 1990;22:801–810.

50. Carter J, Zug KA. Phototherapy for cutaneous T-cell lymphoma: online survey and literature review. *J Am Acad Dermatol.* 2009;60:39–50.

51. Herrmann JJ, Roenigk HH, Hurria A, et al. Treatment of mycosis fungoides with photochemotherapy (PUVA): long-term follow-up. *J Am Acad Dermatol.* 1995;33:234–242.

52. Clark C, Dawe RS, Evans AT, et al. Narrowband TL-01 phototherapy for patch-stage mycosis fungoides. *Arch Dermatol.* 2000;136:748–752.

53. Boztepe G, Sahin S, Ayhan M, et al. Narrowband ultraviolet B phototherapy to clear and maintain clearance in patients with mycosis fungoides. *J Am Acad Dermatol.* 2005;53:242–246.

54. Ponte P, Serrao V, Apetato M. Efficacy of narrowband UVB vs. PUVA in patients with early-stage mycosis fungoides. *J Eur Acad Dermatol Venereol.* 2010;24(6):716–21.

55. Suh KS, Roh HJ, Choi SY, et al. Long-term evaluation of erythema and pigmentation induced by ultraviolet radiations of different wavelengths. *Skin Res Technol.* 2007;13:154–161.

56. Pavlotsky F, Barzilai A, Kasem R. UVB in the management of early stage mycosis fungoides. *J Eur Acad Dermatol Venereol.* 2006;20:565–672.

57. Upjohn E, Foley P, Lane P, et al. Long-term clearance of patch-stage mycosis fungoides with the 308-nm laser. *Clin Exp Dermatol.* 2007;32(2):168–171.

58. Kaye FJ, Bunn Jr PA, Steinber SM, et al. A randomized trial comparing combination electron-beam radiation and chemotherapy with topical therapy in the initial treatment of mycosis fungoides. *N Engl J Med.* 1989;321(26):1784–1790.

59. Hamminga B, Noordijk EM, can Cloten WA. Treatment of mycosis fungoides: total-skin electron-beam irradiation vs. topical mechlorethamine therapy. *Arch Dermatol.* 1982;11:150–153.

60. Chinn DM, Chow S, Kim YH, et al. Total skin electron beam therapy with or without adjuvant topical nitrogen mustard or nitrogen mustard alone as initial treatment of T2 and T3 mycosis fungoides. *Int J Radiat Oncol Biol Phys.* 1999;43(5):951.

61. McKenna KE, Whittaker S, Rhodes LE, et al. Evidence-based practice of photopheresis 1987-2001: a report of a workshop of the British Photodermatology Group and the U.K. Skin Lymphoma Group. *Br J Dermatol.* 2006;154:7–20.

62. Jumbou O, Nguyen JM, Tessier MH, et al. Long-term follow-up in 51 patients with mycosis fungoides and Sézary syndrome treated by interferon-alfa. *Br J Dermatol.* 1999;140:427–431.

63. Stadler R, Otte HG, Luger T, et al. Prospective randomized multicenter clinical trial on the use of interferon-2a plus acitretin versus interferon-2a plus PUVA in patients with cutaneous T-cell lymphoma stages I and II. *Blood.* 1998;92:3578–3581.

64. Abbott RA, Whittaker SJ, Morris SL. Bexarotene therapy for mycosis fungoides and Sézary syndrome. *Br J Dermatol.* 2009;160:1299–1307.

65. Knobler R, Barr ML, Couriel DR, et al. Extracorporeal photopheresis: past, present, and future. *J Am Acad Dermatol.* 2009;61:652–665.

66. Edelson R, Berger C, Gasparro F, et al. Treatment of cutaneous T-cell lymphoma by extracorporeal photochemotherapy. Preliminary results. *N Engl J Med.* 1987;316:297–303.

67. Zic JA. The treatment of cutaneous T-cell lymphoma with photopheresis. *Dermatol Ther.* 2003;16:337–346.

68. Gottlieb SL, Wolfe JT, Fox FE, et al. Treatment of cutaneous T-cell lymphoma with extracorporeal photopheresis monotherapy and in combination with recombinant interferon alfa: a 10-year experience at a single institution. *J Am Acad Dermatol.* 1996;35:946–957.

69. McGinnis KS, Ubriani R, Newton S, et al. The addition of interferon gamma to oral bexarotene therapy with photopheresis for Sézary syndrome. *Arch Dermatol.* 2005;141:1176–1178.

70. Olsen E, Duvic M, Frankel A. Pivotal phase III trial of two dose levels of denileukin diftitox for the treatment of cutaneous T-cell lymphoma. *J Clin Oncol.* 2001;19:376–388.

71. Trautinger F, Knobler R, Willemze R, et al. EORTC consensus recommendations for the treatment of mycosis fungoides/Sézary syndrome. *Eur J Cancer.* 2006;42:1014–1030.

72. Duvic M, Vu J. Update on the treatment of cutaneous T-cell lymphoma (CTCL): focus on vorinostat. *Biologics.* 2007;1(4):377–392.

73. Marks PA, Breslow R. Dimethyl sulfoxide to vorinostat: development of this histone deacetylase inhibitor as an anti-cancer drug. *Nat Biotechnol.* 2007;25:84–90.

74. Olsen E, Kim YH, Kuzel T, et al. Vorinostat (suberoylanilide hydroxamic acid, SAHA) is clinically active in advanced cutaneous T-cell lymphoma (CTCL): results of a phase IIb trial. *J Clin Oncol.* 2006;24:422s.

75. Kennedy GA, Seymour JF, Wolf M, et al. Treatment of patients with advanced mycosis fungoides and Sézary syndrome with alemtuzumab. *Eur J Haematol.* 2003;71:250–256.

76. Querfeld C, Mehta N, Rosen ST, et al. Alemtuzumab for relapsed and refractory erythrodermic cutaneous T-cell lymphoma: a single institution experience from the Robert H. Lurie comprehensive Cancer Center. *Leuk Lymphoma.* 2009;50(12):1969–1976.

77. Schappell DL, Alper JC, McDonald CJ. Treatment of advanced mycosis fungoides and Sézary syndrome with continuous infusions of methotrexate followed by fluorouracil and leucovorin rescue. *Arch Dermatol.* 1995;131(3):307–313.

78. Jidar K, Ingen-Housz-Oro S, Beylot-Barry M, et al. Gemcitabine treatment in cutaneous T-cell lymphoma: a multicentre study of 23 cases. *Br J Dermatol.* 2009;161(3):660–663.

79. Duvic M, Talpur R, Wen S, et al. Phase II evaluation of gemcitabine monotherapy for cutaneous T-cell lymphoma. *Clin Lymphoma Myeloma.* 2006;7(1):51–58.

80. Wollina U, Dummer R, Brockmeyer NH, et al. Multicenter study of pegylated liposomal doxorubicin in patients with cutaneous T-cell lymphoma. *Cancer.* 2003;98(5):993–1001.

81. Pulini S, Rupoli S, Goteri G, et al. Pegylated liposomal doxorubicin in the treatment of primary cutaneous T-cell lymphomas. *Haematologica.* 2007;92(5):686–689.

82. Wu PA, Kim YH, Lavori PW, et al. A meta-analysis of patients receiving allogeneic or autologous hematopoietic stem cell transplant in mycosis fungoides and Sézary syndrome. *Biol Blood Marrow Transplant.* 2009;15:989–990.

83. Guitart J, Wickless SC, Oyama Y, et al. Long-term remission after allogeneic hematopoietic stem cell transplantation for refractory cutaneous T-cell lymphoma. *Arch Dermatol.* 2002;138(10):1359–1365.

84. Guitart J. Combination treatment modalities in cutaneous T-cell lymphoma (CTCL). *Semin Oncol.* 2006;33(1 suppl 3):17–20.

85. Clendenning WE, Rappaport HW. Report of the committee on pathology of cutaneous T cell lymphomas. *Cancer Treat Report.* 1979;63:719–724.

# Dysplastic Nevi

*Holly Kanavy, Jennifer A. Stein, Edward Heilman, Michael K. Miller, David Polsky,*
*and Robert J. Friedman*

## Key Points

- Clinically dysplastic nevi are an important risk factor for development of melanoma.
- The lesion represents a point on a clinicopathological continuum that spans banal nevus at one end and melanoma at the other.
- Individual dysplastic nevi rarely eventuate into melanoma.
- There appears to be a genetic basis for this lesion, the expression of which is under the influence of environmental factors.
- The lesion is readily diagnosed on clinical grounds alone, and histological examination is only necessary when there is clinical suspicion for melanoma.
- Management of patients with dysplastic nevi centers around close surveillance and prevention of advanced melanoma.

## INTRODUCTION

Dysplastic nevi (DN) are a common clinical entity encountered by dermatologists, and have been the source of significant controversy since their initial description over 30 years ago.[1] The clinical relevance of these lesions lies in their well-recognized contribution to an increased risk for melanoma. Studies have demonstrated that DN are reported in up to 34–56% of melanoma cases,[2] and their presence may confer up to a 10-fold increase in melanoma risk.[3]

The biologic nature of DN has yet to be fully elucidated. In the sequential progression model for melanocytic tumors proposed by Clark over 30 years ago, DN represent a point on a continuum that spans from the benign nevus at one end to melanoma at the other. Based on this principle, it has been contended by some that DN are obligate precursor lesions to melanoma. It was at one time proposed that DN and melanoma were pleiotropic effects of a single gene.[4] Genetic studies have since confirmed that this is not the case.[5] Others have refuted the term 'dysplastic nevus', stating that all nevi are abnormal, and what Clark referred to as dysplastic nevi are stable, benign lesions that represent the most common melanocytic nevus in man which do not advance along a stepwise neoplastic progression, but instead are characterized by indolence and regression.[6]

DN remain a highly debated issue and controversial subject in dermatology. While there is controversy regarding the malignant potential of DN, the lesions themselves are benign and there is agreement that they serve as a phenotypic discriminator of those individuals at increased risk for melanoma. As such, recognition of DN is important in the management of patients at risk for melanoma.

## HISTORY

The first reported observation of the dysplastic nevus dates back to 1820 when William Norris described melanoma as a familial syndrome associated with large numbers of moles.[7] In 1952, Edward P. Cawley and colleagues similarly described a family with several cases of cutaneous melanoma and increased numbers of nevi.[8] It was not until 1978, however, that the clinicopathological entity now known as the dysplastic nevus was formally described. W.H. Clark and colleagues examined 58 patients affected by familial melanoma along with spousal controls, and characterized the pigmented lesions in these patients with a distinct set of clinical and histological features. They defined a new disease entity, the B-K mole syndrome, named after two of the patients that contributed to their study.[1] In 1983, Lynch et al. described a family exhibiting a similar phenotype that displayed concordance for malignant melanoma. They termed this syndrome familial atypical multiple mole melanoma (FAMMM) syndrome and noted an inheritance pattern consistent with a simple autosomal dominant factor.[9] In 1980, Elder et al. described 79 melanoma cases that occurred in a non-familial context in patients with multiple abnormal moles, recognizing a sporadic pattern of expression of the phenotype.[10]

Various other names have been applied to the dysplastic nevus, including Clark's nevus[11] and atypical mole,[12] and significant controversy has ensued over the naming of these lesions both clinically and histologically. Due to the lack of a common definition and disagreement over appropriate diagnostic criteria, the National Institutes of Health held a consensus conference in 1992 in order to clarify both the validity and significance of DN, as well as to make recommendations regarding the diagnosis and treatment of DN and early melanoma. It was concluded that the dysplastic nevus is a clinicopathologic entity that the represents an acquired pigmented tumor whose clinical and histologic appearance is different from common moles. The recommendation was to discontinue use of the term 'dysplastic' due to the diversity of its intended meaning by different investigators. Instead, the panel suggested that these lesions be refered to as 'atypical moles', and that histologically they be described as 'nevi with architectural disorder', along with a statement describing the presence and degree of melanocytic cytologic atypia. The committee also proposed that the phenotype observed in members of melanoma-prone families consisting of large numbers of DN be called familial atypical mole and melanoma (FAM-M) syndrome, and that these individuals be screened closely for melanoma.[13] However, this terminology was never fully accepted by the medical community. Over the past 25 years, the term dysplastic nevus has been the most frequently used by clinicians, pathologists and researchers.

## EPIDEMIOLOGY

Population-based studies report that the prevalence of DN lies in the range of 2–18%.[14-18] The importance of the DN lies in its relation to a well-documented increased risk for melanoma (not necessarily arising from the DN), the extent of which has been examined in several studies.[3,18] While the reported odds ratios have been quite variable, it has been consistently demonstrated that there is an increased risk for melanoma with increasing nevus counts. The presence and number of DN most influences this risk.

The estimated magnitude of melanoma risk conferred by DN has varied greatly among studies for several reasons. Major sources of inconsistency between published studies are the lack of a precise, easily reproducible clinical definition for DN (see clinical features section); a variable requirement for histologic confirmation in the diagnosis of DN;[13,19] and lack of universally accepted criteria for the histopathological diagnosis of DN.[20,21] Furthermore, other studies have demonstrated a poor correlation between the clinical and histological diagnoses of atypia,[22-25] raising questions regarding the need for histological confirmation in studies of DN and melanoma risk. Additional factors that may have potentially impacted results of these studies include variability in the presence of other melanoma risk factors, such as sun exposure, in the populations under study.[26-28]

Two extensive reviews of the literature have aided in elucidating more accurate risk estimates in patients with DN. Tucker and Goldstein performed a review of studies in melanoma etiology. They examined the results of several studies reporting odd ratios for melanoma according to DN counts, and found that the results of most studies fell in the range of 2.1 to 7.5.[18] A systematic meta-analysis of all studies published from 1966 to 2002 on risk factors for melanoma revealed similar results.[3] The investigators examined 47 datasets with a total of 10,499 melanoma cases and 14,256 controls with a mean age of 50. Pooled relative risks and confidence intervals were calculated for common and dysplastic nevi, both independently and together. Concerning DN, the relative risk differed depending on study type. Some studies looked at DN dichotomously and found that their presence conferred a 10-fold increased risk for melanoma. Other studies examined relative risk according to the number of dysplastic nevi, and observed an increased risk for each DN counted (Table 22.1). Based on all studies in the meta-analysis the relative risk for

**Table 22.1 Estimates from meta-analysis for atypical naevi and melanoma from case-control studies**

| No. naevi | RR | Lower 95% CI | Upper 95% CI |
|---|---|---|---|
| 0 | 1.00 | | |
| 1 | 1.45 | 1.31 | 1.60 |
| 2 | 2.10 | 1.71 | 2.54 |
| 3 | 3.03 | 2.23 | 4.06 |
| 4 | 4.39 | 2.91 | 6.47 |
| 5 | 6.36 | 3.80 | 10.33 |

RR, relative risk; CI, confidence interval. No. of studies = 13, Heterogeneity v=64.694, P < 0.001.

Modified from Gandini et al.[3]

melanoma in patients with five DN was over 10 times that of individuals with none. When only case–control studies were examined, and cohort studies excluded, a lower relative risk with more narrow confidence intervals for DN was established: the presence of five DN conferred a relative risk of 6.36 for melanoma.[3]

People with DN also tend to have higher numbers of common nevi,[29] and increased numbers of common nevi have been shown to increase a person's risk for melanoma[19,30,31] (Table 22.2). While the reported relative risk for melanoma has ranged widely depending on the population under study, a dose-dependent increase in melanoma risk has been observed, identifying common nevi as an independent risk factor for melanoma apart from other phenotypic risk factors[32-34] and family history.[3,35] Gandini et al. found that compared with people containing fewer than 15 common nevi, those with greater than 100 carry almost seven times the risk for development of melanoma.[3]

## ETIOLOGY AND PATHOGENESIS: GENES, ENVIRONMENT, AND BIOLOGY

There has been considerable investigation into the molecular nature of DN, particularly in relation to melanoma. There is evidence that genetic determinants play a role in the pathogenesis of DN.

**Table 22.2 Pooled Estimates for Risk of Melanoma for an Increasing Number of Common Nevi (Whole Body)**

| Number of Nevi | RR | Lower 95% CI | Upper 95% CI |
|---|---|---|---|
| 0–15 | 1.00 | | |
| 16–40 | 1.47 | 1.36 | 1.59 |
| 41–60 | 2.24 | 1.90 | 2.64 |
| 61–80 | 3.26 | 2.55 | 4.15 |
| 81–100 | 4.74 | 3.44 | 6.65 |
| 101–120 | 6.89 | 4.63 | 10.25 |

Number of studies = 26, P < 0.001.

CI, confidence interval; RR, relative risk.

Modified from Gandini et al.[3]

The first formal genetic analysis was performed by Lynch et al. in 1983. In studying patients and family members affected with the FAMMM syndrome, evidence of an autosomal dominant mode of inheritance was established.[9] This finding has been supported by several other studies.[4,36] Twin studies have also suggested a heritable basis for nevus count.[37-39] A case–control study conducted in a large private dermatology practice by Tucker et al. concluded that the relative risk of having DN was 7.2 in individuals with one or more relatives with DN.[40]

In light of the apparent genetic nature of DN and the close association of DN to familial malignant melanoma, there have been several attempts to assign a role for melanoma susceptibility genes in the development of DN. Bale et al. identified a locus on the short arm of chromosome 1 that appeared to be related to melanoma and DN (CMM/DN locus).[4] They suggested that the DN phenotype might represent the pleiotropic manifestation of a mutation in the 1p36 melanoma gene. However, further studies of this locus failed to demonstrate such an association.[5] A second genetic locus implicated in the DN phenotype was the *CDKN2A* gene on chromosome 9p21, which encodes two cell cycle regulator proteins, p16$^{INK4a}$ and p14$^{ARF}$. Mutations at this site have been identified in melanoma-prone families and have led to its designation as a melanoma susceptibility gene.[41-43] Carriers of the mutation have also been found to have higher nevus counts and nevus densities, suggesting a possible association with nevus count.[44] DN have since been determined to be a risk factor for melanoma independent of *CDKN2A* mutation status,[45] however, and the correlation between mutation status at this site and DN number has been rejected.

Other genes involved in melanoma pathogenesis and susceptibility that have been investigated in relation to DN include the *CDK4* oncogene for which germline mutations have been found in some melanoma families,[46] the *PTEN* tumor supressor gene, and the *BRAF* oncogene. Celebi et al. performed genetic analyses on patients with classic atypical mole syndrome and identified no sequence alterations in these genes.[47]

Phenotypic expression of DN is known to be affected by certain genetic and environmental factors. Overall sun sensitivity, as well as pigmentary characteristics including light skin color, hair and eye color, a tendency to freckle, and propensity to burn, which are genetically determined traits, are strong predictors of nevus development.[28,39,48] Expression of the DN phenotype is accentuated by exposure to UV light. Epidemiologic studies have shown that there is a higher incidence of the DNS phenotype in children who are exposed to greater amounts of UV light.[16,17,26-28] Bataille et al. reported a 6% prevalence of the DN phenotype in Australian children versus 2% in English children, endorsing a role for sun exposure in nevus induction.[26]

Several studies have supported the role for a gene–environment interaction in the pathogenesis of DN. A study was conducted in Vancouver, Canada in 1990, in which children aged 6 to 18 years were examined for nevus counts and phenotypic factors associated with sun sensitivity.

Information regarding UV exposure was recorded. Subjects with fair skin, who tended to burn rather than tan in the sun, and reported a history of numerous or severe sunburns were found to have significantly higher nevus counts than individuals without these characteristics. Subjects who were more likely to tan had fewer nevi, and children who freckled had higher nevus counts than those who did not freckle.[48] Recently, genetic markers related to these factors have been identified by genome-wide association studies.[49,50] Further work is needed to determine how the genes associated with these markers influence the phenotypic expression of the DN phenotype.

Clark proposed a sequential biologic progression model in which DN were described as precursor lesions to melanoma. Many have continued to support this as the biologic basis of DN, citing epidemiologic, histologic, and morphologic evidence. It is known that the presence of DN portends up to a 10-fold increased risk for melanoma,[3] which has led some to conclude that these two entities follow in a stepwise manner. Histologically, it has been noted that there is a degree of cytological and architectural atypia exhibited by DN that is intermediate between banal nevi and melanoma. Electron microscopic studies have revealed that DN with severe dysplasia share several features with radial growth phase melanomas, including: 1) large dysplastic nevus cells; 2) pleomorphic nuclei; 3) well-developed Golgi; 4) abundant and deranged mitochondria; and 5) aberrant melanosomes with deranged structure and irregular melanization.[51]

It has been estimated that approximately 25% of melanoma cases occur in pre-existing nevi, which also points toward this proposed linear relationship between nevi and melanoma. There has, however, been evidence to the contrary.[52] Roesch et al. reported that 75% of melanomas arise de novo with no pre-existing benign melanocytic tumor.[53] It is also important to note regarding such reports of nevus-associated melanomas, that the vast majority of nevi never undergo histologic examination and never eventuate into melanoma. As well, it is known that DN tend to be stable lesions, and either remain unchanged or regress over time.[54] A population-based estimate performed by Tsao et al. concluded that the risk of any particular dysplastic mole transforming into melanoma is 0.0005% (1 in 200,000) in individuals younger than 40 years old. In older individuals, the risk for women was estimated to be 0.009% (1 in 10,800) and for men 0.03% (1 in 3164).[55]

The sequential progression model would also predict that mutations detected in nevi would also be present in melanomas at the same or higher frequencies. However, an analysis of *BRAF* mutations from nevi and early-stage melanomas conducted in the same laboratory found that 82% of nevi contained *BRAF* mutations, whereas only 29% of early melanoma carried a mutation in the gene.[56]

Given all of the above, it is clear that the etiology of DN is complex and involves genetic, phenotypic, and environmental factors. There are likely several genes that play a role in the manifestation of the DN phenotype, and environment appears to play a role in expression of those genes.

## CLINICAL FEATURES

A precise clinical definition for DN is not clearly established. DN are acquired pigmented macules and papules that differ from common nevi in that they exhibit some of the clinical features of melanoma, such as asymmetry, irregular borders and variegated colors (Figs 22.1–22.4). In addition, some authors require DN to have a diameter of 5 mm or larger.[19] It is the degree of each criterion that separates DN from melanoma, although for early melanomas the clinical distinction from DN may be difficult (Fig. 22.2).[57]

When Clark introduced the concept of the dysplastic nevus in 1978, he assigned to the lesion clinical features that set it apart from common nevi. The prototypic lesion was described as being approximately 10 mm in size (5 to 15 mm), with an irregular outline, haphazard color combinations, and a mostly macular morphology with a small palpable (dermal) component. The reported differences between DN (referred to as B-K moles by Clark et al.) and ordinary acquired melanocytic nevi are summarized in Table 22.3.

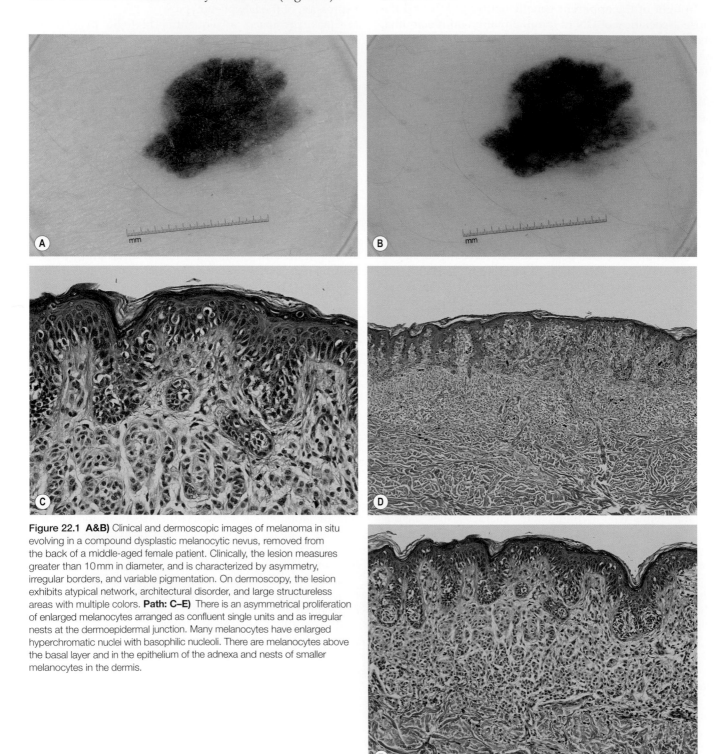

**Figure 22.1  A&B)** Clinical and dermoscopic images of melanoma in situ evolving in a compound dysplastic melanocytic nevus, removed from the back of a middle-aged female patient. Clinically, the lesion measures greater than 10 mm in diameter, and is characterized by asymmetry, irregular borders, and variable pigmentation. On dermoscopy, the lesion exhibits atypical network, architectural disorder, and large structureless areas with multiple colors. **Path: C–E)** There is an asymmetrical proliferation of enlarged melanocytes arranged as confluent single units and as irregular nests at the dermoepidermal junction. Many melanocytes have enlarged hyperchromatic nuclei with basophilic nucleoli. There are melanocytes above the basal layer and in the epithelium of the adnexa and nests of smaller melanocytes in the dermis.

Since the original description by Clark, there have been many attempts to establish a unified clinical definition for DN. Clinical diagnostic criteria set forth by Tucker et al. included a size of 5 mm or greater, being either entirely flat or having a flat component, and at least two of the following: variable pigmentation; irregular, asymmetric outline; and indistinct borders.[19] Kelly et al. used a comparable clinical definition for the DN, classifying DN as pigmented lesions with at least three of five criteria: size greater than 5 mm, irregular pigment distribution, ill-defined or irregular border, and a background of erythema.[58] The NIH con-

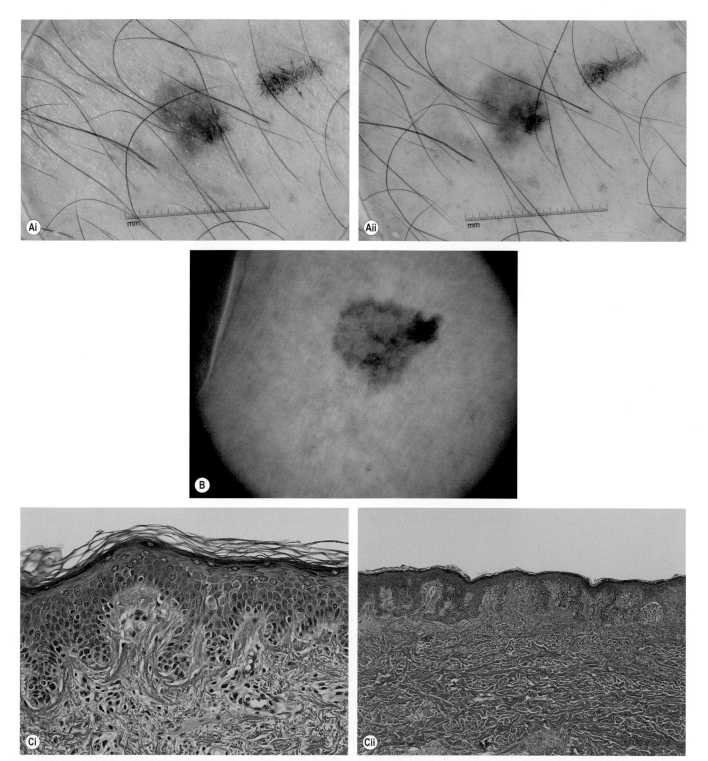

**Figure 22.2** Clinical (**Ai**) and dermoscopic (**Aii**) images of a junctional dysplastic nevus removed from the back a young male patient and **(B)** an invasive melanoma (0.25 mm thickness) removed from the left arm of an elderly female patient. Both lesions display an eccentric focus of darker brown pigmentation. Such similarity in appearance makes differentiation of these lesions difficult. **Path: (C)** High- and low-power photomicrographs of the dysplastic nevus shown in (A) demonstrating a proliferation of slightly enlarged melanocytes arranged as solitary units and predominantly as nests at the dermoepidermal junction. There is confluence of nests, bridging of rete ridges, dermal fibroplasia, proliferation of blood vessels, and a perivascular mononuclear cell infiltrate.

*(Continued)*

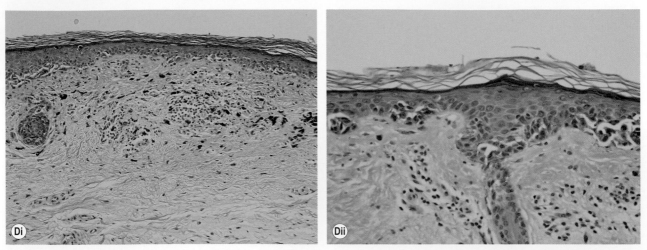

**Figure 22.2—cont'd (D)** High- and low-power photomicrographs of the melanoma shown in (B) demonstrating broad and asymmetrical proliferation of enlarged melanocytes arranged as confluent single units and nests at the dermoepidermal junction and within the epithelium of adnexa, as numerous single units in the upper levels of the epidermis, and as rare small nests and single units within the papillary dermis. There is a focus of dermal fibroplasia with increased numbers of small blood vessels and a perivascular infiltrate of lymphocytes and melanophages.

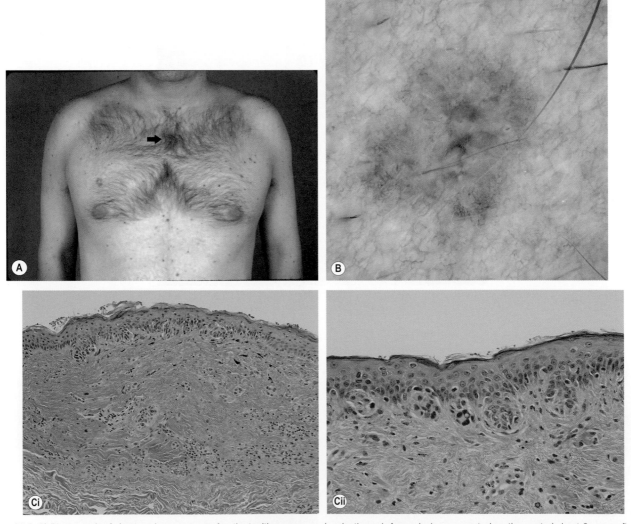

**Figure 22.3 A)** Photograph of chest and upper arms of patient with numerous dysplastic nevi. A new lesion was noted on the central chest 6 years after the photograph was taken, subsequently diagnosed as invasive melanoma (0.72 mm thickness). **B)** Dermoscopic image demonstrates marked lesional heterogeneity and architectural disorder. We observe a fragmented pigment network, structureless areas with possible regression, multiple colors, and polymorphous blood vessels. **Path: C)** There is asymmetrical proliferation of enlarged melanocytes arranged as confluent single units and as irregular at the dermoepidermal junction and predominantly as nests in the papillary dermis and superficial reticular dermis. Melanocytes have enlarged hyperchromatic nuclei and moderate amounts of pale-staining cytoplasm. There are single melanocytes present in the upper levels of the epidermis. There is a perivascular and focal band-like infiltrate predominantly of lymphocytes that extends to the lower portion of the epidermis. There are areas of fibroplasia of the papillary dermis with focal epidermal atrophy and a decreased number of melanocytes.

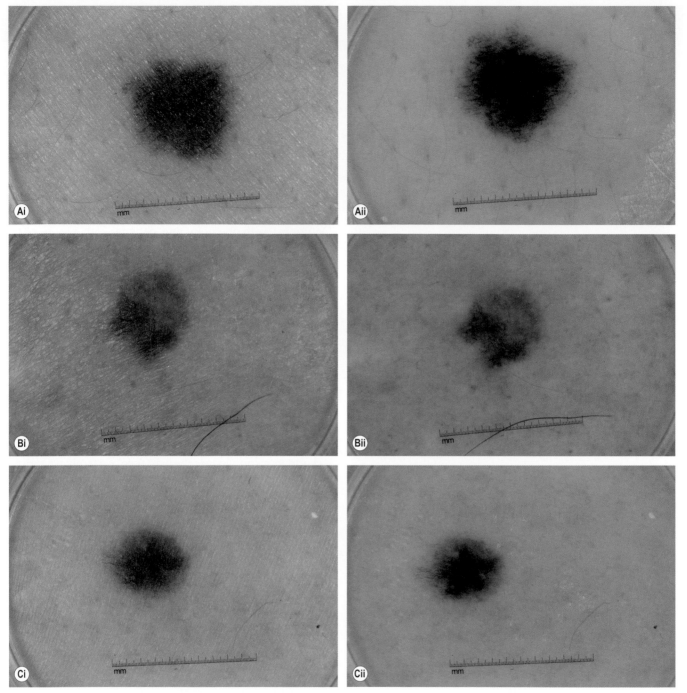

**Figure 22.4 A)** Clinical and dermoscopic images of a compound dysplastic nevus removed from the lower back of a young female patient. Note the variation in pigmentation, creating a dark brown center with a lighter brown border. Dermoscopic features include central globules and a peripheral network pattern.
**B)** Clinical and dermoscopic images of a congenital nevus with dysplastic features removed from the posterior shoulder of a middle-aged male patient. Note the irregular borders and variation in color. Dermoscopically the lesion is characterized by areas of atypical network and structureless areas. **C)** Clinical and dermoscopic images of a moderately dysplastic nevus removed from the chest of a young female patient that became darker during pregnancy. The lesion is clinically characterized by a dark brown center and lighter brown color peripherally. Dermoscopic examination reveals atypical network with variation in color and thickness.

sensus statement,[13] as well as published descriptions from Kopf et al.,[12] contain analogous definitions. A summary of the general clinical features of DN is presented in Table 22.4.

DN may be present anywhere on the skin, including sun-protected areas. They are most commonly seen on the trunk, especially the upper back,[59] but may also be seen on sites such as the buttocks, breast, genital skin, dorsa of feet, and the scalp.[60] DN tend to become clinically apparent during adolescence, although they have been described in prepubertal children,[61] and tend to increase in number into adulthood.[54]

An abundance of DN has been described as part of a clinical syndrome, commonly referred to as dysplastic nevus syndrome (DNS). The defining constituents of the syndrome have varied among different groups (Table 22.5). For

## Table 22.3 Clark's Original Comparison of Acquired Melanocytic Nevi and Dysplastic Nevi ('B-K moles')

| Characteristic | Acquired Melanocytic Nevi | B-K moles |
|---|---|---|
| Distribution of lesions | Sparse on lower extremities; virtually absent on bathing trunk area | Numerous on 'horse collar' area of trunk and upper extremities; present on bathing trunk area and lower extremities |
| Lesion size | Usually <5 mm | 5–10 mm; may be >10 mm |
| Lesion appearance | Regular outline; uniform color | Irregular outline; haphazardly colored |

Modified from Clark WH, Jr., Reimer RR, Greene M, Ainsworth AM, Mastrangelo MJ. Origin of familial malignant melanomas from heritable melanocytic lesions. 'The B-K mole syndrome'. *Arch Dermatol.* 1978 May;114(5):732-8.[1]

## Table 22.4 Summary of Clinical Features of Dysplastic Nevi

| Feature | Clinical Finding |
|---|---|
| Number | Frequently >50–100 |
| Uniformity | Heterogeneous (neighboring nevi differ from each other) |
| Size | ≥5 mm in diameter |
| Color | Variegated: multiple shades of tan, brown, black, red; often with peripheral macular tan zone |
| Elevation | Center is slightly raised; little elevation relative to diameter |
| Perimeter | May be irregular; usually fades into surrounding skin |
| Surface | Often mammillated |
| Symptoms | None |
| Hypertrichosis | Absent |
| Erosion/ulceration | Absent |

Modified from Kopf et al.[12]

patients in whom DN are observed in a familial context, the NIH consensus statement recommended use of the term familial atypical mole melanoma (FAM-M) syndrome, and set forth criteria to be used for its diagnosis[13] which requires histologic confirmation of the DN lesion. More recent studies demonstrated melanoma risk to be associated with clinically recognized DN, making a requirement for histologic confirmation unnecessary.[19]

Newton et al. established a scoring system to identify patients with the atypical mole syndrome (AMS), which was validated in a follow-up study.[62] The five identified features are: 1) 100 or more nevi >2 mm; 2) two or more atypical nevi (defined as a mole >5 mm, with an irregular or blurred edge, and irregular pigmentation); 3) one or more nevi on the anterior scalp; 4) one nevus on the buttocks or two or more on the dorsal feet; and 5) one or more iris nevi. Each

## Table 22.5 Dysplastic Nevus Syndrome: Criteria for Diagnosis

| NIH FAMM | >50 nevi, several atypical<br>Histologic criteria<br>One or more first or second degree relatives |
|---|---|
| Newton | 100 or more >2 mm<br>2 or more clinically atypical nevi<br>1 or more nevi on anterior scalp<br>1 nevus on buttocks or 2 or more on dorsal feet,<br>1 or more iris nevi |
| Kopf CAMS | 100 or more nevi<br>1 or more ≥8 mm<br>1 or more with clinically atypical features |

feature is worth one point and patients with a score of two or higher have AMS.[63] Kopf et al. described the classic atypical mole syndrome, which represents a severe expression of the phenotype. Requirements of this syndrome include the presence of each of the following: 1) 100 or more nevi; 2) one or more nevi 8 mm or greater in diameter; and 3) one or more nevi with clinically atypical features.[12]

Some authors have argued against the use of the term 'dysplastic nevus syndrome'. Ackerman noted that if a syndrome is defined as a constellation of signs and symptoms, then the presence alone of histologically atypical moles does not constitute a syndrome. He reported that in his experience these lesions are extremely common, present in the majority of Caucasians, and therefore most Caucasians would qualify as having the syndrome, reducing its significance.[6] While Ackerman acknowledges the existence of a familial condition characterized by many large DN and cutaneous melanoma, he purports that this clinical entity is extremely rare.

## HISTOLOGY

Dysplastic nevi are commonly classified based on architectural and cytologic features. While there is often agreement on architectural criteria for DN, the classification of cytologic features is more controversial. These cytologic criteria have frequently been reported to lack inter- and even intra-observer reproducibility, and predictive value in regards to clinical behavior.

The 1992 NIH Consensus Conference attempted to set criteria for the diagnosis of DN, but concluded that the use of the term dysplastic nevus should be 'discouraged' both as a clinical and histologic diagnosis. The use of the histologic term 'nevi with architectural disorder' along with an additional comment describing the 'presence and degree of cytologic atypia' was proposed.

Other classification systems using mild, moderate, and severe cytologic dysplasia have subsequently been proposed.[64] Because of difficulties in distinguishing between mild and moderate dysplasia, a low-grade/high-grade distinction was developed.[64,65]

However, none of the published classification schemes have been convincingly shown to provide guidelines for the consistent, reproducible diagnosis and classification of DN, or their associated risk for melanoma. Despite these difficulties, the criteria for the histologic diagnosis of DN are usually grouped into architectural and cytologic features (see Pathology in Figures 22.1–22.4).

**Architectural features,** many of which can be readily identified at low power or scanning power, include: 1) poor circumscription, i.e. epidermal melanocytes present as single cells and nests for a significant distance beyond the dermal component, which is often referred to as a 'shoulder' (Figs 22.5–22.9); 2) lentiginous melanocytic hyperplasia, composed of solitary but also nested melanocytes along the tips and sides of elongated rete ridges, often with bridging nests – as a general rule, melanocytes are confined to the lower portion of the epidermis and are not seen at higher levels (Fig. 22.9); 3) subepidermal fibroplasia, which can be lamellar or concentric and eosinophilic (Figs 22.10 and 22.11); and 4) variable associated dermal lymphohistiocytic inflammatory cell infiltrate. When a dermal component exists, melanocytes are present as nests, strands, and cords, generally in the superficial dermis, but which can

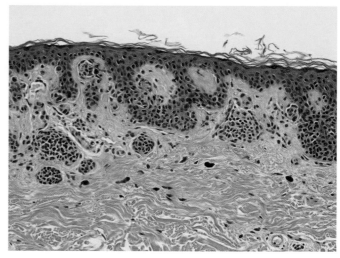

**Figure 22.7** Photomicrograph at higher power exhibits bridging of the rete.

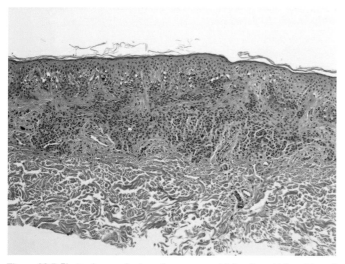

**Figure 22.5** Photomicrograph at medium power exhibits a broad intraepidermal melanocytic proliferation consisting of nested and single melanocytes along the basal layer and along the bases and sides of the rete ridges. Many of the nests vary in size and shape and form confluent bridges between the rete housing the collections of melanocytes. In the dermis there is a band of nevo-melanocytes arranged as nests and strands embedded in the fibrous stroma.

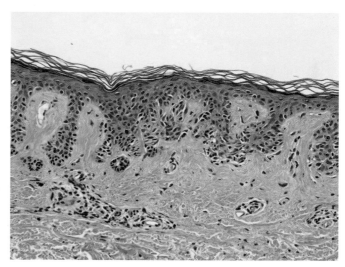

**Figure 22.8** Photomicrograph at higher power exhibits a 'shoulder' proliferation of single and nested melanocytes extending radially beyond the dermal component of the nevus.

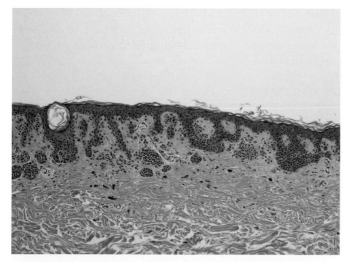

**Figure 22.6** Photomicrograph at medium power exhibits melanocytes arranged as single units and variably shaped nests along the bases and sides of the rete ridges. Bridges are formed by the rete housing the collections of melanocytes.

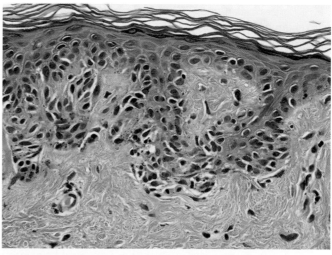

**Figure 22.9** Photomicrograph at highest power exhibits confluent nests of slightly enlarged melanocytes within bridges of elongated rete.

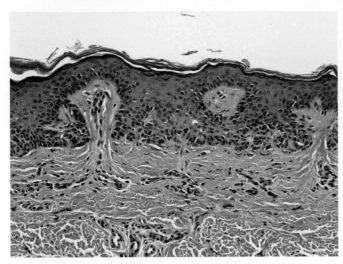

**Figure 22.10** Lamellar fibroplasia within the papillary dermis below elongated rete. There are coarse bundles of collagen and fibroblasts with spindle-shape nuclei arranged in horizontal parallel array.

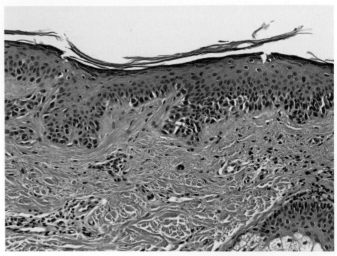

**Figure 22.12** Atypical features within a dysplastic nevus. There are zones in which melanocytes arranged as solitary units predominate and tend towards confluence along the basal layer.

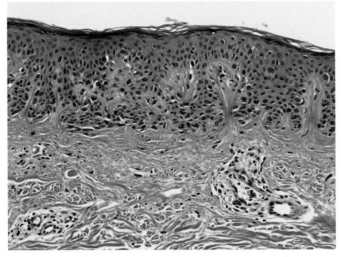

**Figure 22.11** Concentric eosinophilic fibroplasia. Compact collagen fibers outline the elongated rete.

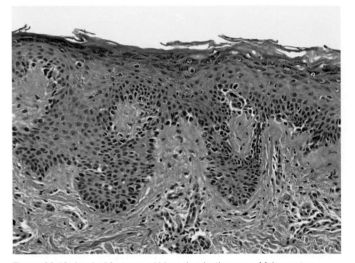

**Figure 22.13** Atypical features within a dysplastic nevus. Melanocytes arranged as solitary units extend to higher levels of the epidermis.

also extend deeply and wrap around adnexal structures and vessels in a congenital pattern.

**Cytologic features** include: 1) random cytologic atypia, i.e. the presence of scattered epithelioid or spindled melanocytes with enlarged, hyperchromatic nuclei and, in some instances, prominent nucleoli; and 2) dermal melanocytes which are generally small (nevoid) to epithelioid in appearance, with at least some maturation with dermal descent. The dermal component can, in some instances, show features of other types of nevi, e.g. congenital, blue, spitzoid, or neuritized.

Problems in reproducibility and predictive behavior of DN arise when the degree of epidermal melanocytic cytologic and/or architectural atypia approaches that seen in malignant melanoma in situ; for example, when solitary or nested epidermal melanocytes exhibit greater cytologic atypia than seen in a 'routine dysplastic nevus', when there are zones in which solitary junctional melanocytes predominate over nested melanocytes, and/or when solitary melanocytes extend to higher levels of the epidermis (Figs 22.12 and 22.13). In many cases such as these, it could be argued that the findings actually represent an evolving melanoma

in situ, arising either de novo or in association with the dysplastic nevus (Figs 22.14–22.16). An additional complicating factor is that, in some instances, cytologic atypia may be present in nevi that lack the architectural features of dysplastic nevi.

## MANAGEMENT

Establishment of guidelines for the management of patients with DN has presented a significant challenge due to the continued controversy over a precise clinicopathologic definition for the lesion and a lack of agreement regarding the degree of risk of melanoma developing in association with individual dysplastic nevi. It has been well documented, however, that patients with DN are at increased risk for melanoma;[3] therefore, the management of these patients centers around early detection of melanoma and prevention of advanced disease. The diagnosis of DN can be made on clinical grounds and does not require histologic confirmation.[2]

DN serve primarily as a phenotypic marker for increased melanoma risk.[55] Therefore, the removal of DN should only

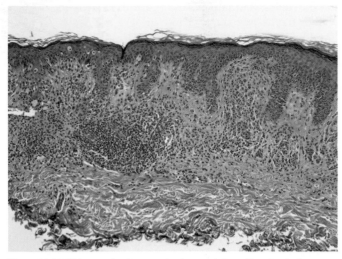

**Figure 22.14** Melanoma in situ occurring in association with a dysplastic nevus. On the right there is a dysplastic nevus and on the left there is a melanoma in situ with pagetoid spread of atypical melanocytes throughout the epidermis.

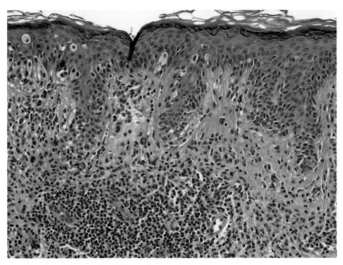

**Figure 22.15** Melanoma in situ occurring in association with a dysplastic nevus. Dysplastic nevus on the right and melanoma in situ on the left.

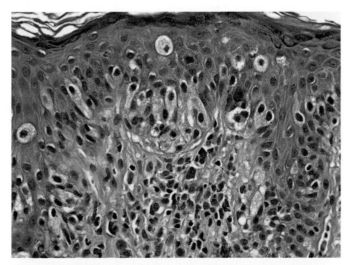

**Figure 22.16** Highest power. Melanoma in situ occurring in association with a dysplastic nevus. Note the pagetoid spread of atypical melanocytes throughout the epidermis.

occur if there is clinical suspicion for melanoma. Once DN are clinically recognized, there are several issues to consider in regard to patient management. These include patient risk stratification; how and when to perform a biopsy; appropriate use of diagnostic aids, including total body photography, dermoscopy, and/or digital imaging devices; and patient counseling.

The first step in the management of the patient with DN is to determine the patient's risk for melanoma. A personal history of melanoma increases a patient's risk for development of a subsequent melanoma by a factor of approximately 8.5.[66] A personal history of non-melanoma skin cancers is also important in risk assessment, and increases the risk for melanoma up to four times.[67] While there is no universally accepted system to assess for melanoma risk according to family history, it is widely accepted that a stronger family history of melanoma predicts a greater likelihood for melanoma[3] and information regarding first and second degree relatives should be recorded. It is important to appreciate, however, that the accuracy of patient-provided family histories is often unreliable, and a reported positive history turns out to be untrue up to 50% of the time.[3]

Immunosuppression also confers increased melanoma risk, so any such conditions or medications should be inquired about and documented.[68–70] The initial visit also provides an opportunity to question patients regarding their history of ultraviolet light exposure, including painful and/or blistering sunburns and indoor tanning, both of which increase the risk for melanoma.[2,67,71,72] Phenotypic traits that are known to confer increased risk for melanoma are also assessed, and include light skin, hair and eye color, sensitivity to sun and inability to tan, freckling tendency, and total body nevus count.[67]

During the initial patient encounter, a thorough cutaneous physical examination should be conducted and should include the intertriginous areas and all non-sun-exposed areas, including the scalp, breasts, buttocks and feet. The clinician will evaluate closely lesions that are particularly concerning to the patient and seek out lesions suspicious for malignancy. In patients with an increased number of melanocytic nevi, the majority of nevi often share a common clinical appearance. Identification of such a 'signature nevus' pattern may be helpful in guiding the examination of such patients.[73] Identification of the signature nevus also aids in the recognition of the so-called 'ugly duckling' lesion, a nevus that stands out as being particularly different in clinical appearance from the patient's other nevi, a potentially worrisome sign. While the 'ugly duckling' most commonly refers to a lesion with increased morphologic atypia, it may also represent a banal-appearing lesion against a background of more clinically dysplastic nevi.[74] Some have suggested a role for biopsy of the most clinically atypical mole at the initial visit in order to define a patient's 'histological baseline',[75] however, there are no data to support the concept that knowledge of a patient's histological baseline aids in patient management.

Evaluation of patients with DN is greatly enhanced by dermoscopic examination (see Chapter 36). Dermoscopy has been shown to increase both the sensitivity and specificity for melanoma diagnosis.[76,77] According to a meta-analysis of 27 studies, dermoscopy increases the diagnostic accuracy of melanoma by 49%.[76] Kittler et al. reported the relative diagnostic odds ratio for melanoma, for dermoscopy compared with naked eye examination, to be 9.0 (95% CI 1.5–54.6, P = 0.03). Although there are no pathognomonic dermoscopic features to distinguish DN from melanoma, there are certain features that help raise the clinical suspicion for melanoma, prompting biopsies where appropriate and helping avoid unneccessary biopsies.[78,79] The benefit of dermoscopy has been demonstrated not only for pigmented lesion specialists, but for use among general dermatologists as well.[79,80]

Once a decision has been made to remove a suspicious pigmented lesion, the manner in which DN are removed is critical to proper diagnosis and future management of the patient. The most important consideration is the ability to provide the pathologist with an adequate specimen for the most accurate diagnosis. Options for biopsy technique include elliptical excision, punch biopsy, shave biopsy, or deep shave saucerization. Removal of the entire lesion should be performed whenever possible with a 2 mm margin of clinically uninvolved skin.[81] The 2 mm margin recommendation is based upon a study conducted by Rigel et al. in which 51 DN were examined. Comparison of the clinically apparent margins of biopsy specimens with histological margins revealed that 95% of lesions excised with 2 mm margins contained clear histological margins.[82]

Even with adequate margins and the opportunity for the pathologist to evaluate the entire lesion, DN still present a diagnostic challenge. Several groups have examined interobserver reproducibility in the histologic diagnoses of melanoma and nevi. Concerning the ability to distinguish these two entities, concordance rates have ranged from 49% to 76%.[83–86] In one study looking to establish a histological grading system for DN according to severity of atypia, concordance rates among experienced dermatopathologists were in the 35–58% range.[87] While much greater agreement can be achieved when pre-determined diagnostic criteria are in place, such universally accepted histopathological criteria are uncommon in clinical practice.[88]

DN with mild or moderate cytologic atypia that have been completely excised or are present focally at the margins typically require no further treatment. For moderately dysplastic nevi that extend to a margin, the dermatopathologist will often recommend complete excision of all remaining or recurrent pigmentation to ensure complete removal of the lesion. For severely dysplastic nevi, some advocate excision with 5 mm margins,[81] while others perform re-excision only if margins are involved or cannot be adequately assessed by the dermatopathologist. A recently published small study of incompletely removed DN found that no melanomas arose within 5 years or longer after biopsy, suggesting that incomplete removal of DN may not pose a significant risk of melanoma to the patient.[89] Larger studies are needed to confirm these preliminary findings.

In patients with increased numbers of melanocytic nevi, there are often atypical lesions that the clinician would like to follow closely rather than remove. For these patients, total body photography may be beneficial to detect new and/or changing melanocytic lesions. Typically, a set of approximately 24 images is obtained of different regions of the skin using standard poses to capture all existing nevi, as well as nevus-free skin.[90] These images are used as a baseline to assess for new or changing lesions. Several reports have provided evidence that total body photography can be valuable in the detection of early melanoma as well as in avoidance of unneccessary biopsies.[58,91,92]

More recently, serial imaging with dermoscopy has shown promise in the management of patients with increased numbers of moles. Sequential dermoscopic images may be obtained over 3-, 6- or 12-month intervals. Several computer-based systems are commercially available for image storage, analysis, and archiving (see Chapter 37). Studies have found these devices may increase the sensitivity for early melanoma detection and reduce the number of unnecessary biopsies.[93–96]

On long-term monitoring (e.g. 12 months), DN may demonstrate either no change or symmetric enlargement without any substantial dermoscopic changes. In contrast, melanomas frequently increase in size and exhibit changes in shape as well as the emergence of new dermoscopic structures.[97] In short-term monitoring (e.g. 3 months, 6 months for face), any lesional change prompts a biopsy, and lesions that remain unchanged may be monitored further or deemed benign.[98] Menzies et al. provided evidence that the sensitivity of short-term dermoscopic monitoring in detection of melanoma was 97.1%.[99] A recent retrospective analysis examined clinical outcome using different follow-up protocols of 3, 6, or 12 months according to the degree of clinical atypia of the patients' nevi. Out of the 600 lesions that underwent monitoring, 54 (9%) were excised. Twelve of the excised lesions were melanomas, ten of which were detected at 3-month follow-up, and two of which were diagnosed at 6 months. The melanoma-to-benign ratio of excised lesions was 1:3.4, which was better than conventional ratios without dermoscopy, which can range as high as 1:18.[100] Patient compliance was 84% for short-term monitoring, 63% for medium-term monitoring, and 30% for long-term monitoring.[96] This study demonstrated the value of both short-term and long-term monitoring in the sensitivity and specificity of melanoma diagnosis in patients with multiple DN.

An important component in the management of patients with DN is periodic follow-up with complete skin examinations. The frequency of follow-up depends on the patient's melanoma risk, comfort level, and ability to perform skin self-examinations. Patients deemed to be at high risk, based on a personal history of melanoma or strong family history and/or very high numbers of atypical nevi, should be seen initially every 3 to 6 months, until both the patient and physician develop confidence in the stability of the patient's nevi. At such a time, the interval between visits may be increased to every 6 to 12 months. Follow-up visits not only allow for monitoring of specific lesions but also provide an opportunity for the clinician to reiterate the importance of self-surveillance and proper sun-protective measures. Because melanoma is exceedingly rare in children, even in melanoma-prone families, screening can be started in the late teens or early twenties and conducted at a frequency dictated by melanoma risk assessment.[101]

Patient counseling is essential in the management of DN. The patient should be made aware that the presence of DN signifies an increased risk for melanoma. The importance of compliance with follow-up examinations must be stressed. Skin self-examination should be emphasized, as patients who perform these examinations have significantly thinner melanomas at diagnosis compared to patients who do not regularly examine their skin;[102] however, for patients with a florid presentation of DN, self-examination may be exceedingly difficult and proper surveillance requires examination by a physician. Although no studies have shown a direct effect of sunscreen use in melanoma prevention, regular use is known to result in less sunburns and the development of fewer nevi in children,[103] two known risk factors for development of melanoma.[104]

Some physicians advocate routine ophthalmological examinations to screen for ocular melanoma in patients with DN. A meta-analysis of this topic revealed an association between uveal melanoma and nevi of the skin and iris. The odds ratio for uveal melanoma in patients with DN was 2.82.[105] Bataille et al. determined that the relative risk for ocular melanoma increases with severity of the DNS phenotype, and recommend ophthalmological screening examinations only in those patients with strong expression of the DNS phenotype, including those with nevi of the iris.[106]

Removal of DN, regardless of the method used, has the potential for leaving the patient with an unsightly scar. This is particularly true of DN on the trunk, where there is a higher risk for hypertrophic scar formation. In attempts to circumvent this issue, other methods for removal have been tried. Medical treatments have included systemic isotretinoin, topical tretinoin with or without hydrocortisone, 5-fluorouracil, and imiquimod.[107-113] None of these treatments have resulted in complete destruction of the nevus, either clinically or histologically.

Laser ablation of DN has been attempted in order to potentially avoid scar formation. To date, no laser consistently results in the complete destruction of melanocytic nevi. Most lasers only ablate melanocytes within the epidermis and papillary dermis, leaving the deeper dermal melanocytes intact. This makes the practitioner unable to monitor treated lesions, and the biologic effect of such laser treatments on DN is not known. It is therefore most prudent to avoid laser treatment of DN.

## CONCLUSIONS

Dysplastic nevi in a patient portend an increased risk for developing melanoma. DN represent a point on the clinico-pathological continuum that spans banal nevus at one end and melanoma at the other. Despite this, individual DN rarely eventuate into melanoma. There appears to be a genetic basis for the lesion, the expression of which is under the influence of environmental factors. The lesion is often diagnosed on clinical grounds alone, and histological examination is only necessary when there is clinical suspicion for melanoma. Management of patients with DN centers around close surveillance and prevention of advanced malignant melanoma.

## FUTURE OUTLOOK

Several non-invasive modalities are currently in development to potentially aid the dermatologist in distinguishing DN from melanoma without requiring a biopsy. These include confocal scanning laser microscopy, reflex transmission imaging using high-resolution ultrasound, optical coherence tomography, and multispectral digital dermoscopy with computer analysis. Genetic testing may also become an important part of management of patients with DN. While there have been several candidate genes identified and investigated as melanoma risk factors, none have proven appropriate for use in routine patient testing. Additional studies are needed to develop clinically useful genetic markers of melanoma risk that will directly enhance DN management.

## REFERENCES

1. Clark Jr WH, Reimer RR, Greene M, et al. Origin of familial malignant melanomas from heritable melanocytic lesions. 'The B-K mole syndrome'. Arch Dermatol. 1978;114(5):732–738.
2. Tucker MA. Melanoma epidemiology. Hematol Oncol Clin North Am. 2009;23(3):383–395 vii.
3. Gandini S, Sera F, Cattaruzza MS, et al. Meta-analysis of risk factors for cutaneous melanoma. I. Common and atypical naevi. Eur J Cancer. 2005;41(1):28–44.
4. Bale SJ, Chakravarti A, Greene MH. Cutaneous malignant melanoma and familial dysplastic nevi: evidence for autosomal dominance and pleiotropy. Am J Hum Genet. 1986;38(2):188–196.
5. Greene MH. The genetics of hereditary melanoma and nevi. 1998 update. Cancer. 1999;86(suppl 11):2464–2477.
6. Ackerman AB. What naevus is dysplastic, a syndrome and the commonest precursor of malignant melanoma? A riddle and an answer. Histopathology. 1988;13(3):241–256.
7. Norris W. A case of fungoid disease. Edinburgh Medical and Surgical Journal. 1820;16:562–565.
8. Cawley EP, Kruse WT, Pinkus HK. Genetic aspects of malignant melanoma. AMA Arch Derm Syphilol. 1952;65(4):440–450.
9. Lynch HT, Fusaro RM, Kimberling WJ, et al. Familial atypical multiple mole-melanoma (FAMMM) syndrome: segregation analysis. J Med Genet. 1983;20(5):342–344.
10. Elder DE, Goldman LI, Goldman SC, et al. Dysplastic nevus syndrome: a phenotypic association of sporadic cutaneous melanoma. Cancer. 1980;46(8):1787–1794.
11. Nollet DJ. Clark's nevus syndrome. Am J Dermatopathol. 1986;8(4):367.
12. Kopf AW, Friedman RJ, Rigel DS. Atypical mole syndrome. J Am Acad Dermatol. 1990;22(1):117–118.
13. NIH Consensus conference. Diagnosis and treatment of early melanoma. JAMA. 1992;268(10):1314–1319.
14. Bataille V, Bishop JA, Sasieni P, et al. Risk of cutaneous melanoma in relation to the numbers, types and sites of naevi: a case-control study. Br J Cancer. 1996;73(12):1605–1611.
15. Cooke KR, Spears GF, Elder DE, et al. Dysplastic naevi in a population-based survey. Cancer. 1989;63(6):1240–1244.
16. Crutcher WA, Sagebiel RW. Prevalence of dysplastic naevi in a community practice. Lancet. 1984;1(8379):729.
17. Sander C, Tschochohei H, Hagedorn M. [Epidemiology of dysplastic nevus]. Hautarzt. 1989;40(12):758–760.
18. Tucker MA, Goldstein AM. Melanoma etiology: where are we? Oncogene. 2003;22(20):3042–3052.
19. Tucker MA, Halpern A, Holly EA, et al. Clinically recognized dysplastic nevi. A central risk factor for cutaneous melanoma. JAMA. 1997;277(18):1439–1444.
20. Duray PH, DerSimonian R, Barnhill R, et al. An analysis of interobserver recognition of the histopathologic features of dysplastic nevi from a mixed group of nevomelanocytic lesions. J Am Acad Dermatol. 1992;27 (5 Pt 1):741–749.
21. Klein LJ, Barr RJ. Histologic atypia in clinically benign nevi. A prospective study. J Am Acad Dermatol. 1990;22(2 Pt 1):275–282.
22. Kelly JW, Crutcher WA, Sagebiel RW. Clinical diagnosis of dysplastic melanocytic nevi. A clinicopathologic correlation. J Am Acad Dermatol. 1986;14(6):1044–1052.
23. Curley RK, Cook MG, Fallowfield ME, et al. Accuracy in clinically evaluating pigmented lesions. BMJ. 1989;299(6690):16–18.
24. Black WC, Hunt WC. Histologic correlations with the clinical diagnosis of dysplastic nevus. Am J Surg Pathol. 1990;14(1):44–52.
25. Annessi G, Cattaruzza MS, Abeni D, et al. Correlation between clinical atypia and histologic dysplasia in acquired melanocytic nevi. J Am Acad Dermatol. 2001;45(1):77–85.
26. Bataille V, Grulich A, Sasieni P, et al. The association between naevi and melanoma in populations with different levels of sun exposure: a joint case-control study of melanoma in the UK and Australia. Br J Cancer. 1998;77(3):505–510.

27. Luther H, Altmeyer P, Garbe C, et al. Increase of melanocytic nevus counts in children during 5 years of follow-up and analysis of associated factors. *Arch Dermatol*. 1996;132(12):1473–1478.

28. Breitbart M, Garbe C, Buttner P, et al. Ultraviolet light exposure, pigmentary traits and the development of melanocytic naevi and cutaneous melanoma. A case-control study of the German Central Malignant Melanoma Registry. *Acta Derm Venereol*. 1997;77(5):374–378.

29. Augustsson A, Stierner U, Suurkula M, et al. Prevalence of common and dysplastic naevi in a Swedish population. *Br J Dermatol*. 1991;124(2):152–156.

30. Grob JJ, Gouvernet J, Aymar D, et al. Count of benign melanocytic nevi as a major indicator of risk for nonfamilial nodular and superficial spreading melanoma. *Cancer*. 1990;66(2):387–395.

31. Weiss J, Bertz J, Jung EG. Malignant melanoma in southern Germany: different predictive value of risk factors for melanoma subtypes. *Dermatologica*. 1991;183(2):109–113.

32. Rodenas JM, Delgado-Rodriguez M, Farinas-Alvarez C, et al. Melanocytic nevi and risk of cutaneous malignant melanoma in southern Spain. *Am J Epidemiol*. 1997;145(11):1020–1029.

33. Carli P, Biggeri A, Giannotti B. Malignant melanoma in Italy: risks associated with common and clinically atypical melanocytic nevi. *J Am Acad Dermatol*. 1995;32(5 Pt 1):734–739.

34. Naldi L, Lorenzo Imberti G, Parazzini F, et al. Pigmentary traits, modalities of sun reaction, history of sunburns, and melanocytic nevi as risk factors for cutaneous malignant melanoma in the Italian population: results of a collaborative case-control study. *Cancer*. 2000;88(12):2703–2710.

35. Ford D, Bliss JM, Swerdlow AJ, et al. Risk of cutaneous melanoma associated with a family history of the disease. The International Melanoma Analysis Group (IMAGE). *Int J Cancer*. 1995;62(4):377–381.

36. Goldstein AM, Tucker MA, Crutcher WA, et al. The inheritance pattern of dysplastic naevi in families of dysplastic naevus patients. *Melanoma Res*. 1993;3(1):15–22.

37. Easton DF, Cox GM, Macdonald AM, et al. Genetic susceptibility to naevi—a twin study. *Br J Cancer*. 1991;64(6):1164–1167.

38. Goldgar DE, Cannon-Albright LA, Meyer LJ, et al. Inheritance of nevus number and size in melanoma and dysplastic nevus syndrome kindreds. *J Natl Cancer Inst*. 1991;83(23):1726–1733.

39. Martin NG, Green AC, Ward PJ. Moliness, p16 and melanoma: a twin study: 090. *Melanoma Res*. 1997;7(suppl 1):S26.

40. Tucker MA, Crutcher WA, Hartge P, et al. Familial and cutaneous features of dysplastic nevi: a case-control study. *J Am Acad Dermatol*. 1993;28(4):558–564.

41. Cannon-Albright LA, Goldgar DE, Meyer LJ, et al. Assignment of a locus for familial melanoma, MLM, to chromosome 9p13-p22. *Science*. 1992;258(5085):1148–1152.

42. Kamb A, Gruis NA, Weaver-Feldhaus J, et al. A cell cycle regulator potentially involved in genesis of many tumor types. *Science*. 1994;264(5157):436–440.

43. Hussussian CJ, Struewing JP, Goldstein AM, et al. Germline p16 mutations in familial melanoma. *Nat Genet*. 1994;8(1):15–21.

44. Cannon-Albright LA, Meyer LJ, Goldgar DE, et al. Penetrance and expressivity of the chromosome 9p melanoma susceptibility locus (MLM). *Cancer Res*. 1994;54(23):6041–6044.

45. Goldstein AM, Martinez M, Tucker MA, et al. Gene-covariate interaction between dysplastic nevi and the CDKN2A gene in American melanoma-prone families. *Cancer Epidemiol Biomarkers Prev*. 2000;9(9):889–894.

46. Udayakumar D, Tsao H. Melanoma genetics: an update on risk-associated genes. *Hematol Oncol Clin North Am*. 2009;23(3):415–429 vii.

47. Celebi JT, Ward KM, Wanner M, et al. Evaluation of germline CDKN2A, ARF, CDK4, PTEN, and BRAF alterations in atypical mole syndrome. *Clin Exp Dermatol*. 2005;30(1):68–70.

48. Gallagher RP, McLean DI, Yang CP, et al. Suntan, sunburn, and pigmentation factors and the frequency of acquired melanocytic nevi in children. Similarities to melanoma: the Vancouver Mole Study. *Arch Dermatol*. 1990;126(6):770–776.

49. Han J, Kraft P, Nan H, et al. A genome-wide association study identifies novel alleles associated with hair color and skin pigmentation. *PLoS Genet*. 2008;4(5):e1000074.

50. Nan H, Kraft P, Qureshi AA, et al. Genome-wide association study of tanning phenotype in a population of European ancestry. *J Invest Dermatol*. 2009;129(9):2250–2257.

51. Langer K, Rappersberger K, Steiner A, et al. The ultrastructure of dysplastic naevi: comparison with superficial spreading melanoma and common naevocellular naevi. *Arch Dermatol Res*. 1990;282(6):353–362.

52. Ackerman AB, Mihara I. Dysplasia, dysplastic melanocytes, dysplastic nevi, the dysplastic nevus syndrome, and the relation between dysplastic nevi and malignant melanomas. *Hum Pathol*. 1985;16(1):87–91.

53. Roesch A, Burgdorf W, Stolz W, et al. Dermatoscopy of "dysplastic nevi": a beacon in diagnostic darkness. *Eur J Dermatol*. 2006;16(5):479–493.

54. Halpern AC, Guerry DT, Elder DE, et al. Natural history of dysplastic nevi. *J Am Acad Dermatol*. 1993;29(1):51–57.

55. Tsao H, Bevona C, Goggins W, et al. The transformation rate of moles (melanocytic nevi) into cutaneous melanoma: a population-based estimate. *Arch Dermatol*. 2003;139(3):282–288.

56. Poynter JN, Elder JT, Fullen DR, et al. BRAF and NRAS mutations in melanoma and melanocytic nevi. *Melanoma Res*. 2006;16(4):267–273.

57. McBride A, Rivers JK, Kopf AW, et al. Clinical features of dysplastic nevi. *Dermatol Clin*. 1991;9(4):717–722.

58. Kelly JW, Yeatman JM, Regalia C, et al. A high incidence of melanoma found in patients with multiple dysplastic naevi by photographic surveillance. *Med J Aust*. 1997;167(4):191–194.

59. Richard MA, Grob JJ, Gouvernet J, et al. Role of sun exposure on nevus. First study in age-sex phenotype-controlled populations. *Arch Dermatol*. 1993;129(10):1280–1285.

60. Mooi WJ. The dysplastic naevus. *J Clin Pathol*. 1997;50(9):711–715.

61. Tucker MA, Greene MH, Clark Jr WH, et al. Dysplastic nevi on the scalp of prepubertal children from melanoma-prone families. *J Pediatr*. 1983;103(1):65–69.

62. Bishop JA, Bradburn M, Bergman W, et al. Teaching non-specialist health care professionals how to identify the atypical mole syndrome phenotype: a multinational study. *Br J Dermatol*. 2000;142(2):331–337.

63. Newton Bishop JA, Bataille V, Pinney E, et al. Family studies in melanoma: identification of the atypical mole syndrome (AMS) phenotype. *Melanoma Res*. 1994;4(4):199–206.

64. Shea CR, Vollmer RT, Prieto VG. Correlating architectural disorder and cytologic atypia in Clark (dysplastic) melanocytic nevi. *Hum Pathol*. 1999;30(5):500–505.

65. Pozo L, Naase M, Cerio R, et al. Critical analysis of histologic criteria for grading atypical (dysplastic) melanocytic nevi. *Am J Clin Pathol*. 2001;115(2):194–204.

66. Kefford RF, Newton Bishop JA, Bergman W, et al. Counseling and DNA testing for individuals perceived to be genetically predisposed to melanoma: a consensus statement of the Melanoma Genetics Consortium. *J Clin Oncol*. 1999;17(10):3245–3251.

67. Gandini S, Sera F, Cattaruzza MS, et al. Meta-analysis of risk factors for cutaneous melanoma: III. Family history, actinic damage and phenotypic factors. *Eur J Cancer*. 2005;41(14):2040–2059.

68. Rhodes AR, Weinstock MA, Fitzpatrick TB, et al. Risk factors for cutaneous melanoma. A practical method of recognizing predisposed individuals. *JAMA*. 1987;258(21):3146–3154.

69. Hollenbeak CS, Todd MM, Billingsley EM, et al. Increased incidence of melanoma in renal transplantation recipients. *Cancer*. 2005;104(9):1962–1967.

70. Le Mire L, Hollowood K, Gray D, et al. Melanomas in renal transplant recipients. *Br J Dermatol*. 2006;154(3):472–477.

71. Ting W, Schultz K, Cac NN, et al. Tanning bed exposure increases the risk of malignant melanoma. *Int J Dermatol*. 2007;46(12):1253–1257.

72. International Agency for Research on Cancer Working Group on artificial ultraviolet (UV) light and skin cancer. The association of use of sunbeds with cutaneous malignant melanoma and other skin cancers: A systematic review. *Int J Cancer*. 2007;120(5):1116–1122.

73. Suh KY, Bolognia JL. Signature nevi. *J Am Acad Dermatol*. 2009;60(3):508–514.

74. Grob JJ, Bonerandi JJ. The 'ugly duckling' sign: identification of the common characteristics of nevi in an individual as a basis for melanoma screening. *Arch Dermatol*. 1998;134(1):103–104.

75. Goodson AG, Grossman D. Strategies for early melanoma detection: approaches to the patient with nevi. *J Am Acad Dermatol*. 2009;60(5):719–735 quiz 36-38.

76. Kittler H, Pehamberger H, Wolff K, et al. Diagnostic accuracy of dermoscopy. *Lancet Oncol*. 2002;3(3):159–165.

77. Vestergaard ME, Macaskill P, Holt PE, et al. Dermoscopy compared with naked eye examination for the diagnosis of primary melanoma: a meta-analysis of studies performed in a clinical setting. *Br J Dermatol*. 2008;159(3):669–676.

78. Salopek TG, Kopf AW, Stefanato CM, et al. Differentiation of atypical moles (dysplastic nevi) from early melanomas by dermoscopy. *Dermatol Clin*. 2001;19(2):337–345.

79. van der Rhee JI, Bergman W, Kukutsch NA. The impact of dermoscopy on the management of pigmented lesions in everyday clinical practice of general dermatologists: a prospective study. *Br J Dermatol*. 2010;162(3):563–567.

80. Terushkin V, Warycha M, Levy M, et al. Analysis of the benign to malignant ratio of lesions biopsied by a general dermatologist before and after the adoption of dermoscopy. *Arch Dermatol*. 2010;146(3):343–344.

81. Culpepper KS, Granter SR, McKee PH. My approach to atypical melanocytic lesions. *J Clin Pathol*. 2004;57(11):1121–1131.

82. Rigel D. *J Dermatol Surg Oncol*. 1985;11:745.

83. Farmer ER, Gonin R, Hanna MP. Discordance in the histopathologic diagnosis of melanoma and melanocytic nevi between expert pathologists. *Hum Pathol*. 1996;27(6):528–531.

84. Corona R, Mele A, Amini M, et al. Interobserver variability on the histopathologic diagnosis of cutaneous melanoma and other pigmented skin lesions. *J Clin Oncol*. 1996;14(4):1218–1223.

85. Urso C, Rongioletti F, Innocenzi D, et al. Interobserver reproducibility of histological features in cutaneous malignant melanoma. *J Clin Pathol.* 2005;58(11):1194–1198.

86. Cerroni L, Kerl H. Tutorial on melanocytic lesions. *Am J Dermatopathol.* 2001;23(3):237–241.

87. Barnhill RL. Malignant melanoma, dysplastic melanocytic nevi, and Spitz tumors. Histologic classification and characteristics. *Clin Plast Surg.* 2000;27(3):331–360 viii.

88. Meyer LJ, Piepkorn M, Goldgar DE, et al. Interobserver concordance in discriminating clinical atypia of melanocytic nevi, and correlations with histologic atypia. *J Am Acad Dermatol.* 1996;34(4):618–625.

89. Kmetz EC, Sanders H, Fisher G, et al. The role of observation in the management of atypical nevi. *South Med J.* 2009;102(1):45–48.

90. Slue W, Kopf AW, Rivers JK. Total-body photographs of dysplastic nevi. *Arch Dermatol.* 1988;124(8):1239–1243.

91. Banky JP, Kelly JW, English DR, et al. Incidence of new and changed nevi and melanomas detected using baseline images and dermoscopy in patients at high risk for melanoma. *Arch Dermatol.* 2005;141(8):998–1006.

92. Feit NE, Dusza SW, Marghoob AA. Melanomas detected with the aid of total cutaneous photography. *Br J Dermatol.* 2004;150(4):706–714.

93. Kittler H, Pehamberger H, Wolff K, et al. Follow-up of melanocytic skin lesions with digital epiluminescence microscopy: patterns of modifications observed in early melanoma, atypical nevi, and common nevi. *J Am Acad Dermatol.* 2000;43(3):467–476.

94. Robinson JK, Nickoloff BJ. Digital epiluminescence microscopy monitoring of high-risk patients. *Arch Dermatol.* 2004;140(1):49–56.

95. Kittler H, Binder M. Risks and benefits of sequential imaging of melanocytic skin lesions in patients with multiple atypical nevi. *Arch Dermatol.* 2001;137(12):1590–1595.

96. Argenziano G, Mordente I, Ferrara G, et al. Dermoscopic monitoring of melanocytic skin lesions: clinical outcome and patient compliance vary according to follow-up protocols. *Br J Dermatol.* 2008;159(2):331–336.

97. Kittler H, Guitera P, Riedl E, et al. Identification of clinically featureless incipient melanoma using sequential dermoscopy imaging. *Arch Dermatol.* 2006;142(9):1113–1119.

98. Menzies SW, Gutenev A, Avramidis M, et al. Short-term digital surface microscopic monitoring of atypical or changing melanocytic lesions. *Arch Dermatol.* 2001;137(12):1583–1589.

99. Menzies SW, Emery J, Staples M, et al. Impact of dermoscopy and short-term sequential digital dermoscopy imaging for the management of pigmented lesions in primary care: a sequential intervention trial. *Br J Dermatol.* 2009;161(6):1270–1277.

100. Carli P, De Giorgi V, Crocetti E, et al. Improvement of malignant/ benign ratio in excised melanocytic lesions in the 'dermoscopy era': a retrospective study 1997–2001. *Br J Dermatol.* 2004;150(4):687–692.

101. Tucker MA, Fraser MC, Goldstein AM, et al. Risk of melanoma and other cancers in melanoma-prone families. *J Invest Dermatol.* 1993;100(3):350S–355S.

102. Berwick M, Begg CB, Fine JA, et al. Screening for cutaneous melanoma by skin self-examination. *J Natl Cancer Inst.* 1996;88(1):17–23.

103. Gallagher RP, Rivers JK, Lee TK, et al. Broad-spectrum sunscreen use and the development of new nevi in white children: a randomized controlled trial. *JAMA.* 2000;283(22):2955–2960.

104. Goldstein AM, Tucker MA. Genetic epidemiology of familial melanoma. *Dermatol Clin.* 1995;13(3):605–612.

105. Weis E, Shah CP, Lajous M, et al. The association of cutaneous and iris nevi with uveal melanoma: a meta-analysis. *Ophthalmology.* 2009;116(3):536–543.e2.

106. Bataille V, Sasieni P, Cuzick J, et al. Risk of ocular melanoma in relation to cutaneous and iris naevi. *Int J Cancer.* 1995;60(5):622–626.

107. Bondi EE, Clark Jr WH, Elder D, et al. Topical chemotherapy of dysplastic melanocytic nevi with 5% fluorouracil. *Arch Dermatol.* 1981;117(2):89–92.

108. Edwards L, Jaffe P. The effect of topical tretinoin on dysplastic nevi. A preliminary trial. *Arch Dermatol.* 1990;126(4):494–499.

109. Halpern AC, Schuchter LM, Elder DE, et al. Effects of topical tretinoin on dysplastic nevi. *J Clin Oncol.* 1994;12(5):1028–1035.

110. Meyskens Jr FL, Edwards L, Levine NS. Role of topical tretinoin in melanoma and dysplastic nevi. *J Am Acad Dermatol.* 1986;15(4 Pt 2):822–825.

111. Stam-Posthuma JJ, Vink J, le Cessie S, et al. Effect of topical tretinoin under occlusion on atypical naevi. *Melanoma Res.* 1998;8(6):539–548.

112. Edwards L, Meyskens F, Levine N. Effect of oral isotretinoin on dysplastic nevi. *J Am Acad Dermatol.* 1989;20(2 Pt 1):257–260.

113. Dusza SW, Delgado R, Busam KJ, et al. Treatment of dysplastic nevi with 5% imiquimod cream, a pilot study. *J Drugs Dermatol.* 2006;5(1):56–62.

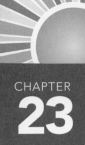

# Congenital Melanocytic Nevi

*Julie V. Schaffer, Harper N. Price, and Seth J. Orlow*

## Key Points

- Congenital melanocytic nevi (CMN) can have medical, cosmetic, and psychological consequences.

- The natural history of CMN may be dynamic and can include development of erosions and proliferative nodules during infancy, changes in pigmentation and topography, neurotization, and spontaneous regression.

- The risk of melanoma arising within a small or medium-sized CMN is low (<1% over a lifetime) and is extremely low before puberty.

- Melanoma develops in approximately 5% of patients with a large CMN, with half of this risk in the first few years of life; primary sites can be extracutaneous (e.g. the central nervous system).

- Both melanoma and neurocutaneous melanocytosis are most likely in patients with CMN that have a projected adult size of >40 cm in diameter, many satellite nevi, and (especially for melanoma risk) a truncal location.

- Management of CMN requires education of patients and parents to reduce unnecessary anxiety and an individualized approach to monitoring and treatment that depends on the size, location, and clinical morphology of the nevus and psychosocial concerns of the family.

## INTRODUCTION

Congenital melanocytic nevi (CMN) are classically defined as melanocytic nevi that are present at birth. A 'tardive' subset of CMN becomes evident during infancy or early childhood, usually before 2 years of age, and has clinical and histological features identical to those of 'true' CMN. The term congenital nevus-like nevus (CNLN) has also been utilized for lesions with clinical and/or histologic features of a CMN when the age of onset is unknown.[1]

A widely used classification system arbitrarily categorizes CMN into three groups according to the largest projected diameter in adulthood: (1) small, <1.5 cm; (2) medium, 1.5–20 cm; and (3) large, >20 cm (Fig. 23.1).[2] The latter size category roughly corresponds to >9 cm on the scalp and >6 cm on the body of a neonate. Because CMN enlarge in proportion to the child's growth, the final diameter can be predicted by estimating a size increase from infancy to adulthood by a factor of 2 on the head and a factor of 3 in other anatomic sites.[3,4] The term 'giant' is often reserved for

CMN with a final diameter of more than 40 cm. Other proposed classification systems for CMN are based upon the surface area or ease of surgical removal of the nevus (e.g. requirement for a skin graft or flap reconstruction to close the defect).

Small and medium-sized CMN can result in cosmetic issues with potential psychosocial impact and often produce anxiety in patients and parents, but the risk of associated melanoma is very low (<1% over a lifetime) and lower still prior to puberty. In contrast, large and/or numerous CMN can reflect a systemic disease process such as neurocutaneous melanocytosis (NCM) and confer a ~5% risk of melanoma that begins during early childhood. The management of patients with CMN must be individualized, with consideration of medical, cosmetic, and psychological concerns.

## EPIDEMIOLOGY

At least one pigmented lesion with the clinical or dermatoscopic features of a melanocytic nevus has been observed in 1–6% of neonates in large series,[5-9] and nevi may be evident at birth more frequently in individuals with darker skin.[7,8] In a recent clinical study, CMN/CNLN measuring ≥6 mm in diameter were observed in 17% of Italian schoolchildren (592/3406).[10] CNLN measuring ≥1.5 cm in diameter, thereby qualifying as medium-sized in the CMN classification, are clinically apparent in 1–4% of older children and adults.[10-13] Large CMN are rare in comparison, occurring in approximately 1 in 20,000 newborns.[14]

Although the vast majority of CMN occur sporadically, at least nine instances of familial clustering of large CMN have been reported.[15] Paradominant inheritance has been proposed as a possible genetic explanation for these observations. In this scenario, a heterozygous germline mutation would not be clinically evident and could be unknowingly transmitted in families until a 'second hit' in the normal copy of the gene occurred during embryogenesis, leading to nevus formation in a patchy (mosaic) distribution.

## PATHOGENESIS AND ETIOLOGY

Activating somatic mutations in genes that encode proteins within the RAS-extracellular signal-regulated kinase (ERK) signaling cascade are known to play a role in melanocytic tumorigenesis. The *BRAF^{V600E}* mutation is found in the majority of small CMN and CNLN, acquired melanocytic nevi, and superficial spreading melanomas. In contrast, more than two-thirds of medium-sized and large CMN

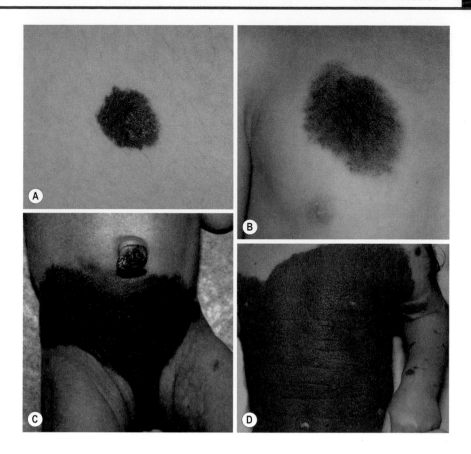

**Figure 23.1** The size range of congenital melanocytic nevi. Small **(A)**, medium-sized **(B)**, large **(C)**, and giant **(D)** congenital melanocytic nevi.

have activating mutations in the *NRAS* proto-oncogene, while *BRAF* mutations are uncommon.[16–18] *NRAS* mutations are also found in a small subset of melanomas (10–30%). This supports the existence of multiple pathways of melanocytic tumorigenesis, with *NRAS* mutations (which also activate phosphatidylinositol-3' signaling) perhaps exerting a stronger growth signal or having different consequences (e.g. with regard to cell migration) during embryogenesis than *BRAF* mutations. Overexpression of hepatocyte growth factor, a promoter of melanocyte proliferation and motility, and post-zygotic mutations in its receptor, the *MET* proto-oncogene, may also be involved in the development of large CMN and NCM.[19] Analysis of gene expression profiles in CMN may help to better understand their pathogenesis.

Both CMN and CNLN, especially those located on the head/neck and trunk (upper back>lower back), tend to have a globular dermatoscopic pattern.[20–22] In contrast, melanocytic nevi that develop in adolescents and adults or on the extremities frequently have a primarily reticular dermatoscopic pattern. It has been hypothesized that CNLN, particularly those with a globular dermatoscopic pattern, are 'programmed' from birth but delayed in becoming clinically apparent.[23] This may reflect a pathway of nevus development in which perturbation of melanoblast migration, which occurs in a cephalad-to-caudal and axial-to-peripheral sequence during embryogenesis, leads to abnormal 'rests' of nevus-precursor melanocytes within the

dermis.[21,23] Of note, incidental microscopic foci of dermal nevic aggregates (measuring ≤1.5 mm, so presumably inapparent clinically) were recently identified in 0.6% (16/2482) of skin excision specimens, most often those from the head/neck (63%) or trunk (25%).[24]

## CLINICAL FEATURES

Although CMN can be round or oval, they frequently have geographic or irregular borders (Fig. 23.2). Giant CMN are sometimes referred to as 'garment' or 'bathing trunk' nevi as a reflection of their distribution pattern (Fig. 23.3). Large and giant CMN are often accompanied by multiple small to medium-sized 'satellite' nevi that can be located anywhere on the skin. Satellite nevi may be present at birth or (especially for smaller lesions) become apparent during early childhood.

The color of CMN can range from tan to black and may be homogeneous or variegated. A CMN's surface may be smooth, mammillated, pebbly, verrucous, or even cerebriform (Fig. 23.4). Hypertrichosis is often evident.

### Natural history

CMN typically increase in size in proportion to the growth of the child, although some lesions grow more or less rapidly. Many CMN undergo additional morphologic changes over time. CMN that begin as flat, evenly pigmented lesions

**247**

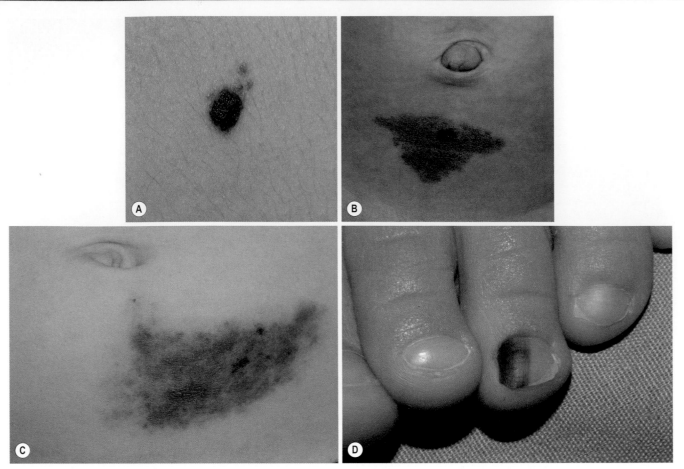

**Figure 23.2** Shapes of small and medium-sized congenital melanocytic nevi. These lesions can have irregular borders and geometric or geographic shapes **(A–C).** They can also present as a broad band of longitudinal melanonychia **(D).**

may become thicker or rugose and develop lighter, darker, mottled, or speckled pigmentation. Superimposed papules and nodules can appear within CMN (Fig. 23.5), and histologic evaluation to exclude the possibility of melanoma is occasionally necessary for focal changes with concerning features such as rapid growth, ulceration, or a black or red color. Dermal melanocytes within CMN frequently undergo 'neurotization' or peripheral nerve sheath differentiation. Clinically, neurotization can manifest as soft nodules (Fig. 23.6A), areas of compressibility and skin laxity, or bulky plexiform neurofibroma-like overgrowth.[25] Neurotized nevi on the scalp sometimes have a cerebriform morphology resembling cutis verticis gyrata, and alopecia may be evident. A decrease in the thickness of the subcutaneous fat underlying a medium-sized or large CMN represents another common observation, and scars occasionally appear without preceding trauma (Fig. 23.6A–C).

The evolution of CMN during the first few months of life can be particularly dynamic. Because of increased skin fragility, erosions or ulcerations may be seen in medium-sized or large CMN at birth or during the first 1–2 weeks of life (Fig. 23.6D).[26] Healing occurs within a few days to weeks. Rapidly growing benign proliferative nodules with

histologic features that mimic melanoma can arise within large CMN during infancy. Comparative genomic hybridization (CGH) of these proliferative nodules tends to show no chromosomal aberrations or only numeric changes (i.e. gains or losses of entire chromosomes) rather than the structural changes (i.e. gains or losses of chromosomal fragments) that characterize the vast majority of melanomas.[27,28] CGH can be performed on DNA extracted from paraffin-embedded tissue. Although costly, it may help to support the benign nature of histologically concerning lesions.

CMN, especially those of smaller size, are usually asymptomatic. However, patients with larger CMN on occasion experience pruritus, paresthesias, temperature sensitivity, and tenderness. The affected skin can become xerotic or eczematized, and the ability to sweat in response to warmer temperatures may be impaired.

## Spontaneous regression

CMN located on the scalp have a peculiar tendency to gradually lighten and regress over time. Complete or almost complete clinical resolution of medium-sized to large CMN on the scalp before the age of 4 years (mean, 30 months) has

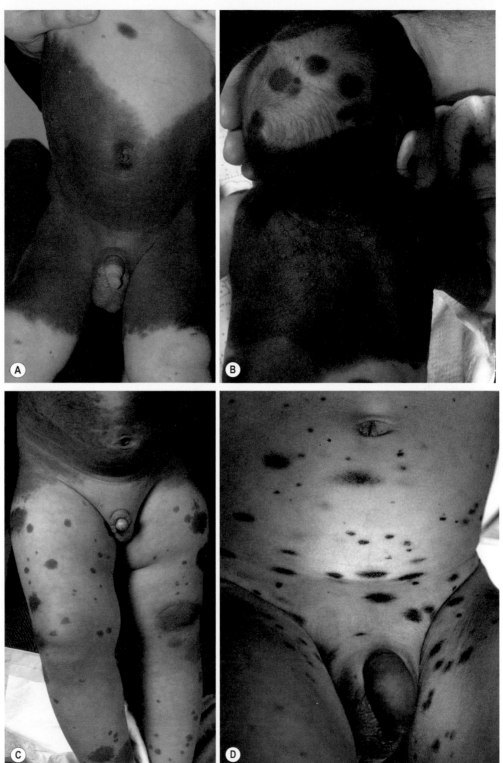

**Figure 23.3** Configurations of large and giant congenital melanocytic nevi. These lesions can have a distribution pattern reminiscent of a garment such as a bathing trunk **(A)** or cape **(B)**. They are often accompanied by multiple, widespread 'satellite' nevi **(C)**, which can also occur in the absence of a large 'mother ship' nevus **(D)**. The presence of numerous nevi represents an important risk factor for neurocutaneous melanocytosis.

been reported in at least seven children.[29,30] Histologic evaluation of two of these CMN revealed residual melanocytes in the deep dermis and within adnexal structures, and there was no evidence of fibrosis or inflammation.[30] Given the low risk of malignant transformation as well as the propensity to undergo regression, the authors are even less likely to recommend removal of CMN from the scalp than from other body locations.

The 'halo' phenomenon represents another means by which CMN can regress (Fig. 23.6E,F). Development of a symmetric or asymmetric depigmented halo around the CMN is followed by lightening and flattening of the nevus over a period of months to years. This process is thought to involve an immune response to melanocytic antigens,[31] and it is occasionally associated with the development of extra-lesional vitiligo.[32] The depigmented halo may be preceded

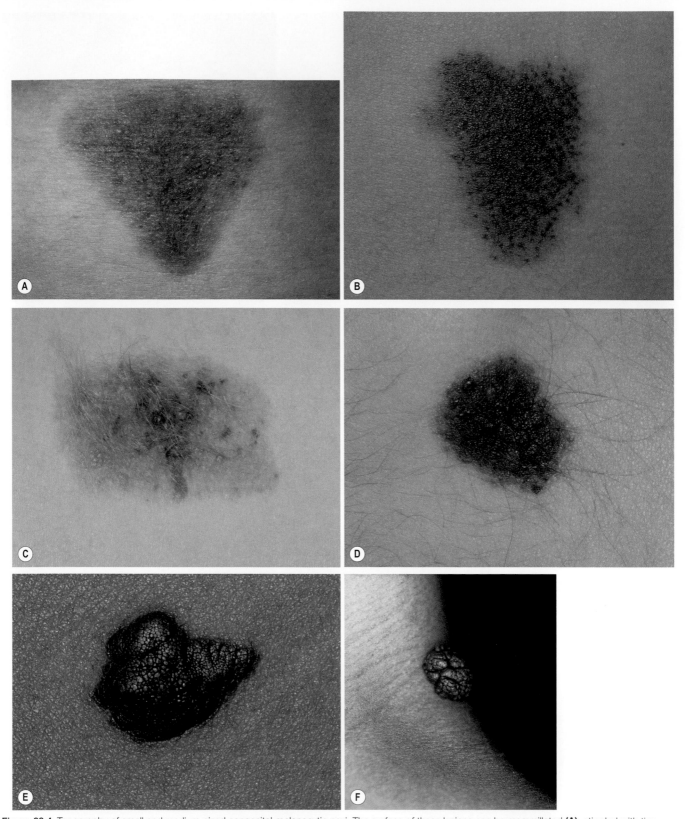

**Figure 23.4** Topography of small and medium-sized congenital melanocytic nevi. The surface of these lesions can be mammillated **(A)**, stippled with tiny follicular papules **(B)**, pebbly **(C,D)**, verrucous **(E)**, or cerebriform **(F)**. Hypertrichosis is often evident **(A,C,D)**.

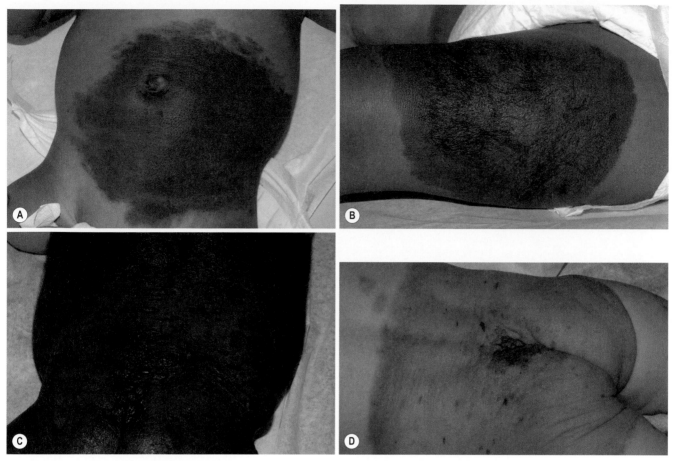

**Figure 23.5** Topography of large congenital melanocytic nevi. Common features include a leathery texture **(A)** and superimposed macules, papules and nodules **(A–D)** as well as hypertrichosis **(B).**

by an inflammatory phase with scaling and crusting; this may exist on a spectrum with the Meyerson phenomenon, a 'halo dermatitis' that is classically not associated with regression of the nevus.[33,34]

The 'desmoplastic hairless hypopigmented' variant of CMN also tends to undergo spontaneous resolution.[35]

These nevi are characterized by woody induration, lack of hair, progressive loss of pigmentation, and intense itching.[35,36] Histologically, dermal fibrosis, diminished or absent hair follicles, and a paucity of nevus cells are observed. The majority of these nevi soften and fade away over time.

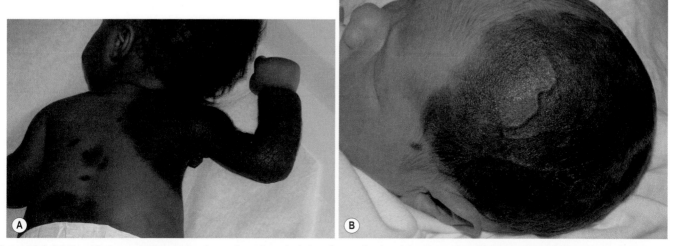

**Figure 23.6** Additional features of congenital melanocytic nevi may include soft neurotized nodules (**A;** see the axilla), lack of underlying subcutaneous fat **(A,B),**

*(Continued)*

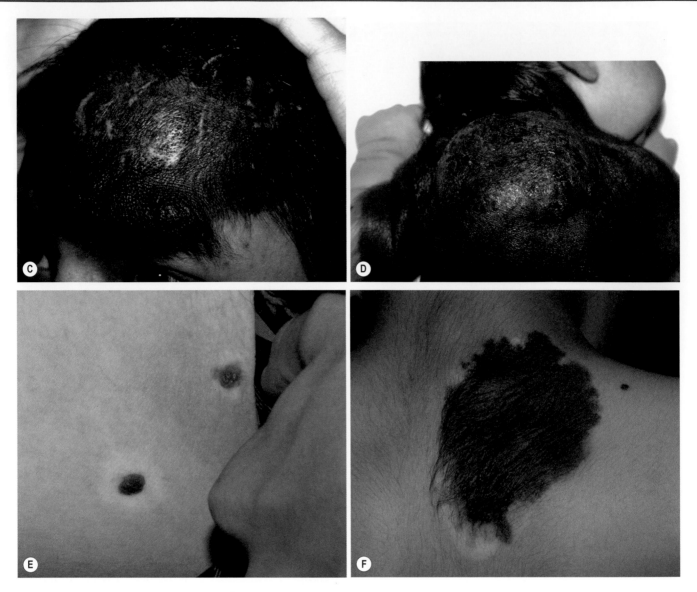

**Figure 23.6—cont'd** spontaneous scar formation **(C)**, erosions and proliferative nodules in the neonatal period **(D)**, and the halo phenomenon **(E,F)**. Note that the development of a halo often heralds lightening of the central nevus **(E)** and that the halo may be asymmetric **(F)**.

## Subtypes of CMN: speckled lentiginous nevi and congenital blue nevi

The 'speckled lentiginous nevus' (SLN) is a subtype of CMN that is evident in 2–3% of adults.[2,37] The tan café-au-lait macule-like background patch of an SLN is usually apparent at birth or during infancy, and superimposed macules and papules develop progressively over time. These 'spots' can range from lentigines to junctional, compound, and intradermal nevi to Spitz and blue nevi, and they may also exhibit hypertrichosis and histologic features of CMN (Fig. 23.7A–E). There are two distinct subtypes of SLN: (1) those with only macular speckles; and (2) those with papular as well as macular speckles.[38] Melanomas have been reported to arise within both macular and papular types of SLN, and the risk is thought to be proportional to the size of the lesion, as in classic CMN.[37,38]

Cellular blue nevi are often congenital. Like dermal melanocytoses, they have a predilection for the scalp, face, dorsal aspects of the distal extremities, and sacral area. Cellular blue nevi typically present as blue-grey to blue-black nodules or plaques with a smooth (Fig. 23.7F) or mammillated surface. Although congenital cellular blue nevi are usually 1–3 cm in diameter, larger lesions can occur and the melanocytes often extend deep into underlying tissues. Localized and disseminated satellite blue nevi have been observed in association with congenital cellular blue nevi.[39] Variants of congenital blue nevi include epithelioid (also referred to as pigmented epithelioid melanocytomas) and pauci-melanotic lesions. Plaque-type blue nevi (favoring the trunk) and neurocristic hamartomas (favoring the scalp) both present as a congenital bluish patch with superimposed blue-black papules and nodules. Neurocristic hamartomas also feature a perifollicular distribution of papules and schwannian differentiation. Melanoma has been reported to arise rarely within congenital cellular blue nevi, especially larger lesions located on the scalp.

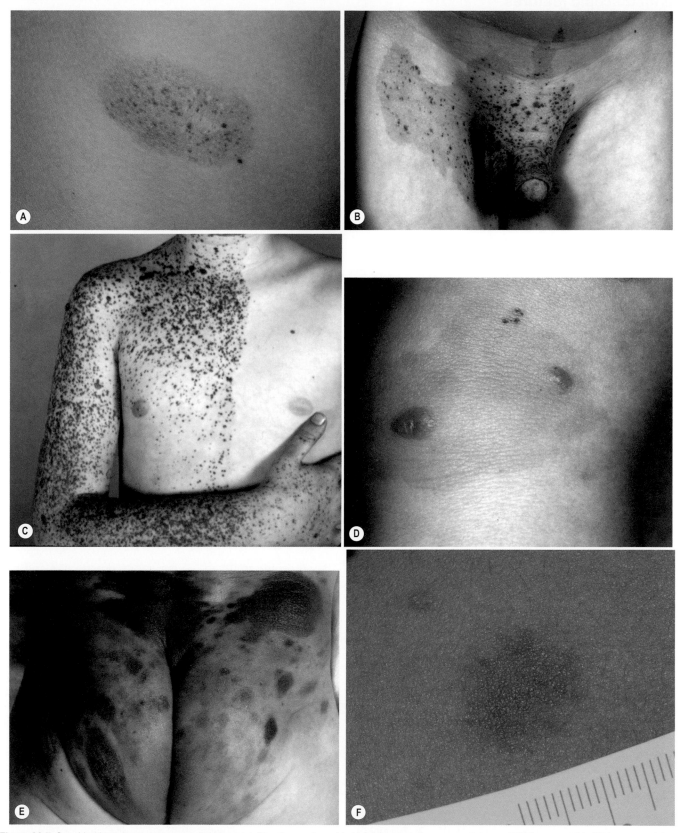

**Figure 23.7** Speckled lentiginous and congenital blue nevi. The shape of speckled lentiginous nevi can range from oval **(A)** to geographic **(B)** to segmental **(C)** with sharp midline demarcation. Superimposed macules and papules can represent Spitz nevi **(D)** and 'classic' congenital melanocytic nevi **(E)** as well as junctional, compound, and dermal nevi. Cellular blue nevi are often congenital and typically measure more than 1 cm in diameter; this lesion was firm to palpation and extended into the subcutis **(F)**.

## Dermatoscopic features

Dermatoscopic examination of CMN can aid in the clinical evaluation of these lesions. Most CMN have one of the following dermatoscopic patterns: (1) reticular (network); (2) globular; (3) reticuloglobular (globules centrally and network peripherally); and (4) diffuse pigmentation with or without remnants of a network or globules.[21] Other common features of CMN include milia-like cysts, hypertrichosis, and perifollicular hyperpigmentation or hypopigmentation. Dermatoscopy can help to characterize and follow subtle focal changes in CMN, thereby facilitating longitudinal observation.

## PATHOLOGY

Although the histologic features of congenital and acquired melanocytic nevi overlap, the following findings are characteristic of CMN: (1) nevus cells arranged 'single file' between collagen bundles; (2) nevus cells in the lower two-thirds of the reticular dermis and subcutaneous tissues; and (3) nevus cells around and within cutaneous appendages, nerves, and vessels.[40] The depth at which nevus cells may be found tends to correlate with the size of the CMN.[41] CMN in infants and young children often exhibit intraepidermal pagetoid spread of nevus cells, but cytologic atypia is usually absent or mild.[42]

Histologic evaluation of neurotized nevi reveals spindle cells with wavy nuclei and tapered ends embedded in a delicate fibrous stroma. 'Nevic corpuscles' reminiscent of neural Wagner–Meissner bodies may also be evident. The clinical and histologic features of neurotized CMN can closely mimic those of neurofibromas. However, although both are S-100 positive, only true neurofibromas typically stain with antibodies directed against Leu-7, glial fibrillary acidic protein, myelin basic protein, and factor XIIIa.[43]

Histologically, cellular blue nevi are characterized by: (1) melanin-rich dendritic dermal melanocytes within a fibrous stroma; and (2) islands of plump, spindle-shaped melanocytes with abundant cytoplasm. In congenital epithelioid blue nevi, melanin-laden, large, polygonal epithelioid melanocytes are found within the dermis and subcutis without a fibrous stroma.

## PATIENT EVALUATION, DIAGNOSIS AND DIFFERENTIAL DIAGNOSIS

History and physical examination are usually sufficient to diagnose a CMN. Parental report of the lesion being present at birth or during the first 2 years of life can help to determine whether a smaller melanocytic nevus is congenital or acquired. The clinical differential diagnosis for a CMN may include a café-au-lait macule, Becker's nevus or smooth muscle hamartoma, variant of dermal melanocytosis (e.g. Mongolian spot, nevus of Ota/Ito), mastocytoma, and plexiform neurofibroma. Dermatoscopy can be useful in distinguishing a CMN from these entities, and histologic evaluation may occasionally be required.

The medical, cosmetic, and psychological ramifications of a CMN vary greatly depending upon its size, location, and clinical appearance (e.g. brown-black, thick, and hairy *versus* tan and thin). Educating patients and parents about the benign nature and expected natural history of CMN is essential to avoid unnecessary anxiety and alleviate unfounded fears. Large CMN and those located in visible sites such as the face often have psychosocial consequences. For example, children with large CMN are more likely to experience depression, display aggressive behavior, and have social problems.[44] Patients and families dealing with such issues may benefit from psychological or family counseling and internet support groups such as Nevus Network (www.nevusnetwork.org) and Nevus Outreach, Inc. (www.nevus.org).

## POTENTIAL COMPLICATIONS

### Risk of melanoma in patients with small and medium-sized nevi

The risk of melanoma occurring within a small or medium-sized CMN is thought to be far less than 1% over a lifetime, but the low frequency has made it difficult for even large studies to establish a more precise estimate of risk (Table 23.1).[45,46,48,50,54,56] For example, no melanomas were observed in three cohort studies including a total of 680 patients with small and/or medium-sized CMN who were followed for a mean of 13.5 years (mean age at entry ~10 years).[45,48,56] Similarly, no patients younger than 20 years of age developed a melanoma within a CMN smaller than 5 cm in diameter over a period of more than 30 years at the New York University Pigmented Lesion Clinics and the Massachusetts General Hospital.[40,58] When melanomas do occur in association with a small or medium-sized CMN, they typically develop after puberty (usually in adulthood) and arise at the dermoepidermal junction (Fig. 23.8), which facilitates early detection. There is no evidence that ultraviolet light plays a role in the development of melanoma within a CMN.

### Risk of melanoma and other malignancies in patients with large CMN

Based on the results of several large, prospective and retrospective cohort studies, the lifetime risk of melanoma in patients with large CMN is currently thought to be approximately 5% (see Table 23.1).[25,45-47,51-54] Previous estimates of considerably higher risk incorporated data from small, retrospective case series emanating from tertiary referral centers, which have inherent selection biases.[59] About half of melanomas in patients with large CMN occur during the first 5 years of life.[47,52,60] However, benign proliferative nodules with histologic features that simulate melanoma may also develop during infancy and represent a possible cause of overestimated risk for this age group. The 39 melanomas in patients with large CMN reported in large studies during the past two decades (see Table 23.1) were diagnosed at a median age of 3.5 years (range, birth to 58 years). These melanomas occurred within CMN on the trunk (27) more often than within CMN on the head/neck (3) or an extremity (1); melanomas also arose in the central nervous system (CNS; 3) and retroperitoneum (2) or from an unknown primary site (3).[25,45-47,51-54] Melanomas tend to develop in the deep dermal or subcutaneous portions of large CMN, making early detection difficult. Rhabdomyosarcomas, liposarcomas, and malignant peripheral nerve sheath tumors have also been reported in association with large CMN.[61]

## Table 23.1 Selected Studies of Melanoma Risk in Congenital Melanocytic Nevi (CMN)*

| Reference | Number of Patients | Mean Age at Entry, Years | Mean Follow-up Time, Years | Number of Patients with Melanoma (% of Total) | Locations of Primary Melanoma |
|---|---|---|---|---|---|
| **Prospective cohort studies of *large* CMN** | | | | | |
| Ruiz-Maldonado et al., 1992 | 80 | 1.7 | 4.7 | 2 (2.5) | All cutaneous/axial |
| Egan et al., 1998 | 46 | 8.4 | 7.3 | 2 (4.3) | All cutaneous/axial |
| Hale et al., 2005 | 170[†] | 1.2 | 5.3 | 4[‡] (2.4) | CNS (2), retroperitoneum (1), unknown (1) |
| **Internet registry-based studies of *large* CMN[§]** | | | | | |
| Bett, 2005 | 861 | NA | (5.6)[¶] | 16 (1.9) Garment CMN: 15/525 (2.9) Head/extremity CMN: 1/336 (0.3) | Cutaneous/axial (14), retroperitoneum (1), unknown (1) |
| Ka et al., 2005 | 379 | 8 | 2–6 | 0 (0) | --- |
| **Retrospective cohort studies of *large* CMN** | | | | | |
| Foster et al., 2001 | 46 | 0.5 | 5 | 0 (0) | --- |
| Lovett et al., 2009 | 52 | 1.3 | 7.4 | 0 (0) | --- |
| **Retrospective cohort study of *medium-sized* CMN** | | | | | |
| Sahin et al., 1998 | 227 | 19 | 6.7 | 0 (0) | --- |
| **Prospective cohort studies of CMN of all sizes** | | | | | |
| Dawson et al., 1996 | 133 | 3.1 | 3.4 | 0 (0) | --- |
| Kinsler et al., 2009 | 349[¶¶] | 2.9 | 9.2 | ≥20 cm CMN: 4[‡]/122 (3.3) 1–19 cm CMN: 0/214 (0) Multiple CMN: 1/13 (7.7) | Cutaneous/axial (2), CNS (2), unknown (1) |
| **Retrospective cohort study of CMN of all sizes** | | | | | |
| Swerdlow et al., 1995 | 265 | (84% <15 y) | 24 | ≥20 cm CMN: 2[‡]/26 (7.6) 5–19 cm CMN: 0/84 (0) 1–4.9 cm CMN: 0/155 (0) | All cutaneous/axial |
| Fernandes et al., 2009 | 74 | 4 | 6 | ≥20 cm CMN: 0/5 (0) <20 cm CMN: 0/69 (0) | --- |
| **Retrospective population-based studies of CMN of all sizes** | | | | | |
| Berg & Lindelöf, 2003 | 3922 | 0 | 10 (median) | 0 (0) | --- |
| Zaal et al., 2005 | 3929 | 19 | 4.7 | >20 cm CMN: 4/320 (1.3) ≤20 cm CMN: 11/3609 (0.3) | Cutaneous/axial (9), cutaneous/extremity (6) |

NA, not available.

* Includes longitudinal studies of ≥40 patients with CMN followed for a mean of ≥3 years that have been published since 1990.[25,45–57]

† Among 35 additional patients who were not followed prospectively, 5 developed melanoma (all within a truncal CMN).

‡ All melanomas developed in association with CMN measuring: ≥39 cm (Hale et al.); >40 cm (Swerdlow et al.); >60 cm (Kinsler et al.)

§ Information was obtained by voluntary report of members of support groups for patients with congenital melanocytic nevi and not confirmed by the physician/medical record.

¶ Melanomas diagnosed prior to entry into the registry were not excluded.

¶¶ Includes 48 patients who were not followed prospectively.

Adapted with permission from Schaffer JV. Pigmented lesions in children: when to worry. Curr Opin Pediatr 2007;19:430-40.

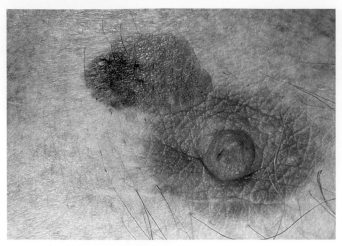

**Figure 23.8** Melanoma arising within a small congenital melanocytic nevus (CMN). This in-situ/minimally invasive melanoma developed at the dermoepidermal junction at the edge of a small CMN in a 70-year-old man. The CMN was present since birth by history and visible in photographs of the patient as a baby. (Courtesy of Ashfaz A Marghoob, MD.)

Factors that increase the likelihood of melanoma include a CMN with a projected adult size of >40 cm in diameter, a truncal location, and numerous (e.g. >20) satellite nevi.[51,52,56,59] Thus far, there have been no well-documented reports of a primary cutaneous melanoma arising within a satellite nevus. However, in an internet registry-based study that lacked physician confirmation of patient information, a young woman was described as having two melanomas, one within her large truncal CMN at age 7 years and one within a satellite nevus on an extremity at age 18 years.[51]

### Risk of neurocutaneous melanocytosis in patients with large and/or multiple CMN

NCM refers to the association of melanocytic nevi with proliferation of benign or malignant melanocytes within the CNS, where melanocytes are physiologically present in the pia mater of the meninges. NCM is divided into symptomatic and symptomatic subsets, and individuals with both cutaneous and CNS melanoma are excluded due to the possible metastatic origin of the CNS lesions.[62] Gadolinium-enhanced magnetic resonance imaging (MRI) of the brain and spine can detect NCM, and it is most sensitive during infancy before progressive myelination potentially obscures the melanin signal.[49] MRI findings of NCM can include areas of brain parenchyma (especially the temporal lobes/amygdala and cerebellum) with increased T1 signal, enhancement of diffusely thickened meninges, and obvious masses.[63] CNS abnormalities such as the Dandy–Walker malformation, posterior fossa cysts, intraspinal lipomas, and a tethered spinal cord have also been described in patients with large CMN.

The presence of numerous CMN, regardless of whether or not there is a 'mother ship' large CMN, represents an important risk factor for NCM.[52,57,64,65] Patients with a large CMN accompanied by satellite nevi account for approximately two-thirds of cases, and those with many small to medium-sized CMN comprise the remaining one-third of cases.[62] Among patients with a large CMN, individuals with >20 satellite nevi are five times more likely to have NCM than

those with ≤20 satellite nevi.[64] An increased risk of NCM has also been observed in patients with CMN that have a final size of >40 cm or (in some but not all studies) a posterior axial location.[64,65]

*Symptomatic NCM* occurs in approximately 4% of patients with high-risk CMN, and the prognosis is poor even in the absence of melanoma.[52,66,67] Patients typically present with hydrocephalus, seizures, and other signs of increased intracranial pressure (e.g. vomiting). Symptoms develop at a median age of 2 years, although patients with a discrete intracranial mass tend to become symptomatic somewhat later, at a median age of 9 years, and are more likely to have focal neurologic deficits.[63] In a recent series, clinical neurologic abnormalities such as developmental delay (motor or cognitive) and abnormal tone were observed in 15% (18/120) of children with high-risk CMN.[65] These findings were more common in boys than girls, and one-quarter of the affected children (5/18) had normal brain MRIs.

*Asymptomatic NCM* can be diagnosed in 5–25% of infants and children with high-risk CMN, based on evidence of CNS melanosis via screening MRI.[49,52,57,65,66] Because of the paucity of longitudinal studies of asymptomatic NCM, the proportion of these patients destined to become symptomatic from NCM is unknown. In one study, 10 patients with asymptomatic NCM diagnosed at a mean age of 6 months were followed for 5 years, and only one individual developed neurologic symptoms.[49]

## MANAGEMENT

### Management of small and medium-sized CMN

Small and medium-sized CMN can be managed on an individual basis, with consideration of the following factors (Table 23.2):

- history of medically worrisome changes
- cosmetic concerns or functional issues
- anxiety level of the patient and parents
- awareness and medical sophistication of the patient and parents
- ease of monitoring, which depends upon the location of the nevus, amount and regularity of pigmentation, thickness and topography, and degree of hypertrichosis.

The authors and others do not recommend routine 'prophylactic' removal of small and medium-sized CMN.[4,40,60,68] One common indication for early surgical excision is a facial CMN with an obviously problematic cosmetic appearance (Fig. 23.9A,B), where the goal is to prevent psychosocial impact during the school-age years. Surgical removal can also be considered for nevi with features that compromise the ability to follow the lesion clinically, such as a thick, extremely rugose or multinodular plaque with irregular dark pigmentation, especially if there are other obstacles to monitoring (e.g. a hidden location, reluctant patient/family).

Periodic evaluation of small and medium-sized CMN is most important after puberty, since the risk of melanoma arising within a small or medium-sized CMN during childhood is negligible. Patients and parents should be instructed to perform (self-) skin examinations and to bring

**Table 23.2 Factors that May Affect the Management of Small and Medium-Sized Congenital Melanocytic Nevi***

| | Features that May Prompt Biopsy or Excision | Features that Favor Observation |
|---|---|---|
| Changes in the nevus | Focal changes with characteristics such as rapid evolution, ulceration, colors (e.g. black or red) not found elsewhere in the nevus, and irregular pigmentation or shape | Changes in color, thickness, topography (e.g. pebbling, verrucosity), or 'speckling' with superimposed macules and papules that occur throughout the nevus or in a symmetric pattern |
| Functional issues | Bulky or protuberant lesion that interferes with daily activities or is irritated/traumatized by clothing/shaving/etc. | |
| Cosmetic concerns | Location on face (> other highly visible areas), especially if: Larger lesion Conspicuous site (e.g. tip of nose) 'Ugly' lesion (e.g. thick, warty, hairy) | Location in a less visible area or a lesion with an appearance that is more cosmetically appealing than the expected surgical scar |
| Anxiety level of patient and parents | Excessively high level of anxiety about the lesion despite counseling | High level of anxiety about surgical procedures |
| Awareness and medical sophistication of patient and parents | Reluctant or unable to periodically evaluate lesion | Willing and able to periodically evaluate lesion |
| Ease of observation: Location Pigmentation Topography Hypertrichosis | Hidden site (e.g. buttock) Black or dark and irregular Thick, multinodular, rugose Very dense | Accessible site Uniformly tan or brown Thin and uniform Minimal |

*When different features point management in opposite directions, the factors can be weighted on an individual basis. For example, patients and parents may choose to monitor nevi in hidden sites or covered with hair on the scalp because they are of little cosmetic concern, whereas nevi on the face are often excised for cosmetic reasons even though they can be more easily observed.

focal changes in color, border, or topography to a physician's attention. Baseline photographs can be helpful, and dermatoscopy represents a useful tool for monitoring focal changes within nevi.

If removal of a small or smaller medium-sized CMN is desired, it can often be accomplished with simple excision and primary closure. Flap reconstruction or serial excision may be necessary for larger lesions or those in challenging locations, and these methods can also improve cosmetic and functional outcomes. Patients and parents should be counseled to have realistic expectations regarding the healing process and resulting scar. If removal is prompted by cosmetic concerns, whether or not the expected scar would represent an improvement over the appearance of the nevus should be considered. Occasionally, a medium-sized CMN cannot be excised without risking functional impairment (Fig. 23.9C). In the absence of anticipated psychosocial or functional issues, it is usually recommended that elective removal of small and medium-sized CMN be delayed until around puberty, when the patient can participate in the decision-making process and tolerate the procedure under local anesthesia.

Laser treatment (see below) may reduce the pigmentation of thin medium-sized CMN that are not amenable to surgical excision because of their anatomic location (e.g. the periorbital area or nasal ala). Hair removal lasers can also reduce the hypertrichosis associated with some CMN.[69]

## Management of large CMN

Early and complete removal of large CMN is often attempted as 'prophylaxis' against the development of melanoma.[4,70] However, it is frequently impossible to fully remove extensive lesions, and nevus cells can involve deeper structures such as fascia and muscle. For example, patients who have undergone 'complete' excision of a large CMN have been reported to develop melanoma underneath skin grafts placed over the surgical defect.[51] Because melanomas can arise in the CNS and other extracutaneous sites, the risk of melanoma would not be eliminated even with complete removal of the nevus. Although a nonsignificant trend toward lower incidence of melanoma has been noted in patients whose large CMN were partially or completely excised,[70] the largest nevi, which have a higher risk of melanoma, are also more likely to be deemed inoperable. Performing an appropriately powered prospective trial to determine the efficacy of prophylactic excision of large CMN in preventing melanoma would be extremely difficult due to the rarity of these lesions, the relatively low incidence of melanoma even without surgical intervention, and the potentially confounding medical and psychosocial factors that contribute to surgical decision making.

When deciding whether or not to pursue surgical intervention for large CMN, treatment-related morbidities and potential complications as well as cosmetic and functional benefits should be considered. Although patients and parents often indicate that scars are cosmetically and socially more acceptable than a large CMN, a recent survey found that those with larger nevi were less likely to feel that their surgical intervention had been worthwhile (Fig. 23.9D).[71,72] Excision of nevi (or portions thereof) that are bulky and cumbersome can be beneficial. However, surgical interventions entail short-term discomfort, limitation of physical activity, and risk of infection, as well as possible long-term complications such as scars that restrict joint mobility. Excision of

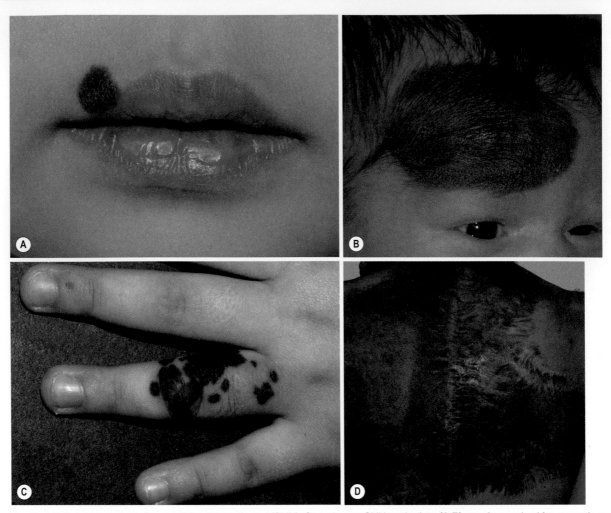

**Figure 23.9** Considerations in the management of congenital melanocytic nevi (CMN). Conspicuous CMN on the face **(A,B)** are often excised for cosmetic and psychosocial reasons. Some medium-sized CMN, such as this circumferential lesion on the finger **(C),** are not amenable to excision without risking functional impairment. Complete excision of giant CMN may not be feasible, and surgeries can result in broad, thick scars with recurrent pigment **(D).**

large CMN is often initiated during the first 2 years of life, with purported advantages of increased skin elasticity and a lower risk of hypertrophic scarring during this period.[4] Unfortunately, pigmentation frequently recurs within or at the edges of scars from these early excisions, likely related to the full extent of CMN not becoming apparent until after 2 years of age.[4,71,72]

Staged excision (down to fascia) with tissue expansion of uninvolved adjacent or distant skin and flap reconstruction are often utilized for large CMN. These methods are relatively well tolerated in young children. Excision followed by skin grafting or the use of artificial skin substitutes or cultured epithelial autographs tends to have inferior aesthetic and functional outcomes.[73]

When surgical excision of large CMN is not feasible, other techniques such as curettage, dermabrasion, and ablative laser therapy (e.g. carbon dioxide or erbium:YAG) may be of cosmetic benefit. These procedures remove only the epidermis and upper portion of the dermis, which is replaced by a layer of scar tissue that may become hypertrophic or result in skin fragility. The best time for treatment is during the neonatal period, when 'active' pigment-producing nevus cells are concentrated in the upper half of the dermis and excessive scarring is less likely.[74] The window for effective

treatment of CMN with curettage, which takes advantage of a temporary neonatal cleavage plane in the upper dermis of these lesions, is limited to the first few weeks of life. Because nevus cells remain in the dermis after these procedures, repigmentation often occurs and melanoma can develop in treated areas.[75]

Controversy exists regarding the use of laser therapy for CMN, as long-term follow-up data are limited. As noted above, laser treatment can be particularly useful for thin facial CMN that are not amenable to surgical intervention. In addition to ablative lasers that non-selectively vaporize tissue, ruby, alexandrite, and Nd:YAG lasers that specifically target melanin within nests of melanocytes (long-pulsed lasers) or melanosomes (Q-switched lasers) have also been employed to treat CMN.[76] Selective lasers have a lower potential for scar formation and can decrease the pigmentation and/or hypertrichosis within CMN, but (as with purely ablative techniques) dermal melanocytes remain under a thin layer of fibroplasias and repigmentation rates are high.[77] A combination of pigment-specific and ablative lasers has also been used.[78] Continued monitoring of the residual nevus is necessary following any type of laser treatment. One case report documented the occurrence of a superficial spreading melanoma at the periphery of a large CMN in a 27-year-old woman whose nevus had been treated with an argon laser 10 years prior.[79]

Regardless of the treatment modalities employed, life-long surveillance of patients with large CMN is necessary. In addition to parent/self skin examination, patients should be followed with periodic total skin examinations by a dermatologist, with the aid of dermatoscopy and baseline photographs; palpation of regional lymph nodes is also recommended. During the examination, palpation of the nevus and scars is essential for detection of firm nodules or focal induration. These and other suspicious changes, such as papules or nodules with rapid growth, foci with colors atypical of the lesion, or ulcers outside of the neonatal period, should be examined histologically. In order to avoid misinterpretation of proliferative nodules and other atypical but benign changes as melanoma, evaluation of biopsy specimens by a dermatopathologist experienced in pigmented lesions is important when concerning histologic features are identified.

## Screening for and management of neurocutaneous melanocytosis

Patients with a large CMN plus satellite nevi or multiple CMN alone can be screened for the presence of NCM with gadolinium-enhanced MRI of the brain and spine during infancy (Fig. 23.10). The ideal time for imaging is during the first 4–6 months of life, prior to myelination that may obscure evidence of melanosis. Such patients should also be followed with serial neurologic examinations and developmental assessment, and those with abnormal clinical or MRI findings can be referred to a pediatric neurologist for further monitoring. Repeat MRI studies are indicated if clinical manifestations develop or, for patients who remain asymptomatic, on an approximately annual basis that can vary depending on the severity and progression of the MRI findings. Evidence of NCM on MRI does not necessarily preclude skin surgery, but aggressive prophylactic removal of CMN should be postponed in patients with symptomatic NCM or asymptomatic disease with particularly worrisome features. In a recent study, 7 of 18 CMN patients with abnormal MRI findings required neurosurgical intervention, suggesting that MRI screening can influence patient care.[65]

## FUTURE OUTLOOK

Large cohort studies have helped to redefine the likelihood of melanoma developing within a large CMN as approximately 5%, with the highest risk in 'giant' truncal lesions, and to confirm the low incidence of melanoma in small and medium-sized CMN. Recent studies have also pointed to the presence of numerous CMN (e.g. satellite nevi) as the primary risk factor for NCM, documented the presence of asymptomatic NCM (based upon MRI evidence of CNS melanosis) in 5–25% of pediatric patients with high-risk CMN, and drawn attention to subtle neurologic abnormalities in patients with large CMN. In the future, additional longitudinal studies of CMN patients will be essential in determining the significance of MRI findings in asymptomatic patients and the effects of surgical interventions on risk of melanoma. In addition, tissue banking will be crucial for molecular studies to elucidate the genetic alterations underlying CMN and associated proliferative nodules and melanomas.

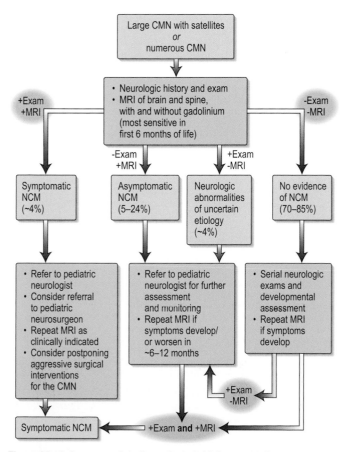

**Figure 23.10** An approach to the patient at risk for neurocutaneous melanocytosis (NCM). CMN, congenital melanocytic nevus; MRI, magnetic resonance imaging.

## REFERENCES

1. Kopf AW, Bart RS, Hennessey P. Congenital nevocytic nevi and malignant melanomas. *J Am Acad Dermatol*. 1979;1:123–130.
2. Kopf AW, Levine LJ, Rigel DS, et al. Prevalence of congenital-nevus-like nevi, nevi spili, and café-au-lait spots. *Arch Dermatol*. 1985;121:766–769.
3. Marghoob AA, Schoenbach SP, Kopf AW, et al. Large congenital melanocytic nevi and the risk for the development of malignant melanoma: a prospective study. *Arch Dermatol*. 1996;132:170–175.
4. Tromberg J, Bauer B, Benvenuto-Adrade C, et al. Congenital nevi needing treatment. *Dermatol Ther*. 2005;18:136–150.
5. Walton RG, Jacobs AH, Cox AJ. Pigmented lesions in newborn infants. *Br J Dermatol*. 1976;95:389–396.
6. Alper JC, Holmes LB. The incidence and significance of birthmarks in a cohort of 4641 newborns. *Pediatr Dermatol*. 1983;1:58–68.
7. Osburn K, Schosser RH, Everett MA. Congenital pigmented and vascular lesions in newborn infants. *J Am Acad Dermatol*. 1987;16:788–792.
8. Rivers JK, Frederiksen PC, Dibdin C. A prevalence survey of dermatoses in the Australian neonate. *J Am Acad Dermatol*. 1990;23:77–81.
9. Boccardi D, Menni S, Ferraroni M, et al. Birthmarks and transient skin lesions in newborns and their relationship to maternal factors: a preliminary report from northern Italy. *Dermatology*. 2007;215:53–58.
10. Gallus S, Naldi L. Oncology Study Group of the Italian Group for Epidemiologic Research in Dermatology. Distribution of congenital melanocytic naevi and congenital naevus-like naevi in a survey of 3406 Italian schoolchildren. *Br J Dermatol*. 2008;159:433–438.
11. Clemmensen OJ, Kroon S. The histology of "congenital features" in early acquired melanocytic nevi. *J Am Acad Dermatol*. 1988;19:742–764.

12. Sigg C, Pelloni F, Schnyder UW. Frequency of congenital nevi, nevi spili and café-au-lait spots and their relation to nevus count and skin complexion in 939 children. *Dermatologica*. 1990;180:118–123.

13. Ingordo V, Gentile C, Iannazzone SS, et al. Congenital melanocytic nevus: an epidemiologic study in Italy. *Dermatology*. 2007;214:227–230.

14. Castilla EE, Dutra MD, Orioli-Parreiras IM. Epidemiology of congenital pigmented naevi: I. Incidence rates and relative frequencies. *Br J Dermatol*. 1982;104:307–315.

15. De Wijn RS, Zaal LH, Hennekam RC, et al. Familial clustering of giant congenital melanocytic nevi. *J Plast Reconstr Aesthet Surg*. 2010;63:906–913.

16. Ichii-Nakato N, Takata M, Takayanagi S, et al. High frequency of BRAF$^{V600E}$ mutation in acquired nevi and small congenital nevi, but low frequency of mutation in medium-sized congenital nevi. *J Invest Dermatol*. 2006;126:2111–2118.

17. Bauer J, Curtin JA, Pinkel D, et al. Congenital melanocytic nevi frequently harbor NRAS mutations but no BRAF mutations. *J Invest Dermatol*. 2007;127:179–182.

18. Dessars B, De Raeve LE, Morandini R, et al. Genotypic and gene expression studies in congenital melanocytic nevi: insight into initial steps of melanotumorigenesis. *J Invest Dermatol*. 2009;129:139–147.

19. Takayama H, Nagashima Y, Hara M, et al. Immunohistochemical detection of the c-met proto-oncogene product in the congenital melanocytic nevus of an infant with neurocutaneous melanosis. *J Am Acad Dermatol*. 2001;44:538–540.

20. Seidenari S, Pellacani G, Martella A, et al. Instrument-, age- and site-dependent variations of dermoscopic patterns of congenital melanocytic naevi: a multicentre study. *Br J Dermatol*. 2006;155:56–61.

21. Changchien L, Dusza SW, Agero AL, et al. Age- and site-specific variation in the dermoscopic patterns of congenital melanocytic nevi: an aid to accurate classification and assessment of melanocytic nevi. *Arch Dermatol*. 2007;143:1007–1014.

22. Scope A, Marghoob AA, Dusza SW, et al. Dermoscopic patterns of naevi in fifth grade children of the Framingham school system. *Br J Dermatol*. 2008;158:1041–1049.

23. Zalaudek I, Hofmann-Wellenhof R, Soyer HP, et al. Naevogenesis: new thoughts based on dermoscopy. *Br J Dermatol*. 2006;154:793–794.

24. Dadzie OE, Goerig R, Bhawan J. Incidental microscopic foci of nevic aggregates in skin. *Am J Dermatopathol*. 2008;30:45–50.

25. Ruiz-Maldonado R, Tamayo L, Laterza AM, et al. Giant pigmented nevi: clinical, histopathologic, and therapeutic considerations. *J Pediatr*. 1992;120:906–911.

26. Giam YC, Williams ML, Leboit PE, et al. Neonatal erosions and ulcerations in giant congenital melanocytic nevi. *Pediatr Dermatol*. 1999;16:354–358.

27. Bastian BC, Xiong J, Frieden IJ, et al. Genetic changes in neoplasms arising in congenital melanocytic nevi: differences between nodular proliferations and melanomas. *Am J Pathol*. 2002;161:1163–1169.

28. Murphy MJ, Jen M, Chang MW, et al. Molecular diagnosis of a benign proliferative nodule developing in a congenital melanocytic nevus in a 3-month-old infant. *J Am Acad Dermatol*. 2008;59:518–523.

29. Strauss RM, Newton Bishop JA. Spontaneous involution of congenital melanocytic nevi of the scalp. *J Am Acad Dermatol*. 2008;58:508–511.

30. Vilarrasa E, Baselga E, Rincon C, et al. Histologic persistence of a congenital melanocytic nevus of the scalp despite clinical involution. *J Am Acad Dermatol*. 2008;59:1091–1092.

31. Tokura Y, Yamanaka K, Wakita H, et al. Halo congenital nevus undergoing spontaneous regression: involvement of T cell immunity in the involution and presence of circulating anti-nevus cell IgM antibodies. *Arch Dermatol*. 1995;130:1036–1041.

32. Stierman SC, Tierney EP, Shwayder TA. Halo congenital nevocellular nevi associated iwth extralesional vitiligo: a case series and review of the literature. *Pediatr Dermatol*. 2009;26:414–424.

33. Patrizi A, Neri I, Sabattini E, et al. Unusual inflammatory and hyperkeratotic halo naevus in children. *Br J Dermatol*. 2005;152:357–360.

34. Rolland S, Kokta V, Marcoux D. Meyerson phenomenon in children: observation in five cases of congenital melanocytic nevi. *Pediatr Dermatol*. 2009;26:292–297.

35. Ruiz-Maldonado R, Orozco-Covarrubias L, Ridaura-Sanz C, et al. Desmoplastic hairless hypopigmented naevus: a variant of giant congenital melanocytic naevus. *Br J Dermatol*. 2003;148:1253–1257.

36. Martin JM, Jorda E, Monteaqudo C, et al. Desmoplastic giant congenital nevus with progressive depigmentation. *J Am Acad Dermatol*. 2007;56:S10–S14.

37. Schaffer JV, Orlow SJ, Lazova R, et al. Speckled lentiginous nevus: within the spectrum of congenital melanocytic nevi. *Arch Dermatol*. 2001;137:172–178.

38. Vidaurri-de la Cruz H, Happle R. Two distinct types of speckled lentiginous nevi characterized by macular versus papular speckles. *Dermatology*. 2006;212:53–58.

39. Serarslan G, Yaldiz M, Verdi M. Giant congenital cellular blue naevus of the scalp with disseminated common blue naevi of the body. *J Eur Acad Dermatol Venereol*. 2009;23:190–191.

40. Tannous ZS, Mihm MC, Sober AJ, et al. Congenital melanocytic nevi: clinical and histopathologic features, risk of melanoma, and clinical management. *J Am Acad Dermatol*. 2005;52:197–203.

41. Barnhill RL, Fleischli M. Histologic features of congenital melanocytic nevi in infants 1 year of age or younger. *J Am Acad Dermatol*. 1995;33:780–785.

42. Haupt HM, Stern JB. Pagetoid melanocytosis. Histologic features in benign and malignant lesions. *Am J Surg Pathol*. 1995;19:792–797.

43. Gray MH, Smoller BR, McNutt NS, et al. Neurofibromas and neurotized melanocytic nevi are immunohistochemically distinct neoplasms. *Am J Dermatopathol*. 1990;12:234–241.

44. Koot HM, de Waard-van der Spek F, Peer CD, et al. Psychosocial sequelae in 29 children with giant congenital melanocytic naevi. *Clin Exp Dermatol*. 2000;25:589–593.

45. Swerdlow AJ, English JS, Qiao Z. The risk of melanoma in patients with congenital nevi: a cohort study. *J Am Acad Dermatol*. 1995;32:595–599.

46. Dawson HA, Atherton DJ, Mayou B. A prospective study of congenital melanocytic naevi: progress report and evaluation after 6 years. *Br J Dermatol*. 1996;134:617–623.

47. Egan CL, Oliveria SA, Elenitsas R, et al. Cutaneous melanoma risk and phenotypic changes in large congenital nevi: a follow-up study of 46 patients. *J Am Acad Dermatol*. 1998;39:923–932.

48. Sahin S, Levin L, Kopf AW, et al. Risk of melanoma in medium-ized congenital melanocytic nevi: a follow-up study. *J Am Acad Dermatol*. 1998;39:428–433.

49. Foster RD, Williams ML, Barkovich AJ, et al. Giant congenital melanocytic nevi: the significance of neurocutaneous melanosis in neurologically asymptomatic children. *Plast Reconstr Surg*. 2001;107:933–941.

50. Berg P, Lindelöf B. Congenital melanocytic naevi and cutaneous melanoma. *Melanoma Res*. 2003;13:441–445.

51. Bett BJ. Large or multiple congenital melanocytic nevi: occurrence of cutaneous melanoma in 1008 persons. *J Am Acad Dermatol*. 2005;52:793–797.

52. Hale EK, Stein J, Ben-Porat L, et al. Association of melanoma and neurocutaneous melanocytosis with large congenital melanocytic naevi: results from the NYU-LCMN registry. *Br J Dermatol*. 2005;152:512–517.

53. Ka VS, Dusza SW, Halpern AC, et al. The association between large congenital melanocytic naevi and cutaneous melanoma: preliminary findings from an Internet-based registry of 379 patients. *Melanoma Res*. 2005;15:61–67.

54. Zaal LH, Mooi WJ, Klip H, et al. Risk of malignant transformation of congenital melanocytic nevi: a retrospective nationwide study from The Netherlands. *Plast Reconstr Surg*. 2005;116:1902–1909.

55. Fernandes NC, Machado JL. Clinical study of congenital melanocytic naevi in the child and adolescent. *An Bras Dermatol*. 2009;84:129–135.

56. Kinsler VA, Birley J, Atherton DJ. Great Ormond Street Hospital for Children Registry for congenital melanocytic naevi: prospective study 1988-2007. Part 1-epidemiology, phenotype and outcomes. *Br J Dermatol*. 2009;160:143–150.

57. Lovett A, Maari C, Decarie JC, et al. Large congenital melanocytic nevi and neurocutaneous melanocytosis: one pediatric center's experience. *J Am Acad Dermatol*. 2009;61:766–774.

58. Scalzo DA, Hida CA, Toth G, et al. Childhood melanoma: a clinicopathological study of 22 cases. *Melanoma Res*. 1997;7:63–68.

59. Krengel S, Hauschild A, Schafer T. Melanoma risk in congenital melanocytic naevi: a systematic review. *Br J Dermatol*. 2006;155:1–8.

60. Marghoob AA. Congenital melanocytic nevi. Evaluation and management. *Dermatol Clin*. 2002;20:607–616.

61. Gruson LM, Orlow SJ, Schaffer JV. Phacomatosis pigmentokeratotica associated with hemihypertrophy and a rhabdomyosarcoma of the abdominal wall. *J Am Acad Dermatol*. 2006;55:S16–S20.

62. Kadonaga JN, Frieden IJ. Neurocutaneous melanosis: definition and review of the literature. *J Am Acad Dermatol*. 1991;24:747–755.

63. Schaffer JV, McNiff JM, Bolognia JL. Cerebral mass due to neurocutaneous melanosis: eight years later. *Pediatr Dermatol*. 2001;18:369–377.

64. Marghoob AA, Dusza S, Oliveria S, et al. Number of satellite nevi as a correlate for neurocutaneous melanocytosis in patients with large congenital melanocytic nevi. *Arch Dermatol*. 2004;140:171–175.

65. Kinsler VA, Chong WK, Aylett SE, et al. Complications of congenital melanocytic naevi in children: analysis of 16 years' experience and clinical practice. *Br J Dermatol*. 2008;159:907–914.

66. Agero AL, Benvenuto-Andrade C, Dusza SW, et al. Asymptomatic neurocutaneous melanocytosis inpatients with large congenital melanocytic nevi: a study of cases from an Internet-based registry. *J Am Acad Dermatol*. 2005;53:959–965.

67. Bett BJ. Large or multiple congenital melanocytic nevi: occurrence of neurocutaneous melanocytosis in 1008 persons. *J Am Acad Dermatol*. 2006;54:767–777.

68. Makkar HS, Frieden IJ. Congenital melanocytic nevi: an update for the pediatrician. *Curr Opin Pediatr*. 2002;14:397–403.

69. Rajpar SF, Hague JS, Abdullah A, et al. Hair removal with the long-pulse alexandrite and long-pulse Nd:YAG lasers is safe and well tolerated in children. *Clin Exp Dermatol*. 2009;34:684–687.

70. Marghoob AA, Agero AL, Benvenuto-Andrade C, et al. Large congenital melanocytic nevi, risk of cutaneous melanoma, and prophylactic surgery. *J Am Acad Dermatol.* 2006;54:868–873.

71. Kinsler VA, Birley J, Atherton DJ. Great Ormond Street Hospital for Children Registry for Congenital Melanocytic Naevi: prospective study 1988-2007. Part 2–Evaluation of treatments. *Br J Dermatol.* 2009;160:387–392.

72. Mérigou D, Prey S, Niamba P, et al. Management of congenital nevi at a dermatologic surgical paediatric outpatient clinic: consequences of an audit survey 1990-1997. *Dermatology.* 2009;218:126–133.

73. Earle SA, Marshall DM. Management of giant congential nevi with artificial skin substitutes in children. *J Craniofac Surg.* 2005;16:904–907.

74. De Raeve LE, Claes A, Ruiter DJ, et al. Distinct phenotypic changes between the superficial and deep component of giant congenital melanocytic naevi: a rationale for curettage. *Br J Dermatol.* 2006;154:485–492.

75. Dragieva G, Hafner J, Künzi W, et al. Malignant melanoma in a large congenital melanocytic nevus 9 years after dermabrasion in childhood. *Dermatology.* 2006;212:208–209.

76. Kishi K, Okabe K, Ninomiya R, et al. Early serial X-switched ruby laser therapy for medium-sized to giant congenital melanocytic naevi. *Br J Dermatol.* 2009;161:345–352.

77. Imayama S, Ueda S. Long- and short-term histological observations of congenital nevi treated with the normal-mode ruby laser. *Arch Dermatol.* 1999;135:1211–1218.

78. Dave R, Mahaffey PJ. Combined early treatment of congenital melanocytic naevus with carbon dioxide and Nd:YAG lasers. *Br J Plast Surg.* 2004;57:720–724.

79. Woodrow SL, Burrows NP. Malignant melanoma occurring at the periphery of a giant congenital naevus previously treated with laser therapy. *Br J Dermatol.* 2003;149:886–888.

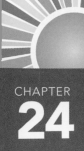

CHAPTER
# 24

# The Many Faces of Melanoma

*Darrell S. Rigel*

The incidence of malignant melanoma continues to increase at an alarming rate. In the US, melanoma is the only major cancer where incidence is still rising and the reported incidence of melanoma may be lower than the actual rates.[1,2] In 2010, the lifetime risk for an American developing invasive malignant melanoma was 1 in 58 and, should the current rate of increase continue, will be 1 in 50 by the year 2015 (Fig. 24.1).[3]

Melanoma is the most clear-cut form of cancer where early detection is a critical factor influencing survival. Patients diagnosed with melanoma in its earliest phase have an almost 100% chance of surviving their disease, while those with advanced disease at the time of diagnosis have an extremely poor prognosis. With incidence rates for this cancer continuing to rise, the importance of the clinician being able to recognize melanoma as early as possible has become even more essential.

However, melanoma can present clinically with many faces, from the early flat lesions often described using the ABCDE system (**A**symmetry, **B**order Irregularity, **C**olor variegation, **D**iameter >6 mm and **E**volving)[4] to more advanced lesions demonstrating elevation, ulceration and bleeding. The purpose of the atlas is to depict many of the typical (and not as typical) presentations of melanoma to help enhance the reader's diagnostic skills for earlier detection of this cancer.

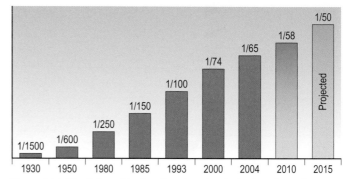

**Figure 24.1** The lifetime risk of an American developing invasive melanoma by year.

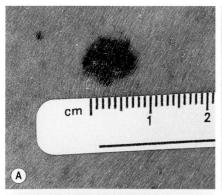

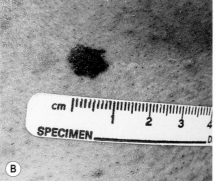

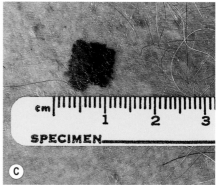

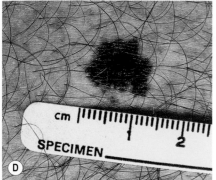

**Figure 24.2** Early melanomas displaying the ABCD signs. (Images courtesy of New York University Department of Dermatology.)

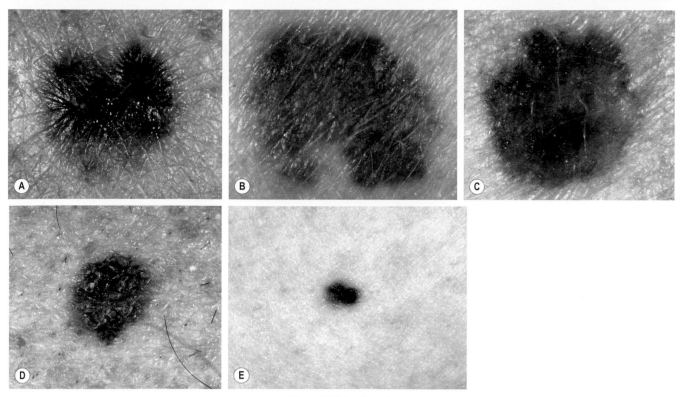

**Figure 24.3** In-situ melanomas.

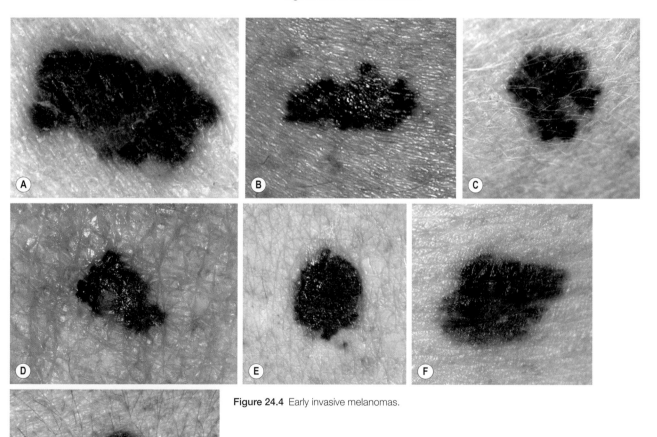

**Figure 24.4** Early invasive melanomas.

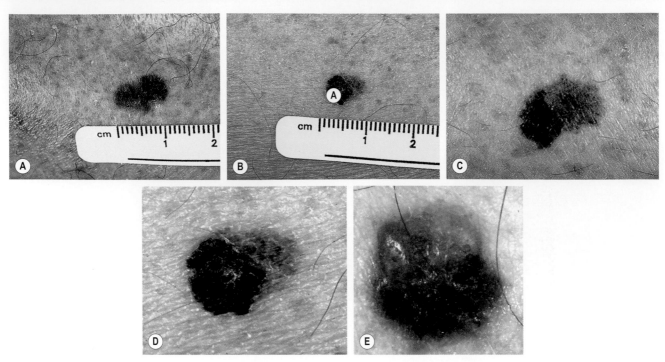

Figure 24.5 Melanoma arising in a pre-existing nevus. (A,B: Images courtesy of New York University Department of Dermatology.)

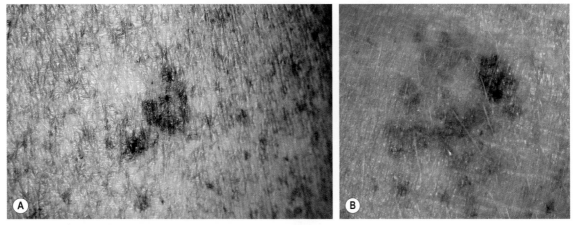

Figure 24.6 Desmoplastic melanomas with typical subtle presentation.

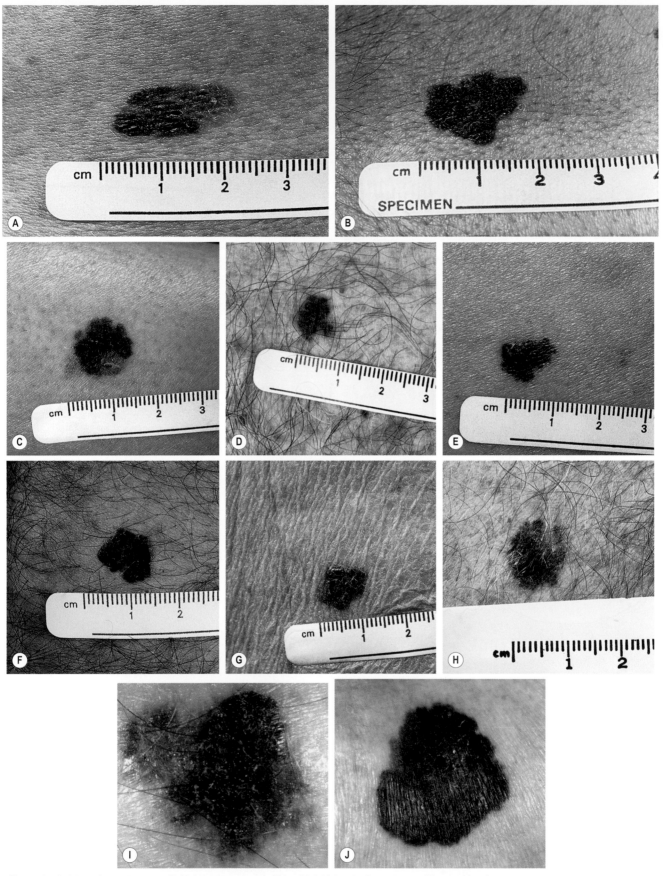

**Figure 24.7** Advancing melanomas. (A-H: Images courtesy of New York University Department of Dermatology.)

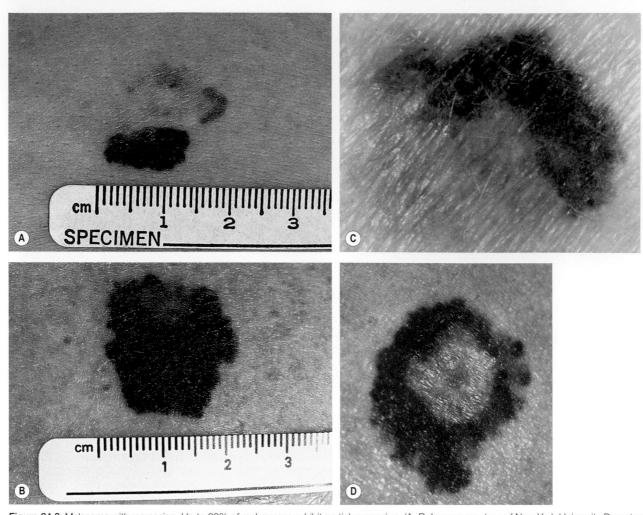

**Figure 24.8** Melanoma with regression. Up to 20% of melanomas exhibit partial regression. (A, B: Images courtesy of New York University Department of Dermatology.)

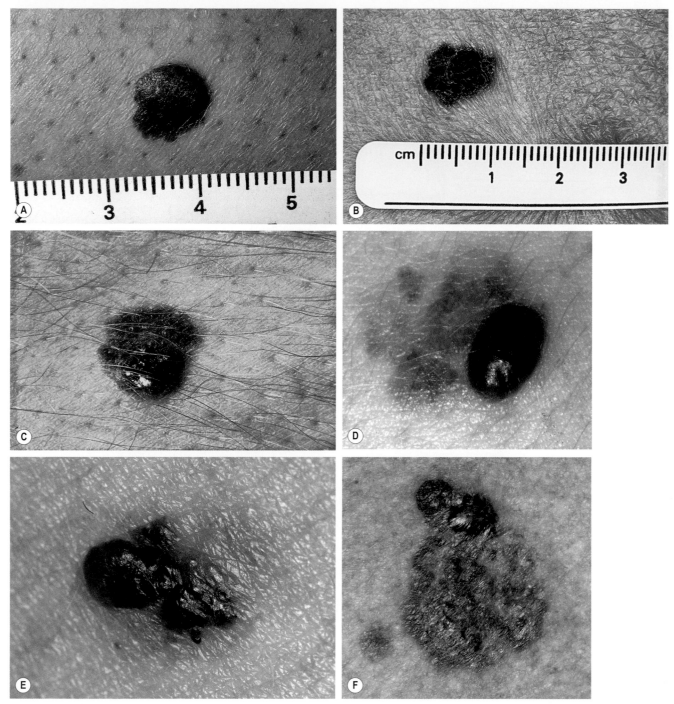

**Figure 24.9** Nodular melanomas. (A-C: Images courtesy of New York University Department of Dermatology.)

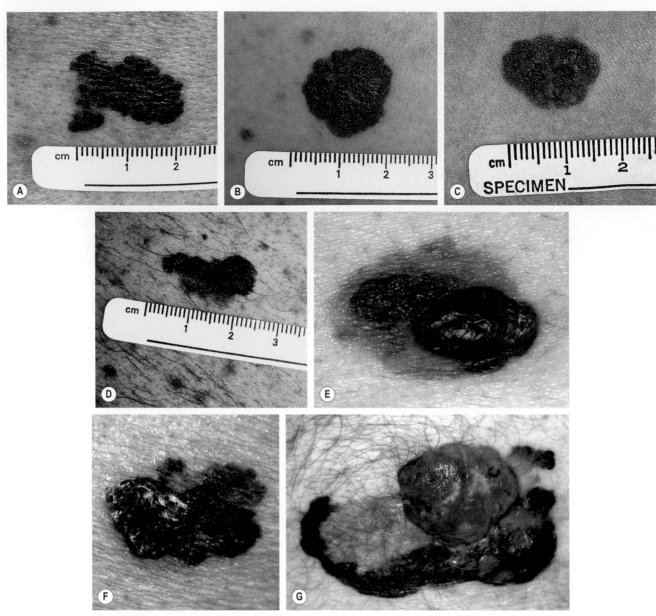

**Figure 24.10** Later presentations of melanoma. (10 A-D, F, image courtesy of New York University Department of Dermatology.)

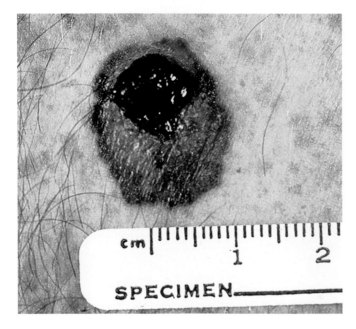

**Figure 24.11** Melanoma with clinical ulceration (presence of this factor significantly worsens prognosis). (Image courtesy of New York University Department of Dermatology.)

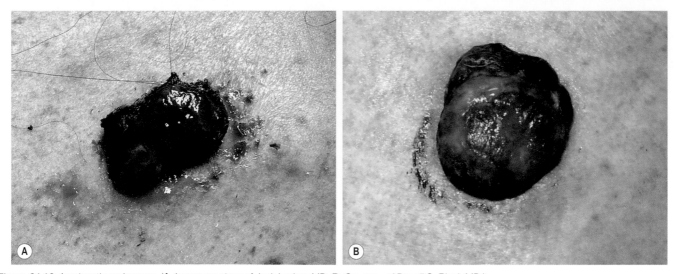

**Figure 24.12** Amelanotic melanoma. (**A,** image courtesy of Jack Lesher, MD. **B,** Courtesy of Darrell S. Rigel, MD.)

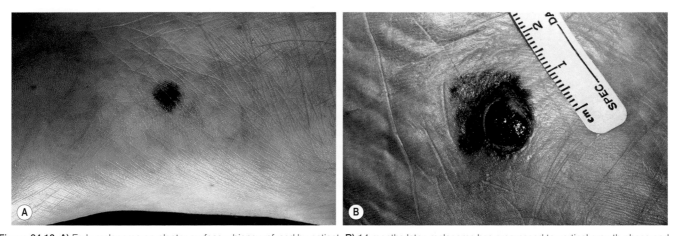

**Figure 24.13 A)** Early melanoma on plantar surface – biopsy refused by patient. **B)** 14 months later, melanoma has progressed to vertical growth phase and nodule. Patient expired 4 months later. (Images courtesy of New York University Department of Dermatology.)

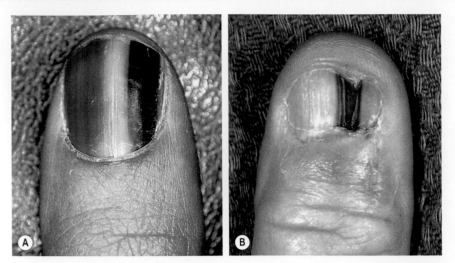

**Figure 24.14** Melanoma arising in nail. Note subtle pigment in proximal nail fold (Hutchinson's sign).

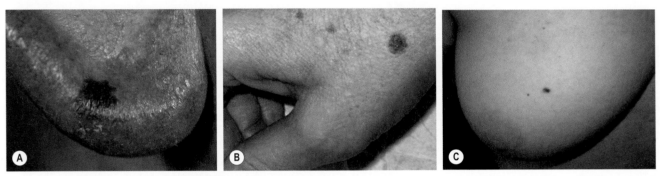

**Figure 24.15** Melanoma in unusual places. **A)** Invasive melanoma on earlobe. **B)** Invasive melanoma on base of thumb. **C)** In-situ melanoma on breast. (Courtesy of Darrell S. Rigel, MD)

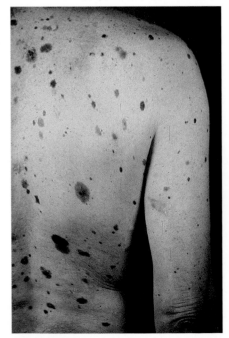

**Figure 24.16** Patient with history of multiple primary melanomas with 'classic' dysplastic nevus syndrome. (Image courtesy of New York University Department of Dermatology.)

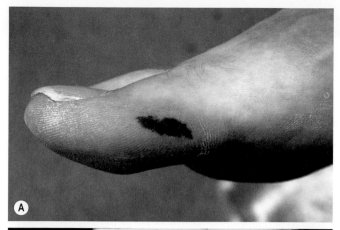

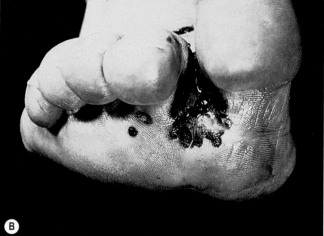

**Figure 24.17 A)** Early melanoma on toe. **B)** More advanced melanoma on the foot. (Image courtesy of New York University Department of Dermatology.)

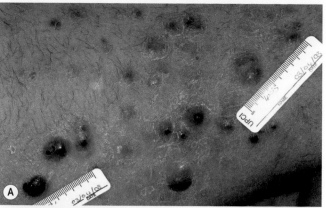

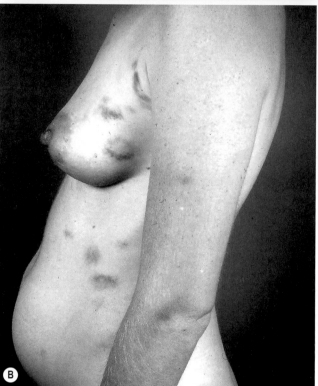

**Figure 24.18 A)** Metastatic melanoma on a thigh. **B)** Metastatic melanoma in a pregnant woman. (Image courtesy of New York University Department of Dermatology.)

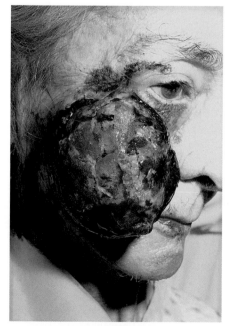

**Figure 24.19** Advanced melanoma (52 mm in thickness) of the cheek. (Image courtesy of New York University Department of Dermatology.)

## REFERENCES

1.  Merlino LA, Sullivan KJ, Whitaker DC, et al. The independent pathology laboratory as a reporting source for cutaneous melanoma incidence in Iowa, 1977–1994. *J Am Acad Dermatol.* 1997;37(4):578–585.

2.  Cockburn M, Swetter SM, Peng D, et al. Melanoma underreporting: why does it happen, how big is the problem, and how do we fix it? *J Am Acad Dermatol.* 2008;59(6):1081–1085.

3.  Rigel DS. Trends in dermatology: melanoma incidence. *Arch Dermatol.* 2010;146(3):318.

4.  Robinson JK, Ortiz S. Use of photographs illustrating ABCDE criteria in skin self-examination. *Arch Dermatol.* 2009;145(3):332–333.

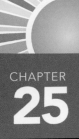

# The Importance of Early Detection of Melanoma, Physician and Self-Examination

*Julie E. Russak, Darrell S. Rigel, and Robert J. Friedman*

---

## Key Points

- The incidence of melanoma has been increasing faster than that of any other cancer in the United States.

- Early detection of melanoma is critical for better patient survival.

- Many early melanomas can be recognized with the help of the ABCDEs, and new evolving techniques using complex computer algorithms will augment the effectiveness of early diagnosis.

- Public and professional education, regular full-body skin examination by the clinician, and self-examination of the skin are vitally important public health components for reducing deaths from melanoma.

## INTRODUCTION

Melanoma is an increasingly important public health problem in the United States and worldwide. The incidence of melanoma has been increasing faster than that of any other cancer in the United States.[1] US invasive melanoma incidence increased 3.1% (p<0.001) annually from 1992. Statistically significant increases are occurring for all histologic subtypes and thicknesses, including those greater than 4 mm. Invasive melanoma currently is the fifth most common cancer in men and the seventh most frequently found cancer in women in the US. A total of 68,180 newly diagnosed cases of invasive melanoma and 46,770 cases of in-situ melanoma were expected in 2010.[2] At current rates, the lifetime risk of an American developing invasive melanoma is 1 in 59 overall and 1 in 37 for Caucasian men and 1 in 56 for Caucasian women. This contrasts dramatically with a lifetime risk of 1 in 1500 for Americans born in 1935.[3] Melanoma is also the most fatal of skin cancers, accounting for 79% of all skin cancer deaths.[4]

The importance of diagnosing melanoma early in its evolution cannot be understated. Since prognosis in melanoma is directly proportional to the depth of the neoplasm, detection of melanoma early in its evolution is of critical importance in saving lives. Melanoma initially grows horizontally within the epidermis (melanoma in situ). In time, it then penetrates into the dermis ('invasive melanoma').[5] The vertical depth of the melanoma (measured downward from stratum granulosum) has been shown in multivariate analyses to be the factor that best correlates with prognosis. Therefore, more accurate and effective early diagnosis leading to earlier treatment is critical to successful management.

Fortunately, there has been steady improvement in melanoma survival over decades, with the 5-year survival for invasive melanoma rising from 82% in 1979 to 92% in 2002.[6] Since the primary treatment modality of cutaneous melanoma, surgical excision, has not changed substantially over the past several decades, the improved 5-year survival rate can be primarily attributed to earlier detection.

Earlier detection and therapy also leads to decreased cost of therapy. An estimated 90% of costs spent on melanoma therapy in the US are related to those with advanced disease.[7] Therefore, a significant saving in healthcare cost can be realized if melanoma can be detected in an earlier, more easily treatable phase.

The standard method to evaluate a skin growth to rule out melanoma is biopsy followed by histopathological examination. The challenge lies in identifying the appropriate 'spot(s)' on patients who have multiple lesions that have the highest probability for being melanoma. Such lesions should be biopsied and their histopathology appropriately evaluated at the earliest possible time in their evolution. Through education of both healthcare professionals and the lay public as to methods of identifying melanoma, routine physician-driven total cutaneous examinations, and through the teaching of patient self-examination, physicians can play a significant role in reducing deaths from melanoma.

## HISTORY OF MELANOMA DIAGNOSIS

A century ago, melanoma was often not diagnosed until metastatic disease was present. However, diagnostic accuracy has significantly improved over the past 30 years where there has been a significant evolution in the diagnosis of early melanoma[8] (Table 25.1). Several factors have contributed to a marked improvement in detection of cutaneous melanomas at an early, curable stage. Prior to the 1980s, there had been little change in identifying melanoma as the diagnosis was made by identifying gross clinical features. Melanomas were often recognized only when they were large, ulcerated and fungating (see Chapter 24 for clinical presentations). By that time, prognosis was poor. Overall melanoma incidence and mortality continued to increase in the United States and elsewhere, making the early recognition of melanoma a critical public health priority.[9]

The goal for every clinician involved in melanoma diagnosis is to strive to increase the ability to detect melanoma at the earliest stage in its development and to promptly remove it. Historically, there are much data to support the fact that melanomas early in their development (in situ or

Table 25.1 Evolution of Melanoma Diagnosis

| Years | Diagnostic Features | Factors |
|---|---|---|
| 1960–70s | Gross symptoms | Bleeding, ulceration |
| 1980s | Clinical | ABCDs |
| 1990s | Subsurface | Dermoscopy |
| 2000s | Digital | Computer-aided analysis |

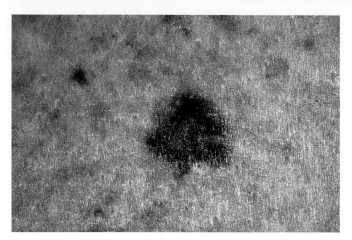

**Figure 25.1** Malignant melanoma, in situ, chest, illustrating significant clinical asymmetry, along with border irregularity and subtle variability in color. The lesion measures 7.2 mm in diameter.

very thin lesions) have an excellent prognosis.[10] Alexander Breslow in 1970 was the first to show that metastases generally did not occur in lesions <0.76 mm in thickness.[11] The fact that early melanomas have excellent prognoses has been repeatedly confirmed by many investigators.[12]

## CLINICAL CONSIDERATIONS

### Important factors in early diagnosis of melanoma

In order for the clinician to make a clinical diagnosis of a possible melanoma, he/she must have a high index of suspicion for melanoma and a thorough knowledge of:

- the clinical features of early melanomas (Chapter 24)
- the clinical features of common pigmented lesions that must be differentiated from melanoma
- the characteristics and clinical features of variants of clinically atypical melanocytic nevi (i.e. dysplastic nevi) which may be more commonly seen in association with a higher risk for and/or together with melanoma (Chapters 22 and 23)
- other factors that increase the risk for a patient developing melanoma: e.g. personal and/or family history of melanoma, history of other non-melanoma skin cancer, presence of dysplastic nevi, presence of many (>100) melanocytic nevi, intermittent sun exposure and sunburn history, history of tanning-booth exposure, especially in childhood/adolescence, red/blonde hair, light eyes, fair complexion, freckling, etc (Chapters 5 and 6).

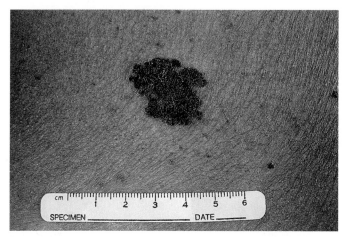

**Figure 25.2** Malignant melanoma, predominantly in situ, but focally measuring approximately 0.22 mm in greatest thickness, trunk, illustrating classic border irregularity, coupled with lesion asymmetry and very subtle play in color from dark brown/black to medium brown. The lesion measures about 13 mm in greatest diameter. (Image courtesy of New York University Department of Dermatology.)

### Clinical characteristics of early melanoma

In 1985, recognizing the critical need to educate physicians and the lay public to recognize melanoma in its early clinical presentation, our group at New York University devised the *ABCD* acronym (*A*symmetry, *B*order irregularity, *C*olor variegation, *D*iameter >6 mm).[13,14]

That study[13] demonstrated that most early melanomas demonstrate the following features:

- *Asymmetry* – they generally cannot be easily divided in half and have one half look like the other (Fig. 25.1).
- *Border irregularity* – the borders of most early melanomas are irregularly shaped (Fig. 25.2).
- *Color variability* – most early melanomas have a play in color ranging from subtle nuances of tans and browns, to areas of black, and, more rarely, red, white (regression) and blue (deeper pigment) (Fig. 25.3). Keep in mind,

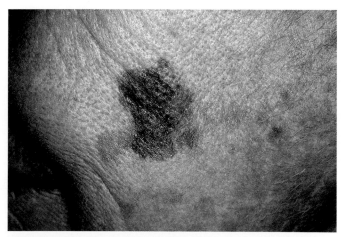

**Figure 25.3** Malignant melanoma, predominantly in situ of face, illustrating a play in color from tan to brown with a focal amelanotic (pink/red) component. There was a focal dermal component to this lesion measuring about 0.18 mm in thickness. The lesion is quite large, measuring over 20 mm in diameter. It also exhibits lesion asymmetry and border irregularity. (Image courtesy of New York University Department of Dermatology.)

most amelanotic melanomas will lack the play in color usually seen in pigmented melanomas. Sometimes, however, there may be some subtle pigmentation within the lesion which helps the observer in making a diagnosis.

■ *Diameter* – most early melanomas when they are clinically readily identified are >6 mm in diameter (Fig. 25.4).

It is important to remember that all melanomas have a microscopic origin of one or more neoplastic melanocytes. For this reason, there is a stage in the early evolution of melanoma where one or more of the ABCD criteria may be lacking. The most common missing criterion will be the D, in that a few melanomas will have diameters 6 mm or less. Therefore, a good clue to an otherwise atypical pigmented lesion is remembering that malignant neoplasms change over time. Even in a smaller lesion, *a change in diameter over time in the presence of other clinically atypical features should arouse the observer's index of suspicion.*

The ABCD criteria were intended as a simple tool that could be implemented in daily life, a mnemonic 'as easy as ABC', to alert both the layperson and healthcare professionals to the clinical features of early melanoma. Based on our experience evaluating patients in the Melanoma Cooperative Group at New York University School of Medicine, we found that asymmetry, border irregularity, and color variegation were consistently associated with lesion diameter greater than 6 mm in early melanoma lesions. These observations led to the addition of D to the A, B and C criteria. Recent studies have reconfirmed that this diameter guideline of larger than 6 mm remains a useful parameter for clinical diagnosis.[15]

The ABCDs were intended to help describe a subset of melanomas, namely early, thin tumors that might otherwise be confused with benign pigmented lesions.[10,16] Therefore, both elevated and ulcerated lesions were excluded in the initial analysis because we sought to elucidate features of early melanoma. Pigmented skin lesions

that were ulcerated without a history of antecedent trauma would have already been highly suspicious for advanced melanoma and would have required biopsy regardless of other features. Also, it should be emphasized that the criteria were developed to assist non-dermatologists in differentiating common moles from cancer and were not meant to provide a comprehensive template for the recognition of all melanomas.

The ABCD criteria have subsequently been verified in multiple studies documenting their diagnostic accuracy in clinical practice.[17-19] The sensitivity and specificity of these criteria vary when used singly or in combination: sensitivity ranges from 57% to 90% and specificity from 59% to 90%.[20] Barnhill et al. investigated interobserver variability and reported moderate but statistically significant agreement in most clinical features, including irregular borders and multiple colors, among four physician evaluators,[21] and interrater reliability and objectivity for these criteria has been demonstrated by others.[22] The combination of reliable sensitivity and specificity in addition to adequate interobserver concordance in the application of the ABCD criteria supports the ongoing utility of this screening instrument in clinical medicine.

The importance of lesion evolution as a cardinal feature of cutaneous melanoma is also well supported.[23] The need to recognize lesion change in our acronym was met by our revising the *ABCDs* through the addition of 'E' for 'Evolving'.[11] This substantially enhanced the ability of physicians and laypersons to recognize melanomas at earlier stages. 'E' for Evolving is especially important for the diagnosis of nodular melanomas, which frequently present as smaller lesions that are at more advanced stages (i.e. thicker tumors) where early recognition is even more critical.[24] The *ABCDE* is a simple, succinct, and memorable tool, which has been demonstrated to effectively educate the public, the non-dermatologist as well as the dermatology medical community about the key features of melanoma including lesion change.[25]

These now well-known parameters of Asymmetry, Border irregularity, Color variegation, Diameter greater than 6 mm and Evolving have been used worldwide by groups such as the American Cancer Society, American Academy of Dermatology, and others, and have been featured in the lay press to provide simple parameters for evaluation and identification of pigmented lesions that may need to be further examined. It should be noted that not all melanomas have all five *ABCDE* features. It is the combination of features (e.g. ABC, A+C, and the like) that render cutaneous lesions most suspicious for early melanoma.

Other melanoma early diagnosis paradigms have been developed to enhance early diagnosis. The most recognized of these is the Glasgow seven-point checklist that includes three major criteria (change in size, shape, color) and four minor criteria (sensory change, diameter of 7 mm or greater, inflammation, crusting or bleeding).[26] The Glasgow checklist has been less widely adopted than the *ABCDE* criteria possibly due to its greater complexity. The 'ugly duckling' sign is another clinical approach, in which a pigmented lesion that 'looks different than all of its neighbors' may be suspicious for melanoma.[27] This sign has been shown to be sensitive for melanoma detection, even for non-dermatologists.[28]

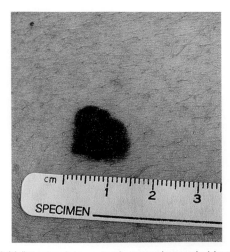

**Figure 25.4** Malignant melanoma, trunk, measuring nearly 14 mm in diameter. The lesion was present for at least 2 years and was slowly growing. It measures about 0.4 mm in greatest thickness, with a sizeable component of the lesion still in situ. It too exhibits subtle asymmetry and border irregularity. There are subtle variations in pigmentation from brown to dark brown. (Image courtesy of New York University Department of Dermatology.)

The clinically diagnostic features of early malignant melanoma are relatively similar regardless of anatomic site,[29,30] despite current hypotheses that melanoma from different body sites may have different etiologies.[31]

The clinician must keep in mind that while the clinical features of early melanoma to be described are generally present in most lesions, there are exceptions that need to be recognized.

The early clinical diagnosis of melanoma has its basis not only in the clinical appearance of the lesion (physical examination), but also in the history and symptomatology. Change in a pre-existing melanocytic lesion or the development of a new pigmented lesion later in life (after the age of 40) are also important features which should alert the patient to seek medical care, and the physician to use his or her skills and ancillary technologies to rule out the possibility of a melanoma. Other clinically suspicious signs seen in pigmented lesions that are suggestive for melanoma are illustrated in Table 25.2.

## PATIENT EVALUATION, DIAGNOSIS AND DIFFERENTIAL DIAGNOSIS

### Common benign pigmented lesions

The most frequently encountered pigmented lesions are simple lentigines, 'common moles' (i.e. melanocytic nevi – junctional, compound, intradermal), solar lentigines, and seborrheic keratoses.

### Simple lentigo

A simple lentigo is a small (1 to 5 mm) pigmented lesion. It is the initial stage of development of a common mole. The simple lentigo is a sharply defined, brown to black pigmented macule with regular or jagged edges that may appear anywhere on the surface of the skin. The pigmentation oftentimes has a reticulated (net-like) pattern. Such a lesion generally arises in childhood, but may also appear later in life with increased amount of sun exposure. Some simple lentigines are clinically indistinguishable from junctional nevi.

| Table 25.2 Clinical Signs Suggestive of Malignant Melanoma |
| --- |
| **Change in color** – specially multiple shades of dark brown or black; red, white and blue; spread of color from the edge of the lesion into surrounding skin |
| **Change in size** – especially sudden or continuous enlargement |
| **Change in shape** – especially development of irregular margins |
| **Change in elevation** – especially sudden elevation of a previously macular pigmented lesion |
| **Change in surface** – especially scaliness, erosion, oozing, crusting, ulceration, bleeding |
| **Change in surrounding skin** – especially redness, swelling, satellite pigmentations |
| **Change in sensation** – especially itching, tenderness, pain |
| **Change in consistency** – especially softening or friability |

### Junctional nevus

A junctional nevus is generally a small (<6 mm) well-circumscribed, pigmented lesion with a smooth surface, and uniform pigmentation ranging from light brown to brown to darker brown or even black. It may appear on any skin surface, but usually is seen on areas exposed to sun. A junctional nevus usually arises in childhood, but may develop during adolescence and young adulthood. It may persist throughout adulthood in a junctional position or may develop into a compound or intradermal nevus as its cells proliferate and extend into the dermis. Rarely do junctional nevi develop in people over the age of 40. The development of a macular, pigmented lesion in someone older than 40 years should alert the physician and patient to the possibility that it is an early malignant melanoma.

### Compound nevus

A compound nevus is generally a well-circumscribed, small (<6 mm) raised papule which is mostly uniformly pigmented with a range of color from skin-colored to tan to brown with either a rough or smooth surface. It may have excess hair associated with it (which sometimes indicates a congenital origin). It usually develops in late childhood, adolescence, or early adulthood.

### Intradermal nevus

The intradermal nevus is generally a small (up to 6 mm) well-circumscribed papule with generally uniform pigmentation from skin-colored to tan to various shades of brown. The surface may be smooth or rough. They, too, may have excess hair.

### Solar lentigo

A solar lentigo is generally a uniform tan to brown macule, known to the lay public as a 'liver spot'. It is found on sun-exposed skin in people with significantly sun-damaged skin. Common sites include the face, chest, and dorsa of the hands.

### Seborrheic keratosis

A seborrheic keratosis is generally a verrucous, round to ovoid, variably raised, light to darker brown to sometimes black, sharply demarcated papule or plaque that varies in diameter from a few millimeters to several centimeters. The surface is usually 'dull' or 'warty' and oftentimes has a stuck-on appearance. Seborrheic keratoses are often found on the face, neck and trunk. They are composed predominantly of proliferating keratinocytes (epidermal cells) and are not primarily melanocytic in origin (Fig. 25.5).

It is also important to consider the age of the patient when making a differential diagnosis of a clinically pigmented lesion. It is rare for a child to develop a melanoma,[32] although such may be the case more frequently in familial melanoma. Other circumstances where melanomas are seen in childhood are those in which the melanoma arises in association with a congenital nevus (usually of the giant type).[33] Ephelides (freckles), simple lentigines and junctional nevi are the most commonly identified pigmented lesions in children. A rarer variant of melanocytic nevus, the Spitz nevus, can also be found in children. This lesion,

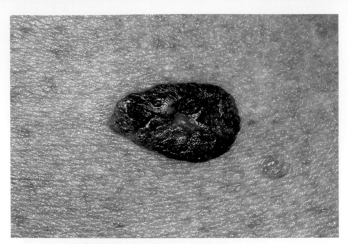

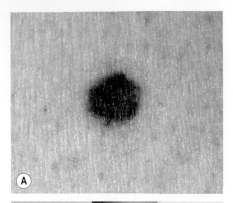

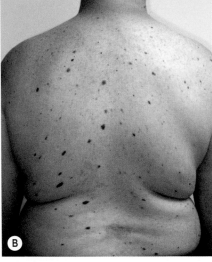

**Figure 25.5** The seborrheic keratosis ('wax-like rough spot') is commonly found in older persons. They are typically well demarcated, uniformly brown papules/plaques.

**Figure 25.6 A)** Typical dysplastic nevus demonstrating uneven color with symmetry. **B)** Typical dysplastic nevus patient presentation with multiple lesions..

if removed, shares some features in common with melanoma and should be diagnosed only by pathologists having extensive experience with this type of nevus. Compound nevi generally develop in later childhood and adolescence, while intradermal nevi more commonly develop in young adulthood. The non-melanocytic pigmented lesions of the skin which can sometimes simulate melanoma, namely the solar lentigo and seborrheic keratosis, usually develop later in life (>35).

Melanoma is rare in childhood and increases with advancing age.[34,35] While the mean age for presentation of melanoma is about 50, any new pigmented lesion not fulfilling the criteria for diagnosis of the previously noted benign pigmented lesions in patients >40 should be a suspect for melanoma or a dysplastic nevus.[3]

## Potential precursor lesions of malignant melanoma

### Atypical (dysplastic) nevi

Dysplastic nevi are acquired pigmented lesions of the skin. Dysplastic nevi are typically larger than ordinary nevi, generally ranging from 6 to 12 mm or more in diameter. They usually have both macular and elevated (pebbly, papular, nodular, or plaque) components. The borders of dysplastic nevi, unlike those of common nevi, are often irregular and frequently so ill-defined that they fade imperceptibly into the surrounding skin (Fig. 25.6).

Dysplastic nevi usually are variegated in color, ranging from tan to dark brown, at times with a prominent pink component. These lesions may appear anywhere on the body, especially on the sun-exposed areas of the trunk and extremities. However, they may also occur on sun-protected areas like the breasts, pubic area, buttocks, and scalp.[36] Young adults generally have an average of 25 common melanocytic nevi, whereas individuals with dysplastic nevi may have more than 100 lesions. Common melanocytic nevi usually do not develop after the age of 40, whereas dysplastic nevi generally begin in adolescence and continue to appear throughout life. Dysplastic nevi may be familial or sporadic (see Chapter 22).

Melanomas may arise in dysplastic nevi (Fig. 25.7). Dysplastic nevi are also markers for increased melanoma risk in general, and persons with these lesions should be considered for extra surveillance. Overall, patients with dysplastic nevi have a reported lifetime risk for malignant melanoma of approximately 5–10%, compared with the risk of about 1.2% for the general population.[37] The risk of developing malignant melanoma is greater for those with one or more relatives with a history of dysplastic nevi.[38,39] Lifetime risk of malignant melanoma approaches a reported 100% for those patients with dysplastic nevi who have both two or more first-degree relatives with cutaneous malignant melanomas and two or more with dysplastic nevi. Melanomas in such individuals may arise either within the dysplastic nevi or de novo in normal-appearing skin.

## The clinical examination

The first step in the evaluation and examination of the skin centers on a thorough history which includes the following:

- general medical history
- personal or family history of skin cancer, including melanoma
- personal or family history of increased number of nevi (>100)
- personal or family history of atypical (*dysplastic*) nevi

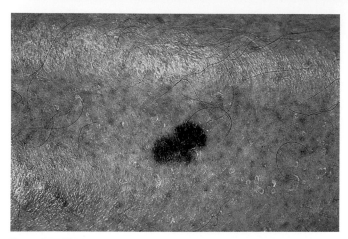

**Figure 25.7** This 7-mm pigmented lesion had its beginnings with the uniformly brown pigmented lesion at the left lower portion of this clinical photograph. The darker brown, slightly asymmetric lesion with irregular borders at the upper right edge of the photograph developed over the past 5 or 6 months. Biopsy revealed a very early melanoma in situ arising in association with a compound melanocytic nevus having features of so-called dysplastic nevus.

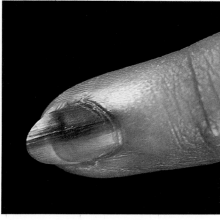

**Figure 25.8** Melanonychia striata with subtle Hutchinson's sign at proximal nail fold. This melanoma in situ (on biopsy) is a clear exception to the ABCD rule. The clue to the diagnosis is a longitudinal band of pigmentation (of varying color in this patient) which has increased (historically) in width over time. The presence of a Hutchinson sign is key to making the diagnosis of melanoma (vs nevus) in this patient. The biopsy should be taken from the nail matrix.

- pharmaceutical history
- social history, including sun exposure/sunburns during childhood and young adult life versus sun exposure currently.

## Physical examination of the skin

The equipment required for physical examination of the skin consists of: 1) examination table (preferably one that allows the patient to lie flat); 2) source of bright light, 3) magnifying lens (2–4×); and 4) dermatoscope (for those physicians adept at dermoscopy). The patient should be placed on the examination table with proper draping in place. When appropriate, it is advisable to have a nurse present during the examination of sensitive areas of the body. The patient should lie on the examination table and the entire anterior surface of the body, including the intertriginous areas, should be closely examined for the presence of any skin cancers/ pigmented lesions. If the female patient wishes, examination of the genital areas can be done by their gynecologist with the understanding that the gynecologist will report any findings to the physician responsible for the skin examination.

Next, examine the entire posterior aspect of the body (including the intertriginous areas). The feet and hands should also be thoroughly examined, including areas between the toes and fingers. Be sure to examine the nailbeds for any evidence of skin cancer, including any abnormal pigmentation such as melanonychia striata (Fig. 25.8), which may indicate a nail matrix-based melanoma.

The scalp should also be thoroughly examined. There are two methods for thoroughly examining the scalp. One uses an ordinary blow dryer on a cool setting to better visualize the scalp. The other method, the 'digital-visual' examination, uses the fingers to separate the hair and to palpate the scalp for any palpable lesions, coupled with a thorough visual examination of the surface of the scalp.

Any suspicious lesions should be carefully evaluated. Baseline total body imaging for patients having many atypical nevi and/or a family history of melanoma is helpful both for the patient and for the examining physician in terms of identifying new or changing pigmented lesions. In such cases, dermoscopy can also be used to help in the clinical classification of any pigmented lesion in question.

Any lesion suggestive of melanoma is subject to biopsy in toto. A complete annual examination of the skin by a physician is recommended for everyone, supplemented by more frequent physician-based examinations for those patients at higher risk for melanoma (personal history of melanoma, personal/family history of *dysplastic nevi* and family history of melanoma). Further, in such patients, it is recommended that a comprehensive program of patient education including monthly skin self-examination be considered.

The clinical diagnosis of melanoma is based not only on the clinical appearance of a lesion (physical examination), but also on the history and symptomatology. Change in a pre-existing melanocytic lesion or the development of a new pigmented lesion later in life (after the age of 40) are important features which should alert the patient to seek medical care, and the physician to use their skills and ancillary technologies to rule out the possibility of a melanoma.

## Self-examination of the skin

It is important for the high-risk patient to be a partner in their early-melanoma detection efforts.[40] Routine self-examination of the skin (SSE) achieves that goal and is inexpensive (free), non-invasive, and lacks any danger. Performed correctly, the self-examination process reinforces the educational experience which occurs in the physicians' office at the time of the semi-annual or annual total cutaneous exam (Figs 25.9–25.16).

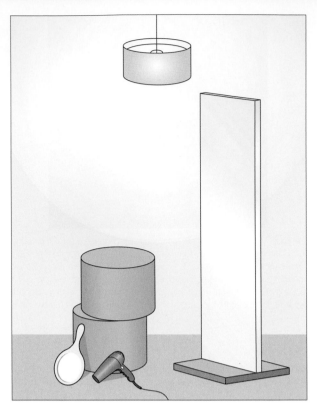

**Figure 25.9** Make sure the room is well lit and that you have nearby a full-length mirror, a handheld mirror, a handheld blow dryer and two chairs or stools. Undress completely. (Adapted from Friedman RJ, et al. Early detection of malignant melanoma: the role of physician-examination and self-examination of the skin. *CA Cancer J Clin.* 1985; 35:130–151.)

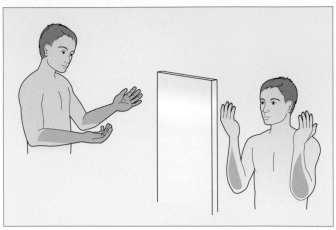

**Figure 25.10** Left: Hold your hands with the palms face up, as shown in the drawing. Look at your palms, fingers, spaces between the fingers, and forearms. Then turn your hands over and examine the backs of your hands, fingers, spaces between the fingers, fingernails, and forearms. Right: Now position yourself in front of the full-length mirror. Hold up your arms, bent at the elbows, with your palms facing you. In the mirror, look at the backs of your forearms and elbow. (Adapted from Friedman RJ, et al. Early detection of malignant melanoma: the role of physician-examination and self-examination of the skin. *CA Cancer J Clin.* 1985;35:130–151.)

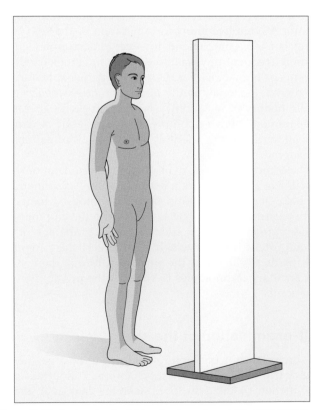

**Figure 25.11** Again using the full-length mirror, observe the entire front of your body. In turn, look at your face, neck, and arms. Turn your palms to face the mirror and look at your upper arms. Then look at your chest and abdomen, pubic area, thighs and lower legs. (Adapted from Friedman RJ, et al. Early detection of malignant melanoma: the role of physician-examination and self-examination of the skin. *CA Cancer J Clin.* 1985;35:130–151.)

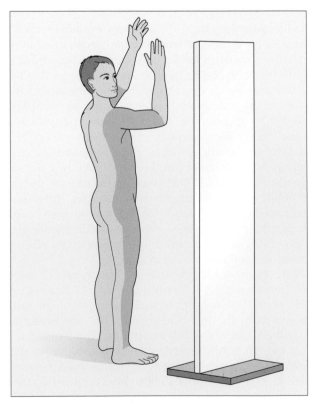

**Figure 25.12** Still standing in front of the mirror, lift your arms over your head with the palms facing each other. Turn so that your right side is facing the mirror and look at the entire side of your body – your hands and arms, underarms, sides of your trunk, thighs, and lower legs. Then turn and repeat the process with your left side. (Adapted from Friedman RJ, et al. Early detection of malignant melanoma: the role of physician-examination and self-examination of the skin. *CA Cancer J Clin.* 1985;35:130–151.)

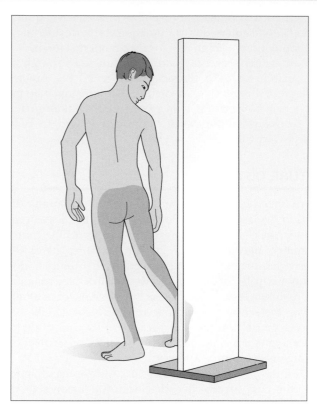

**Figure 25.13** With your back toward the full-length mirror, look at your buttocks and the backs of your thighs and lower legs. (Adapted from Friedman RJ, et al. Early detection of malignant melanoma: the role of physician-examination and self-examination of the skin. *CA Cancer J Clin.* 1985;35:130–151.)

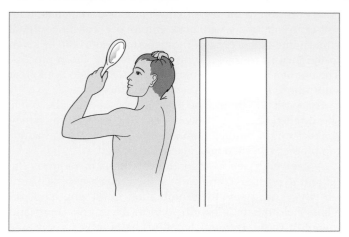

**Figure 25.15** Use the handheld mirror and the full-length mirror to look at your scalp. Because the scalp is difficult to examine, we suggest you also use a handheld blow dryer turned to a cool setting, to lift the hair from the scalp. While some people find it easy to hold the mirror in one hand and the dryer in the other while looking in the full-length mirror, many do not. For the scalp examination in particular, then, you might ask your spouse or a friend to assist you. (Adapted from Friedman RJ, et al. Early detection of malignant melanoma: the role of physician-examination and self-examination of the skin. *CA Cancer J Clin.* 1985; 35:130–151.)

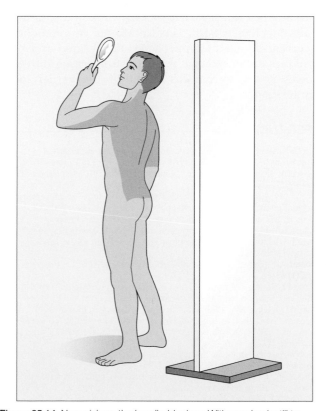

**Figure 25.14** Now pick up the handheld mirror. With your back still to the full-length mirror, examine the back of your neck, and your back and buttocks. Also examine the backs of your arms in this way. Some areas are hard to see, and you may find it helpful to ask your spouse or a friend to assist you. (Adapted from Friedman RJ, et al. Early detection of malignant melanoma: the role of physician-examination and self-examination of the skin. *CA Cancer J Clin.* 1985; 35:130–151.)

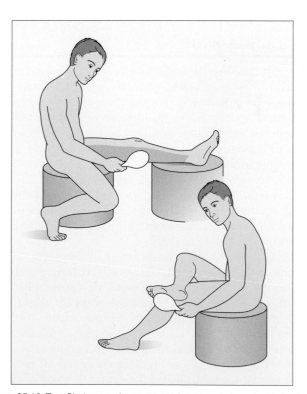

**Figure 25.16** Top: Sit down and prop up one leg on a chair or stool in front of you as shown. Using the handheld mirror, examine the inside of the propped-up leg, beginning at the groin area and moving the mirror down the leg to your foot. Repeat the procedure for your other leg. Bottom: Still sitting, cross one leg over the other. Use the handheld mirror to examine the top of your foot, the toes, toenails, and spaces between the toes. Then look at the sole or bottom of your foot. Repeat the procedure for the other foot. (Adapted from Friedman RJ, et al. Early detection of malignant melanoma: the role of physician-examination and self-examination of the skin. *CA Cancer J Clin.* 1985;35:130–151.)

In addition to the use of visual aids and information on self-examination, when also employing baseline digital clinical imaging, a copy of these digital images can be given to the patient for use during the self-examination process. The use of a visual benchmark has been found to be of great importance in terms of patient compliance.

All patients should be encouraged to call the office should they detect any new or changing lesions which they suspect might be melanoma. Earlier intervention, including biopsy, can then take place if indicated.

A thorough self-examination of the skin requires the patient to undress completely and, in the absence of a *partner* who can assist in the examination, a full-length mirror, a handheld mirror, a handheld blow dryer, two chairs and a well-lit room. Immediately after bathing is a good time for the examination. In women, we recommend that the self-examination occur at the same time that they are practicing self-examination of the breast.

The first few times that the patient performs SSE they should spend some time inspecting the entire surface of their skin. With experience, however, the self-examination should take but a few minutes. To visualize parts of the skin surface that may otherwise be difficult to see (e.g. some areas of the back, scalp and buttocks), the patient may find it helpful to elicit the help of a partner. The self-examination process should be done in a stepwise fashion, as illustrated in Figures 25.9–25.16. The patient should be advised to see their healthcare professional if there are any newly discovered or significantly changing lesions.

## MASS SCREENINGS

Mass skin cancer screenings have been undertaken in multiple countries to enhance secondary prevention and public education (Chapter 7). Formal volunteer programs that have been sponsored by groups such as the American Academy of Dermatology, American Cancer Society, Skin Cancer Foundation and others have screened over 2 million people in the US since 1985 and thousands of clinically presumptive melanomas have been detected.[41] The first Monday in May has been recognized in the US as Melanoma Monday with associated public education events undertaken each year.[42] Additional programs have effectively been conducted worldwide.[43]

The specific recommended intervals for screening of persons at risk are varied and remain controversial. The American Cancer Society recommends cancer check-up including skin examination every 3 years for those aged 20–39 and annually after age 40. The American Academy of Dermatology, Skin Cancer Foundation, and the 1992 National Institutes of Health Consensus Conference on Early Melanoma recommend annual screening for all patients. The National Cancer Institute encourages routine examination of the skin, with particular emphasis on high-risk groups. The U.S. Preventive Services Task Force (USPSTF), American Academy of Family Physicians, and American College of Obstetrics and Gynecology recommend screening only for high-risk populations with a family or personal history of skin cancer, increased occupational or recreational exposure to sunlight, or clinical evidence of precursor lesions.

The American College of Preventive Medicine recommends periodic total cutaneous examinations be performed targeting populations at high risk for malignant melanoma.

Skin cancer screening can be conducted through self-examination or by a physician. However, the American College of Preventive Medicine recommends that practitioners who perform skin examinations undergo training to assure high-quality examinations and to reduce unnecessary biopsies.[44]

## FUTURE OUTLOOK

There have been significant advances in melanoma diagnosis in the last 25 years. Beginning with the development of the ABCDs, through current attempts using complex computer algorithms and genetic markers, all of these approaches have augmented the clinician's ability to detect melanoma in its earliest form. However, all of these techniques still require a 'good eye' to select the lesions for evaluation among the sea of lesions that are prevalent. Unlike other cancers which are internal, because of its cutaneous location malignant melanoma has the potential to be diagnosed through non-invasive approaches.

Despite all of the advances in melanoma diagnosis over the past several decades, accurate lesion selection, timely recognition, detection and treatment of melanoma remain critical. To be successful we must be able to recognize melanoma in its earliest form. As Neville Davis so eloquently stated'…unlike other cancers, which are generally hidden from view, malignant melanoma writes its message in the skin with its own ink and it is there for all of us to see. Some see, but do not comprehend.'[45] As current diagnostic approaches are refined and new techniques enhanced, we will hopefully reach our goal to lower mortality from this cancer through earlier, more accurate diagnosis.

## REFERENCES

1. Linos E, Swetter SM, Cockburn MG, et al. Increasing burden of melanoma in the United States. *J Invest Dermatol.* 2009;129(7):1666–1674.
2. Jemal A, Siegel R, Xu J, Ward E. Cancer statistics, 2010. *CA Cancer J Clin.* 2010;60(5):277–300.
3. Kopf AW, Rigel DS, Friedman RJ. The rising incidence and mortality rate of malignant melanoma. *J Dermatol Surg Oncol.* 1982;8(9):760–761.
4. American Cancer Society. *Skin cancer.* 2005. www.cancer.org.
5. Clark Jr WH, Elder DE, Guerry 4th D, et al. Model predicting survival in stage I melanoma based on tumor progression. *J Natl Cancer Inst.* 1989;81(24):1893–1904.
6. Jemal A, Siegel R, Ward E, et al. Cancer statistics, 2007. *CA Cancer J Clin.* 2007;57(1):43–66.
7. Tsao H, Rogers GS, Sober AJ. An estimate of the annual direct cost of treating cutaneous melanoma. *J Am Acad Dermatol.* 1998;38(5 Pt 1):669–680.
8. Grin CM, Kopf AW, Welkovich B, et al. Accuracy in the clinical diagnosis of malignant melanoma. *Arch Dermatol.* 1990;126(6):763–766.
9. Bevona C, Sober AJ. Melanoma incidence trends. *Dermatol Clin.* 2002;20:589–595.
10. Sober AJ, Fitzpatrick TB, Mihm Jr MC, et al. Early recognition of cutaneous melanoma. *JAMA.* 1979;242:2795–2799.
11. Breslow A. Thickness, cross sectional area and depth of invasion in the prognosis of cutaneous melanoma. *Ann Surg.* 1970;172:902–908.
12. Balch CM, Milton GW, Shaw HM, et al. *Cutaneous Melanoma. Clinical Management and Treatment Results Worldwide.* Philadelphia, PA: JB Lippincott; 1985.
13. Friedman RJ, Rigel DS, Kopf AW. Early detection of malignant melanoma: the role of physician examination and self-examination of the skin. *CA Cancer J Clin.* 1985;35:130–151.
14. Rigel DS, Friedman RJ. The rationale of the ABCDs of early melanoma. *J Am Acad Dermatol.* 1993;29:1060–1061.

3. There is no lower threshold of tumor burden defining the presence of regional nodal metastasis. Based on a consensus that volume of regional metastatic tumor deposits <0.2 mm in diameter (an empiric lower threshold previously used by the AJCC for defining nodal metastasis in breast cancer patients) is clinically significant in melanoma patients, nodal tumor deposits of any size are included in staging nodal disease. An evidence-based lower threshold of clinically insignificant nodal metastases has not yet been defined.

4. Survival estimates for patients with intralymphatic regional metastases (i.e. satellites and in-transit metastases) are somewhat better than for the remaining cohort of stage IIIB patients; nonetheless, the current stage definition for intralymphatic regional metastasis has been retained, since this stage grouping represents the closest statistical fit.

5. The prognostic significance of microsatellites remains controversial. This uncommon feature has been retained in the N2c category, largely because previous published studies were insufficient to substantiate revision of the definitions used in the 6th edition of the staging manual.

6. The site of distant metastases remains the primary component of the M category (non-visceral, M1a [cutaneous, subcutaneous, distant nodal]; lung, M1b; and visceral metastasis, M1c). An elevated serum lactic dehydrogenase (LDH) level remains a powerful adverse predictor of survival; patients with an increased LDH are all categorized as M1c, regardless of the sites of distant disease.

7. No subgroups of stage IV melanoma are recommended.

8. The definition of metastatic melanoma from an unknown primary site was clarified; isolated metastases arising in lymph nodes, skin, and subcutaneous tissues are categorized as stage III rather than stage IV.

9. Lymphatic mapping and sentinel lymph node (SLN) biopsy are important components of melanoma staging and should be used (or at least discussed with the patient) in defining occult stage III disease among patients who present with clinical stages IB and II melanoma.

The 7th edition melanoma staging system TNM categories are defined in Table 26.1 and the stage groupings in Table 26.2.[6] These revisions are based on the updated AJCC collaborative melanoma database that contained prospective data on over 50,000 patients with stages I–III melanoma, and nearly 10,000 patients with stage IV melanoma. Interestingly, 5-year survival rates over the 5-year interval between this and the prior staging system demonstrate some increase in survival, likely due to the improvements in melanoma staging (i.e. more widespread use of sentinel node biopsy for patients with T1b–T4 lesions) and treatment (Table 26.3). Serving as an introduction to melanoma staging and prognosis, the overall heterogeneity of survival among patients with varying stages of disease is illustrated by the survival estimates for patients with stages I to IV melanoma (Fig. 26.1).

### Table 26.1 TNM Staging Categories for Cutaneous Melanoma (7th edition)

| T Classification | Thickness | Ulceration Status |
|---|---|---|
| Tis | NA | NA |
| T1 | ≤1.00 mm | a: w/o ulceration and mitosis <1/mm$^2$ <br> b: with ulceration or mitoses ≥1/mm$^2$ |
| T2 | 1.01–2.0 mm | a: w/o ulceration <br> b: with ulceration |
| T3 | 2.01–4.0 mm | a: w/o ulceration <br> b: with ulceration |
| T4 | >4.0 mm | a: w/o ulceration <br> b: with ulceration |

| N Classification | # of Metastatic Nodes | Nodal Metastatic Burden |
|---|---|---|
| N0 | 0 | NA |
| N1 | 1 | a: micrometastasis* <br> b: macrometastasis† |
| N2 | 2–3 | a: micrometastasis* <br> b: macrometastasis† <br> c: in-transit met(s)/satellite(s) without metastatic nodes |
| N3 | 4+ metastatic nodes, or matted nodes, or in-transit metastases/satellites with metastatic nodes | |

| M Classification | Site | Serum LDH |
|---|---|---|
| M0 | No distant metastases | NA |
| M1a | Distant skin, subcutaneous, or nodal metastases | Normal |
| M1b | Lung metastases | Normal |
| M1c | All other visceral metastases <br> Any distant metastasis | Normal <br> Elevated |

NA, not applicable; LDH, lactate dehydrogenase.

*Micrometastases are diagnosed after sentinel lymph node biopsy.

†Macrometastases are defined as clinically detectable nodal metastases confirmed pathologically.

From Balch CM, Gershenwald JE, Soong S, et al. JCO 27(36): 6199-206, 2009.

## PROGNOSTIC FACTORS IN PRIMARY MELANOMA (STAGES I AND II)

The overall prognosis for patients who present with localized melanoma without regional lymph node or distant metastases is generally favorable (Fig. 26.1A,B).[5] In the AJCC analysis, among 25,734 patients with localized

## Table 26.2 Anatomic Stage Groupings for Cutaneous Melanoma (7th Edition)

| | Clinical Staging* | | | | Pathologic Staging† | | |
|---|---|---|---|---|---|---|---|
| | T | N | M | | T | N | M |
| 0 | Tis | N0 | M0 | 0 | Tis | N0 | M0 |
| IA | T1a | N0 | M0 | IA | T1a | N0 | M0 |
| IB | T1b | N0 | M0 | IB | T1b | N0 | M0 |
| | T2a | N0 | M0 | | T2a | N0 | M0 |
| IIA | T2b | N0 | M0 | IIA | T2b | N0 | M0 |
| | T3a | N0 | M0 | | T3a | N0 | M0 |
| IIB | T3b | N0 | M0 | IIB | T3b | N0 | M0 |
| | T4a | N0 | M0 | | T4a | N0 | M0 |
| IIC | T4b | N0 | M0 | IIC | T4b | N0 | M0 |
| III | Any T | N > N0 | M0 | IIIA | T1–4a | N1a | M0 |
| | | | | | T1–4a | N2a | M0 |
| | | | | IIIB | T1–4b | N1a | M0 |
| | | | | | T1–4b | N2a | M0 |
| | | | | | T1–4a | N1b | M0 |
| | | | | | T1–4a | N2b | M0 |
| | | | | | T1–4a | N2c | M0 |
| | | | | IIIC | T1–4b | N1b | M0 |
| | | | | | T1–4b | N2b | M0 |
| | | | | | T1–4b | N2c | M0 |
| | | | | | Any T | N3 | M0 |
| IV | Any T | Any N | M1 | IV | Any T | Any N | M1 |

*Clinical staging includes microstaging of the primary melanoma and clinical/radiologic evaluation for metastases. By convention, it should be used after complete excision of the primary melanoma with clinical assessment for regional and distant metastases.

†Pathologic staging includes microstaging of the primary melanoma and pathologic information about the regional lymph nodes after partial (i.e. sentinel lymph node biopsy) or complete lymphadenectomy. Pathologic stage 0 or stage IA patients are the exception; they do not require pathologic evaluation of their lymph nodes.

Source: From Balch CM, Gershenwald JE, Soong S, et al, JCO 27(36): 6199-206, 200.

## Table 26.3 AJCC Collaborative Melanoma Database: 5-Year Survival Rates by T Classification Comparing Outcomes Published in the 6th and 7th Edition of the AJCC Cancer Staging Manual

| | 5-Year Survival Rate (SE) | | | |
|---|---|---|---|---|
| | 6th Edition (2001) | | 7th Edition SLN Subset* | |
| T Classification | % ± SE | (n) | % ± SE | (n) |
| T1a | 95 ± 0.4 | 4150 | 97 ± 0.2 | 9452 |
| T1b | 91 ± 1.0 | 1380 | 95 ± 1.5 | 597 |
| T2a | 89 ± 0.7 | 3285 | 95 ± 0.6 | 2842 |
| T2b | 77 ± 1.7 | 958 | 86 ± 2.0 | 614 |
| T3a | 79 ± 1.2 | 1717 | 85 ± 1.5 | 1158 |
| T3b | 63 ± 1.5 | 1523 | 76 ± 2.5 | 677 |
| T4a | 67 ± 2.4 | 563 | 76 ± 3.6 | 338 |
| T4b | 45 ± 1.9 | 978 | 67 ± 3.6 | 386 |

SE, standard error.

*Patients staged based on sentinel node staging for T1b–T4.

Adapted from Balch CM: Melanoma of the Skin, in Greene FL, Page DL, Fleming ID, et al (eds): AJCC Cancer Staging Manual (ed 6th). New York, Springer Verlag, 2002 and Balch CM: Melanoma of the Skin, in Greene FL, Page DL, Fleming ID, et al (eds): AJCC Cancer Staging Manual (ed 7th). New York, Springer Verlag, 2009.

## Tumor thickness

One of the earliest descriptions of tumor thickness was published by Breslow[7] in 1970, when he theorized that primary melanoma tumor volume correlates with prognosis. Realizing that accurate and reproducible tumor volume measurements are essential yet difficult to perform, he reasoned that the maximal thickness of the primary melanoma (measured from the granular layer to the deepest component of the tumor using an ocular micrometer) (Fig. 26.2) would be an accurate, reproducible surrogate for tumor volume and a significant predictor of prognosis. This concept has since been validated in multiple studies, including the AJCC analysis.[4–8] In the 7th edition AJCC staging system, the cutoff points for tumor thickness strata remain at 1 mm, 2 mm, and 4 mm on the basis of prior statistical modeling,[9] the lack of naturally occurring break points in the analysis,[4] and utility as thresholds for clinical decision-making (Tables 26.1 and 26.2). To date, tumor thickness remains the most powerful primary tumor-derived prognostic factor in melanoma.

When a patient presents with a lesion suggestive of melanoma, biopsy followed by histologic examination is essential. While specific biopsy techniques are addressed elsewhere, full-thickness biopsy into the subcutaneous tissue must be performed to permit proper microstaging of the lesion. In this setting, shave biopsies are generally discouraged, since failure to obtain a full-thickness specimen may result in inaccurate microstaging if melanoma is diagnosed.

## Primary tumor ulceration

Primary tumor ulceration has also been recognized as an important predictor of survival in clinically node-nega-

melanoma (documented clinically or pathologically), tumor thickness and ulceration were the dominant independent predictors of survival (Table 26.4).[5] Similar results were obtained in the cohort of 9883 patients without clinical evidence of nodal metastases at initial presentation, whose regional nodes were pathologically staged primarily by sentinel node biopsy (Table 26.5).[5] In this latter group, nodal status was the most significant independent predictor, and level of invasion was no longer a predictor of outcome.

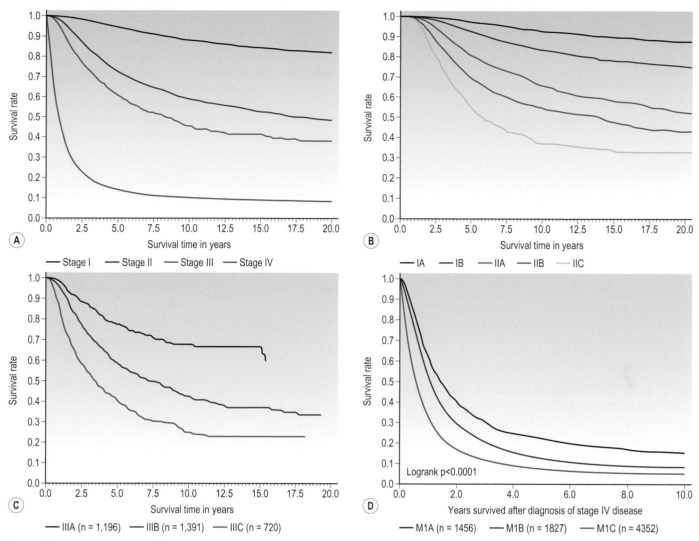

**Figure 26.1** 2009 American Joint Committee on Cancer (AJCC) melanoma staging system. **A)** Survival curves for patients with localized melanoma (stages I and II), regional metastases (stage III), and distant metastases (stage IV). The differences between the curves are highly significant (p<0.0001). **B)** Stage I/II survival by substage groupings for stages I and II melanoma. **C)** Stage III melanoma by substage. **D)** Stage IV melanoma survival by site of distant metastases (*Note – LDH level NOT included in this graph). The numbers in parentheses are the numbers of patients from the AJCC 2008 melanoma staging database used to calculate the survival rates. (Balch CM. Melanoma of the skin. In: Edge SB, Byrd DR, Compton CC, et al., eds. *AJCC Cancer Staging Manual*. 7th ed. New York: Springer Verlag; 2009.)

**Table 26.4 AJCC 2008 Melanoma Database: Cox Regression Analysis for Patients without Evidence of Nodal or Distant Metastases (1 DF)**

| Variable | Without Mitotic Rate in Model (N=25,754) | | | With Mitotic Rate in Model (N=10,233) | | |
|---|---|---|---|---|---|---|
| | Chi-Square | P | HR (5% CI) | Chi-Square | P | HR (95% CI) |
| Tumor thickness | 420.1 | <0.0001 | 1.35 (1.31–1.39) | 84.6 | <0.0001 | 1.25 (1.91–1.31) |
| Ulceration | 257.3 | <0.0001 | 1.93 (1.78–2.10) | 47.2 | <0.0001 | 1.56 (1.38–1.78) |
| Clark level | 46.3 | <0.0001 | 1.22 (1.16–1.30) | 8.2 | 0.0041 | 1.15 (1.04–1.26) |
| Mitotic rate | – | – | – | 79.1 | <0.0001 | 1.26 (1.20–1.32) |
| Site | 75.6 | <0.0001 | 1.41 (1.30–1.52) | 29.1 | <0.0001 | 1.38 (1.23–1.54) |
| Gender | 46.5 | <0.0001 | 0.76 (0.71–0.83) | 32.4 | <0.0001 | 0.70 (0.62–0.79) |
| Age | 90.0 | <0.0001 | 1.16 (1.13–1.20) | 40.8 | <0.0001 | 1.16 (1.11–1.22) |

CI, confidence interval; DF, degree of freedom; HR, hazard ratio, P, probability.

Source: Adapted from Gershenwald JE, Balch CM, Soong S, et al: Prognostic factors and natural history of melanoma, in Balch CM, Soong SJ, Sober AJ, et al (eds): Cutaneous Melanoma (ed 5th). St. Louis, Quality Medical Publishing, Inc., 2009.

Table 26.5 AJCC 2008 Melanoma Database: Cox Regression Analysis for 9883 Melanoma Patients without Clinical Evidence of Nodal or Distant Metastases whose Regional Lymph Nodes were Pathologically Staged after Sentinel or Elective Lymphadenectomy (1 DF)

| Variable | Chi-Square | Hazard Ratio (95% CI) | P |
|---|---|---|---|
| Nodal status | 222.5 | 2.52 (2.23–2.84) | <0.0001 |
| Thickness | 162.1 | 1.33 (1.27–1.38) | <0.0001 |
| Ulceration | 113.4 | 1.93 (1.71– 2.18) | <0.0001 |
| Site | 36.1 | 1.45 (1.28–1.63) | <0.0001 |
| Age | 47.6 | 1.20 (1.14–1.26) | <0.0001 |
| Gender | 11.3 | 0.80 (0.71–0.91) | 0.0008 |
| Clark level | 2.1 | 1.11 (0.96–1.29) | 0.1512 |

CI, confidence interval; DF, degree of freedom; P, probability.

Source: Adapted from Gershenwald JE, Balch CM, Soong S, et al: Prognostic factors and natural history of melanoma, in Balch CM, Soong SJ, Sober AJ, et al (eds): Cutaneous Melanoma (ed 5th). St. Louis, Quality Medical Publishing, Inc., 2009.

tive patients.[4] Ulceration is defined as the absence of an intact epidermis (i.e. loss of continuity of the overlying epithelium) overlying the primary tumor on histologic examination[1,5,10,11] and is a reproducibly identifiable feature of melanoma (Fig. 26.3).

Numerous studies have shown that patients with ulcerated primaries have a higher likelihood of metastases and a worse prognosis compared to patients with non-ulcerated tumors when controlled for tumor thickness.[4,6,10,11] Although the biological basis of ulceration remains speculative, it may be related to the inherent aggressiveness of the tumor itself or possibly other stromal factors, such as angiogenic support. As noted in both the 2001 and the 2008 AJCC prognostic factor analyses, patients with ulcerated primaries had outcomes approximately the same as those of patients in the next-higher tumor thickness stratum whose lesions were not ulcerated (Fig. 26.4).[1,3,6]

In the AJCC T classification, ulceration at each tumor thickness level is categorized as either absent or present. Spatz et al.[12] developed a clear definition of histologic criteria for traumatic ulceration, an important contribution since this form of ulceration has no prognostic value, but non-trau-

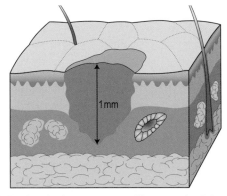

Figure 26.2 Breslow depth measurement. The tumor depth is measured from the granular layer to the deepest portion of the tumor.

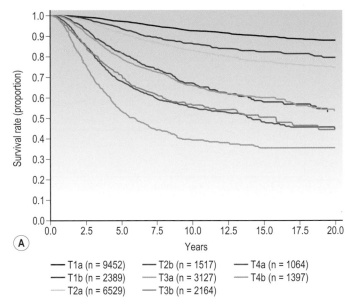

Figure 26.4 Survival curves from the AJCC melanoma staging database comparing the different T categories. (From Balch CM, Gershenwald JE et al. Final version of 2009 AJCC melanoma staging and classification. *J Clin Oncol.* 27(36): 6199-206, 2009.)

Legend (Figure 26.4):
— T1a (n = 9452)   — T2b (n = 1517)   — T4a (n = 1064)
— T1b (n = 2389)   — T3a (n = 3127)   — T4b (n = 1397)
— T2a (n = 6529)   — T3b (n = 2164)

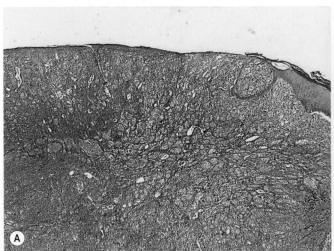

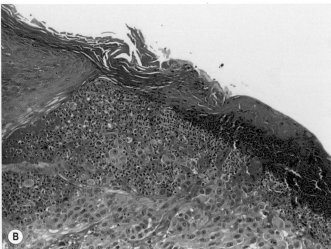

Figure 26.3 Ulceration. Photomicrographs illustrating (A) low-power and (B) high-power views of ulceration. (Images courtesy of Dr Martin Mihm.)

matic ulceration has independent prognostic significance. The incidence of ulceration among primary tumors is quite heterogenous, ranging from approximately 3% in patients with T1 lesions to 57% among those with T4 melanoma.[13]

Importantly, ulceration is a primary tumor feature that also carries independent prognostic significance in patients with stage III (regional node) disease (see below).[4,6] Ulceration has been included in the AJCC staging system for melanoma since 2002.[1,5,6]

## Mitotic rate

Accumulating evidence supports the notion that primary tumor mitotic rate is an important independent prognostic factor in patients with cutaneous melanoma. In 1983, Schmoeckel et al. found a correlation between mitotic rate and prognosis. In the largest single institution study to date, the Sydney Melanoma Unit determined by Cox multivariate analysis that tumor mitotic rate (expressed as the number of mitoses/mm$^2$) was the second most powerful independent prognostic factor after tumor thickness,[14] an observation also noted by others investigators.[15-20]

As a result of numerous studies showing an inverse association between primary tumor mitotic rate and survival, this factor was included for the first time in the 2008 AJCC collaborative melanoma database analysis. The number of mitoses/mm$^2$ correlated strongly with tumor thickness.[21] By univariate analysis, there was a significant inverse correlation between the number of mitoses/mm$^2$ (using the so-called 'hot spot' approach) and survival. Remarkably, among the 11,664 patients with stage I or II melanoma in whom mitotic rate was known, it was the second most powerful independent adverse predictor of survival (Table 26.4).[6] Tumor ulceration remained highly significant, whereas level of invasion maintained only borderline significance. Among patients with T1 (i.e. 'thin') melanomas, the presence of at least 1 mitosis/mm$^2$ was an independent adverse predictor of survival, and contributed to the decision to include mitotic rate as a primary tumor (T-category) criterion for patients with thin melanoma (Tables 26.1, 26.2, and 26.6).[5]

Standardized assessment of tumor mitotic rate using the 'hot spot' method (expressed as mitoses/mm$^2$) is now recommended by the AJCC as a required element of the primary tumor pathology report.[5] The recommended approach to mitotic rate measurement is detailed in the 7th edition *AJCC Cancer Staging Manual*.[5] This involves finding the so-called 'hot spot' by identifying the area in the dermis containing the greatest concentration of mitotic figures. After counting the mitoses in the hot spot, the mitoses in adjacent fields are counted until an area corresponding to 1 mm$^2$ has been assessed. Usually this will mean assessment of four high-power fields at 400× magnification, but calibration of individual microscopes is required since field sizes may vary considerably. If no hot spot can be identified and mitoses are sparse and/or randomly distributed throughout the tumor, then a single mitosis is selected, and beginning with the count in that field, the mitoses in adjacent fields are counted until an area of 1 mm$^2$ has been assessed. All mitotic rate results should be reported as mitoses/mm$^2$. When the invasive component of a melanoma is <1 mm$^2$ in area, the mitotic rate can be reported as ≥1/mm$^2$ (if at least 1 mitosis is identified) or 0/mm$^2$ (if no mitoses are identified).

## Clark level of invasion

In 1969, Clark and colleagues[22] described the histologic classification of melanoma by its level of invasion into the dermis or subcutaneous tissue. Five categories of invasion analogous to the current five Clark levels were described (Fig. 26.5). However, the prognostic significance and reproducibility of Clark level have been debated. In most,[23] but not all,[24] comparative studies, including analyses of large prospective databases,[9] tumor thickness was shown to be a more powerful prognostic factor and more reproducible measurement than the Clark level.

More recent analyses have confirmed the importance of tumor thickness as a prognostic factor and found that level of invasion was significant only for melanoma lesions ≤1 mm in thickness. Similarly, in the 2002 AJCC database analysis,[4] the level of invasion had greater prognostic significance than ulceration only for tumors ≤1 mm. While Clark level was included in the 2002 staging system for T1 lesions only, it has been supplanted by mitotic rate as a primary criterion for T1b melanoma (with ulceration) in the 7th edition melanoma staging system (except in those rare instances when mitotic rate cannot be determined) since it was not found to be prognostic when both mitotic rate and ulceration were in the model.[5,6]

Table 26.6 Survival Rates for 4861 T1 Melanoma Patients (≤1.00 mm) Subgrouped by Thickness and Mitotic Rate of the Primary Melanoma

| Thickness (mm) | Mitosis per mm$^2$ | N | Survival Rate ± SE | |
| --- | --- | --- | --- | --- |
| | | | 5-Year | 10-Year |
| 0.01–0.50 | <1.0 | 1194 | 99.1 ± 0.4 | 97.4 ± 8.6 |
| 0.01–0.50 | ≥1.0 | 327 | 97.0 ± 1.2 | 95.2 ± 1.7 |
| 0.51–1.00 | <1.0 | 1472 | 97.7 ± 0.5 | 93.0 ± 1.0 |
| 0.51–1.00 | ≥1.0 | 1868 | 93.5 ± 0.6 | 87.1 ± 1.2 |

Source: Adapted from Gershenwald JE, Balch CM, Soong S, et al: Prognostic factors and natural history of melanoma, in Balch CM, Soong SJ, Sober AJ, et al (eds): Cutaneous Melanoma (ed 5th). St. Louis, Quality Medical Publishing, Inc., 2009.

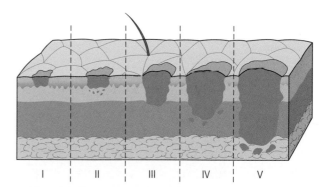

**Figure 26.5** Clark level measurement. Level I tumors are confined to the epidermis. Level II tumors penetrate into the papillary dermis. Level III tumors fill the papillary dermis. Level IV tumors extend into the reticular dermis. Level V tumors invade the subcutis.

## Other factors

Age, sex, primary tumor site, regression, growth phase, and tumor-infiltrating lymphocytes have also been associated with prognosis in at least some studies.[13]

In general, older patients present with thicker primary tumors and are more likely to present with an ulcerated primary with increased mitotic rate. By AJCC multivariate Cox analyses, patient age retained independent prognostic significance, even when accounting for tumor thickness, ulceration, and mitotic activity (Table 26.5). Paradoxically, as patient age increases, the probablity of SLN metastasis declines.

When nodal status is included in the AJCC multivariate models for patients with primary melanoma (Table 26.5), the relative impact of patient gender pales in comparision to that of tumor thickness, ulceration, and mitotic rate.

In addition to patient age, anatomic location of the primary melanoma correlated significantly with survival in an AJCC analysis of patients with stage I and II localized disease.[13] Lesions located on the head, neck and trunk had a risk ratio of 1.34 (95% CI 1.22–1.46) compared with those located on the extremities. Other studies have also demonstrated the importance of anatomic location.[25,26]

Clark et al. extended earlier observations and proposed that melanomas could be biologically distinguished based on their pattern of growth into those in radial growth phase (RGP), associated with low metastatic potential, and those in vertical growth phase (VGP), associated with greater metastatic potential (Fig. 26.6).[27] This potential factor was not formally included in the recent AJCC analysis and its role as a predictor of survival in this era is being explored.

Tumor-infiltrating lymphocytes (TILs) were originally classified as brisk, non-brisk, or absent (Fig. 26.7).[28] TILs, when brisk, are thought to represent a vigorous host response to the primary tumor and, thus, a better prognosis. Although some studies have demonstrated correlation between TIL status and survival,[29] multivariate assessment of this potential prognostic factor is currently in evolution.

Although histologic evidence of regression has been observed in up to 20% of primary melanomas, its impact on recurrence and survival remain unclear.[19]

Although melanomas arising during pregnancy may be thicker at presentation compared to non-pregnancy-associated tumors, they are not necessarily associated with a worse prognosis[30,31] (see Chapter 29).

## Stage I and II groupings

In the 2009 AJCC melanoma staging system, primary melanomas without evidence of nodal or distant metastases are grouped into stage I or II stratified by primary tumor characteristics comprising the T classification (Tables 26.1 and 26.2; Figs 26.1 and 26.4). A notable observation in this stage grouping is that the presence of primary tumor ulceration 'upstages' a patient's survival to that of a patient with a non-ulcerated melanoma of the next-highest tumor thickness category[5] (Table 26.2, Fig. 26.4); current stage groupings (IA–IIB) are summarized in Table 26.2.[5]

## REGIONAL DISEASE

### N classification (stage III)

Regional lymph nodes represent the most common first site of metastasis in patients with melanoma. In the 2002 AJCC melanoma staging system and representing a departure from prior staging systems, four criteria were established as significant prognostic factors for survival in patients with regional metastases and these have been maintained in the 2009 system: 1) the number of lymph nodes that contain metastases, 2) microscopic versus macroscopic nodal tumor burden, 3) the presence of satellite or in-transit metastases, and 4) the presence or absence of primary tumor

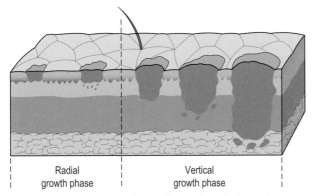

Radial growth phase | Vertical growth phase

**Figure 26.6** Melanoma growth phases. Tumors in vertical growth phase have a higher metastatic potential.

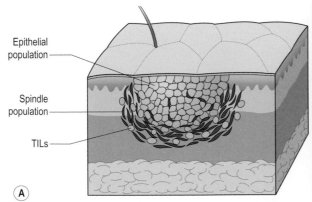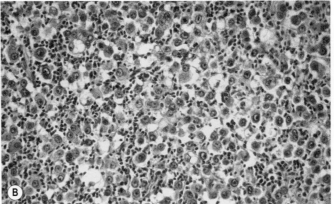

Epithelial population

Spindle population

TILs

(A) (B)

**Figure 26.7** Tumor-infiltrating lymphocytes: **A)** an illustrated example of lymphocytic infiltration which is peripheral but non-brisk; **B)** a photomicrograph showing a brisk lymphocytic infiltrate. (Image courtesy of Dr Martin Mihm.)

ulceration[1,5,6] (Tables 26.1 and 26.2). Reflecting the prognostic importance of these criteria, pathologic evaluation of regional lymph nodes is required to determine a pathologic stage in all patients except those with T0 (i.e. melanoma in situ) or T1a disease.[3,5]

## Number of involved lymph nodes

Based on earlier staging systems, nodal size (3 cm cutpoint in the 1997 AJCC staging system)[2] was the principal stratification criterion. The number of involved lymph nodes was the most important predictor of survival in the more recent multivariate analyses for patients with nodal disease[9,32,33] and represents a principal component of the N classification.[5] The best statistical grouping for involved lymph nodes was again noted to be 1 versus 2 to 3 versus 4 or more. [5,6]

## Regional lymph node tumor burden

Another important prognostic factor in the AJCC N-classification analysis was regional lymph node tumor burden, empirically defined as microscopic versus macroscopic. Microscopic tumor burden was defined as nodal metastases that were pathologically detected (commonly by SLN biopsy – see below) yet clinically occult. Macroscopic tumor burden was defined as nodal metastases that were clinically identified and pathologically confirmed. In the recent AJCC analysis, 5-year survival rates for patients with macroscopic nodal disease (43%) were significantly worse than rates for patients with microscopic nodal disease (67%, P<0.001) (see also Table 26.7).[5]

## Evolution of stage III disease

The technique of lymphatic mapping and SLN biopsy has been shown to be highly accurate in representing the status of the regional nodal basin (Fig. 26.8).[34-38] Based on its prognostic significance, this approach has become a standard of care for staging clinically negative regional lymph node basins in patients deemed to have sufficient risk of occult nodal metastasis.[39] In nearly all melanoma centers worldwide, SLN biopsy is routinely offered to patients with primary cutaneous melanoma whose primary tumor thickness is at least 1 mm. Among the very prevalent group of patients whose primary tumors are less than 1 mm, in many centers, various clinicopathologic factors have been employed in an attempt to identify patients in this overall favorable risk group who may be at increased risk of harboring microscopic stage III disease and for whom SLN biopsy may be warranted.[40]

The AJCC melanoma staging system currently recommends SLN biopsy for patients with T1b and greater melanoma (including patients with thick primaries). It is important to note that while roughly half of patients with stage III disease in the 2002 AJCC analysis had microscopic disease, 81% of patients with stage III disease in the current AJCC analysis had only microscopic nodal disease, the majority of whom were staged using this technique (Table 26.7).[41] This approach has also led to a significant shift in prognosis of patients with melanoma metastatic to regional lymph nodes, as survival is notably better in patients with micrometastases compared to patients with macrometastases.

**Table 26.7 Five-Year Survival Rates for Stage III (Nodal Metastases) Patients Stratified by Number of Metastatic Nodes, Primary Tumor Ulceration, and Nodal Tumor Burden (Microscopic or Macroscopic) (n=2313)**

| Primary Tumor Ulceration | No. of Nodal Micrometastases % ± S.E. | | | No. of Nodal Macrometastases % ± S.E. | | |
|---|---|---|---|---|---|---|
| | 1 | 2–3 | ≥4 | 1 | 2–3 | ≥4 |
| Absent | 81.5 ± 1.9 (777) | 73.2 ± 3.7 (246) | 38.0 ± 8.5 (46) | 51.6 ± 7.2 (75) | 46.6 ± 7.9 (67) | 45.4 ± 9.1 (50) |
| Present | 56.6 ± 2.9 (531) | 53.9 ± 4.2 (223) | 34.0 ± 8.3 (49) | 49.4 ± 6.2 (88) | 37.7 ± 6.2 (93) | 29.2 ± 6.7 (68) |

Source: Balch CM, Gershenwald JE, Soong SJ, et al: Multivariate analysis of prognostic factors among 2313 patients with stage III melanoma: comparison of nodal micrometastases versus macrometastases. *J Clin Oncol.* 2009, *In press.*

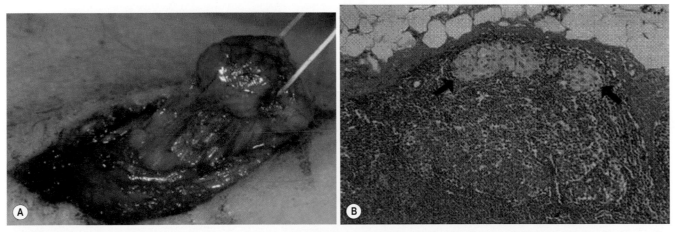

**Figure 26.8 A)** Intraoperative identification of a sentinel lymph node (SLN). Intradermal injection of a vital blue dye around the intact melanoma or biopsy site leads to uptake of the dye by the lymphatic system and transport of the dye to the draining regional nodal basins, thereby allowing for identification of SLNs. Note isosulfan blue-stained afferent lymphatic vessel leading to blue-stained SLN. (Courtesy of Jeffrey E. Gershenwald, MD. Copyright retained by the author and the U.T. M. D. Anderson Cancer Center). **B)** Example of SLN metastasis (hematoxylin & eosin). (From Gershenwald JE, Colome MI, Lee JE, et al: Patterns of recurrence following a negative sentinel lymph node biopsy in 243 patients with stage I or II melanoma. *J Clin Oncol.* 1998; 16:2253-60.)

## Satellite and in-transit disease

Conceptually, in-transit and satellite metastases have been described as recurrent locoregional disease found in the dermis or subcutaneous tissue between the primary melanoma and the regional lymph node basin (Fig. 26.9). Both satellite and in-transit disease represent manifestations of intralymphatic tumor dissemination, and beginning with the 2002 AJCC melanoma staging system, were merged with regional nodes into the N category (Tables 26.1 and 26.2; Fig. 26.3) to better reflect this biological continuum. In many studies, including the 2008 AJCC analysis, patients with satellite or in-transit disease (AJCC 5-year survival 69%, N2c) had a prognosis relatively similar to that of patients with nodal metastases.[5,6,9,42-44] Therefore, the designation N2c is included in the N2 classification for in-transit or satellite metastases in the absence of nodal metastases. Melanomas with both nodal and in-transit or satellite metastases are classified as N3 disease, since this extent of disease is associated with worse survival (AJCC 5-year survival 33%, N3) (Tables 26.1 and 26.2). This pattern of recurrence is unique to melanoma and is reported to occur in 3% to 12% of melanoma cases.[45] Although the molecular deter-minants and pathophysiology of in-transit disease are not well defined, such events most likely represent an intralymphatic manifestation of melanoma metastases.

In a study from The University of Texas M. D. Anderson Cancer Center, patients with a positive SLN had a significantly higher rate of in-transit metastases (12%) than patients with a negative SLN (3.5%).[45] Regional nodal metastases occur in about two-thirds of patients with in-transit disease and, if present, are associated with lower survival rates.

## Primary tumor ulceration

Ulceration of the primary tumor was included in the stage III classification beginning in 2002 because it independently predicted survival in patients with nodal metastases;[4,5,9,46,47] the presence of an ulcerated primary melanoma in patients with stage III disease upstages a patient's survival to that of a patient with a non-ulcerated melanoma in a higher nodal tumor burden category (Table 26.2).[6]

## Other variables

Multivariate AJCC analyses revealed distinct patterns of independent predictors when patients were stratified by

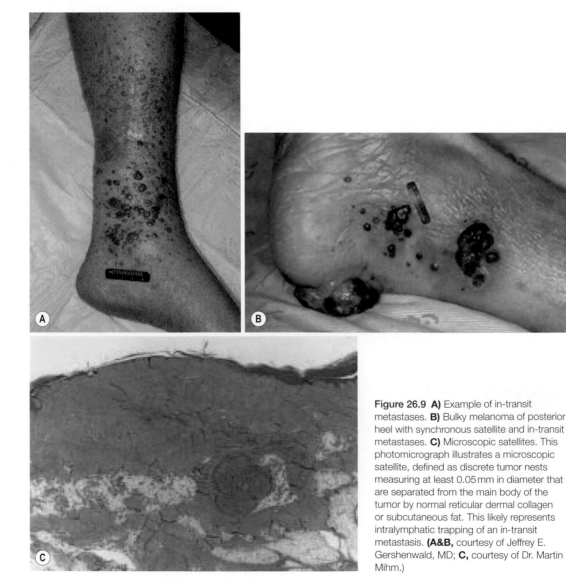

**Figure 26.9 A)** Example of in-transit metastases. **B)** Bulky melanoma of posterior heel with synchronous satellite and in-transit metastases. **C)** Microscopic satellites. This photomicrograph illustrates a microscopic satellite, defined as discrete tumor nests measuring at least 0.05 mm in diameter that are separated from the main body of the tumor by normal reticular dermal collagen or subcutaneous fat. This likely represents intralymphatic trapping of an in-transit metastasis. **(A&B,** courtesy of Jeffrey E. Gershenwald, MD; **C,** courtesy of Dr. Martin Mihm.)

tumor burden. In 1072 patients with nodal micrometastases, number of involved lymph nodes, primary tumor thickness, ulceration, mitotic rate, and anatomic site of primary (but not Clark level) all correlated with survival; in contrast, none of these histopathologic features independently predicted survival in 268 patients with macrometastases.[41]

## Stage III groupings

Because of the significant heterogeneity of prognoses among patients with stage III disease, three substages were defined: IIIA, IIIB, and IIIC (Table 26.2, Fig. 26.1C).[3,5] The 5-year survival rates for patients with stages IIIA, IIIB, and IIIC disease are 78%, 59%, and 40%, respectively (Fig. 26.1C). The heterogeneity of stage III melanoma patients with regional metastases is well illustrated in Table 26.7, most notably among patients with nodal micrometastases (5-year survival 29.2–81.5%).

## Additional considerations – local recurrence, satellites, and in-transit metastasis

### Local recurrence versus satellites

Classically, true local recurrence implies the regrowth of incompletely excised melanoma and should be distinguished from clinical satellitosis and/or in-transit disease. However, since most melanoma patients who develop local recurrences have had wide local excision with relatively extensive negative margins, local recurrence after wide excision likely more accurately represents a form of lymphatic metastasis that is distinct from regrowth of primary tumor that was incompletely excised.[9] This is supported by the similar prognosis for patients with 'local recurrence'[44,48,49] compared with that for patients with satellite, in-transit,[44,48,50] and/or regional lymph node metastases,[12,18,51-57] supporting the concept that these are probably manifestations of the same disease process – i.e. lymphatic dissemination.

True local recurrence is defined as recurrence at the primary tumor site, within or contiguous with the scar, and is most likely the result of incomplete excision of the primary tumor. This finding is uncommon and may often, more appropriately, be considered persistence of the primary tumor.[58,59] Since the prognosis after a true local recurrence is significantly better than that associated with in-transit disease (see the next section), correct classification is important in treatment planning.

### Microscopic satellitosis and in-transit metastases

Microscopic satellites are defined as discrete tumor nests measuring at least 0.05mm in diameter that are separated from the main body of the tumor by normal reticular dermal collagen or subcutaneous fat (Fig. 26.9C). While this histologic finding has been variably considered to be either a feature of the primary tumor or manifestation of intralymphatic metastasis, it is included in this discussion of regional disease since prognostically it is similar to that of clinical satellites and in-transit metastases.[43] Based on the observation by Buzaid et al.[9] that patients with either satel-

litosis, in-transit metastases, or both, had similar survival using a graphic overlay technique, both the 2002 and 2009 AJCC melanoma staging systems group clinical and microscopic satellitosis with in-transit metastases (i.e. as stage IIIB).[1,5,6]

## Clinical relevance of submicroscopic disease

Molecular techniques such as reverse transcriptase polymerase chain reaction (RT-PCR) have been explored to detect submicroscopic disease in SLNs that might not be detectable by even contemporary conventional histologic methods.[60-68] Early studies with limited follow-up have suggested that the prognosis of patients with an SLN that is RT-PCR-positive but histologically negative is worse than that of patients who have negative results by all techniques; however, after longer follow-up in two of these studies, there was no difference in recurrence rates between patients in the two groups.[69,70] Taken together, these data suggest that the clinical utility of RT-PCR SLN staging is not yet clear.[66,71] Despite the absence of survival impact from these longer-term follow-up studies, investigators at the JWCI reported intriguing data to support the possibility that these approaches may be used to identify submicroscopic disease[72,73] and are addressing this hypothesis in the Multicenter Selective Lymphadenectomy Trial-II (MSLT-II). Nonetheless, RT-PCR remains investigational and should not be used to direct adjuvant therapy or completion lymph node dissection at this time.[69,70]

### DISTANT METASTASES

Patients with stage IV melanoma generally have a poor prognosis with a median survival from the time of initial stage IV diagnosis of 6–7.5 months and an associated 5-year survival of less than 10%.[13,74-77] Recent prognostic factor analyses have, however, identified several independent factors that predict survival in the overall poor-prognosis group.[76-78] In an effort to significantly expand previous stage IV analyses, the AJCC developed a first-in-kind international AJCC stage IV database in 2008 in which more than 9000 patients with stage IV melanoma were compiled (Fig. 26.1A,D).

In patients with distant disease, the site or sites of metastases and serum levels of LDH are used to delineate the M categories into three groups: M1a, M1b, and M1c, with 1-year survival rates of 62% for M1a, 53% for M1b, and 33% for M1c melanoma.[5] Patients with distant metastasis in the skin, subcutaneous tissue, or distant lymph nodes are categorized as M1a if their LDH level is normal, and have a relatively better prognosis compared to patients with disease located in other anatomic sites. Patients with metastases to the lung are categorized as M1b based on an 'intermediate' stage IV prognosis. Patients with metastases to any other visceral sites, or a combination of any site with an elevated serum LDH, are designated as M1c and are associated with the shortest survival estimates. While LDH levels have definite prognostic significance in known metastatic disease, the benefit of screening LDH levels for patients with localized disease, if any, has not been established.

Building on the initial experience of the 2002 AJCC melanoma database analysis, the international AJCC 2008 stage IV database demonstrated that survival differences among skin, subcutaneous and distant lymph node metastases (M1a), versus lung metastases (M1b), versus other visceral sites of metastases (M1c) were maintained and were also independently associated with survival by multivariate Cox regression analysis that included elevated LDH level as an important independent adverse predictor of survival. These data support the current AJCC stage IV staging system.[79] Other predictors of survival in patients with stage IV disease include site of distant metastasis, number of metastatic sites, and number of metastases and performance status.[74-77,80] It is anticipated that ongoing analyses will identify additional prognostic factors that may also facilitate design and analysis of melanoma clinical trials and potentially calibrate therapeutic intensity to metastatic risk.

## METASTATIC MELANOMA TO LYMPH NODES FROM AN UNKNOWN PRIMARY SITE

Although the majority of patients with metastatic melanoma initially present with a known primary, no identifiable primary tumor and no history of a primary melanoma is identified in 2–9% of patients who present with evidence of melanoma nodal metastasis. The most frequent site of nodal involvment when a primary site is not identified is the axilla (47%), followed by the neck and groin.[13] Cormier et al.[81] conducted a retrospective analysis of consecutive patients with melanoma from an unknown primary (MUP) (n=71) who underwent surgical resection for metastasis to regional lymph nodes and were classified by N category after lymph node dissection was performed. In multivariate analyses, MUP was identified as a favorable prognostic factor for overall survival, supporting previous reports that demonstrated similar survival rates in patients with an unknown primary site compared to patients matched according to nodal metastasis having a known primary site.[74] More recently, the favorable survival profile in patients with MUP was also noted in a study of 262 patients with MUP by researchers at the John Wayne Cancer Institute.[82]

The relatively favorable survival profile of patients with MUP suggests that patients with MUP have a natural history that is relatively similar to if not better than that of many patients with stage III disease.[5] The inability to identify the primary tumor in patients with metastatic melanoma to lymph nodes after a thorough search does not appear to be an adverse prognostic factor; accordingly, if an appropriate staging work-up does not reveal any other sites of metastases, these patients are now considered AJCC stage III and should be considered for a surgical approach as well as stage III adjuvant therapy protocols.[81] Of note, patients who present with skin or subcutaneous metastases without a known primary should also be presumed to be regional (i.e. stage III instead of stage IV) if appropriate staging work-up does not reveal sites of distant metastasis and pathology review by an experienced melanoma pathologist confirms the lesion is not a variant of a primary melanoma.[6]

## FUTURE OUTLOOK

The absence of dependable biomarkers to gauge prognosis and response to therapy has limited the speed with which new agents can be evaluated, especially for adjuvant therapeutic trials. While LDH levels have been associated with poor prognosis in patients with metastatic melanoma and have therefore been incorporated into the staging system as described above, its non-specific nature does not allow LDH levels to be followed as a biomarker during therapy. A number of studies have evaluated various potential biomarkers, including methods to detect circulating DNA and PCR of circulating mononuclear cells for the expression of tumor antigens such as MART-1 and gp100. Work has also been performed evaluating serum S100B levels in melanoma patients. In one study evaluating stage IIB and III melanoma patients, S100B levels were found to correlate with relapse and death.[83] Lower S100B values at baseline and over 1 year of follow-up were associated with longer survival when compared to patients with low levels at baseline that increased to high levels during the follow-up period. In a meta-analysis including 22 studies (3393 stage I to IV cutaneous melanoma patients),[84] serum S100B levels were associated with poorer survival (hazard ratio 2.23 [p<0.0001]). While S100B and LDH may add to prognostic information, biomarkers that can be followed to assess response to therapy are needed. Reliable biomarkers may ultimately enhance prognostic assessment, facilitate selection of patients for specific therapies, and contribute to the evaluation of new agents. Perhaps the melanoma community's first glimmers of this potential reality include the identification of somatic kit and B-RAF mutations that have led to the first cadre of melanoma targeted therapy trials currently underway.

These and other data[85] clearly demonstrate advances in our understanding of the genetic basis for melanocytic transformation.[85] Overall, these findings may be leveraged in the future to improve the classification of melanoma, possibly leading to an improved ability to predict outcome and, by identification of new targets for anti-tumor therapy, response to therapy, too.[85]

As its incidence continues to increase, melanoma remains a growing public health concern. Insights into genetic aberrations in melanoma provide the unique opportunity to refine our approach to melanoma classification by defining patient subsets based on biology, and has the potential to evolve into better diagnostic, prognostic, and therapeutic approaches for this disease.

The 7th edition of the *AJCC Cancer Staging Manual* reflects a contemporary understanding of relevant prognostic factors based on a comprehensive database analysis. While this analysis largely validated the prior staging system, notable lessons learned include the importance of mitotic rate in primary melanoma, the evolution and tremendous heterogeneity of stage III disease, and insights regarding stage IV disease.

It is probable that multiple known and as yet unknown prognostic factors may further define heterogeneity in clinical course and outcome for patients with early-stage melanoma. Going forward, rapidly maturing technologies may make possible a genomic approach to melanoma classification – in both the primary and metastases alike – potentially allowing the identification of candidate genetic markers or expression profiles that might be important for diagnosis, prognostic assessment, and even identification of therapeutic targets and response to therapy.

## REFERENCES

1. Balch CM, Buzaid AC, Soong SJ, et al. Final version of the American Joint Committee on Cancer staging system for cutaneous melanoma. *J Clin Oncol.* 2001;19:3635–3648.
2. Gershenwald JE, Buzaid AC, Ross MI. Classification and staging of melanoma. *Hematol Oncol Clin North Am.* 1998;12:737–765.
3. Balch CM. Melanoma of the skin. In: Greene FL, Page DL, Fleming ID, et al., eds. AJCC Cancer Staging Manual. 6th ed. New York: Springer Verlag; 2002.
4. Balch CM, Soong SJ, Gershenwald JE, et al. Prognostic factors analysis of 17,600 melanoma patients: validation of the American Joint Committee on Cancer melanoma staging system. *J Clin Oncol.* 2001;19:3622–3634.
5. Balch CM. Melanoma of the skin. In: Edge SB, Byrd DR, Compton CC, et al., eds. AJCC *Cancer Staging Manual.* 7th ed. New York: Springer Verlag; 2009.
6. Balch CM, Gershenwald JE, Soong SJ, et al. Final version of 2009 AJCC melanoma staging and classification. *J Clin Oncol.* 2009;27:6199–6206.
7. Breslow A. Thickness, cross-sectional areas and depth of invasion in the prognosis of cutaneous melanoma. *Ann Surg.* 1970;172:902–908.
8. Balch C, Soong S, Ross M, et al. Long-term results of a multi-institutional randomized trial comparing prognostic factors and surgical results for intermediate thickness melanomas (1.0 to 4.0 mm). Intergroup Melanoma Surgical Trial. *Ann Surg Oncol.* 2000;7:87–97.
9. Buzaid AC, Ross MI, Balch CM, et al. Critical analysis of the current American Joint Committee on Cancer staging system for cutaneous melanoma and proposal of a new staging system. *J Clin Oncol.* 1997;15:1039–1051.
10. Balch CM, Wilkerson JA, Murad TM, et al. The prognostic significance of ulceration of cutaneous melanoma. *Cancer.* 1980;45:3012–3017.
11. McGovern VJ, Shaw HM, Milton GW, et al. Ulceration and prognosis in cutaneous malignant melanoma. *Histopathology.* 1982;6:399–407.
12. Spatz A, Cook MG, Elder DE, et al. Interobserver reproducibility of ulceration assessment in primary cutaneous melanomas. *Eur J Cancer.* 2003;39:1861–1865.
13. Gershenwald JE, Balch CM, Soong S, et al. Prognostic factors and natural history of melanoma. In: Balch CM, Soong SJ, Sober AJ, et al., eds. Cutaneous Melanoma. 5th ed. St. Louis: Quality Medical Publishing; 2009.
14. Azzola MF, Shaw HM, Thompson JF, et al. Tumor mitotic rate is a more powerful prognostic indicator than ulceration in patients with primary cutaneous melanoma: an analysis of 3661 patients from a single center. *Cancer.* 2003;97:1488–1498.
15. Nagore E, Oliver V, Botella-Estrada R, et al. Prognostic factors in localized invasive cutaneous melanoma: high value of mitotic rate, vascular invasion and microscopic satellitosis. *Melanoma Res.* 2005;15:169–177.
16. Lasithiotakis KG, Leiter U, Eigentler T, et al. Improvement of overall survival of patients with cutaneous melanoma in Germany, 1976-2001: which factors contributed? *Cancer.* 2007;109:1174–1182.
17. Zogakis TG, Essner R, Wang HJ, et al. Natural history of melanoma in 773 patients with tumor-negative sentinel lymph nodes. *Ann Surg Oncol.* 2007;14:1604–1611.
18. Barnhill RL, Katzen J, Spatz A, et al. The importance of mitotic rate as a prognostic factor for localized cutaneous melanoma. *J Cutan Pathol.* 2005;32:268–273.
19. Busam KJ. The prognostic importance of tumor mitotic rate for patients with primary cutaneous melanoma. *Ann Surg Oncol.* 2004;11:360–361.
20. Gimotty PA, Elder DE, Fraker DL, et al. Identification of high-risk patients among those diagnosed with thin cutaneous melanomas. *J Clin Oncol.* 2007;25:1129–1134.
21. Balch CM, Gershenwald JE, Soong S, et al. Melanoma staging and classification. In: Balch CM, Soong SJ, Sober AJ, et al, eds. Cutaneous Melanoma. 5th ed. St. Louis: Quality Medical Publishing; 2009:65–85.
22. Clark Jr WH, From L, Bernardino EA, et al. The histogenesis and biologic behavior of primary human malignant melanomas of the skin. *Cancer Res.* 1969;29:705–727.
23. Vollmer RT. Malignant melanoma. A multivariate analysis of prognostic factors. *Pathol Annu.* 1989;24(Pt 1):383–407.
24. Morton DL, Davtyan DG, Wanek LA, et al. Multivariate analysis of the relationship between survival and the microstage of primary melanoma by Clark level and Breslow thickness. *Cancer.* 1993;71:3737–3743.
25. Garbe C, Buttner P, Bertz J, et al. Primary cutaneous melanoma. Prognostic classification of anatomic location. *Cancer.* 1995;75:2492–2498.
26. Schuchter L, Schultz DJ, Synnestvedt M, et al. A prognostic model for predicting 10-year survival in patients with primary melanoma. The Pigmented Lesion Group [see comments]. *Ann Intern Med.* 1996;125:369–375.
27. Clark Jr WH, Elder DE, Van Horn M. The biologic forms of malignant melanoma. *Hum Pathol.* 1986;17:443–450.
28. Clark Jr WH, Elder DE, Guerry D, et al. Model predicting survival in stage I melanoma based on tumor progression. *J Natl Cancer Inst.* 1989;81:1893–1904.
29. Mraz-Gernhard S, Sagebiel RW, Kashani-Sabet M, et al. Prediction of sentinel lymph node micrometastasis by histological features in primary cutaneous malignant melanoma. *Arch Dermatol.* 1998;134:983–987.
30. MacKie RM, Bufalino R, Morabito A, et al. Lack of effect of pregnancy on outcome of melanoma. For The World Health Organisation Melanoma Programme. *Lancet.* 1991;337:653–655.
31. Travers RL, Sober AJ, Berwick M, et al. Increased thickness of pregnancy-associated melanoma. *Br J Dermatol.* 1995;132:876–883.
32. Gershenwald JE, Colome MI, Lee JE, et al. Patterns of recurrence following a negative sentinel lymph node biopsy in 243 patients with stage I or II melanoma. *J Clin Oncol.* 1998;16:2253–2260.
33. Gershenwald JE, Fischer D, Buzaid AC. Clinical classification and staging. *Clin Plast Surg.* 2000;27:361–376.
34. Morton DL, Wen DR, Wong JH, et al. Technical details of intraoperative lymphatic mapping for early stage melanoma. *Arch Surg.* 1992;127:392–399.
35. Gershenwald J, Thompson W, Mansfield P, et al. Multi-institutional melanoma lymphatic mapping experience: the prognostic value of sentinel lymph node status in 612 stage I or II melanoma patients. *J Clin Oncol.* 1999;17:976–983.
36. Morton DL, Thompson JF, Cochran AJ, et al. Sentinel-node biopsy or nodal observation in melanoma. *N Engl J Med.* 2006;355:1307–1317.
37. Morton DL, Thompson JF, Essner R, et al. Validation of the accuracy of intraoperative lymphatic mapping and sentinel lymphadenectomy for early-stage melanoma. *Ann Surg.* 1999;230:453–465.
38. Thompson JF, McCarthy WH, Bosch CM, et al. Sentinel lymph node status as an indicator of the presence of metastatic melanoma in regional lymph nodes. *Melanoma Res.* 1995;5:255–260.
39. Balch CM, Morton DL, Gershenwald JE, et al. Sentinel node biopsy and standard of care for melanoma. *J Am Acad Dermatol.* 2009;60:872–875.
40. Andtbacka RH, Gershenwald JE. The role of sentinel lymph node biopsy in patients with thin melanoma. *J Natl Compr Canc Netw.* 2009;7:308–317.
41. Balch CM, Gershenwald JE, Soong SJ, et al. Multivariate analysis of prognostic factors among 2313 patients with stage III melanoma: comparison of nodal micrometastases versus macrometastases. *J Clin Oncol.* 2010;28:2452–2459.
42. Cascinelli N, Belli F, Santinami M, et al. Sentinel lymph node biopsy in cutaneous melanoma: the WHO Melanoma Program experience. *Ann Surg Oncol.* 2000;7:469–474.
43. Haffner AC, Garbe C, Burg G, et al. The prognosis of primary and metastasising melanoma. An evaluation of the TNM classification in 2,495 patients. *Br J Cancer.* 1992;66:856–861.
44. Karakousis CP, Temple DF, Moore R, et al. Prognostic parameters in recurrent malignant melanoma. *Cancer.* 1983;52:575–579.
45. Pawlik TM, Ross MI, Johnson MM, et al. Predictors and natural history of in-transit melanoma after sentinel lymphadenectomy. *Ann Surg Oncol.* 2005;12:587–596.
46. Balch C, Soong S, Murad T, et al. A multifactorial analysis of melanoma: prognostic factors in melanoma patients with lymph node metastases (stage II). *Ann Surg.* 1981;193:377–388.
47. Gershenwald JE, Thompson W, Mansfield PF, et al. Multi-institutional melanoma lymphatic mapping experience: the prognostic value of sentinel lymph node status in 612 stage I or II melanoma patients. *J Clin Oncol.* 1999;17:976–983.
48. Cascinelli N, Bufalino R, Marolda R, et al. Regional non-nodal metastases of cutaneous melanoma. *Eur J Surg Oncol.* 1986;12:175–180.
49. Reintgen DS, Vollmer R, Tso CY, et al. Prognosis for recurrent stage I malignant melanoma. *Arch Surg.* 1987;122:1338–1342.
50. Roses DF, Karp NS, Oratz R, et al. Survival with regional and distant metastases from cutaneous malignant melanoma. *Surg Gynecol Obstet.* 1991;172:262–268.
51. Balch CM, Soong S, Ross MI, et al. Long-term results of a multi-institutional randomized trial comparing prognostic factors and surgical results for intermediate thickness melanomas (1.0 to 4.0 mm). Intergroup Melanoma Surgical Trial. *Ann Surg Oncol.* 2000;7:87–97.
52. Balch CM, Urist MM, Karakousis CP, et al. Efficacy of 2-cm surgical margins for intermediate-thickness melanomas (1 to 4 mm). Results of a multi-institutional randomized surgical trial. *Ann Surg.* 1993;218:262–267.
53. Leon P, Daly JM, Synnestvedt M, et al. The prognostic implications of microscopic satellites in patients with clinical stage I melanoma. *Arch Surg.* 1991;126:1461–1468.
54. Ringborg U, Andersson R, Eldh J, et al. Resection margins of 2 versus 5 cm for cutaneous malignant melanoma with a tumor thickness of 0.8 to 2.0 mm: randomized study by the Swedish Melanoma Study Group. *Cancer.* 1996;77:1809–1814.
55. Sondak VK, Taylor JM, Sabel MS, et al. Mitotic rate and younger age are predictors of sentinel lymph node positivity: lessons learned from the generation of a probabilistic model. *Ann Surg Oncol.* 2004;11:247–258.

56. Thomas JM, Newton-Bishop J, A'Hern R, et al. Excision margins in high-risk malignant melanoma. *N Engl J Med.* 2004;350:757–766.

57. Veronesi U, Cascinelli N. Narrow excision (1-cm margin). A safe procedure for thin cutaneous melanoma. *Arch Surg.* 1991;126:438–441.

58. Wolf IH, Richtig E, Kopera D, et al. Locoregional cutaneous metastases of malignant melanoma and their management. *Dermatol Surg.* 2004;30:244–247.

59. Yu LL, Heenan PJ. The morphological features of locally recurrent melanoma and cutaneous metastases of melanoma. *Hum Pathol.* 1999;30:551–555.

60. Goydos JS, Patel KN, Shih WJ, et al. Patterns of recurrence in patients with melanoma and histologically negative but RT-PCR-positive sentinel lymph nodes. *J Am Coll Surg.* 2003;196:196–204.

61. Goydos JS, Ravikumar TS, Germino FJ, et al. Minimally invasive staging of patients with melanoma: sentinel lymphadenectomy and detection of the melanoma-specific proteins MART-1 and tyrosinase by reverse transcriptase polymerase chain reaction. *J Am Coll Surg.* 1998;187:182–188; discussion 188-190.

62. Reintgen D, Albertini J, Berman C, et al. Accurate nodal staging of malignant melanoma. *Cancer Control.* 1995;2:405–414.

63. Ribuffo D, Gradilone A, Vonella M, et al. Prognostic significance of reverse transcriptase-polymerase chain reaction-negative sentinel nodes in malignant melanoma. *Ann Surg Oncol.* 2003;10:396–402.

64. Shivers SC, Wang X, Li W, et al. Molecular staging of malignant melanoma: correlation with clinical outcome. *JAMA.* 1998;280:1410–1415.

65. Wang X, Heller R, VanVoorhis N, et al. Detection of submicroscopic lymph node metastases with polymerase chain reaction in patients with malignant melanoma. *Ann Surg.* 1994;220:768–774.

66. Chapman PB. Detection of melanoma cells in sentinel lymph nodes by PCR is not yet ready for prime time. *Pigment Cell Res.* 2007;20:343–344.

67. Mocellin S, Hoon DS, Pilati P, et al. Sentinel lymph node molecular ultrastaging in patients with melanoma: a systematic review and meta-analysis of prognosis. *J Clin Oncol.* 2007;25:1588–1595.

68. Smith B, Selby P, Southgate J, et al. Detection of melanoma cells in peripheral blood by means of reverse transcriptase and polymerase chain reaction. *Lancet.* 1991;338:1227–1229.

69. Kammula U, Ghossein R, Bhattacharya S, et al. Serial follow-up and the prognostic significance of reverse transcriptase-polymerase chain reaction-staged sentinel lymph nodes from melanoma patients. *J Clin Oncol.* 2004;22:3989–3996.

70. Scoggins CR, Ross MI, Reintgen DS, et al. Prospective multi-institutional study of reverse transcriptase polymerase chain reaction for molecular staging of melanoma. *J Clin Oncol.* 2006;24:2849–2857.

71. Tatlidil C, Parkhill WS, Giacomantonio CA, et al. Detection of tyrosinase mRNA in the sentinel lymph nodes of melanoma patients is not a predictor of short-term disease recurrence. *Mod Pathol.* 2007;20:427–434.

72. Hoon DS, Wang W, Dale PS, et al. Detection of occult melanoma cells in blood with a multiple-marker polymerase chain reaction assay. *J Clin Oncol.* 1995;13:2109–2116.

73. Takeuchi H, Morton DL, Kuo C, et al. Prognostic significance of molecular upstaging of paraffin-embedded sentinel lymph nodes in melanoma patients. *J Clin Oncol.* 2004;22:2671–2680.

74. Balch CM. Cutaneous Melanoma. 2nd ed. Philadelphia: JB Lippincott; 1992.

75. Barth A, Wanek LA, Morton DL. Prognostic factors in 1,521 melanoma patients with distant metastases. *J Am Coll Surg.* 1995;181:193–201.

76. Manola J, Atkins M, Ibrahim J, et al. Prognostic factors in metastatic melanoma: a pooled analysis of Eastern Cooperative Oncology Group trials. *J Clin Oncol.* 2000;18:3782–3793.

77. Unger JM, Flaherty LE, Liu PY, et al. Gender and other survival predictors in patients with metastatic melanoma on Southwest Oncology Group trials. *Cancer.* 2001;91:1148–1155.

78. Van Der Esch EP, Cascinelli N, Preda F, et al. Stage I melanoma of the skin: evaluation of prognosis according to histologic characteristics. *Cancer.* 1981;48:1668–1673.

79. Gershenwald JE, Morton DL, Thompson JF, et al. *Staging and prognostic factors for stage IV melanoma: initial results of an American Joint Committee on Cancer (AJCC) international evidence-based assessment of 4895 melanoma patients.* Chicago, IL: 44th Annual Meeting of the American Society of Clinical Oncology; 2008.

80. Eton O, Legha SS, Moon TE, et al. Prognostic factors for survival of patients treated systemically for disseminated melanoma. *J Clin Oncol.* 1998;16:1103–1111.

81. Cormier JN, Xing Y, Feng L, et al. Metastatic melanoma to lymph nodes in patients with unknown primary sites. *Cancer.* 2006;106:2012–2020.

82. Lee CC, Faries MB, Wanek LA, et al. Improved survival after lymphadenectomy for nodal metastasis from an unknown primary melanoma. *J Clin Oncol.* 2008;26:535–541.

83. Tarhini AA, Stuckert J, Lee S, et al. Prognostic significance of serum S100B protein in high-risk surgically resected melanoma patients participating in Intergroup Trial ECOG 1694. *J Clin Oncol.* 2009;27:38–44.

84. Mocellin S, Zavagno G, Nitti D. The prognostic value of serum S100B in patients with cutaneous melanoma: a meta-analysis. *Int J Cancer.* 2008;123:2370–2376.

85. Bastian BC, Pinkel D, Viros A. Genetics and molecular pathology. In: Balch CM, Milton GW, Soong SJ, eds. *Cutaneous Melanoma.* 5th ed. St. Louis: Quality Medical Publishing; 2009:807–820.

# Pathology of Melanoma: Interpretation and New Concepts

*Carlos Ricotti, Jennifer Cather, and Clay J. Cockerell*

## Key Points

- It is essential that clinicians understand the appropriate methods for biopsy of lesions that are highly suspect for melanoma to enhance accurate diagnosis.

- Histopathologists who diagnose cutaneous melanoma must be aware of the many different histologic variants and the simulators of melanoma.

- Special stains and other techniques are valuable adjuncts to routine histology but no individual stain or special technique alone can distinguish between a benign nevus and melanoma.

- The ability to assess melanoma prognosis based on histologic features alone is somewhat limited.

- Breslow thickness remains the most reliable individual histological prognostic factor.

## INTRODUCTION

The clinical analysis of pigmented lesions typically results in sampling of the lesion for microscopic examination to determine whether the lesion is benign or malignant. The diagnosis of melanoma is established on pathological grounds using cytological and architectural features observed under the microscope that when grouped are known as 'criteria' that allow for definitive diagnosis. Though most melanocytic proliferations can be classified as either benign or malignant using routine histopathology, there are lesions that demonstrate 'conflicting' criteria making definitive diagnosis difficult.

Adjunctive clinical tools such as dermoscopy have improved detection.[1] Management of 'suspicious' pigmented lesions requires appropriate sampling so that accurate pathological diagnosis and staging can be rendered.

Recently there has been a surge of sophisticated molecular techniques developed for the diagnosis of melanoma, but although the published data are somewhat promising, these have yet to substitute for routine histopathological diagnosis.[2]

## HISTOLOGIC DIAGNOSIS OF MELANOMA

### Natural history of melanoma: histologic aspects

Although some controversy exists about how melanoma develops and evolves, a pathway proposed by Ackerman is considered by many to be the most valid.[3,4] Accordingly,

an oncogenic stimulus such as ultraviolet irradiation affects melanocytes in the epidermis at the dermoepidermal junction (DEJ) resulting in neoplastic transformation. These altered melanocytes begin to proliferate initially as solitary units at the DEJ and manifest histologically as scattered, single hyperchromatic cells with a cleft or halo surrounding them. Clinically, there may be only a very light tan macule or it may be undetectable (Fig. 27.1).

Over time, these melanocytes become more numerous and coalesce forming small nests confined to the DEJ. There may also be involvement of adnexal structures such as acrotrichia and acrosyringia. At this point, there is often a tan to brown macule ranging from 3 to 4 mm in diameter but it is usually not significantly atypical (Fig. 27.2). As the lesion progresses, more nests of atypical melanocytes develop at the DEJ and solitary atypical melanocytes ascend to the upper portions of the epidermis.[5] In time, nests also extend above the DEJ. Clinically, such lesions may appear darker brown and shades of black may be seen which correlates with the presence of melanin in the upper levels of the epidermis and cornified layer (Fig. 27.3). Some of the architectural features of melanoma may begin to be visible at this time, namely asymmetry and irregular borders.

As the lesion progresses, there is more involvement of the epidermis with nests and single atypical melanocytes throughout and involving the adnexal structures. Neoplastic melanocytes also enter the papillary dermis, initially in small foci, but over time it becomes more extensively involved, filled and expanded (Figs 27.4 and 27.5). At this stage, lesions are usually greater than 6 mm in diameter and demonstrate the 'ABCDE' clinical features of melanoma in most cases. Most lesions at this stage are still macular or only slightly elevated although skin markings are often obliterated.

Subsequently, lesions may progress to involve deeper structures such as the reticular dermis and subcutaneous fat. This may be accompanied by additional clinical features including nodule formation, ulceration and colors such as red, blue and white, the latter associated with regression. These features signify more advanced lesions and worse prognosis.[6,7] Finally, metastasis may develop. Usually, regional lymph nodes are involved first although local 'satellite' cutaneous metastasis may be the initial manifestation of metastatic disease.

Different clinical and histologic manifestations are seen depending on which sites are involved. In cutaneous metastases of melanoma, histologically there are aggregates of atypical neoplastic melanocytes in the dermis usually

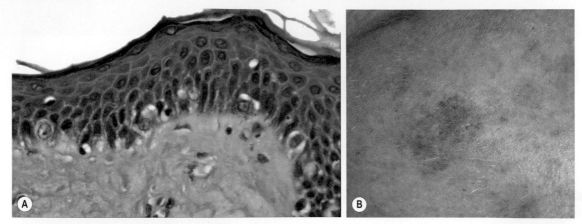

**Figure 27.1** Natural history of melanoma. Melanoma begins with a proliferation of slightly atypical melanocytes arranged as solitary units at the dermoepidermal junction, usually on sun-damaged skin as depicted here **(A)**. The distance between melanocytes varies. Atypical melanocytes are manifest as small, hyperchromatic cells with clear haloes surrounding them (H&E, original magnification ×100.) Clinically, there may be no lesion visible or only a very faint tan macule, as in this photograph **(B)**.

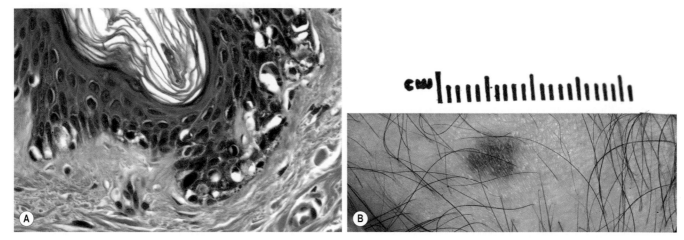

**Figure 27.2** Natural history of melanoma. As melanoma evolves, the number of atypical melanocytes increases, their nuclei become more atypical and melanocytes are present above the dermoepidermal junction and within the epithelium of adnexal structures **(A)**. Clinically, these are usually tan macules, usually up to 4 mm in diameter. They may be quite nondescript and, as such, biopsies may not be performed at this stage **(B)**. (H&E, original magnification ×100.)

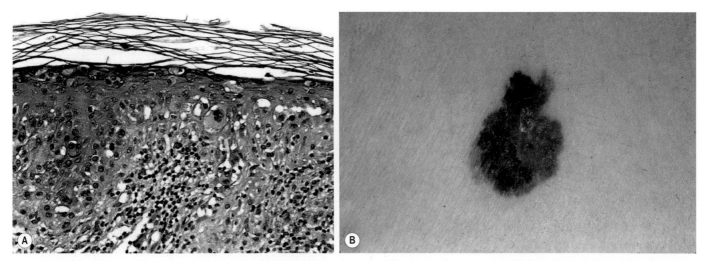

**Figure 27.3** Natural history of melanoma. In time, nests of atypical melanocytes form at the dermoepidermal junction that are distributed non-uniformly and begin to coalesce. More atypical melanocytes, both singly and in nests, are present throughout the epidermis, giving rise to the 'buckshot scatter' pattern **(A)**. Clinically, these lesions are usually tan with foci of black, have irregular borders and are usually greater than 6 mm in diameter **(B)**. This represents melanoma in situ. (H&E, original magnification ×100.)

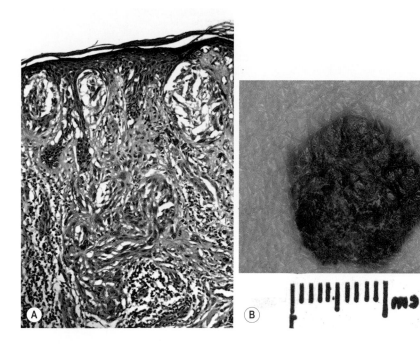

**Figure 27.4** Natural history of melanoma. In this melanoma, although most of the atypical melanocytes are present throughout the epidermis, there is a small nest of atypical melanocytes in the papillary dermis **(A)**. Clinically, this represents melanoma with early dermal involvement and would usually have an appearance that has been described by the mnemonic 'ABCD' **(B)**. (H&E, original magnification ×100.)

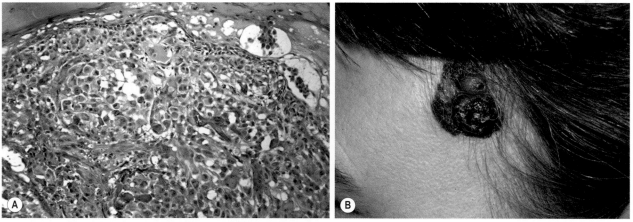

**Figure 27.5** Natural history of melanoma. In this lesion, there are extensive nests of melanocytes in the dermis that vary in size and shape and are confluent. Melanocytes are more atypical. Neoplastic melanocytes in the epidermis are confluent **(A)**. Clinically such lesions are readily recognizable as melanoma in the vast majority of cases **(B)**. When the dermis is involved extensively, the prognosis is poorer. (H&E, original magnification ×100.)

without contiguity with the epidermis (Fig. 27.6). There may also be involvement of the superficial papillary dermis in so-called 'epidermotropic' metastases. Blood vessels and lymphatics also often contain neoplastic cells and there may be involvement of nerves. Clinically, these may appear as intracutaneous or subcutaneous nodules that range in color from that of normal skin to jet black. When lymph nodes are involved, clinically there are usually one or more firm nodules that develop in a lymph node chain or group that may be fixed to underlying structures. Histologically, there is usually replacement of the lymph node architecture by atypical neoplastic melanocytes.

Although this pathway describes melanoma that develops de novo, approximately 25% of melanomas develop in association with nevi (Fig. 27.7).[8] This has led some investigators to propose a pathway that describes 'precursor' lesions. However, melanoma may arise in virtually any melanocytic nevus, especially giant congenital nevi, so it

remains important for clinicians to evaluate all nevi carefully for changes that may signal the development of melanoma within them.

Clark et al. described a model of progression of melanoma where a 'radial' growth phase is followed by a 'vertical' growth phase.[9] The radial growth phase is characterized by malignant melanocytes proliferating in the epidermis and papillary dermis at which time the cells purportedly do not have the ability to metastasize. These same cells were shown to have limited capacity for growth in cell culture.[10,11] Melanomas in this phase have been considered to be biologically less aggressive than those of the so-called 'vertical growth phase' in which there is more extensive involvement of the dermis. Melanocytes from lesions in this phase have the capacity for immortality in cell culture.[11] However, there are significant exceptions to this model, including nodular melanomas that have a very short or no radial growth phase and metastasizing thin melanomas without a vertical growth phase.[8,12]

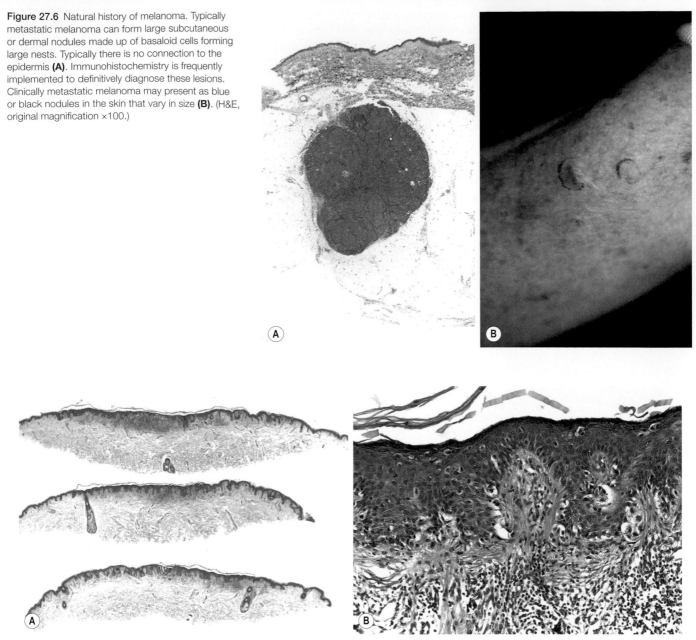

**Figure 27.6** Natural history of melanoma. Typically metastatic melanoma can form large subcutaneous or dermal nodules made up of basaloid cells forming large nests. Typically there is no connection to the epidermis **(A)**. Immunohistochemistry is frequently implemented to definitively diagnose these lesions. Clinically metastatic melanoma may present as blue or black nodules in the skin that vary in size **(B)**. (H&E, original magnification ×100.)

**Figure 27.7** Melanoma in situ arising in a compound 'dysplastic' nevus. **(A)** At low power (×4 magnification) there is a slightly asymmetrical melanocytic proliferation present at the dermoepidermal junction as well as within the dermis. In this image there is horizontal bridging between adjacent epidermal rete ridges. At low power one also appreciates a focal lymphocytic infiltrate present within the melanocytic proliferation. **(B)** At higher power (magnification ×100) there are scattered large atypical melanocytes present above the dermoepidermal junction, going into the granular layer.

Recent studies using comparative genomic hybridization have demonstrated that cells from acrolentiginous melanoma demonstrate genotypic features of metastatic melanoma while confined to the epidermis.[13,14] In addition, it is not clear whether some 'radial' growth phase melanoma cells that were cultured were nevus cells. Finally, the determination of when the 'radial' growth phase ends and the 'vertical' growth phase begins is a subjective determination based on evaluation of histologic sections which can be prone to sampling and interpretation errors. As such, the assignment of radial and vertical growth phases for melanoma has fallen into disfavor.[15]

Molecular studies suggest that some 'dysplastic' nevi may represent intermediate lesions in a multi-step melanoma tumorigenesis pathway.[16,17] Alterations of some tumor suppressor genes, oncogenes, mismatch repair proteins, extracellular matrix proteins, and growth factors are common to both lesions. However, such work remains controversial and speculative and most workers still consider 'dysplastic' nevi to be markers for the development of melanoma in some patients rather than true precursors.

## Appropriate biopsy technique

Appropriate clinical examination, lesion selection and the resulting method of choice for sampling are important steps for accurate pathological diagnosis (see Chapter 40).

Examination of a patient with a pigmented lesion should include a full skin evaluation and determination of family and personal risk factors for melanoma. Patients with many nevi, especially dysplastic nevi, present a particular clinical challenge in that they may have numerous lesions that fulfill the 'ABCDE' criteria for the clinical diagnosis of melanoma. These patients present with the 'signature' nevus phenomenon in which a given individual develops multiple similarly appearing nevi that display a biologically benign phenotype even though they may appear clinically atypical.[18] In this subset of patients, it is important to recognize lesions that appear significantly different and atypical and perform a biopsy of such lesions.

The American Academy of Dermatology Guidelines/ Outcomes Committee for Cutaneous Melanoma and the National Comprehensive Cancer Network have published information outlining initial management of melanocytic lesions suspected of being melanoma.[19,20] Classic teaching is that excision of the entire lesion should be performed. However, there are a number of problems with this recommendation. First, many lesions are located in cosmetically sensitive areas and primary excision may be mutilating or impossible. Second, and perhaps more important, there are many lesions that may simulate melanoma clinically (such as pigmented basal cell carcinoma, squamous cell carcinoma and seborrheic keratosis among others). Given the large number of such lesions, excision of all lesions that could theoretically represent melanoma would be impossible. There are no good studies to quantify what qualifies a lesion to be suspected as, but not diagnostic of, melanoma, by a clinician. We recommend that lesions with a greater than 50% chance of being melanoma based on clinical and/or dermoscopic examination be considered for primary excision where possible. However, in the other 50%, other time-honored accepted biopsy techniques can be utilized. These include saucerization or deep shave, broad punch and incisional techniques. The choice of an incorrect or inappropriate technique can compromise microscopic evaluation for diagnosis.[21,22]

Optimizing cosmetic outcome with a superficial shave or small-diameter punch biopsy is not recommended when suspicion of melanoma is high. These techniques may fail to sample diagnostic areas, especially in clinically suspected melanomas. Many of the histologic criteria of melanoma are architectural, such as breadth, symmetry and circumscription, and therefore biopsies should be of sufficient breadth and depth to allow for assessment of these features.

A full-thickness incisional biopsy is an accepted form of sampling for a lesion that would normally be a candidate for primary excision yet is on an anatomic site that would prove difficult for excision or is a large lesion. This method involves performing an ellipse within the lesion that attempts to sample a significant portion of it, especially encompassing areas that are elevated or black. Most of these provide a sample that is diagnostic, although clinicians should realize that a subsequent re-biopsy may be required if the sample is not adequate for either diagnosis.

Punch biopsies represent either an excision, if the entire lesion is removed with the punch, or a form of an incision, if only a part of the lesion is removed. While a punch excision is obviously an excellent biopsy technique, punches taken of broad lesions may be prone to sampling error and should be performed with caution especially when less than 5–6 mm in diameter (Fig. 27.8). Multiple small punches may also not be optimal and may be associated with sampling error.

Some have postulated that partial incisional or shave biopsies of intact primary melanomas may increase the rate of sentinel lymph node (SLN) micrometastases. Martin et al. evaluated 2164 patients with melanoma and concluded that biopsy technique did not affect incidence of SLN metastasis, locoregional recurrence, or overall survival for patients who underwent excisional versus incisional versus shave biopsy.[23]

Since the most important prognostic factor for melanoma is thickness (Breslow depth) of the lesion, a non-representative biopsy could potentially yield false information on which treatment planning is based. A retrospective review of 145 cutaneous melanomas demonstrated that initial diagnostic biopsies performed using non-excisional saucerization or punch technique provided specimens that allowed for 88% accuracy of assessment of Breslow depth when compared with the Breslow depth determined on the re-excision specimen. Saucerization biopsies were more accurate than punch biopsies less than 5 mm in diameter for melanomas less than 1 mm thick. Therefore, saucerization biopsy is preferable to superficial shave or punch biopsy for primary cutaneous melanoma when an initial sample is taken for diagnosis.[24]

Additionally, Hsu and Cockerell reviewed 1123 histologically proven cutaneous melanomas and found significant diagnostic discrepancy between initial punch biopsies and re-excision specimens. While excisional biopsy and saucerization shave biopsy demonstrated near 100% accuracy, punch technique was only 86.5% accurate.[25] Due to the inherent intralesional heterogeneity of cutaneous melanoma, small punch biopsies may not always obtain representative specimens and may subject the patient to a significant risk of misdiagnosis.

## Histopathologic criteria for melanoma

Currently the histologic diagnosis of melanoma is based on a constellation of cytological and architectural microscopic features referred to as 'criteria' for diagnosis. Histological criteria represent a constellation of findings observed microscopically that are highly specific and sensitive for the diagnosis of melanoma. Other histological findings that may be observed in melanoma are referred to as 'clues' to diagnosis and are used along with criteria to establish a definitive diagnosis.

A 'unifying concept' regarding the histologic classification of melanomas based on both architectural and cytologic features has been proposed by Ackerman.[3] The three cardinal architectural characteristics of melanoma include large dimensions of the lesion (diameter >6 mm), asymmetry, and poor circumscription. While a valuable criterion, asymmetry may be difficult to appreciate in early lesions. Other features include predominance of single melanocytes over nests of melanocytes in the epidermis, extensive involvement of adnexal epithelium by atypical melanocytes, presence of atypical melanocytes throughout the entire thickness of the epidermis (pagetoid spread), and irregularity in size and shape of nests of melanocytes (Fig. 27.9). Variability in the size and spacing between nests of melanocytes, patchy inflammation, and irregular pigment distribution throughout a lesion are other findings that may be present. Pagetoid

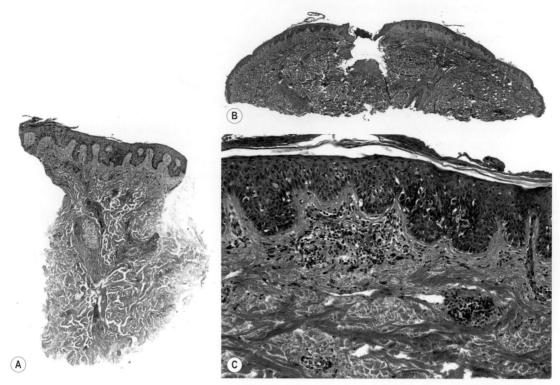

**Figure 27.8** Melanocytic lesions may be difficult to interpret when only a portion of the lesion is sampled with 'punch' biopsy technique. **A)** Low-power view of the punch biopsy (×2 magnification) shows budding epidermal rete with increased pigmentation and only few melanocytes observed above the dermoepidermal junction. **B)** The lesion was re-sampled using a broad saucerization technique. At ×2 magnification there is a central ulcer from the previous punch biopsy performed and laterally there is a melanocytic proliferation. **C)** Laterally to the central ulcer there are scattered melanocytes above the dermoepidermal junction representative of early melanoma in situ (×100 magnification).

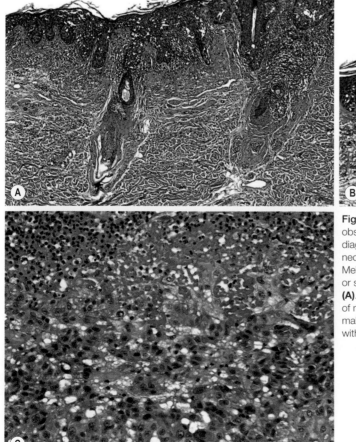

**Figure 27.9** Histological criteria represent a constellation of findings observed microscopically that are highly specific and sensitive for the diagnosis of melanoma. In this section we appreciate 'pagetoid' spread of neoplastic cells throughout the epidermis and involving follicular epithelium. Melanocytic proliferation involving adnexal structures such as hair follicles or sweat ducts is a commonly used criterion for the diagnosis of melanoma **(A)**. Ascent of solitary atypical melanocytes is characteristic of most forms of melanoma (pagetoid spread) **(B)**. Tumoral necrosis if present can assist in making the diagnosis and is a marker of worse prognosis when associated with overlying ulceration in melanoma **(C)**.

spread is a highly sensitive histological finding of melanoma, especially when observed in the setting of other criteria or extensive solar elastosis. Characteristic findings of melanoma in the dermis include coalescence of nests of melanocytes into sheets and lack of maturation, which refers to failure of cells to become smaller with increasing depth.

Cytologically, melanocytes in melanoma may assume a number of different morphologies and may be small round, large round, pagetoid, balloon, oval, spindle, multinucleate or dendritic. There may be variable cytologic atypia ranging from virtually none in some melanoma in situ, some desmoplastic melanomas (DMM) and early acrolentiginous or mucosal melanoma, to frank anaplasia. When atypical, there is cellular pleomorphism with variability in cell size and shape, prominent chromatin, large nucleoli and reversal of the nuclear:cytoplasmic ratio. There may be increased mitotic activity although absence of mitotic activity may also be observed. Mitotic figures, especially if atypical, numerous and in deeper portions of a lesion, is a sign of melanoma with rare exceptions. Other features include lack of maturation and the presence of necrotic melanocytes. Necrosis en masse of large areas of a melanocytic lesion also is virtually diagnostic of melanoma.

## Pathologic features of different clinical forms of cutaneous melanoma

### Superficial spreading melanoma (SSM)

This histologic variant by definition demonstrates a horizontally oriented lesion in which there is pagetoid spread of melanocytes throughout the epidermis. Architecturally, melanocytic nests show varying asymmetry in distribution, size and shape and tend to confluence. Cytologically, neoplastic melanocytes are large with abundant pale cytoplasm that contains variable amounts of melanin. Nuclear pleomorphism and mitoses are commonly observed. Up to 20–25% of SSM are associated with a pre-existing melanocytic nevus.

### Melanoma in situ

Melanoma in situ is a term used to define melanoma that is confined to the epidermis. It may be applied to any of the classically described subtypes of melanoma. It is a useful term in that it conveys information about prognosis by its very nature, namely that it is curable following appropriate early surgical therapy. The most common subtype, lentigo maligna, is present on sun-damaged skin of older individuals.

Melanoma in situ is characterized histologically by an increased number of atypical melanocytes arranged singly and in nests distributed irregularly at the DEJ and above it (Fig. 27.10). They involve a broad area of the epidermis, and in contrast to junctional nevi and lentigines, the epidermis is often thin and there may be effacement of epidermal retia. Atypical melanocytes are often present in cutaneous adnexal structures. Solar elastosis is a common finding and is an important clue to the diagnosis of melanoma in situ in the setting of melanocytic hyperplasia. There may be a lichenoid infiltrate of lymphocytes in the superficial papillary dermis that may obscure the

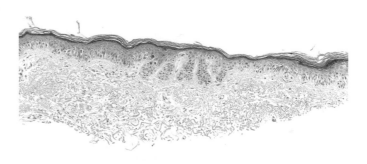

**Figure 27.10** Lentigo maligna. There is a proliferation of atypical melanocytes with effacement of rete ridges at the dermoepidermal junction as well as thinning of the epidermis. Within the dermis there is extensive solar elastosis as a result of sun (ultraviolet light) damage. (×40 magnification.)

melanocytic proliferation in the epidermis and impart features similar to a benign lichenoid keratosis, which is a histologic pitfall that may lead to misdiagnosis.

The histologic evaluation of margin status following excision of these lesions may be difficult because of diffuse melanocytic proliferation that is present in the background skin of these patients as a consequence of longstanding sun damage.[26] In contrast to persistent melanoma, the number of melanocytes per unit area is less and nests of melanocytes are not seen. In some cases, however, the distinction may be impossible without clinical correlation.

### Nodular melanoma

This variant of melanoma refers to lesions with a predominant dermal component, often with a relatively minimal intraepidermal component. In some cases, the dermal component extends laterally further than the epidermal component (Fig. 27.11). While some individuals consider this to represent a true variant, others consider it as a more advanced form of melanoma of any subtype which has become nodular as a consequence of evolution. As virtually all melanomas progress through an in situ stage, if left untreated, they may progress to involve the dermis and may form papules or nodules clinically. There is one form of nodular melanoma known as 'early' nodular melanoma, however, that involves the dermis at a relatively early point in time in contrast to others that tend to remain confined to the epidermis for a significant part of their evolution.[27,28]

### Acrolentiginous melanoma

These lesions tend to have a greater number of dendritic melanocytes with dendrites extending to the upper levels of the epidermis on volar skin. Initially, the degree of cytologic atypia may be minimal. Later, melanocytes may become more spindle or pagetoid in appearance with prominent pleomorphism and subsequently involve the deeper dermis (Fig. 27.12).[13]

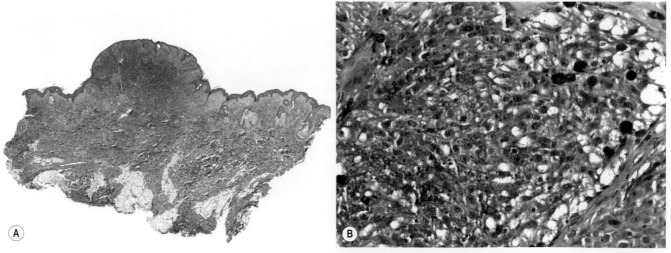

**Figure 27.11** Nodular melanoma. **A)** In this excision specimen there is a large dense nodular mass of melanocytes expanding the dermis with an asymmetric distribution of melanin (×2 magnification). **B)** At higher magnification, there are heavily pigmented atypical melanocytes with mitotic figures and apoptotic bodies present within the lesion.

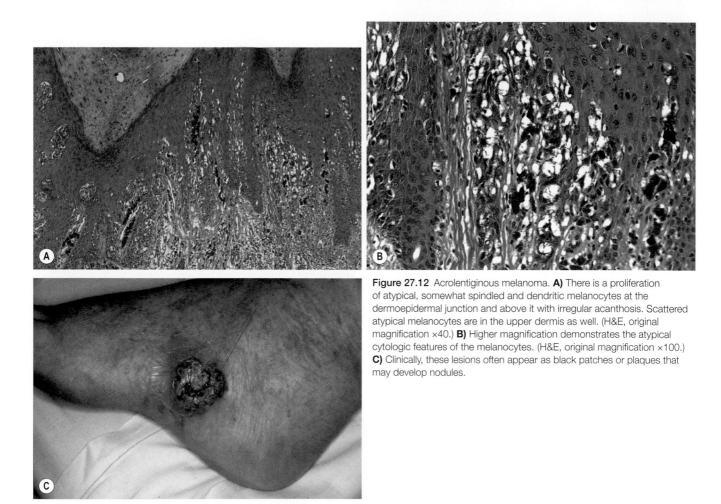

**Figure 27.12** Acrolentiginous melanoma. **A)** There is a proliferation of atypical, somewhat spindled and dendritic melanocytes at the dermoepidermal junction and above it with irregular acanthosis. Scattered atypical melanocytes are in the upper dermis as well. (H&E, original magnification ×40.) **B)** Higher magnification demonstrates the atypical cytologic features of the melanocytes. (H&E, original magnification ×100.) **C)** Clinically, these lesions often appear as black patches or plaques that may develop nodules.

## Desmoplastic melanoma

Desmoplastic melanoma (DMM) represents less than 1% of all variants of melanoma. It usually presents as a slightly pigmented or skin-colored to pink indurated papule, nodule or plaque on sun-exposed skin (Fig. 27.13). Typically they affect the head and neck region, appear later in adult life and are more commonly seen in men. Up to

70% of cases are misdiagnosed clinically, often described as 'fibroma', 'squamous cell carcinoma' or 'scar'.[29] As a result of its banal histologic appearance and its clinically non-descript morphology, it is often misdiagnosed both clinically and histologically and is a common source of litigation.

There are several histologic variants of DMM shown and described in Figure 27.14. All tend to be large, poorly

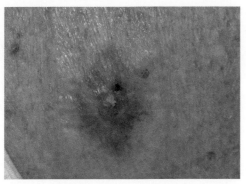

Figure 27.13 Clinical photograph of a desmoplastic melanoma (DMM). This lesion was present on the upper back. Frequently these lesions are clinically misdiagnosed as scar, squamous cell carcinoma or basal cell carcinomas. The nondescript nature of this lesion is characteristic of DMM.

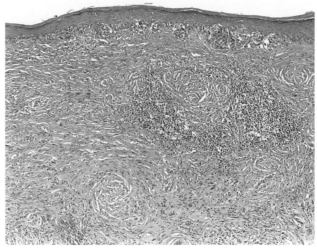

Figure 27.15 Melanoma in situ is commonly observed in desmoplastic melanoma, and is a helpful clue to its diagnosis. This lesion shows large nests of melanocytes at the dermoepidermal junction along with scattered atypical melanocytes present throughout the epidermis. Underneath in the dermis there is a moderately cellular spindle cell tumor forming ill-defined fascicles (×20 magnification).

demarcated neoplasms involving the full thickness of the dermis, sometimes with a slightly raised central nodule. Most lesions have a component of melanoma in situ in the overlying epidermis but this may be absent in 20% of cases (Fig. 27.15). They can arise in association with a pre-existing melanoma of another type, often lentigo maligna, although they may arise de novo. Perineural involvement is evident in up to 35% and is responsible for recurrence and spread along nerves (Fig. 27.16). Cytologically, neoplastic cells consist of spindle-shaped melanocytes with variable pleomorphism and hyperchromatic nuclei although there may be minimal to absent atypia. Neoplastic cells may appear small and monomorphous with scant cytoplasm and have a low mitotic index (<1/mm²). Two common histologic clues used to assist in the diagnosis of DMM are the presence of pigment within cells and the presence of nodular aggregates of lymphocytes scattered throughout the dermis (Fig. 27.17).

Traditionally, DMM have been thought of as having a better prognosis when compared to other types of

melanoma of equivalent Breslow depth. Several reports have contradicted this finding, suggesting that case-matched control patients with melanoma matched for tumor thickness have similar survival rates to patients with DMM. In light of these findings, several authors have proposed that DMM with prominent fibrosis (pure subtype) are unlikely to disseminate to regional lymph nodes and are associated with a favorable outcome when compared with those with mixed desmoplasia or other melanoma variants.[30,31]

Immunohistochemistry (Table 27.1) is often necessary to distinguish DMM from other entities included in the histologic differential diagnosis as the spindle cells may be

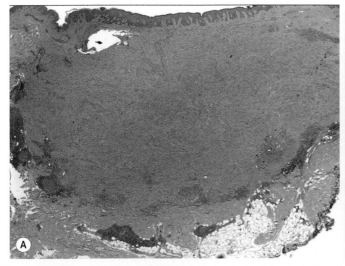
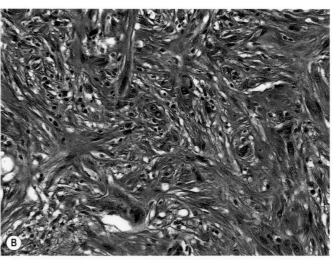

Figure 27.14 There have been several histological variants of desmoplastic melanoma described. One common form has features of a scar or fibroma. A) At low magnification (×2 magnification), there is a proliferation of spindle-shaped cells admixed with collagen and blood vessels in the dermis. Commonly they have a lymphocytic infiltrate present within the lesion as well as associated melanoma in situ. Spindled cells show large atypical morphology as shown in Figure 27.15. B) Another variant is comprised of abundant strikingly atypical spindle and/or epithelioid cells arranged in sheets or fascicles. This variant contains abundant pleomorphic cells with hyperchromatic and bizarre nuclei (×40 magnification). A third histological variant not depicted in this figure may demonstrate minimal atypia and may simulate a neurofibroma or neural proliferation.

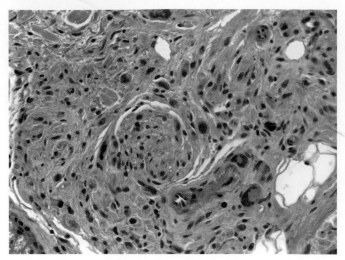

Figure 27.16 A common histologic finding in desmoplastic melanoma is perineural involvement. Neoplastic cells are arranged in a concentric fashion around cutaneous nerves.

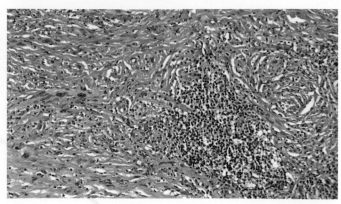

Figure 27.17 A patchy lymphocytic infiltrate is often present and is a helpful clue to the diagnosis of desmoplastic melanoma (×40 magnification). This is also observed in Figure 27.14A at lower magnification.

poorly differentiated. S100 protein is the most useful stain as it is almost uniformly positive although occasionally only weakly. Stains for MART-1 and HMB-45 antigen are negative in most DMM although a few reports have demonstrated focal positive staining.[32]

## Verrucous melanoma

Verrucous melanoma is a variant described as a hyperkeratotic pigmented lesion, usually on an extremity (71%). Clinically, they are usually misdiagnosed as benign lesions such as seborrheic keratosis, verruca, nevus and Spitz nevus.

This lesion is often considered a variant of superficial spreading melanoma and is characterized by having

## Table 27.1 Commonly Used Immunohistochemical Markers for Melanoma

| Marker | Cell Type/Tumor Recognized (Staining) | End Protein Product/Recognized Protein/Epitope | Staining Pattern | Note |
|---|---|---|---|---|
| S100 protein | Melanocytes, cells derived from neural crest cells, and tumors derived from: Langerhans cells, nerve sheath cells, adipocytes, antigen-presenting dendritic cells | 21 kDa acidic calcium binding protein | Nuclear and cytoplasmic | DMM = usually positive |
| HMB-45 | Melanocytes, clear cell sarcoma of soft parts, angiomyolipomas, lymphangioleiomyomatosis, sweat gland tumors, renal cell carcinoma with t(6,11)(p21;q12) | Glycoprotein gp100 | Cytoplasmic | DMM = typically negative |
| MART-1/MelanA | Melanocytes, angiomyolipomas, lymphangioleiomyomatosis, adrenal cortical tumors, gonadal steroid tumors | MART-1: Melanoma antigen recognized by T cells (melanA represents the gene) | Cytoplasmic and/or nuclear | DMM = typically negative |
| Tyrosinase | Melanocytes, some angiomyolipomas, pigmented nerve sheath tumors | Enzyme in melanin synthesis | Cytoplasmic | DMM = typically negative |
| MITF | Melanocytes, reports of staining histiocytes, fibroblasts, lymphocytes and mast cells. Spindle cell tumors, angiomyolipomas, rarely breast and renal cancer | Microphthalmia-associated transcription factor | Nuclear | DMM = typically negative |
| NKIC3 (CD63) | Melanocytes, histiocytes, eosinophils, dendritic cells, mast cells, endothelial cells, cellular neurothekeomas, medullary thyroid cancer, granular cell tumor, neuroendocrine tumors, neurofibromas, schwannomas. Reports of staining in several internal malignancies including bladder and colorectal | 25–110 kD glycoprotein | Peripheral cytoplasmic membrane staining | Cellular neurothekeomas tend to be NKI/C3 positive, and S100, HMB-45, MART-1 negative |

DMM = desmoplastic melanoma

Sensitivity/specificity of melanocyte markers

Sensitivity:
S100 protein (97–00%) > HMB-45 (69–93%) = MART-1 (75–92%) = Tyrosinase (84–94%) = MITF (81–100%)

Specificity:
HMB-45 (95–100%) = Mart-1 (88–100%) = Tyrosinase (94–100%) > S100 protein (75–87%)

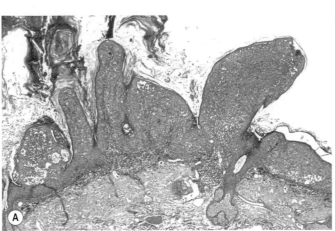 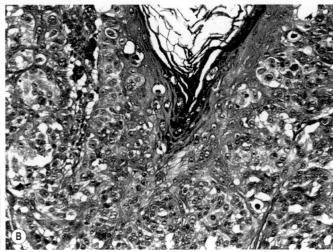

Figure 27.18 Verrucous melanoma. **A)** At low magnification, marked verrucous hyperplasia of the epidermis is seen, simulating a verruca or epithelial neoplasm. Nests of melanocytes fill the dermis. (H&E, original magnification ×20.) **B)** At higher magnification, the atypia of the melanocytes is readily appreciated. (H&E, original magnification ×100.)

an exophytic papillomatous growth pattern (Fig. 27.18).[33] Pseudo-epitheliomatous hyperplasia and overlying hyperkeratosis are prominent features which may obscure the underlying melanoma cells. Blessing et al. reviewed 20 cases and found 10% had been given erroneous diagnosis; however, eight patients suffered metastases and seven died of their disease.[34] The Breslow depth and Clark's level may be difficult to determine given the papillomatous architecture. Kuehnl-Petzoldt et al. reported that reliable Clark's levels could be assigned in only two-thirds of these neoplasms.[35] It is important to recognize this variant as it may easily be confused with squamous cell carcinoma or other benign epithelial proliferations.

## Animal melanoma

The lesions are comprised of sheets of heavily pigmented epithelioid or spindle cells with numerous melanophages in the dermis. Mitoses are infrequent but present upon careful inspection. The amount of pigment present may render evaluation of the cytology of the cells difficult. They may be confused with heavily pigmented blue nevi although the diffuse architecture, asymmetry, presence of scattered mitoses and deep extension are features that allow the diagnosis to be rendered.[36] It has recently been suggested that the term pigmented epithelioid melanocytoma be used rather than animal melanoma for this entity.[37] Its 'less aggressive' nature, when compared to other types of melanoma, has been suggested by both clinical and molecular studies examining this variant.[38,39]

## Nevoid melanoma

At scanning magnification, architecturally, these lesions resemble ordinary compound or dermal nevi; however, subtle pleomorphism and impaired maturation (pseudomaturation), asymmetry, as well as mitoses are clues that aid in the diagnosis (Fig. 27.19). Histologically, some have divided nevoid melanomas into two large groups: nevoid small cell melanoma and a larger cell variant resembling Spitz nevi.[40] Inflammatory cell infiltrates commonly found

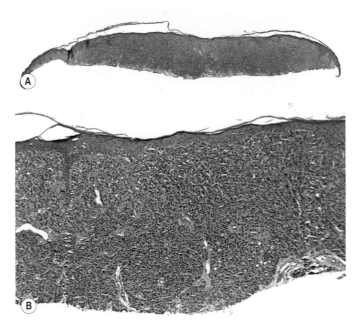

Figure 27.19 Nevoid melanoma. **A)** At low power, the architecture of this lesion appears regular and symmetrical. There appears to be a slightly dense melanocytic infiltrate (×2 magnification). **B)** On higher power, there are scattered melanocytes above the dermoepidermal junction and nests in the dermis which differ in size and shape. As in this lesion, they frequently do not have pigment. Pseudomaturation, a clue to the diagnosis of nevoid melanoma, can be observed in this image (×20 magnification).

in other types of melanoma are usually absent in this variant. 'Pseudomaturation' or the appearance of progressively smaller melanocytes at the deeper aspects of the lesion is not uncommon. In true maturation of melanocytes in nevi, both the cytoplasm and nuclei of the cells are in the deeper portions of lesions. In pseudomaturation, although the cytoplasm is less voluminous in deeper melanocytes, the nuclei retain their size. A clue to diagnosis of this variant is the irregular size and shape of dermal melanocytic nests. Such lesions in the past have been referred to as 'borderline melanoma' or 'minimal deviation melanoma' but those terms are no longer used.[41]

## Malignant blue 'nevus'

Malignant blue nevus is a misnomer that refers to either de-novo melanoma that simulates a cellular blue nevus or a melanoma that arises in association with or from a cellular blue nevus. Most lesions are present for many years prior to diagnosis and may elude suspicion because they tend to grow slowly and involve the deep dermis rather than the epidermis.[42]

Individual cells in this entity are epithelioid or spindle in shape and demonstrate mitoses, necrosis, nuclear atypia, pleomorphism, hyperchromasia, and prominent nucleoli. Pigmented dendritic cells are seen in virtually all lesions (Fig. 27.20).

## 'Spitzoid' melanoma

Spitz's nevus and 'spitzoid' melanoma are known histologic simulators of one another. These lesions share features of large size of nevus cells and their nuclei. Cells may be epithelioid or spindle in shape. Though many times difficult to distinguish, histologic clues that favor melanoma are ulceration, necrosis en masse, asymmetry, failure of maturation, deep mitoses (and high mitotic index >2/mm$^2$), and lack of Kamino bodies (Fig. 27.21).[43,44] Furthermore, 'spitzoid' lesions in adults should be considered melanoma if there are virtually any features more consistent with the diagnosis of melanoma, while the reverse is true of similar lesions in children, especially prepubertal children.

## Spindle cell melanoma

Some melanomas may be characterized by a proliferation of spindle-shaped melanocytes arranged in fascicles and sheets yet they do not demonstrate the diffuse and deep nature of the so-called sarcomatoid melanoma or of DMM. Many of these lesions still demonstrate features that suggest melanoma, such as involvement of the epidermis, pagetoid spread of melanocytes, nesting and melanin (Fig. 27.22). However, because they are poorly differentiated, these lesions must be

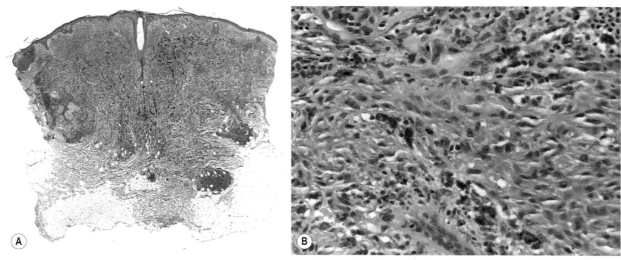

**Figure 27.20** Malignant 'blue' nevus or blue nevus-'like' melanoma. **A)** At low-power magnification, the lesion exhibits a striking architectural and cytological resemblance to cellular blue nevus. In this section, note the lymphoid aggregates at the periphery of the tumor; this can be utilized as a clue to diagnosis. **B)** Higher-power magnification shows markedly increased nuclear atypia, mitotic figures and increased cellular pleomorphism (×100 magnification).

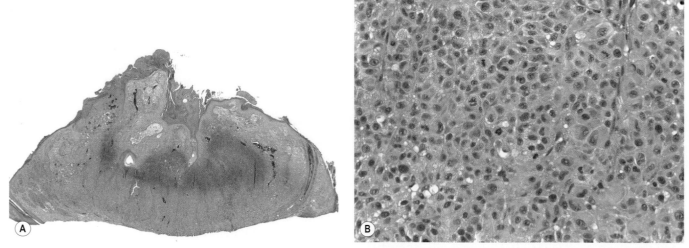

**Figure 27.21** Spitzoid melanoma. **A)** On low-power magnification, Spitzoid melanomas tend to be thick and large, some with a verrucous morphology. The basal portion of the lesion appears to push into the dermis and the epidermis may form a collarette surrounding the tumor. As found in Spitz nevi, edema and telangiectasias in the upper dermis may be observed. **B)** Melanocytes are variably enlarged, and nests contain pleomorphic cells with mitotic activity throughout the lesion.

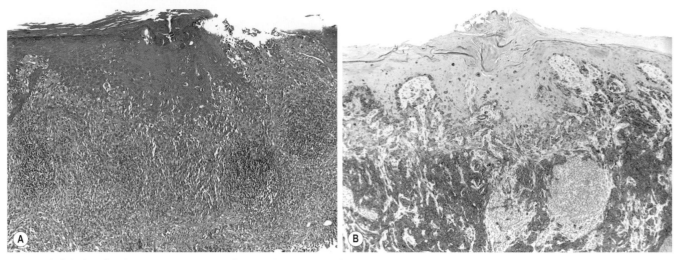

Figure 27.22 Spindle cell melanomas may mimic squamous cell carcinomas. **A)** At ×10 magnification, there is the appearance of pseudoepitheliomatous hyperplasia of keratinocytes with a brisk host response at the dermoepidermal junction. **B)** MART-1 staining of this specimen shows a diffuse proliferation of atypical melanocytes present throughout the thickness of the epidermis and invading deep into the reticular dermis.

distinguished from other malignant neoplasms of the skin that may demonstrate a spindle cell morphology, including spindle cell squamous cell carcinoma and atypical fibroxanthoma. As with the other poorly differentiated variants of melanoma, immunoperoxidase stains are required to render a precise diagnosis.

## Melanoma in children

Melanoma is quite rare in children (prepubertal) and its incidence is estimated to be between 0.1 and 0.4 per 100,000.[45] The diagnosis should only be made when virtually every feature of melanoma is present both clinically and histologically.

Most melanomas in children arise from large or giant congenital nevi, in patients with xeroderma pigmentosum or in those with familial dysplastic nevus syndrome.[46,47] On occasion the melanomas may be of transplacental origin.[48] They have histologic features that are identical with melanomas in adults. The histologic diagnosis is more difficult when the lesions demonstrate 'spitzoid' morphology as most such lesions represent Spitz's nevus. When 'spitzoid' lesions in children demonstrate poor maturation, mitoses near their bases, and have wide as well as deep areas the diagnosis of melanoma should be strongly considered.[49]

## Challenges in the histologic diagnosis of cutaneous melanoma

There are a number of problems that may cause difficulty in the diagnosis of melanoma other than those described above. Some of these represent 'simulators' of melanoma while others are issues associated with certain settings in which melanoma may develop or may be altered by other factors.

### Nevi on 'special' sites

Melanocytic nevi located on certain body sites may closely simulate melanoma. It is important not to overdiagnose melanoma in these circumstances. Some of these sites include the breast, the scalp (especially in children), the ear,

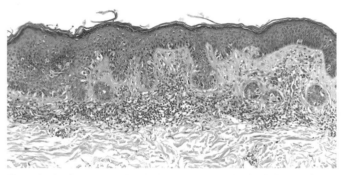

Figure 27.23 Compound 'dysplastic' nevus on special site (pubic area). There is a symmetrical proliferation of nests and individual melanocytes at the dermoepidermal junction and in the upper dermis. Individual melanocytes are larger than usual and have abundant cytoplasm. There may be slight pagetoid spread of melanocytes though no mitotic figures are present. This is a common melanoma simulator. (H&E, ×100 magnification.)

the umbilicus, the perineal and genital area, and flexural sites such as the axilla, neck, popliteal and antecubital fossa (Fig. 27.23). Features that may cause difficulty in diagnosis include large size of individual melanocytes, large nests of melanocytes, and slight pagetoid spread of melanocytes in the epidermis.[50,51] Although these lesions may demonstrate these features, they do not usually have cytologic atypia or mitoses, and if mitotic figures (especially atypical ones) are seen, the diagnosis of melanoma should be considered.

### Congenital nevi biopsied in neonates and young children

Congenital nevi biopsied shortly after birth up to 2 to 3 years of age may simulate melanoma due to pagetoid spread of melanocytes throughout the epidermis and large size of melanocytes with abundant cytoplasm.[52] This is thought to be a consequence of migration of evolving nevus cells (melanoblasts) through the epidermis. As congenital nevi mature, the single cells in the epidermis become arranged as nests and then become situated at the dermoepidermal junction and in the dermis. Although there is a prominent intraepidermal melanocytic proliferation, there are also nests of typical appearing melanocytes in the dermis between and among collagen bundles and around adnexal structures characteristic of a congenital nevus beneath the epidermal component. Of interest, when evaluating congenital nevi in adults, the junctional component may demonstrate a proliferation of single melanocytes with relatively abundant cytoplasm that may cause confusion in diagnosis. Clinical correlation is also valuable in making an accurate diagnosis.[53]

## Congenital melanoblastic proliferation

Occasionally in congenital nevi, there may be relatively large nodular aggregations of small melanocytes that are hyperchromatic. Such proliferations may simulate melanoma because of pleomorphism and the presence of mitoses. The key to the diagnosis is that the process is virtually always symmetrical and well circumscribed and demonstrates evidence of maturation. Furthermore, this lesion is usually always present at birth and matures with age, some undergoing complete regression.[53]

## Persistent (recurrent) nevi

Melanocytic nevi that have recurred after a previous procedure such as incomplete removal after biopsy or trauma may develop histologic features that simulate melanoma ('pseudomelanoma').[54] Melanocytes in the epidermis may be large, may coalesce forming irregular nests, and may be present at all levels of the epidermis including the granular and cornified layer. Occasional mitotic figures may be seen although this is relatively uncommon. There is also scar tissue in the dermis and the atypical changes are confined to the epidermis directly over the scar (Fig. 27.24). If the melanocytic proliferation extends beyond the margin of the scar, the diagnosis of melanoma should be considered. There may also be nests of normal-appearing nevus cells in the dermis beneath or within the scar which is a clue to the diagnosis. Clinical correlation is important as the changes may simulate melanoma quite closely and it is often valuable to review histologic sections from the prior biopsy if possible. If not, it might be reasonable to recommend conservative re-excision. Caution should be exercised in diagnosing any previously biopsied lesion as melanoma until evaluating prior biopsy specimens to avoid medicolegal liability.

## Single cell melanocytic proliferations

Any proliferation of single melanocytes in the epidermis may simulate melanoma in situ as it begins in this fashion. Single melanocytic proliferation may be observed in a number of different settings, including overlying congenital nevi (Fig. 27.25), on sun-damaged skin, on the eyelid, in the epidermis overlying fibrous papules, within solar lentigines and on mucocutaneous sites such as in the nail unit. Thus, prior to a definitive diagnosis of melanoma based on melanocyte ascent through the epidermis, other differential diagnostic possibilities should be entertained (Table 27.2). Melanocyte ascent in benign melanocytic proliferations do not demonstrate the density of melanocytes that is seen in melanoma in situ, melanocytes uncommonly exhibit cytological atypia, and ascent of melanocytes tends to be central

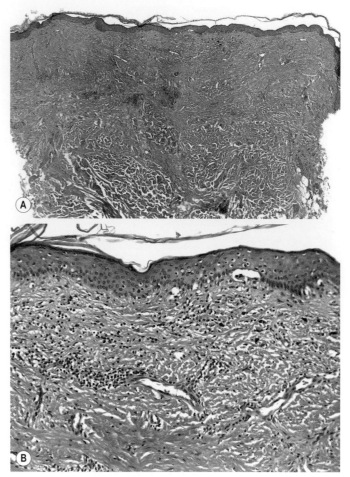

**Figure 27.24** Persistent (recurrent) nevus. **A)** There is often evidence of residual nevus in the specimen and the unusual features are confined to the epidermis directly overlying the scar and not to the side of it. **B)** Melanocytes overlying the scar of a previously biopsied nevus are often large, somewhat atypical and may demonstrate pagetoid spread, thereby simulating melanoma. The presence of a scar in the dermis should prompt the review of prior records and biopsy specimens when possible. In this case, there was a history of a previously biopsied 'dysplastic' nevus at this site. (**A:** ×2 magnification, **B:** ×40 magnification.)

to the lesion rather than at its lateral margins. Furthermore, in coincidental melanocytic proliferation, there are usually no nests. Clinical correlation is extremely valuable as most of these lesions demonstrate either an obvious benign lesion such as a congenital nevus or no visible pigmented lesion.[55,56]

## Completely regressed melanoma

As a result of the host response, melanoma may undergo regression. Histologically there is a characteristic pattern of dermal fibrosis in the upper dermis with telangiectases, lymphocytes and abundant melanophages. The stroma is fibromucinous and differs from fibroplasia seen in scars. The fibrosis is broad, asymmetrically distributed and mirrors the original melanoma that was present previously. There may be scattered single melanocytes remaining in the epidermis or a few nests of atypical melanocytes in the fibrotic dermis although there may be no residual melanocytes (Fig. 27.26).[57–59]

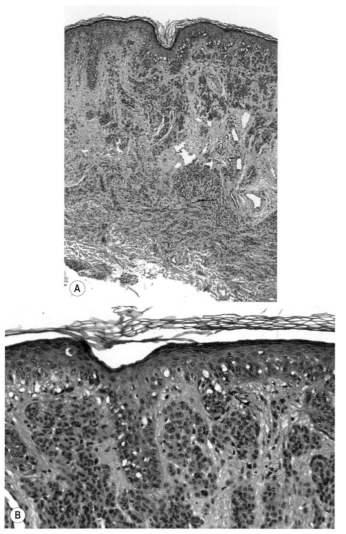

**Figure 27.25** Congenital nevus with intraepidermal melanocytic proliferation. **A)** Proliferations of single melanocytes are often seen in the epidermis overlying the dermal component of congenital nevi, which may simulate melanoma in situ. (H&E, ×20) **B)** The density of epidermal melanocytes is less than that seen in melanoma and they are virtually always seen overlying the dermal nevus component. (H&E, ×100.)

| Table 27.2 Histologic Differential of Upward Migration of Single Melanocytes Within the Epidermis |
| --- |
| **Melanoma** |
| **Benign melanocyte ascent:** |
| Recurrent nevi |
| Traumatized nevi |
| Irritated and 'sunburn' nevi |
| Nevi on 'special sites' including acral nevi |
| Congenital nevi |
| Melanocytic hyperplasia on sun-damaged skin/overlying fibrous papule |
| Spitz nevi |
| Melanocytic hyperplasia at the excision site of a previous benign melanocytic proliferation or melanoma |
| **Pagetoid spread in melanoma simulators (non-melanocytic):** |
| Extramammary and mammary Paget's |
| Pagetoid reticulosis |
| Cutaneous lymphoma |
| Pigmented Bowen's disease and pigmented actinic keratosis |
| Intraepidermal Merkel cell carcinoma |
| Squamous cell carcinoma |

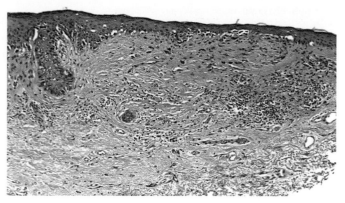

**Figure 27.26** Melanoma with partial regression. There is the presence of melanoma in situ with a focal dermal melanocytic nest to the right of the image. There is a patchy inflammatory infiltrate and the presence of melanophages within the papillary dermis. The stroma is fibromucinous. (H&E, ×100.)

## Metastatic melanoma

Most metastases of melanoma are characterized by atypical melanocytes in the deep dermis or subcutis either in nodules or diffusely in cords and strands. Occasionally, melanoma may involve the superficial dermis as well as the epidermis. These lesions may be quite small, which may cause confusion with nevi or primary melanoma. They are often as deep as they are broad and melanocytes are atypical with mitoses seen throughout.

Another form of metastatic melanoma is characterized by atypical but delicate pigmented spindle or dendritic melanocytes showing mitotic activity in the dermis. These may simulate blue nevi (Fig. 27.27).

Microscopic satellite lesions may be present within a section of a large melanoma and likely are a form of micrometastases. These are usually present in the deep dermis, subcutaneous tissue or within vessels and histologically appear as a small focus of grouped melanoma cells (> 0.05 mm) separated by normal tissue from the primary melanoma mass (Fig. 27.28). These may represent vascular invasion, true dermal/subcutaneous tissue metastasis or extensions of the primary tumor mass that is not contiguous in the sections reviewed.[60,61]

## 'Atypical' melanocytic proliferations

On occasion, melanocytic lesions that resemble 'dysplastic' nevi, Spitz nevi, blue nevi, and deep penetrating nevi present with histological features that may be observed in both nevi and melanoma so that an unequivocal diagnosis may not be able to be rendered.[62] Furthermore, correlation of clinical and pathological findings may be insufficient to determine the exact biological potential of these lesions.

Lesions that most commonly pose difficulty in diagnosis have been termed 'atypical' spitzoid melanocytic lesions, 'atypical' blue nevus-like lesions, and melanocytic tumors of uncertain/unknown biologic potential.[63] These may demonstrate criteria of both benignity and malignancy so that application of the standard criteria for diagnosis simply cannot be applied as in most conventional lesions. Obviously, when the pathologist has difficulty in rendering a precise diagnosis, there may be confusion on the part of

**Figure 27.27** Metastatic pigmented melanoma mimicking a blue nevus. The history of a previous melanoma is obviously an important clue to the diagnosis of this entity. **A)** At low power there is a dense pigmented proliferation of melanocytes with a few lymphoid aggregates. (H&E, ×2.) **B)** Higher power reveals cellular pleomorphism as well as mitotic figures deep into the lesion. (H&E, ×100.)

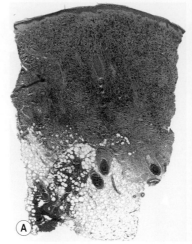

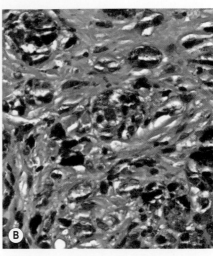

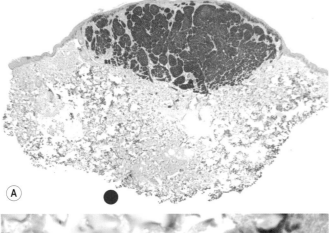

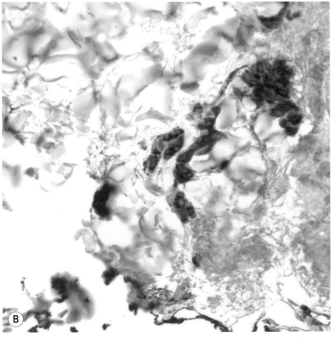

**Figure 27.28** MART-1 immunohistochemical staining of a nodular melanoma with a microscopic satellite ('microsatellite'). (MART-1, alkaline phosphatase method.) **A)** Low-power magnification shows staining of a nodular melanoma in the superficial dermis. At the bottom left of the biopsy specimen there is a red dot highlighting the microsatellite lesion. (H&E, ×2.) **B)** At ×100 magnification, a small collection of melanocytes is observed more than 0.05 mm from the primary tumor mass.

the treating clinician as to how to interpret such a result and how to manage the patient with this type of lesion.[64]

Currently there are no evidence-based guidelines for the management of these 'atypical' melanocytic lesions. Clinical information regarding age, sex, medical history, family history, anatomic location and risk factors for melanoma should be taken into account. If an 'atypical spitzoid lesion' is diagnosed in a child, it is almost certainly a benign process and the patient can be followed. However, in adults, because the malignant potential of such a lesion remains uncertain, most clinicians and patients decide to treat more aggressively to avoid under-treating a potentially lethal malignancy. These patients are frequently managed in a similar fashion to melanoma patients, with wide excision of the primary lesion and, in some cases, performance of sentinel lymph node biopsy.

'Atypical' spitzoid neoplasms of unknown biological potential (or 'atypical' spitzoid melanocytic neoplasms) have been the most extensively studied. Recently, a review of 67 cases of 'atypical spitzoid melanocytic' lesions that were excised completely and in which patients underwent subsequent SLN biopsies revealed that 27 subjects had lymph nodes that contained melanocytic neoplasm.[65] The authors described the histopathology of the nodes in all cases and described one case with more than 10% of the nodal surface area effaced by melanocytes. In spite of lymph node involvement, all patients survived with a mean follow-up of 3.5 years. The authors' approach to management of such patients is to counsel the patient regarding the meaning of the diagnosis and to recommend excision with a 1-cm margin to prevent local recurrence. SLN is recommended for patients with lesions greater than 1 mm in depth or greater than 0.75 mm in depth if the lesion has histological features that suggest a more aggressive biologic behavior such as abundant mitoses or necrosis. Although positive lymph node biopsies do not necessarily predict a poor outcome, negative results are reassuring to the patient.

Molecular techniques such as comparative genome hybridization and fluorescence in-situ hybridization have helped elucidate some of the chromosomal fingerprints and mutations that may improve the diagnostic accuracy of Spitz nevi, 'atypical' spitzoid melanocytic proliferations and 'spitzoid' melanomas. Although these ancillary molecular techniques show promise, currently there is no consensus algorithm for their use and they have yet to replace clinical and histopathologic correlation for definitive diagnosis.

## Techniques to improve accuracy of histopathologic diagnosis of melanoma

### Special stains and immunohistochemical stains

For poorly differentiated lesions that may represent melanocytic lesions or amelanotic melanomas, a silver stain such as the Fontana–Masson stain for melanin in conjunction with specialized immunohistochemical stains may be useful. Table 27.1 lists the important aspects of different immunohistochemical markers used in assisting in the definitive diagnosis of melanocytic tumors. Stains directed against S100 protein are the most sensitive marker for melanocytic lesions and are useful in determining melanocytic differentiation in the appropriate setting (Fig. 27.29). Commercially available antibodies to S100 protein are typically specific to S100B polypeptide chains.

Recently, efforts have been made to use differential staining patterns to different S100 polypeptide chains in melanocytic neoplasms to differentiate between Spitz nevi and melanoma. Ribé and McNutt examined S100 protein expression in 42 Spitz nevi and 105 melanomas.[66] All of the Spitz nevi stained with monoclonal antibodies to S100A6 whereas only 35 of the 105 melanomas were similarly stained. While promising, these results are not specific enough for this marker to be used to reliably differentiate between these two lesions.

A pan-melanoma antigen cocktail containing HMB-45, MART-1 and tyrosinase has a high sensitivity for all forms of melanoma and is a complementary marker to polyclonal S100 protein.[67] Cells that stain positively for S100 protein are not specific for melanocytic cells as this marker is expressed in other cells. This assumes special importance when attempting to differentiate DMM from scar tissue. Chorny and Barr found positive S100 staining in 9 of 10 scars from previously biopsied non-melanocytic neoplasms in the spindle cell component.[68] Scars from re-excision of previously biopsied nevomelanocytic lesions also stain for S100 protein.

Although useful in assisting in differentiating benign melanocytic proliferations from melanoma, immunohistochemistry is an adjuvant tool and does not substitute for clinical and routine pathological evaluation of melanocytic tumors.

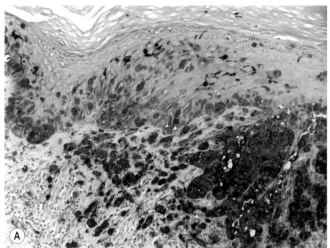

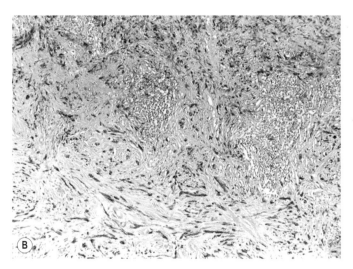

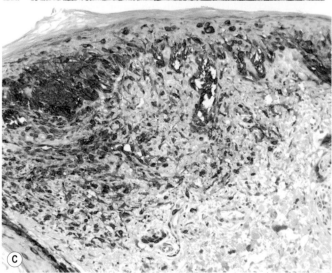

**Figure 27.29** Immunohistochemical staining of melanoma. **A)** Immunoreactivity for S100 protein is shown both in Langerhans cells in the epidermis and in melanoma cells in both the epidermis and dermis. Langerhans cells appear dendritic and are present in the mid epidermis. (S100 immunostain, streptavidin alkaline phosphatase, original magnification ×100.) **B)** S100 labeling spindled melanocytes in a case of desmoplastic melanoma which are commonly MART-1 negative. **C)** MART-1 stain highlights melanocytes in this melanoma, but does not highlight Langerhans cells. MART-1 is more specific than S100 protein staining but less sensitive in certain cases. Immunohistochemical stains with specific melanocyte markers will also stain benign nevi and staining patterns should be evaluated in the context of routine histological observations.

## Proliferation markers

A number of different malignancies have been found to have proliferation markers that may aid in the diagnosis and prognosis of melanocytic neoplasms. Several studies have investigated the role of melanocytic cellular antigens as markers of proliferation. Ki-67 is a nuclear antigen expressed during periods of cellular growth. However, this antigen is not expressed during non-proliferating stages (G0 and early G1). Antibodies to Ki-67 have been used to label melanocytes in an effort to correlate the rate of proliferation with presumed histologic malignancy.

Smolle et al. examined 25 melanocytic skin tumors using antibodies to Ki-67 on fresh frozen tissue. Using the parameter of 'growth fraction' (percentage of positively stained nuclei to total nuclei), statistically significant differences were found between nevi, primary melanomas and malignant melanomas.[69] Similarly, Li et al. used MIB1, another antibody to Ki-67, which is able to stain nuclear antigen on formalin-fixed, paraffin-embedded specimens and therefore is potentially useful in archival tissues.[70] Seventy-two lesions (including compound nevi, dysplastic nevi, Spitz nevi and malignant melanomas) were retrospectively evaluated using MIB1 staining. Using the percentage of positively stained cells, the researchers were able to discriminate between benign lesions and melanomas with statistical significance. Staining for Ki-67 may be considered as an adjunctive technique and should not be viewed as a more important criterion for diagnosis than others such as routine histologic findings.

## Histologic evaluation of staging and prognosis

The revised AJCC melanoma staging system presents several new criteria used to establish prognosis (Table 27.3). For the first time, mitotic rate (number of mitoses/mm²) is included. The data that were reviewed suggest that in patients with localized disease, tumor thickness, mitotic rate and ulceration are the most important histological prognostic indicators.

### Breslow's depth

In 1970, Alexander Breslow evaluated melanoma excision specimens obtained from 98 patients. After 5 years, 71 of the patients remained disease free while 27 developed metastatic or recurrent disease. An ocular micrometer was used to measure from the skin surface to the deepest level of extension of the tumor. There was no recurrence or metastasis in those patients whose maximum tumor thickness was less than 0.76 mm (n=38).[71] Breslow thickness, defined as the depth from the granular layer to the deepest level of neoplasm, has subsequently been determined by multiple studies to be the most important prognostic indicator of survival in primary cutaneous melanomas.[6,72] Extension of melanoma surrounding skin appendages such as hair follicles should not be included in measuring Breslow thickness.

As with any technique, there are a number of limitations. In some areas such as near volar skin, the epidermis may be quite thick and contribute significantly to this measurement, imparting an artificially higher value than if the lesion were present on another site. Conversely, at sites where the skin is very thin such as the eyelid, thin lesions may extend into the deep dermis or subcutis and the level of involvement may artifactually portend a worse prognosis than would otherwise be expected. Furthermore, thickness measurements are subjective and can vary between histopathologists. This can be a consequence of the section that was cut or even in variation between microscopes. It should also be remembered that re-excision specimens may reveal areas that are thicker than in the original biopsy specimen. Thus, although thickness measurements provide important information, their absolute values should not be overemphasized. For example, there is virtually no significance between a lesion of 1.0 mm in thickness and one that is 1.2 mm in thickness. Recommendations for using melanoma thickness in TNM categories and stage groupings in the current AJCC groupings remain unchanged.

### Clark's levels

In 1969, Clark et al. proposed a schema whereby melanoma was described by its anatomical depth of involvement (Table 27.4).[73] In the current AJCC staging system, the Clark's level of invasion has been replaced with mitotic rate for defining of T1b melanomas.

### Ulceration

Ulceration is defined histologically as loss of epidermis and some of the dermis. In 1980, Balch et al.[74] found that the presence of ulceration reduced 5-year survival from 80% to 55% for patients with stage I melanoma and from 53% to 12% for patients with stage II melanoma. These trends remained when corrected for thickness as ulceration is virtually always confined to thicker melanomas.[75]

There are, however, a number of problems with ulceration as a prognostic variable. The definition of ulceration as applied to melanoma is highly subjective. True ulceration in a neoplasm is a manifestation of the lesion outgrowing its blood supply and is almost always associated with zones of necrosis (Fig. 27.30). Such neoplasms are almost always quite thick and highly proliferative and, as such, have higher metastatic potential.

The current use of ulceration as a prognostic variable is also problematic in that it does not define the extent of ulceration of a lesion and does not discriminate between lesions that may have been previously traumatized or biopsied. Furthermore, no recommendations have been made with respect to how much of a lesion needs to be evaluated to search for ulceration. When ulceration occurs in a subset of thick, nodular lesions and when it is extensive, it is a marker of a more aggressive lesion. It is not present in thin or in-situ lesions and caution is advised in reporting tiny, microscopic foci of ulceration or erosion that may have been induced by trauma or a prior procedure as that may impart a worse prognosis to a patient when it is not truly indicated.

## Table 27.3 2009 AJCC Melanoma Staging Classification

### A. TNM Staging for Melanoma (Clinical Staging):

|  | T | N | M |
|---|---|---|---|
| 0 | Tis | N0 | M0 |
| IA | T1a | N0 | M0 |
| IB | T1b<br>T2a | N0<br>N0 | M0<br>M0 |
| IIA | T2b<br>T3a | N0<br>N0 | M0<br>M0 |
| IIB | T3b<br>T4a | N0<br>N0 | M0<br>M0 |
| IIC | T4b | N0 | M0 |
| III | Any T | N > N0 | M0 |
| IV | Any T | Any N | M1 |

### B. TNM Staging Categories for Melanoma

| Classification | Thickness | Ulceration/Mitosis |
|---|---|---|
| **T** | | |
| Tis | NA | NA |
| T1 | ≤ 1.00 | a. Without ulceration and mitosis <1/mm²<br>b. With ulceration or mitoses ≥1/mm² |
| T2 | 1.01–2.00 | a. Without ulceration<br>b. With ulceration |
| T3 | 2.01–4.00 | a. Without ulceration<br>b. With ulceration |
| T4 | >4.00 | a. Without ulceration<br>b. With ulceration |
| **N** | **No. of Metastatic Nodes** | **Nodal Metastatic Burden** |
| N0 | 0 | NA |
| | 1 | a. Micrometastasis<br>b. Macrometastasis |
| | 2–3 | a. Micrometastasis<br>b. Macrometastasis<br>c. In-transit metastases / satellites without metastatic nodes |
| | 4+ metastatic nodes or matted nodes, or in-transit metastases/satellites with metastatic nodes | |
| **M** | **Site** | **Serum LDH** |
| M0 | No distant metastases | NA |
| M1a | Distant skin, subcutaneous or nodal metastases | Normal |
| M1b | Lung metastases | Normal |
| M1c | All other visceral metastases<br>Any distant metastasis | Normal<br>Elevated |

Modified from: Balch CM, Gershenwald JE, Soong SJ, et al. Final version of 2009 AJCC melanoma staging and classification. *J Clin Oncol.* 2009;27(36): 6199-6206.

| Table 27.4 Clark's Levels | |
|---|---|
| I | Confined to the epidermis (in situ) |
| II | Neoplasm to the papillary dermis, but not filling the papillary dermis |
| III | Neoplasm extending to the level of the junction between the papillary and reticular dermis (filling the papillary dermis) |
| IV | Neoplasm extending into the reticular dermis |
| V | Neoplasm extending into the subcutaneous fat |

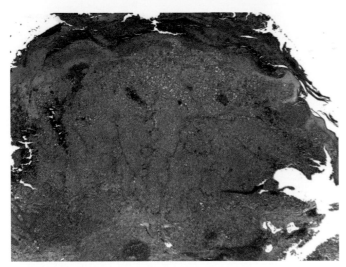

**Figure 27.30** Ulceration in melanoma. This thick melanoma demonstrates ulceration with marked necrosis. It is important to distinguish ulceration from excoriation or biopsy-related erosion as this does not represent true ulceration, which is a manifestation of the neoplasm outgrowing its blood supply. True ulceration tends to have worse prognosis.

## Tumor-infiltrating lymphocytes

In 1989, Clark et al. demonstrated that tumor-infiltrating lymphocytes were independent predictors of 8-year survival.[76] Infiltrating-lymphocyte patterns are described as 'brisk', 'non-brisk' and 'absent'. A 'brisk' infiltrating-lymphocyte pattern, defined as a dense infiltrate of lymphocytes within and surrounding the neoplasm, was associated with improved prognosis. Tuthill et al. later confirmed these findings.[77] However, there has been criticism regarding lack of histologic criteria and standardization in evaluating tumor-infiltrating lymphocytes and it is not routinely included in pathology reports of melanoma today.

## Regression

Regression is defined as host response destruction of melanoma cells with replacement by fibrous tissue, blood vessels and melanophages. Guitart and co-workers performed a case–control study of 43 cases to investigate the histological characteristics associated with metastasizing thin melanomas.[78] Extensive regression was found in 42% of the cases versus 5% of the controls. Another study examined 103 patients with thin melanomas (≤0.76 mm).[57] Of the 103 patients, 30 had histologic evidence of partial regression. Six of the patients with regression died of metastatic

disease. All of these six patients had greater than 77% regression. The remaining 24 patients in the partial regression group remained alive at the end of the 3-year study and most had regression of less than 50% (mean, 29.9%). No metastasis occurred in the 73 patients who had thin melanomas without regression. There is speculation that these lesions are thin because they have undergone regression and may have once represented deeper and therefore more aggressive melanomas.

Complete regression of melanoma has been shown to be associated with metastatic disease and worsened prognosis. In contrast, thick lesions with partial regression have been reported to be associated with an improved prognosis.[57-59]

## Mitotic rate

Mitotic rate is a new addition to the seventh edition (2009) TNM staging system for melanoma. The data from the AJCC melanoma staging database showed that mitotic rate was the second most powerful predictor of survival after tumor thickness in localized melanomas 1 mm or less in thickness. In thin melanomas the most significant correlation with survival was identified as a threshold of at least 1 mitosis per square millimeter. In non-ulcerated localized melanomas 1 mm or less in thickness (stage I) with a mitotic rate $<1/mm^2$, 10-year survival was 95%; this fell to 88% in cases with a mitotic rate $>1/mm^2$. As a result of these findings, in the seventh edition, the AJCC Melanoma Staging Committee has replaced Clark's level with mitotic rate for defining T1 tumors. Survival was not significantly altered by mitotic rate in ulcerated thin localized melanomas.

Though the association of mitotic rate and survival is well documented and is now part of the new staging system, it does present several practical problems. Localized melanomas 1 mm or less in thickness are frequently too small to accurately calculate mitotic activity. When calculating mitotic rate, the pathologist requires five high-power fields, which simply may not be visible in small shave specimens. Furthermore, in larger lesions there is currently no consensus regarding high-power fields from which mitotic rate should be calculated. Should these be from the most mitotically active regions or selected at random? Unfortunately, these recommendations have been put forth when more study is clearly indicated.

The primary criterion for defining T1b melanomas is now mitotic rate rather than level of invasion. All patients with microscopic nodal metastases, regardless of extent of tumor burden, are classified as stage III.

## Histologic satellite metastases of melanoma

Patients with melanoma and histological evidence of microscopic satellite metastases have a 5-year disease-free survival of approximately 36%. Patients without satellites have a survival rate of 89%.[79] The AJCC Melanoma Staging Committee has recommended that this feature be recognized as a sign of early lymphatic metastases and be retained in the category of N2c melanoma.

Because of the significant subjectivity in assigning prognosis based on histologic variables, histologic features should be used as general guidelines only. Furthermore, as none are as reliable as tumor thickness, many dermatopathologists do not routinely include them in pathology reports.

## Sentinel lymph node biopsy

Several groups have studied the importance of SLN biopsies for determining prognosis in patients with melanoma (Chapter 50).[80,81] Statius Muller et al. evaluated 263 patients with stage I or II melanoma who had undergone SLN biopsy. Tumor-positive nodes were found in 20% of the patients. The 5-year disease-free survival rate was 49% in node-positive patients, as compared with 91% in the tumor-free SLN group. As such, SLN status was found to be the most powerful predictor of survival for melanoma patients.[82] Thus, the presence of a biopsy demonstrating SLN positivity for melanoma correlates with a worsened prognosis and is an indication that metastasis has occurred from the primary neoplasm.[83,84]

Molecular staging has also been performed on SLN tissue. Of 114 patients with stage I or II melanoma who underwent SLN biopsy and were followed an average of 28 months, 23 (20%) had pathologically positive SLNs which were also RT-PCR positive for tyrosinase messenger-RNA, a sign of metastatic melanoma. Forty-seven of the 91 histologically negative lymph nodes were RT-PCR positive. There was a recurrence rate among 14 (61%) of the 23 patients who were both pathologically and RT-PCR positive and a recurrence rate among 1 (2%) of 44 patients who were both pathologically and RT-PCR negative. For patients who were upstaged by the molecular assay (pathologically negative, RT-PCR positive), there was a recurrence rate among 6 (13%) of 47 patients. In both univariate and multivariate regression analyses, the histological and RT-PCR status of the SLNs were the best predictors of disease-free survival.[85,86]

When examining SLN, benign intraparenchymal nevus cells in clusters of only a few cells up to 2.1-mm aggregates may occasionally be noted. These benign melanocytes lack mitotic figures and lymphatic or vascular involvement. Additionally, the nevus cell aggregates express S100 protein and/or MART-1 but not gp100 protein (HMB-45) or Ki-67 (<1%). The utilization of immunohistochemistry for the detection of nodal micrometastasis has been recommended where appropriate.

Kelley and Cockerell have proposed that sentinel lymphadenectomy be considered in patients with melanocytic neoplasms of uncertain behavior that are 1.0 mm or more in thickness. If excised lymph nodes were found to contain atypical melanocytes, specifically effacing large areas of the sampled lymph node with atypical cells, the suspicion of malignancy would be greater and careful follow-up and possibly additional therapy would be recommended. Performing SLN biopsy also remains controversial in melanomas <1.0 mm in thickness.[87]

## FUTURE OUTLOOK

A key challenge regarding the diagnosis and treatment of melanoma still lies at the histologic level where the diagnosis is often first made. There may be significant difficulty in rendering an accurate diagnosis of melanoma histologically. Furthermore, the ability to prognosticate based on the histologic findings of the primary lesion is limited.

In the future, techniques may be available that allow for more accurate diagnoses to be rendered quickly using biometric assays and techniques that can be used in conjunction with routine histology. In addition, techniques will likely be developed that allow for more accurate prediction of prognosis and likelihood of metastasis based on features such as the genotype of the melanoma coupled with immunologic profiles of the patient.

## REFERENCES

1. McGovern TW, Litaker MS. Clinical predictors of malignant pigmented lesions: a comparison of the Glasgow seven-point checklist and the American Cancer Society's ABCDs of pigmented lesions. *J Dermatol Surg Oncol.* 1992;18:22–26.
2. Blokx WA, van Dijk MC, Ruiter DJ. Molecular cytogenetics of cutaneous melanocytic lesions – diagnostic, prognostic and therapeutic aspects. *Histopathology.* 2010;56(1):121–132.
3. Ackerman AB. Malignant melanoma: a unifying concept. *Hum Pathol.* 1980;11(6):591–595.
4. Ackerman AB, David KM. A unifying concept of malignant melanoma: biologic aspects. *Hum Pathol.* 1986;17(5):438–440.
5. Bono A, Bartoli C, Moglia D, et al. Small melanomas: a clinical study on 270 consecutive cases of cutaneous melanoma. *Melanoma Res.* 1999;9(6):583–586.
6. Balch CM, Gershenwald JE, Soong SJ, et al. Final version of 2009 AJCC melanoma staging and classification. *J Clin Oncol.* 2009;27(36):6199–6206.
7. Balch CM, Soong SJ, Gershenwald JE, et al. Prognostic factors analysis of 17,600 melanoma patients: validation of the American Joint Committee on Cancer melanoma staging system. *J Clin Oncol.* 2001;19(16):3622–3634.
8. Clark Jr WH, Elder DE, Guerry 4th D, et al. A study of tumor progression: the precursor lesions of superficial spreading and nodular melanoma. *Hum Pathol.* 1984;15(12):1147–1165.
9. Clark Jr WH, Elder DE, Van Horn M. The biologic forms of malignant melanoma. *Hum Pathol.* 1986;17(5):443–450.
10. Elder DE, Guerry 4th D, Epstein MN, et al. Invasive malignant melanomas lacking competence for metastasis. *Am J Dermatopathol.* 1984;6(suppl):55–61.
11. Herlyn M, Clark WH, Rodeck U, et al. Biology of tumor progression in human melanocytes. *Lab Invest.* 1987;56(5):461–474.
12. Barnhill RL, Mihm Jr MC. The histopathology of cutaneous malignant melanoma. *Semin Diagn Pathol.* 1993;10(1):47–75.
13. Ashida A, Takata M, Murata H, et al. Pathological activation of KIT in metastatic tumors of acral and mucosal melanomas. *Int J Cancer.* 2009;124(4):862–868.
14. Su WP. Malignant melanoma: basic approach to clinicopathologic correlation. *Mayo Clin Proc.* 1997;72(3):267–272.
15. Abramova L, Slingluff Jr CL, Patterson JW. Problems in the interpretation of apparent "radial growth phase" malignant melanomas that metastasize. *J Cutan Pathol.* 2002;29(7):407–414.
16. Caporaso N, Greene MH, Tsai S, et al. Cytogenetics in hereditary malignant melanoma and dysplastic nevus syndrome: is dysplastic nevus syndrome a chromosome instability disorder? *Cancer Genet Cytogenet.* 1987;24(2):299–314.
17. Hussein MR, Wood GS. Molecular aspects of melanocytic dysplastic nevi. *J Mol Diagn.* 2002;4(2):71–80.
18. Suh KY, Bolognia JL. Signature nevi. *J Am Acad Dermatol.* 2009;60(3):508–514.
19. Sober AJ, Chuang TY, Duvic M, et al. Guidelines of care for primary cutaneous melanoma. *J Am Acad Dermatol.* 2001;45:579–586.
20. Houghton AN, Coit DG, Daud A, et al. NCCN Clinical Practice Guidelines in Oncology: Melanoma. *J Natl Compr Canc Netw.* 2006;4:666–684.
21. Marghoob AA, Terushkin V, Dusza SW, et al. Dermatologists, general practitioners, and the best method to biopsy suspect melanocytic neoplasms. *Arch Dermatol.* 2010;146(3):325–328.
22. Tran KT, Wright NA, Cockerell CJ. Biopsy of the pigmented lesion – when and how. *J Am Acad Dermatol.* 2008;59(5):852–871.
23. Martin 2nd RC, Scoggins CR, Ross MI, et al. Is incisional biopsy of melanoma harmful? *Am J Surg.* 2005;190(6):913–917.
24. Ng PC, Barzilai DA, Ismail SA, et al. Evaluating invasive cutaneous melanoma: is the initial biopsy representative of the final depth? *J Am Acad Dermatol.* 2003;48(3):420–424.
25. Hsu M, Cockerell CJ. *Punch biopsy of melanocytic neoplasms: a poorly recognized pitfall in the diagnosis of cutaneous malignant melanoma.* In press. 2009

26. Florell SR, Boucher KM, Leachman SA, et al. Histopathologic recognition of involved margins of lentigo maligna excised by staged excision; an interobserver comparison study. *Arch Dermatol.* 2003;139(5):595–604.

27. Heenan PJ. Nodular melanoma is not a distinct entity. *Arch Dermatol.* 2003;139(3):387.

28. Chamberlain AJ, Fritschi L, Giles GG, et al. Nodular type and older age as the most significant associations of thick melanoma in Victoria, Australia. *Arch Dermatol.* 2002;138(5):609–614.

29. de Almeida LS, Requena L, Rütten A, et al. Desmoplastic malignant melanoma: a clinicopathologic analysis of 113 cases. *Am J Dermatopathol.* 2008;30(3):207–215.

30. Livestro DP, Muzikansky A, Kaine EM, et al. Biology of desmoplastic melanoma: a case-control comparison with other melanomas. *J Clin Oncol.* 2005;23(27):6739–6746.

31. Hawkins WG, Busam KJ, Ben-Porat L, et al. Desmoplastic melanoma: a pathologically and clinically distinct form of cutaneous melanoma. *Ann Surg Oncol.* 2005;12(3):207–213.

32. Kucher C, Zhang PJ, Pasha T, et al. Expression of Melan-A and Ki-67 in desmoplastic melanoma and desmoplastic nevi. *Am J Dermatopathol.* 2004;26(6):452–457.

33. Steiner A, Konrad K, Pehamberger H, et al. Verrucous malignant melanoma. *Arch Dermatol.* 1988;124(10):1534–1537.

34. Blessing K, Evans AT, al-Nafussi A. Verrucous naevoid and keratotic malignant melanoma: a clinico-pathological study of 20 cases. *Histopathology.* 1993;23(5):453–458.

35. Kuehnl-Petzoldt C, Berger H, Wiebelt H. Verrucous keratotic variations of malignant melanoma: a clinicopathological study. *Am J Dermatopathol.* 1982;4(5):403–410.

36. Crowson AN, Magro CM, Mihm Jr MC. Malignant melanoma with prominent pigment synthesis: "animal type" melanoma – a clinical and histological study of six cases with a consideration of other melanocytic neoplasms with prominent pigment synthesis. *Hum Pathol.* 1999;30(5):543–550.

37. Zembowicz A, Carney JA, Mihm MC. Pigmented epithelioid melanocytoma: a low-grade melanocytic tumor with metastatic potential indistinguishable from animal-type melanoma and epithelioid blue nevus. *Am J Surg Pathol.* 2004;28(1):31–40.

38. Clemente C, Bettio D, Venci A, et al. A fluorescence in situ hybridization (FISH) procedure to assist in differentiating benign from malignant melanocytic lesions. *Pathologica.* 2009;101(5):169–174.

39. Lim C, Murali R, McCarthy SW, et al. Pigmented epithelioid melanocytoma: a recently described melanocytic tumour of low malignant potential. *Pathology.* 2010;42(3):284–286.

40. Weedon D. In: *Skin Pathology.* 2nd ed.2002: Edinburgh: Churchill Livingstone; 828.

41. Zembowicz A, McCusker M, Chiarelli C, et al. Morphological analysis of nevoid melanoma: a study of 20 cases with a review of the literature. *Am J Dermatopathol.* 2001;23(3):167–175.

42. Mones JM, Ackerman AB. "Atypical" blue nevus, "malignant" blue nevus, and "metastasizing" blue nevus: a critique in historical perspective of three concepts flawed fatally. *Am J Dermatopathol.* 2004;26(5):407–430.

43. Walsh N, Crotty K, Palmer A, et al. Spitz nevus versus spitzoid malignant melanoma: an evaluation of the current distinguishing histopathologic criteria. *Hum Pathol.* 1998;29:1105–1112.

44. Crotty KA, Scolyer RA, Li L, et al. Spitz naevus versus Spitzoid melanoma: when and how can they be distinguished? *Pathology.* 2002;34(1):6–12.

45. Horner MJ, Ries LAG, Krapcho M, et al., eds. *SEER Cancer Statistics Review.* Bethesda, MD: National Cancer Institute; 1975-2006. http://seer.cancer.gov/csr/1975_2006/results_merged/sect_16_melanoma_skin.pdf.

46. Richardson SK, Tannous ZS, Mihm Jr MC. Congenital and infantile melanoma: review of the literature and report of an uncommon variant, pigment-synthesizing melanoma. *J Am Acad Dermatol.* 2002;47(1):77–90.

47. Hamre MR, Chuba P, Bakhshi S, et al. Cutaneous melanoma in childhood and adolescence. *Pediatr Hematol Oncol.* 2002;19(5):309–317.

48. Alexander A, Samlowski WE, Grossman D, et al. Metastatic melanoma in pregnancy: risk of transplacental metastases in the infant. *J Clin Oncol.* 2003;21(11):2179–2186.

49. Paradela S, Fonseca E, Pita S, et al. Spitzoid melanoma in children: clinicopathological study and application of immunohistochemistry as an adjunct diagnostic tool. *J Cutan Pathol.* 2009;36(7):740–752.

50. Haupt HM, Stern JB. Pagetoid melanocytosis. Histologic features in benign and malignant lesions. *Am J Surg Pathol.* 1995;19:792–797.

51. Elder DE. Precursors to melanoma and their mimics: nevi of special sites. *Mod Pathol.* 2006;19(suppl 2):S4–S20.

52. Cullity G. Intra-epithelial changes in childhood nevi simulating malignant melanoma. *Pathology.* 1984;16(3):307–311.

53. Leech SN, Bell H, Leonard N, et al. Neonatal giant congenital nevi with proliferative nodules: a clinicopathologic study and literature review of neonatal melanoma. *Arch Dermatol.* 2004;140(1):83–88.

54. Kornberg R, Ackerman AB. Pseudomelanoma: recurrent melanocytic nevus following partial surgical removal. *Arch Dermatol.* 1975;111(12):1588–1590.

55. Petronic-Rosic V, Shea CR, Krausz T. Pagetoid melanocytosis: when is it significant? *Pathology.* 2004;36(5):435–444.

56. Stern JB, Haupt HM. Pagetoid melanocytosis: tease or tocsin? *Semin Diagn Pathol.* 1998;15(3):225–229.

57. Ronan SG, Eng AM, Briele HA, et al. Thin malignant melanomas with regression and metastases. *Arch Dermatol.* 1987;123:1326–1330.

58. Cooper PH, Wanebo HJ, Hagar RW. Regression in thin malignant melanoma. *Arch Dermatol.* 1985;121:1127–1131.

59. Sondergaard K, Schou G. Therapeutic and clinicopathological factors in the survival of 1,469 patients with primary cutaneous malignant melanoma in clinical stage I. A multivariate regression analysis. *Virchows Arch A Pathol Anat Histopathol.* 1985;408:249–258.

60. Plaza JA, Torres-Cabala C, Evans H, et al. Cutaneous metastases of malignant melanoma: a clinicopathologic study of 192 cases with emphasis on the morphologic spectrum. *Am J Dermatopathol.* 2010;32(2):129–136.

61. Harrist TJ, Rigel DS, Day Jr CL, et al. "Microscopic satellites" are more highly associated with regional lymph node metastases than is primary melanoma thickness. *Cancer.* 1984;53(10):2183–2187.

62. Cerroni L, Barnhill R, Elder D, et al. Melanocytic tumors of uncertain malignant potential: results of a tutorial held at the XXIX Symposium of the International Society of Dermatopathology in Graz, October 2008. *Am J Surg Pathol.* 2010;34(3):314–326.

63. Barnhill RL, Argenyi Z, Berwick M, et al. Atypical cellular blue nevi (cellular blue nevi with atypical features): lack of consensus for diagnosis and distinction from cellular blue nevi and malignant melanoma ("malignant blue nevus"). *Am J Surg Pathol.* 2008;32(1):36–44.

64. Elder DE, Xu X. The approach to the patient with a difficult melanocytic lesion. *Pathology.* 2004;36(5):428–434.

65. Ludgate MW, Fullen DR, Lee J, et al. The atypical Spitz tumor of uncertain biologic potential: a series of 67 patients from a single institution. *Cancer.* 2009;115(3):631–641.

66. Ribé A, McNutt NS. S100A6 protein expression is different in Spitz nevi and melanomas. *Mod Pathol.* 2003;16(5):505–511.

67. Orchard G. Evaluation of melanocytic neoplasms: application of a pan-melanoma antibody cocktail. *Br J Biomed Sci.* 2002;59(4):196–202.

68. Chorny JA, Barr RJ. S100 positive spindle cells in scars: a diagnostic pitfall in the re-excision of desmoplastic melanoma. *Am J Dermatopathol.* 2002;24(4):309–312.

69. Smolle J, Soyer HP, Kerl H. Proliferation activity of cutaneous melanocytic tumors defined by Ki-67 monoclonal antibody. *Am J Dermatopathol.* 1989;11(4):301–307.

70. Li LX, Crotty KA, McCarthy SW, et al. A zonal comparison of MIB1-Ki67 immunoreactivity in benign and malignant melanocytic lesions. *Am J Dermatopathol.* 2000;22(6):489–495.

71. Breslow A. Thickness, cross-sectional areas and depth of invasion in the prognosis of cutaneous melanoma. *Ann Surg.* 1970;172(5):902–908.

72. Barnhill RL, Fine JA, Roush GC, et al. Predicting five-year outcome for patients with cutaneous melanoma in a population-based study. *Cancer.* 1996;78(3):427–432.

73. Clark Jr WH, From L, Bernardino EA, et al. The histogenesis and biologic behavior of primary human malignant melanomas of the skin. *Cancer Res.* 1969;29(3):705–727.

74. Balch CM, Wilkerson JA, Murad TM, et al. The prognostic significance of ulceration of cutaneous melanoma. *Cancer.* 1980;45(12):3012–3017.

75. Balch CM, Soong SJ, Gershenwald JE, et al. Prognostic factors analysis of 17,600 melanoma patients: validation of the American Joint Committee on Cancer melanoma staging system. *J Clin Oncol.* 2001;19(16):3622–3634.

76. Clark Jr WH, Elder DE, Guerry 4th D, et al. Model predicting survival in stage I melanoma based on tumor progression. *J Natl Cancer Inst.* 1989;81(24):1893–1904.

77. Tuthill RJ, Unger JM, Liu PY, et al. Southwest Oncology Group. Risk assessment in localized primary cutaneous melanoma: a Southwest Oncology Group study evaluating nine factors and a test of the Clark logistic regression prediction model. *Am J Clin Pathol.* 2002;118(4):504–511.

78. Guitart J, Lowe L, Piepkorn M, et al. Histological characteristics of metastasizing thin melanomas: a case-control study of 43 cases. *Arch Dermatol.* 2002;138(5):603–608.

79. Day Jr CL, Harrist TJ, Gorstein F, et al. Malignant melanoma. Prognostic significance of "microscopic satellites" in the reticular dermis and subcutaneous fat. *Ann Surg.* 1981;194(1):108–112.

**80.** Cochran AJ, Wen DR, Morton DL. Management of the regional lymph nodes in patients with cutaneous malignant melanoma. *World J Surg.* 1992;16(2):214–221.

**81.** Rousseau Jr DL, Ross MI, Johnson MM, et al. Revised American Joint Committee on Cancer staging criteria accurately predict sentinel lymph node positivity in clinically node-negative melanoma patients. *Ann Surg Oncol.* 2003;10(5):569–574.

**82.** Statius Muller MG, van Leeuwen PA, de Lange-de Klerk ES, et al. The sentinel lymph node status is an important factor for predicting clinical outcome in patients with Stage I or II cutaneous melanoma. *Cancer.* 2001;91(12):2401–2408.

**83.** Gershenwald JE, Thompson W, Mansfield PF, et al. Multi-institutional melanoma lymphatic mapping experience: the prognostic value of sentinel lymph node status in 612 stage I or II melanoma patients. *J Clin Oncol.* 1999;17(3):976–983.

**84.** Vuylsteke RJ, van Leeuwen PA, Statius Muller MG, et al. Clinical outcome of stage I/II melanoma patients after selective sentinel lymph node dissection: long-term follow-up results. *J Clin Oncol.* 2003;21(6):1057–1065.

**85.** Shivers SC, Wang X, Li W, et al. Molecular staging of malignant melanoma: correlation with clinical outcome. *JAMA.* 1998;280(16): 1410–1415.

**86.** Goydos JS, Patel KN, Shih WJ, et al. Patterns of recurrence in patients with melanoma and histologically negative of RT-PCR positive sentinel lymph nodes. *J Am Coll Surg.* 2003;97(2):196–205.

**87.** Kelley SW, Cockerell CJ. Sentinel lymph node biopsy as an adjunct to management of histologically difficult to diagnose melanocytic lesions: a proposal. *J Am Acad Dermatol.* 2000;42(3):527–530.

# Management of the Patient with Melanoma

*Jacqueline M. Goulart and Allan C. Halpern*

## Key Points

- Melanoma management should be tailored to the needs of each individual patient.

- Surgical excision is the cornerstone of melanoma management.

- Sentinel lymph node biopsy is currently a staging and prognostic tool in the management of melanoma.

- Adjuvant therapy should be considered in patients at high risk of recurrence.

- Single drug chemotherapy remains the standard treatment for advanced metastatic disease. Clinical trials should be strongly considered for patients with metastatic melanoma.

- Regular follow-up, skin self-examinations, and sun protection are important for patients with a history of melanoma and their family members.

## INTRODUCTION

### Existing guidelines

Melanoma is increasingly recognized as a major public health concern due to a continued rise in incidence and mortality over the past few decades.[1] Optimal management of a patient diagnosed with melanoma remains challenging, and the most effective strategies for reducing morbidity and mortality rely on prevention and early detection.[2] A multifaceted approach is employed when deciding management of the primary site, staging procedures, adjuvant therapy, and follow-up.

Several guidelines for melanoma management have been set forth by different organizations, including the National Comprehensive Cancer Network (NCCN), American Academy of Dermatology, Society of Surgical Oncology, and the British Association of Dermatologists.[2a,3–6] The NCCN guidelines have been most recently updated and a practical representation of their recommendations on staging and initial management for common scenarios is provided in Figure 28.1. The significant variations among these different published guidelines highlight the absence of a single 'evidence-based' approach for managing melanoma patients. Therefore, treatment should be tailored to the needs of each individual patient. This chapter presents a generalized approach to the diagnostic and staging work-up for melanoma, surgical management, adjuvant treatment, and post-treatment surveillance, and more detailed descriptions of each of these components.

Detailed discussions concerning the various stage-specific treatment modalities, including current practice, recent advances, and controversies, may be found in subsequent chapters.

## MANAGEMENT

### Initial assessment

The diagnosis of melanoma begins with a biopsy of the suspected primary lesion. Ideally, an excisional biopsy is performed where appropriate to avoid sampling error and to obtain the most precise diagnostic and prognostic information. However, full-thickness incisional and shave biopsies are often performed, especially when the index of suspicion is low or if the lesion is large and/or impractical to excise completely. While concern has been raised about trauma inducing tumor cell metastasis, multiple studies suggest that incising a melanoma does not result in a worse prognosis.[7] Shave biopsy is a convenient and commonly utilized technique that often accurately represents the depth of lesion for thin melanomas, still some specimens may have positive deep margins complicating accurate microstaging and treatment recommendations.[8] Once a histopathologic diagnosis has been established, attention should be given to the prognostic attributes of the lesion (see Chapter 26), such as thickness, ulceration, and mitotic rate, as well as the age and overall medical condition of the patient. Work-up, treatment, and follow-up recommendations are guided by the stage of the patient's disease.

Clinical staging of a melanoma patient requires a thorough history and physical examination. A problem-oriented physical examination should include a complete skin and lymph node examination and assessment of any abnormalities detected on a thorough review of systems. Suspicious signs, symptoms, and physical findings (e.g. in-transit metastases, satellite lesions, and palpable lymph nodes) may warrant additional laboratory studies, imaging, and histological confirmation. The American Joint Committee on Cancer (AJCC) melanoma staging system takes into account the status of lymph node involvement for those who undergo lymphatic mapping.[9] The AJCC stage groupings and subsequent survival data are provided in Table 28.1. Tumor cell mitotic rate has been shown to be an independent prognostic factor for melanoma survival and has been added to the next iteration of the staging system.[10,11] More comprehensive staging criteria will improve the accuracy of prognostic and survival information. This is especially true for thin melanomas, which

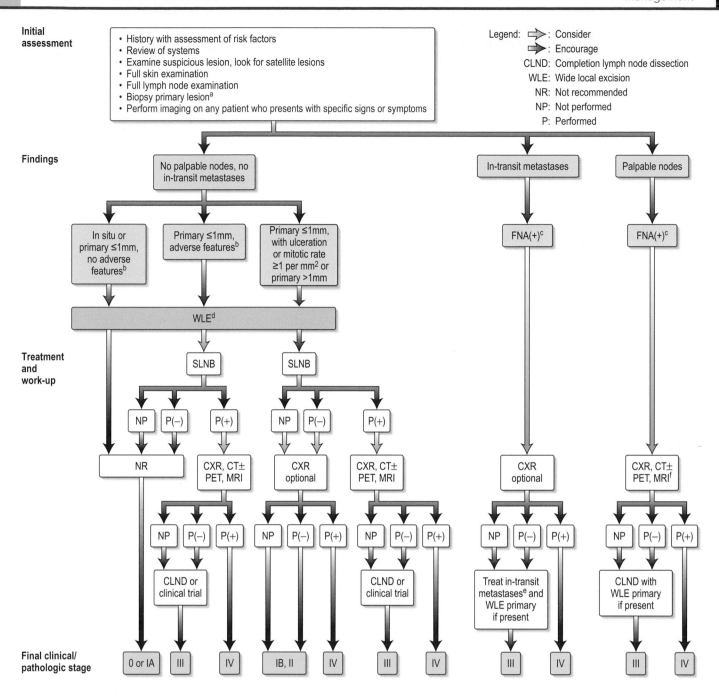

**Initial assessment**

- History with assessment of risk factors
- Review of systems
- Examine suspicious lesion, look for satellite lesions
- Full skin examination
- Full lymph node examination
- Biopsy primary lesion[a]
- Perform imaging on any patient who presents with specific signs or symptoms

Legend: ⇒ : Consider
⇒ : Encourage
CLND: Completion lymph node dissection
WLE: Wide local excision
NR: Not recommended
NP: Not performed
P: Performed

**Findings**

- No palpable nodes, no in-transit metastases
- In-transit metastases
- Palpable nodes

- In situ or primary ≤1mm, no adverse features[b]
- Primary ≤1mm, adverse features[b]
- Primary ≤1mm, with ulceration or mitotic rate ≥1 per mm$^2$ or primary >1mm
- FNA(+)[c]
- FNA(+)[c]

**Treatment and work-up**

WLE[d]

SLNB — SLNB

NP | P(−) | P(+)     NP | P(−) | P(+)

NR     CXR, CT± PET, MRI     CXR optional     CXR, CT± PET, MRI     CXR optional     CXR, CT± PET, MRI[f]

NP | P(−) | P(+)   NP | P(−) | P(+)   NP | P(−) | P(+)   NP | P(−) | P(+)   NP | P(−) | P(+)

CLND or clinical trial     CLND or clinical trial     Treat in-transit metastases[e] and WLE primary if present     CLND with WLE primary if present

**Final clinical/pathologic stage**

0 or IA | III | IV     IB, II | IV     III | IV     III | IV     III | IV

[a] Complete removal of lesion at initial biopsy is highly preferable. If biopsy is inadequate to provide information for prognosis then re-biopsy. Prognostic information includes: Breslow thickness, ulceration status, dermal mitotic rate, mitotic rate, deep and peripheral margin status, microsatellitosis, Clark level.

[b] Adverse features include ≥ 0.75 mm thick, positive deep margins, lymphovascular invasion, or Clark Level IV.

[c] FNA preferred, if feasible, or biopsy. If FNA negative, perform open biopsy. If open biopsy negative, proceed with treatment as per features of primary.

[d] For lesions with significant metastatic potential for which WLE will result in significant cosmetic or functional impairment, consider extent-of-disease work-up prior to undertaking surgery.

[e] The recommended treatment for in-transit metastases is surgical excision when feasible with consideration of SLNB; alternatives include intralesional injection, topical imiquimod, laser ablation, hyperthermic isolated limb perfusion/isolated limb infusion, clinical trial, radiation therapy and systemic therapy.

[f] Pelvic CT indicated if inguinofemoral nodes positive.

**Figure 28.1** Schema for staging and initial management of melanoma based on NCCN guidelines.[2a] Footnotes reproduced with permission from the **NCCN Clinical Practice Guidelines in Oncology (NCCN Guidelines™) for Melanoma V.1.2011.** © 2010 National Comprehensive Cancer Network, Inc. All rights reserved. The NCCN Guidelines™ and illustrations herein may not be reproduced in any form for any purpose without the express written permission of the NCCN. To view the most recent and complete version of the NCCN Guidelines, go online to HYPERLINK "http://www.nccn.org/"NCCN.org. NATIONAL COMPREHENSIVE CANCER NETWORK®, NCCN®, NCCN GUIDELINES™, and all other NCCN Content are trademarks owned by the National Comprehensive Cancer Network, Inc.

## Table 28.1 Survival Data for Melanoma by AJCC Stage

| Stage | Criteria | Survival (%) 5-year |
|---|---|---|
| In situ (0) | No invasive component | |
| IA | ≤1.0 mm with no ulceration, <1 mitosis/mm² | 97 |
| IB | <1.0 mm with ulceration or ≥ 1 mitosis/mm² 1.01–2.0 mm with no ulceration | 90 |
| IIA | 1.01–2.0 mm with ulceration 2.01–4.0 mm, no ulceration | 79–82 |
| IIB | 2.01–4.0 mm with ulceration >4.0 mm, no ulceration | 68–71 |
| IIC | >4.0 mm with ulceration | 53 |
| IIIA | Non-ulcerated primary tumor (T1–T4a) with ≤3 nodal micromets | 78 |
| IIIB | Non-ulcerated primary tumor (T1–T4a) with ≤3 macromets Any primary tumor (T1–T4b) with ≤3 nodal micromets Any T with in-transit or satellite | 59 |
| IIIC | Any T with ≤3 macromets Any T with ≥4 nodes | 40 |
| IV M1a | Distant skin, subcutaneous or nodal mets with normal LDH | |
| IV M1b | Lung metastasis with normal LDH | <20 5-year survival for all IV M1 categories |
| IV M1c | All other visceral metastasis with normal LDH. Any distant metastasis with elevated LDH | |

Stage I, II – worse prognosis with ulceration, increasing thickness, age, axial location, being male.

Stage III – worse with increasing number of nodes, macrometastasis, and ulceration of primary tumor.

Stage IV – depends on site, but differences are minimal.

Mets to the lung only has 1-year survival advantage over other visceral mets.

Adapted from Edge SB, Byrd DR, Compton CC, et al. Melanoma of the skin. In: AJCC Cancer Staging Manual. 7th ed. New York, NY: Springer; 2009:325-340.

represent the majority of melanoma diagnoses. The use of additional prognostic criteria has shown that survival for thin melanoma varies beyond the risk groupings predicted by current AJCC criteria, as shown in Table 28.2.[12]

## Extent-of-disease work-up

Once the prognostic attributes of the primary lesion and clinical stage have been established, baseline laboratory tests and imaging studies may be considered. Patients with melanomas ≤1.0 mm do not need specific blood work or imaging studies to search for occult metastases. For patients with melanomas >1.0 mm, laboratory values including complete blood count (CBC), lactic dehydrogenase (LDH),

and other liver function tests have been suggested by some guidelines to be included in the initial work-up. These studies have very low yield, and are therefore not strongly recommended. In patients with more advanced stages of disease, LDH levels may be used to monitor the progression or recurrence of metastatic disease. Elevated serum LDH is an independent and highly significant predictor of survival outcome among patients with stage IV disease and should be obtained at the time stage IV disease is documented.[9] However, elevated LDH can be quite non-specific and other common causes must be ruled out. For this reason, elevated serum LDH is considered an indication of metastatic disease when obtained on two separate occasions, at least 24 hours apart. LDH testing is relatively inexpensive and provides a baseline for future reference when followed as a marker for disease activity in patients with stage IV disease. There is little evidence to support the utility of this test in the initial work-up of early stage melanoma.

Serum level of S100B has recently been investigated as a tumor marker predictive of recurrence. Results have been encouraging in some studies but not found to be consistently of value.[13-15] More information is needed before the routine use of this serum marker is recommended and for which stage of disease. Routine imaging studies are not indicated in patients with stage I or II disease. Baseline radiologic and nuclear imaging studies may be useful in evaluating disease progression and guiding the management of stage III and IV patients who have nodal or metastatic disease. Chest X-ray, CT scans, and more recently PET scans are commonly used to evaluate specific signs or symptoms, but are considered low yield when used for screening (see Chapter 56).[3]

## Surgical management

The cornerstone of treatment for primary melanoma is excisional surgery with margins based on Breslow thickness (see Chapter 49). Generally accepted surgical margins for excision are listed in Table 28.3. Excision of large and/or deep lesions with appropriate margins often requires a complex closure (Fig. 28.2) (see also Chapter 51). Margins may be modified to accommodate individual anatomic or cosmetic considerations. Adjustments may also be made depending on the type of melanoma. For example, the preferred treatment for lentigo maligna is complete surgical excision; however, these lesions are frequently large in size and commonly occur on the face of elderly patients (Fig. 28.3). Such cases warrant consideration of radiation therapy, cryotherapy, topical therapy, or observation.

For patients with thin melanomas ≤1.0 mm without negative prognostic attributes such as ulceration or mitotic rate ≥1 per mm² or extensive regression, wide local excision is sufficient treatment. For patients with thin melanomas ≤1.0 mm with negative prognostic attributes, or intermediate and thick lesions >1.0 mm with clinical evidence of nodal involvement, lymphatic mapping with sentinel lymph node biopsy (SLNB) should be encouraged in conjunction with wide local excision (see Chapter 50). Lymphatic mapping may also be considered for patients with thinner melanomas with high-risk characteristics that have yet to be consistently reported, but include Clark level IV or ≥ 0.75 mm thick evidence of extensive regression, positive deep margins, or evidence of lymphovascular

**Table 28.2** Survival Variation in Patients with Non-Ulcerated Thin (≤1 mm) Melanomas Using (A) Expanded AJCC Criteria with Class-Specific 10-year Survival Rates for Surveillance, Epidemiology, and End Results (SEER; n = 26,291) and Pigmented Lesion Group (PLG) Patients (n = 2389) and (B) New Prognostic Tree with Class-Specific 10-year Survival Rates for Pigmented Lesion Group (PLG) (n = 2361)

**A.**

| Group | Level (Stage) | Thickness | Level | Age | Site | Gender | SEER 10-year Survival Rate (%) | PLG 10-year Survival Rate (%) |
|---|---|---|---|---|---|---|---|---|
| 1 | II/III T1a (IA) | ≤0.78 | II | <60 | --------------- | ---------- | 99.0 | 99.6 |
| 2 | | | | ≥60 | --------------- | ---------- | 97.5 | 97.7 |
| 3 | | | III | ---------- | Other | ---------- | 96.8 | 95.7 |
| 4 | | | | ---------- | Scalp, head, neck | ---------- | 92.1 | 89.5 |
| 5 | | >0.78 | -------- | ---------- | --------------- | Female | 95.6 | 92.5 |
| 6 | | | -------- | ---------- | --------------- | Male | 90.6 | 90.6 |
| 7 | IV/V T1b (IB) | --------- | -------- | ---------- | --------------- | ---------- | 91.4 | 92.2 |

**B.**

| Group | Level | Mitogenicity | Gender | PLG 10-year Survival Rate (%) |
|---|---|---|---|---|
| A | II | --------------- | Female | 100.0 |
| B | | --------------- | Male | 98.5 |
| C | III and IV | Non-mitogenic | ------------ | 96.7 |
| D | | Mitogenic | Female | 94.3 |
| E | | Mitogenic | Male | 83.4 |

Adapted from Gimotty PA, Elder DE, Fraker DL, et al. Identification of high-risk patients among those diagnosed with thin cutaneous melanomas. J Clin Oncol. 2007;25(9):1129-1134.

**Table 28.3** Recommended Surgical Margins for Melanoma

| Tumor Thickness | Recommended Margins |
|---|---|
| In situ | 0.5 cm |
| <1.0 mm | 1.0 cm |
| 1.01–2.0 mm | 1.0–2.0 cm |
| ≥2.01 mm | 2.0 cm |

Adapted from the NCCN Guidelines Version 1.2011Melanoma, pp ME1-4.

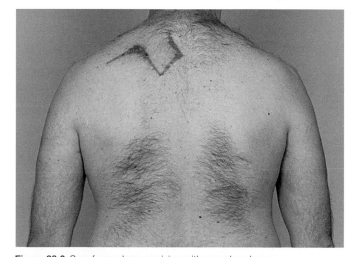

**Figure 28.2** Scar from a large excision with complex closure.

invasion.[3,16] Decreasing patient age has also been associated with increased likelihood of sentinel node (SN) positivity, though this stands in contrast to the observation that increasing age is a negative prognostic indicator.[17] Patients with clinical evidence of regional lymph node metastases are evaluated with fine needle aspiration or lymph node biopsy; therapeutic lymphadenectomy is performed subsequent to histologically confirmed metastases.

Lymph node status in general is an excellent prognostic indicator of recurrence and survival, with the number of positive regional nodes noted on dissection relating directly to prognosis. Figure 28.4 depicts the prognostic stratification achieved by lymph node status. Lymphatic mapping with SLNB is useful in identifying patients with positive SNs for early therapeutic lymph node dissection, also known as completion lymph node dissection (CLND), which has largely replaced elective lymph node dissections.

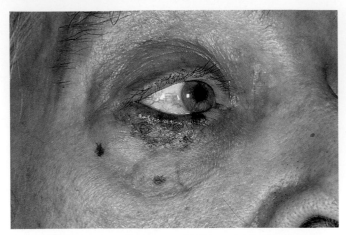

**Figure 28.3** Melanoma on the lower eyelid. This anatomical location precludes excision with suggested margins.

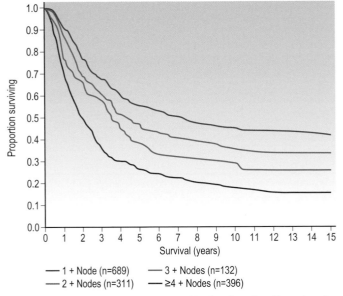

— 1 + Node (n=689)     — 3 + Nodes (n=132)
— 2 + Nodes (n=311)     — ≥4 + Nodes (n=396)

**Figure 28.4** Survival versus number of positive lymph nodes. (Reproduced from Balch CM et al. Prognostic factors analysis of 17,600 melanoma patients: validation of the American Joint Committee on Cancer melanoma staging system. J Clin Oncol 2001;19:3622–3634. Reprinted with permission from the American Society of Clinical Oncology.)

SLNB provides information for pathologic staging and serves to stratify patients for therapy. Patients with micrometastasis found on SLNB are candidates for clinical trials or adjuvant therapy with interferon-α (IFN). Approximately 20% of SNs are positive for melanoma, ranging from 10.6% to 58.7% in the literature.[18] Efforts to improve the sensitivity for detecting positive nodes have been focused on identifying micrometastasis and effectively ultrastaging the SN. Such enhanced pathologic analysis is done with immunostains for specific tumor markers as well as reverse transcriptase–polymerase chain reaction (RT-PCR). However, the resulting increased sensitivity is of equivocal value for predicting recurrence and overall survival.[18] Patients who do not have evidence of melanoma in the SN are spared additional surgery; however, a negative sentinel node is not a perfect predictor of prognosis. Even in the presence of a negative node, there is still a 10–15% chance of locoregional recurrence.[18] In terms of overall survival, while

sentinel node status is an important component of staging, it is only one of multiple prognostic attributes.

The therapeutic value of SLNB has been hotly debated. The large international Multicenter Selective Lymphadenectomy Trial found no effect on survival in the overall study population based on the primary randomization criteria. However, a subset analysis comparing SN-positive patients in the treatment arm to patients who went on to develop nodal disease in the observation arm has been reported as support, albeit controversial, for a survival advantage associated with SLNB.[19,20] Several trials are evaluating the role for CLND and adjuvant IFN in SN-positive patients. Preliminary results have not supported the value of treatment over observation after SLNB.[21–23] Alternative methods of evaluating regional lymph node basins are under investigation, such as ultrasound screening and lymphoscintigraphy with ultrasound-guided fine needle aspiration. These techniques, while compromising sensitivity, could provide less invasive and more specific alternatives to SLNB and also have the potential to enhance observation after SLNB if CLND is deferred.[23,24]

## Adjuvant therapy

Adjuvant therapy should be considered for patients at high risk for recurrence, particularly those with thick primary tumors and/or positive lymph nodes (see Chapter 53). Multiple approaches to adjuvant therapy have been studied, including chemotherapy, immunotherapy, and vaccine therapy. Randomized studies of adjuvant treatment using Bacillus Calmette-Guérin (BCG), *Corynebacterium parvum*, dacarbazine (DTIC), levamisole, vitamin A, or megestrol acetate, alone or in combination, have generally failed to show any benefit in disease-free or overall survival. Small subsets of isolated positive results have not been corroborated.[25]

High-dose IFN is FDA-approved for the adjuvant treatment of melanoma. Pooled data from updated analyses of several pivotal trials involving high-dose IFN revealed consistent increases in relapse-free survival but not overall survival.[26] High-dose IFN has significant toxicity, which must be weighed heavily in the face of minimal survival benefit. Attempts to reduce toxicity have prompted numerous studies of varying IFN doses, preparations and regimens. When several of these studies were analyzed by independent patient data, improved relapse-free survival was not found to be associated with dose and conclusions about dose could not be drawn.[27] Further, individual trials with lower-dose preparations, such as with pegylated IFN, still resulted in decreased health-related quality of life.[28]

Retrospective analyses of some of the larger randomized interferon trials have suggested that the patients with ulcerated primary melanomas are the patients who may benefit most. These data are currently viewed as hypothesis-generating rather than influencing current practice. To that end, the EORTC trials group in Europe is currently investigating this observation in a large phase III randomized trial in an effort to identify a target patient population for IFN therapy.

Alternative adjuvant therapy modalities have been studied, including vaccine and radiation therapy. Initial studies demonstrated regression of melanoma in response to vaccine therapy. As a result, the role for vaccines in adjuvant therapies has been rigorously pursued, despite repeated failure to reproduce a treatment benefit.[29] More promising is adjuvant therapy with radiation, which has been shown to control regional recurrence after lymphadenectomy in high-risk patients and those with extracapsular nodal disease. Reports indicate that radiation therapy has an acceptable level of toxicity, though an effect on overall survival has not been demonstrated.[30]

## Management of the patient with metastatic disease

Metastatic melanoma has a poor prognosis and while new treatment options are being studied aggressively, they remain experimental (see Chapter 57). Patients are typically treated with conventional chemotherapy or are enlisted in clinical trials, which often result in improved short-term survival but rarely alter overall survival.

The treatment modality for metastatic melanoma varies by the extent of disease. Limited in-transit metastatic disease can be managed with excision, carbon dioxide laser ablation, intralesional immunotherapy with BCG or IFN, or topical treatment with imiquimod or dinitrochlorobenzene. These have all been shown to be effective in local control of limited in-transit disease. Hyperthermic isolated limb perfusion (HILP) is a treatment option for patients with more extensive in-transit metastatic disease. Several agents have been studied for regional perfusion; however, melphalan is the drug of choice for HILP. Isolated limb infusion has been studied more recently as a minimally invasive alternative to HILP, and while neither has been associated with significant improvement in overall survival, both are effective in controlling local recurrence and can have dramatic palliative effects and avoid the need for amputation in some patients with extensive limb involvement.[31] Radiation therapy can alternatively provide palliation in this setting when the recurrent process is of a more limited scope, albeit less effectively.

In patients with distant metastases, curative resection of relatively stable remote nodal and soft tissue lesions, as well as isolated visceral lesions, should be considered. In symptomatic patients, palliative resection may also be appropriate. Prolonged survival among some patients treated with surgical resection of limited liver, pulmonary, or brain metastases has been reported.[32] The lung is the most common visceral site of metastasis that is potentially curable with the resection of isolated lesions. Palliative radiation therapy is an option in the setting of inoperable brain metastases, prolonging survival by 1–2 months.

Systemic chemotherapy with DTIC remains the mainstay of therapy for patients with extensive distant metastatic disease. Response rates are generally low (7.5–12.1%) and median duration of responses approaches 1 year.[33] Complete responses are rare, usually less than 5%. Temozolomide, an oral analog of DTIC with improved bioavailability and CNS penetration, has similar response rates to DTIC. Several combination chemotherapy and hormonal modulator regimens, notably the Dartmouth regimen, have been evaluated over the years. None have demonstrated consistent improvements in survival compared to single agent DTIC, and often the combination regimens have worse toxicity.[34]

The association between improved outcome and the spontaneous development of leukoderma in melanoma patients served as the initial stimulus for decades of research in immunotherapy as treatment for metastatic melanoma. IFN and IL-2 have been studied alone or as combination immunotherapy. Used as single agent therapy, high-dose IL-2 is associated with a reported response rate of 16% in selected patients, with 6% of patients achieving a complete response and more than half of these alive and disease-free 2 years later.[33] When immunotherapy is used in combination with chemotherapy ('biochemotherapy') initial response rates are consistently improved; however, meta-analysis has shown that overall survival is not affected.[33] The latest advance in immunotherapy is the use of monoclonal antibodies as immunomodulators. Ipilimumab is a human monoclonal antibody against cytotoxic T-lymphocyte antigen-4 (CTLA-4), which negatively regulates the T-cell response. Blocking CTLA-4 results in sustained T-cell activation and enhances the natural anti-tumor response of the immune system. Results from recent trials are promising and have demonstrated increased overall survival, which improved further with the addition of DTIC.[35,36] As with other immunotherapies, response to ipilimumab has been associated with the development of autoimmunity, a feature that may serve as a prognostic indicator for patients treated with this modality.

Vaccine therapy in metastatic disease has often proven to be no more effective than with adjuvant therapy (see Chapter 54). Despite many vaccine trials, the objective response rate remains poor. While melanoma is thought to be an immunogenic tumor, the poor vaccine response may be due to low numbers of circulating T cells directed at tumor antigens, difficulty infiltrating the tumor, and minimal activation once localized.[37] One method for increasing the number of tumor-directed T cells is with adoptive cell therapy of autologous tumor-infiltrating lymphocytes. This has been performed successfully after lymphodepletion and more recently after total body radiation, with much higher response rates than achieved with immunotherapy or immunomodulator therapy alone.[38]

## Follow-up

There are many opinions on the appropriate follow-up regimen for melanoma patients, though certain basic principles are generally applicable. Photoprotection, including the proper use of sunscreens, sun-protective clothing, sunglasses, and hats, should be highly encouraged for patients and their families (Chapter 9), while taking care to maintain appropriate vitamin D levels (Chapter 60).[39] Regular skin examinations are of paramount importance for patients with melanoma. Approximately 0.2–8.6% of melanoma patients will develop subsequent primary melanomas, the majority occurring within the first year or two of initial diagnosis.[40] All patients should be instructed in self-examination and return for routine physician surveillance for additional primary lesions. One retrospective study concluded that skin self-examination has the potential to reduce melanoma mortality by 63%.[41] Patient education on skin self-examination includes information on how to recognize a suspicious

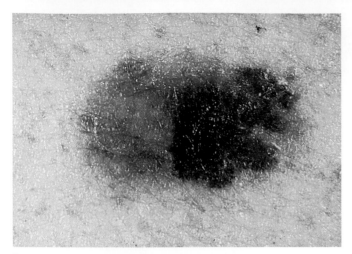

**Figure 28.5** Melanoma arising from a dysplastic nevus.

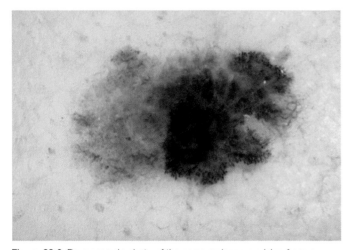

**Figure 28.6** Dermoscopic photo of the same melanoma arising from a dysplastic nevus.

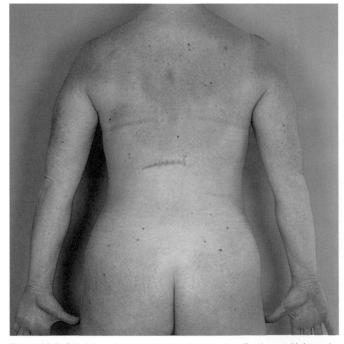

**Figure 28.7** One image from total body photographs allowing multiple nevi to be followed for changes.

lesion and instruction on how to perform a thorough total body skin examination. The majority of new lesions arise de novo, though roughly 25% transform from existing nevi (Figs 28.5 and 28.6).[42]

Individuals with very prominent and/or atypical nevi may benefit from having their cutaneous surface photographed (see Chapter 61). These photographs serve as a baseline to which future skin examinations can be compared (Fig. 28.7). They can assist in the detection of up to 74% of melanomas by facilitating recognition of subtle changes in size, shape and color.[43] Any new, changing, or symptomatic pigmented lesions should be examined closely and possibly biopsied. Imaging is increasingly integrated into melanoma surveillance, and various techniques, such as photography and dermoscopy, have become more widely used while new technologies, like 3-D total body imaging and confocal microscopy, are being studied.[44]

Patients with invasive primary malignant melanoma need regular follow-up for assessment of metastasis.[45] A thorough review of systems and physical examination including lymph node examination should be performed on all follow-up visits. Initially, patients with melanoma should be followed closely every 2–6 months depending on the prognostic attributes. Although recurrences can occur at any time, even as far out as 10–20 years from the primary, the greatest risk is in the 2 years following diagnosis. Therefore, surveillance is most important in the period immediately following treatment. After those first two years, if the patient remains free of disease, the interval between follow-up visits can be spaced out to between 6 months and 1 year, depending on individual risk factors. Time to recurrence for patients with node-negative disease varies inversely with the thickness of the primary tumor. Thus, patients with thin melanomas can potentially recur years after initial diagnosis, though other factors, such as an elevated tumor mitotic index, can identify a thin melanoma as high risk necessitating closer follow-up.[12] Every patient with a history of melanoma should be examined at least yearly for life.

Follow-up laboratory and imaging studies are guided by history, review of systems and symptoms, as well as findings on physical examination. Fifty percent of recurrences are found on physical examination or may produce symptoms that are revealed on review of systems.[45] The first site of metastasis is most commonly the skin and subcutaneous and distant lymph nodes, followed by lung, liver, and brain.[46] For patients who undergo SLNB, first recurrence is most often systemic, followed by in-transit disease, regional nodal failure, and local; this pattern of recurrence is seen regardless of SLNB status, though those with positive SLNB recur earlier.[47] The addition of lymph node sonography to surveillance can result in detecting one-third of melanomas not yet palpable on physical examination.[48] A much smaller percentage of metastases are found on abdominal sonography and chest X-ray. Symptom-guided regional CT has proven to be the most useful in detecting recurrences, especially in stage III and IV disease. For patients with stage IB–IV, routine screening blood work for LDH and hematocrit may be performed on a case-by-case basis but is generally considered low yield and not recommended.[3]

It is also of great importance to provide psychosocial support for a patient diagnosed with melanoma. It is a serious, potentially fatal cancer that can be a source of intense anxiety and fear for the patient and his or her family. Counseling may be adjusted according to prognosis; in general, men and older patients have a worse prognosis than women and younger patients. Frequent follow-up visits in the period immediately after diagnosis can provide reassurance and comfort from careful surveillance.

## FUTURE OUTLOOK

### Improved risk stratification

As more cellular and molecular prognostic factors are identified, patients with melanoma will be better stratified, leading to improved initial and follow-up regimens. Genetic testing for inherited predisposition to melanoma is currently available as a research tool but which still has limited clinical utility (see Chapter 30). Two major melanoma susceptibility genes, CDKN2A and CDK4, have been identified to date. The CDKN2A gene located on chromosome 9p21 encodes two cell cycle regulatory proteins, p16$^{INK4A}$ and p14$^{ARF}$. Inherited mutations in these genes confer an increased risk of melanoma for carriers. However, only a very small percentage (less than 1–2%) of all melanomas can be attributed to inherited mutations in these genes. It is most likely in individuals from high-risk families with a strong family history (three or more affected members). Even among these families, fewer than half will have the mutation. It is argued that for those from high-risk families, a negative genetic test would be reassuring. However, some non-carriers may develop a false sense of security and become lax with surveillance though they may still develop melanoma and could have higher risk than the general population. On the other hand, a positive test requires interpretation of the uncertain penetrance of the mutation. Some identified as gene carriers may never develop melanoma but would suffer from over-biopsying and increased anxiety.[49]

Testing for DNA status does not change prevention counseling, surveillance, or management of patients and their families at this point and, as such, genetic screening for melanoma susceptibility genes cannot be recommended. It can be anticipated that ongoing trials will lead to improved risk stratification for melanoma based on genotype. However, until this occurs, general efforts in prevention and early detection must rely on phenotypic risk factors, such as skin color or type, nevus pattern, and evidence of sun damage.

Molecular therapies targeting genetic subsets of melanoma are on the horizon (Chapter 55). Current classification systems for melanoma subsets are of limited value in terms of directing clinical management for tumors of equivalent stage. Attempts at correlating oncogenic mutations with histomorphologic or phenotypic characteristics have opened the door for classifying melanomas by genetic association and developing molecularly targeted treatment. The most promising is BRAF, which is mutated in 60% of melanomas and is associated with a distinct histologic morphology.[50] In patients with this type of tumor, preliminary studies with B-raf kinase inhibitors have induced tumor regression.[51] Research is ongoing to identify other genetic mutations that are involved in the remaining minority of melanomas. The KIT mutation is found in a smaller subset of melanomas characterized by their acral and mucosal distribution as well as strong association with chronic sun-damaged skin. Studies are underway to evaluate the role for imatinib, a tyrosine kinase inhibitor with action against c-kit, in melanoma patients who have been screened for this mutation.[52] Uveal melanoma has recently been linked to a GNAQ mutation, presenting yet another opportunity for targeted therapy.[53] The presence of MAGE-3 is another potential target for therapy. Approximately 65% of melanoma tumors express this antigen and it has been shown to be a negative prognostic marker compared to MAGE-3-negative patients. A vaccine therapy has been developed against this antigen and is currently being investigated as an adjuvant therapy for macroscopic node-positive patients in a phase III prospective randomized trial. As the genetic basis for melanoma is better understood and melanoma types better categorized, it is expected that more effective focused therapies can be developed and implemented.

## REFERENCES

1. Jemal A, Siegel R, Xu J, et al. Cancer statistics, 2010. CA Cancer J Clin. 2010;60(5):277–300.
2. Rigel DS, Carucci JA. Malignant melanoma: prevention, early detection, and treatment in the 21st century. CA Cancer J Clin. 2000;50(4):215–236; quiz 37-40.
2a. Cited with permission from the NCCN Clinical Practice Guidelines in Oncology (NCCN Guidelines™) for Melanoma V.1.2011. © 2010 National Comprehensive Cancer Network, Inc. All rights reserved. The NCCN Guidelines™ and illustrations herein may not be reproduced in any form for any purpose without the express written permission of the NCCN. To view the most recent and complete version of the NCCN Guidelines, go online to HYPERLINK "http://www.nccn.org/"NCCN.org. NATIONAL COMPREHENSIVE CANCER NETWORK®, NCCN®, NCCN GUIDELINES™, and all other NCCN Content are trademarks owned by the National Comprehensive Cancer Network, Inc.
3. Coit DG, Andtbacka R, Bichakjian CK, et al. Melanoma. J Natl Compr Canc Netw. 2009;7(3):250–275.
4. Coit D, Wallack M, Balch C. Society of Surgical Oncology practice guidelines. Melanoma surgical practice guidelines. Oncology (Williston Park). 1997;11(9):1317–1323.
5. Roberts DL, Anstey AV, Barlow RJ, et al. U.K. guidelines for the management of cutaneous melanoma. Br J Dermatol. 2002;146(1):7–17.
6. Sober AJ, Chuang TY, Duvic M, et al. Guidelines of care for primary cutaneous melanoma. J Am Acad Dermatol. 2001;45(4):579–586.
7. Martin 2nd RC, Scoggins CR, Ross MI, et al. Is incisional biopsy of melanoma harmful? Am J Surg. 2005;190(6):913–917.
8. Stell VH, Norton HJ, Smith KS, et al. Method of biopsy and incidence of positive margins in primary melanoma. Ann Surg Oncol. 2007;14(2):893–898.
9. Balch CM, Gershenwald JE, Soong SJ, et al. Final version of 2009 AJCC melanoma staging and classification. J Clin Oncol. 2009;27(36):6199–6206.
10. Azzola MF, Shaw HM, Thompson JF, et al. Tumor mitotic rate is a more powerful prognostic indicator than ulceration in patients with primary cutaneous melanoma: an analysis of 3661 patients from a single center. Cancer. 2003;97(6):1488–1498.
11. Barnhill R, Katzen J, Spatz A, et al. The importance of mitotic rate as a prognostic factor for localized cutaneous melanoma. J Cutan Pathol. 2005;32(4):268–273.
12. Gimotty PA, Elder DE, Fraker DL, et al. Identification of high-risk patients among those diagnosed with thin cutaneous melanomas. J Clin Oncol. 2007;25(9):1129–1134.
13. Egberts F, Hitscler WN, Weichenthal M, et al. Prospective monitoring of adjuvant treatment in high-risk melanoma patients: lactate dehydrogenase and protein S-100B as indicators of relapse. Melanoma Res. 2009;19(1):31–35.
14. Tarhini AA, Stuckert J, Lee S, et al. Prognostic significance of serum S100B protein in high-risk surgically resected melanoma patients participating in Intergroup Trial ECOG 1694. J Clin Oncol. 2009;27:38–44.
15. Mocellin S, Zavagno G, Nitti D. The prognostic value of serum S100B in patients with cutaneous melanoma: a meta-analysis. Int J Cancer. 2008;123:2370–2376.

16. Wong S, Brady M, Busam K, et al. Results of sentinel lymph node biopsy in patients with thin melanoma. *Ann Surg Oncol*. 2006;13(3):302–309.
17. Sondak V, Taylor J, Sabel M, et al. Mitotic rate and younger age are predictors of sentinel lymph node positivity: lessons learned from the generation of a probabilistic model. *Ann Surg Oncol*. 2004;11(3):247–258.
18. Mocellin S, Hoon DS, Pilati P, et al. Sentinel lymph node molecular ultrastaging in patients with melanoma: a systematic review and meta-analysis of prognosis. *J Clin Oncol*. 2007;25(12):1588–1595.
19. Morton DL, Thompson JF, Cochran AJ, et al. Sentinel-node biopsy or nodal observation in melanoma. *N Engl J Med*. 2006;355(13):1307–1317.
20. Thomas J. Concerns relating to the conduct and statistical analysis of the Multicenter Selective Lymphadenectomy Trial (MSLT-1) in patients with melanoma. *J Plast Reconstr Aesthet Surg*. 2009;62(4):442–446.
21. McMasters K, Ross M, Reintgen D, et al. Final results of the Sunbelt Melanoma Trial. *J Clin Oncol*. 2008;26(May 20 suppl): abstr 9003.
22. Reintgen D, Jakub J, Pendas S, et al. The staging of malignant melanoma and the Florida Melanoma Trial. *Ann Surg Oncol*. 2004;11(suppl 3):186S–191S.
23. Thompson J, Shaw H. Sentinel node mapping for melanoma: results of trials and current applications. *Surg Oncol Clin N Am*. 2007;16(1):35–54.
24. Voit C, Van Akkooi A, Schafer-Hesterberg G, et al. Role of ultrasound (US) and US-guided fine needle aspiration cytology (US-FNAC) prior to sentinel lymph node biopsy (SLNB) in 500 melanoma patients: reduction of need for SNLB by high US-FNAC SN positive identification rate. 2007 ASCO Annual Meeting Proceedings Part I. *J Clin Oncol*. 2007;25: abstr 8512.
25. Agarwala SS, Kirkwood JM. Adjuvant therapy of melanoma. *Semin Surg Oncol*. 1998;14(4):302–310.
26. Kirkwood JM, Manola J, Ibrahim J, et al. A pooled analysis of eastern cooperative oncology group and intergroup trials of adjuvant high-dose interferon for melanoma. *Clin Cancer Res*. 2004;10(5):1670–1677.
27. Wheatley K, Ives N, Eggermont A, et al. Interferon-{alpha} as adjuvant therapy for melanoma: an individual patient data meta-analysis of randomised trials. *J Clin Oncol*. 2007;25(June 20 suppl): Abstr 8526.
28. Bottomley A, Coens C, Suciu S, et al. Adjuvant therapy with pegylated interferon alfa-2b versus observation in resected stage III melanoma: a phase III randomized controlled trial of health-related quality of life and symptoms by the European Organisation for Research and Treatment of Cancer Melanoma Group. *J Clin Oncol*. 2009;27(18):2916–2923.
29. Eggermont AM, Testori A, Marsden J, et al. Utility of adjuvant systemic therapy in melanoma. *Ann Oncol*. 2009;20(suppl 6):vi30–vi34.
30. Henderson MA, Burmeister B, Thompson JF, et al. Adjuvant radiotherapy and regional lymph node field control in melanoma patients after lymphadenectomy: results of an intergroup randomized trial (ANZMTG 01.02/TROG 02.01). *J Clin Oncol (Meeting Abstracts)*. 2009;27(15S): LBA9084.
31. Beasley GM, Kahn L, Tyler DS. Current clinical and research approaches to optimizing regional chemotherapy: novel strategies generated through a better understanding of drug pharmacokinetics, drug resistance, and the development of clinically relevant animal models. *Surg Oncol Clin N Am*. 2008;17(4):731–758, vii–viii.
32. Young SE, Martinez SR, Essner R. The role of surgery in treatment of stage IV melanoma. *J Surg Oncol*. 2006;94(4):344–351.
33. Ives NJ, Stowe RL, Lorigan P, et al. Chemotherapy compared with biochemotherapy for the treatment of metastatic melanoma: a meta-analysis of 18 trials involving 2,621 patients. *J Clin Oncol*. 2007;25(34):5426–5434.
34. Eggermont A, Kirkwood J. Re-evaluating the role of dacarbazine in metastatic melanoma: what have we learned in 30 years? *Eur J Cancer*. 2004;40(12):1825–1836.

35. Hersh E, Weber J, Powderly J, et al. Long-term survival of patients (pts) with advanced melanoma treated with ipilimumab with or without dacarbazine. *J Clin Oncol (Meeting Abstracts)*. 2009;27(15S):9038.
36. Hodi FS, O'Day SJ, McDermott DF, et al. "Improved survival with ipilimumab in patients with metastatic melanoma." *N Engl J Med*. 363(8):711–23.
37. Rosenberg SA, Yang JC, Restifo NP. Cancer immunotherapy: moving beyond current vaccines. *Nat Med*. 2004;10(9):909–915.
38. Dudley ME, Yang JC, Sherry R, et al. Adoptive cell therapy for patients with metastatic melanoma: evaluation of intensive myeloablative chemoradiation preparative regimens. *J Clin Oncol*. 2008;26(32):5233–5239.
39. Newton-Bishop JA, Beswick S, Randerson-Moor J, et al. Serum 25-hydroxyvitamin D3 levels are associated with Breslow thickness at presentation and survival from melanoma. *J Clin Oncol*. 2009;27(32):5439–5444.
40. Ferrone CR, Ben Porat L, Panageas KS, et al. Clinicopathological features of and risk factors for multiple primary melanomas. *JAMA*. 2005;294(13):1647–1654.
41. Berwick M, Begg CB, Fine JA, et al. Screening for cutaneous melanoma by skin self-examination. *J Natl Cancer Inst*. 1996;88(1):17–23.
42. Bevona C, Goggins W, Quinn T, et al. Cutaneous melanomas associated with nevi. *Arch Dermatol*. 2003;139(12):1620–1624.
43. Feit N, Dusza S, Marghoob A. Melanomas detected with the aid of total cutaneous photography. *Br J Dermatol*. 2004;150(4):706.
44. Psaty EL, Halpern AC. Current and emerging technologies in melanoma diagnosis: the state of the art. *Clin Dermatol*. 2009;27(1):35–45.
45. Garbe C, Paul A, Kohler-Spath H, et al. Prospective evaluation of a follow-up schedule in cutaneous melanoma patients: recommendations for an effective follow-up strategy. *J Clin Oncol*. 2003;21(3):520–529.
46. Balch CM, Soong SJ, Murad TM, et al. A multifactorial analysis of melanoma. IV. Prognostic factors in 200 melanoma patients with distant metastases (stage III). *J Clin Oncol*. 1983;1(2):126–134.
47. Dalal K, Patel A, Brady M, et al. Patterns of first-recurrence and post-recurrence survival in patients with primary cutaneous melanoma after sentinel lymph node biopsy. *Ann Surg Oncol*. 2007;14(6):1934–1942.
48. Blum A, Schlagenhauff B, Stroebel W, et al. Ultrasound examination of regional lymph nodes significantly improves early detection of locoregional metastases during the follow-up of patients with cutaneous melanoma: results of a prospective study of 1288 patients. *Cancer*. 2000;88(11):2534.
49. Newton Bishop J, Gruis N, eds. Genetics: What Advice for Patients Who Present With a Family History of Melanoma? *Semin Oncol* 34(6):452–459.
50. Viros A, Fridlyand J, Bauer J, et al. Improving melanoma classification by integrating genetic and morphologic features. *PLoS Med*. 2008;5(6):e120.
51. Flaherty K, Puzanov I, Sosman J, et al. Phase I study of PLX4032: proof of concept for V600E BRAF mutation as a therapeutic target in human cancer. *J Clin Oncol (Meeting Abstracts)*. 2009;27(15S):9000.
52. Carvajal RD, Chapman PB, Wolchok JD, et al. A phase II study of imatinib mesylate (IM) for patients with advanced melanoma harboring somatic alterations of KIT. *J Clin Oncol (Meeting Abstracts)*. 2009;27(15S):9001.
53. Van Raamsdonk CD, Bezrookove V, Green G, et al. Frequent somatic mutations of GNAQ in uveal melanoma and blue naevi. *Nature*. 2009;457(7229):599–602.

# Pregnancy and Melanoma

*Marcia S. Driscoll and Jane M. Grant-Kels*

## Key Points

- Pregnancy does not have an adverse effect on the prognosis of patients with stage I/II melanoma.
- There is some evidence that pregnant patients are diagnosed with thicker melanomas compared with non-pregnant controls, but this finding needs further study.
- Although estrogen receptor β expression has been observed in melanomas diagnosed in pregnant patients, clinical relevance needs to be elucidated.
- Recommendations for these patients regarding future pregnancies should be based on the prognostic factors for the given tumor.

## INTRODUCTION

There has been significant controversy regarding the relationship between pregnancy and malignant melanoma (MM). The origin of this concern arises from case reports published over the past 50 years, suggesting a poor prognosis for women developing MM during pregnancy and observations that MM may be a hormonally responsive tumor. This has become an increasingly important issue as more women delay childbearing until the fourth or even fifth decade of life. As the age-specific incidence of MM increases during these decades, a rising incidence of MM during pregnancy may be seen in the coming years.

## HISTORY

The controversy concerning the influence of pregnancy on the prognosis of MM began with multiple case reports dating back to 1951. Pack and Scharnagel[1] reviewed 1050 cases of MM and reported that of 10 patients diagnosed with MM during pregnancy, five died within 30 months of diagnosis. Another 11 patients noted changes in nevi during pregnancy and were subsequently diagnosed with MM in the postpartum period. Two of these women died of widely metastatic disease within 3 years and one was noted to have probable brain metastases. These investigators concluded that 'some benign nevi are incited to undergo malignant degeneration during pregnancy . . . such melanomas grow with unusual rapidity and metastasize widely . . . the prognosis of pregnant women with melanoma is bad and few cures are obtained'. In 1954, Byrd and McGanity[2] stated that the risk of pregnancy, in women with a history of MM, was

significant enough to 'justify surgical sterilization in those women who were amenable to terminating their child bearing career'.

In addition to case reports, there were observations which supported a relationship between hormones and MM, including: the rare occurrence of MM before puberty, the increasing incidence of MM during the childbearing years, the darkening and enlargement of nevi during pregnancy, the presence of receptors for estrogen and progesterone in some MMs, the augmentation of MM cell growth in tissue culture on addition of steroid hormones, and the enhancement of MM growth in mice after administration of estrogen. Over the past several years, data from recent laboratory and clinical studies have been unable to substantiate most of the above hypotheses and observations. However, recent data concerning estrogen receptor β expression in MMs raises some new questions about hormonal effects on MM.

## EPIDEMIOLOGY

One-third of women with MM are of childbearing age at the time of diagnosis. The incidence of MM during pregnancy is estimated as 2.6 cases per 1000 births.[3] MM is one of the most common cancers diagnosed during pregnancy, representing 8% of all malignancies occurring during pregnancy. A recent Norwegian registry-based cohort study observed that MM was the most frequent malignancy diagnosed during pregnancy, representing 160 of 516 (31%) malignancies.[4] A Swedish study reported that MM represented 24.5% of all malignancies diagnosed during pregnancy.[5] MM is the most likely tumor to metastasize to the placenta, although this is still a rare occurrence. If transplacental metastases occur, there is an estimated 25% risk that the fetus will be affected.[6]

## PATHOGENESIS AND ETIOLOGY

Although it has been hypothesized that there may be some factor associated with pregnancy that could affect MM cell proliferation and/or the induction of angiogenesis, no specific pregnancy-related hormones or migratory fetal cells have been identified.

Numerous investigators have studied the binding of estrogen, progesterone, androgens and glucocorticoids to MM in tissue culture utilizing various techniques. If binding did occur, it was at a low level and most of the binding seen in MM was not to true receptors. Recent laboratory studies utilizing monoclonal antibody techniques, which are likely to have greater specificity than the previous studies, did not detect estrogen receptors (ER) in benign nevi, primary MM, metastatic MM, or pregnancy-associated MM.[7-9] These initially-described ERs are now referred to as ERα. Recently, a second form of ER (ERβ) has been described.[10,11] This has incited new investigations into ERβ expression in MMs. Investigators have detected ERβ expression in both benign melanocytic lesions and MMs using immunohistochemical techniques,[12] and immunohistochemical analysis as well as real-time reverse transcriptase–polymerase chain reaction.[13] They observed decreased expression of ERβ in thicker MMs and in a small number of metastatic MMs. Further investigations are required to determine the relevance of ERβ expression in MMs.

Two groups of melanoma investigators[14,15] have studied placenta growth factor (PlGF), a member of the platelet-derived growth factor family. While both groups found that human melanoma cell lines secrete PlGF, only one group[14] observed MM cell proliferation in response to PlGF.

In addition to laboratory investigations, endocrine manipulation with anti-estrogens, such as tamoxifen, has been ineffective in the treatment of patients with MM.

Likewise, several epidemiologic studies have not demonstrated an increased risk for MM in women who have taken oral contraceptive pills.[16]

## CLINICAL FEATURES AND PROGNOSIS

### Influence of pregnancy on the prognosis of MM

Several case–control studies have shown no significant difference in survival rates in women diagnosed with localized MM (American Joint Committee on Cancer [AJCC] stage I or II) while pregnant compared with non-pregnant women with MM.[17-22] Three recent large population-based studies provide additional evidence for a lack of effect on prognosis in women diagnosed with MM during pregnancy.[4,23,24]

Six case-control studies, which all demonstrated no consequence of pregnancy on survival from MM, have been described in detail in a previous review[25] (Table 29.1). However, two studies[17,20] observed that the disease-free interval (DFI) was significantly shortened in patients diagnosed during pregnancy, attributable to a shortened time to nodal metastases. These investigators postulated that

**Table 29.1 Malignant Melanoma During Pregnancy: Case–Control Studies**

| Authors | Patients (n) | Control Groups | AJCC Stage of Disease | Mean Thickness of Primary Lesion (mm) | Duration of Follow-up | Effect of Pregnancy on Survival | Effect of Pregnancy on Disease-Free Interval (DFI) |
|---|---|---|---|---|---|---|---|
| Reintgen et al.[17] | 58 | Not pregnant at time of dx or within 5 years of dx (n=585) | I or II | Study group: 1.90 Controls: 1.51 SD not stated | 5 years (mean) | No | Yes (shorter DFI in study group, P=0.04) |
| McManamny et al.[18] | 23 | Not pregnant at time of dx or after dx (n=243) | I or II | Study group: 1.62 (survived); 2.62 (died) Controls: 1.72 (survived); 3.96 (died) | 2 months–20 years | No | No |
| Wong et al.[19] | 66 | Controls: Not pregnant at time of dx (n-=619) Matched controls: Not pregnant at time of dx and matched for age, tumor thickness, site of primary lesion, and histopathologic type (n=66) | I or II | Study group: 1.24 Controls: 1.28 Matched controls: 1.06 SD not stated | Not stated | No | Actuarial DFI curves not generated. Study group: 37.7 months. Matched controls: 27.3 months. SD not stated |
| Slinguff et al.[20] | 88 | Not pregnant at time of dx (n=79) | I or II | Study group: 1.87 Controls: 1.75 SD not stated | 6 years (mean) | No | Yes (shorter DFI in study group, P=0.039) |
| | 100 | Not pregnant at time of dx (n=86) | All stages | Study group: 2.17 Controls: 1.52 SD, P=0.052 | 6 years (mean) | No | Yes (shorter DFI in study group, P=0.028) |
| MacKie et al.[21] | 92 | Not pregnant at time of dx (n=143) | I or II | Study group: 2.38 Controls: 1.96 SD, P=0.002 | Not stated | No | No |
| Daryanani et al.[22] | 46 | Not pregnant at time of dx (n = 368) | I or II | Study group: 2.0 Control: 1.7 NS | 9 years | No | No |

AJCC, American Joint Committee on Cancer; dx, diagnosis; SD, significant difference; NS, not significantly different.

the shortened DFI, without effect on overall survival, either was due to insufficient duration of patient follow-up or that pregnancy increases risk for recurrence of MM without an effect on survival.

The most recently published case-control study followed 46 women diagnosed with MM during pregnancy for approximately 10 years after diagnosis. There was no significant difference in overall survival rates for patients with stage I or stage II MM compared with the control group of non-pregnant patients. The pregnant women did have thicker melanomas at the time of diagnosis but this difference was not statistically significant.[22]

Three large population-based studies from Sweden, California, and Norway all consistently demonstrated a lack of repercussion of pregnancy on the prognosis of MM[4,23,24] (Table 29.2). Some limitations to these large studies include incomplete data on Breslow depth, the grouping of all stages of melanoma together in two analyses,[4,23] and bunching of patients diagnosed with MM during pregnancy along with those diagnosed up to 1 year postpartum.[24] Lens et al.[23] analyzed data from the Swedish National and Regional Registries in their retrospective cohort study. When accounting for important prognostic factors, pregnancy was not a significant prognostic factor in overall survival in pregnant patients diagnosed with MM. O'Meara et al.[24] evaluated records from the California Cancer Registry and identified cases of 'pregnancy-associated melanoma' (women diagnosed with melanoma during pregnancy or within 1 year postpartum) from 1991 to 1999. There was no significant difference in survival when 289 patients with localized disease were compared to 1716 controls.

A recent Norwegian population-based cohort study evaluated cause-specific survival for women diagnosed with various types of cancer during pregnancy or lactation.[4] MM was the most common malignancy diagnosed during pregnancy or lactation. When 160 cases were compared to 4460 non-pregnant controls, MM was the only cancer in which pregnancy appeared to increase one's risk of death. On further analysis, the pregnant women had significantly more MMs in anatomic sites that portend a poorer prognosis (head, neck, trunk) compared to controls. Once the investigators adjusted for this difference, the hazard ratio was reduced. The investigators concluded that pregnancy likely did not adversely affect the prognosis for those diagnosed with MM.

Two controlled studies[21,26] addressed the effect of *prior* pregnancies on the prognosis of MM. There was no significant difference in prognosis for women with melanoma who had prior pregnancies compared with those who had never been pregnant. Three controlled studies[17,21,23] addressed the effect of *subsequent* pregnancies on the prognosis of MM. These studies found no significant difference in survival or in DFI (in the two studies in which this was evaluated) in women who became pregnant after being diagnosed with MM compared to women who did not have a subsequent pregnancy.

## Table 29.2 Malignant Melanoma During Pregnancy: Population-Based Studies

| Authors | Patients (n) | Control Groups | AJCC Stage of Disease | Mean Thickness of Primary Lesion (mm) | Duration of Follow-up | Effect of Pregnancy on Survival |
|---|---|---|---|---|---|---|
| Lens et al.[23] | 185 | Not pregnant at time of dx or within 5 years of dx (n=5348) | All | Study group: 1.28 Controls: 1.07 NS between groups | 11,6 years (median) | **No** HR=1.08 (95% CI 0.60–1.93) |
| O'Meara et al.[24] | | Not pregnant at time of dx or after dx: | All | **Localized MM** during pregnancy: Study group: 0.77 Controls: 0.81 NS between groups | Not stated | **No** – Kaplan–Meier survival distributions showed NS for localized MM NS for all stages MM |
| | **Localized MM** = 289 | **Localized MM** (n=1716) | | **Regional/remote MM** during pregnancy: Study group: 1.45 Controls: 2.41 NS between groups | | |
| | **All stages MM** = 303 | **All stages MM** (n=1799) | | **All stages MM** during pregnancy: Not stated | | |
| Stensheim et al.[4] | 160 | Not pregnant at time of dx or after dx (n=4460) | All | Thickness not stated, but NS between groups | 11.9 years (median) | **No** – slight increase in risk of cause-specific death HR=1.52 (95% CI 1.01–2.31), but adjustment for anatomic location decreased HR such that authors concluded no adverse effect on survival |

AJCC, American Joint Committee on Cancer; CI, confidence interval; dx, diagnosis; HR, hazard ratio; SD, significant difference; NS, not significantly different.

Based on the above controlled studies, pregnancy before, after, or during the time of diagnosis of stage I or II MM does not appear to influence overall survival.

## Features of MM and nevi during pregnancy

Three studies[20,21,27] have observed a significantly increased tumor thickness in pregnancy-associated MM. There may be a still-unidentified specific pregnancy-related hormone that accelerates MM growth. A delay in diagnosis of MM during pregnancy due to the unsubstantiated reports that nevi typically darken and enlarge during pregnancy may also play a role.

Few studies have investigated changes in nevi during pregnancy. In two studies that addressed this issue, the changes were reported by the patients themselves and most of these changes occurred in non-melanocytic lesions rather than in melanocytic nevi.[28,29] There are two prospective evaluations of changes in nevi during pregnancy: one in patients with the dysplastic nevus syndrome (DNS)[30] and one in women who did not have DNS.[31] In the women without DNS, changes in nevi on the backs of pregnant women were studied from the first to third trimester, utilizing photography. Of 129 identified nevi, eight (6.2%) changed from the first to third trimester: four nevi increased by 1 mm and four decreased by 1mm.[31] When 17 patients with DNS were evaluated over the course of 22 pregnancies, serving as their own controls, the rate of clinical change of nevi was 3.9 times higher during pregnancy compared to when they were not pregnant.[30] Patients with numerous atypical nevi may have a higher risk for change and an enhanced risk of developing MM.[32]

Recent studies on changes in nevi during pregnancy have utilized dermoscopy[33,34] and spectrophotometric intracutaneous analysis (SIA).[35] Zampino and colleagues[33] prospectively studied nevi on the backs of 47 women throughout pregnancy and at about 6 months postpartum. Three observers evaluated dermoscopic images of 86 individual nevi for changes based on total dermatoscopic score (TDS) based on the Stolz ABCD rule[36] and on a broad range of criteria (described in detail by the investigators). Although there was a mean increase in TDS over the course of pregnancy, the change in TDS was statistically significant for only one of three observers. This study showed no significant change in the size of nevi over the course of pregnancy, consistent with the earlier study utilizing photography.[31] Changes in diameter and structure of nevi may be seen over the course of pregnancy, but these findings may be due to expansion of the skin during pregnancy.[34] Other studies demonstrated that pregnancy does not significantly influence the appearance of nevi.[35]

Larger prospective studies need to be performed, but one should not assume that changes in nevi during pregnancy are physiologic. Biopsy of changing nevi during pregnancy should not be delayed.

## Placental and fetal metastases

MM in the newborn can develop: (1) through transplacental spread (metastasis to the fetus), (2) within a large congenital nevus, (3) as part of neurocutaneous melanosis, or (4) de novo in the skin. When considering all types of cancer, MM is the most common maternal malignancy to metastasize to the placenta or fetus, but only a small number of these cases have been reported.[37-39] Twenty-eight cases of MM that metastasized to the placenta have been reported: Alexander et al.[40] described 27 of these cases in detail, with one additional case reported in 2008. Metastasis to the placenta may be underreported, because all placentas do not routinely undergo histologic examination and numerous sections of the placenta may be required to detect foci of MM.[40] Metastasis to the placenta occurred only in pregnant women who had widely metastatic MM. In addition, it should be emphasized that metastasis to the placenta does not necessarily result in metastasis to the fetus. Alexander and colleagues[40] estimated that in those cases with placental metastases, only 22% of newborns will be affected. Invasion of the chorionic villi does not predict fetal involvement. In the ten cases where intravillous invasion was observed, only two developed MM.

## PATIENT EVALUATION AND DIAGNOSIS

In general, the evaluation of the pregnant patient with MM is similar to that for the non-pregnant patient. However, there are some special concerns that must be addressed to protect the wellbeing of the fetus.

Since the early diagnosis and treatment of MM is crucial to improved prognosis and survival, biopsy of suspicious pigmented lesions during pregnancy should not be delayed. In patients with multiple dysplastic nevi (atypical-mole syndrome), photographic documentation at the beginning of pregnancy can be helpful in establishing a baseline for subsequent comparison throughout the pregnancy. Follow-up visits each trimester are often recommended to detect any changes.

Once the diagnosis of MM is made, a wide excision under local anesthesia is indicated. Local anesthesia utilizing lidocaine is safe during pregnancy. The use of lidocaine *with epinephrine (adrenaline)* is safe if used cautiously.[41] Avoidance of general anesthesia is advised during pregnancy.

If the tumor is associated with a high risk for recurrence or metastasis, then sentinel lymph node mapping and biopsy (SLN) should be considered. There is controversy concerning the safety of SLN in pregnancy. Squatrito and Harlow[42] recommended the use of the blue dye technique alone and avoidance of the radiolabeled technique during pregnancy if the nodal drainage basin is predictable. In contrast, Nicklas and Baker[43] felt that the amount of radiation associated with the technetium tracer is very small and that this technique could be used safely in pregnancy. SLN is sometimes done with radiocolloid alone because of the concern of anaphylactic reactions to blue dye.[44] A small case series of six pregnant patients diagnosed with MM had SLN. All the patients tolerated the procedure well, regardless of technique (two received radiocolloid alone, two blue dye alone, and two had the combination of radiocolloid and blue dye).[45]

In pregnant patients where there is high risk for distant metastases, imaging studies should be considered. Radiographs of the chest can be performed safely in pregnant patients with appropriate shielding. Ultrasonography may also be safely used. However, CT scanning with IV contrast is generally not recommended in early pregnancy because of the risk of brain injury to the fetus. This risk is highest between 8 and 15 weeks of gestation.[46] While MRI has been considered relatively safe, avoidance in the first trimester is recommended because radiofrequency fields used may cause heating of fetal tissues.[42]

## PATHOLOGY

It is important that the placenta of pregnant women with MM be examined grossly as well as leveled and examined microscopically for the presence of metastases. Multiple sections are required to detect small foci of tumor.[38]

## TREATMENT

In general, the recommendations for the pregnant melanoma patient should be based on the same prognostic factors established for the non-pregnant patient. Treatment of the pregnant patient with stage I or II MM should include wide excision and consideration of sentinel lymph node biopsy. In contrast, the treatment regimen for the pregnant patient with advanced disease (stages III, IV) needs to be individualized (Fig. 29.1) and take into consideration the safety of the fetus. While the benefits of interferon for MM are continually debated, this treatment has been safely used during pregnancy. In contrast, the use of chemotherapy has been associated with an increased incidence of spontaneous abortion in the first month of pregnancy and with an increased risk of mental retardation when used later in pregnancy. A recent review of 22 cases of MM in women with AJCC stage III and IV observed that surgical procedures, such as complete lymph node dissection or subcutaneous metastasis removal, were the easiest and safest to use, while chemotherapy use was limited.[47]

## Subsequent pregnancy, oral contraceptives and hormone replacement therapy

Should a woman postpone or avoid a subsequent pregnancy after the diagnosis of MM? To date, there is no evidence that

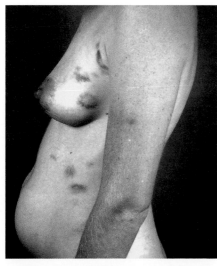

**Figure 29.1** Pregnant patient with MM metastases.

pregnancy has an adverse effect on MM outcome. When advising an MM patient whether to become pregnant, one must consider her prognosis for that given MM and her life expectancy. If the patient has been diagnosed with a tumor with a high risk for recurrence, a waiting period of 2–3 years is reasonable as the majority of recurrences will occur during this time. If, however, a patient is diagnosed with an early, thin MM, then there is less reason to delay a subsequent pregnancy.

How should women with a history of MM diagnosed during pregnancy be advised concerning the use of oral contraceptives (OCs) or hormone replacement therapy (HRT)? Most of the studies concerning exogenous hormones and MM focus on the relationship between exposure to OCs and the incidence of MM. Only one[48] of 17 studies showed a significantly increased risk for development of MM in patients who had ever taken OCs.[16,48-63] There were several studies[49-53] that found an increased risk for MM in specific subsets of patients. All of the studies suggesting an increased risk for MM in women taking OCs had inadequate controls for potential confounding variables, such as sun exposure, and/or included a small number of cases.

There are few studies that address the incidence of MM in patients taking HRT. Most of these studies[48,50,53,57,60,64,65] have not found an enhanced risk for MM in patients taking HRT.

Unfortunately, studies on the impact of OCs or HRT on the prognosis of patients who have MM are limited.[66-68] Shaw and colleagues[66] reported a slightly, but not significantly, better 5-year survival rate in 113 patients with MM who were taking OCs compared with 237 patients not taking OCs. These investigators failed to address tumor thickness in their analysis and there were more patients with regional and distant metastases among non-users of OCs.

Mackie and Bray[67] published a study of 206 women with a history of MM: 83 of the patients received HRT and 123 never took HRT after diagnosis. There was no adverse effect of HRT on prognosis. Rather, there was a suggestion that those who took HRT may have had an improved outcome.

Based on existing evidence, exogenous hormones do not appear to influence the development of MM or to adversely affect prognosis. This evidence, combined with the lack of effect of endogenous hormones (in pregnancy) on the prognosis of MM, suggests that women with MM who have a strong medical indication for OCs or HRT and do not have reasonable alternatives, should not have OCs or HRT withheld.

## FUTURE OUTLOOK

Presently, one-third of MMs occur in women of childbearing age. This number will rise as more women choose to defer pregnancy. Although there have been multiple studies published in the last 5–10 years showing a lack of influence on pregnancy on the prognosis of MM, current management recommendations are based upon a limited number of studies and conflicting data. The expression of ERβ receptors in melanocytic lesions will hopefully lead to more clinically relevant investigations. Future studies in this important area are needed to better define the association between MM, pregnancy, and hormones, to develop more evidence-based recommendations.

# REFERENCES

1. Pack GT, Scharnagel IM. The prognosis for malignant melanoma in the pregnant woman. *Cancer.* 1951;4:324–334.
2. Byrd BF, McGanity WJ. The effect of pregnancy on the clinical course of malignant melanoma. *South Med J.* 1954;47:196–200.
3. Pavlidis NA. Coexistence of pregnancy and malignancy. *Oncologist.* 2002;7:279–287.
4. Stensheim H, Møller B, van Dijk T, et al. Cause-specific survival for women diagnosed with cancer during pregnancy or lactation: a registry-based cohort study. *J Clin Oncol.* 2009;27:45–51.
5. Mathiason L, Berg G. Malignant melanoma, the most common cancer type, first appearing during pregnancy. *Lakartidningen.* 1989;86:2845–2848.
6. Anderson JF, Kent S, Machin GA. Maternal malignant melanoma with placental metastases: a case report with literature review. *Pediatr Pathol.* 1989;9:35–42.
7. Flowers JL, Seigler HF, McCarty KS, et al. Absence of estrogen receptors in human melanoma as evaluated by a monoclonal antiestrogen receptor antibody. *Arch Dermatol.* 1987;123:764–765.
8. Lecavalier MA, From L, Gaid N. Absence of estrogen receptors in dysplastic nevi and malignant melanoma. *J Am Acad Dermatol.* 1990;23:242–246.
9. Duncan LM, Travers RL, Koerner FC, et al. Estrogen and progesterone receptor analysis in pregnancy-associated melanoma: absence of immunohistochemically detectable hormone receptors. *Hum Pathol.* 1994;25:36–41.
10. Kuiper GG, Enmark E, Massi D, et al. Cloning of a novel receptor expressed in rat prostate and ovary. *Proc Natl Acad Sci U S A.* 1996;93:5925–5930.
11. Mosselman S, Polman J, Dijkema R. Identification and characterization of a novel human estrogen receptor. *FEBS Lett.* 1996;392:49–53.
12. Schmidt AN, Nanney LB, Boyd AS, et al. Oestrogen receptor-beta expression in melanocytic lesions. *Exp Dermatol.* 2006;15:971–980.
13. de Giorgi V, Mavilia C, Massi D, et al. Estrogen receptor expression in cutaneous melanoma. *Arch Dermatol.* 2009;145:30–36.
14. Lacal PM, Failla CM, Pagani E, et al. Human melanoma cells secrete and respond to placenta growth factor and vascular endothelial growth factor. *J Invest Dermatol.* 2000;115:1000–1007.
15. Graeven U, Rodeck U, Karpinski S, et al. Expression patterns of placenta growth factor in human melanocytic cell lines. *J Invest Dermatol.* 2000;115:118–123.
16. Holly EA, Cress RD, Ahn DK. Cutaneous melanoma in women. III. Reproductive factors and oral contraceptive use. *Am J Epidemiol.* 1995;141:943–950.
17. Reintgen DS, McCarty KS, Vollmer R, et al. Malignant melanoma and pregnancy. *Cancer.* 1985;55:1340–1344.
18. McManamny DS, Moss ALH, Pocock PV, et al. Melanoma and pregnancy: a long term follow-up. *Br J Obstet Gynecol.* 1989;96:1419–1423.
19. Wong JH, Stern EE, Kopald KH, et al. Prognostic significance of pregnancy in stage I melanoma. *Arch Surg.* 1989;124:1227–1231.
20. Slinguff Jr CL, Reintgen DS, Vollmer RT, et al. Malignant melanoma arising during pregnancy: a study of 100 patients. *Ann Surg.* 1990;211:552–559.
21. MacKie RM, Bufalino R, Morabito A, et al. Lack of effect of pregnancy on outcome of melanoma. *Lancet.* 1991;337:653–655.
22. Daryanani D, Plukker JT, De Hullu JA, et al. Pregnancy and early-stage melanoma. *Cancer.* 2003;97:2248–2253.
23. Lens MB, Rosdahl I, Ahlbom A, et al. Effect of pregnancy on survival in women with cutaneous malignant melanoma. *J Clin Oncol.* 2004;22:4369–4375.
24. O'Meara AT, Cress R, Xing G, et al. Malignant melanoma in pregnancy: a population-based evaluation. *Cancer.* 2005;103:1217–1226.
25. Driscoll MS, Grant-Kels JM. Melanoma and pregnancy. *G Ital Dermatol Venereol.* 2008;143:251–257.
26. Bork K, Brauninger W. Prior pregnancy and melanoma survival. *Arch Dermatol.* 1986;122:1097.
27. Travers RL, Sober AJ, Berwick M, et al. Increased thickness of pregnancy-associated melanoma. *Br J Dermatol.* 1995;132:876–883.
28. Foucar E, Bentley TJ, Laube DW, et al. A histopathologic examination of nevocellular nevi in pregnancy. *Arch Dermatol.* 1985;121:350–354.
29. Sanchez JL, Figueroa LD, Rodriguez E. Behavior of melanocytic nevi during pregnancy. *Arch Dermatol.* 1984;6(suppl 1):89–91.
30. Ellis DL. Pregnancy and sex steroid hormone effects on nevi of patients with the dysplastic nevus syndrome. *J Am Acad Dermatol.* 1991;25:467–482.
31. Pennoyer JW, Grin CM, Driscoll MS, et al. Changes in size of melanocytic nevi during pregnancy. *J Am Acad Dermatol.* 1997;36:378–382.
32. Tucker MA, Fraser MC, Goldstein AM, et al. A natural history of melanomas and dysplastic nevi: an atlas of lesions in melanoma-prone families. *Cancer.* 2002;94:3192–3209.
33. Zampino MR, Corazza M, Costantino D, et al. Are melanocytic nevi influenced by pregnancy? A dermatoscopic evaluation. *Dermatol Surg.* 2006;32:1497–1504.
34. Aktürk AS, Bilen N, Bayrämgürler D, et al. Dermoscopy is a suitable method for the observation of the pregnancy-related changes in melanocytic nevi. *J Eur Acad Dermatol Venereol.* 2007;21:1086–1090.
35. Wyon Y, Synnerstad I, Fredrikson M, et al. Spectrophotometric analysis of melanocytic naevi during pregnancy. *Acta Derm Venereol.* 2007;87:231–237.
36. Stolz W, Riemann A, Cognetta AB. ABCD rule of dermoscopy: a new practical method of early recognition of malignant melanoma. *Eur J Dermatol.* 1994;4:521–527.
37. Ferreira CM, Maceira JM, Coelho JM. Melanoma and pregnancy with placental metastases. Report of a case. *Am J Dermatopathol.* 1998;20:403–407.
38. Baergen RN, Johnson D, Moore T, et al. Maternal melanoma metastatic to the placenta: a case report and review of the literature. *Arch Pathol Lab Med.* 1997;121:508–511.
39. Alexander A, Harris RM, Grossman D, et al. Vulvar melanoma: diffuse melanosis and metastasis to the placenta. *J Am Acad Dermatol.* 2004;50:293–298.
40. Alexander A, Samlowski WE, Grossman D, et al. Metastatic melanoma in pregnancy: risk of transplacental metastases in the infant. *J Clin Oncol.* 2003;21:2179–2186.
41. Driscoll MS, Grant-Kels JM. Hormones, nevi, and melanoma: an approach to the patient. *J Am Acad Dermatol.* 2007;57:919–931.
42. Squatrito RC, Harlow SP. Melanoma complicating pregnancy. *Obstet Gynecol Clin North Am.* 1998;25:407–416.
43. Nicklas AH, Baker ME. Imaging strategies in the pregnant cancer patient. *Semin Oncol.* 2000;27:623–632.
44. Schwartz JL, Mozurkewich EL, Johnson TM. Current management of patients with melanoma who are pregnant, want to get pregnant, or do not want to get pregnant. *Cancer.* 2003;97:2130–2133.
45. Mondi MM, Cueca RE, Ollila DW, et al. Sentinel lymph node biopsy during pregnancy: initial clinical experience. *Ann Surg Oncol.* 2007;14:218–221.
46. Shapiro RL. Surgical approaches to malignant melanoma. Practical guidelines. *Dermatol Clin.* 2002;20:681–699.
47. Pagès C, Robert C, Thomas L, et al. Management and outcome of metastatic melanoma during pregnancy. *Br J Dermatol.* 2010;162:274–281.
48. Beral V, Ramcharan S, Faris R. Malignant melanoma and oral contraceptive use among women in California. *Br J Cancer.* 1977;36:804–809.
49. Adam SA, Sheaves SA, Wright NH, et al. A case–control study of the possible association between oral contraceptives and malignant melanoma. *Br J Cancer.* 1981;44:45–50.
50. Holly EA, Weiss NS, Liff JM. Cutaneous melanoma in relation to exogenous hormones and reproductive factors. *J Natl Cancer Inst.* 1983;70:827–831.
51. Lê MG, Cabanes PA, Desvignes V, et al. Oral contraceptive use and the risk of cutaneous malignant melanoma in a case–control study of French women. *Cancer Causes Control.* 1992;3:199–205.
52. Palmer JR, Rosenberg L, Strom BL, et al. Oral contraceptive use and risk of cutaneous malignant melanoma. *Cancer Causes Control.* 1992;3:547–554.
53. Beral V, Evans S, Shaw H, et al. Oral contraceptive use and malignant melanoma in Australia. *Br J Cancer.* 1984;50:681–685.
54. Hannaford PC, Villard-Mackintosh L, Vessey MP, et al. Oral contraceptives and malignant melanoma. *Br J Cancer.* 1991;63:430–433.
55. Zanetti R, Franceschi S, Rosso S, et al. Cutaneous malignant melanoma in females: the role of hormonal and reproductive factors. *Int J Epidemiol.* 1990;19:522–526.
56. Osterlind A, Tucker MA, Stone BJ, et al. The Danish case–control study of cutaneous malignant melanoma. III. Hormonal and reproductive factors in women. *Int J Cancer.* 1988;42:821–824.
57. Gallagher RP, Elwood JM, Hill GB, et al. Reproductive factors, oral contraceptives and risk of malignant melanoma: Western Canada melanoma study. *Br J Cancer.* 1985;52:901–907.
58. Green A, Bain C. Hormonal factors and melanoma in women. *Med J Aust.* 1985;142:446–448.
59. Helmrich SP, Rosenberg L, Kaufman DW, et al. Lack of an elevated risk of malignant melanoma in relation to oral contraceptive use. *J Natl Cancer Inst.* 1984;72:617–620.
60. Holman CDJ, Armstrong BK, Heenan PJ. Cutaneous malignant melanoma in females: exogenous sex hormones and reproductive factors. *Br J Cancer.* 1984;50:673–680.
61. Bain C, Hennekens CH, Speizer FE, et al. Oral contraceptive use and malignant melanoma. *J Natl Cancer Inst.* 1982;68:537–539.
62. Westerdahl J, Jonsson N, Ingvar C, et al. Risk of malignant melanoma in relation to drug intake, alcohol, smoking and hormonal factors. *Br J Cancer.* 1996;73:1126–1131.
63. Smith MA, Fine JA, Barnhill RL, et al. Hormonal and reproductive influences and risk of melanoma in women. *Int J Epidemiol.* 1998;27:751–757.

64. Persson I, Yuen J, Berkvist L, et al. Cancer incidence and mortality in women receiving estrogen and estrogen-progestin replacement therapy: long-term follow-up of a Swedish cohort. *Int J Cancer*. 1996;67:327–332.

65. Naldi L, Altieri A, Imberti GL, et al. Cutaneous malignant melanoma in women. Phenotypic characteristics, sun exposure, and hormonal factors: a case-control study from Italy. *Ann Epidemiol*. 2005;15:545–550.

66. Shaw HM, Milton GW, Farago G, et al. Endocrine influences on survival from malignant melanoma. *Cancer*. 1976;42:669–677.

67. Mackie RM, Bray CA. Hormone replacement therapy after surgery for Stage 1 or 2 cutaneous melanoma. *Br J Cancer*. 2004;90:770–772.

68. Mackie RM. Pregnancy and exogenous hormones in patients with cutaneous malignant melanoma. *Curr Opin Oncol*. 1999;11:129–131.

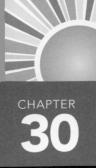

# Genetic Testing for Melanoma

*Wendy Kohlmann and Sancy A. Leachman*

## Key Points

- Approximately 10% of melanomas occur in family clusters.

- In North American populations, mutations in the *CDKN2A* gene are associated with up to a 76% lifetime risk for melanoma. *CDKN2A* may also increase the risk for pancreatic cancer to as much as 25%.

- Clinical genetic testing is available to identify families with mutations in the *CDKN2A* gene.

- In moderate to high melanoma incidence areas, referral for genetic counseling and testing should be considered for: (1) individuals with three or more primary invasive melanomas; (2) families with at least one invasive melanoma and two or more other diagnoses of invasive melanoma and/or pancreatic cancer.

- Carriers of a deleterious *CDKN2A* mutation should receive aggressive melanoma surveillance and be educated about the risk for pancreatic cancer, including the possibility of participating in a pancreatic cancer surveillance program.

## INTRODUCTION

Approximately 10% of melanomas present in familial clusters[1] (Fig. 30.1). Aggregation of melanoma in a family may occur due to a combination of shared environmental exposure and genetic factors. Melanoma risk factors are summarized in Table 30.1. A recent study has found that approximately 40% of risk in families is due to shared variants in genes associated with pigmentation.[2] While shared phenotypic features and environmental exposures accounts for a significant amount of familial melanoma risk, rare families harbor mutations in highly penetrant cancer predisposition genes. Patients who have inherited predisposition for melanoma are at 30–70-fold higher risk of developing melanoma than the general population.[3]

To date, two high penetrance genes definitively associated with hereditary melanoma, cyclin-dependent kinase inhibitor 2A (*CDKN2A*) on chromosome 19p21 and cyclin-dependent kinase 4 (*CDK4*) on chromosome 12q14, have been identified.[4] Mutations in *CDKN2A* account for approximately 20–40% of hereditary melanoma, and 0.2–1% of all melanomas[5–7] (Fig. 30.1). Mutations in *CDK4* are rare and have been reported in fewer than fifteen families worldwide, leaving *CDKN2A* as the most significant melanoma predisposition gene identified thus far.

An efficient method for identifying this subset of particularly high-risk patients is needed so that additional clinical resources can be devoted to their care, even in fast-paced outpatient practices. Genetic testing is one mechanism by which high-risk patients and their families can be quickly identified. While *CDKN2A* was identified in 1994,[8,9] incorporation of hereditary melanoma genetic testing into clinical practice has lagged behind that of other cancer predisposition genes such as *BRCA1/BRCA2* (hereditary breast/ovarian cancer) and *MSH2/MLH1* (Lynch syndrome – hereditary colon cancer). Recent studies suggest a strong interest in genetic testing among families with a history of melanoma, and that receiving genetic test results with appropriate education and counseling may help promote positive screening and behavioral changes among high-risk individuals.[10–12] In order to address this growing demand for genetic services for hereditary melanoma, an international consortium recently published guidelines for appropriately identifying patients who are candidates for genetic counseling and testing for hereditary melanoma.[13] In this chapter we will summarize current information about *CDKN2A*, the process of identifying high-risk families and incorporating genetic testing into clinical practice.

## GENE IDENTIFICATION

*CDKN2A* is a tumor suppressor gene that regulates cellular proliferation and growth by inhibiting RB (retinoblastoma protein) phosphorylation and entry into the cell cycle.[14–16] *CDKN2A* produces two protein products, p16^INK4a, which is transcribed from exons 1α, 2, and 3, and p14^ARF, which is transcribed from an alternate reading frame and includes exons 1β, 2, and 3. Depending on the location, mutations in *CDKN2A* may disrupt one or both of the proteins produced by this gene. Most mutations that have been found to cause a risk for melanoma affect p16^INK4a, and at least one study has suggested that mutations which affect both proteins may be more penetrant.[6] However, rare mutations which only affect p14^ARF have also been reported to segregate with the melanoma diagnoses in families, establishing it as an independent bona fide melanoma predisposition gene.[4,6] Inheriting a deleterious mutation in one copy of *CDKN2A* is sufficient to cause an individual to have a melanoma predisposition. Parents who have a mutation in the *CDKN2A* gene will have a 50% chance of passing on the mutated allele and a 50% chance of passing on the functional copy of the gene with each offspring.

*CDKN2A* mutation penetrance estimates vary between populations and geographic regions due to gene–gene and

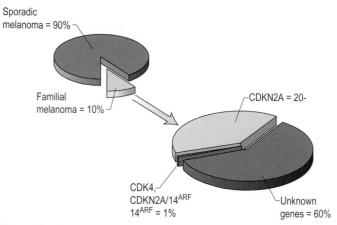

**Figure 30.1** Prevalence of hereditary melanoma and of *p16* mutation in hereditary melanoma.

## Table 30.1 Risk Factors for Cutaneous Melanoma[38–40]

| Risk Factor | Estimated Relative Risk* |
|---|---|
| Skin type I (fair skin) | 1.4 |
| Freckling | 2–3 |
| Blue eyes | 1.6 |
| Red hair | 2.4–4 |
| History of blistering sunburns | 2–3 |
| ≥6 atypical nevi | 6.3 |
| ≥10 dysplastic nevi | 12 |
| 100 or more nevi* | 3.1–16.5 |
| Family history of melanoma† | 2–3 |
| Previous primary cutaneous melanoma | 8.5 |
| Member of melanoma-prone family‡ | Up to 35–70 |

*Relative risk in the United Kingdom population.

†One or more affected first-degree relatives.

‡Multiple affected relatives on the same side of the family.

gene–environment interactions. Studies of families ascertained on the basis of multiple cases have demonstrated penetrance estimates of 91%, 76%, and 58% in Australia, the United States, and Europe, respectively.[17] Penetrance estimates are greatest in areas with high background rates of melanoma. This is likely because there are additional factors such as high ultraviolet radiation (UV) intensity and other shared genetic factors which work synergistically with the *CDKN2A* gene to increase melanoma risk. One of the best-studied genetic interactions is between *CDKN2A* and *MC1R*. Box et al. found the penetrance of *CDKN2A* mutations increased from 50% to 84% when inherited with a *MC1R* variant.[18] Other genetic factors that contribute to incomplete penetrance have not yet been well defined. Yang et al. conducted an association study looking for potential *CDKN2A* interactions with 152 genes associated with pigmentation, DNA repair, apoptosis, and immune response. The only significant association identified was with *IL9* (a gene involved with Th1:Th2 immune pathway), but several other candidate genes showed possible interactions that may become more evident with a larger sample size.[19] Further studies are needed to characterize the gene–environment interactions that contribute to the differing melanoma risk estimates. Population-based studies have resulted in lower, but still significant, risk estimates. Begg et al. estimated a 28% risk for melanoma to age 80 in a population-based sample.[7] However, for patients presenting in a clinical setting, penetrance estimates based on multiple case families are likely to be the most appropriate estimates to use for counseling when they are referred based on family history.

In addition to predisposing to melanoma, *CDKN2A* mutations are also associated with an increased risk for pancreatic cancer in some families. GenoMEL, an international melanoma genetics consortium, found that 28% of *CDKN2A* families had diagnoses of pancreatic cancer, compared to 6% of families without mutations. However, when data were evaluated by country, no excess risk of pancreatic cancer was seen in Australian families.[20] Therefore, the nature of the association between *CDKN2A* and pancreatic cancer is still incompletely understood. Studies of families with *CDKN2A* mutations exhibiting pancreatic cancer have found that the risk to age 80 may be as high as 25%.[21]

## GENETIC TESTING IN CLINICAL PRACTICE

There are several required steps for incorporating genetic testing into clinical practice, including identification of high-risk patients, providing genetic counseling, appropriately ordering genetic testing, interpreting results and incorporating findings into management recommendations. All of these steps can be time-intensive and referral to a local genetic counseling resource may be the most efficient approach for providing patients with these services. Table 30.2 provides a list of online resources for identifying cancer genetic services.

### Patient selection criteria

Because *CDKN2A* mutations are a rare cause of melanoma, routine testing of all melanoma patients is not an efficient or appropriate approach for identifying high-risk families. Recently, an international consortium established guidelines for identifying candidates for referral for genetic counseling and potential testing. Just as *CDKN2A* penetrance varies by region, the likelihood of detecting a mutation also varies. In very high melanoma incidence areas there is a greater chance that melanoma may cluster in a family due to other factors, and therefore more diagnoses in a family are required to suggest the presence of a *CDKN2A* mutation. In areas where melanoma is rare, fewer cases are needed to raise the possibility of a *CDKN2A* mutation. Therefore, criteria for genetic counseling and testing referral need to be tailored to the patterns of melanoma development in specific areas (Table 30.3). In moderate to high melanoma incidence areas, referral for genetic services is recommended for individuals with three or more invasive

### Table 30.2 Directories of Genetic Counseling, Genetic Testing, and Research Resources

| Resource | Website | Services |
|---|---|---|
| National Society of Genetic Counselors | www.nsgc.org | International directory of genetic counselors that is searchable by location and specialty |
| National Cancer Institute Cancer Genetics Service Directory | www.cancer.gov/search/geneticsservices/ | Directory of clinical cancer genetic services that is searchable by location and specialty |
| GeneTests | www.genetests.org | International directory of clinical and research laboratories providing genetic testing<br>Directory of genetics clinics |
| GenoMEL | www.genomel.org | International melanoma research consortium |

### Table 30.3 Criteria for Referral for Genetic Services Based on Geographic or Population Background Melanoma Incidence[13]

| Moderate to High Melanoma Incidence Areas* | Low Melanoma Incidence Areas* |
|---|---|
| Individuals with three or more (synchronous or metachronous) primary melanomas† | Individuals with two or more (synchronous or metachronous) primary melanomas† |
| Families with a diagnosis of melanoma and two or more first- or second-degree relatives‡ with melanoma and/or pancreatic cancer | Families with a diagnosis of melanoma and one or more first- or second-degree relatives‡ with melanoma and/or pancreatic cancer |

*Moderate to high melanoma incidence areas include Australia, North America, and Northern Europe, while most other areas of the world have low melanoma incidence. However, clinicians must use clinical judgment and take into consideration a patient's ethnic background, sun exposure, and other melanoma risk factors when evaluating a family history.

†This table refers to pathologically confirmed invasive melanoma.

‡Relatives should be on the same side of the family.

primary melanomas (synchronous cases) and/or families with a diagnosis of an invasive melanoma plus two or more additional cases of invasive melanoma and/or pancreatic cancer in first- or second-degree relatives (metachronous cases). In low melanoma incidence areas, individuals with two primary melanomas or families with an invasive melanoma and one or more additional diagnoses of melanoma or pancreatic cancer are sufficient to warrant referral. Current studies of CDKN2A have focused on cases with invasive melanoma. The relationship of CDKN2A mutations to melanoma in situ or lentigo maligna has been less well described and it is not currently possible to make express recommendations for in-situ disease.

Taking a thorough family history is a crucial step in identifying high-risk families. A family history should include information on parents, siblings, children, aunts, uncles, grandparents and cousins. All cancer diagnoses in the family should be elicited since the presence of pancreatic cancer is a strong predictor of CDKN2A mutation identification. Aitken et al. found that approximately 40% of proxy reports of melanoma diagnoses by first-degree relatives are inaccurate.[22] The most common error is misreporting basal or squamous cell carcinomas as melanoma. Reported family history tends to be even less accurate for more distantly related family members. Confirming verbal reports with medical records, particularly pathology reports, provides the most accurate basis for risk assessment.

## Genetic counseling and informed consent

Genetic counseling is recommended prior to genetic testing. Genetic counseling is an interactive process intended to help patients make an informed decision about testing and to prepare them to understand the implications of their results. Pre-test counseling should include the likelihood of detecting a mutation, sensitivity and specificity of the test, potential outcomes, implication of the test results for management, implications for family members, and discussion of current legal protections regarding genetic discrimination. Ideally, patients deciding to proceed with testing will sign a written informed consent (Fig. 30.2).

Genetic discrimination has been a theoretical concern associated with genetic testing though actual reports of discrimination have been rare. In 2008, the Genetic Information Nondiscrimination Act (GINA) was signed into law in the United States in order to ensure basic protections against the use of genetic information by health insurers and employers. GINA prohibits group and private health insurers from using genetic information to determine eligibility for coverage or in setting premiums, and employers cannot use genetic information when making hiring decisions. However, GINA does not require that insurers cover the costs of genetic testing or related services, and it also does not prohibit the use of medical history information, such as a melanoma diagnosis, from being considered by insurers. At present there are no specific laws addressing the use of the genetic information by life or disability insurers.[23]

## Testing factors

Most CDKN2A mutations occur in exons 1α and 2, and the majority of mutations are missense mutations, but mutations in the 5' and 3' untranslated regions (UTRs), and small insertions and deletions have also been identified.[6,24] Large deletions and rearrangements are rare.[25] Several clinical laboratories offer clinical testing which includes sequencing of the coding exons as well at the 5' and 3' UTR regions. This test will include some of the sequence which codes for p14[ARF], but complete sequencing of exon 1β is not included. Testing for large genetic rearrangements usually needs to be ordered as a separate test and is less readily available. A worldwide resource for locating clinical genetic testing laboratories is available at http://www.genetests.org[26] (Table 30.3).

Ideally, genetic testing should be performed first in a family member who has had melanoma or pancreatic cancer, in order to increase the likelihood of finding a mutation if one is present in the family. When testing the first person in the family, there are three possible outcomes from testing.

**1. Pathogenic mutation is identified:** This result confirms the presence of a *CDKN2A* mutation in the family, and allows for other at-risk relatives to be tested for the specific mutation. Once a mutation has been identified, other family members can be tested for the specific mutation with very high accuracy and for a much lower cost than the cost of testing the initial proband (approximately $850 for full analysis, and $350 for mutation-specific testing). Patients should be encouraged to share results with relatives, so they will have the option to be tested. Since children who inherit a *CDKN2A* mutation are at increased risk for melanoma, genetic testing may be considered for children 10 year of age and older in order to determine if they are at risk and in need of additional screening.

The melanoma risk for family members who test negative is greatly reduced, but their risk may still be slightly higher than the background population risk.[27] This is because highly penetrant *CDKN2A* families likely have additional genetic factors or environmental exposures contributing to their risk. Therefore, relatives testing negative still need to be counseled about the potential for residual risk and the need for screening.

**2. No mutation is identified:** This result does not rule out an increased risk, but rather means that current technology was not able to pinpoint the specific genetic alteration that has conferred the high risk for melanoma. In these situations it is important that patients be properly counseled about this result to avoid being falsely reassured by the lack of an identified mutation. Increased screening and UV protection will still be recommended for all family members on the basis of family history.

---

### CONSENT TO TEST FOR CDKN2A GENE FOR MELANOMA SUSCEPTIBILITY

You have requested laboratory testing to look for a gene change that increases the risk for developing melanoma skin cancer, and possibly other types of cancer. The gene that will be analyzed is called CDKN2A (also called p16). The genetic test is called DNA sequencing and is done on a blood sample. If you are found to have inherited a mutation in this gene (a change in the gene that makes in work incorrectly), it may help explain why you have developed cancer or may mean that you will develop cancer in the future, although the test cannot usually predict if or when this will happen. You have been counseled regarding the risks, limitations and benefits of knowing your test results and have had your questions answered. Following are some of the key points that have been shared during that discussion:

**ABOUT THE TEST**

The test is done from a small sample of your blood. Blood is drawn by placing a small needle into a vein in the arm. The risks of blood drawing are minimal and include superficial bruising, bleeding from the site of the puncture, and uneasiness associated with needles. The laboratory used for this test is a clinical laboratory approved by the Clinical Laboratories Improvement Amendment. Every effort is made to assure quality control in the laboratory, but undetected laboratory errors can occur.

**POSSIBLE RESULTS OF THE TEST**

There are three possible results to this test:

1. A significant mutation is found in the CDKN2A gene.
   This type of gene change is associated with an increased risk of developing melanoma and possibly pancreatic cancer.
2. A change of unknown significance is found in the CDKN2A gene.
   At this time we do not know whether these types of changes alter the risk of developing melanoma or other cancers.
3. No evidence of a mutation is found in the CDKN2A gene. In this case, it is possible that a) the CDKN2A gene is not functioning properly, but a mutation cannot be detected by the current test; b) there is a gene mutation in another, as yet unidentified, melanoma susceptibility gene; c) that no inherited risk for melanoma is present and the melanomas in you or your family were due to other causes.

**RISKS OF THE TEST**

In addition to the physical risk of drawing blood, which is described above, there may also be emotional or social risks associated with genetic testing.
- Emotional risks include the psychological stress that may come from knowing your DNA results. Finding that you do not carry the gene mutation can produce guilt as well as joy. Finding that you do carry the gene mutation can cause feelings of depression, futility, and distress. Finding that you carry the gene may also cause feelings of guilt about the possibility of passing the mutation on to your children.
- Social risks include the possibility of employment or insurance discrimination. Federal laws such as the Genetic Information Nondiscrimination Act prohibit the use of information from genetic testing by health insurers or employers. However, there are not laws which restrict the use of this information by life or disability insurers.

**LIMITATIONS OF THE TEST**

The decision to test this particular gene has been made based on information that you have provided about your personal and family's medical history. If this information is incomplete or inaccurate, the wrong gene may be tested, and negative test results may be falsely reassuring. Also, other genes can cause inherited cancer. It is possible that the cancer in your family is caused by a mutation in a different gene, and in that case, this test will not detect it.

Sometimes testing may be unable to find a mutation in a gene, even when one is present. Therefore, negative test results do not mean that your risk of cancer, specifically melanoma, is zero. In fact, if a mutation is not found, your and your family's risk of cancer would continue to be assessed based on your family and personal history. In addition, test results of uncertain significance can occur, meaning that it is unknown whether or not the change is a true mutation causing an increased cancer risk of cancer.

**Figure 30.2** Example consent for DNA testing of *CDKN2A*.

*(Continued)*

Our understanding about cancer syndromes and their management is changing rapidly. There is still uncertainty about the medical recommendations for people who have CDKN2A mutations. The CDKN2A gene is just one of many factors influencing melanoma risk, and we are still learning how CDKN2A gene mutations interact with these other factors. The best treatment or prevention options for people who test positive may not yet be known, but when you learn your results, specific current information will also be provided to you.

**BENEFITS OF THE TEST**

The benefits of testing include better knowledge about your risk of melanoma and possibly pancreatic cancer, and the opportunity to use this information in your future health care planning as we learn more about how to best care for people who carry CDKN2A mutations as well as those who do not (see above limitations to this test). Finding that you carry the gene mutation may help you take measures to prevent cancer or reduce the severity of cancer in the future, such as having more frequent skin examinations with your doctor, checking your own skin more regularly, or limiting your sun exposure.

If this test is able to identify an inherited CDKN2A gene mutation in you, other family members would also be at risk for carrying this mutation and testing would be available to identify whether or not they have inherited the mutation or not.

**LEARNING YOUR RESULTS**

The information obtained from your genetic test will only be told to you by a physician or genetic counselor. Your genetic information will be kept confidential, and no information about your genetic test will be released to anyone without your written permission. We encourage you to share this genetic information with the doctor who will be providing your routine health care.

**VOLUNTARY NATURE OF THE TEST**

Participation in genetic testing is completely voluntary. Not having this test will involve no penalty or loss of benefits to which you are otherwise entitled. Even after the test is complete, you may choose to not learn your test results, and you will still receive the same standard of care that you otherwise would have received.

**FINANCIAL RESPONSIBILITY:**

Genetic testing for the CDKN2A gene is $_____ for the first member of your family. If a genetic mutation is found, testing for each additional family member is $_____. _____(Laboratory Name) will bill you directly for the cost of the testing. Your health care plan may not fully cover payment for this testing. You will be personally responsible for paying for the test.

You will be given a copy of this signed and dated consent form.

With the above information, and after having the chance to have all of my questions answered to my satisfaction, I request that my blood be drawn for genetic testing of the CDKN2A melanoma susceptibility gene.

Signature: _____    Witness: _____
Date: _____    Date: _____

**Physician's/Counselor's Statement:**

I have explained DNA testing to this person. I have addressed the items outlined above, and I have given them the opportunity to have their questions answered.

Signature: _____    Date: _____

**Figure 30.2—cont'd.**

For high-risk families without an identified mutation, additional testing to look for large deletions or rearrangements in *CDKN2A* or testing of *CDK4* and *CDKN2A/p14*[ARF] on a research basis may be considered, but the yield will likely be very low.[28]

### 3. Variant of uncertain significance is identified:
Not all variations in the genetic code will result in loss or disruption of gene function. Sometimes clinical laboratories do not have sufficient data to classify a specific variant as deleterious or benign. The IARC Unclassified Genetic Variants Working Group has proposed a classification system for variants which includes five categories: 1) definitely pathogenic; 2) likely pathogenic; 3) uncertain; 4) likely not pathogenic; and 5) definitely no clinical significance.[29] Laboratories may take into account several lines of evidence when classifying variants, including previous published reports, computer-based models which predict the effect of a variant based on the effect on the protein and conservation between species, segregation analysis, and functional studies. A laboratory may be interested in testing other family members for a variant of uncertain significance to aid in the classification of the variant, but this information should not be used to modify the relatives' melanoma risk. Some laboratories may update clinicians once a variant has been reclassified, but most do not routinely do this. Only once a variant has been classified as deleterious or likely deleterious is it appropriate to use that information to determine risk of other family members.[29]

## Adjusting management in persons with positive findings

At this time there are no specific data evaluating approaches for managing melanoma risk in this population. However, recommendations based on expert opinion include performing monthly self-skin examinations (SSE) as well as having a total-body skin examination (TBSE) every 6 to 12 months by a dermatologist.[30] Photographs may be helpful for documenting the distribution and appearance of nevi. Also, due to the significant a priori risk for melanoma, clinicians should have a low threshold for biopsy of suspicious lesions. While the average age of melanoma onset in CDKN2A families is 35 years, very early onset cases have been reported and screening is recommended to begin between 10 to 12 years of age for children with CDKN2A mutations.[17,30] While the exact mechanism of UV exposure on melanoma risk is uncertain, counseling should include discussion of lifestyle changes that can be made to minimize UV exposure. Precautionary behaviors include minimizing outdoor activities during peak UV intensity hours, wearing protective clothing and sunglasses, and appropriate application of sunscreen.[31,32]

Because of the multifactorial nature of melanoma risk, families without mutations or those who test negative for a family mutation will still be at some increased risk for melanoma.[17,27] Screening with clinical and self-skin examinations and implementing protective behaviors while in the sun should still be advised. However, knowledge of genetic status may allow dermatologists to tailor screening by delaying or reducing the frequency of TBSE for those found to not carry a mutation.[27]

Due to the increased risk for pancreatic cancer, screening has been suggested for CDKN2A mutation carriers.[33] However, proven methods for early detection have been elusive. At this time there are only a few centers with expertise in pancreatic cancer screening, and participation in a research study is the ideal approach for accessing pancreatic cancer screening. Approaches under investigation include imaging with CT or magnetic resonance imaging with magnetic resonance cholangiopancreatography (MRI/MRCP), tumor biomarkers (e.g. CA19-9), and examination by endoscopic ultrasound (EUS) beginning at age 50 (or 10 years younger than earliest pancreatic cancer in the family).[34] If abnormalities are found on imaging, a biopsy may be performed. When advanced pathological histology is identified in an individual who has a CDKN2A mutation, partial or complete pancreatectomy may be considered. Though also not proven to prevent pancreatic cancer, patients should be counseled about modifiable risk factors such as smoking cessation and maintenance of healthy body weight.

### Patient behavioral changes post testing

Studies of patients undergoing genetic testing for other hereditary cancer syndromes have demonstrated that learning one's genetic status can promote adherence to screening measures or facilitate decisions about prophylactic surgery. For example, adherence to colon cancer screening in families with mutations in the mismatch repair genes which cause Lynch syndrome prevented increased mortality due to colon cancer.[35] However, currently there have been very few studies on the outcome of genetic testing for hereditary melanoma.

Kasparian and colleagues did not find clinically significant levels of distress, depression or anxiety among individuals receiving genetic testing for hereditary melanoma. However, some patients were concerned about the implications for family members.[36] Perceived benefits of genetic testing include a desire to help research, to learn about children's risk, and to help take personal steps to reduce risk.[37]

A study by Aspinwall et al. looked at the impact of receiving CDKN2A test results on screening intentions.[10] This study compared pre- and post-test screening intentions among members of hereditary melanoma families. At baseline, 78% of those with a previous melanoma had had a TBSE, while only 40% of those without melanoma had a previous TBSE. After receiving genetic test results, 97% of unaffected individuals who tested positive intended to undergo TBSE. Learning that one carried a mutation predisposing to melanoma stimulated this group to raise their screening intentions up to the level typically seen in melanoma patients. The group testing negative for CDKN2A mutations also increased their intended level of TBSE screening to 65%. Among unaffected individuals who tested positive for a mutation, the percentage performing SSE at least once a month went from 36% to 100% after receiving test results.

A unique aspect of CDKN2A mutation testing is that routine UV exposure is likely to play a role in risk. This means that daily behaviors might be important in mitigating the associated risk. Management of other hereditary cancer syndromes predominantly focuses on making a one-time decision about prophylactic surgery or adherence to an annual screening program. CDKN2A mutation carriers are recommended to take steps on a daily basis to minimize their amount of UV exposure. Aspinwall and colleagues also looked at the impact of receiving CDKN2A genetic testing results on sun-safe behaviors.[11] Following reporting of genetic test results, intentions for photoprotection increased among both those testing positive and those testing negative. Overall, 33% of participants indicated using one or more new photoprotective behaviors.

## FUTURE OUTLOOK

Reports of short-term outcomes of genetic testing are very encouraging and indicate that information from genetic testing may have greater impact on behavior than family history alone. However, continued long-term follow-up studies are needed to determine if these positive changes are maintained over time. It is unlikely that any single event is sufficient to maintain a lifetime of behavior change and ongoing reinforcement of the patient's risk status and management recommendations is likely necessary. Also, current studies have included extensive pre- and post-test counseling as part of the testing process. There may be fewer positive behavioral gains and greater potential for negative psychosocial consequences in the absence of appropriate education and counseling.

CDKN2A currently accounts for only a portion of hereditary melanoma. There are likely other predisposing genes yet to be identified, and research is continuing to narrow down the regions of the genome that may contain these genes. Melanoma genetics is likely to continue to be complicated by the fact that multiple gene–gene and gene–environment interactions contribute to risk, and ongoing research is needed to delineate these relationships. Collaborations between the dermatology, melanoma and genetic counseling communities will be necessary to develop the optimal methods for translating genetic advances into clinical care.

**339**

## REFERENCES

1. Florell SR, Boucher KM, Garibotti G, et al. Population-based analysis of prognostic factors and survival in familial melanoma. *J Clin Oncol.* 2005;23:7168–7177.
2. Duffy D, Zhao Z, Sturm R, et al. Multiple pigmentation gene polymorphisms account for a substantial proportion of risk of cutaneous malignant melanoma. *J Invest Dermatol.* 2010;130:520–528.
3. Kefford RF, Newton Bishop JA, Bergman W, et al. Counseling and DNA testing for individuals perceived to be genetically predisposed to melanoma: a consensus statement of the Melanoma Genetics Consortium. *J Clin Oncol.* 1999;17:3245–3251.
4. Meyer K, Guldberg P. Genetic risk factors for melanoma. *Hum Genet.* 2009;120:499–510.
5. Aitken J, Welch J, Duffy D, et al. CDKN2A variants in a population-based sample of Queensland families with melanoma. *J Natl Cancer Inst.* 1999;91:446–452.
6. Berwick M, Orlow I, Hummer A, et al. The prevalence of CDKN2A germ-line mutations and relative risk for cutaneous malignant melanoma: an international population-based study. *Cancer Epidemiol Biomarkers Prev.* 2006;15:1520–1525.
7. Begg CB, Orlow I, Hummer AJ, et al. Lifetime risk of melanoma in CDKN2A mutation carriers in a population-based sample. *J Natl Cancer Inst.* 2005;97:1507–1515.
8. Kamb A, Shattuck-Eidens D, Eeles R, et al. Analysis of the p16 gene (CDKN2) as a candidate for the chromosome 9p melanoma susceptibility locus. *Nat Genet.* 1994;8:23–26.
9. Hussussian C, Struewing J, Goldstein A, et al. Germline p16 mutations in familial melanoma. *Nat Genet.* 1994;8:15–21.
10. Aspinwall L, Leaf S, Dola E, et al. CDKN2A/p16 genetic test reporting improves early detection intentions and practices in high-risk melanoma families. *Cancer Epidemiol Biomarkers Prev.* 2008;17:1510–1519.
11. Aspinwall L, Leaf S, Kohlmann W, et al. Patterns of photoprotection following CDKN2A/p16 genetic test reporting and counseling. *J Am Acad Dermatol.* 2009;60:745–757.
12. Kasparian N, Meiser B, Butow P, et al. Anticipated uptake of genetic testing for familial melanoma in an Australian sample: an exploratory study. *Psychooncology.* 2007;16:69–78.
13. Leachman S, Carucci J, Kohlmann W, et al. Selection criteria for genetic assessment of patients with familial melanoma. *J Am Acad Dermatol.* 2009;61:677.e1–677.e14.
14. Ruas M, Peters G. The p16INK4a/CDKN2A tumor suppressor and its relatives. *Biochim Biophys Acta.* 1998;1378:F115–F177.
15. Cannon-Albright L, Goldgar D, Neuhausen S, et al. Localization of the 9p melanoma susceptibility locus (MLM) to a 2-cM region between D9S736 and D9S171. *Genomics.* 1994;23:265–268.
16. Sviderskaya E, Gray-Schopfer V, Hill S, et al. p16/cyclin-dependent kinase inhibitor 2A deficiency in human melanocyte senescence, apoptosis, and immortalization: possible implications for melanoma progression. *J Natl Cancer Inst.* 2003;95:723–732.
17. Bishop DT, Demenais F, Goldstein AM, et al. Geographical variation in the penetrance of CDKN2A mutations for melanoma. *J Natl Cancer Inst.* 2002;94:894–903.
18. Box NF, Duffy DL, Chen W, et al. MC1R genotype modifies risk of melanoma in families segregating CDKN2A mutations. *Am J Hum Genet.* 2001;69:765–773.
19. Yang X, Pfeiffer R, Wheeler W, et al. Identification of modifier genes for cutaneous malignant melanoma in melanoma-prone families with and without *CDKN2A* mutations. *Int J Cancer.* 2009;125:2912–2917.
20. Goldstein AM, Chan M, Harland M, et al. High-risk melanoma susceptibility genes and pancreatic cancer, neural system tumors, and uveal melanoma across GenoMEL. *Cancer Res.* 2006;66:9818–9828.
21. de Snoo F, Bishop D, Bergman W, et al. Increased risk of cancer other than melanoma in CDKN2A founder mutation (p16-Leiden)-positive melanoma families. *Clin Cancer Res.* 2008;14:7151–7157.
22. Aitken JF, Youl P, Green A, et al. Accuracy of case-reported family history of melanoma in Queensland, Australia. *Melanoma Res.* 1996;6:313–317.
23. Hudson K, Holohan M, Collins F. Keeping pace with the times—the Genetic Information Nondiscrimination Act of 2008. *N Engl J Med.* 2008;358:2661–2663.
24. Harland M, Goldstein A, Kukalizch K, et al. A comparison of CDKN2A mutation detection within the Melanoma Genetics Consortium (GenoMEL). *Eur J Cancer.* 2008;44:1269–1274.
25. Laud K, Marian C, Avril M, et al. Comprehensive analysis of CDKN2A (p16INK4A/p14ARF) and CDKN2B genes in 53 melanoma index cases considered to be a heightened risk of melanoma. *J Med Genet.* 2006;43:39–47.
26. *GeneTests: Medical Genetics Information Resource (database online).* 1993–2009 U. o. W. Copyright editor. Seattle.
27. Hansen CB, Wadge LM, Lowstuter K, et al. Clinical germline genetic testing for melanoma. *Lancet Oncol.* 2004;5:314–319.
28. Goldstein AM, Struewing JP, Chidambaram, et al. Genotype-phenotype relationships in U.S. melanoma-prone families with CDKN2A and CDK4 mutations. *J Natl Cancer Inst.* 2000;92:1006–1010.
29. Plon S, Eccles D, Easton D, et al. Sequence variant classification and reporting: recommendations for improving the interpretation of cancer susceptibility genetic test results. *Hum Mutat.* 2008;29:1282–1291.
30. Kefford R, Bishop J, Tucker M, et al. Genetic testing for melanoma. *Lancet Oncol.* 2002;3:653–654.
31. Diffey B. Sunscreens and melanoma: the future looks bright. *Dermatology.* 2005;153:378–381.
32. English D. Armstrong B. Melanocytic nevi in children. *Am J Epidemiol.* 1994;139:367–392.
33. Parker JF, Florell SR, Alexander A, et al. Pancreatic carcinoma surveillance in patients with familial melanoma. *Arch Dermatol.* 2003;139:1019–1025.
34. Canto MI, Goggins M, Hruban RH, et al. Screening for early pancreatic neoplasia in high-risk individuals: a prospective controlled study. *Clin Gastroenterol Hepatol.* 2006;4:766–781 quiz 665.
35. Jarvinen H, Renkonen-Sinisalo L, Aktan-Collan K, et al. Ten years after mutation testing for Lynch syndrome: cancer incidence and outcome in mutation-positive and mutation negative families. *J Clin Oncol.* 2009;27:4793–4797.
36. Kasparian N, Meiser B, Butow P, et al. Predictors of psychological distress among individuals with a strong family history of malignant melanoma. *Clin Genet.* 2008;73:121–131.
37. Kasparian N, Meiser B, Butow P, et al. Genetic testing for melanoma risk: a prospective cohort study of uptake and outcomes among Australian families. *Genet Med.* 2009;11:265–278.
38. Gandini S, Sera F, Cattaruzza M, et al. Meta-analysis of risk factors for cutaneous melanoma: I. common and atypical nevi. *Eur J Cancer.* 2005;41:28–44.
39. Gandini S, Sera F, Cattaruzza M, et al. Meta-analysis of risk factors for cutaneous melanoma: II. sun exposure. *Eur J Cancer.* 2005;41:45–60.
40. Gandini S, Sera F, Cattaruzza M, et al. Meta-analysis of risk factors for cutaneous melanoma: III. family history, actinic damage and phenotypic factors. *Eur J Cancer.* 2005;41:2040–2059.

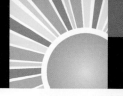

# Spitz Nevus

*Philip E. LeBoit*

## Key Points

- Spitz nevi can be clinically and histopathologically distinguished from melanoma in a large majority of cases.

- Spitz nevi are predominantly seen in children and young adults, but recent studies have shown a broader age range than was previously appreciated.

- Spitz nevi are classically solitary, well circumscribed pink papules, but large, deeply pigmented, verrucous and other variations in appearance can occur.

- Spitz can be junctional, compound or dermal, and are composed of large oval, polygonal or fusiform melanocytes.

- Kamino bodies can be seen in Spitz nevi, and while not pathognomonic, are very rarely large, well formed or multiple in melanoma.

## HISTORY

Sophie Spitz, a pathologist at Memorial Sloan Kettering, published a series of 13 patients in 1948, under the title 'Melanomas of childhood'.[1] While there had been some previous observations of lesions that were probably Spitz nevi, her paper is generally credited with outlining the entity, even if she viewed it in 1948 as a form of melanoma. She noted a variety of clinical appearances, from small to large lesions, some smooth and some verrucous. She observed no differences histopathologically between 'melanoma of childhood' and melanomas in adults, save for the presence of giant cells in the former group.

A concise description of the histopathologic features of 'melanomas' of childhood did not emerge for years. Spitz and Allen re-evaluated similar cases, concluding that the 'melanomas' in question were actually benign.[2] The term 'spindle and epithelioid cell nevus' came into common use a few years later, reflecting the dominant cell types found in these lesions.[3]

Progressively more detailed observations, most notably those by Paniago-Perreira, Maize and Ackerman in 1978,[4] established some criteria for differentiating Spitz nevi from melanoma. A. Bernard Ackerman, who trained initially as a dermatologist before specializing as a dermatopathologist, brought more of a clinical bent than previous observers, and some of his criteria (e.g. circumscription and symmetry in Spitz nevi) reflect the correlates of clinical observations. The last two decades of the twentieth century, and the first decade of the twenty-first century, saw detailed morphologic studies of Spitz nevus and of its many variants. In 1989, a paper by Smith and colleagues from the Armed Forces Institute of Pathology cast doubt on the idea that there was a clean dichotomy between Spitz nevus and melanoma,[5] but the benign/malignant paradigm dominated most articles, textbooks and clinical practice. The last several years have seen increasing questioning of this paradigm, and the limitations of clinical and histopathologic criteria in the differential diagnosis.[6,7]

## CLINICAL FEATURES

The clinical features of Spitz nevus were overly simplified in early reports, ignoring the diverse appearances that Spitz noted. Also, because Spitz noted that children with melanoma had a more favorable course than adults, her nevus was initially believed to only occur in children. Spitz and Allen later did note the occurrence of their lesion in adults, and this observation was expanded in a series by Weedon and Little.[8] An accurate assessment of the age distribution of Spitz nevus did not come for many years, probably because identical lesions in middle-aged and older adults were diagnosed as melanoma.[9]

The clinical diversity of Spitz nevus is remarkable. Lesions vary in size, with some stabilizing after reaching a few millimeters in diameter (Fig. 31.1A–E) while others grow to several centimeters. Most have sharp, even borders, and are symmetrical. Their surfaces vary from smooth to warty and scaly. They vary from bright red (lesions of this appearance are mistaken for hemangiomas) to tan, brown and nearly black. Usually, only one color is present, unlike the case in melanoma. The near-black lesions are often pigmented spindle cell, or Reed's, nevi. Reed's nevi seem to be a distinctive clinicopathologic form of Spitz nevi (see below).[10] Rare Spitz nevi elicit a halo reaction, and are surrounded by a collar of depigmented skin.[11]

## PATHOLOGY

The first recognizable pathology stage in Spitz nevus seems to be an intraepidermal proliferation of enlarged single melanocytes. Lesions in which single cells predominate over nested ones are usually only a few millimeters in diameter, and correspond to lightly pigmented macules. The melanocytes have abundant evenly stained eosinophilic cytoplasm and enlarged but monomorphous vesicular nuclei with small central nuclei. The cells are separated from adjacent keratinocytes by clefts. Such lesions have been termed 'pagetoid' Spitz nevi if some cells are scattered above the junction.[12] It is often difficult to be certain about the diagnosis, as many of the more specific findings seen in more developed lesions are not yet present.

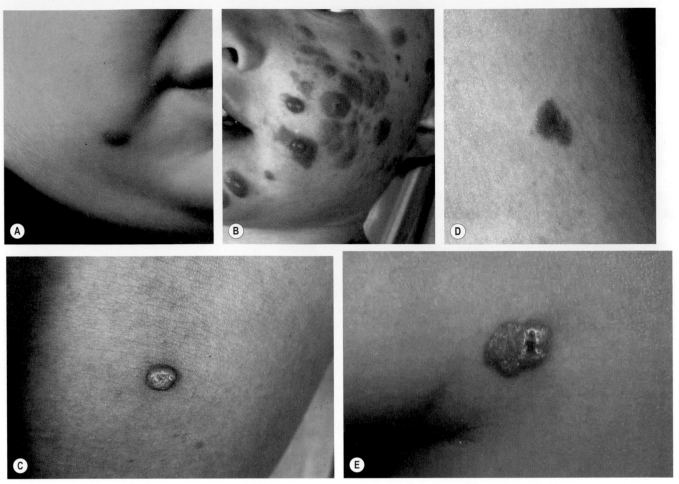

**Figure 31.1 A)** Typical presentation with solitary red brown nodule on face of young boy. **B)** Multiple agminated red brown papules on the face. **C)** Rarer presentation with scaly surface. **D)** Spitz nevus with irregular shape. **E)** Spitz nevus on the knee of a 3-year-old. Note that this papule has sharp borders, but is not round. While many Spitz nevi have this appearance, a great deal of heterogeneity is present. (A-D, Courtesy of Carlos Riccoti, MD).

The next stage in the evolution of a junctional Spitz nevus usually combines the formation of nests along the junctional zone and thickening of the epidermis containing the lesion. Just as individual cells are surrounded by clefts, nests are too. The thickened epidermis has an accentuated granular layer, and can be covered by compact hyperkeratosis. These epidermal changes span the breadth of many lesions, and cause the surface to be slightly elevated over that of the adjacent epidermis.

As junctional nests enlarge and become more numerous, they often demarcate the edges of Spitz nevi. As a result, lesions often 'end with a nest' rather than with single cells. At the same stage of development as the predominance of nests, one may encounter Kamino bodies.[13] These are generally absent at the single cell stage. Kamino bodies are masses of basement membrane and other proteins.[14] They have a dull eosinophilic appearance, and vary from tiny droplets to large scalloped masses, surrounded by crescentic keratinocytes with shrunken nuclei (Fig. 31.2). Kamino bodies are sometimes confused with necrotic keratinocytes, which have a more refractile and more deeply eosinophilic appearance. The initial suggestion by Kamino that apoptotic cells may contribute to the globules is not supported by nick end-labeling studies.[15] Kamino bodies can be

identified by special and immunoperoxidase stains. They are PAS-D positive, stain the same color as collagen does in trichromes stain, and stain for type IV collagen and laminin in immunoperoxidase stains.

A dermal component is evident in most Spitz nevi over 4 mm in diameter. This usually appears in the center of the lesion, and at first involves just the papillary dermis. The constituent cells resemble those at the junction in thin lesions. As Spitz nevi become thicker, the dermal component acquires a more characteristic pattern. The superficial nests are usually larger than deep ones, and the superficial cells are usually larger than ones at the base of the lesion. These features are components of maturation, as are diminished amounts of cytoplasm, smaller nuclei and smaller nucleoli. Nucleoli vary in their hue depending on exactly how hematoxylin and eosin stains are balanced, but most nucleoli in Spitz nevi are basophilic, and those at the bases of lesions certainly are. The bases of Spitz nevi are usually relatively even, and either flat or wedge-shaped. The resultant silhouette is thus usually symmetrical (Fig. 31.3). Some compound and intradermal Spitz nevi have small collections of cells positioned between thickened collagen bundles, and are termed desmoplastic Spitz nevi.[16] In such cases, the thickened collagen bundles often encompass the entire

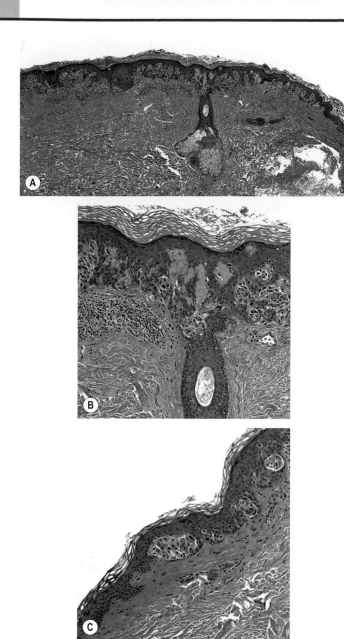

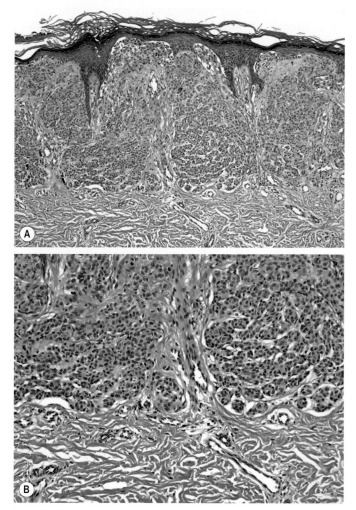

Figure 31.3 A compound Spitz nevus. The lesion has a flat base, and a domed surface, with a predominance of nests at the junction **(A).** The sizes both of nests and of the melanocytes that comprise them diminish toward the flat base of the lesion **(B).**

Figure 31.2 A junctional Spitz nevus. At scanning magnification, the lesion is symmetrical and well circumscribed **(A).** There is epidermal hyperplasia, with many large eosinophilic globules, or Kamino bodies **(B).** These have scalloped borders, with crescent-shaped keratinocytes at their edges. The lesion 'ends with a nest', but a few single melanocytes are positioned above the basal layer just internal to the peripheral-most nest **(C).**

population of melanocytes, and the edge of the fibrotic area demarcates the edge of the lesion. This is not the case in most melanomas, especially desmoplastic melanoma. A minority of desmoplastic Spitz nevi have strikingly dilated vessels, and are termed 'angiomatous' Spitz nevi.

The epidermis above well-developed junctional, compound and most dermal Spitz nevi is hyperplastic and hyperkeratotic. The finding of a thinned epidermis with confluent nests of melanocytes apposed to it is called consumption of the epidermis. This finding supports the diagnosis of melanoma, rather than Spitz nevus.[17] In diagnostically ambiguous lesions, the finding of consumption of the epidermis correlates with the presence of aberrations associated with melanoma.

Some Spitz nevi lack a junctional component, and are entirely, or nearly entirely, dermal. The spectrum of morphologic findings outlined above thus suggests a progression from junctional to compound to intradermal stages. Occasional cases have a dermal component with a periadnexal distribution, as seen in congenital nevi. In some cases this population consists of small, round melanocytes (and represents a combined nevus), but in others Spitz cells are present around adnexa.

Mitoses are present in all of the stages of Spitz nevus. In junctional lesions, occasional mitotic figures can be present in junctional nests. The finding of three or more mitotic figures in a 4-mm biopsy specimen of a junctional lesion makes it worth reconsidering the diagnosis. It should be noted, however, that most examples of melanoma in situ do not contain mitoses. In compound Spitz nevi, mitoses can be seen in the junctional component, and in the upper cells of the dermal component. Deep mitoses, especially those within a high power microscopic field (400×) of the deep edge of the lesion, constitute a reason to re-think a diagnosis of Spitz nevus.[18] Pyknotic nuclei, the significance of which is unknown, can be mistaken for mitotic figures.

It may be that many pyknotic nuclei are a finding against the diagnosis of Spitz nevus, but one can see clusters of pyknotic cells in lesions that have been subjected to forceps compression.

## Variants of Spitz nevus

There are a number of well-established variants of Spitz nevus. While the diagnosis of many cases of the standard forms of Spitz nevus (e.g. junctional, compound, dermal) is within the ambit of general pathologists, the variants are uncommon, and it is unlikely that a general pathologist will have enough experience to recognize most of them reliably. Consultation with a dermatopathologist expert in melanocytic lesions is prudent for most pathologists and many dermatopathologists in trying to come to grips with variant appearances. Variants of Spitz nevus are listed in Table 31.1.

One of the most important variants, pigmented spindle cell (or Reed's) nevus, is common enough to deserve special comment. The clinical lesions are deeply pigmented (Fig. 31.4). The thighs of women in their 30s and 40s are a particularly common site. Pigmented spindle cell nevi are dark brown, flattish and are usually well demarcated from surrounding skin. They have a distinctive dermatoscopic appearance, with large globules that radiate from a central focus (a starburst pattern).[19] Experienced clinicians can recognize them readily, but they alarm many unsophisticated dermatologists who equate deep pigmentation with risk of malignancy. The melanocytes that make up a pigmented spindle cell nevus typically have less cytoplasm than do those of a conventional Spitz nevus, and smaller nuclei. The cells are of uniform size, and the nuclei are monomorphous. Small pigmented spindle cell nevi are often poorly circumscribed, suggesting that they are rapidly growing, and may have some melanocytes positioned above the junction. With this exception, most pigmented spindle cell nevi are well-circumscribed lesions with many of the architectural findings of Spitz nevi – e.g. they are symmetrical, well circumscribed and have a flat base. Like conventional Spitz nevi, nests predominate over single melanocytes along the junction. Most lesions 'stop' abruptly at the papillary/reticular dermal interface, without dispersion from nests to single cells as occurs in conventional Spitz nevus. Kamino bodies may be present (Fig. 31.5). The junctional nests of pigmented spindle cell nevus often have vertically oriented melanocytes, while nests in the papillary dermis may be horizontally oriented. In most conventional Spitz nevi, the nests in the superficial dermis diminish in size, and appear to disperse within the upper reticular dermis. In pigmented spindle cell nevus, a flat base at the papillary/

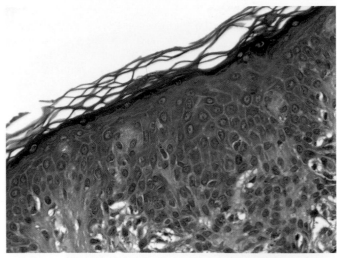

**Figure 31.4** A pigmented spindle cell nevus, presenting as a dark macule with slightly uneven edges.

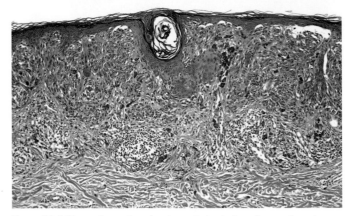

**Figure 31.5** The melanocytes of a pigmented spindle cell nevus have less cytoplasm than do those of conventional Spitz nevi, and their nuclei are usually more monomorphous.

reticular dermal interface is common. The cells at the base of a pigmented spindle cell nevus are often small and may appear round, either because they are, or because they are fusiform but horizontally oriented and are cut *en face*.

Combined Spitz nevus is among the most difficult differential diagnoses in dermatopathology.[20] Combined nevi contain melanocytes of different types, from small, round cells ('ordinary nevus') to dendritic (blue nevus). In some combined nevi, the different populations of melanocytes are topographically separate, while in others, they are mixed. Spitzoid cells can also be a component of a combined nevus. Combined Spitz nevi make up a large proportion of cases sent to consultants, as they can be difficult to distinguish from melanomas that arise in pre-existing nevi. In the cases in which the spitzoid component is separate, the architectural features are usually those of a symmetrical and well-circumscribed lesion, and maturation may be present. Even if the overall lesion is asymmetrical, the spitzoid component usually maintains bilateral symmetry. One particular pattern of combined Spitz nevus features a centrally positioned spitzoid component, surrounded on either side by small, round melanocytes. This arrangement contrasts with that found in most melanomas that arise in pre-existent nevi, in which the melanoma arises on one side or the other.

| Table 31.1 Variants of Spitz nevus |
| --- |
| Pigmented spindle cell (Reed) nevus |
| Spitz nevus with halo reaction |
| Angiomatoid Spitz nevus |
| Hyalinizing Spitz nevus |
| Polypoid Spitz nevus |
| Combined Spitz nevus |
| Persistent/recurrent Spitz nevus |
| Acral Spitz nevus |

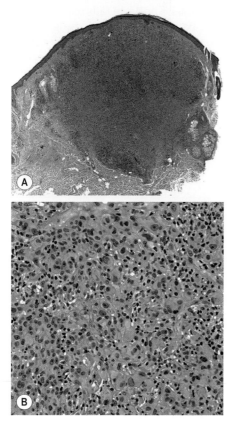

**Figure 31.6** Combined Spitz nevi are usually asymmetrical, as the two components are often topographically separate **(A)**. There are many lymphocytes within the areas of spitzoid cells, a finding that can verge in some cases on a halo reaction **(B)**.

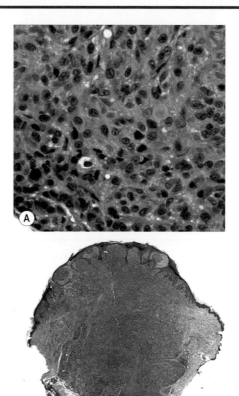

**Figure 31.7** Spitzoid melanoma of childhood often presents with a vertically oriented, smooth bordered silhouette **(A)**. The cells of this lesion have no tendency to disperse with descent, and deep mitoses are present **(B)**.

Maturation with descent is found in most combined Spitz nevi. In some combined Spitz nevi where the spitzoid component is deep in the lesion, maturation may be absent (Fig. 31.6). Mitotic figures can occur in combined lesions, but the presence of more than a few of them is cautionary.

Halo reactions occur in some Spitz nevi. Many of these are combined Spitz nevi, with the lymphocytic infiltrate directed against the spitzoid portion. In halo Spitz nevi, the lymphocytes are evenly distributed throughout the spitzoid population (Fig. 31.7). The finding of a nodule of large melanocytes that is spared by the lymphocytic infiltrate favors melanoma. A peculiar cytologic change occurs in many halo Spitz nevi, in cells that have lymphocytes directly apposed to them. These melanocytes have eccentric nuclei with clumped chromatin (resembling the clock-face nuclei of plasma cells) and ground glass-like cytoplasm.

Spitz nevi can occur on acral skin and can have distinctive features. Conventional acral nevi are one form of 'nevi of special sites'. Special sites are those at which nevi can have some of the histopathologic traits of melanoma. Acral nevi differ in appearance depending on the plane of section in which they are cut. Those sectioned perpendicular to dermatoglyphic ridges are well circumscribed, while those cut parallel to the ridges appear poorly circumscribed. One can see single melanocytes scattered above the junction beneath sulci superficiales (the furrows between fingerprint ridges). Columns of pigmented cornified cells also are present above sulci superficiales, resulting in the 'pigmented furrow pattern' seen with dermoscopy of acral nevi. These same findings can occur with acral Spitz nevi. Because acral Spitz nevi feature large melanocytes and pagetoid scatter, they are particularly prone to be misdiagnosed as melanoma. It is worth keeping in mind that the cells of acral melanomas seldom have much cytoplasm until the lesions become quite broad. Those of narrow lesions, and at the edges of broad ones, often have hyperchromatic, angulated nuclei and scant cytoplasm. This contrasts with the large vesicular nuclei and abundant cytoplasm seen throughout acral Spitz nevi. The dermal component in acral Spitz nevus is not distinctive.

Persistent or recurrent Spitz nevi pose particular problems. The regrowth of nevi following incomplete removal often leads to several features simulating melanoma. These include asymmetry, as one part of the nevus can be replaced by scar. Melanocytes in the dermis, especially those in adnexa, can ascend to repopulate the epidermis, resulting in an intraepidermal component with some features of melanoma in situ. These can include confluence of melanocytes along the junction, a predominance of single melanocytes over nests, and scatter of single melanocytes above the dermal–epidermal junction. Some findings that enable the recognition of junctional regrowth are architectural and some are cytologic. The architectural feature of greatest importance is that the area simulating melanoma in situ is positioned directly above the center of the scar, with the greatest concentration of cells centrally. The cells of intraepidermal regrowth often have much more intensely pigmented cytoplasm than do those of the subjacent dermal component, or even those of the nevus prior to the biopsy.

The same findings can occur in Spitz nevi that regrow following incomplete removal. In such cases, the large size of the constituent melanocytes often results in a diagnosis of melanoma, especially if the pathologist analyzing the lesion is unaware of the previous biopsy, or does not have access to sections from the initial biopsy. In addition to this pattern, which is similar to that of persistent or recurrent conventional nevi, two other patterns can complicate the regrowth of incompletely removed Spitz nevi. In one, nodular aggregates of spitzoid cells appear in the dermis. The second affects desmoplastic Spitz nevus, and results in regrowth with a pattern similar to that of the initial lesion.

## DIFFERENTIATION FROM MELANOMA

As noted above, many authors have delineated diagnostic criteria to distinguish between Spitz nevus, a benign lesion, and melanoma. An increasingly sophisticated array of morphologic findings has been employed in an attempt to define the most difficult cases. Those in which metastases supervene have been held to be due to failure to correctly apply criteria, or to a need to develop better criteria. The criteria that the author uses for this differential diagnosis vary for the stage of Spitz nevus, and also vary if a variant is in question. The most useful criteria for the general differential diagnosis of Spitz nevus and melanoma are outlined in Table 31.2 (architectural criteria) and Table 31.3 (cytological criteria). These cannot be applied to all cases, especially with variants. No one knows how much to weight each criterion, or what combinations of criteria are meaningful. 'Experience' is a nebulous concept, but may reflect the fact that successful consultants avoid misdiagnosis by instinctively weighing and combining criteria.

The dichotomous paradigm fails to explain how the most expert dermatopathologists fail to recognize some lesions as melanoma. While some failures, even by experts, are due to inattention to microscopic details, in other cases the mistake may seem inexplicable. Mounting evidence suggests that these 'mistakes' are due to biology and not error.

Most pathologists readily accept the concept of low-grade malignancy in many organ systems. Among vascular neoplasms, two entities – epithelioid hemangioendothelioma and retiform hemangioendothelioma – are regarded as distinct from conventional angiosarcoma.[21] The latter is often fatal, while the first two neoplasms, if they occur in the skin and are recognized early, are usually cured by complete excision. With melanoma, the distinction between Clark's histogenetic types – lentigo maligna, superficial spreading, nodular and acral-lentiginous melanoma – have been largely morphologic, thought to reflect different pathogeneses and epidemiologic settings, rather than significantly different prognoses. When one says 'Spitz nevus vs melanoma', one usually means one of these forms of melanoma in an adult.

There is mounting evidence that there is a low-grade form of melanoma that overlaps morphologically with Spitz nevus. An early observation in this vein was that of Smith et al.[5] The 32 patients in their report had lesions that were judged to have findings beyond those of Spitz nevi, while having a composition of cells that were remarkably similar to them. The findings included ulceration, stromal plasma cells, deep mitoses, and, most notably, lesions that, rather than dispersing as they grew into the deep dermis or subcutis, formed large protruding masses. Six of their patients had evidence of metastasis, in three from findings from elective lymph node dissection. None of the patients had developed distant metastases when the report was published. The authors called these lesions 'malignant Spitz nevus', a choice that drew criticism as a contradiction in terms.

In the ensuing decades, a number of subsequent publications have forwarded the proposal that a category of

| Table 31.2 Spitz nevus vs Melanoma – Architectural Features, with Exceptions | |
|---|---|
| **Spitz nevus** | **Melanoma** |
| Symmetrical contour (a) | Asymmetrical contour |
| Well circumscribed (b) | Poorly circumscribed |
| Base even (usually flat or wedge-shaped) | Base uneven |
| Nests along junction discrete | Nests along junction confluent |
| Nests at each stratum of the dermis of similar size | Nests at each stratum of the dermis of different size |
| No consumption of the epidermis | Consumption of the epidermis |
| Pagetoid scatter, if present, in center of lesion (c) | Pagetoid scatter can be at edge of lesion |
| Pigmentation even from side to side (d) | Pigmentation irregular from side to side |
| Pigmentation, if present, diminishes toward base | Deep portion of lesion may be pigmented |
| Mitoses superficial | Mitoses superficial and deep |

Exceptions: (a) combined Spitz nevus; (b) early junctional Spitz nevus; (c) pagetoid spread in early junctional Spitz nevus; (d) combined Spitz/blue nevus and combined pigmented spindle cell nevus.

| Table 31.3 Spitz nevus vs Melanoma – Cytologic Features and Exceptions | |
|---|---|
| **Spitz nevus** | **Melanoma** |
| Large but monomorphous nuclei (a) | Large but often pleomorphic nuclei throughout the lesion |
| Maturation with descent commonly | Maturation with descent rarely (b) |
| Nucleoli small to large | Eosinophilic macronucleoli, sometimes |
| Chromatin around nuclei membranes even, especially at the base of the lesion | Chromatin around nuclei membranes uneven, even at the base of the lesion |
| Cytoplasm homogeneous | Vacuolated cytoplasm with finely divided melanin (c) |

Exceptions: (a) the superficial cells of Spitz nevus are often pleomorphic; (b) so-called pseudomaturation can occur in melanoma; (c) large melanocytes with dusty melanin in pale, vacuolated cytoplasm can occur in foci of Spitz nevi, but can occasionally predominate, especially in dark-skinned patients.

melanocytic neoplasms intermediate between Spitz nevus and melanoma exists. The terms used have included Spitz tumor, atypical Spitz tumor, minimum deviation melanoma of the Spitz type, and MELTUMP (melanocytic tumor of unknown malignant potential). Some have proposed grading such lesions in search of criteria that predict behavior, rather than a fixation on a specific diagnosis, which may not actually reflect the prognosis of the lesion.[7] One study in which a panel of expert observers evaluated criteria rather than diagnosis found that among a group of MELTUMPs, the presence of several and especially deep mitotic figures and an inflammatory infiltrate correlated with widespread metastasis.[22] It is important that generalists looking at studies such as this one do not misinterpret them as showing that all spitzoid lesions are diagnostically ambiguous and only need to be evaluated for these few criteria.

The realization that low-grade spitzoid melanoma might exist, and might explain the failure of diagnostic criteria in some cases, has been propelled by the advent of sentinel lymph node biopsy. This technique was initially applied to unequivocal melanoma, in the hope of delineating patients who would benefit from lymph node dissection. Some surgeons later began to use it in borderline cases, assuming that if there were enlarged melanocytes in sentinel nodes, the diagnosis should be changed to melanoma. To Ackerman, the finding of large melanocytes in a lymph node in the same region as a questionable melanocytic neoplasm was strong evidence that the lesion in question was melanoma.[23] The finding that small collections of spitzoid melanocytes could be found in the nodes of patients seemingly having Spitz nevi that had been misdiagnosed as melanoma complicated the matter further by raising the possibility of benign metastasis.[24] Pathologists have long been aware of Müllerian rests and benign breast tissue involving lymph nodes. Even nodal nevi may represent benign metastases rather than aberrant migration.

Given spitzoid cells in small numbers in a node, without knowing more of the primary lesion, one must be cautious. Limited involvement of a lymph node draining a Spitz nevus may thus represent 'benign metastasis'. A second scenario that could result in spitzoid cells involving a node is if the primary lesion were a low-grade spitzoid melanoma. A third is that the cells derive from a fully malignant melanoma, whose mimicry of Spitz nevus is only morphologic. Considering these alternatives, the chances of a sentinel lymph node providing meaningful diagnostic or prognostic information in a case in which the primary lesion is ambiguous diminish. Only if a node contains large aggregations, and especially if mitotic figures are present, can the findings be used to establish the diagnosis of melanoma. Many clinicians, regrettably, regard a sentinel node containing small deposits of spitzoid cells as evidence of metastatic melanoma.[25]

## Immunohistochemical and molecular features

For many years, little difference could be found between Spitz nevus and melanoma beyond light microscopy. Increasingly, small differences in the immunohistochemical features of the two neoplasms are emerging, and it is possible that these may one day be exploited, perhaps in combination to enable immunohistochemical testing.

While Spitz nevi can have rapidly proliferating cells, some studies have shown a gradient among Ki-67+ nuclei, with fewer proliferating cells toward the base of the lesion in Spitz nevi than in melanoma.[26] The protein product of the tumor suppressor gene *p16* is retained in Spitz nevi but lost in many melanomas.[27] The overlap is not sufficient, however, to use this as a free-standing diagnostic test. Cyclin D1 or bcl-1 is strongly expressed throughout the full thickness of the lesion in many melanomas (reflecting gains involving chromosome 11q). Some melanomas have diminished staining for bcl-1 toward the base of the lesion, as do most Spitz nevi.[28,29]

More distinct differences seem to be emerging with the application of molecular techniques such as comparative genomic hybridization (CGH). Conventional melanomas feature gains or losses in about 95% of cases. Spitz nevi, in contrast, lack chromosomal gains or losses in 80% of cases. A gain of 11p is present in about 20% of cases.[30] This gain seems to be due to the formation of an isochromosome in which two copies of 11p are linked by a centromere. Spitz nevi that have this aberration seem more apt to be deeply infiltrative lesions, to have cells with particularly pale cytoplasm and delicate, sharply defined cytoplasmic membranes, and to carry mutations in *HRAS*;[29] a melanoma with an isolated gain of 11p has not yet been reported, making this marker very specific for Spitz nevus, but not very sensitive. Array-based CGH takes about 2 weeks to perform, can use paraffin-embedded tissue, but is not widely available at the time of writing.

The initiating mutations in many types of nevi and melanoma have been delineated in recent years. *BRAF*, *HRAS*, *NRAS* and *GNAQ* are important oncogenes that are part of, or impact, the MAP-kinase pathway, regulating the entry of cells into the cell cycle. Mutations at these loci give rise to nevi, with second hits, in some cases, resulting in melanoma.[31] While *HRAS* mutations occur in a minority of Spitz nevi, *BRAF* mutations (found in most acquired nevi) are rare, and the initiating mutation in most Spitz nevi has still not been found.[32]

## Challenges in differential diagnosis

The distinction between melanoma and Spitz nevus is one of the most difficult in pathology, and for the reasons noted above, it may not be obtainable in some cases. Unequivocal Spitz nevi, Spitz nevi with atypical histopathologic features, low-grade spitzoid melanoma, and high-grade melanomas with a morphologic resemblance to Spitz nevus may lie on a morphologic continuum due to their overlapping features. The most common scenarios that lead to misdiagnosis are related to 'under-diagnosis', e.g. failure to recognize melanoma. Contributory factors include:

- poorly prepared slides
- failure to recognize that a spitzoid lesion in severely sun-damaged skin is exceptional and bears closer scrutiny
- partial biopsy of a larger lesion
- non-representative biopsy of a combined Spitz nevus
- over-reliance on the age of the patient.

## MANAGEMENT CONSIDERATIONS

Spitz nevi are benign neoplasms that theoretically need no further treatment. However, there is no consensus on the management of Spitz nevi. This lack of uniformity in treating Spitz nevi is in part due to the difficulty, in some cases, in distinguishing these lesions from melanoma. Also, Spitz nevi can occur in young children, in whom general anesthesia can be necessary for removal, and in locations (e.g. the nose) in which complete removal can be disfiguring. A decision on whether to completely excise a Spitz nevus needs to take into account the skill of the histopathologist making the diagnosis, their level of certainty, the adequacy of the specimen, the site, and the age of the patient.[33]

## FUTURE OUTLOOK

The many recent contributions to the literature (a PubMed search of Spitz nevus, gene and 2009 yielded 28 hits) suggest that further progress in better understanding the challenges of Spitz nevi will be rapid. Up until the last decade, it could be argued that therapy for melanoma beyond complete excision with clean margins was completely unproven. With the common practice of sentinel lymph node biopsy for melanomas over 1 mm in thickness, an argument can be made that the failure to recognize a Spitz nevus deprives a patient of prognostic, if not therapeutic, benefit.

Targeted therapy of melanoma with *c-KIT, BRAF* and other oncogene inhibitors is currently in clinical trials, and will likely enter routine clinical practice in the near future. While this is currently limited to metastatic disease, it is only a matter of time before high-risk primary lesions are treated with these agents. It will become even more important that Spitz nevi are recognized for what they are, and that patients with them are not subjected to needless procedures and therapies.

## REFERENCES

1. Spitz S. Melanomas of childhood. *Am J Pathol.* 1948;24(3):591–609.
2. Allen AC, Spitz S. Histogenesis and clinicopathologic correlation of nevi and malignant melanomas; current status. *AMA Arch Derm Syphilol.* 1954;69(2):150–171.
3. Kernen JA, Ackerman LV. Spindle cell nevi and epithelioid cell nevi (so-called juvenile melanomas) in children and adults: a clinicopathological study of 27 cases. *Cancer.* 1960;13:612–625.
4. Paniago-Pereira C, Maize JC, Ackerman AB. Nevus of large spindle and/or epithelioid cells (Spitz nevus). *Arch Dermatol.* 1978;114(12):1811–1823.
5. Smith KJ, Barrett TL, Skelton HG, et al. Spindle cell and epithelioid cell nevi with atypia and metastasis (malignant Spitz nevus). *Am J Surg Pathol.* 1989;13(11):931–939.
6. Cerroni L. A new perspective for Spitz tumors? *Am J Dermatopathol.* 2005;27(4):366–367.
7. Barnhill RL. The Spitzoid lesion: rethinking Spitz tumors, atypical variants, 'Spitzoid melanoma' and risk assessment. *Mod Pathol.* 2006;19(Suppl 2):S21–S33.
8. Weedon D, Little JH. Spindle and epithelioid cell nevi in children and adults. A review of 211 cases of the Spitz nevus. *Cancer.* 1977;40(1):217–225.

9. Cesinaro AM, Foroni M, Sighinolfi P, et al. Spitz nevus is relatively frequent in adults: a clinico-pathologic study of 247 cases related to patient's age. *Am J Dermatopathol.* 2005;27(6):469–475.
10. Sagebiel RW, Chinn EK, Egbert BM. Pigmented spindle cell nevus. Clinical and histologic review of 90 cases. *Am J Surg Pathol.* 1984;8(9):645–653.
11. Harvell JD, Meehan SA, LeBoit PE. Spitz nevi with halo reaction: a histopathologic study of 17 cases. *J Cutan Pathol.* 1997;24(10):611–619.
12. Busam KJ, Barnhill RL. Pagetoid Spitz nevus. Intraepidermal Spitz tumor with prominent pagetoid spread. *Am J Surg Pathol.* 1995;19(9):1061–1067.
13. Kamino H, Flotte TJ, Misheloff E, et al. Eosinophilic globules in Spitz nevi. New findings and a diagnostic sign. *Am J Dermatopathol.* 1979;1(4):319–324.
14. Skelton HG, Miller ML, Lupton GP, et al. Eosinophilic globules in spindle cell and epithelioid cell nevi: composition and possible origin. *Am J Dermatopathol.* 1998;20(6):547–550.
15. Wesselmann U, Becker LR, Bröcker EB, et al. Eosinophilic globules in Spitz nevi: no evidence for apoptosis. *Am J Dermatopathol.* 1998;20(6):551–554.
16. Requena C, Requena L, Kutzner H, et al. Spitz nevus: a clinicopathological study of 349 cases. *Am J Dermatopathol.* 2009;31(2):107–116.
17. Hantschke M, Bastian BC, LeBoit PE. Consumption of the epidermis: a diagnostic criterion for the differential diagnosis of melanoma and Spitz nevus. *Am J Surg Pathol.* 2004;28(12):1621–1625.
18. Crotty KA, McCarthy SW, Palmer AA, et al. Malignant melanoma in childhood: a clinicopathologic study of 13 cases and comparison with Spitz nevi. *World J Surg.* 1992;16(2):179–185.
19. Pizzichetta MA, Argenziano G, Grandi G, et al. Morphologic changes of a pigmented Spitz nevus assessed by dermoscopy. *J Am Acad Dermatol.* 2002;47(1):137–139.
20. Pulitzer DR, Martin PC, Cohen AP, et al. Histologic classification of the combined nevus. Analysis of the variable expression of melanocytic nevi. *Am J Surg Pathol.* 1991;15(12):1111–1122.
21. Nayler SJ, Rubin BP, Calonje E, et al. Composite hemangioendothelioma: a complex, low-grade vascular lesion mimicking angiosarcoma. *Am J Surg Pathol.* 2000;24(3):352–361.
22. Cerroni L, Barnhill R, Elder D, et al. Melanocytic tumors of uncertain malignant potential: results of a tutorial held at the XXIX Symposium of the International Society of Dermatopathology in Graz, October 2008. *Am J Surg Pathol.* 2010;34(3):314–326.
23. Mones JM, Ackerman AB. "Atypical" Spitz nevus, "malignant" Spitz nevus, and "metastasizing" Spitz nevus: a critique in historical perspective of three concepts flawed fatally. *Am J Dermatopathol.* 2004;26(4):310–333.
24. LeBoit PE. What do these cells prove? *Am J Dermatopathol.* 2003;25(4):355–356.
25. Busam KJ, Pulitzer M. Sentinel lymph node biopsy for patients with diagnostically controversial Spitzoid melanocytic tumors? *Adv Anat Pathol.* 2008;15(5):253–262.
26. Bergman R, Malkin L, Sabo E, et al. MIB-1 monoclonal antibody to determine proliferative activity of Ki-67 antigen as an adjunct to the histopathologic differential diagnosis of Spitz nevi. *J Am Acad Dermatol.* 2001;44(3):500–504.
27. Hilliard NJ, Krahl D, Sellheyer K. p16 expression differentiates between desmoplastic Spitz nevus and desmoplastic melanoma. *J Cutan Pathol.* 2009;36(7):753–759.
28. Nagasaka T, Lai R, Medeiros LJ, et al. Cyclin D1 overexpression in Spitz nevi: an immunohistochemical study. *Am J Dermatopathol.* 1999;21(2):115–120.
29. Maldonado JL, Timmerman L, Fridlyand J, et al. Mechanisms of cell-cycle arrest in Spitz nevi with constitutive activation of the MAP-kinase pathway. *Am J Pathol.* 2004;164(5):1783–1787.
30. Bastian BC, Wesselmann U, Pinkel D, et al. Molecular cytogenetic analysis of Spitz nevi shows clear differences to melanoma. *J Invest Dermatol.* 1999;113(6):1065–1069.
31. LeBoit P. Safe Spitz and its alternatives. *Pediatr Dermatol.* 2002;19(2):163–165.
32. Indsto JO, Kumar S, Wang L, et al. Low prevalence of RAS-RAF-activating mutations in Spitz melanocytic nevi compared with other melanocytic lesions. *J Cutan Pathol.* 2007;34(6):448–455.
33. Gelbard SN, Tripp JM, Marghoob AA, et al. Management of Spitz nevi: a survey of dermatologists in the United States. *J Am Acad Dermatol.* 2002;47(2):224–230.

# Cutaneous Carcinogenesis Related to Dermatologic Therapy

*Rebecca Kleinerman, Allison P. Weinkle, and Mark G. Lebwohl*

## Key Points

- Potential risks and benefits associated with phototherapy and drug therapy should be discussed with all patients.

- Screening examinations should be performed prior to prescribing a therapy with carcinogenic risk.

- Attention must be paid to treatment interactions that may increase carcinogenesis when multiple medications are prescribed.

## INTRODUCTION

Any systemic treatment is associated with the risk of systemic side effects. The prudent physician must use caution when prescribing such therapy and is obliged to be alert that the therapy does not pose an additional significant risk to the patient. The clinician must weigh the benefits of the treatment or medication against its potential adverse effects by carefully assessing drug associations and toxicities. Regardless of the care taken, adverse effects may never completely be avoided given the imperfect nature of medical risk reduction and the unpredictability of the human body. It is important to minimize the untoward consequences of the pharmacotherapy and phototherapy used that may increase cutaneous carcinogenesis.

## POTENTIAL MECHANISMS OF DRUG-RELATED CARCINOGENESIS

Skin cancer represents a breach in the defense mechanisms necessary to ensure that proliferation and differentiation of skin cells occur within bounds. The disruptions of these mechanisms, environmental or programmed, may take the form of new promoters that invite unregulated cell growth or the loss of suppressors to prevent such growth, creating cells which lose their original confinement, invade and disrupt surrounding tissues.

Mutations of the *p53* tumor suppressor gene are among the most frequent abnormalities found in the genome of human cancers. The *p53* gene has a regulatory role in activating DNA repair, holding the cell cycle at the G1/S phase, and initiating apoptosis, all of which prevent mutation and subsequent carcinogenesis.[1] In the functional cell, *p53* products are continuously degraded and kept at low levels. However, *p53* expression becomes activated in response to a number of stress types, such as ultraviolet light (UV), ionizing radiation (IR), or chemically induced DNA damage. There are three cellular pathways that provoke the functioning *p53* system. IR induces the first pathway by activating two protein kinases, ataxia telangiectasia-mutated (ATM) and *CHK2* checkpoint homolog.[2] The second pathway results from abnormal growth signals, particularly from the expression of the proteins *RAS* and Bcl-2.[3,4] The third path is prompted by ultraviolet light, chemotherapeutic agents and kinase inhibitors, and is not dependent on *Chk2, p14* or *ATM*. Data show that *p53* mutations are present in approximately 56% of human basal cell carcinomas (BCC), 40–60% of squamous cell carcinomas (SCC), and 10% of malignant melanomas (MM).[5,6]

The hedgehog signaling pathway is also vital to proper cellular differentiation. Regulatory errors or mutations in the hedgehog pathway are associated with carcinogenesis as well as prenatal defects. Central to this cascade lies a tumor suppressor gene called patched (Ptc). In the normally functioning cell, Ptc prevents a molecule called smoothened (Smo) from initiating growth signals. When hedgehog (Hh) proteins bind to the Ptc–Smo complex, Smo separates from Ptc, enabling it to activate a transcription factor named Gli. Gli then migrates into the nucleus, where it influences a variety of target genes. It has been found that Hh augments the cell's capacity for long-term growth.[7] Misregulated Hh may also induce the Bcl-2 pathway, creating anti-apoptotic products that promote that aberrant growth and eventually tumorigenesis.[8] The hedgehog pathway is especially implicated in the formation of BCC, both genetic and sporadic.[9] Recent data demonstrate that the expression of Gli1 in basal cells is likely to induce BCC formation.[10] There is also evidence that the Ptc gene may be mutated in cutaneous SCC.[11]

Thus, it is helpful to understand the molecular basis for skin cancer as a background for the comprehension of drug and physical treatment-induced tumorigenesis, since all of the therapies discussed here are thought to exert their potentially harmful effects at the molecular level.

## THERAPIES ASSOCIATED WITH INCREASED SKIN CANCER RISK

(Table 32.1)

## I. Therapeutic radiation

### Phototherapy

Phototherapy has been a traditional dermatologic treatment for over 75 years. It is divided into two basic modalities: UVA treatment, with wavelengths between 320 nm and 400 nm,

**Table 32.1 Therapeutic Carcinogenic Risks**

| Therapy | SCC | BCC | MM | Other |
|---|---|---|---|---|
| PUVA | + Stern,[13] Stern,[14] Stern,[19] Studinberg,[21] Kreimer-Erlacher[16] | + Studniberg [21] | + Stern,[17] Kreimer-Erlacher[16] | |
| UVB (Broadband) | + Ishigaki[23] (Note: animal study) − Weischer[24] | − Weischer[24] | + De Fabo[22] (Note: animal study) | |
| UVB (Narrowband) | − Weischer, [24] Hearn[28] + Kunisada[26] (Note: animal study) | − Weischer,[24] Hearn[28] + Kunisada[26] (Note: animal study) | − Hearn[28] + Robinson[27] (Note: animal study) | |
| Methotrexate | | + Dybdahl[30] (*suggestive of*) | + Buchbinder[29] | + Increased risk of non-Hodgkin lymphoma: Buchbinder[29] + Increased risk of EBV-associated lymphoma: Paul,[31] Hsiao[32] |
| Cyclosporin | − Vakeva[34] (*short term*) + Paul[37] (*long term; pts in study on concurrent PUVA*) | − Vakeva[34] (*short term*) | − Vakeva[34] (*short term*) + Arellano,[39] Zavos,[40] Merot,[41] Hodi[42] (*cases; suggestive of*) | − Lymphoma: Vakeva[34] (*short term*) + Lymphoma: Kirby,[35] Koo[36] (*cases; short term*) |
| Azathioprine | + Bottomley,[52] Nachbar[53] (*cases; suggestive of*),Guenova[51] | + Harwood[54] (*suggestive of*) | + Jensen[56] | + Kaposi sarcoma: Jensen[56] + Lymphoma: Ehrenfeld[57] + Merkel cell carcinoma: Gooptu[58] |
| Mycophenolate mofetil | − Epinette[62] + Gulamhusein[63] (*case; suggestive of*) | | | |
| Topical calcineurin inhibitors | − Naylor,[70] Margolis[71] + Niwa[66] (Note: animal study) | − Naylor,[70] Margolis[71] + Niwa[66] (Note: animal study) | | − Lymphoma: Arellano,[72] Schneeweiss[73] |
| TNF-α blockers | − Klareskog,[76] Lebwohl[77] (*5-year follow-up*) + Chakravarty,[78] Wolfe,[79] Smith,[74] Esser[75] (*cases; suggestive of*) | − Klareskog[76] (*5-year follow-up*) + Chakravarty,[78] Wolfe[79] | + Bongartz,[81] Wolfe,[79] Khan,[82] Fulchiero[83] | + Lymphoma: Wolfe,[86] Geborek,[85] Adams,[88] Berthelot,[89] Dalle[90] (*cases; suggestive of*) − Lymphoma: Wolfe[87] |
| T-cell modulators | − Perlmutter[91] | − Perlmutter[91] | − Perlmutter[91] | + Lymphoma: Schmidt[92] (*case; suggestive of*) |

often given in conjunction with a photosensitizing chemical, and UVB treatment, with wavelengths between 280 and 320 nm. Both UVA and UVB therapy have many indications in dermatology.

PUVA photochemotherapy represents the interaction between psoralen (P), a photosensitizing organic chemical, and ultraviolet A radiation. It is largely agreed that PUVA limits keratinocyte proliferation by creating photoadducts that cross-link DNA helices and inhibit DNA replication.[12] PUVA further imparts selective cytotoxicity and immunosuppression, reducing the number of T cells and antigen-presenting cells in the skin.[12] Keratinocyte turnover is slowed, thereby improving hyperproliferative disorders. PUVA has been used as an effective treatment in diseases such as psoriasis, vitiligo, certain neoplastic dermatoses, intractable pruritus, and papulosquamous dermatoses. Numerous clinical trials have documented PUVA's carcinogenic potential.[13,14] Data suggest that PUVA-induced

carcinogenesis occurs by way of mutations in *p53* and *Ha-ras*.[15,16] PUVA has been implicated in the development of SCC, BCC and MM (Figs 32.1 and 32.2). A dose-dependent effect with respect to all three of these neoplasms has been suggested.[17,18] A 5.7-year prospective study of 1380 patients treated with PUVA revealed a dose-dependent risk of SCC, specifically that the risk 22 months after the first treatment was 12.8 times higher in patients exposed to the high dose compared to the low dose PUVA.[19] Research on the risk of melanoma after long-term exposure to PUVA demonstrated that 15 years after photochemotherapy initiation, an increased MM risk was observed in a cohort of 1380 PUVA-treated patients, with this risk directly proportional to the number of treatments provided.[17] A recent study in the same cohort found that PUVA-treated patients with high UVB exposure levels had a greater susceptibility to non-melanoma skin cancer (NMSC) than did those without additional high UVB exposure.[20] Methotrexate is not

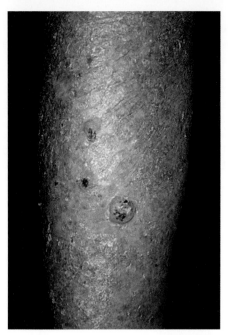

**Figure 32.1** Keratoacanthoma and squamous cell carcinomas in a patient treated with PUVA.

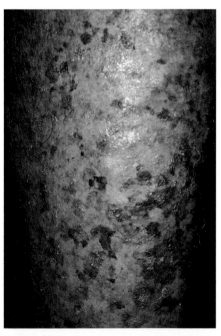

**Figure 32.2** PUVA lentigines: an increase in skin pigmentation caused by PUVA.

contraindicated in conjunction with PUVA treatment, but caution should be demonstrated with the administration of both therapies.[21]

Broadband ultraviolet B radiation (BB-UVB) represents the entire spectrum of wavelengths between 280 nm and 320 nm. Narrowband UVB radiation (NB-UVB) represents near monochromatic radiation around 311 nm. In the 1970s, BB-UVB, given at doses meant to create minimal erythema, was established as a safe and effective treatment for the mild forms of psoriasis. UVB phototherapy creates pyrimidine dimers within DNA, suppressing DNA replication. There are concerns about possible carcinogenesis associated with

UVB therapy as animal models have suggested that UVB is involved in the initiation of melanoma as well as non-melanoma skin cancer.[22,23] However, clinical attempts to demonstrate an increase in skin cancers in patients treated with UVB have not been successful.[24] This may be because of the conservative guidelines of treatment, i.e. the face and genitals are covered, doses are increased gradually to avoid burns, and UVB therapy is withheld should burns occur. In the mid-1980s, fluorescent bulbs were developed that emitted NB-UVB, now thought to be have a stronger efficacy profile than BB-UVB for a number of dermatoses, including psoriasis, atopic dermatitis, mycosis fungoides and vitiligo.[25] Animal studies, however, have shown an increased risk of carcinogenesis with NB-UVB compared with BB-UVB.[26] Animal models have further linked NB-UVB with the development of MM.[27] Despite the preclinical evidence, a recent large retrospective study of 3867 patients treated with a median of 29 NB-UVB sessions concluded that there was no increased risk of any type of skin cancer associated with NB-UVB.[28] These authors continue to follow a cohort with over 100 NB-UVB treatment sessions to determine if there is a delayed incidence peak associated with a large number of treatment sessions.

## II. Chemotherapy and immunosuppressive agents

*Methotrexate (MTX)*, a folic acid antagonist, is used in dermatology to treat a number of inflammatory, neoplastic, and autoimmune diseases. The beneficial effect of MTX in many of these disorders is thought to be related to its ability to inhibit inflammatory cells and suppress the hyperproliferation of keratinocytes. Much of what we know about the risk of cutaneous malignancy in association with MTX therapy comes from the rheumatologic literature, as MTX has long had a place in the treatment of collagen vascular diseases. Buchbinder et al. examined the incidence of malignancy in a population of 459 patients with rheumatoid arthritis who were treated with MTX for an average of 9.3 years.[29] The authors noted a 50% increased risk of malignancy in this population compared to the general population, with a threefold increase in the incidence of melanoma and a fivefold increase in the risk of non-Hodgkin lymphoma. Based upon these data, careful skin cancer screenings are indicated in patients on MTX therapy. The authors were unable to quantify the risk of NMSC since this was not recorded in their patient database. Other studies suggest that an increased risk of NMSC is found in psoriasis patients treated with MTX, perhaps related to a limited ability to enact proper DNA repair.[30] Additionally, there are data to suggest an increased risk for lymphoma, both cutaneous and extracutaneous, in patients treated with MTX. This may be an Epstein-Barr virus (EBV)-induced phenomenon.[31,32] In a retrospective review of patients with mycosis fungoides treated with MTX, an increased transformation to large cell lymphoma was noted, a malignancy which confers a worse prognosis.[33]

*Cyclosporin (CsA)* is an immunosuppressive that acts by inhibiting interleukin-2 (IL-2) formation, decreasing the number of activated CD4 and CD8 T lymphocytes present in the epidermis, and concomitantly reducing the secretion of proinflammatory cytokines. Like MTX, CsA has been used for inflammatory, neoplastic, and autoimmune disorders in dermatology. The long-term use of CsA carries concerns for the development of renal failure, lymphoproliferative disease, and both cutaneous and internal malignancy. The short-term use of CsA, however, is regarded as relatively safe. A Finnish retrospective study of the short-term risk of malignancy in 272 patients treated with CsA for a median period of 8 months and followed for a median period of 10.9 years did not detect any increase in the incidence of skin cancer or lymphoma.[34] Only case series[35,36] have reported patients who developed lymphoma on short-term CsA. In one of these,[35] when the CsA was stopped, the lymphoma regressed. Another reported that a patient treated with CsA for 6 months subsequently developed lymphoma and died.[36] Of note, this patient had a long history of treatment with a number of other oral immunosuppressive treatments. The most rigorous data regarding the use of CsA and the risk of malignancy come from a 5-year cohort study of transplant patients conducted by Paul et al.[37] The authors observed that CsA used for over 2 years was associated with an increased risk of SCC.[37] The concurrent use of CsA and PUVA or other immunosuppressive treatment has also been said to increase the risk of SCC, and clinicians must be aware of this additional risk.[38] With regard to MM, there are several cases suggesting that CsA may contribute to tumorigenesis, and one suggests that withdrawal of CsA may have a hand in promoting regression of the tumor.[39-42] However, in several of the published cases that link CsA to melanoma, the patients described were adjunctively treated with low-dose prednisone and other immunosuppressives.[40,41] There is new laboratory evidence to suggest, in fact, that CsA, alone or in combination with bacterial derived immunotoxins or interferon, may have an anti-tumor effect, inducing apoptosis in malignant melanoma cells both in vitro and in vivo.[43-45] Older studies in animal models had suggested the opposite, i.e., that CsA may upmodulate the metastatic potential of melanoma cells.[46] More work, clinically correlated, is needed before this question can be resolved.

*Azathioprine* is an anti-inflammatory and immunosuppressive drug used in dermatology. Its active metabolite, a purine analog, inhibits DNA and RNA synthesis, decreasing T-cell activity and antibody production by B cells. Azathioprine has been used, variably, to treat psoriasis, atopic dermatitis, bullous disorders, vasculitides, sarcoid, connective tissue disorders, and pyoderma gangrenosum. Azathioprine has long been identified as a carcinogen based on initial studies in the organ transplant population.[47] O'Donovan et al., in initial and confirmatory studies, clarified the mechanism by which azathioprine induces mutagenesis.[48] The authors demonstrated that azathioprine, which is metabolized to 6-thioguanine, intercalates in DNA and creates a DNA sequence that induces chronic oxidative stress, carcinogenicity, and a *p53* response.[48,49] Moreover, the incorporated product is selectively reactive to UVA, and works synergistically with UVA to increase mutagenicity.[50] Organ transplant patients treated with azathioprine are said to have a 50–250-fold increase in the risk of cutaneous squamous cell carcinoma over 20 years.[48,51] Dermatologic cases have also reported a

relationship between aggressive SCC and azathioprine.[52,53] Recent work has further shown that azathioprine-treated patients were much more likely to have PTCH mutations in basal cells on non-sun-exposed skin, implying that azathioprine may have a hand in non-UV-related BCCs.[54] A large-scale evaluation of organ transplant recipients in a temperate climate over a 21-year period, most receiving azathioprine and corticosteroids, demonstrated that there was a 61% cumulative risk of skin cancer at 20 years' time, with a ratio of SCC/BCC at 3.2/1.[55] Other studies in the transplant population have indicated an increased relative risk for melanoma and Kaposi sarcoma[56] (Fig. 32.3). Merkel cell carcinoma and lymphoma have also been reported in association with azathioprine.[57,58]

*Mycophenolate mofetil (MMF)* acts by inhibiting de novo purine synthesis, suppressing T and B lymphocyte proliferation. Like the other immunosuppressive drugs discussed, it is used for selected inflammatory and neoplastic disorders in dermatology. The data implicating MMF in cutaneous carcinogenesis are not as strong as the findings related to several of the immunosuppressive medications previously discussed. A comparative study indicated that the incidence of skin cancer in renal transplant patients on MMF was lower than that of patients on azathioprine at 3 years' time, though statistical significance was not achieved.[59] The study also found that the incidence of skin cancer in patients on a higher dose of MMF was statistically significantly lower than that of patients on a lower dose of MMF at the 3-year endpoint.[59] Research has suggested that MMF may in fact have anti-tumor effects that are more substantial in vitro than in vivo, related to the drug's bioavailability.[60] A study asserted that MMF in the post-transplantation period was associated with a 27% adjusted risk reduction for the development of malignancy.[61] A study that followed 76 psoriasis patients treated with MMF for 52–670 weeks, observed that there were a total of seven malignant neoplasms discovered over a 13-year period, three of which were BCCs. This did not vary from the incidence of BCC in the general population.[62] Cases from the rheumatologic literature have suggested that MMF may be implicated in the development of SCC in patients treated with MMF for systemic scleroderma, as indicated by regression of the tumor in one patient when

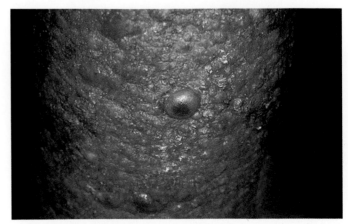

**Figure 32.3** Kaposi sarcoma: ecchymotic-like macules that evolve into papules, nodules and tumors that are violaceous, red, pink or tan can occur in patients on immunosuppressive medications.

the medication was stopped.[63] However, more data are needed to support such a link. To our knowledge, MMF has not been reported in conjunction with the development of other malignant skin neoplasms.

*Topical calcineurin inhibitors (TCIs)* are a family of compounds that bind cytosolic proteins known as immunophillins, inhibiting calcineurin phosphatase activity and preventing cytokine production and T-cell activation.[64] They were FDA approved in 2000 and 2001 for atopic dermatitis, and are used in a number of other inflammatory dermatoses in which topical steroids may be undesirable. The use of systemic calcineurin inhibitors in transplant patients has been determined to pose an increased risk of carcinogenesis.[65] Consequently, the carcinogenic risk of TCI therapy is of concern. A number of studies have investigated this risk. One such effort examined the incidence of skin tumors in 117 mice following treatment with topical tacrolimus in conjunction with a tumor initiator and promoter.[66] Tumorigenesis was found to be markedly greater in topical tacrolimus-treated mice, primarily with an increase in papillomas, which are uncommon benign neoplasms, but also with SCC representing 8.5% of the tumors.[66] The incidence of SCC was equivalent to that in the untreated subgroup of mice, exposed to the tumor initiator and promoter alone. Critics have further remarked that the mice were housed together in group accommodations, which may have confounded the study, given scratching and mechanical irritation of the skin is tumorigenic in mice.[67,68] A more recent study, examining the effect of TCIs on hairless mouse epidermis, observed a statistically significant decrease in thymine dimers (UVB photoproducts) in the epidermis of mice pretreated with 1% pimecrolimus cream and 0.1% tacrolimus ointment, at 48 hours after UVB irradiation.[69] The authors suggest that, in contrast to the previous study, TCIs may in fact exert a filter effect, preventing UVB mutagenesis in DNA. Clinically, two other studies have been published that undermine any association between TCI use and an increased risk of NMSC.[70,71] One of those studies collected data from 9813 adult and pediatric patients using 0.03% or 0.01% tacrolimus ointment twice daily, with 1718 patient-years of follow-up included for those patients over 40 years of age. No increase in the incidence of NMSC above that of the general population was noted.[70] The other study surveyed patients between 2002 and 2005 with a diagnosis of dermatitis. Margolis et al. determined that a significantly greater proportion of patients who had not been exposed to TCIs developed NMSC, and in fact, the odds ratio for developing NMSC decreased as the dosage of the drug increased.[71] To our knowledge, there are no data to support an association between TCIs and melanoma. The question of a possible relationship between TCIs and lymphoma, both cutaneous and extracutaneous, has been raised, in light of post-marketing animal studies in which lymphoma occurred in monkeys subjected to 30 times the maximum recommended human dose and in mice who were treated with long-term continuous TCI therapy, reaching systemic levels of the medication. This work elicited a black-box warning statement from the FDA. While long-term safety data with regard to TCIs are yet unavailable, short-term clinical data have not established this connection. In a 2007 study, Arellano et al., following a large cohort of patients with atopic dermatitis treated with either TCIs or topical steroids, found that the development of lymphoma better correlated with the severity of the atopic dermatitis rather than the class of topical medication used, and that the odds ratio for the development of lymphoma was lower in the TCI group than in the topical steroid group.[72] A 2009 epidemiologic study by Schneeweiss et al. also failed to show an increased incidence of lymphoma in TCI users relative to users of other topical agents when examined over 1.3 years. The population examined, however, did have an increased incidence of lymphoma as compared to the general population.[73]

## III. Biologic agents

Biologic agents represent a relatively new genre of bioengineered systemic medications that target ultra-specific aspects of the inflammatory response. There are four biologic agents currently approved for use in clinical dermatology, with others on the horizon. These medications exert an effect either by preventing the action of pro-inflammatory cytokines or by modulating the T-cell response to inflammatory signals. As such, they alter the immune response, raising concern that the physiologic immune surveillance mechanisms necessary to detect and prevent the development of cutaneous malignancy might also be affected. As with many systemic immunomodulators, biologic agents are also used in rheumatology, and a significant part of the information regarding the risk of cutaneous carcinogenesis associated with the biologics arises from the rheumatologic literature.

The anti-tumor necrosis factor-α (anti-TNF-α) agents include the biologics etanercept, adalimumab and infliximab. These are structurally variable compounds that bind soluble TNF-α (etanercept) or soluble and membrane bound TNF-α (adalimumab, infliximab). All three medications are approved for the treatment of psoriasis and psoriatic arthritis. Adalimumab and infliximab are approved for inflammatory bowel disease. While case reports have been suggestive of an increased risk of NMSC in patients treated with these agents,[74,75] there are certain caveats in assessing the inferences to be drawn from these cases (multiple prior immunosuppressive medications in the patients described, significant UV exposure), and the data from larger studies are less clear. An open-label study from the rheumatologic literature examining the safety and efficacy of etanercept in 549 patients with rheumatoid arthritis who were not treated with other disease-modifying agents found that there was no increased risk of skin cancer within the 5-year follow-up period.[76] A retrospective examination of the clinical trials database of etanercept patients found that in a total of 1442 patients with rheumatoid arthritis followed for 4257 patient-years of etanercept exposure, the incidence of SCC was comparable to that in the general population.[77] However, a cohort study of 15,789 rheumatoid arthritis patients compared with 3639 osteoarthritis patients found that there was an increased risk of NMSC in patients with rheumatoid arthritis (hazard ratio 1.19). This suggested that while the disease state alone may predispose to the development of NMSC, there may also be an increased incidence of NMSC in patients on TNF-α antagonists (hazard ratio 1.24).[78] Another study, examining the risk of malignancy associated with biologic treatment for rheumatoid arthritis, observed that there was an increased relative risk of NMSC in patients on etanercept (1.2) as well as infliximab (1.7).[79] Recent articles agree that the relationship between the TNF-α antagonists and the development of NMSC has yet to be elucidated, and, in the interim, regular skin screening is warranted in patients on these drugs.[80]

The relationship between the TNF-α blockers and the development of melanoma merits concern. A systematic meta-analysis investigating the risk of malignancy and infection associated with anti-TNF-α treatment (including infliximab and adalimumab) in the rheumatoid arthritis population found that a pooled odds ratio for malignancy was 3.3, with a dose-dependent effect noted.[81] This study was criticized for excluding etanercept and was not normalized for duration of therapy, disease severity, or concomitant treatments. Wolfe et al. also found an increased relative risk for melanoma in rheumatoid arthritis patients on both etanercept and infliximab, (2.4 and 2.6, respectively.).[79] Additionally, several case reports have chronicled the development of melanomas after biologic therapy. Khan et al. described a 70-year-old patient with a long history of occupational sun exposure, previously treated with methotrexate for rheumatoid arthritis for a period of 5 years, who developed a melanoma on the scalp 1 year after starting infliximab for worsening rheumatoid arthritis.[82] Of note, this patient also had significant exposure to additional carcinogens, including UV light and methotrexate, the latter of which independently confers an increased risk of melanoma. Fulchiero et al. reported two cases of late local recurrence of melanoma, 6 and 9 years after surgical treatment, within 6 months after anti-TNF-α therapy was initiated.[83] Prior therapy in these patients was not discussed. With support from the transplant literature,[84] the evidence suggests that there is a genuine need for caution in prescribing such immunosuppressive therapies to patients with a history of melanoma.

The development of both cutaneous and systemic T-cell lymphoma has been described following anti-TNF-α therapy. There are data for and against a causal relationship with the drug therapy in a population of patients whose immune dysregulation may already place them at a higher risk for lymphoma.[85-87] Isolated case reports regarding the development of cutaneous lymphoma following anti-TNF-α therapy have been published. Adams et al. documented the development of Sézary syndrome and anaplastic large cell lymphoma 18 and 4 months after commencing therapy with etanercept and infliximab, respectively.[88] Berthelot et al. reported the development of atypical CD8+ cutaneous T-cell lymphoma after infliximab for severe rheumatoid arthritis.[89] Dalle et al. reported the rapid development of a mycosis fungoides-associated follicular mucinosis in the context of adalimumab therapy.[90] Some authors have suggested that suppressing TNF-α may inhibit apoptotic pathways, permitting atypical lymphoma cells to grow.[88]

The T-cell modulator alefacept, the first biologic to be approved for the treatment of psoriasis, has been examined in a long-term safety trial. No higher risk of malignancy than that expected in the psoriatic population was found.[91] To our knowledge, only a single report associates alefacept with the development of a large T-cell lymphoma arising as the transformation of mycosis fungoides 3 months after 7 weeks of therapy with the drug.[92] Of note, the patient had been treated with prednisone, acitretin, methotrexate and etanercept in the recent past, making the correlation with alefacept suspect.

## FUTURE OUTLOOK

With continued medical research, new physical and pharmacotherapies will certainly be developed. Some of these therapies will correlate with an increased risk of developing skin cancer. Clinicians must continue to be alert to the carcinogenic potential of longstanding conventional as well as new treatments. Patients on these therapies will require regular skin cancer screening, and a high index of suspicion will be necessary to detect neoplasms in these patients in their earliest stages of development.

## REFERENCES

1. Levine AJ, Momand J, Finlay CA. The p53 tumour suppressor gene. *Nature.* 1991;351:453–456.
2. Carr AM. Cell cycle. Piecing together the p53 puzzle. *Science.* 2000;287:1765–1766.
3. de Gruijl FR, van Kranen HJ, Mullenders LH. UV-induced DNA damage, repair, mutations and oncogenic pathways in skin cancer. *J Photochem Photobiol B.* 2001;63:19–27.
4. Wikonkal NM, Berg RJ, van Haselen CW, et al. bcl-2 vs p53 protein expression and apoptotic rate in human nonmelanoma skin cancers. *Arch Dermatol.* 1997;133:599–602.
5. Sarasin A, Giglia-Mari G. p53 gene mutations in human skin cancers. *Exp Dermatol.* 2002;11(suppl 1):44–47.
6. Lacour JP. Carcinogenesis of basal cell carcinomas: genetics and molecular mechanisms. *Br J Dermatol.* 2002;146(suppl 61):17–19.
7. Fan H, Khavari PA. Sonic hedgehog opposes epithelial cell cycle arrest. *J Cell Biol.* 1999;147:71–76.
8. Fan H, Oro AE, Scott MP, et al. Induction of basal cell carcinoma features in transgenic human skin expressing Sonic Hedgehog. *Nat Med.* 1997;3:788–792.
9. Ling G, Ahmadian A, Persson A, et al. PATCHED and p53 gene alterations in sporadic and hereditary basal cell cancer. *Oncogene.* 2001;20:7770–7778.
10. Dahmane N, Lee J, Robins P, et al. Activation of the transcription factor Gli1 and the Sonic hedgehog signalling pathway in skin tumours. *Nature.* 1997;389:876–881.
11. Ping XL, Ratner D, Zhang H, et al. PTCH mutations in squamous cell carcinoma of the skin. *J Invest Dermatol.* 2001;116:614–616.
12. Luftl M, Rocken M, Plewig G, et al. PUVA inhibits DNA replication, but not gene transcription at nonlethal dosages. *J Invest Dermatol.* 1998;111:399–405.
13. Stern RS, Lunder EJ. Risk of squamous cell carcinoma and methoxsalen (psoralen) and UV-A radiation (PUVA). A meta-analysis. *Arch Dermatol.* 1998;134:1582–1585.
14. Stern RS, Liebman EJ, Vakeva L. Oral psoralen and ultraviolet-A light (PUVA) treatment of psoriasis and persistent risk of nonmelanoma skin cancer. PUVA Follow-up Study. *J Natl Cancer Inst.* 1998;90:1278–1284.
15. Stern RS, Bolshakov S, Nataraj AJ, et al. p53 mutation in nonmelanoma skin cancers occurring in psoralen ultraviolet a-treated patients: evidence for heterogeneity and field cancerization. *J Invest Dermatol.* 2002;119:522–526.
16. Kreimer-Erlacher H, Seidl H, Back B, et al. High mutation frequency at Ha-ras exons 1–4 in squamous cell carcinomas from PUVA-treated psoriasis patients. *Photochem Photobiol.* 2001;74:323–330.
17. Stern RS, Nichols KT, Vakeva LH. Malignant melanoma in patients treated for psoriasis with methoxsalen (psoralen) and ultraviolet A radiation (PUVA). The PUVA Follow-Up Study. *N Engl J Med.* 1997;336:1041–1045.
18. McKenna KE, Patterson CC, Handley J, et al. Cutaneous neoplasia following PUVA therapy for psoriasis. *Br J Dermatol.* 1996;134:639–642.
19. Stern RS, Laird N, Melski J, et al. Cutaneous squamous-cell carcinoma in patients treated with PUVA. *N Engl J Med.* 1984;310:1156–1161.
20. Lim JL, Stern RS. High levels of ultraviolet B exposure increase the risk of non-melanoma skin cancer in psoralen and ultraviolet A-treated patients. *J Invest Dermatol.* 2005;124:505–513.

21. Studniberg HM, Weller P. PUVA, UVB, psoriasis, and nonmelanoma skin cancer. *J Am Acad Dermatol*. 1993;29:1013–1022.

22. De Fabo EC, Noonan FP, Fears T, et al. Ultraviolet B but not ultraviolet A radiation initiates melanoma. *Cancer Res*. 2004;64:6372–6376.

23. Ishigaki Y, Suzuki F, Hayakawa J, et al. An UVB-carcinogenesis model with KSN nude mice. *J Radiat Res (Tokyo)*. 1998;39:73–81.

24. Weischer M, Blum A, Eberhard F, et al. No evidence for increased skin cancer risk in psoriasis patients treated with broadband or narrowband UVB phototherapy: a first retrospective study. *Acta Derm Venereol*. 2004;84:370–374.

25. Lebwohl M. Should we switch from combination UVA/UVB phototherapy units to narrowband UVB? *Photodermatol Photoimmunol Photomed*. 2002;18:44–46; discussion 7–9.

26. Kunisada M, Kumimoto H, Ishizaki K, et al. Narrow-band UVB induces more carcinogenic skin tumors than broad-band UVB through the formation of cyclobutane pyrimidine dimer. *J Invest Dermatol*. 2007;127:2865–2871.

27. Robinson ES, Hubbard GB, Dooley TP. Metastatic melanoma in an adult opossum (Monodelphis domestica) after short-term intermittent UVB exposure. *Arch Dermatol Res*. 2000;292:469–471.

28. Hearn RM, Kerr AC, Rahim KF, et al. Incidence of skin cancers in 3867 patients treated with narrow-band ultraviolet B phototherapy. *Br J Dermatol*. 2008;159:931–935.

29. Buchbinder R, Barber M, Heuzenroeder L, et al. Incidence of melanoma and other malignancies among rheumatoid arthritis patients treated with methotrexate. *Arthritis Rheum*. 2008;59:794–799.

30. Dybdahl M, Frentz G, Vogel U, et al. Low DNA repair is a risk factor in skin carcinogenesis: a study of basal cell carcinoma in psoriasis patients. *Mutat Res*. 1999;433:15–22.

31. Paul C, Le Tourneau A, Cayuela JM, et al. Epstein-Barr virus-associated lymphoproliferative disease during methotrexate therapy for psoriasis. *Arch Dermatol*. 1997;133:867–871.

32. Hsiao SC, Ichinohasama R, Lin SH, et al. EBV-associated diffuse large B-cell lymphoma in a psoriatic treated with methotrexate. *Pathol Res Pract*. 2009;205:43–49.

33. Abd-el-Baki J, Demierre MF, Li N, et al. Transformation in mycosis fungoides: the role of methotrexate. *J Cutan Med Surg*. 2002;6:109–116.

34. Vakeva L, Reitamo S, Pukkala E, et al. Long-term follow-up of cancer risk in patients treated with short-term cyclosporine. *Acta Derm Venereol*. 2008;88:117–120.

35. Kirby B, Owen CM, Blewitt RW, et al. Cutaneous T-cell lymphoma developing in a patient on cyclosporin therapy. *J Am Acad Dermatol*. 2002;47:S165–S167.

36. Koo JY, Kadonaga JN, Wintroub BV, et al. The development of B-cell lymphoma in a patient with psoriasis treated with cyclosporine. *J Am Acad Dermatol*. 1992;26:836–840.

37. Paul CF, Ho VC, McGeown C, et al. Risk of malignancies in psoriasis patients treated with cyclosporine: a 5 y cohort study. *J Invest Dermatol*. 2003;120:211–216.

38. Marcil I, Stern RS. Squamous-cell cancer of the skin in patients given PUVA and ciclosporin: nested cohort crossover study. *Lancet*. 2001;358:1042–1045.

39. Arellano F, Krupp PF. Cutaneous malignant melanoma occurring after cyclosporin A therapy. *Br J Dermatol*. 1991;124:611.

40. Zavos G, Papaconstantinou I, Chrisostomidis C, et al. Metastatic melanoma within a transplanted kidney: a case report. *Transplant Proc*. 2004;36:1411–1412.

41. Merot Y, Miescher PA, Balsiger F, et al. Cutaneous malignant melanomas occurring under cyclosporin A therapy: a report of two cases. *Br J Dermatol*. 1990;123:237–239.

42. Hodi FS, Granter S, Antin J. Withdrawal of immunosuppression contributing to the remission of malignant melanoma: a case report. *Cancer Immun*. 2005;5:7.

43. Ciechomska I, Legat M, Golab J, et al. Cyclosporine A and its non-immunosuppressive derivative NIM811 induce apoptosis of malignant melanoma cells in in vitro and in vivo studies. *Int J Cancer*. 2005;117:59–67.

44. Schwenkert M, Birkholz K, Schwemmlein M, et al. A single chain immunotoxin, targeting the melanoma-associated chondroitin sulfate proteoglycan, is a potent inducer of apoptosis in cultured human melanoma cells. *Melanoma Res*. 2008;18:73–84.

45. Charak BS, Brown EG, Mazumder A. Induction of antitumor effect by treatment with cyclosporine A plus interferon-gamma after chemotherapy: role of cytotoxic cells. *J Immunother Emphasis Tumor Immunol*. 1995;17:131–140.

46. Boyano MD, de Galdeano AG, Garcia-Vazquez MD, et al. Cyclosporin A upmodulates the alpha-subunit of the interleukin-2 receptor and the metastatic ability of murine B16F10 melanoma cells. *Invasion Metastasis*. 1998;18:122–133.

47. National Toxicology Program. Azathioprine. *Rep Carcinog*. 2002;10:23–24.

48. O'Donovan P, Perrett CM, Zhang X, et al. Azathioprine and UVA light generate mutagenic oxidative DNA damage. *Science*. 2005;309:1871–1874.

49. Zhang X, Jeffs G, Ren X, et al. Novel DNA lesions generated by the interaction between therapeutic thiopurines and UVA light. *DNA Repair (Amst)*. 2007;6:344–354.

50. Perrett CM, Walker SL, O'Donovan P, et al. Azathioprine treatment photosensitizes human skin to ultraviolet A radiation. *Br J Dermatol*. 2008;159:198–204.

51. Guenova E, Lichte V, Hoetzenecker W, et al. Nodular malignant melanoma and multiple cutaneous neoplasms under immunosuppression with azathioprine. *Melanoma Res*. 2009;19:271–273.

52. Bottomley WW, Ford G, Cunliffe WJ, et al. Aggressive squamous cell carcinomas developing in patients receiving long-term azathioprine. *Br J Dermatol*. 1995;133:460–462.

53. Nachbar F, Stolz W, Volkenandt M, et al. Squamous cell carcinoma in localized scleroderma following immunosuppressive therapy with azathioprine. *Acta Derm Venereol*. 1993;73:217–219.

54. Harwood CA, Attard NR, O'Donovan P, et al. PTCH mutations in basal cell carcinomas from azathioprine-treated organ transplant recipients. *Br J Cancer*. 2008;99:1276–1284.

55. Bordea C, Wojnarowska F, Millard PR, et al. Skin cancers in renal-transplant recipients occur more frequently than previously recognized in a temperate climate. *Transplantation*. 2004;77:574–579.

56. Jensen P, Hansen S, Moller B, et al. Skin cancer in kidney and heart transplant recipients and different long-term immunosuppressive therapy regimens. *J Am Acad Dermatol*. 1999;40:177–186.

57. Ehrenfeld M, Abu-Shakra M, Buskila D, et al. The dual association between lymphoma and autoimmunity. *Blood Cells Mol Dis*. 2001;27:750–756.

58. Gooptu C, Woollons A, Ross J, et al. Merkel cell carcinoma arising after therapeutic immunosuppression. *Br J Dermatol*. 1997;137:637–641.

59. Wang K, Zhang H, Li Y, et al. Safety of mycophenolate mofetil versus azathioprine in renal transplantation: a systematic review. *Transplant Proc*. 2004;36:2068–2070.

60. Koehl GE, Wagner F, Stoeltzing O, et al. Mycophenolate mofetil inhibits tumor growth and angiogenesis in vitro but has variable antitumor effects in vivo, possibly related to bioavailability. *Transplantation*. 2007;83:607–614.

61. O'Neill JO, Edwards LB, Taylor DO. Mycophenolate mofetil and risk of developing malignancy after orthotopic heart transplantation: analysis of the transplant registry of the International Society for Heart and Lung Transplantation. *J Heart Lung Transplant*. 2006;25:1186–1191.

62. Epinette WW, Parker CM, Jones EL. Mycophenolic acid for psoriasis. A review of pharmacology, long-term efficacy, and safety. *J Am Acad Dermatol*. 1987;17:962–971.

63. Gulamhusein A, Pope JE. Squamous cell carcinomas in 2 patients with diffuse scleroderma treated with mycophenolate mofetil. *J Rheumatol*. 2009;36:460–462.

64. Hanifin JM, Chan S. Biochemical and immunologic mechanisms in atopic dermatitis: new targets for emerging therapies. *J Am Acad Dermatol*. 1999;41:72–77.

65. Berardinelli L, Messa PG, Pozzoli E, et al. Malignancies in 2,753 kidney recipients transplanted during a 39-year experience. *Transplant Proc*. 2009;41:1231–1232.

66. Niwa Y, Terashima T, Sumi H. Topical application of the immunosuppressant tacrolimus accelerates carcinogenesis in mouse skin. *Br J Dermatol*. 2003;149:960–967.

67. Ring J, Mohrenschlager M, Henkel V. The US FDA 'black box' warning for topical calcineurin inhibitors: an ongoing controversy. *Drug Saf*. 2008;31:185–198.

68. Siegsmund M, Wayss K, Amtmann E. Activation of latent papillomavirus genomes by chronic mechanical irritation. *J Gen Virol*. 1991;72(Pt 11):2787–2789.

69. Tran C, Lubbe J, Sorg O, et al. Topical calcineurin inhibitors decrease the production of UVB-induced thymine dimers from hairless mouse epidermis. *Dermatology*. 2005;211:341–347.

70. Naylor M, Elmets C, Jaracz E, et al. Non-melanoma skin cancer in patients with atopic dermatitis treated with topical tacrolimus. *J Dermatolog Treat*. 2005;16:149–153.

71. Margolis DJ, Hoffstad O, Bilker W. Lack of association between exposure to topical calcineurin inhibitors and skin cancer in adults. *Dermatology*. 2007;214:289–295.

72. Arellano FM, Wentworth CE, Arana A, et al. Risk of lymphoma following exposure to calcineurin inhibitors and topical steroids in patients with atopic dermatitis. *J Invest Dermatol*. 2007;127:808–816.

73. Schneeweiss S, Doherty M, Zhu S, et al. Topical treatments with pimecrolimus, tacrolimus and medium- to high-potency corticosteroids, and risk of lymphoma. *Dermatology*. 2009;219:7–21.

74. Smith KJ, Skelton HG. Rapid onset of cutaneous squamous cell carcinoma in patients with rheumatoid arthritis after starting tumor necrosis factor alpha receptor IgG1-Fc fusion complex therapy. *J Am Acad Dermatol*. 2001;45:953–956.

75. Esser AC, Abril A, Fayne S, et al. Acute development of multiple keratoacanthomas and squamous cell carcinomas after treatment with infliximab. *J Am Acad Dermatol*. 2004;50:S75–S77.

76. Klareskog L, Gaubitz M, Rodriguez-Valverde V, et al. A long-term, open-label trial of the safety and efficacy of etanercept (Enbrel) in patients with rheumatoid arthritis not treated with other disease-modifying antirheumatic drugs. *Ann Rheum Dis*. 2006;65:1578–1584.

77. Lebwohl M, Blum R, Berkowitz E, et al. No evidence for increased risk of cutaneous squamous cell carcinoma in patients with rheumatoid arthritis receiving etanercept for up to 5 years. *Arch Dermatol.* 2005;141:861–864.

78. Chakravarty EF, Michaud K, Wolfe F. Skin cancer, rheumatoid arthritis, and tumor necrosis factor inhibitors. *J Rheumatol.* 2005;32:2130–2135.

79. Wolfe F, Michaud K. Biologic treatment of rheumatoid arthritis and the risk of malignancy: analyses from a large US observational study. *Arthritis Rheum.* 2007;56:2886–2895.

80. Moustou AE, Matekovits A, Dessinioti C, et al. Cutaneous side effects of anti-tumor necrosis factor biologic therapy: a clinical review. *J Am Acad Dermatol.* 2009;61:486–504.

81. Bongartz T, Sutton AJ, Sweeting MJ, et al. Anti-TNF antibody therapy in rheumatoid arthritis and the risk of serious infections and malignancies: systematic review and meta-analysis of rare harmful effects in randomized controlled trials. *JAMA.* 2006;295:2275–2285.

82. Khan I, Rahman L, McKenna DB. Primary cutaneous melanoma: a complication of infliximab treatment? *Clin Exp Dermatol.* 2009;34:524–526.

83. Fulchiero Jr GJ, Salvaggio H, Drabick JJ, et al. Eruptive latent metastatic melanomas after initiation of antitumor necrosis factor therapies. *J Am Acad Dermatol.* 2007;56:S65–S67.

84. Penn I. Malignant melanoma in organ allograft recipients. *Transplantation.* 1996;61:274–278.

85. Geborek P, Bladstrom A, Turesson C, et al. Tumour necrosis factor blockers do not increase overall tumour risk in patients with rheumatoid arthritis, but may be associated with an increased risk of lymphomas. *Ann Rheum Dis.* 2005;64:699–703.

86. Wolfe F, Michaud K. Lymphoma in rheumatoid arthritis: the effect of methotrexate and anti-tumor necrosis factor therapy in 18,572 patients. *Arthritis Rheum.* 2004;50:1740–1751.

87. Wolfe F, Michaud K. The effect of methotrexate and anti-tumor necrosis factor therapy on the risk of lymphoma in rheumatoid arthritis in 19,562 patients during 89,710 person-years of observation. *Arthritis Rheum.* 2007;56:1433–1439.

88. Adams AE, Zwicker J, Curiel C, et al. Aggressive cutaneous T-cell lymphomas after TNFalpha blockade. *J Am Acad Dermatol.* 2004;51:660–662.

89. Berthelot C, Cather J, Jones D, et al. Atypical CD8+ cutaneous T-cell lymphoma after immunomodulatory therapy. *Clin Lymphoma Myeloma.* 2006;6:329–332.

90. Dalle S, Balme B, Berger F, et al. Mycosis fungoides-associated follicular mucinosis under adalimumab. *Br J Dermatol.* 2005;153:207–208.

91. Perlmutter A, Cather J, Franks B, et al. Alefacept revisited: our 3-year clinical experience in 200 patients with chronic plaque psoriasis. *J Am Acad Dermatol.* 2008;58:116–124.

92. Schmidt A, Robbins J, Zic J. Transformed mycosis fungoides developing after treatment with alefacept. *J Am Acad Dermatol.* 2005;53:355–356.

# Genetic Disorders Predisposing to Skin Malignancy

*Courtney Schadt and Jo-David Fine*

## Key Points

- Several genodermatoses have a predisposition for the development of one or more types of skin cancers. Internal malignancies may also arise in a few.

- These diseases are caused by mutations in over 30 genes which normally function as tumor suppressors, repair of UV-damaged DNA, telomere length regulation, maintenance of cutaneous structural integrity, and susceptibility to mutagenesis by specific human papillomaviruses.

- Multidisciplinary management includes early diagnosis, photoprotection, surveillance for cutaneous and internal malignancies, definitive surgical care, and genetic counseling.

## BASAL CELL NEVUS SYNDROME

### Introduction

Basal cell nevus syndrome (BCNS, MIM #109400; nevoid basal cell carcinoma syndrome; Gorlin or Gorlin–Goltz syndrome), a rare autosomal dominant condition, is characterized by the presence of multiple basal cell carcinomas (BCCs), palmoplantar pits, odontogenic keratocysts, and skeletal abnormalities.

### History

In 1960, Gorlin and Goltz described a syndrome of multiple basal cell epitheliomas, jaw cysts, and bifid ribs.[1] Since then, numerous additional clinical findings, including medulloblastoma, palmoplantar pits, ovarian carcinoma, and frontal bossing, have been reported.

### Epidemiology

Prevalence estimates range from 1:56,000 to 1:164,000.[2,3]

### Pathogenesis and etiology

The BCNS gene, a tumor suppressor gene, was mapped to chromosome 9q22.3-q31 in 1992.[4-6] Subsequent studies identified the gene as *PATCHED* (PTCH), a transmembrane receptor in the sonic hedgehog pathway, similar to Drosophila patched involvement in fly development.[7-9] The hedgehog pathway is fundamental in human growth and development, including neural tube, skeleton, limbs, craniofacial structures, and skin.[9] Loss of heterozygosity for genetic markers in this region has been detected in 50% of sporadic BCCs, supporting its role as a tumor suppressor gene. Mutations in *PTCH1* and *PTCH2* have been identified in BCNS.[7-10] The PTCH protein inhibits the smoothened protein in the absence of hedgehog. With hedgehog binding, smoothened is released, and through the transcription factor Gli, multiple downstream target genes involved in cell proliferation are expressed. With *PTCH* mutations, loss of negative autoregulation leads to increased transcription of non-functional PTCH mRNA, in addition to a constitutively active smoothened.[11]

### Clinical features

The characteristic skin finding in this syndrome, BCCs, typically appears between puberty and age 35.[12] These may occur as early as 2 years of life,[12] and are influenced by ethnicity. In one study, 38% of black patients developed BCCs versus 80% of Caucasians.[13] BCCs can number from a few to thousands (Fig. 33.1) and can be mistaken for skin tags, nevi, hemangiomas, or molluscum contagiosum.[14] Most involve the face, back, or chest. Although only rarely invasive, they may occur following radiation for medulloblastoma and lead to death.[13] A major cutaneous finding is palmoplantar pitting (Figs 33.2 and 33.3), seen in up to 87% of patients and as early as 5 months of life.[13] Milia may also be intermixed with BCCs, and epidermal cysts are seen in a majority of patients.[2,14]

Odontogenic keratocysts of the jaw usually develop during the first decade and peak in the second or third decades. They are most often detected on routine dental check-ups and can be seen in over 80% of patients, more often in the mandible. While they almost never cause symptoms unless secondarily infected, they can displace developing permanent teeth and affect expansion of the jaws.[14]

Musculoskeletal abnormalities are quite common and include fused, splayed, hypoplastic, or bifid ribs (in approximately 60%), kyphoscoliosis, spina bifida occulta, malformations of the occipitovertebral junction, and enlarged occipitofrontal circumference with frontal bossing and macrocephaly (Fig. 33.4).[12,14] Other features include highly arched eyebrows, high arched palate, narrow sloping shoulder, immobile thumbs, cleft lip and palate, and low pitched voice.[2,13]

Medulloblastoma has been reported in very young children with BCNS, with an incidence estimated as 3.5%.[3]

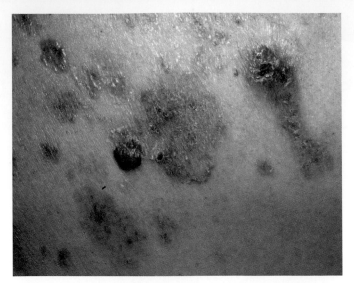

Figure 33.1 Widespread BCCs on the back of a patient with BCNS.

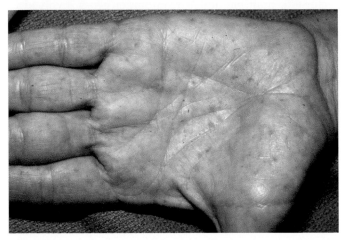

Figure 33.2 Numerous shallow pits are present on the palm of a patient with BCNS.

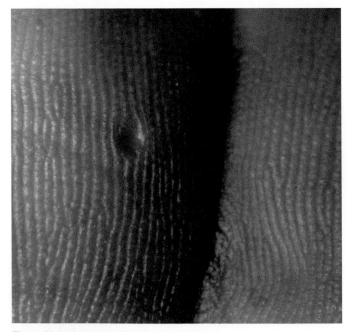

Figure 33.3 Higher magnification of a palmar pit.

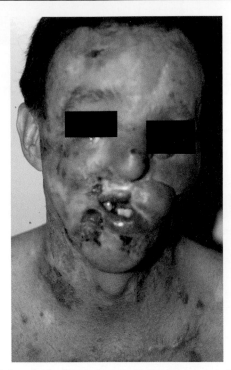

Figure 33.4 A markedly disfigured adult with BCNS, demonstrating frontal bossing, the presence of numerous BCCs on the face, neck, and upper chest, and post-surgical scarring.

Radiation therapy for this tumor can markedly affect the onset, number, and biological aggressiveness of BCCs.[13] Other reported brain tumors include meningiomas, craniopharyngioma, astrocytoma, and cysts in the brain.[14] Falx cerebri calcification occurs relatively early in life and is detectable in at least 85% of patients.[12]

## Patient evaluation, diagnosis, and differential diagnosis

Major and minor diagnostic criteria for BCNS are summarized in Table 33.1. In a patient with multiple BCCs, other diagnoses to consider include Bazex–Dupré–Christol and Rombo syndromes (see below).

Dermatological evaluation of patients with BCNS is recommended every 2–3 months, particularly during adolescence. Beginning at age 8, patients should have a panoramic radiograph of the jaws every year, with complete removal of any odontogenic keratocysts. Other tests to consider are annual magnetic resonance imaging from infancy through age 8, to evaluate for medulloblastoma; periodic chest radiography to screen for cardiac fibromas; and radiographic studies to detect calcification of the falx cerebri and rib anomalies.[14]

## Pathology

BCCs seen in BCNS are indistinguishable from those seen sporadically.

## Treatment

There is a paucity of studies evaluating treatment of the numerous BCCs in BCNS. It has been recommended that superficial BCCs without follicular involvement

## Table 33.1 Diagnostic Criteria for BCNS

Diagnosis of BCNS is made in the presence of two major or one major and two minor criteria:

Major criteria:
1. More then two BCCs or one under the age of 20 years
2. Odontogenic keratocysts of the jaw proven by histology
3. Three or more palmar or plantar pits
4. Bilamellar calcification of the falx cerebri
5. Bifid, fused or markedly splayed ribs
6. First-degree relative with NBCC syndrome

Minor criteria
Any one of the following features:
1. Macrocephaly determined after adjustment for height
2. Congenital malformations: cleft lip or palate, frontal bossing, 'coarse face', moderate or severe hypertelorism
3. Other skeletal abnormalities: Sprengel deformity, marked pectus deformity, marked syndactyly of the digits
4. Radiological abnormalities: bridging of the sella turcica, vertebral anomalies such as hemivertebrae, fusion or elongation of the vertebral bodies, modeling defects of the hands and feet, or flame-shaped lucencies of the hands or feet
5. Ovarian fibroma
6. Medulloblastoma

Modified from Kimonis VE, Goldstein AM, Pastakia B. Clinical manifestations in 105 persons with nevoid basal cell carcinoma syndrome. *Am J Med Genet*. 1997;69:299–308.

be managed by total body application of 0.1% tretinoin cream and 5% 5-fluorouracil cream twice daily.[15] More invasive lesions should be curetted or excised, with Mohs micrographic surgery employed for indicated lesions. One report of four patients with BCNS described successful treatment of the majority of superficial and nodular BCCs with imiquimod when used five times a week for 8–14 weeks.[16]

A randomized placebo-controlled trial of 981 patients with a history of BCC (not BCNS) evaluated the daily use of 10 mg isotretinoin versus placebo in the prevention of BCCs.[17] Patients enrolled had a history of at least two previous BCCs and were treated for 36 months. No difference was seen in the development of subsequent BCCs. No trials have evaluated isotretinoin in patients with BCNS. One case report showed a decrease in the number of new BCCs in a patient treated with 0.4 mg/kg/day of isotretinoin over 4 years, compared to 0.2 mg/kg/day.[18] A case report on the combined use of isotretinoin and intralesional interferon alfa failed to demonstrate synergism or effective clearance of BCCs in one patient.[19]

Case reports of the use of carbon dioxide laser resurfacing and topical and systemic photodynamic therapy have reported some efficacy.[20-22]

## INHERITED EPIDERMOLYSIS BULLOSA

### Introduction

Inherited epidermolysis bullosa (EB) encompasses over 30 different diseases, each of which has a distinctive phenotype and/or genotype.[23,24] This heterogeneous group of genodermatoses has as its unifying feature the development of blisters following minimal or seemingly insignificant traction on the skin. Four major EB types – EB simplex (EBS), junctional EB (JEB), dystrophic EB (DEB), Kindler syndrome – are separated on the basis of the ultrastructural level in which blisters form.[23]

### History

The name epidermolysis bullosa was first used by Köbner in 1886,[25] although individual cases were previously reported under other names, based on confusion with several other unrelated acquired blistering diseases, including pemphigus.

### Epidemiology

The overall incidence and prevalence of EB, based on data from the American National EB Registry, is 19 per 1 million live births and 8 per 1 million individuals, respectively.[26] With rare exceptions, similar rates have been observed elsewhere in the world. There are no gender or racial predilections.

### Pathogenesis and etiology

With rare exceptions, EBS is transmitted as an autosomal dominant disease (as is dominant dystrophic EB), whereas JEB (with only one possible exception) and recessive dystrophic EB are autosomal recessive disorders. Each EB type and subtype results from mutations in genes encoding specific structural proteins within keratinocytes or the dermoepidermal junction (DEJ).[23] Their presence leads to mechanical instability within specific structures (i.e. keratin filaments; hemidesmosomes; anchoring fibrils) residing within the skin. Mutations in the genes (*KRT5*; *KRT14*) encoding keratins 5 and 14 account for all but a few EBS subtypes. Most JEB subtypes are associated with mutations in laminin 332, a three-chained macromolecule present in both the hemidesmosome and the underlying anchoring filaments. Other genes that may result in JEB phenotypes are those encoding type XVII collagen, plectin, and integrin, mutations in the latter of which are accompanied by pyloric atresia. All subtypes of DEB are caused by mutations within the type VII collagen gene (*COL7A*). Although strong phenotype–genotype correlations do not exist for every EB subtype, in general those autosomal recessive EB patients having the most severe cutaneous and extracutaneous disease manifestations possess mutations that result in homozygous or compound heterozygous premature termination codons. Mouse models of JEB and recessive DEB (RDEB) suggest that mutations in the genes encoding laminin 332 and type VII collagen[27,28] play an important role in promotion and invasiveness of SCCs.

### Clinical features

All subtypes of EB are characterized by the presence of mechanically fragile skin, recurrent blisters or erosions, and poorly healing crusted wounds. Whereas the four major EB types are distinguished by their mode of transmission and antigenic and ultrastructural findings (see Pathology), individual EB subtypes are separated primarily on the basis of their clinical phenotype (both cutaneous and extracutaneous), as well as distribution (localized; generalized; inverse) and relative severity of skin involvement.[23] As will be discussed, with only rare exceptions are skin cancers a concern in inherited EB.

The only unique cutaneous finding in EB – and seen only in EBS, Dowling–Meara type (EBS-DM) – is herpetiform-grouped blisters. Other cutaneous findings, pertinent to those EB subtypes prone to develop skin cancers, have been recently summarized.[23]

Severe generalized JEB and DEB patients frequently have involvement of multiple extracutaneous tissues.[29,30] Some have an increased risk of death during childhood and early to mid adulthood,[31] due to failure to thrive, sepsis, and acute airway obstruction. By adulthood, the most common causes of death in RDEB patients are metastatic SCC (see below) and renal failure (cumulative lifetime risk of approximately 12%).

Skin cancers, both non-melanoma (SCC; BCC) and melanoma, arise in much higher frequency in selected EB subtypes.[32] Patients with RDEB-sev gen are at highest risk for developing potentially life-threatening SCCs. These usually histologically well-differentiated tumors tend to develop on the extremities in areas of chronic non-healing wounds or scars and have a predilection for local recurrence and regional or distant metastasis. Arising as early as about age 13, the cumulative risks of SCCs in this EB subtype are 7.4%, 26.7%, 51.7%, 73.6%, and 90.1% by ages 20, 25, 30, 40, and 50, respectively (Fig. 33.5). Identical appearing SCCs arise in lower frequency in generalized mitis RDEB (RDEB-gen mitis; non-Hallopeau–Siemens RDEB), inverse RDEB, and Herlitz JEB. Despite wide surgical excision with clear margins, the majority of patients with RDEB-sev gen eventually develop additional SCCs, with a cumulative risk of

mortality from metastases of 12.7%, 42.3%, 57.2%, 81.0%, and 87.3% by ages 20, 30, 35, 40, and 45, respectively. Lower mortality risks occur in other RDEB subtypes and JEB.

BCCs arise in higher frequency only in EBS-DM, with a cumulative risk of 43.6% by age 55. These tumors, however, act biologically identical to those arising in the non-EB Caucasian population. There is also a surprisingly high cumulative risk of cutaneous melanoma arising in RDEB-sev gen (plateauing at 2.5% by age 12).

## Patient evaluation, diagnosis, and differential diagnosis

The diagnosis of EB is usually readily made on the basis of clinical findings alone.[33] The diagnosis may be confirmed by transmission electron microscopy (TEM) or immunofluorescence antigenic mapping (IAM), the latter to include staining of skin specimens with specific monoclonal antibodies. Subclassification is based on combinations of clinical and laboratory findings. Mutational analysis is available commercially for most EB subtypes, although this technique is used primarily for the determination of the mode of transmission and for prenatal diagnosis.

## Pathology

The major four EB types are distinguished by the ultrastructural level in which blisters arise, via either TEM or IAM, but not reliably by routine light microscopy. Some structures are reduced in number, embryonic in appearance, or undetectable in specific EB types or subtypes (i.e. hemidesmosomes and subbasal dense plates in JEB, particularly Herlitz JEB; anchoring fibrils in RDEB). Other subtypes may be defined by the presence of unusual ultrastructural findings (e.g. clumped tonofilaments in EBS-DM). Differential staining patterns with monoclonal antibodies can be used to distinguish among some of the EB subtypes, although there are limitations in specificity and specificity.[34] Prototypic patients with RDEB-sev gen and RDEB-gen mitis lack or have reduced staining of type VII collagen along the dermoepidermal junction, respectively, with anti-type VII collagen monoclonal antibody. Similarly, anti-laminin 332 monoclonal antibody lacks or has markedly reduced staining of the dermoepidermal junction in Herlitz and non-Herlitz JEB skin, respectively.[23]

## Treatment

In the absence of an effective cure, the treatment of EB remains focused on the prevention of blisters, promotion of wound healing, nutritional supplementation, and medical or surgical intervention of specific extracutaneous complications, to include excision of skin cancers.

## XERODERMA PIGMENTOSUM

## Introduction

Xeroderma pigmentosum (XP) is an autosomal recessive disease that is characterized by defective nucleotide excision repair (NER).[35-37] Initially believed to be a single disease, XP

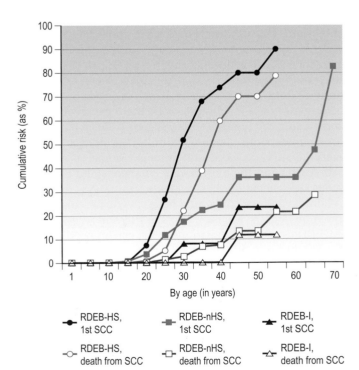

**Figure 33.5** Cumulative risks of the first SCC and death from any SCC in RDEB. (Reproduced from Fine JD et al., *J Am Acad Dermatol.* 2009;60(2):203–211, by permission of the publisher.)

Legend:
- RDEB-HS, 1st SCC
- RDEB-nHS, 1st SCC
- RDEB-I, 1st SCC
- RDEB-HS, death from SCC
- RDEB-nHS, death from SCC
- RDEB-I, death from SCC

now encompasses several closely related entities, each of which is associated with skin photosensitivity, premature photoaging, and a marked tendency for the development of precancerous and cancerous lesions.

## History

Xeroderma pigmentosa was described by Kaposi and Hebra in the early 1870s. Defective DNA repair was first reported in XP by Cleaver in 1968.[38] Since then, XP has been subdivided into several different groups, based on distinguishing laboratory characteristics, to include identification of mutations in several different genes.

## Epidemiology

The prevalence of XP in the United States and in Western Europe is estimated at 1 per million and 2.3 per million, respectively.[35,39] The frequency of silent carriers may be as high as 1 in 500. A much higher prevalence (1 in 40,000) has been reported in Japan.

## Pathogenesis and etiology

XP was the first human disease found to be the result of defective NER. Others include cerebro-oculo-facio-skeletal syndrome, mild ultraviolet-sensitive syndrome, trichothiodystrophy (TTD), Cockayne syndrome (CS), and patients with symptoms of both XP and either CS or TTD.[35] Murine knockout models of XP, following exposure to UV or chemical carcinogens, reproduce the clinical finding of a markedly increased risk of skin cancers. Some mice also develop internal malignancies.

XP patients were originally separated into seven repair-deficient complementation groups (XPA–XPG) (MIM # 278700, 610651, 278720, 278730, 278740, 278760, 278780) based on differences in the ability of cultured XP fibroblasts to undergo NER following exposure to UV radiation. One subtype of XP, XP-V (MIM# 278750), actually has normal NER but lacks a low-fidelity-polymerase (Polη) that results in excessive UV-induced mutagenesis and skin cancers. These different complementation groups have more recently been shown to result from the presence of mutations in distinct genes (XPA–XPV) located on different chromosomes.

BCCs, SCCs, and melanomas arising in XP have been shown to be associated with UV-associated mutations in the genes encoding for patched protein in the hedgehog pathway, *p53*, and the PTEN ('phosphatase and tensin homologue') tumor suppressor gene, respectively.[40–42]

## Clinical features

Most XP patients demonstrate marked sunlight sensitivity within the first 1–2 years of life. Earliest skin findings include severe sunburning, blistering, and freckling. Skin cancers (both non-melanoma and melanoma) develop early, with an overall incidence of skin cancer in those under the age of 20 that is 1000 to 2000 times higher than that seen within the general population.[35] Multiple skin cancers are the norm in these patients, with a mean age of

onset of less than 10 years. SCCs also arise on the tongue and anterior portions of the oral cavity. Mutations in some XP genes (XPA, XPB, XPG) are also associated with neurological degeneration. An early finding in XP patients is sensorineural deafness. Ocular manifestations include photophobia, chronic UV light-induced conjunctivitis, conjunctival growths (pingueculae; pterygia), keratitis, corneal opacities, diminished vision, and ectropion formation.

The lifespan of some patients (for example, those with XPA in Japan) may be foreshortened. Solid tumors that have been reported in XP include those arising in the lung, breast, uterus, stomach, pancreas, kidney, and testicle. Reported CNS tumors include medulloblastoma, astrocytoma, and glioma.

## Patient evaluation, diagnosis, and differential diagnosis

XP patients (with the exception of those with XPV) have been subclassified on the basis of NER findings in UV-treated fibroblasts in cell culture. Identical studies can be performed prenatally on amniotic cells and trophoblasts. Diagnosis can also be confirmed via mutational analysis. Silent heterozygous carriers can be identified by mutational analysis if the diagnosis has been previously confirmed molecularly in an affected family member.

## Pathology

The histologic findings in tumors arising in XP skin are identical to those seen in cancers arising in the normal population.

## Treatment

Aggressive photoprotection, beginning in early childhood, is the mainstay of care in XP patients. Patients should also be counseled to avoid exposure to any other known carcinogens, photosensitizing drugs, or cancer-associated habits (i.e. smoking). Meticulous surveillance for cancers (cutaneous; intraoral; internal) is extremely important. Proven malignancies may be treated by conventional surgical techniques. Precancerous actinic keratoses should be treated with cryotherapy, 5-fluorouracil, or imiquimod. Data also suggest the potential chemopreventive value of systemic retinoids in XP.

## MUIR–TORRE SYNDROME

### Introduction

Muir–Torre Syndrome (MTS, MIM #158320) is a rare autosomal dominant condition characterized by sebaceous neoplasms and internal malignancy.[43]

### History

In 1967 Muir described a patient who had carcinomas of the colon and duodenum, intestinal polyps, facial keratoacanthomas, and sebaceous adenomas.[44] Torre subsequently presented a patient in 1968 who had more than 100 skin tumors, including sebaceous adenomas, sebaceous carcinomas, and BCCs with sebaceous differentiation on the face, trunk, and scalp, as well as two gastrointestinal carcinomas and an intestinal polyp.[45] Fahmy et al. later suggested the name Muir–Torre syndrome to describe this constellation of findings.[46]

## Epidemiology

MTS is inherited as an autosomal dominant trait with high penetrance and variable expression. Median age (in years) at diagnosis and the appearance of skin lesions is 55 and 53, respectively, and for detection of the initial visceral neoplasm is 50.[43,47]

## Pathogenesis and etiology

MTS is a phenotypic variant of hereditary non-polyposis colorectal cancer (HNPCC), given its similar genetic origin and clinical characteristics.[48] Germline mutations of mismatch repair genes, most commonly hMSH2 but also hMLH1 and hMLH6, lead to microsatellite instability, and are detectable in the majority of MTS lesions.[49-52] MTS may represent the more full phenotypic expression of HNPCC.[48] It has been suggested that there are two subgroups of MTS patients. Those with microsatellite instability have earlier onset of colorectal cancer, greater numbers of visceral and skin tumors, and a strong family history. Those with microsatellite-stable neoplasms have late-onset cancers and a less pronounced family history.[51,53]

## Clinical features

The typical presentation of MTS is the presence of a sebaceous tumor and a low-grade visceral malignancy. A summary of published cases demonstrated that sebaceous tumors appeared before the internal malignancy in 22%, concurrently in 6%, and after the internal malignancy in 56% of patients.[48] The temporal relationship was unknown in 15%. Nearly half of MTS patients have more than one primary malignancy.[47] Gastrointestinal tumors are the most common internal malignancy, followed by those arising in urogenital tissues. Colorectal cancers arising in MTS are often proximally located, and are detected a decade earlier (median age 50 years) than those arising in the general population.[47] Seventeen of 44 sebaceous carcinomas in a large review of cases were of the meibomian gland.[48] Most of these sebaceous neoplasms develop on the head and neck, but they also can arise elsewhere.[51] In one series, keratoacanthomas were reported in 48% of patients.

## Patient evaluation, diagnosis, and differential diagnosis

Diagnostic criteria (Table 33.2) include the presence of at least one sebaceous adenoma, epithelioma or carcinoma (which excludes sebaceous hyperplasia and nevus sebaceus of Jadassohn) and at least one visceral cancer.[43,54] Patients may have only a solitary sebaceous neoplasm or hundreds. Incomplete clinical manifestations have been reported,

### Table 33.2 Diagnostic Criteria* for Muir–Torre Syndrome

| Group A |
| --- |
| Sebaceous adenoma |
| Sebaceous epithelioma |
| Sebaceous carcinoma |
| Keratoacanthoma with sebaceous differentiation |

| Group B |
| --- |
| Visceral malignancy |

| Group C |
| --- |
| Multiple keratoacanthomas |
| Multiple visceral malignancies |
| Family history of Muir–Torre syndrome |

*Diagnosis requires one criterion from group A and group B, or all three from group C, in the absence of other predisposing factors, such as radiotherapy for childhood retinoblastoma associated with eyelid sebaceous carcinoma, AIDS, and Kaposi sarcoma (in which case neither the Kaposi sarcoma nor a lymphoma should count as the visceral malignancy) or nevus sebaceus (in which neoplasms such as sebaceous epithelioma are predisposed to develop).

Modified from Michaelsson G, Olsson E, Westermark P. The Rombo syndrome: a familial disorder with vermiculate atrophoderma, milia, hpotrichosis, trichoepitheliomas, basal cell carcinomas and peripheral vasodilation with cyanosis. *Acta Derm Venereol.* 1981;61:497–503.

such as in patients on immunosuppressive medications, in family members of patients with MTS, and in cases of keratoacanthoma with visceral malignancy in the absence of sebaceous tumors.[43,51]

MTS is unique in the presence of sebaceous neoplasms. Conditions having multiple eruptive keratoacanthomas such as Ferguson–Smith and Grzybowski syndromes should be considered in the differential diagnosis. Gardner's syndrome can be easily distinguished from MTS since it is associated with colonic polyps and epidermal inclusion cysts, not sebaceous, tumors.

## Pathology

The histological features of sebaceous adenomas in MTS patients are identical to those seen in the general population.

## Treatment

Identification of a sebaceous neoplasm, even solitary, suggests the need for further screening for a possible internal malignancy.[55] Patients with MTS need regular monitoring for the development of cutaneous neoplasms, in addition to visceral malignancy. Sebaceous neoplasms should be excised or treated with Mohs micrographic surgery. Oral isotretinoin may be effective, as seen in two patients treated with low maintenance dosage who did not develop any new lesions while on therapy.[56] It has been recommended that MTS patients have annual colonoscopy, beginning at age 25.[43]

## EPIDERMODYSPLASIA VERRUCIFORMIS

Epidermodysplasia verruciformis (EV) is a rare genetic disease characterized by susceptibility to specific human papillomavirus (HPV) genotypes, with possible progression to SCC (see Chapter 19).

# OTHER GENETIC CONDITIONS ASSOCIATED WITH SKIN CANCERS

## Dyskeratosis congenita

Dyskeratosis congenita (DKC; Zinsser-Engman-Cole syndrome; MIM #305000, 127550, 224230), first described in 1904, is characterized by reticulate hyperpigmentation, premalignant leukoplakia, and nail dystrophy, in addition to multiple systemic abnormalities.[57] Most cases are inherited in an X-linked recessive manner, but autosomal dominant and autosomal recessive cases have been reported.[57]

## Pathogenesis and etiology

The X-linked recessive form of DKC is caused by mutations in the DKC1 gene, which was mapped to Xq28 and encodes dyskerin.[58] Patients with DKC have abnormally short telomeres, and DKC1 is involved in telomere length regulation.[59] The autosomal dominant form is associated with mutations in the RNA subunit of telomerase (TERC), the telomerase enzyme (TERT), and a component of the shelterin telomere protection complex (TINF2) genes.[60-62] The autosomal recessive form is associated with mutations in NOLA3 and NOLA2 genes, which are involved in telomerase regulation.[63,64]

## Clinical features

Reticulate pigmentation is usually the first cutaneous manifestation, and can be initially limited to the neck, chest, and proximal limbs. Other findings include nail dystrophy, thinning or early graying of hair, hyperkeratosis of the palms and soles, adermatoglyphia, and acrocyanosis.[59] Hematologic complications include bone marrow failure, myelodysplastic syndrome, and leukemia. Oral findings include leukoplakia, erythematous patches, brown/black patches, short tooth roots, and enlarged dental pulp. Additional systemic manifestations include esophageal stenosis, lacrimal duct obstruction, pulmonary fibrosis, cerebellar hypoplasia, osteoporosis, and gynecologic masses.[59] Bone marrow failure is the major cause of death, in addition to malignancy and pulmonary complications.[57]

A crude rate of 9.4% has been estimated for the development of all types of malignancies, with a median age at diagnosis of 29 years.[65] The crude death rate of those with cancer was 58%, and the median survival ages were 42 years for all patients and 39 and 46 years for those having or lacking cancer, respectively. The most frequent cancers were SCCs of the head and neck (mostly tongue), followed by cutaneous SCCs, anorectal cancer, stomach, lung, esophageal SCC, and Hodgkin disease. Acute myelogenous leukemia has also been reported.

## Patient evaluation, diagnosis, and differential diagnosis

The diagnosis of DKC can be challenging. Flow fluorescence in-situ hybridization can detect very short telomere length in addition to silent mutation carriers.[66] It has been shown to be sensitive and specific in distinguishing DKC patients from unaffected family members.[59] DKC needs to be distinguished from Fanconi's anemia, a disorder with dyspigmentation, hematologic abnormalities, and increased risk of malignancy. Fanconi's anemia differs from DKC by many clinical findings, including some of the types of associated malignancies, bony defects, renal and cardiac malformations, and the character of dyspigmentation.

## Treatment

Close surveillance of mucosal surfaces and skin, and strict photoprotection, are recommended, as well as monitoring for possible bone marrow failure. Regular dental, gynecologic, and otolaryngological examinations, and pulmonary function testing, should be performed.[59] Treatment with G-CSF and erythropoietin has been helpful in some patients, but hematopoeitic stem cell transplantation is the only definitive treatment for marrow failure.[59]

## Bazex–Dupré–Christol, Rombo, and Scleroatrophic syndromes

Bazex–Dupré–Christol syndrome (Bazex syndrome; MIM #301845), an X-linked dominant syndrome, is characterized by follicular atrophoderma with multiple BCCs, hypotrichosis (primarily head and neck), and hypohidrosis.[67] The gene has been linked to chromosome Xq24-q27.[68] Additional features include milia, twisted flattened hair shafts, skin hyperpigmentation, unusual facies (including pinched nose) and trichoepitheliomas.[67-70] Of note, follicular atrophoderma has also been described in X-linked dominant chondrodysplasia punctata.[68] Trichoepitheliomas may arise in this disease in childhood; BCCs have been diagnosed in the third and fourth decades and may resemble skin tags.[67,69]

Rombo syndrome (MIM #180730), an autosomal dominant disease, is characterized by vermiculate atrophoderma, BCCs, trichoepitheliomas, and acrocyanosis.[71] Its molecular basis is as yet unknown. Vermiculate atrophoderma causes the facial skin to appear coarse, grainy, and worm-eaten from the presence of follicular atrophy and yellowish papules. This may also occur on the upper chest, back, lateral and extensor arms. Hypotrichosis may be scattered diffusely. Pronounced cyanosis is seen in the lips, hands, and feet. Both vermiculate atrophoderma and cyanosis develop by ages 7 to 10. BCCs develop during middle age and may arise from trichoepitheliomas.[72]

Scleroatrophic syndrome of Huriez (sclerotylosis, scleroatrophic and keratotic dermatosis of limbs; Huriez syndrome; MIM #181600) is an autosomal dominant disease characterized by congenital atrophy of the distal extremities, palmoplantar keratoderma, and hypoplastic nail changes.[73,74] Hands are disproportionately small, with patchy reticulate erythema on the dorsum of the hands and feet, and with scleroatrophy of the digits. Palmoplantar hyperkeratosis is mild and is usually easily distinguishable from other hereditary keratodermas.[74] Nails can be hypoplastic, with ridging, distal splitting, and V-shaped notches.[74,75] Additional clinical features include poikiloderma-like changes on the nose, flexion contractures of the fifth digits, telangiectasias on the lips, and palmar nodules.[75] Aggressive SCCs, with early metastasis, develop in approximately 13%, typically in the third to fourth decade of life, with a 5% mortality rate.[74,76] The gene has been linked to chromosome 4q2371. It has been hypothesized that skin fragility leads to chronic scarring, predisposing to cancer, as seen in Marjolin's

### Table 33.3 Genetic Diseases Predisposing to Skin Malignancies

| Disease | Mode of Inheritance | Cutaneous Malignancies | Internal Malignancies* | Gene or Chromosome |
|---|---|---|---|---|
| Basal cell nevus syndrome | AD | BCC | Yes[1] | PTCH1, PTCH2 |
| Bazex–Dupre–Christol syndrome | XL dominant | BCC | No | Chromosome Xq24-X27 |
| Dyskeratosis congenita | XL recessive > AD or AR | SCC | Yes[2] | DKC1, TERC, TERT, TINF2, NOLA2, NOLA3 |
| EB, junctional (JEB) | AR[†] | SCC | No | LAMA3, LAMB3, LAMC2, COL17A |
| EB, recessive (RDEB) | AR | SCC (RDEB-sev gen > RDEB-gen mitis > RDEB-inversa MM (RDEB-sev gen) | No | COL7A |
| EB, simplex, Dowling-Meara variant (EBS-DM) | AD | BCC | No | K5, K14 |
| Epidermodysplasia verruciformis | AR | SCC | No | EV1, EVER1, EVER2 |
| Familial atypical mole-melanoma (FAMMM) syndrome | AD | MM | Yes[3] | CDKN2A, CDK4 |
| Ferguson–Smith syndrome | AD | Keratoacanthoma | No | Chromosome 9q22-q31 |
| Muir–Torre syndrome | AD | Sebaceous carcinoma, keratoacanthoma | Yes[4] | hMSH2, hMLH1, hMLH6 |
| Oculocutaneous albinism | AR; rare AD | SCC > BCC and MM | No | TYR, TPRP1, OCA2, MATP |
| Rombo syndrome | AD | BCC | No | Unknown |
| Scleroatrophy of Huriez | AD | SCC | No | Chromosome 4q23 |
| Xeroderma pigmentosum | AR | BCC, SCC, MM | No | XPA-G, XP-V |

AD, autosomal dominant; AR, autosomal recessive; XL, X-linked; BCC, basal cell carcinoma; SCC, squamous cell carcinoma; MM, malignant melanoma; EB, epidermolysis bullosa; JEB, junctional EB; RDEB, recessive dystrophic EB.

* Excluding oral cavity.

† One case of JEB with AD transmission has been recently reported.

[1] medulloblastoma

[2] anorectal; gastric; esophageal; lung; Hodgkin disease; myelodysplasia; leukemia

[3] pancreatic cancer

[4] gastrointestinal; urogenital

ulcers.[77] A complete absence of epidermal Langerhans cells in affected skin has been observed, suggesting that these patients are more susceptible to malignant degeneration via decreased cutaneous immunosurveillance.[74]

Table 33.3 summarizes other genetic diseases predisposed to develop skin cancers.

## FUTURE OUTLOOK

The results of a recent phase I clinical trial evaluating the use of GDC-0449 (a small-molecule inhibitor of smoothened for BCNS) in patients with locally advanced or metastatic BCCs has demonstrated a response.[78] This could provide an additional therapeutic option for patients with BCNS. Intensive research is also currently focused on wound healing, carcinogenesis, and gene replacement or, in the case of autosomal dominant diseases, gene inactivation.

A truly effective therapy in XP will likely require molecular correction of the affected gene. Further definition of the molecular basis of these diseases will improve our understanding and hopefully lead to additional therapeutic options.

Future advances in chemoprevention may also have a positive impact on reducing the risk of carcinogenesis in these diseases.

## REFERENCES

1. Gorlin RJ, Goltz RW. Multiple nevoid basal-cell epithelioma, jaw cysts and bifid rib. A syndrome. *N Engl J Med.* 1960;262:908–912.
2. Shanley S, Ratcliffe J, Hockey A. Nevoid basal cell carcinoma syndrome: review of 118 affected individuals. *Am J Med Genet.* 1994;50:282–290.
3. Evans DG, Frandon PA, Burnell LD, et al. The incidence of Gorlin syndrome in 173 consecutive cases of medulloblastoma. *Br J Cancer.* 1991;64:959–961.

4. Gailani MR, Bale SJ, Leffell DJ. Developmental defects in Gorlin syndrome related to a putative tumor suppressor gene on chromosome 9. *Cell.* 1992;69:111–117.

5. Farndon PA, Del Mastro RG, Evans DG, et al. Location of gene for Gorlin syndrome. *Lancet.* 1992;339:581–582.

6. Reis A, Kuster W, Linss G. Localisation of gene for naevoid basal-cell carcinoma syndrome. *Lancet.* 1992;339:617.

7. Hahn H, Christiansen J, Wicking C. A mammalian patched homolog is expressed in target tissues of sonic hedgehog and maps to a region associated with developmental abnormalities. *J Biol Chem.* 1996;271:12125–12128.

8. Hahn H, Wicking C, Zaphiropoulous PG. Mutations of the human homolog of Drosophilia patched in the nevoid basal cell carcinoma syndrome. *Cell.* 1996;85:841–851.

9. Johnson RL, Rothman AL, Xie J. Human homolog of patched, a candidate gene for the basal cell nevus syndrome. *Science.* 1996;272:1668–1671.

10. Smyth I, Narang MA, Evans T. Isolation and characterization of human patched 2 (PTCH2), a putative tumour suppressor gene in basal cell carcinoma and medulloblastoma on chromosome 1p32. *Hum Mol Genet.* 1999;8:291–297.

11. Wicking C, Smyth I, Bale A. The hedgehog signalling pathway in tumorigenesis and development. *Oncogene.* 1999;18:7844–7851.

12. Gorlin RJ. Nevoid basal-cell carcinoma sydrome. *Medicine (Baltimore).* 1987;66:98–113.

13. Kimonis VE, Goldstein AM, Pastakia B. Clinical manifestations in 105 persons with nevoid basal cell carcinoma syndrome. *Am J Med Genet.* 1997;69:299–308.

14. Gorlin RJ. Nevoid basal cell carcinoma syndrome. *Dermatol Clin.* 1995;13:113–125.

15. Strange PR, Lang PGJ. Long-term management of basal cell nevus syndrome with topical tretinoin and 5-fluorouracil. *J Am Acad Dermatol.* 1992;27:842–845.

16. Micali G, Lacarrubba F, Nasca MR, et al. The use of imiquimod 5% cream for the treatment of basal cell carcinoma as observed in Gorlin's syndrome. *Clin Exp Dermatol.* 2003;28(suppl 1):19–23.

17. Tangrea JA, Edwards BK, Taylor PR. Long-term therapy with low-dose isotretinoin for prevention of basal cell carcinoma: a multicenter clinical trial. Isotretinoin-Basal Cell Carcinoma Study Group. *J Natl Cancer Inst.* 1992;84:328–332.

18. Goldberg LH, Hsu SH, Alcalay J. Effectiveness of isotretinoin in preventing the appearance of basal cell carcinomas in basal cell nevus syndrome. *J Am Acad Dermatol.* 1989;21:144–145.

19. Sollitto RB, DIGiovanni JJ. Failure of interferon alfa and isotretinoin combination therapy in the nevoid basal cell carcinoma syndrome. *Arch Dermatol.* 1996;132:94–95.

20. Doctoroff A, Oberlender SA, Purcell SM. Full-face carbon dioxide laser resurfacing in the management of a patient with the nevoid basal cell carcinoma syndrome. *Dermatol Surg.* 2003;29:1236–1240.

21. Itkin A, Gilchrest BA. Delta-aminolevulinic acid and blue light photodynamic therapy for treatment of multiple basal cell carcinomas in two patients with nevoid basal cell carcinoma syndrome. *Dermatol Surg.* 2004;30:1054–1061.

22. Madan V, Loncaster JA, Allan D. Nodular basal cell carcinoma in Gorlin's syndrome treated with systemic photodynamic therapy and interstitial optical fiber diffuser laser. *J Am Acad Dermatol.* 2006;55:586–589.

23. Fine J-D, Eady RAJ, Bauer JA, et al. The classification of inherited epidermolysis bullosa (EB): report of the Third International Consensus Meeting on Diagnosis and Classification of EB. *J Am Acad Dermatol.* 2008;58(6):931–950.

24. Fine J-D, Hintner H. *Life with Epidermolysis Bullosa: Etiology, Diagnosis, and Multidisciplinary Care and Therapy.* Vienna: Springer Verlag; 2009.

25. Koebner H. Hereditare Anlage zur Blasenbildung (epidermolysis bullosa hereditaria). *Dtsch Med Wochenschr.* 1886;12:21–22.

26. Fine JD, Johnson LB, Suchindran C, et al. The epidemiology of inherited EB: findings within American, Canadian, and European study populations. In: Fine JD, Bauer EA, McGuire J, et al., eds. *Epidermolysis Bullosa: Clinical, Epidemiologic, and Laboratory Advances, and the Findings of the National Epidermolysis Bullosa Registry.* Baltimore: Johns Hopkins University Press; 1999:101–113.

27. Ortiz-Urda S, Garcia J, Green CL, et al. Type VII collagen is required for Ras-driven human epidermal tumorigenesis. *Science.* 2005;307:1773–1776.

28. Pourreyron C, Cox G, Mao X, et al. Patients with recessive dystrophic epidermolysis bullosa develop squamous-cell carcinoma regardless of type VII collagen expression. *J Invest Dermatol.* 2007;127:2438–2444.

29. Fine JD, Mellerio J. Extracutaneous manifestations and complications of inherited epidermolysis bullosa: Part II. Other organs. *J Am Acad Dermatol.* 2009;61(3):387–402.

30. Fine JD, Mellerio J. Extracutaneous manifestations and complications of inherited epidermolysis bullosa: Part I. Epithelial associated tissues. *J Am Acad Dermatol.* 2009;61(3):367–384.

31. Fine J-D, Johnson LB, Weiner M, et al. Cause-specific risks of childhood death in inherited epidermolysis bullosa. *J Pediatr.* 2008;152(2):276–280.

32. Fine J-D, Johnson LB, Weiner M, et al. Inherited epidermolysis bullosa (EB) and the risk of life-threatening skin-derived cancers: experience of the National EB Registry,1986–2006. *J Am Acad Dermatol.* 2009;60:203–211.

33. Fine J-D, Eady RAJ, Bauer EA, et al. Revised classification system for inherited epidermolysis bullosa: report of the Second International Consensus Meeting on diagnosis and classification of epidermolysis bullosa. *J Am Acad Dermatol.* 2000;42:1051–1066.

34. Fine JD, Smith LT. Non-molecular diagnostic testing of inherited epidermolysis bullosa: current techniques, major findings, and relative sensitivity and specificity. In: Fine JD, Bauer EA, McGuire J, et al., eds. *Epidermolysis Bullosa: Clinical, Epidemiologic, and Laboratory Advances, and the Findings of the National Epidermolysis Bullosa Registry.* Baltimore: Johns Hopkins University Press; 1999:48–78.

35. Cleaver JE, Lam ET, Revet I. Disorders of nucleotide excision repair: the genetic and molecular basis of heterogeneity. *Nat Genet.* 2009;10:756–768.

36. Reardon JT, Sancar A. Nucleotide excision repair. *Prog Nucleic Acid Res Mol Biol.* 2005;79:183–235.

37. Kraemer KH, Patronas NJ, Schiffmann R, et al. Xeroderma pigmentosum, trichothiodystrophy and Cockayne syndrome: a complex genotype-phenotype relationship. *Neuroscience.* 2007;145:1388–1396.

38. Cleaver JE. Defective repair replication in xeroderma pigmentosum. *Nature.* 1968;218:652–656.

39. Kleijer WJ, Laugel V, Berneburg M, et al. Incidence of DNA repair deficiency disorders in western Europe: xeroderma pigmentosum, Cockayne syndrome and trichothiodystrophy. *DNA Repair (Amst).* 2008;7:744–750.

40. D'Errico M, Calcagnile A, Canzona F, et al. UV mutation signature in tumor suppressor genes involved in skin carcinogenesis in xeroderma pigmentosum patients. *Oncogene.* 2000;19:463–467.

41. Wang Y, DIGiovanni JJ, Stern JB, et al. Evidence of ultraviolet type mutations in xeroderma pigmentosum melanomas. *Proc Natl Acad Sci USA.* 2009;106:6279–6284.

42. Ziegler A, Leffell DJ, Kunala S, et al. Mutation hotspots due to sunlight in the p53 gene of nonmelanoma skin cancers. *Proc Natl Acad Sci USA.* 1993;90:4216–4220.

43. Schwartz RA, Torre DP. The Muir-Torre syndrome: a 25-year retrospect. *J Am Acad Dermatol.* 1995;33:90–104.

44. Muir EG, Bell AJ, Barlow KA. Multiple primary carcinomata of the colon, duodenum, and larynx associated with kerato-acanthomata of the face. *Br J Surg.* 1967;54:191–195.

45. Torre D. Multiple sebaceous tumors. *Arch Dermatol.* 1968;98:549–551.

46. Fahmy A, Burgdorf WH, Schosser RH, et al. Muir-Torre syndrome: report of a case and reevaluation of the dermatopathologic features. *Cancer.* 1982;49:1898–1903.

47. Cohen PR, Kohn SR, Kurzrock R. Association of sebaceous gland tumors and internal malignancy: the Muir-Torre syndrome. *Am J Med.* 1991;90:606–613.

48. Akhtar S, Oza KK, Khan SA, et al. Muir-Torre syndrome: case report of a patient with concurrent jejunal and ureteral cancer and a review of the literature. *J Am Acad Dermatol.* 1999;41:681–686.

49. Kruse R, Lamberti C, Wang Y. Is the mismatch repair deficient type of Muir-Torre syndrome confined to mutations in the hMSH2 gene? *Hum Genet.* 1996;98:747–750.

50. Bapat B, Xia L, Madlensky L. The genetic basis of Muir-Torre syndrome includes the hMLH1 locus. *Am J Hum Genet.* 1996;59:736–739.

51. Ponti G, Losi L, Di Gregorio C. Identification of Muir-Torre syndrome among patients with sebaceous tumors and keratoacanthomas: role of clinical features, microsatellite instability, and immunohistochemistry. *Cancer.* 2005;103:1018–1025.

52. Mangold E, Rahner N, Friedrichs N. MSH6 mutation in Muir-Torre syndrome: could this be a rare finding? *Br J Dermatol.* 2007;156:158–162.

53. Honchel R, Halling KC, Schaid DJ, et al. Microsatellite instability in Muir-Torre syndrome. *Cancer Res.* 54;54:1159–1163.

54. Eisen DB, Michael DJ. Sebaceous lesions and their associated syndromes: Part II. *J Am Acad Dermatol.* 2009;61:563–578.

55. Rothenberg J, Lambert WC, Vail JTJ, et al. The Muir-Torre (Torre's) syndrome: the significance of a solitary sebaceous tumor. *J Am Acad Dermatol.* 1990;12:475–480.

56. Spielvogel RL, DeVillez RL, Roberts LC. Oral isotretinoin therapy for familial Muir-Torre syndrome. *J Am Acad Dermatol.* 1985;12:475–480.

57. Dokal I. Dyskeratosis congenita in all its forms. *Br J Haematol.* 2000;110:768–779.

58. Connor JM, Gatherer D, Gray FC, et al. Assignment of the gene for dyskeratosis congenita to Xq28. *Hum Genet.* 1986;72:348–351.

59. Savage SA, Dokal I, Armanios M. Dyskeratosis congenita: the first NIH clinical research workshop. *Pediatr Blood Cancer.* 2009;53:520–523.

60. Vulliamy T, Marrone A, Goldman F. The RNA component of telomerase is mutated in autosomal dominant dyskeratosis congenita. *Nature.* 2001;413:432–435.

61. Armanios M, Chen JL, Chang YP. Haploinsufficiency of telomerase reverse transcriptase leads to anticipation in autosomal dominant dyskeratosis congenita. *Proc Natl Acad Sci USA.* 2005;102:15960–15964.

62. Savage SA, Giri N, Baerlocher GM, et al. TINF2, a component of the shelterin telomere protection complex, is mutated in dyskeratosis congenita. *Am J Hum Genet.* 2008;82:501–509.

63. Waine AJ, Vulliamy T, Marrone A. Genetic heterogeneity in autosomal recessive dyskeratosis congenita with one subtype due to mutations in the telomerase-associated protein NOP10. *Hum Mol Genet.* 2007;16:1619–1629.

64. Vulliamy T, Beswick R, Kirwan M. Mutations in the telomerase component NHP2 cause the premature ageing syndrome dyskeratosis congenita. *Proc Natl Acad Sci USA*. 2008;105:8073–8078.

65. Alter BP, Giri N, Savage SA, et al. Cancer in dyskeratosis congenita. *Blood*. 2009;113:6549–6557.

66. Alter BP, Baerlocher GM, Savage SA. Very short telomere length by flow fluorescence in situ hybridization identifies patients with dyskeratosis congenita. *Blood*. 2007;110:1439–1447.

67. Castori M, Castiglia D, Passarelli F, et al. Bazex-Dupre-Christol syndrome: an ectodermal dysplasia with skin appendage neoplasms. *Eur J Med Genet*. 2009;52:250–255.

68. Vabres P, Lacombe D, Rabinowitz LG. The gene for Bazex-Dupre-Christol syndrome maps to chromosome Xq. *J Invest Dermatol*. 1995;105:87–91.

69. Gould DJ, Barker DJ. Follicular atrophoderma with multiple basal cell carcinomas (Bazex). *Br J Dermatol*. 1978;99:431–435.

70. Goeteyn M, Geerts ML, Kint A, et al. The Bazex-Dupre-Christol syndrome. *Arch Dermatol*. 1994;130:337–342.

71. Michaelsson G, Olsson E, Westermark P. The Rombo syndrome: a familial disorder with vermiculate atrophoderma, milia, hypotrichosis, trichoepitheliomas, basal cell carcinomas and peripheral vasodilation with cyanosis. *Acta Derm Venereol*. 1981;61:497–503.

72. Ashinoff R, Jacobson M, Belsito DV. Rombo syndrome: a second case report and review. *J Am Acad Dermatol*. 1993;28:1011–1014.

73. Huriez C, Agache P, Bombart M, et al. Spinocellular epitheliomas in congenital cutaneous atrophy in 2 families with high cancer morbidity. *Bull Soc Fr Derm Syph*. 1963;70:24–28.

74. Hamm H, Traupe H, Brocker E-B, et al. The scleroatrophic syndrome of Huriez: a cancer-prone genodermatosis. *Br J Dermatol*. 1996;134:512–518.

75. Kavanagh GM, Jardine PE, Peachey RD, et al. The scleroatrophic syndrome of Huriez. *Br J Dermatol*. 1997;137:114–118.

76. Delaporte E, N'Guyen-Mailfer C, Janin A. Keratoderma with scleroatrophy of the extremities or sclerotylosis (Huriez syndrome): a reappraisal. *Br J Dermatol*. 1995;133:409–416.

77. Lee YA, Stevens HP, Delaporte E, et al. A gene for an autosomal dominant scleroatrophic syndrome predisposing to skin cancer (Huriez syndrome) maps to chromosome 4q23. *Am J Hum Genet*. 2000;66:326–330.

78. Von Hoff DD, LoRusso PM, Rudin CM. Inhibition of hedgehog pathway in advanced basal-cell carcinoma. *N Engl J Med*. 2009;361:1164–1172.

# Dermatologic Manifestations of Internal Malignancy

*Diana D. Antonovich, Bruce H. Thiers, and Jeffrey P. Callen*

## Key Points

- Internal malignancy can involve the skin either directly or indirectly.
- Direct involvement is defined as tumor metastatic to the skin.
- Indirect involvement refers to changes in the skin that suggest the possibility of an underlying malignancy.
- Patients with direct involvement should be assumed to have an underlying neoplasm and must be evaluated accordingly.
- Patients with indirect involvement may not have an underlying neoplasm when first evaluated, but must be monitored for its possible future development.

## INTRODUCTION

The skin, the largest organ in the body, often mirrors changes occurring within the organism it envelops. A wide spectrum of inflammatory, proliferative, metabolic, and neoplastic diseases may affect the skin in association with an underlying malignancy. This chapter will focus on these changes, known collectively as the skin signs of internal malignancy. Internal cancer may affect the skin both directly and indirectly.[1] Direct involvement may be defined as the actual presence of malignant cells within the skin and includes neoplasms that often first become manifested in the skin, but eventually affect internal organs (such as mycosis fungoides), visceral neoplasms metastatic to the skin (such as the Sister Joseph nodule of gastric carcinoma), and tumors arising within or below the skin that ultimately spread to the cutaneous surface (such as mammary and extramammary Paget disease). Indirect involvement of the skin in cancer patients implies the absence of tumor cells within the skin. This group includes (1) inherited syndromes associated with skin manifestations and an increased incidence of systemic neoplasia, (2) cutaneous changes resulting from hormone secretion by tumors, and (3) a wide spectrum of proliferative and inflammatory disorders occurring in conjunction with internal malignancy.

## HISTORY

In the original text *Cancer of the Skin*, Curth outlined a set of criteria that could be used to analyze the relationship between an internal malignancy and a cutaneous disorder.[2] Curth's postulates, as Callen has subsequently labeled

them, consist of five characteristics: (1) a concurrent onset – the malignancy is discovered when the skin disease occurs; (2) a parallel course – if the malignancy is removed or successfully treated, the skin disease remits, and when the malignancy recurs, the cutaneous disease also recurs; (3) a uniform malignancy – there is a specific tumor cell type or site associated with the skin disease; (4) a statistical association – based on sound case-control studies there is a significantly more frequent occurrence of malignancy in a patient with a cutaneous disease; and (5) a genetic association. These criteria are extremely useful and should be satisfied before a link between an internal neoplasm and a specific skin change can be assumed.

## INHERITED SYNDROMES ASSOCIATED WITH INTERNAL MALIGNANCY

Many familial cancer syndromes have prominent dermatologic features. When characteristic skin findings are encountered, a thorough review of systems and family history should be undertaken. Genetic testing and counseling is a central component of patient management. Multidisciplinary care is often required. This topic has been extensively reviewed elsewhere and is summarized in Table 34.1.[3,4]

## SKIN CHANGES RESULTING FROM HORMONE-SECRETING TUMORS

Ectopic humoral syndromes are best understood in context of the APUD cell system (i.e. cells with a capacity of *a*mino *p*recursor *u*ptake and *d*ecarboxylation). These cells, which may have a common origin from the neural crest, can secrete a variety of biologically active amines and polypeptide hormones. Neoplastic proliferation of these cells may result in characteristic symptom complexes associated with specific cutaneous changes.

### Ectopic ACTH-producing tumors

Ectopic ACTH-producing tumors account for 10–15% of cases of Cushing syndrome, presenting with many typical signs of the syndrome, including hypertension, hypokalemia, and myasthenia gravis-like profound proximal muscle weakness.[5] However, intense hyperpigmentation (Fig. 34.10), occurring in only 6–10% of patients with Cushing's disease, is especially common in the setting of ectopic ACTH production and should alert the clinician to the possibility of a hormone-secreting tumor.[6] Although the cause of hyperpigmentation

## Table 34.1 Inherited Syndromes Associated with Internal Malignancy

| Disease | Inheritance, Genetic Defect | Clinical Findings | Associated Malignancy* |
|---|---|---|---|
| Cowden syndrome | AD, *PTEN* | Tricholemmomas (Fig. 34.1), 'cobblestone' oral papillomas, acral keratoses, macrocephaly, fibrocystic breast disease | Breast, thyroid |
| Gardner syndrome | AD, *APC* (adenomatous polyposis coli) | Epidermoid cysts (Fig. 34.2), osteomas, congenital hypertrophy of retinal pigment, gastrointestinal adenomatous polyps | Colorectal |
| Peutz–Jeghers syndrome | AD, *STK11* (serine/threonine kinase 11) | Brown-black macules (Figs 34.3, 34.4) on lips, oral mucosa, nails, palms, soles, hamartomatous gastrointestinal polyps, intussusception | Gastrointestinal, reproductive organs, breast, pancreas |
| Muir–Torre syndrome | AD, *MSH-2, MLH-1* | Sebaceous gland tumors (Fig. 34.5) | Gastrointestinal, genitourinary |
| Howel–Evans syndrome | AD, *TOC* (tylosis (o) esophageal cancer) | Palmoplantar hyperkeratosis over pressure points | Esophageal |
| Birt–Hogg–Dubé syndrome | AD, *BHD* | Fibrofolliculomas (Fig. 34.6), trichodiscomas, achrocordons, pulmonary cysts, spontaneous pneumothorax | Renal |
| Hereditary leiomyomatosis renal cell cancer syndrome | AD, *FH* (fumarate hydratase) | Cutaneous and uterine leiomyomas | Renal (papillary renal cell) |
| Multiple mucosal neuromas syndrome (MEN 2b) | AD, *RET* | Lip and oral cavity neuromas (Fig. 34.7), thick lips, marfanoid habitus, megacolon, pheochromocytoma | Thyroid (medullary) |
| Multiple endocrine neoplasia type 1 (Werner syndrome) | AD | Collagenomas, lipomas, angiofibromas, hypopigmented 'confetti-like' macules, CALMs, benign neoplasms of the pituitary, parathyroid, and pancreas | Pancreatic |
| Multiple endocrine neoplasia type 2a (Sipple syndrome) | AD | Notalgia paresthetica, macular/lichen amyloidosis, benign parathyroid tumors or hyperplasia, pheochromocytoma | Thyroid (medullary) |
| Bloom syndrome | AR, *RecQL3* helicase | Photosensitivity (Fig. 34.8), telangiectasia, CALMs, cheilitis, immunodeficiency | Leukemia, lymphoma, gastrointestinal |
| Ataxia-telangiectasia | AR, *ATM* | Skin and bulbar telangiectasia (Fig. 34.9), ataxia, elevated prenatal alpha-fetoprotein, immunodeficiency, sinopulmonary infections | Lymphoma, breast (heterozygote carriers) |
| Wiskott–Aldrich syndrome | X-linked AR, *WAS* | Eczematous dermatitis, petechiae, recurrent infections, bloody diarrhea, immunodeficiency | Lymphoma |
| Chédiak–Higashi syndrome | AR, *LYST* | Silvery light hair, light grayish skin, immunodeficiency, recurrent infections | Lymphoma, lymphoma-like phase |
| Griscelli syndrome | AR, *myosin5a, Rab27a* | Pigmentary loss, immunodeficiency, recurrent infections | Lymphoma-like phase |
| Werner syndrome | AR, *RecQL2* helicase | Sclerodermoid, hyperkeratosis and ulcerations over bony prominences, accelerated aging | Fibrosarcoma, osteosarcoma |
| Rothmund–Thomson syndrome | AR, *RecQL4* helicase | Photosensitivity, poikiloderma, acral keratoses, skeletal abnormalities | Osteosarcoma, fibrosacoma |
| Nevoid basal cell syndrome | AR, *PTCH1* | Multiple basal cell carcinomas, palmoplantar pits, odontogenic cysts, calcified falx cerebri | Fibrosarcoma, medulloblastoma |
| Neurofibromatosis type I | AD | CALMs, axillary freckling, neurofibromas, Lisch nodules | Rhabdomyosarcoma, neurofibrosarcoma, Wilms' tumor, juvenile myelomonocytic leukemia (in children with concomitant juvenile xanthogranulomas) |

AD, autosomal dominant; AR, autosomal recessive; CALMs, café-au-lait macules.

*Those listed represent only the most common associated malignancies.

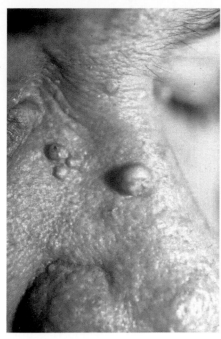

Figure 34.1 Cowden syndrome. Multiple tricholemmomas, few have a wart-like appearance.

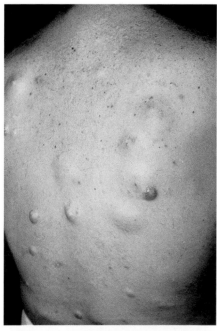

Figure 34.2 Gardner syndrome. Multiple epidermoid cysts.

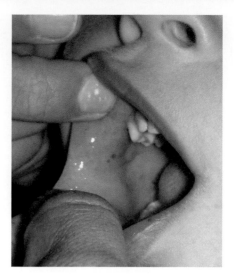

Figure 34.3 Peutz–Jeghers syndrome. Multiple brown macules on the buccal mucosa and vermillion lip.

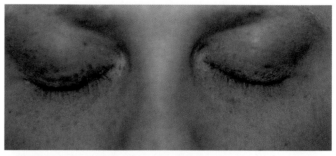

Figure 34.4 Peutz–Jeghers syndrome. Multiple periorbital brown macules.

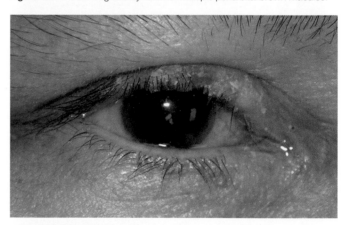

Figure 34.5 Muir–Torre syndrome. Sebaceous carcinoma involving the upper eyelid. Note associated loss of eyelashes. (Image courtesy of Dr. Joel Cook, Charleston, SC.)

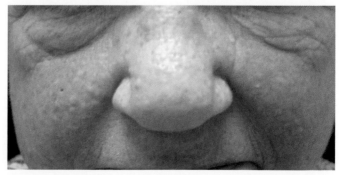

Figure 34.6 Birt–Hogg–Dubé syndrome. Multiple monomorphous flesh-colored fibrofolliculomas.

is unclear, it may be related to tumor production of the peptide β-lipotropin, which contains within its sequence of 91 amino acids, the 22 amino acid sequence of β-melanocyte stimulating hormone (MSH). Serum ACTH levels are usually very elevated. Bronchopulmonary tumors, particularly oat cell carcinoma, are most often associated with ectopic ACTH production, although other malignancies have been reported.

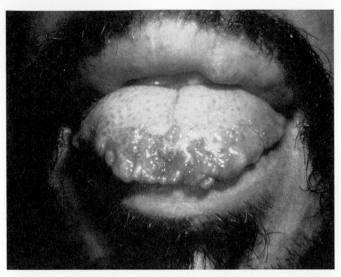

**Figure 34.7** Multiple mucosal neuromas syndrome. Multiple neuromas on the tongue.

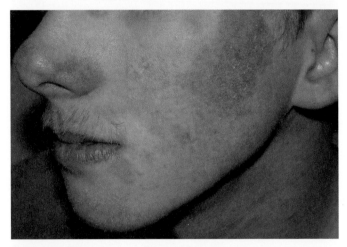

**Figure 34.8** Bloom syndrome. Photodistributed telangiectasia and scaly plaques. (Image courtesy of Dr. Joel Cook, Charleston, SC.)

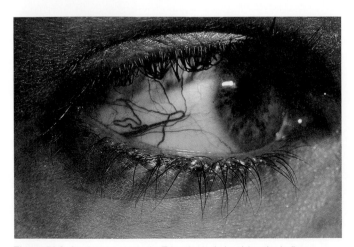

**Figure 34.9** Ataxia-telangiectasia. Telangiectasia involving the bulbar conjunctiva.

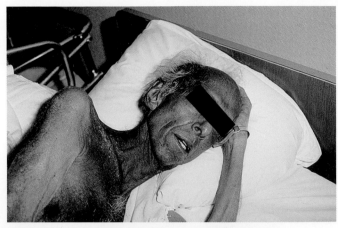

**Figure 34.10** Ectopic ACTH syndrome. Diffuse hyperpigmentation. (Image courtesy of Dr. Donald Lookingbill, Jacksonville, FL.)

## Carcinoid syndrome

The carcinoid syndrome is another example of a humoral syndrome associated with a non-endocrine tumor. Elevated serotonin levels are characteristic, but multiple vasoactive molecules contribute to the syndrome's numerous systemic symptoms. The most striking cutaneous manifestations are episodes of flushing, initially lasting 10 to 30 minutes and involving only the upper half of the body; as the flush resolves, gyrate and serpiginous patterns may be noted. With successive attacks, more extensive areas may be affected and the redness takes on a cyanotic quality, eventually leading to a more permanent facial cyanotic flush with associated telangiectasia, resembling rosacea (Fig. 34.11). Persistent edema and erythema of the face may result in leonine facies. A pellagra-like picture that has been noted in some patients may be due to abnormal tryptophan metabolism. Systemic symptoms associated with

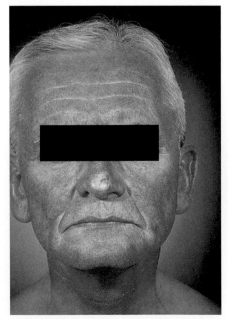

**Figure 34.11** Carcinoid syndrome. Persistent facial erythema. (Image courtesy of Dr. Walter Lobitz, Portland, OR.)

cutaneous flushing include abdominal pain with explosive watery diarrhea, shortness of breath, palpitations, and hypertension.

Carcinoid tumors are usually found in the appendix or small intestine; extraintestinal carcinoids may arise in the bile ducts, pancreas, stomach, ovaries, testis, or bronchi. The carcinoid syndrome occurs primarily with intestinal carcinoids metastatic to the liver or with extraintestinal tumors; flushing attacks can be provoked by palpation of hepatic or abdominal metastases or by alcohol ingestion, enemas, emotional stress, or sudden changes in body temperature. When the syndrome is associated with bronchial adenomas of the carcinoid variety, the flushing is more prolonged and often associated with fever, marked anxiety, disorientation, sweating, salivation and lacrimation. Elevated 24-hour urine 5-hydroxyindoleacetic acid (5-HIAA), a metabolite of serotonin, is a useful marker for diagnosis. The somatostatin analog, octreotide, may be used for symptomatic control.[7]

## Glucagonoma syndrome

The glucagonoma syndrome is associated with an APUDoma involving the glucagon-secreting alpha cell of the pancreas.[8] The characteristic cutaneous eruption, necrolytic migratory erythema, usually occurs on the abdomen, perineum, thighs, buttocks (Fig. 34.12), and groin, and may be mistaken for intertrigo. Patches of intense erythema with irregular outlines expand and coalesce, resulting in circinate or polycyclic configurations. Superficial vesicles on the surface rupture quickly to form crusts, but new vesicles may continue to develop along the active margins. An eczema craquelé-like appearance may be noted. Angular cheilitis and glossitis are additional features. Patients may be hyperglycemic and ill-appearing. The syndrome shares features with acrodermatitis enteropathica; deficiency of zinc, amino acids, and essential fatty acid levels occurs in some cases. Nutritional supplementation can improve cutaneous involvement; however,

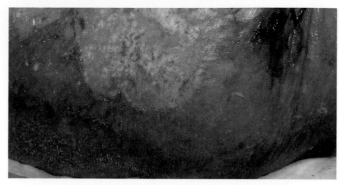

Figure 34.12 Necrolytic migratory erythema. Large erosion involving the buttocks. (Image courtesy of Dr. Marta Hampton, Charleston, SC.)

complete tumor resection is necessary for cure. The overall prognosis is poor as approximately 50% of cases are metastatic at the time of diagnosis.

The three clinical patterns of familial multiple endocrine neoplasia discussed above are also examples of polyglandular endocrine disorders involving the APUD cell system.

## PROLIFERATIVE AND INFLAMMATORY DERMATOSES ASSOCIATED WITH INTERNAL MALIGANCY (Table 34.2)

Many of the conditions discussed in this section are nonspecific and have been reported both in association with and in the absence of underlying malignant disease. Malignancy is most often only one of a number of possible provoking factors.

## Hypertrichosis lanuginosa acquisita

The association of acquired hypertrichosis lanuginosa (malignant down) with cancer is among the most consistent. The hair growth is extensive, non-pigmented, silky, fine

### Table 34.2 Proliferative and Inflammatory Dermatoses Associated with Internal Malignancy

| Dermatoses | Findings | Associated Malignancy* |
|---|---|---|
| Hypertrichosis lanuginosa acquisita | Extensive lanugo hair | Women – colorectal, lung, breast<br>Men – lung, colorectal |
| Acanthosis nigricans | Flexural velvety hyperpigmentation, oral cavity papillomatous change, +/- tripe palms | Intra-abdominal adenocarcinoma, gastric most commonly |
| Tripe palms | Diffuse palmar ridging | Lung gastric adenocarcinoma if in setting of acanthosis nigricans |
| Sign of Leser–Trélat | Sudden-onset multiple seborrheic keratoses | Gastrointestinal |
| Bazex syndrome (acrokeratosis paraneoplastica) | Violaceous psoriasiform plaques on fingers, toes, nose, helices<br>Nail dystrophy | Aerodigestive tract |
| Primary systemic amyloidosis | Protein AL deposition in multiple organs, facial perioroficial waxy papules, 'pinch purpura', macroglossia | Multiple myeloma |
| Scleromyxedema | IgG lambda paraprotein Waxy lichenoid papules on face, neck, upper trunk, upper extremities<br>Multiorgan system involvement | Multiple myeloma |

*(Continued)*

**Table 34.2 Proliferative and inflammatory dermatoses associated with internal malignancy—Cont'd**

| Dermatoses | Findings | Associated Malignancy* |
|---|---|---|
| Sweet syndrome (acute febrile neutrophilic dermatoses) | Violaceous pseudovesicular plaques on face, neck, upper extremities<br>Fever<br>Neutrophilia | Hematologic, particularly acute myelogenous leukemia |
| Pyoderma gangrenosum | Deep ulcerations with undermined dusky border, pseudovesicular plaques | Hematologic, particularly acute myelogenous leukemia |
| Paraneoplastic pemphigus | Polymorphous cutaneous eruption that may be lichenoid, bullous, or erosive<br>Mucosal involvement<br>Bronchiolitis obliterans | Non-Hodgkin lymphoma, chronic lymphocytic leukemia |
| Anti-epiligrin cicatricial pemphigoid | Painful mucosal erosions, eyes and oral cavity<br>Scarring, blindness | Solid tumors |
| Dermatomyositis | Heliotrope rash, Gottron's papules, photosensitivity, periungual erythema, cuticular overgrowth, poikiloderma<br>Proximal muscle weakness | Women – ovarian, breast. Men… lung, prostate |
| Extramammary Paget disease | Erythematous scaly plaque, erosions, involving groin, axillae, perianal areas | Gastrointestinal, urogenital, apocrine carcinoma |
| Multicentric reticulohistiocytosis | Flesh-colored to brownish nodules involving hands and face<br>Destructive polyarthritis | Cervical, gastric, breast, bronchial, hematologic |
| Necrobiotic xanthogranuloma | Yellow-orange noduloplaques, periorbital, trunk, extremities<br>IgG kappa paraprotein<br>Multisystem disorder | Myeloma, leukemia, lymphoma |
| Erythema gyratum repens | Figurate erythema with scaly 'wood-grain' appearance | Bronchial carcinoma > breast, uterine, prostate, gastrointestinal, myeloma |
| Exaggerated insect bite reaction | Papulonodular or vesiculobullous<br>Exposed sites | Chronic lymphocytic leukemia |

*Those listed represent only the most common associated malignancies.

lanugo hair, typically involving the face (Fig. 34.13), neck, trunk, and sometimes the extremities. Acanthosis nigricans, painful glossitis, and swollen fungiform papillae on the anterior tongue may accompany the cutaneous changes. Women are disproportionately affected. Colorectal cancer followed by lung and breast cancers are the most common associated malignancies in women; for men, lung followed by colorectal cancers are the most common. Hematologic, genitourinary, pancreatic, gallbladder, and soft tissue sarcoma are malignancies that have also been reported.[9] Occurrence is usually late in the course of the cancer but may rarely be a presenting sign. Other causes of hypertrichosis, such as porphyria cutanea tarda, anorexia nervosa, endocrinopathy, and medication reaction, must be ruled out.

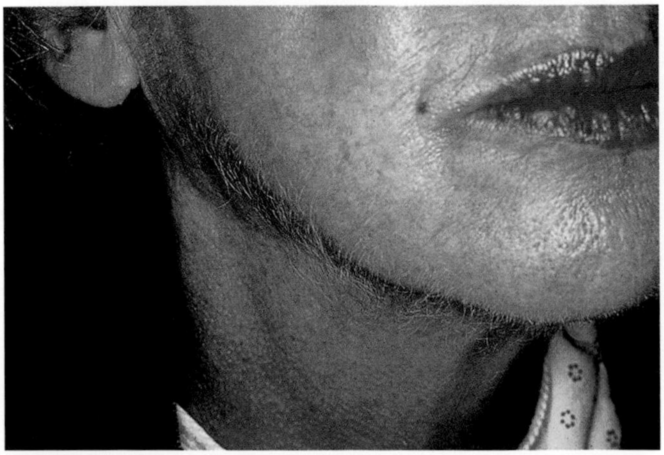

## Acanthosis nigricans

Acanthosis nigricans is perhaps the best known of the cutaneous markers of internal malignancy. Flexural areas, especially the axillae, groin and neck, are most commonly involved; the skin has a hyperpigmented velvety appearance and in severe cases can become quite verrucous (Fig. 34.14). Papillomatous changes may be noted in the oral cavity and hyperkeratosis in a rugose pattern may develop on the palms (tripe palms) and dorsal surfaces of large joints. Oral acanthosis nigricans is more strongly correlated with underlying malignancy.[10] The cutaneous changes can occur before, coincident with (60%), or after the discovery of the underlying malignancy, which most often is an adenocarcinoma, most commonly of the stomach, but almost always in the abdominal cavity.[11] Acanthosis nigricans is idiopathic or associated with benign conditions (familial, obesity, endocrine dysfunction) in the vast majority of cases, therefore, a detailed history must be included in the evaluation of all affected patients. The possibility of underlying cancer should be strongly considered in any non-obese adult who develops acanthosis nigricans in the absence of

**Figure 34.13** Acquired hypertrichosis lanuginosa. Excessive non-pigmented hair on the face.

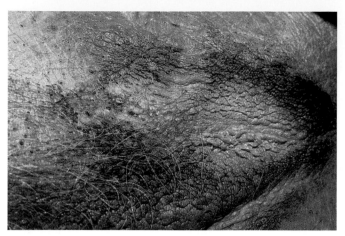

**Figure 34.14** Acanthosis nigricans. Flexural verrucous hyperpigmented plaque. (Image courtesy of Dr. Frederic Stearns, Tulsa, OK.)

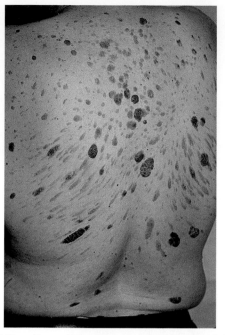

**Figure 34.15** Sign of Leser–Trélat. Numerous truncal seborrheic keratoses.

a recognizable endocrinopathy, particularly if of abrupt onset with rapid progression. Such an individual requires an extensive gastrointestinal evaluation.

## Tripe palms

Tripe palms refers to a diffuse, thickened, ridged appearance to the palms. The name originates from the condition's resemblance to the surface of the bovine stomach. Its presence is strongly associated with an underlying malignancy affecting the lung. It may also occur in the setting of acanthosis nigricans, in which case the most common associated malignancy is gastric adenocarcinoma. There is speculation that tripe palms merely represents site-specific acanthosis nigricans; the two conditions are similar histopathologically. In 60% of cases, tripe palms predate the diagnosis of the underlying cancer.[12]

## Sign of Leser–Trélat

The sign of Leser–Trélat refers to the sudden appearance and/or rapid increase in size of multiple seborrheic keratoses (Fig. 34.15), most often associated with carcinoma of the gastrointestinal tract.[13] Hematologic and reproductive organ malignancies have also been associated. Pruritus is a reported feature in 43% of patients. Because some of these patients have coexistent acanthosis nigricans and the malignancy is often an adenocarcinoma of gastrointestinal origin, some propose that this condition may represent a generalized variant of acanthosis nigricans. Given the frequency with which multiple seborrheic keratoses are seen in older individuals, the sign of Leser–Trélat as a true paraneoplastic marker has been challenged.

## Bazex syndrome (acrokeratosis paraneoplastica)

Patients with Bazex syndrome develop erythematous to violaceous psoriasiform plaques predominantly involving the fingers (Fig. 34.16), toes, nose, and helices. The nails are typically dystrophic and the palms are hyperkeratotic. Progression may result in more widespread involvement. The syndrome is universally associated with an under-lying

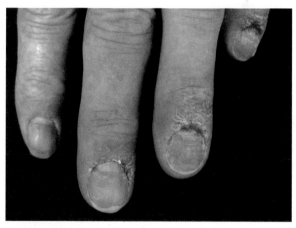

**Figure 34.16** Bazex syndrome. Erythematous to violaceous psoriasiform plaques and nail dystrophy.

malignancy, mostly squamous cell carcinomas of the 'aerodigestive' tract, and its course parallels that of the cancer. In 20% of cases the skin findings are coincident with the cancer, while predating it in 60%.[14]

## Primary systemic amyloidosis

Primary systemic amyloidosis is characterized by the deposition of protein AL, comprised of light chains, into multiple organs, including heart, gastrointestinal tract, nerves, and skin. Cutaneous involvement is reported in 25–40% of cases.[15] Shiny, smooth, waxy papules favor facial periorificial areas but may be found elsewhere (Fig. 34.17). Amyloid infiltration of blood vessels results in fragility manifesting as 'pinch purpura' around the eyes, oral cavity, and areas subject to trauma. Bullous amyloidosis is characterized by hemorrhagic blisters and is a rare finding. Macroglossia affects 20% of patients (Fig. 34.18). Patients with primary systemic amyloidosis almost always have an underlying plasma cell dyscrasia, with multiple myeloma occurring

**373**

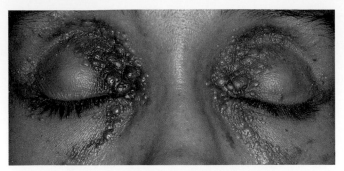

Figure 34.17 Primary systemic amyloidosis. Periorbital smooth, waxy papules and pinch purpura. (Image courtesy of Dr. Ross Pollack, Charleston, SC.)

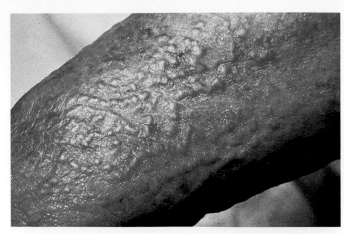

Figure 34.19 Scleromyxedema. Multiple linearly arranged waxy papules.

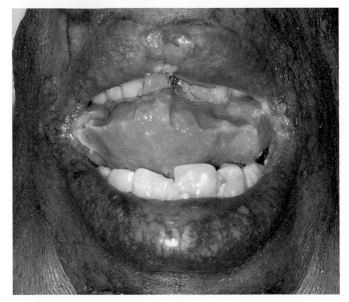

Figure 34.18 Primary systemic amyloidosis. Macroglossia. (Image courtesy of Dr. Ross Pollack, Charleston, SC.)

in approximately 13–16%.[16] The prognosis is poor but may improve with chemotherapy including melphalan and stem cell transplantation.

## Scleromyxedema

Scleromyxedema, a cutaneous mucinosis representing the generalized variant of lichen myxedematosus, has been associated with a serum monoclonal paraprotein in 80% of cases.[16–19] The paraprotein is usually of the IgG class and almost always possesses light chains of the lambda type. Clinically, the disorder appears as a generalized eruption of 2–3-mm waxy lichenoid papules, often in a linear arrangement (Fig. 34.19); lesions are most common on the hands, elbows, forearms, upper trunk, face and neck, but may be found anywhere. Induration of the underlying tissue may resemble scleroderma and result in tightening. Mucin deposition in forehead skin may be disfiguring and lead to longitudinal furrowing reminiscent of leonine facies. Systemic involvement involving multiple organ systems, including gastrointestinal, pulmonary, musculoskeletal, and CNS, may occur. Infiltration of the esophagus produces dysphagia. No correlation appears to exist between the levels of the

paraprotein and the extent or progression of the skin disease. Only a minority of patients have overt myeloma or a detectable plasma cell dyscrasia. Thus, the role of plasma cells or the paraprotein in the pathogenesis of scleromyxedema remains unclear. Nevertheless, affected patients should be screened with urine and serum protein electrophoresis and immunofixation electrophoresis. Thyroid dysfunction should be ruled out. The disease course tends to be chronic and progressive and treatment-resistant.

## Sweet syndrome (acute febrile neutrophilic dermatosas)

Numerous potential triggers for Sweet syndrome have been reported including: pregnancy, infection, inflammatory bowel disease, medication, and underlying malignancy in approximately 20% of cases. Hematologic malignancies are the most common associated cancer, accounting for 85%, particularly acute myelogenous leukemia. Solid tumors have also been reported with the syndrome.[20] Clinical presentation includes acute onset of violaceous, dusky, pseudovesicular plaques involving the face, upper extremities, and neck (Figs 34.20 and 34.21). Fever, malaise and neutrophilia accompany the cutaneous eruption, which histologically

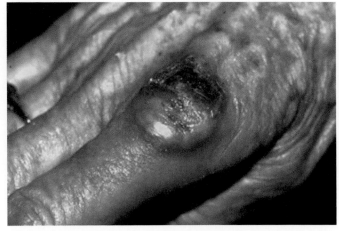

Figure 34.20 Sweet syndrome. Violaceous pseudovesicular plaque on the dorsal hand.

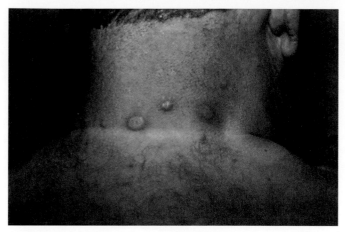

**Figure 34.21** Sweet syndrome. Pseudovesicular papules and plaques on the neck.

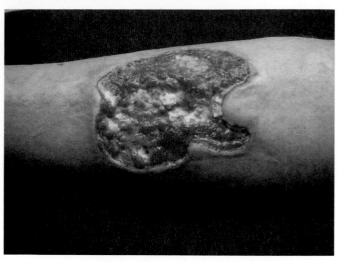

**Figure 34.22** Pyoderma gangrenosum. Deep, undermined ulcer with a dusky border involving the lower extremity.

shows a dense dermal neutrophilic infiltrate. Features that may aid in distinguishing malignancy-associated Sweet syndrome include: extensive involvement, bullous or ulcerative lesions, oral involvement, absence of neutrophilia, and the presence of anemia, thrombocytopenia, or neutropenia.[21] Patients with cytopenias may benefit from bone marrow evaluation. Cutaneous involvement readily responds to treatment with systemic corticosteroids.

## Pyoderma gangrenosum

Pyoderma gangrenosum is a neutrophilic ulcerative dermatosis often occurring in association with underlying illness, including inflammatory bowel disease, rheumatologic and hematologic disorders. Several clinical variants exist. The atypical bullous form is more closely associated with hematologic disease or underlying malignancy, occurring in as many as 27% of cases.[22] While acute myelogenous leukemia is most common, other proliferative hematologic disorders and solid tumors are also associated. Lesions of atypical bullous pyoderma gangrenosum tend to be superficial and vesiculobullous affecting the face, neck, and dorsal hands, unlike the deeper, undermined ulcers on the lower extremities characteristic of classic pyoderma gangrenosum (Fig. 34.22). Pyoderma gangrenosum has been associated with a monoclonal gammopathy, mostly IgA, in up to 18% of patients.[23,24] Multiple myeloma is rarely associated.[24] Some suggest that pyoderma gangrenosum may be related to Sweet syndrome. As with Sweet syndrome, affected patients should have a careful hematologic evaluation, and bone marrow biopsy is indicated in select patients.

## Immunobullous disorders

*Paraneoplastic pemphigus* (PNP) by definition manifests in association with underlying neoplasia, both benign and malignant. Non-Hodgkin lymphoma occurs most commonly, in approximately 40% of cases, followed by chronic lymphocytic leukemia, and Castleman disease.[25] Castleman disease is more common in children with PNP. Other related tumors are thymoma, sarcoma, and lung cancer. Waldenström's macroglobulinemia has also been reported

in the setting of PNP. In 50% of cases the diagnosis of malignancy predates the mucocutaneous findings.[26] A polymorphous cutaneous eruption is characteristic; skin lesions may be erythema multiforme-like, lichenoid, bullous, or erosive. Mucosal involvement may be severe, affecting the eyes, oral cavity, and genitalia. Bronchiolitis obliterans is increasingly reported as a cause of mortality.[27] The removal of benign tumors results in resolution of the mucocutaneous lesions. Overall, the prognosis is poor.

*Anti-epiligrin cicatricial pemphigoid* (AECP) is a subtype of mucous membrane pemphigoid manifesting autoantibodies that target laminin-5 (epiligrin). Like other subtypes of cicatricial pemphigoid, AECP affects the mucosal surfaces, particularly the conjunctiva and oral cavity (Fig. 34.23); painful erosions may lead to scarring and blindness. Additionally, AECP is reported to carry an increased relative risk of internal malignancy.[28] Cancers reported with AECP have primarily been solid tumors, particularly adenocarcinoma, often diagnosed within the first year of the onset of cutaneous lesions. A more recent report suggests that the relative risk of AECP-associated malignancy may be lower than initially proposed.[29]

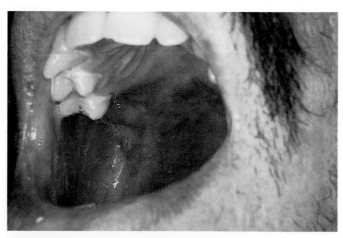

**Figure 34.23** Anti-epiligrin cicatricial pemphigoid. Multiple erosions involving the palate. (Image courtesy of Dr. Kim Yancey, Milwaukee, WI.)

The proposed association of bullous pemphigoid with malignancy probably reflects the tendency of both of these conditions to occur in the elderly rather than any true association. Individuals with dermatitis herpetiformis may have an increased relative risk of intestinal lymphoma similar to that noted in patients with celiac disease alone.[30] Epidermolysis bullosa acquisita has also very rarely been reported in patients with lymphoreticular tumors.

## Dermatomyositis

Pathognomonic clinical manifestations include an edematous, violaceous eruption of the upper eyelids (heliotrope rash) and atrophic scaly papules over bony prominences (Gottron papules) (Fig. 34.24); photosensitivity, malar erythema, proximal muscle weakness, poikiloderma (Fig. 34.25) and periungual telangiectasias are important, although less specific, findings. Approximately 10–30% of adult patients with dermatomyositis have an associated malignancy.[31] The neoplasm may occur before, concurrent with, or after the diagnosis of dermatomyositis. An awareness of this potential should alert the physician to carefully evaluate all dermatomyositis patients for malignancy. Dermatomyositis is not specific for any particular site or cell type of cancer; however, in Western countries, ovarian and breast carcinoma in women and lung and prostate carcinoma in men are overrepresented. The risk of developing cancer is highest in the first 3 years after the diagnosis of dermatomyositis.[32] Raynaud's phenomenon, pulmonary fibrosis or features of scleroderma, when they occur in an adult with dermatomyositis, suggest an overlap syndrome, a variant that is much less frequently associated with malignant disease. Childhood dermatomyositis is not associated with malignancy. Screening for malignancy should be done at the time of presentation, and annually for the 3 years that follow.[33] In all patients, screening should include computed tomography (CT) of the chest and abdomen, rectal examination and stool hematest. For women, screening should include pelvic examination with ultrasound and CT as well as mammography. A prostate-specific antigen level should be determined in men.

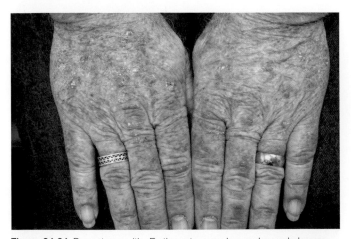

**Figure 34.24** Dermatomyositis. Erythematous scaly papules and plaques, periungual erythema, and cuticular overgrowth.

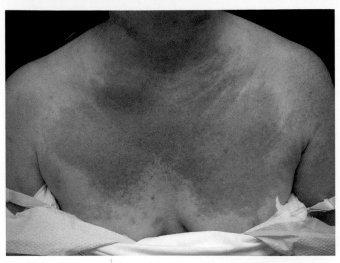

**Figure 34.25** Dermatomyositis. Violaceous poikilodermatous plaque.

## Cutaneous leukocytoclastic vasculitis

A purported association between cutaneous leukocytoclastic vasculitis and cancer has not been proven, although numerous individual case reports have related various vasculitic syndromes to malignancy, particularly lymphoproliferative disorders but also solid tumors.[34] Often, the patient with coexistent neoplastic disease has the malignancy at the time of diagnosis of the vasculitis. In other cases, release of tumor antigens into the circulation, such as after radiation therapy or chemotherapy, may be the inciting event. A parallel course between the tumor and the vasculitis has not been evident except in a few instances.

## Extramammary Paget disease

Extramammary Paget disease manifests as an erythematous, scaly, sometimes eroded plaque affecting the groin, axillae, or perianal area (Fig. 34.26). Its presence should alert the clinician to the possibility of an underlying, non-contiguous, gastrointestinal, urogenital, or apocrine carcinoma. In most cases extramammary Paget disease is a primary intraepithelial adenocarcinoma unrelated to an underlying cancer. Approximately 25% of cases are associated with an underlying cancer.[35] Perianal lesions are more likely to be associated with secondary malignancy, particularly colorectal cancer.

## Multicentric reticulohistiocytosis

Multicentric reticulohistiocytosis is characterized by the combination of destructive polyarthritis and the appearance of multiple flesh-colored to brownish nodules involving the hands, including periungual sites, and face. Approximately 20–25% of cases have an associated malignancy. An array of cancers have been reported, including cervical, gastric, breast, bronchial, and hematologic malignancies.[36,37] The diagnosis of cancer usually postdates the onset of skin lesions.

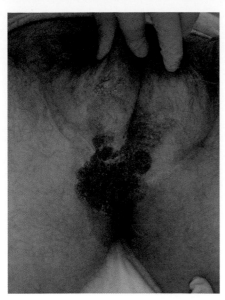

Figure 34.26 Extramammary Paget disease. Large eroded plaque.

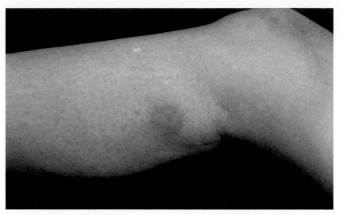

Figure 34.28 Exaggerated insect bite reaction. Erythematous indurated plaque on the lower extremity.

## Necrobiotic xanthogranuloma

Necrobiotic xanthogranuloma is a chronic, potentially multisystem disorder. Cutaneous lesions appear as yellow-orange indurated noduloplaques with a predilection for the periorbital area followed by the trunk and extremities. The upper airway, lungs, heart, and eyes may also be affected. Eighty percent of cases are associated with a monoclonal gammopathy, usually IgG kappa type.[38] Myeloma, leukemia, and lymphoma have been reported to occur in association and may be diagnosed years after the onset of cutaneous lesions.

## Erythema gyratum repens

Erythema gyratum repens is a rare figurate erythema with striking cutaneous findings. Multiple wavy urticarial bands with a fine scale migrate over the cutaneous surface, giving it an appearance similar to the grain of wood (Fig. 34.27). Approximately 80% of cases are malignancy associated. Bronchial carcinoma is the most common, followed by breast, bladder, uterine, prostate, gastrointestinal, and myeloma.[39,40] Erythema gyratum repens may rarely occur in association with inflammatory dermatoses. The skin eruption predates the diagnosis of malignancy in 80% of cases, by months to years.[41] Exhaustive cancer screening is required at presentation, and ongoing surveillance if a malignancy is not initially detected.

## Exaggerated insect bite reaction

Exaggerated insect bite reactions may be a sign of hematologic malignancy, particularly chronic lymphocytic leukemia (CLL).[42] The characteristic lesions are indurated papulonodules (Fig. 34.28) or vesiculobullous, occurring on exposed areas, more commonly during the spring and summer. The reaction can be severe and persistent, requiring systemic corticosteroids for clearance. Mosquitoes are typically the offending arthropod. Affected patients may not be able to recall the initiating arthropod assault. No clear relationship exists between the state of the underlying malignancy and the presence or severity of the cutaneous reaction.[43] Exaggerated arthropod reactions may develop prior to the diagnosis of malignancy, as CLL is generally a low-grade cancer in its initial stage and patients may otherwise be asymptomatic. Individuals presenting with exaggerated insect bite reactions should be questioned regarding the presence of constitutional symptoms and complete blood cell count with differential should be obtained.

## FUTURE OUTLOOK

The dermatologist can play an integral role in cancer diagnosis by recognizing cutaneous manifestations of internal malignancy. Better recognition of these signs may lead to earlier diagnosis and hopefully improve the prognosis of affected patients.

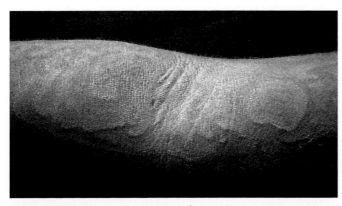

Figure 34.27 Erythema gyratum repens. Concentric scaly bands resulting in wood-grain appearance.

# REFERENCES

1. Thiers BH. Dermatologic manifestations of internal cancer. *CA Cancer J Clin*. 1986;36(3):130–138.
2. Curth HO. Skin lesions and internal carcinoma. In: Andrade R, Gumport SL, Popkin GL, eds. *Cancer of the Skin*. Philadlphia: WB Saunders; 1976:1308–1309.
3. Somoano B, Tsao H. Genodermatoses with cutaneous tumors and internal malignancies. *Dermatol Clin*. 2008;26:69–87.
4. Spitz JL. *Genodermatoses: A Clinical Guide to Genetic Skin Disorders*. 2nd ed. Philadelphia: Lippincott Williams & Williams; 2005.
5. Hernandez I, Espinosa-de-los M, Mendoza V, et al. Ectopic ACTH-secreting syndrome: a single center experience with a high prevalence of occult tumor. *Arch Med Res*. 2006;37(8):976–980.
6. Torpy DJ, Mullen N, Ilias I, et al. Association of hypertension and hypokalemia with Cushing's syndrome caused by ectopic ACTH secretion: a series of 58 cases. *Ann N Y Acad Sci*. 2002;970:134–144.
7. Maroun J, Kocha W, Kvols L, et al. Guidelines for the diagnosis and management of carcinoid tumours. Part I: The gastrointestinal tract. A statement from a Canadian National Carcinoid Expert Group. *Curr Oncol*. 2006;13:67–76.
8. Seng J, Wang B, Ma D, et al. Glucagonoma syndrome: diagnosis and treatment. *J Am Acad Dermatol*. 2003;48:297–298.
9. Slee PH, van der Waal RI, Schagen van Leeuwen JH, et al. Paraneoplastic hypertrichosis lanuginosa acquisita: uncommon or overlooked? *Br J Dermatol*. 2007;157(6):1087–1092.
10. Ramirez-Amador V, Esquivel-Pedraza L, Caballero-Mendoza E, et al. Oral manifestations as a hallmark of malignant acanthosis nigricans. *J Oral Pathol Med*. 1999;28:278–281.
11. Yeh JS, Munn SE, Plunkett TA, et al. Coexistence of acanthosis nigricans and the sign of Leser-Trelat in a patient with gastric adenocarcinoma: a case report and literature review. *J Am Acad Dermatol*. 2000;42:357–362.
12. Cohen PR, Grossman ME, Almeida L, et al. Tripe palms and malignancy. *J Clin Oncol*. 1989;7:669–678.
13. Schwartz RA. Sign of Leser-Trelat. *J Am Acad Dermatol*. 1996;35(1):88–95.
14. Kurzrock R, Cohen PR. Cutaneous paraneoplastic syndromes in solid tumors. *Am J Med*. 1995;99:662–671.
15. Silverstein SR. Primary, systemic amyloidosis and the dermatologist: where classic skin lesions may provide the clue for early diagnosis. *Dermatol Online J*. 2005;11(1):5.
16. Daoud MS, Lust JA, Kyle RA, et al. Monoclonal gammopathies and associated skin disorders. *J Am Acad Dermatol*. 1999;40(4):507–525.
17. Pomann JJ, Rudner EJ. Scleromyxedema revisited. *Int J Dermatol*. 2003;42(1):31–35.
18. Jackson EM, English 3rd JC. Diffuse cutaneous mucinosis. *Dermatol Clin*. 2002;20(3):493–501.
19. Mori Y, Kahari VM, Varga J. Scleroderma-like cutaneous syndromes. *Curr Rheumatol Rep*. 2002;4(2):113–122.
20. Sobol UA, Sherman KL, Smith K, et al. Sweet's syndrome with neurologic manifestations in a patient with esophageal adenocarcinoma: a case report and review of the literature. *Int J Dermatol*. 2009;48(10):1062–1065.
21. Bourke JF, Keohane S, Long CC, et al. Sweet's syndrome and malignancy in the U.K. *Br J Dermatol*. 1997;137(4):609–613.
22. Bennett ML, Jackson JM, Jorizzo JL, et al. Pyoderma gangrenosum. A comparison of typical and atypical forms with an emphasis on time to remission. Case review of 86 patients from 2 institutions. *Medicine (Baltimore)*. 2000;79:37–46.
23. Ahmad K, Ramsay B. Pyoderma gangrenosum associated with subcorneal pustular dermatosis and IgA myeloma. *Clin Exp Dermatol*. 2009;34(1):46–48.
24. Ruocco E, Sangiuliano S, Gravina AG, et al. Pyoderma gangrenosum: an updated review. *J Eur Acad Dermatol Venereol*. 2009;23(9):1008–1017.
25. Kaplan I, Hodak E, Ackerman L, et al. Neoplasms associated with paraneoplastic pemphigus: a review with emphasis on non-hematologic malignancy and oral mucosal manifestations. *Oral Oncol*. 2004;40(6):553–562.
26. Sklavounou A, Laskaris G. Paraneoplastic pemphigus: a review. *Oral Oncol*. 1998;34:437–440.
27. Zhu X, Zhang B. Paraneoplastic pemphigus. *J Dermatol*. 2007;34(8):503–511.
28. Egan CA, Lazarova Z, Darling TN, et al. Anti-epiligrin cicatricial pemphigoid: clinical findings, immunopathogenesis, and significant associations. *Medicine (Baltimore)*. 2003;82(3):177–186.
29. Letko E, Gurcan HM, Papaliodis GN, et al. Relative risk for cancer in mucous membrane pemphigoid associated with antibodies to the beta4 integrin subunit. *Clin Exp Dermatol*. 2007;32(6):637–641.
30. Askling J, Linet M, Gridley G, et al. Cancer incidence in a population-based cohort of individuals hospitalized with celiac disease or dermatitis herpetiformis. *Gastroenterology*. 2002;123(5):1428–1435.
31. Andras C, Ponyi A, Constantin T, et al. Dermatomyositis and polymyositis associated with malignancy: a 21-year retrospective study. *J Rheumatol*. 2008;35:438–444.
32. Stockton D, Doherty VR, Brewster DH. Risk of cancer in patients with dermatomyositis or polymyositis and follow-up implications: a Scottish population-based cohort study. *Br J Cancer*. 2001;85(1):41–45.
33. Callen JP. Collagen vascular diseases. *J Am Acad Dermatol*. 2004;51:427–439.
34. Fain O, Hamidou M, Cacoub P, et al. Vasculitides associated with malignancies: analysis of sixty patients. *Arthritis Rheum*. 2007;57:1473–1480.
35. Chanda J. Extramammary Paget's disease: prognosis and relationship to internal malignancy. *J Am Acad Dermatol*. 1985;13(6):1009–1014.
36. Snow JL, Muller SA. Malignancy-associated multicentric reticulohistiocytosis: a clinical, histological, and immunophenotypic study. *Br J Dermatol*. 1995;133(1):71–76.
37. Kishikawa T, Miyashita T, Fujiwara E, et al. Multicentric reticulohistiocytosis associated with ovarian cancer. *Mod Rheumatol*. 2007;17(5):422–425.
38. Spicknall KE, Mehregan DA. Necrobiotic xanthogranuloma. *Int J Dermatol*. 2009;48(1):1–10.
39. Eubanks LE, McBurney E, Reed R. Erythema gyratum repens. *Am J Med Sci*. 2001;321:302–305.
40. Kleyn CE, Lai-Cheong JE, Bell HK. Cutaneous manifestations of internal malignancy: diagnosis and management. *Am J Clin Dermatol*. 2006;7(2):71–84.
41. Chung VQ, Moschella SL, Zembowicz A. Clinical and pathologic findings of paraneoplastic dermatoses. *J Am Acad Dermatol*. 2006;54(5):745–762.
42. Barzilai A, Shpiro D, Goldberg I, et al. Insect bite-like reaction in patients with hematologic malignant neoplasms. *Arch Dermatol*. 1999;135(12):1503–1507.
43. Cocuroccia B, Gisondi P, Gubinelli E, et al. An itchy vesiculobullous eruption in a patient with chronic lymphocytic leukemia. *Int J Clin Pract*. 2004;58(12):1177–1179.

# Dermatologic Manifestations of Systemic Oncologic Therapy of Cutaneous Malignancies

*Beth McLellan, Caroline Robert, and Mario E. Lacouture*

## Key Points

- Developments in cancer therapy led to significant improvement in patient survival and increased awareness of the associated dermatologic side effects.

- Dermatologic side effects can be emotionally difficult for patients and cause disruption in cancer treatment, underscoring the importance of recognition and treatment.

- Targeted therapies are becoming important in the treatment of cancers of the skin and soft tissues.

- In most patients, EGFR inhibitors cause a characteristic papulopustular eruption. Improved outcomes may be associated with increasing severity of the eruption.

## HISTORY

After the discovery of micrometastases in the 1960s, combined systemic modality treatment with chemotherapy became standard cancer treatment.[1] Recently, targeted therapies have led to a significant decline in mortality from cancer and an increasing number of dermatologic side effects. This chapter will focus on dermatologic side effects that develop from systemic agents and radiation used to treat skin and soft tissue malignancies (Table 35.1).

## CUTANEOUS MANIFESTATIONS OF SKIN CANCER SYSTEMIC THERAPY

### Alopecia

Chemotherapy-induced alopecia (CIA), one of the most common and distressing side effects, occurs in 65% of patients, with 47% considering it the most traumatic side effect of chemotherapy.[2] Fear of hair loss would cause 8% of patients to decline chemotherapy. Although clinical patterns can vary, hair loss is usually acute, diffuse and of dystrophic anagen effluvium type. The onset is usually 1–3 weeks after beginning chemotherapy and is complete at 1–2 months. Doxorubicin causes alopecia in 60–100% of patients and paclitaxel in more than 80%. Other agents that usually cause alopecia include daunorubicin and docetaxel.

Although CIA is usually reversible, there is a 3–6-month delay of regrowth, which may be incomplete. In 65% of patients, there is a change in the color and/or texture of the new hair. Persistent alopecia after use of taxanes has been reported.[3] Topical minoxidil and growth factor AS101 can shorten the duration of CIA but do not prevent it.[4] Scalp cooling has shown a significant benefit in preventing alopecia, especially in cases of anthracyclines and taxanes. Using a cooling cap, cold air, or liquid during chemotherapy infusion may work by inducing vasoconstriction, thereby decreasing biochemical activity and cellular drug uptake. The putative risk of scalp metastases when scalp cooling is used has not been established.[5]

## Hand–foot syndrome (palmoplantar erythrodysesthesia)

Hand–foot syndrome can be caused by pegylated liposomal doxorubicin, continuous-infusion doxorubicin, cytarabine, floxuridine, high-dose interleukin-2, docetaxel, 5-fluorouracil (5-FU) and its prodrug capecitabine, vinorelbine, and gemcitabine. Symptoms begin 2–12 days after administration of the drug. The skin becomes erythematous and edematous, followed by dryness, scaling, and associated burning pain (Fig. 35.1). Blisters and ulcerations can develop in advanced cases.[6]

Like for many chemotherapeutic side effects, the mechanism is unknown, but several theories have been proposed. Increased toxicity in the palms and soles may be related to the high turnover rate of this skin, high density of sweat glands, absence of folliculo-sebaceous units, thickened stratum corneum, wide dermal papillae, and increased trauma and friction. Some studies have supported the theory that the chemotherapeutic is excreted in the sweat and the increased number of eccrine glands on the palms and soles may increase the toxicity in these areas.[7]

Therapies such as cooling, topical dimethylsulfoxide, oral and topical steroids, topical urea and vitamin E, and oral pyridoxine may be effective, although data are limited.[8] Small trials have described benefit of urea-containing moisturizers, oral vitamin E supplements, and celecoxib in patients receiving capecitabine.[9–11]

## Mucositis

Most patients rate mucositis as their worst side effect from chemotherapy. Part of the profound impact on quality of life of mucositis is impaired adequate nutrition, and increased risk of infection and sepsis.[12] The rapidly dividing tissue of the mucosa of the aerodigestive tract is a frequent target of chemotherapy. Palifermin, a recombinant keratinocyte growth factor, decreases the incidence, duration, and severity of oral mucosal lesions in patients but has an unclear role in improved nutrition and survival.[13] Cryotherapy using

## Table 35.1 Dermatologic Malignancies and Agents Being Employed on or off Label

| Drug Class | Cancers Treated |
|---|---|
| EGFR inhibitors | Recurrent or metastatic BCC and SCC |
| Multikinase inhibitors | Angiosarcoma, malignant melanoma |
| Taxanes | Kaposi sarcoma, malignant melanoma |
| Anthracyclines | Merkel cell carcinoma, cutaneous B-cell lymphoma, Kaposi sarcoma, soft tissue sarcomas, and mycosis fungoides |
| Alkylating agents | Soft tissue sarcomas, melanoma |
| Multitargeted kinase inhibitors | DFSP, desmoid tumor, certain types of mastocytosis, Kaposi sarcoma |
| Immunokines | Mycosis fungoides, malignant melanoma |
| Bleomycin | SCC, Kaposi sarcoma, mycosis fungoides, malignant melanoma |

BCC, basal cell carcinoma; SCC, squamous cell carcinoma; DFSP, dermatofibrosarcoma protuberans.

crushed ice during infusion of bolus 5-FU[14] and low-level laser resurfacing may be effective.

## Morbilliform eruption

A mildly pruritic morbilliform (maculopapular) eruption of the upper body is caused by doxorubicin, cytarabine, gemcitabine, and taxanes. This eruption is not a type I allergic reaction. Histology shows a mixed infiltrate with eosinophils. Topical and/or oral corticosteroids can be used, as well as premedication with corticosteroids, antihistamines, and acetaminophen.[15]

## Nails

Nail-growth slowing, onychoptosis, Beau's lines, nail hyperpigmentation, leukonychias, onycholysis, and subungual

hemorrhages can be seen with chemotherapies including alkylating agents, taxanes, anthracyclines, and bleomycin.[16]

## Neutrophilic eccrine hidradenitis

Neutrophilic eccrine hydradenitis, which occurs 2 to 20 days after the onset of treatment, can be observed with anthracyclines and bleomycin. It appears as erythematous papules on the superior part of the body. Pathology shows eccrine gland and epithelial necrosis and a dense neutrophilic infiltrate. It usually does not recur when the chemotherapy is reintroduced.

## CHEMOTHERAPEUTIC AGENTS THAT LEAD TO DERMATOLOGIC MANIFESTATIONS

## Epidermal growth factor receptor inhibitors

Epidermal growth factor receptor inhibitors (EGFRIs) have been used for metastatic basal cell carcinoma and recurrent and metastatic squamous cell carcinoma although they are not yet approved for these indications. They have been approved by regulatory agencies for the treatment of lung, pancreatic, colorectal, and head and neck cancers.[17] Frequent and severe papulopustular eruption is associated with increased tumor response and longer median survival, thus, cessation of EGFRI treatment due to papulopustular eruption should be avoided.[18]

A papulopustular eruption is seen in 45–100% of patients receiving EGFRIs and can have a significant physical and emotional strain on the patient. The eruption occurs mainly in sebaceous skin, including the scalp, face, and upper trunk, and consists of follicularly based papules and pustules (Fig. 35.2). Because this eruption lacks comedones, the term 'acneiform' is not a clinically accurate description. The eruption starts 8–10 days after initiation of chemotherapy, peaks at 2 weeks, and resolves 8–10 weeks after treatment cessation.[19] Secondary impetiginization occurs in up to 38% of patients.[20] Histopathology shows a suppurative perifollicular inflammation. In 10–17% of patients, the eruption can

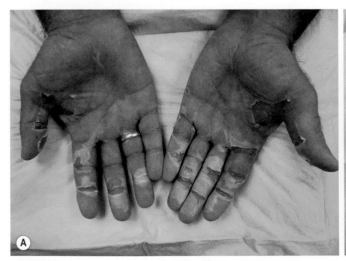
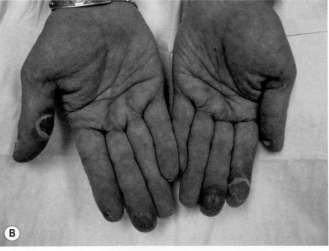

**Figure 35.1** Hand–foot syndrome induced by **(A)** liposomal doxorubicin and **(B)** a multitargeted kinase inhibitor (sorafenib or sunitinib). From Cancer Management: A Multidisciplinary Approach, 11th edition. Pazdur R, Wagman L, Camphausen K, et al. (eds). Copyright 2008, All rights reserved.

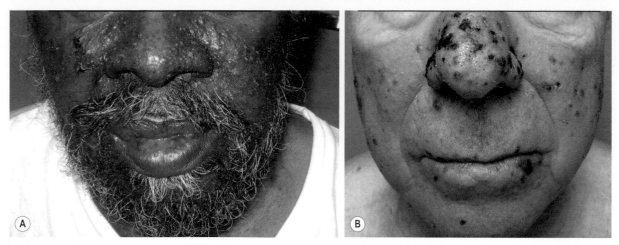

**Figure 35.2** Papulopustular eruption caused by EGFRI in **(A)** pustular stage and **(B)** crusted stage. **B** from Cancer Management: A Multidisciplinary Approach, 11th edition. Pazdur R, Wagman L, Camphausen K, et al. (eds). Copyright 2008, All rights reserved.

be severe enough to interrupt treatment, and 32% of oncologists will stop anti-EGFR therapy due to rash alone.[21]

In addition, 10–20% of patients receiving EGFRIs develop nail changes, including onychoschizia, paronychia, and periungual pyogenic granulomas. Hair changes due to EGFRIs include trichomegaly of the eyelashes and eyebrows, facial hirsutism, and alopecia of the scalp and body. Xerosis and pruritus develop in 58% of patients (Fig. 35.3).[22,23]

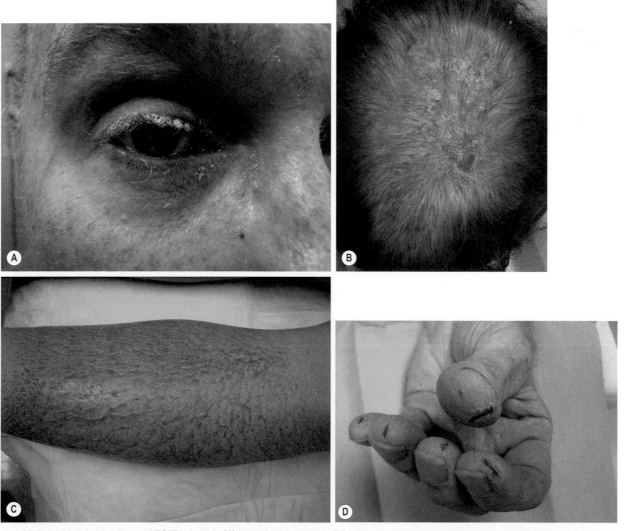

**Figure 35.3** Additional side effects of EGFRIs include **(A)** eyelash trichomegaly, **(B)** inflammatory alopecia, **(C)** xerosis, and **(D)** fissures. From Cancer Management: A Multidisciplinary Approach, 11th edition. Pazdur R, Wagman L, Camphausen K, et al. (eds). Copyright 2008, All rights reserved.

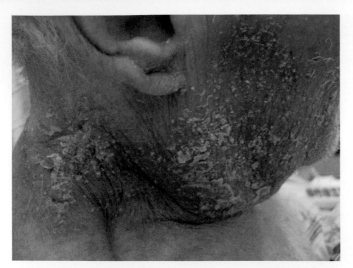

**Figure 35.4** Radiation dermatitis in a patient treated with EGFRI (cetuximab) and radiotherapy. From Cancer Management: A Multidisciplinary Approach, 11th edition. Pazdur R, Wagman L, Camphausen K, et al. (eds). Copyright 2008, All rights reserved.

EGFRIs, when used concurrently with radiation therapy, increase the risk of radiation dermatitis[24] (Fig. 35.4).

The EGFR, which is expressed in the basal layer of normal skin, is important to keratinocyte function. Inhibition of this receptor causes immediate abnormalities in keratinocyte growth and migration, including apoptosis, increased cell attachment and differentiation, and inflammation.[25]

There are limited data regarding best treatments for the papulopustular eruption. Based on the histological findings of neutrophilic infiltrates and bacterial colonies, topical/oral corticosteroids and antibiotics may be effective. Keratolytics and petroleum jelly can be used for removal of crusts and debris. Secondary infections should be cultured and treated appropriately. Severe, recurrent, or refractory rash may be treated with systemic agents including tetracycline, doxycycline, or minocycline and low-dose retinoids (isotretinoin or acitretin). As sunlight can exacerbate the eruption, sunscreens should be encouraged.[22] Prophylactic oral tetracycline, doxycycline, or minocycline alone or in combination with a sunscreen and topical hydrocortisone have been shown to reduce grade ≥2 papulopustular eruption by more than 50%.[26-28]

## Multikinase (VEGFR) inhibitors

Sorafenib, an inhibitor of vascular endothelial growth factor receptor-1, -2, and -3; platelet-derived growth factor receptor-α and –β; and the Raf/MEK/ERK pathway, has been tested in treatment of angiosarcoma and is in trials for metastatic melanoma. The most common dermatologic side effects from sorafenib include hand–foot skin reaction (HFSR), facial erythema, splinter subungual hemorrhages, alopecia, pruritus, and xerosis. Most dermatologic symptoms arise in the first 6 weeks after treatment.[29] Among 144 patients treated with sorafenib for metastatic or recurrent sarcomas, 75% of dose reductions were due to dermatologic toxicities.[30]

HFSR, which is seen in 60% of patients receiving sorafenib, is associated with painful erythema on the palms and soles that can be associated with tingling and heat intolerance.

The HFSR caused by sorafenib is typically more localized than the acral erythema seen with other chemotherapies. Keratoderma over pressure areas can also be seen. Treatment includes cotton socks, gel inserts, and soft shoes to avoid pressure points. Temperature extremes, pressure, and friction should be avoided.[31] Removal of calluses and proper orthotics can prevent HSFR. Topical moisturizers and keratolytics have shown anecdotal benefit. High-potency topical steroids such as clobetasol 0.05% can be applied to erythematous areas and topical lidocaine to painful areas. If patients develop pain and swelling that disrupts their activities of daily living, ulcerations, blisters, and/or desquamation, dose modification or interruption of therapy may be necessary.[32]

Facial erythema occurs 1–2 weeks after treatment and can be preceded by a scalp eruption which is clinically similar to seborrheic dermatitis. It is usually self-limited and can be treated symptomatically with emollients, topical steroids, and topical antifungals.

Subungual splinter hemorrhages develop in more than 60% of patients taking sorafenib. They occur after 1–2 weeks of treatment and grow out with the nail. These lesions might be due to the antiangiogenic effects of sorafenib. Other less common dermatologic side effects reported due to sorafenib include xerosis, eruptive benign nevi, eruptive keratoacanthomas, and exanthema.[31]

## Taxanes

Paclitaxel, a mitotic inhibitor, is FDA-approved for treatment of Kaposi sarcoma and can be used in the treatment of melanoma. It causes alopecia in 55–96% of patients and mucositis in 5–45%.[33] Patients receiving paclitaxel are usually premedicated with dexamethasone, diphenhydramine, and cimetidine to prevent a hypersensitivity reaction.[34] Taxanes induce nail changes in about 25% of patients, including discoloration, paronychia, ridging, Beau's lines, and onycholysis. Specially designed gel-containing frozen gloves and socks have been shown to reduce nail toxicity when utilized during agent infusion.[35] Less common effects of paclitaxel are erythema multiforme (EM), including one reported case of photo-distributed EM, IV site changes, pustular dermatosis, photosensitive dermatoses (including subacute cutaneous lupus erythematosus), urticaria, and scleroderma-like reaction.[34]

## Anthracyclines

Pegylated liposomal doxorubicin (PLD) is used in the treatment of Merkel cell carcinoma, cutaneous B- and T-cell lymphomas, Kaposi sarcoma, and soft tissue sarcomas. The most common cutaneous side effect is hand–foot syndrome (HFS), which is seen in 45% of patients. This reaction can be dose-limiting and therapy with PLD is permanently discontinued in 4–7% of patients because of HFS.[36] Although data are limited, treatment options including oral pyridoxine, regional cooling, oral corticosteroids, topical dimethylsuphoxide, IV amifostine, and antioxidative ointment are being investigated.[37] Oral dexamethasone (8 mg bid for 5 days) decreases the need for dosage adjustment due to grade 2 HFS.[38] In addition, 10% of the patients develop a diffuse follicular eruption most prominent on the lateral limbs, 8% experience an intertrigo-like eruption, and 5% show melanotic macules.[39] Inflammation of actinic keratoses has also been described.[40]

## Alkylating agents

In 159 cycles of ifosfamide in 34 patients, 8.8% developed a severe acute cutaneous allergic reaction.[41] A rare side effect of ifosfamide, which is currently used to treat soft tissue sarcomas, is hyperpigmentation in the nails, dorsal hands and feet.[42]

Temozolomide, which is in phase I trials to treat melanoma, infrequently induces skin side effects and rash. One case of an extensive desquamative eruption has been described.[43] Dacarbazine, a related alkylating agent also used to melanoma, can cause photosensitivity, and sunscreen should be encouraged.[44]

## Multitargeted kinase inhibitors

Imatinib mesylate is an oral medication that inhibits the Abelson cytoplasmic tyrosine kinase (Abl) and two type III receptor tyrosine kinases, c-Kit and platelet-derived growth factor receptor (PDGFR). It has been approved by the US FDA for treatment of dermatofibrosarcoma protuberans (DFSP) and may play a role in treatment of aggressive fibromatosis (desmoid tumor),[45] certain types of mastocytosis, and Kaposi sarcoma.[46] Additionally, imatinib mesylate is under investigation for treatment of advanced KIT-mutated melanoma.[45] In 9.5–69% of treated patients, dermatologic side effects occur. One of the most frequent side effects is edema, commonly periorbital, which occurs in 54–76% of treated patients. Other side effects are: a) severe generalized skin eruptions rarely leading to erythroderma, Stevens–Johnson syndrome, and toxic epidermal necrolysis (TEN); b) acute generalized exanthematous pustulosis and mycosis fungoides-like reactions; c) lichenoid eruptions on the skin and oral mucosa; and d) papulosquamous eruptions including pityriasis rosea and psoriasis.[47]

Focal and generalized hypopigmentation of the skin and repigmentation of the hair has been seen following imatinib use. Conversely, dasatinib and sunitinib can cause depigmentation of the hair. The differences in effects on hair color may be related to differences between the drugs in their effects on c Kit signaling. Hair pigmentary changes are reversible.[48,49]

## Bleomycin

Bleomycin is FDA-approved for the treatment of squamous cell carcinoma and has been used intravenously and intralesionally in the treatment of Kaposi sarcoma and melanoma. In most tissues, bleomycin hydrolase inactivates the drug, but because this enzyme is not present in the lungs and skin, a variety of dose-dependent cutaneous toxicities have been observed at doses between 200 and 300 U. A characteristic cutaneous side effect of bleomycin is flagellate erythema, which appears as erythematous and violaceous linear streaks on the trunk in 8–66% of patients and occurs hours to months after bleomycin administration. Systemic sclerodermatous changes have been seen in patients after receiving bleomycin, and bleomycin-induced dermal sclerosis has been used as a mouse model for scleroderma.

Neutrophilic eccrine hidradenitis is associated with combination chemotherapy regimens including bleomycin and also cytarabine, doxorubicin, vincristine, cisplatin, and dacarbazine. It causes erythematous plaques and nodules characterized by neutrophilic infiltrates in the eccrine glands. Acute generalized exanthematous pustulosis, Stevens–Johnson syndrome, nail pigmentation, and alopecia are other side effects of bleomycin.[50]

## Immunokines

High-dose IL-2, interferon (IFN)-β, and IFN-α are used in treatment of metastatic melanoma and cutaneous T-cell lymphomas. In a study of 270 patients receiving high-dose IL-2 for melanoma, 10% developed rash and 6% developed an exfoliative dermatitis.[51] IFN-α can induce lichen planus, possibly through the induction of CD8$^+$ T cells. It also can cause vitiligo, alopecia, and changes in hair color.[52]

## RADIATION DERMATITIS

Incidence of acute radiation dermatitis depends on the dose of radiation as well as concurrent medications (i.e. various chemotherapy agents will act as radiosensitizers in tumors as well as neighboring skin). It presents with erythema which progresses and peaks 1–2 weeks after completing treatment. Severe forms are characterized by bullae, desquamation, and necrosis. When used from the first day of radiation therapy until 3 weeks after completion, high-potency topical steroids are superior to emollient cream in preventing acute radiation dermatitis.[53] Patients should be encouraged to gently wash their skin during radiation therapy using a mild soap. Other preventive agents that have been investigated with mixed results include sucralfate cream, Biafine, ascorbic acid, aloe vera, chamomile cream, almond ointment, and polymer adhesive skin sealant. General recommendations regarding treatment of existing acute radiation dermatitis are barrier creams in cases without skin breakdown and low-dose corticosteroids for reduction of itching and irritation.[54,55] Non-aluminum-containing deodorants do not cause increased dermatitis in cases of axillary lymph node radiation.[56]

Chronic radiodermatitis is characterized by atrophy, scaling, dyspigmentation, telangiectasias, and alopecia. Alexandrite epilation laser has been used for treatment of the hyperpigmentation and pulse dye laser for treatment of telangiectasias.[57] Hyperbaric oxygen therapy has been used to alleviate pain associated with the erythema, edema, or lymphedema. Keratolytic and emollient agents are useful for the scaling and xerosis.

An erythematous rash located on previously irradiated skin areas (months to 15 years previously) can occur in the hours or days following chemotherapy administration and is known as radiation recall. The mechanism underlying this phenomenon is obscure.

## FUTURE OUTLOOK

Many of the dermatologic and mucosal side effects associated with cancer treatment play a significant role in a patient's experience with cancer and it is becoming increasingly important for the physician to aggressively recognize and treat these side effects, not only to improve patient quality of life but also to minimize treatment disruptions which may affect clinical outcome. Rapid access to a dermatologist and close communication with the treating oncologist are increasingly important to ensure that the most appropriate care is given. These observations have led to the establishment of interdisciplinary clinical programs focused on the management of dermatologic side effects in cancer patients.[58]

It is noteworthy that the majority of the data available for the management of these untoward events has been derived from existing information for clinically similar conditions with a distinct etiology. With increasing significance of these toxicities, principally the EGFRI-induced eruption, trials specific to this patient population are underway and hopefully will provide management strategies based on controlled data. In addition, improvements in the grading system utilized in oncology clinical trials, the Common Terminology Criteria for Adverse Events (CTCAE) version 4.0, have been implemented.[59] Dermatologists will have a unique and important role in the care of cancer patients and survivors.

## REFERENCES

1. Devita Jr VT, Chu E. A history of cancer chemotherapy. *Cancer Res*. 2008;68:8643–8653.
2. Mols F, van den Hurk CJ, Vingerhoets AJ, et al. Scalp cooling to prevent chemotherapy-induced hair loss: practical and clinical considerations. *Support Care Cancer*. 2009;17:181–189.
3. Prevezas C, Matard B, Pinquier L, et al. Irreversible and severe alopecia following docetaxel or paclitaxel cytotoxic therapy for breast cancer. *Br J Dermatol*. 2009;160:883–885.
4. Wang J, Lu Z, Au JL. Protection against chemotherapy-induced alopecia. *Pharm Res*. 2006;23:2505–2514.
5. Trüeb RM. Chemotherapy-induced alopecia. *Semin Cutan Med Surg*. 2009;28:11–14.
6. Lorusso D, Di Stefano A, Carone V, et al. Pegylated liposomal doxorubicin-related palmar-plantar erythrodysesthesia ('hand-foot' syndrome). *Ann Oncol*. 2007;18:1159–1164.
7. Martschick A, Sehouli J, Patzelt A, et al. The pathogenetic mechanism of anthracycline-induced palmar-plantar erythrodysesthesia. *Anticancer Res*. 2009;29:2307–2313.
8. von Moos R, Thuerlimann BJK, Aapro M, et al. Pegylated liposomal doxorubicin-associated hand-foot syndrome: recommendations of an international panel of experts. *Eur J Cancer*. 2008;44:781–790.
9. Pendharkar D, Goyal H. Novel & effective management of capecitabine induced hand foot syndrome [abstract]. *J Clin Oncol*. 2004;22(14S):8105.
10. Yamamoto D, Yamamoto C, Tanaka K. Novel and effective management of capecitabine induced hand foot syndrome [abstract]. *J Clin Oncol*. 2008;26(suppl):734s.
11. Lin EH, Morris J, Chau NK, et al. Celecoxib attenuated capecitabine induced hand-and-foot syndrome (HFS) and diarrhea and improved time to tumor progression in metastatic colorectal cancer (MCRC). *Proc Am Soc Clin Oncol*. 2002;21: (abstr 2364).
12. Sorensen JB, Skovsgaard T, Bork E, et al. Double-blind, placebo-controlled, randomized study of chlorhexidine prophylaxis for 5-fluorouracil-based chemotherapy-induced oral mucositis with nonblinded randomized comparison to oral cooling (cryotherapy) in gastrointestinal malignancies. *Cancer*. 2008;112:1600–1606.
13. Barasch A, Epstein J, Tilashalski K. Palifermin for management of treatment-induced oral mucositis in cancer patients. *Biologics*. 2009;3:111–116.
14. Peterson DE, Bensadoun RJ, Roila F, EMSO Guidelines Working Group. Management of oral and gastrointestinal mucositis: ESMO clinical recommendations. *Ann Oncol*. 2008;19:ii122–ii125.
15. Agha R, Kinahan K, Bennett CL, et al. Dermatologic challenges in cancer patients and survivors. *Oncology (Williston Park)*. 2007;21:1462–1472.
16. Gilbar P, Hain A, Peereboom VM. Nail toxicity induced by cancer chemotherapy. *J Oncol Pharm Pract*. 2009;15:143–155.
17. Caron J, Dereure O, Kerob D, et al. Metastatic basal cell carcinoma: report of two cases treated with cetuximab. *Br J Dermatol*. 2009;161:702–703.
18. Li T, Perez-Soler R. Skin toxicities associated with epidermal growth factor receptor inhibitors. *Target Oncol*. 2009;4:107–119.
19. Boone SL, Rademaker A, Liu D, et al. Impact and management of skin toxicity associated with anti-epidermal growth factor receptor therapy. *Oncology*. 2007;72:152–159.
20. Eilers Jr RE, West DP, Ortiz S, et al. *Dermatologic infections complicate epidermal growth factor receptor inhibitor (EGFRI) therapy in cancer patients.* Poster session presented at: 67th Annual Meeting of the American Academy of Dermatology, 6-10 March, San Francisco, CA; 2009.
21. Burtness B, Anadkat M, Basti S, et al. NCCN Task Force Report: Management of dermatologic and other toxicities associated with EGFR inhibition in patients with cancer. *J Natl Compr Canc Netw*. 2009;7:S5–S21.
22. Osio A, Mateus C, Soria JC, et al. Cutaneous side-effects in patients on long-term treatment with epidermal growth factor receptor inhibitors. *Br J Dermatol*. 2009;161:515–521.
23. Roé E, García Muret MP, Marcuello E, et al. Description and management of cutaneous side effects during cetuximab or erlotinib treatments: a prospective study of 30 patients. *J Am Acad Dermatol*. 2006;55:429–437.
24. Tejwani A, Wu S, Jia Y, et al. Increased risk of high-grade dermatologic toxicities with radiation plus epidermal growth factor receptor inhibitor therapy. *Cancer*. 2009;115:1286–1299.
25. Lacouture ME. Mechanisms of cutaneous toxicities to EGFR inhibitors. *Nat Rev Cancer*. 2006;6:803–812.
26. Scope A, Agero ALC, Dusza SW, et al. Randomized double-blind trial of prophylactic oral minocycline and topical tazarotene for cetuximab-associated acne-like eruption. *J Clin Oncol*. 2007;25:5390–5396.
27. Jatoi A, Rowland K, Sloan JA, et al. Results of a placebo-controlled trial from the North Central Cancer Treatment Group (N03CB). *Cancer*. 2008;113:847–853.
28. Lacouture ME, Mitchell EP, Shearer H, et al. Impact of pre-emptive skin toxicity (ST) treatment (tx) on panitumumab (pmab)-related skin toxicities and quality of life (QOL) in patients (pts) with metastatic colorectal cancer (mCRC): Results from STEPP. *ASCO abstract*. 291, 2009.
29. Robert C, Mateus C, Spatz A, et al. Dermatologic symptoms associated with the multikinase inhibitor sorafenib. *J Am Acad Dermatol*. 2009;60:299–305.
30. Maki RG, D'Adamo DR, Keohan ML, et al. Phase II study of sorafenib in patients with metastatic or recurrent sarcomas. *J Clin Oncol*. 2009;27:3133–3140.
31. Chu D, Lacouture ME, Fillos T, et al. Risk of hand-foot skin reaction with sorafenib: a systematic review and meta-analysis. *Acta Oncol*. 2008;47:176–186.
32. Lacouture ME, Wu S, Robert C, et al. Evolving strategies for the management of hand-foot skin reaction associated with the multitargeted kinase inhibitors sorafenib and sunitinib. *Oncologist*. 2008;3:1001–1011.
33. Paclitaxel. In: *DrugDex® System [Internet database]*. Greenwood Village, Colo: Thomson Reuters (Healthcare) Inc; Updated periodically.
34. Cohen PR. Photodistributed erythema multiforme: paclitaxel-related, photosensitive conditions in patients with cancer. *J Drugs Dermatol*. 2009;8:61–64.
35. Winther D, Saunte DM, Knap M, et al. Nail changes due to docetaxel – a neglected side effect and nuisance for the patient. *Support Care Cancer*. 2007;15:1191–1197.
36. Von Moos R, Thuerlimann BJ, Aapro M, et al. Pegylated liposomal doxorubicin-associated hand-foot syndrome: recommendations of an international panel of experts. *Eur J Cancer*. 2008;44:781–790.
37. Mangana J, Zipser MC, Conrad C, et al. Skin problems associated with pegylated liposomal doxorubicin – more than palmoplantar erythrodysesthesia syndrome. *Eur J Dermatol*. 2008;8:566–570.
38. Drake RD, Lin WM, King M, et al. Oral dexamethasone attenuates Doxil-induced palmar-plantar erythrodysesthesias in patients with recurrent gynecologic malignancies. *Gynecol Oncol*. 2004;94:320–324.
39. Lotem M, Hubert A, Lyass O, et al. Skin toxic effects of polyethylene glycol-coated liposomal doxorubicin. *Arch Dermatol*. 2000;136:1475–1480.
40. Ilyas EN, Grana G, Green JJ. Inflammatory actinic keratoses secondary to systemic chemotherapy. *Cutis*. 2005;75:167–168.
41. Cartei G, Clocchiatti L, Sacco C, et al. Dose finding of ifosfamide administered with a chronic two-week continuous infusion. *Oncology*. 2003;65(suppl 2):31–36.
42. Teresi ME, Murry DJ, Cornelius AS. Ifosfamide-induced hyperpigmentation. *Cancer*. 1993;71:2873–2875.
43. Pick AM, Neff WJ, Nystrom KK. Temozolomide-induced desquamative skin rash in a patient with metastatic melanoma. *Pharmacotherapy*. 2008;28:406–409.
44. Yung CW, Winston EM, Lorincz AL. Dacarbazine-induced photosensitivity reaction. *J Am Acad Dermatol*. 1981;4:541–543.
45. Duffaud F, Le Cesne A. Imatinib in the treatment of solid tumours. *Targ Oncol*. 2009;4:45–56.
46. Scheinfeld N. A comprehensive review of imatinib mesylate (Gleevec) for dermatological diseases. *J Drugs Dermatol*. 2006;5:117–122.

**47.** Scheinfeld N. Imatinib mesylate and dermatology part 2: a review of the cutaneous side effects of imatinib mesylate. *J Drugs Dermatol.* 2006;5:228–231.

**48.** Sun A, Akin RS, Cobos E, et al. Hair depigmentation during chemotherapy with dasatinib, a dual Bcr-Abl/Src family tyrosine kinase inhibitor. *J Drugs Dermatol.* 2009;8:395–398.

**49.** Hartmann JT, Kanz L. Sunitinib and periodic hair depigmentation due to temporary c-KIT inhibition. *Arch Dermatol.* 2008;144:1525–1526.

**50.** Yamamoto T. Bleomycin and the skin. *Br J Dermatol.* 2006;155:869–875.

**51.** Atkins MB, Lotze MT, Dutcher JP, et al. High-dose recombinant interleukin 2 therapy for patients with metastatic melanoma: analysis of 270 patients treated between 1985 and 1993. *J Clin Oncol.* 1999;7:2106–2116.

**52.** Asarch A, Gottlieb AB, Lee J, et al. Lichen planus-like eruptions: an emerging side effect of tumor necrosis factor-α antagonists. *J Am Acad Dermatol.* 2009;61:104–111.

**53.** Boström A, Lindman H, Swartling C, et al. Potent corticosteroid cream (mometasone furoate) significantly reduces acute radiation dermatitis: results from a double-blind, randomized study. *Radiother Oncol.* 2001;59:257–265.

**54.** Schmuth M, Wimmer MA, Hofer S, et al. Topical corticosteroid therapy for acute radiation dermatitis: a prospective, randomized, double-blind study. *Br J Dermatol.* 2002;146:983–991.

**55.** Bolderston A, Lloyd NS, Wong RG, et al. Supportive Care Guidelines Group of Cancer Care Ontario Program in Evidence-Based Care. The prevention and management of acute skin reactions related to radiation therapy: a systematic review and practice guideline. *Support Care Cancer.* 2006;14:802–817.

**56.** Theberge V, Harel F, Dagnault A. Use of axillary deodorant and effect on acute skin toxicity during radiotherapy for breast cancer: a prospective randomized noninferiority trial. *Int J Radiat Oncol Biol Phys.* 2009;75(4):1048–1052.

**57.** Santos-Juanes J, Coto-Segura P, Galache Osuna C, et al. Treatment of hyperpigmentation component in chronic radiodermatitis with alexandrite epilation laser. *Br J Dermatol.* 2009;160:210–211.

**58.** Lacouture ME, Basti S, Patel J, et al. The SERIES clinic: an interdisciplinary approach to the management of toxicities of EGFR inhibitors. *J Support Oncol.* 2006;4:236–238.

**59.** U.S. Department of Health and Human Services. *Common Terminology Criteria for Adverse Events (CTCAE) v 4.0.* 2009. < http://ctep.cancer.gov/protocoldevelopment/electronic_applications/docs/ctcaev4.pdf >; Accessed 25.10.09.

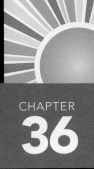

# The Dermoscopic Patterns of Melanoma and Non-Melanoma Skin Cancer

*Steven Q. Wang, Margaret C. Oliviero, and Harold S. Rabinovitz*

## Key Points

- Dermoscopy is a non-invasive technique that enhances diagnosis of pigmented and other skin lesions.

- This technique allows for the analysis of subsurface structures to determine malignancy.

- Although diagnostic accuracy may decrease in health professionals first learning the technique, in the hands of experienced users this approach can significantly improve the ability to correctly diagnose skin cancers without biopsy.

## INTRODUCTION

Dermoscopy (also known as epiluminescence microscopy or dermoscopy) is a method of using a handheld microscope to examine skin lesions. It is an in-vivo, non-invasive technique that permits clinicians to better visualize cellular structures in the epidermis, dermoepidermal junction, and dermis; in contrast to naked-eye inspection, where clinicians may only detect the gross morphological features of the lesions, such as size, shape, colors, elevations or ulcerations. The development of dermoscopy has led to the recognition of a number of new morphologic structures that can improve diagnostic accuracy[1,2] and confidence level for both pigmented and non-pigmented skin lesions.

The introduction of dermoscopy to clinical dermatology is largely credited to Rona MacKie in 1971,[3,4] who first demonstrated its clinical utility in differentiating benign versus malignant pigmented skin lesions. Since then, clinicians and researchers have worked to better define the diagnostic features and criteria associated with an array of pigmented and non-pigmented skin lesions. Over the past two decades, there has been nearly a 20-fold increase in the number of scientific publications in this field. The number of clinicians worldwide who use dermoscopy has also risen at a dramatic rate. In the United States, only 5% of surveyed dermatologists used this diagnostic technique in their daily practice in 1995, and the rate quickly jumped to 23% in 2002.[5] In the latest survey, the rate of adoption in the US is now 60%.[6]

## DERMOSCOPIC EQUIPMENT

Currently, there are two major categories of dermoscopes available in the market (Table 36.1). The first is the non-polarized (NPD) dermoscope. This device contains light-emitting diodes for illumination and is equipped with a 10× to 20× magnification lens (Fig. 36.1A). A liquid interface (ideally with refraction index equal to that of skin) is required, and direct contact of the skin with the glass plate of the dermoscope is needed. Different immersion liquids include water, mineral oil, alcohol or gel (i.e. ultrasound gel, antibacterial gel). Alcohol is widely used as it is more hygienic and can reduce the risk of bacterial contamination.[7] For examining nail apparatus, ultrasound or antibacterial gels are the liquids of choice.[8,9] The viscous nature of gels prevents them from rolling off the convex nail surface. The setup of skin–liquid–glass interface decreases light reflection and increases refraction. By minimizing glare, the stratum corneum appears more translucent and deeper structures in the skin can be visualized.

The second type of dermoscope is the polarized device (PD). This type of device was introduced to the clinical arena in 2000. It uses two polarizers to achieve cross-polarization. Under this condition, the polarizers allow the dermoscope to preferentially capture the backscattered light from the deeper levels of the skin. The major advantage of PD is obviating the need for any fluid or direct contact with the skin and permitting clinicians to quickly scan lesions during the examination (Fig. 36.1B). Some of the PD devices allow the user to toggle between contact and non-contact PD mode. A new scope is now commercially available that permits the user to choose between PD and NPD mode.

In general, the dermoscopic image qualities from PD and NPD are relatively similar, but a few important differences exist (Table 36.1).[10] Epidermal structures, such as comedo-like openings and milia-like cysts, are better seen with the NPD. As mentioned above, PD devices obviate the need for direct contact between the skin and the glass plate, therefore reducing the compression effects associated with the NPDs. Consequently, blood vessels and red color areas corresponding to vascular changes are better seen under PD. Improved visualization of vessel morphology has aided the diagnosis of hypomelanotic and amelanotic melanoma, squamous cell cancer, and other inflammatory dermatologic conditions. The differences between NPD and PD are minor, and both types of devices provide complementary information. However, it is important to note that these small subtleties can impact the diagnostic accuracy and confidence level, especially for beginners.[11] Hence, it is important to know which types of dermoscopes one is using in the diagnostic process.

Table 36.1 Differences in Colors and Dermoscopic Structures Seen Between Non-Polarized Dermoscopy (NPD) and Polarized Dermoscopy (PD)

| Colors and Structures | NPD | PD |
|---|---|---|
| **Colors** | | |
| Melanin | + | ++ |
| Red/pink | + | +++ |
| Blue-white due to orthokeratosis | +++ | + |
| Blue-white due to regression | +++ | ++ |
| **Structures** | | |
| Peppering | +++ | ++ |
| Chrysalis or white scar | +/− | +++ |
| Vessels | + | +++ |
| Milia cyst | +++ | +/− |

## BASAL CELL CARCINOMA

The clinical presentation of basal cell carcinoma (BCC) varies from erythematous patches to dark nodules. As a result, differential diagnoses for BCC can be extensive, and dermoscopy can help the clinician improve the diagnostic accuracy for both pigmented and non-pigmented BCCs.

## Pigmented BCCs

Pigmented BCCs are not uncommon. With the aid of dermoscopy, light brown, dark brown or black pigmentation can be seen in different subtypes of BCCs, such as superficial, nodular or infiltrative types. These colors are due to the deposition of free melanin, melanocytes or melanophages in the dermis and dermal–epidemal junction. Depending on the depth of these pigmentation sources, different colors are seen. Furthermore, knowledge of the basic histological patterns of BCCs can enhance knowledge regarding the dermoscopic structures and patterns seen in association with pigmented BCCs. Histologically, BCC tumors are commonly present as clusters or islands of basaloid cells in the dermis or the dermoepidermal junction. The peripheries of these tumor islands are lined with palisading cells. The presence of free melanin or melanophages within these tumor islands produces the pigmentation. The different dermoscopic structures correlate to (1) the shape and size of the tumor islands and (2) the variation in the amount and distribution of the melanin pigment. Pigmentation found in small islands of tumors may be seen as multiple blue-gray globules under dermoscopy. The presence of large amounts of pigmentation seen in a large cluster of tumors may correspond to the ovoid nests.

Many dermoscopic features associated with pigmented BCCs have been described.[12-15] These features are listed in Table 36.2, and Figures 36.2 and 36.3 illustrate some of these in dermoscopic images of BCCs. The majority of these dermoscopic structures were described by Menzies et al.,[14] when the investigators examined 426 lesions and reviewed 45 dermoscopic structures to select out the critical dermoscopic features that distinguish pigmented BCCs from other pigmented skin lesions. This analysis yielded a very practical diagnostic method with a sensitivity of 93% and specificity of 89–92%. A comparable level of sensitivity and specificity results were reported by Peris and co-workers,[15] who independently validated this diagnostic method in their patient population.

## Non-pigmented BCCs

The introduction of PD enhanced the ability of clinicians to identify and appreciate key dermoscopic features associated with non-pigmented BCCs. Polarized dermoscopes

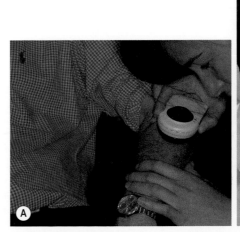
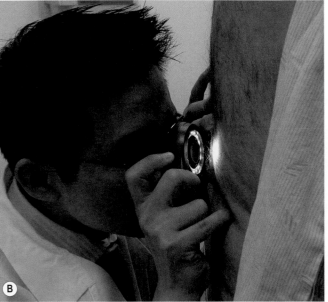

**Figure 36.1** The use of non-polarized **(A)** and polarized **(B)** dermoscopes in skin examination. (Courtesy of Harold S. Rabinovitz, MD).

### Table 36.2 Dermoscopic Structures of Pigmented and Non-Pigmented Basal Cell Cancer

| Dermoscopic Structures | Description |
|---|---|
| Large blue-gray ovoid nests | The nests are defined as confluent or nearly confluent, well-circumscribed, pigmented ovoid or elongated areas that are not closely connected to the pigmented tumor body. Nests are larger than globules |
| Multiple blue-gray globules | These are well-defined round or oval structures, larger than dots, but smaller than large ovoid nests. They are blue-gray in color |
| Leaf-like areas | These areas are defined as discrete, bulbous extensions connected at a base area, forming a leaf-like pattern. They are usually brown or gray-blue in color |
| Spoke-wheel areas | These are well-defined radial projections surrounding a central point. The projections have tan, blue or gray color, and the central point usually is dark brown, blue or black. This structure is very specific for BCCs |
| Arborizing telangiectasia (serpentine branched vessels) | These are multiple branching blood vessels in a tree-like pattern. These are often appreciated in non-pigmented BCCs, and are rarely seen in nevi, melanomas and other benign pigmented skin lesions |
| Ulceration | Ulceration may appear as congealed blood. It is important to rule out a previous history of trauma for ulceration to be a valid feature |
| Small fine telangiectasia* | Small-diameter vessels have length <1 mm; few branches |
| Shiny white to red areas* | Areas with white to red, translucent to opaque appearance |

*Dermoscopic structures associated with non-pigmented basal cell cancer.

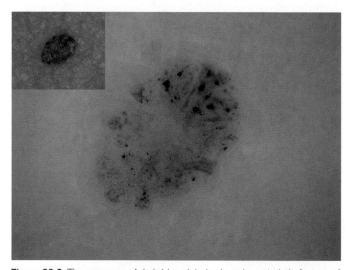

**Figure 36.2** The presence of dark-blue globules is a characteristic feature of pigmented basal cell carcinoma. (Courtesy of Harold S. Rabinovitz, MD).

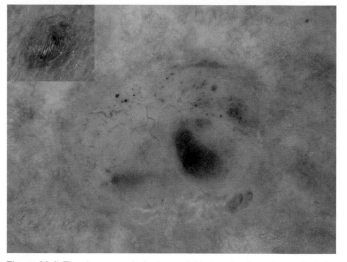

**Figure 36.3** The dermoscopic features of this basal cell carcinoma include serpentine branched blood vessels (arborizing vessels) on a pink-white background, with blue and brown globules, as well as blue and brown ovoid nests. (Courtesy of Harold S. Rabinovitz, MD).

allow visualization of deeper skin structures, such as small caliber-sized blood vessels in the dermis. In addition, polarized dermoscopes do not require contact between the skin and the scope and do not compress the vessels.

Two key dermoscopic features that are helpful to diagnose non-pigmented BCCs are (1) small fine telangiectasias (SFTs) and (2) shiny white to red areas (Table 36.2). The small fine telangiectasias, often serpentine in appearance, have a length < 1 mm. Unlike the arborizing vessels (large-diameter vessels, often serpentine in appearance), small fine telangiectasias have few branches, and are distributed irregularly within the whitish area. Shiny white-to-red structureless areas have translucent to opaque appearance (Fig. 36.4). Aside from these two features, ulcerations and arborizing (serpentine) vessels can also be present. In 2005, Giacomel et al.[13] looked at 24 superficial and non-pigmented

BCCs. They noted that the shiny white-red areas were seen in 100% of the lesions, SFTs in 92%, ulceration in 71%, and arborizing (serpentine) vessels in 8%.

## SQUAMOUS CELL CARCINOMA

Clinical presentation of squamous cell cancer (SCC) ranges from sharply demarcated, erythematous and scaly plaques to rapidly growing and tender nodules. The differential diagnosis includes a range of skin disorders, such as actinic keratosis, basal cell cancer, amelanotic melanoma, psoriasis, warts, and clear cell acanthoma.

Dermoscopy allows the visualization of vascular structures and/or small amount of pigmentation within the SCC

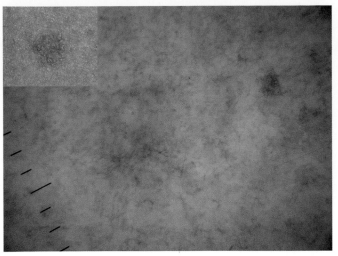

**Figure 36.4** This superficial basal cell carcinoma is characterized by a pink-white area and thin-diameter serpentine branched vessels. (Courtesy of Harold S. Rabinovitz, MD).

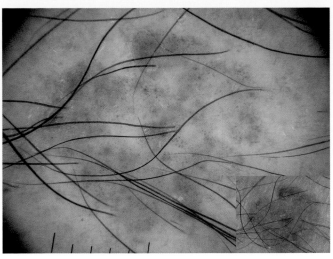

**Figure 36.6** This squamous cell carcinoma in situ is characterized by diffuse vessels as red dots and a fine scale. (Courtesy of Harold S. Rabinovitz, MD).

that are not visible to the naked eye. The presence of distinct vessel morphologies provides a key clue for diagnosing early SCCs, especially in-situ lesions. Similar to what is seen in BCC, vessel morphologies in SCC are better visualized with PDs. Dermoscopic structures commonly found in SCCs include glomerular (coiled) vessels, dotted vessels[16,17] and scales (Figs 36.5 and 36.6). Glomerular vessels are so-named because of their resemblance to the capillaries seen in the glomerular unit of the kidney. On a casual glance, glomerular vessels may be mistaken for dotted vessels. However, upon close inspection, the glomerular vessels are larger in size, always forming tortuous loops. Histologically, it corresponds to the presence of grouped and dilated capillaries winding spirally in the dermal papillae. The presence of glomerular vessels is most commonly seen in SCC in situ. However, this type of vessel may occasionally be seen with psoriasis and porokeratosis. The glomerular (coiled) vessels are never seen in melanocytic lesions. Glomerular vessels

and scales were seen in nearly 90% of cases of SCC in situ in one series studied.[17] Diffuse dotted vessels are the other common vascular feature seen in SCC in situ. Dotted vessels can also be seen in clear cell acanthoma, porokeratosis, Spitz nevus, and melanoma. For clear cell acanthoma, the dotted vessels are distributed in a 'string of pearls' arrangement.[18] For melanoma and atypical melanocytic nevi, dotted vessels have focal distribution.

Additional, but not as specific, structures seen in pigmented SCC in situ include brown dots/globules, structureless pigmentation, streaks, pigmented network, and ulceration.[17] In another retrospective case review, Cameron et al.[19] also confirmed the observation of coiled vessels and dots in pigmented Bowen's disease. More importantly, the investigators observed that the dots and vessels are frequently arranged in linear distribution, a key difference from the dots seen in melanocytic lesions. However, it is important to emphasize that the presence of these dermoscopic structures (i.e. brown dots) may pose a challenge for the differential diagnosis. According to the two-step algorithm in the pattern analysis, the presence of pigmented network and globules should make the observers pursue the melanocytic pathway. Hence, when scales and glomerular vessels are present in conjunction with dermoscopic structures associated with melanocytic lesions (i.e. pigmented network and globules), the differential diagnosis of SCCs needs to be entertained, especially when the dots are arranged in linear fashion.

## MELANOMA

Early melanoma (MM) detection is the key to ensuring a good prognosis. However, accurately diagnosing MM is challenging, especially for atypical or dysplastic nevi, because atypical nevi share some or all of the ABCD features of MM. Dermoscopy can help to better differentiate MMs from benign nevi. A number of diagnostic algorithms and approaches have been described with the aim of teaching novices to correctly diagnose melanoma (see Table 36.3 for the sensitivity and specificity of each algorithm). In general,

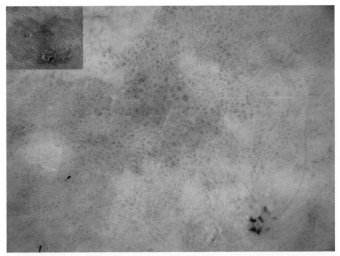

**Figure 36.5** This squamous cell carcinoma is characterized clinically by a red-brown scaly plaque. Dermoscopically it is characterized by diffuse coiled vessels (glomerular) and a fine scale. (Courtesy of Harold S. Rabinovitz, MD).

### Table 36.3 Comparison of Sensitivity and Specificity of Dermoscopy Algorithms

| Dermoscopy Diagnostic Algorithm | Sensitivity | Specificity |
|---|---|---|
| Pattern analysis*[25] | 100% | 87.7% |
| ABCD*[25] | 96.3% | 70.4% |
| Seven-point checklist*[25] | 96.3% | 72.8% |
| CASH[23] | 98% | 68% |
| Menzies*[25] | 96.3% | 72.8% |

*Sensitivity and specificity results from the 2003 Internet Consensus Meeting.

the algorithms can be classified as score-based (e.g. ABCD rule of dermoscopy,[20] CASH, or seven-point checklist[21]) or Gestalt-based (e.g. pattern analysis).

## ABCD rule of dermoscopy

This was the first score-based system, developed by German physicians,[22] to quantitatively diagnose melanoma from benign melanocytic lesions. Stolz et al.[22] reviewed 31 dermoscopic features from 151 melanocytic lesions. The investigators identified four critical criteria: (1) Asymmetry, (2) Border sharpness, (3) Color, and (4) Dermoscopic structures (Table 36.4). This method has a sensitivity of 92.8% and specificity of 90% in diagnosing melanomas.[20]

Asymmetry score is defined by first bisecting a lesion with two 90° axes that are designed to yield the lowest possible asymmetry score. Asymmetry is calculated according to the contour, colors and dermoscopic structures on either side of each axis. If the lesion is symmetrical in both axes, the lesion has a score of 0. If there is asymmetry in one axis, the score is 1. If asymmetry is present in both axes, then the score is 2. Melanoma tends to have a high asymmetry score.

Border score is defined as the sharp or abrupt cut-off of the pigmented structures at the periphery of a lesion. To determine the border score, the lesion is first divided into eight segments, and the presence or absence of sharp cut-off of the pigmented structures is scored for each of the eight sections. The maximum border score is 8, and the minimum score is 0. Melanoma tends to have a higher score.

Color score is defined by the number of six colors present in a lesion. The six colors are white, red, light brown, dark brown, blue-gray, and black. The value of the color score ranges from 1 to 6. In the original analysis,[22] 85% of the melanomas in the study were found to have more than three colors, and 40% had five or six colors.

Dermoscopic structure score is defined by the presence of five structures. These are: structureless areas, pigment network, branched streaks, dots, and globules. The structureless area must be at least 10% of the total lesion. The initial study[22] showed that 90% of the benign melanocytic nevi had fewer than three structures, and 73% of the melanomas had more than four structures.

To differentiate melanomas from benign melanocytic nevi, the individual scores from each of the ABCD categories are combined to yield a total dermoscopy score (TDS; Table 36.5). TDS ranges from 1 to 8.9. A benign lesion has a score from 1 to 4.75, and a malignant lesion has a score >5.45. A suspicious lesion, such as severely atypical nevi or early melanoma in situ, has a score ranging from 4.75 to 5.45.

## Seven-point checklist

This is an another score-based approach, first described by Argenziano et al.[21] in 1998. This algorithm relies on the presence or absence of seven specific dermoscopic criteria. The initial study showed this algorithm has a sensitivity of 85–93% and specificity of 45–48% when applied by non-experts.

Compared to the ABCD dermoscopy rule, the seven-point checklist is more streamlined and requires less mathematical computation. The seven dermoscopic criteria in

### Table 36.4 ABCD Rule of Dermoscopy

| Parameter | Definition | Points |
|---|---|---|
| A = Asymmetry | Symmetry is measured based on the contour, colors and dermoscopic structures within a lesion | 0 = symmetry in 2 axes<br>1 = symmetry in 1 axis<br>2 = asymmetry in 2 axes |
| B = Border sharpness | Lesion is divided in 8 equal segments. One point is assigned for each segment with sharp border | Range 0 to 8<br>0 = no segment of the lesions with sharp demarcated borders<br>8 = the entire border of the lesions ends abruptly at the periphery |
| C = Colors | Light brown, dark brown, black, red, white, blue-gray. | Range 1 to 6 |
| D = Dermoscopy structures | Pigmented network, dots, globules, branched streaks, structureless area | Range 1 to 5 |

### Table 36.5 Total Dermoscopy Score of the ABCD Rule

| Parameter | Points | Coefficient Factor | Score |
|---|---|---|---|
| Asymmetry | 0 to 2 | × 1.3 | 0 to 2.6 |
| Border sharpness | 0 to 8 | × 0.1 | 0 to 0.8 |
| Colors | 1 to 6 | × 0.5 | 0.5 to 3.0 |
| Dermoscopic structures | 1 to 5 | × 0.5 | 0.5 to 2.5 |
| Total dermoscopy score (TDS): | | | 1 to 8.9 |

## Table 36.6 The Seven-Point Checklist

| Dermoscopic Structure | Definition | Score |
|---|---|---|
| **Major criteria** | | |
| Atypical pigmented network | Network with irregular holes and line thickness<br>Networks can have multiple colors<br>Found often in focal areas of the lesion | 2 |
| Blue-white veil | Confluent blue pigmentation covered by a white 'ground-glass' haze, yielding an image of blue-white veil<br>The edge of the veil is not sharply demarcated<br>The structure cannot occupy the entire lesion | 2 |
| Atypical vessels | Linear irregular or dotted vessels dispersed in a focal area of the lesion | 2 |
| **Minor criteria** | | |
| Irregular streaks | These include pseudopods, streaks, radial streaming | 1 |
| Dots or globules | Dots are round/oval structures < 0.1 mm Globules are round/oval structures > 0.1 mm<br>***To be scored, the dots/globules must be haphazardly or irregularly distributed*** | 1 |
| Blotches | An aggregate of dark brown or black pigmentation within the lesion<br>***To be scored, the blotches must be haphazardly or irregularly distributed*** | 1 |
| Regression structures | Presence of white areas, blue areas, and combination of both<br>White area needs to be whiter than the surrounding skin<br>Blue area is marked by multiple blue dots or 'peppering' | 1 |

the checklist are divided into three major and four minor criteria (Table 36.6). The dermoscopic structures in the major criteria include: (1) atypical pigmented network, (2) atypical vascular pattern, (3) blue-white veil. Structures in the minor criteria are (1) irregular streaks, (2) irregular pigmentation, (3) irregular dots/globules, and (4) regression area.

To score a lesion, the presence or absence of each of the seven dermoscopic criteria is first determined. Two points are assigned for the presence of each major criterion, and one point is assigned for the presence of each minor criterion. The final score of the lesion is calculated by simple addition of the individual scores from the major and minor categories. A minimum total score of 3 is needed for the diagnosis of melanoma, and a lesion with a score of less than 3 is a non-melanoma.

## CASH algorithm

This dermoscopic algorithm was created by clinicians in the United States, where the investigators analyzed 131 MMs and 194 benign melanocytic lesions.[23] Like the aforementioned algorithms, the CASH method focuses on the color, symmetry and dermoscopic structures (i.e. homogeneity or heterogeneity) of a lesion. The major addition is the inclusion of architectural order versus disorder. Benign lesions are thought to grow in a controlled manner and have a well-organized (i.e. ordered) arrangement of the dermoscopic structures. In contrast, cells in malignant lesions no longer communicate with each other and therefore grow in uncontrollable proliferation. Dermoscopic appearances of malignant lesions are architecturally disordered. The CASH algorithm has a sensitivity of 98% and specificity of 68% in differentiating MM from benign melanocytic lesions.[23]

## Table 36.7 Cash Algorithm

| Parameter | Points |
|---|---|
| C = Colors | 1 point for each of the following colors: light brown, dark brown, black, red, white, blue |
| A = Architectural disorder | 0 = none/mild<br>1 = moderate<br>2 = significant |
| S = Symmetry | 0 = symmetry in 2 axes<br>1 = symmetry in 1 axis<br>2 = asymmetry in 2 axes |
| H = Homogeneity/Heterogeneity | 1 point for each of the following dermoscopic structures: pigmented network, dots/globules, streaks/pseudopods, blue-white veil, regression structures, blotches, polymorphous vessels |

A description of the CASH criteria and scoring system is shown in Table 36.7. Briefly, points are assigned as follows: colors (1 point each for light brown, dark brown, black, red, white, blue); architectural disorder (0=none/mild, 1=moderate, 2=significant); symmetry (0=symmetry in two axes, 1=symmetry in one axis, 2=no symmetry in two axes); and homogeneity/heterogeneity based on the number of seven dermoscopic structures (i.e. network; dots/globules; streaks/pseudopods; blue-white veil; regression; blotches; polymorphous blood vessels.) A total score for a lesion is calculated by adding the individual scores from each of the CASH categories. The possible score ranges from 2 to 17. A total score of ≥8 favors the diagnosis of melanoma.[23]

## Menzies method

This is the work from Australia, and it was first published in 1996.[24] In developing this system, the investigators reviewed 72 dermoscopic features of 159 benign and 62 malignant melanocytic lesions, and identified 11 important criteria. In the initial study,[24] this method had a sensitivity of 92% and specificity of 71% in classifying melanomas. For a lesion to be diagnosed as melanoma, it must have neither of the two negative features and one or more of the nine positive features. These negative and positive features are listed in Table 36.8.

In contrast to the ABCD rule of dermoscopy, seven-point checklist and CASH algorithm, the Menzies method does not use a score-based approach. It is a simplified variation of the pattern-analysis approach. Nevertheless, like the score-based algorithms, the Menzies method also focuses on the importance of symmetry, colors, and the presence or absence of certain dermoscopic structures.

## Pattern analysis

Pattern analysis is the approach most frequently used by experts in the clinical setting to distinguish melanoma from benign moles[1,25] mainly because expert dermoscopists can come to a diagnostic conclusion within a few seconds. However, this is also the most difficult approach to teach a novice, mainly because it requires both knowledge and experience, and diagnostic acumen may degrade temporarily in the early learning process. We will attempt to teach pattern analysis by comparing the classic patterns of benign melanocytic nevi, those of obvious melanoma, and those of atypical nevi.

### Dermoscopic pattern of benign melanocytic nevi

Recognizing the patterns of benign nevi is a valuable first step to identifying melanoma. If a lesion fits one of the classic dermoscopic patterns of benign nevi and does not have any local features of melanoma, then it is very likely that this lesion is not a melanoma. Conversely, if a lesion does not fit into any patterns associated with benign nevi and has local features suggestive of melanoma, then the index of suspicion for melanoma should be raised.

Dermoscopic patterns of benign nevi have consistent features (Table 36.9). In general, benign nevi have fewer (<3) colors and fewer numbers of dermoscopic structures. Benign lesions are symmetric in colors, shape and the distribution of dermoscopic structures. Most benign pigmented lesions have at least one axis of symmetry. In addition, the dermoscopic structures (networks, globules) of benign nevi are uniform and are of similar shape, size and color. Lastly, benign nevi are architecturally organized, a key concept described in the CASH algorithm.[23] Most benign nevi have an organized layout, as opposed to the disorganized layout seen in melanoma.

There are nine typical dermoscopic patterns of benign melanocytic nevi that have been well described. These patterns include: (1) diffuse reticular network, (2) patchy reticular network, (3) peripheral reticular network with central hypopigmentation, (4) peripheral reticular network with central hyperpigmentation, (5) peripheral reticular network with central globules, (6) globular, (7) peripheral globules with central reticular network or starburst, (8) homogeneous, and (9) multicomponent patterns[26] (Fig. 36.7).

These nine patterns are derived from three basic dermoscopic structures: (1) reticular network, (2) globules, and (3) homogeneous areas. Benign nevi may have only one structure or have a combination of all three structures.[27] The detailed description and schematic illustration of each pattern are listed in Table 36.9 and illustrated in Figures 36.7–36.16. In general, lesions that resemble these benign patterns and do not exhibit any local features of melanoma are benign.

## Dermoscopic patterns of melanoma

Classic dermoscopic patterns of melanoma share little or no similarity with the motifs and patterns described in benign nevi. The global motifs for melanoma are diametrically opposite to those associated with benign nevi. Melanomas have multiple colors (>3) and many dermoscopic structures. Most melanomas display asymmetry in at least one axis, and most have two axes of asymmetry. Again, it is important to emphasize that symmetry is judged by shape, color, and dermoscopic structures. If a lesion is symmetrical in shape and asymmetrical in the distribution of dermoscopic structures, this lesion should still be ranked as asymmetrical. In contrast to the case in benign nevi, the shape and size of the dermoscopic structures are not uniform, and the structures are arranged in a haphazard distribution. In terms of architectural order, the dermoscopic patterns of melanoma are chaotic and disorganized.

In terms of specific dermoscopic patterns of melanoma, in contradistinction to limited variants seen in benign nevi, there are multiple patterns that can be found. The presence of many patterns should not be a surprise if one considers the biological activity of melanoma cells. As a result, it is not possible to describe all the infinite variations of different dermoscopic patterns of melanomas. For novices without extensive training, the following guideline may be helpful. Melanomas are lesions that (1) do not fit into any of the aforementioned nine benign dermoscopic patterns associated with nevi, (2) have asymmetry, non-uniformity, and architectural disorder, and (3) have any of the local

| Table 36.8 The Menzies Method |
| --- |
| **Negative features** |
| • Symmetry of pigmentation patterns<br>• Presence of only one color |
| **Positive features** |
| • Blue-white veil<br>• Multiple brown dots<br>• Pseudopods<br>• Radial streaming<br>• Scar-like pigmentation<br>• Peripheral black dots/globules<br>• Multiple (5–6) colors<br>• Multiple blue-gray dots<br>• Broadened network |

## Table 36.9 Benign Dermoscopic Patterns of Melanocytic Nevi

| Benign Pattern | Description |
|---|---|
| Diffuse reticular network | Uniform network distributed diffusely and throughout the lesion. The line of network represents the presence of melanocytes or pigmented keratinocytes along the epidermal rete ridges. The holes in the network represent the dermal papillae |
| Patchy reticular network | Patches of uniform network scattered throughout the lesion. There are structureless areas interspersed among the patches of network |
| Peripheral reticular network with central hypopigmentation | Uniform network is located at the periphery and surrounding a central structureless or light-brown homogeneous area |
| Peripheral reticular network with central hyperpigmentation | Uniform network is located at the periphery and surrounding a central darkly pigmented and homogeneous area. There may also be a small number of dots present in the center or overlying the network lines |
| Peripheral reticular network with central globules | Uniform network is located at the periphery and surrounding a cluster of globules in the center of the lesion |
| Globular | Uniform globules are the predominant feature. The globules correspond to nests of melanocytes. Depending on the depth of these nests, the globules can be either light brown, dark brown or black in color. Close proximity and juxtaposition of these globules can form a 'cobble-stoned'-appearing pattern |
| Homogeneous pattern | Brown homogeneous pigment throughout the entire lesion. On occasion one may see a few globules and/or remnants of a network |
| Peripheral globular with central reticular network or centrally homogeneous area (this pattern also includes the starburst pattern) | A rim of uniformly distributed globules surrounding an area of network. This pattern is frequently seen in growing nevi. If instead of seeing globules one sees pseudopods around the periphery of the lesion (starburst pattern), then the most likely diagnosis is a Spitz nevus |
| Symmetric multicomponent | Combination of three or more structures distributed symmetrically. Multicomponent lesions should always be viewed with caution. Only if the structures are completely symmetrically distributed should one consider this a benign pattern |

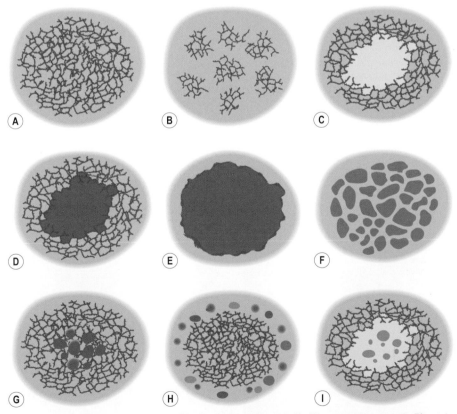

**Figure 36.7** Cartoon illustration of the nine dermoscopic patterns of benign melanocytic nevi: **A)** diffuse reticular network, **B)** patchy reticular network, **C)** peripheral reticular network with central hypopigmentation, **D)** peripheral reticular network with central hyperpigmentation, **E)** homogeneous, **F)** globular, **G)** peripheral reticular network with central globules, **H)** peripheral globular with central reticular network, and **I)** multicomponent.

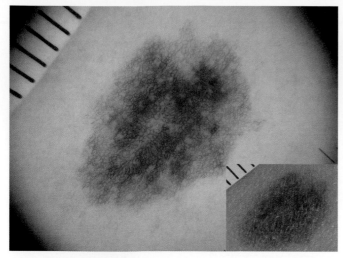

**Figure 36.8** A benign melanocytic nevus with diffuse reticular network pattern. (Courtesy of Harold S. Rabinovitz, MD).

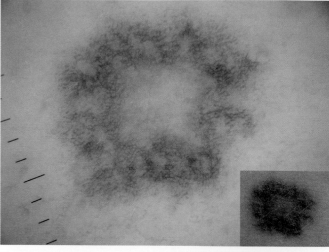

**Figure 36.11** This reticular homogeneous pattern is characterized by a symmetrical hypopigmented structureless area (homogeneous) and a uniform network at the periphery. (Courtesy of Harold S. Rabinovitz, MD).

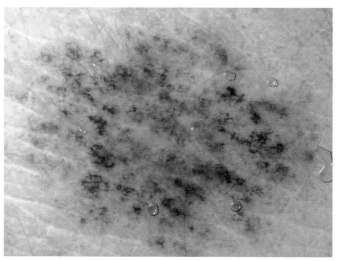

**Figure 36.9** This patchy network is characteristic of a junctional Clark's nevus or a junctional dysplastic nevus with mild atypia. (Courtesy of Harold S. Rabinovitz, MD).

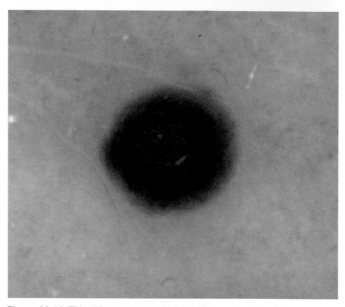

**Figure 36.12** This diffuse homogeneous pattern is characterized by a blue structureless area and is characteristic of a blue nevus. (Courtesy of Harold S. Rabinovitz, MD).

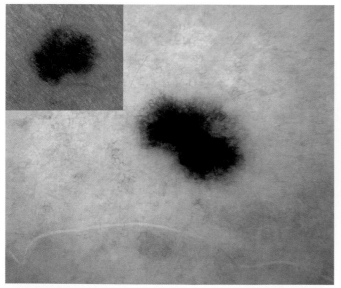

**Figure 36.10** This reticular homogeneous pattern is characterized by a symmetrical hyperpigmented structureless area (homogeneous) and a uniform network at the periphery. (Courtesy of Harold S. Rabinovitz, MD).

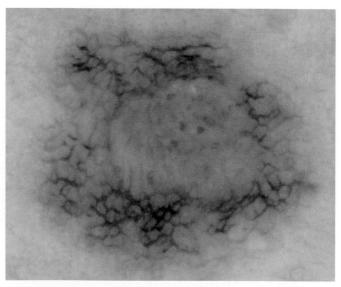

**Figure 36.13** The reticular-globular pattern is characterized by central globules with a uniform network at the periphery. These are commonly seen in congenital nevi and in nevi with congenital-like features. (Courtesy of Harold S. Rabinovitz, MD).

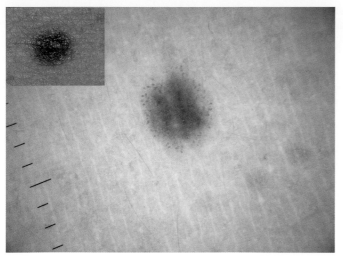

Figure 36.14 The reticular-globular pattern with peripheral globules is characterized by a uniform network with globules that are symmetrically rimming the lesion along the periphery. This type of nevus is commonly seen in children and is suggestive of enlarging melanocytic nevi. (Courtesy of Harold S. Rabinovitz, MD).

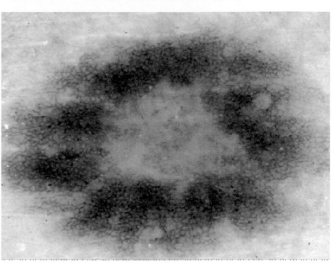

Figure 36.16 The multicomponent pattern is characterized by a network, globules, and structureless areas. These lesions tend to be symmetrical in pattern and are most commonly seen with congenital nevi. (Courtesy of Harold S. Rabinovitz, MD).

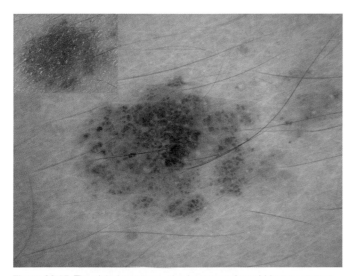

Figure 36.15 The globular pattern, also known as the cobblestone pattern, is characterized by diffuse globules throughout the lesion. These are commonly seen in congenital nevi, superficial or intradermal type. (Courtesy of Harold S. Rabinovitz, MD).

features associated with melanoma (Table 36.10). Figures 36.17–36.27 illustrate examples of dermoscopic patterns of frank melanomas.

The contrast and comparison between the dermoscopic patterns of benign melanocytic nevi and melanoma has also been described as 'the beauty and the beast' sign.[28] The 'beauty' connotes the dermoscopic patterns of benign nevi revealing symmetry and engendering a sense of ease in the observer. The 'beast' refers to the features and patterns of melanomas, most of which reveal asymmetry and engender a sense of unease in the viewer. In essence, the dermoscopic diagnosis of melanoma relies on the understanding of the benign patterns seen in melanocytic nevi.

## Dermoscopic patterns of atypical nevi

The differentiation of melanoma from common and atypical melanocytic nevi can be a challenge. It is sometimes difficult to discriminate some melanomas from melanocytic nevi, and this task is especially challenging when differentiating melanoma in situ from atypical nevi based on clinical and histologic criteria. These lesions have indeterminate dermoscopic patterns and fall into a category where the diagnosis is not obvious. Most of the lesions in this 'gray' category are atypical nevi (e.g. high-grade dysplastic nevi, atypical Spitz nevi, Clark nevi with unusual features, and congenital nevi with unconventional features) or early melanomas.

In general, the dermoscopic patterns of atypical nevi fall between the two extremes: the benign nevi and the obvious melanomas. These lesions do not fit into one of the nine patterns associated with benign melanocytic nevi (Figs 36.28–36.30). They may have either one or two axes of asymmetry, multiple colors and dermoscopic structures. These lesions may or may not have any of the significant dermoscopic features seen in melanoma. Clinical management of these lesions with equivocal patterns includes biopsy or monitoring using serial imaging.[29,30] Short-term mole monitoring is based on the premise that biologically active melanomas will display dermoscopic changes over a 3-month period and benign nevi will not show any change. The decision to biopsy versus monitoring depends on a number of factors. The patient's own history and observation are important elements in the diagnostic consideration. Lesions with symptoms of pain, bleeding, itching or change are significant concerns. Lesions that appear different (via either clinical or dermoscopic examination) from their neighbors, the 'ugly duckling sign',[31,32] should be considered for biopsy.

### Table 36.10 Dermoscopic Structures Commonly Seen in Melanomas

| Structure | Description |
| --- | --- |
| Atypical network (including branched streaks) | Black, brown or gray network with focal irregular mesh with thick lines and different sized holes. The lines represent the melanocytes and melanin along the rete ridges, and the holes represent the dermal papillae. Branched streaks represent remnants of pigmented rete ridges resulting from bridging of nests of melanocytes at the dermoepidermal junction |
| Streaks (includes pseudopods and radial streaming) | Linear pigmented projections at the periphery of the lesion. When these linear structures terminate with a bulbous projection, they are called pseudopods. Histologically they represent confluent junctional nests of melanocytes |
| Atypical dots and globules | Black, brown or gray dots or globules, varied in size and distributed haphazardly within the lesions. They frequently occur at the periphery of the lesion and are not associated with the network. Histologically, black dots represent melanin in the stratum corneum, gray dots represent melanin free in the dermis or within melanophages, and brown dots represent small nevomelanocytic nests at the tips of the rete ridges. Brown globules represent larger nevomelanocytic nests along the dermoepidermal junction or in the dermis |
| Negative or reverse pigment network | The lines of the network appear lighter (almost white) in color compared to the holes, which are darker in color. Histologically this probably represents narrow and hypopigmented rete ridges accompanied by the presence of large melanocytic nests within a widened papillary dermis |
| Off-center blotch | A blotch is a darkly pigmented area in which one cannot discern any structures. Histologically it represents large concentrations of melanin in the epidermis and/or dermis |
| Blue-white veil overlying flat (macular) areas and/or the presence of blue-gray granules (peppering) | Irregular, confluent, gray-blue to whitish blue pigmentation overlying flat areas within the lesion. Histologically this represents regression. One can also see peppering which represents melanin or melanophages in the papillary dermis. If the regression is complete, then one will see a white scar-like area instead |
| Blue-white veil overlying raised areas | Irregular, confluent, blue-white hazy pigmentation overlying raised areas within the lesion. Histologically it represents melanocytes in the dermis together with compact orthokeratosis |
| Vascular structures | Presence of different shaped blood vessels can be seen in melanoma. The most common are dotted, linear irregular and polymorphous vessels |

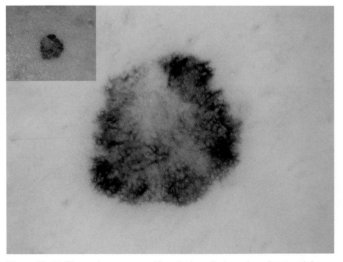

**Figure 36.17** The melanoma-specific criterion of a broadened network is seen with this melanoma in situ. (Courtesy of Harold S. Rabinovitz, MD).

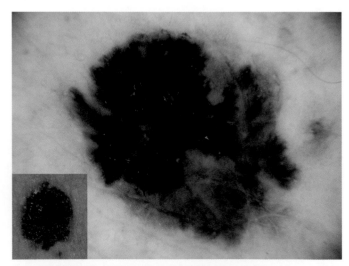

**Figure 36.18** The blue-white veil is characterized by a dark-blue area with a superimposed white haze. This feature is most commonly seen in invasive or thick melanomas. (Courtesy of Harold S. Rabinovitz, MD).

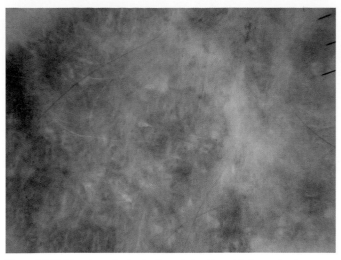

**Figure 36.19** The chrysalis sign is characterized by white linear streaks running orthogonally and is a feature seen with melanomas. Polarized light accentuates the chrysalis-like features. (Courtesy of Harold S. Rabinovitz, MD).

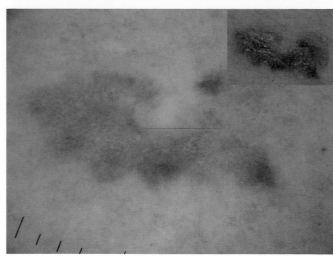

**Figure 36.22** A negative pigmented network is the reverse of a pigmented network and is a helpful clue in diagnosing melanoma. (Courtesy of Harold S. Rabinovitz, MD).

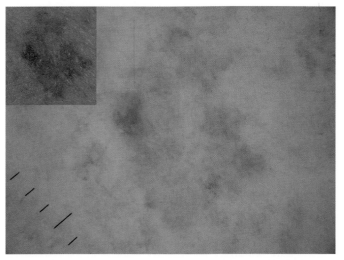

**Figure 36.20** Light-brown structureless area greater than 10% of the periphery of the lesion is a helpful sign in identifying subtle melanomas. (Courtesy of Harold S. Rabinovitz, MD).

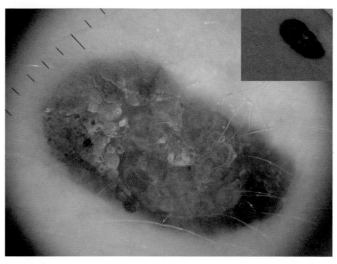

**Figure 36.23** This invasive melanoma has dots and globules asymmetrically focally distributed at one periphery. (Courtesy of Harold S. Rabinovitz, MD).

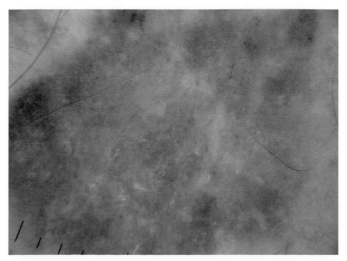

**Figure 36.21** In this melanoma, there are the multiple colors of blue, red, brown, white, pink and gray. (Courtesy of Harold S. Rabinovitz, MD).

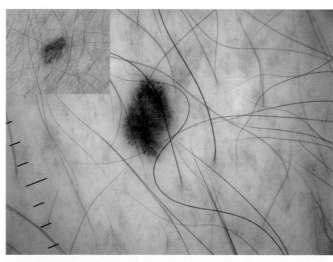

**Figure 36.24** This early melanoma has pseudopods irregularly distributed at the periphery. (Courtesy of Harold S. Rabinovitz, MD).

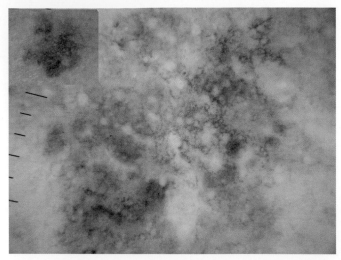

**Figure 36.25** Gray dots/granules, also known as peppering, are features of dermoscopic regression. These are commonly seen with melanomas on sun-damaged skin. (Courtesy of Harold S. Rabinovitz, MD).

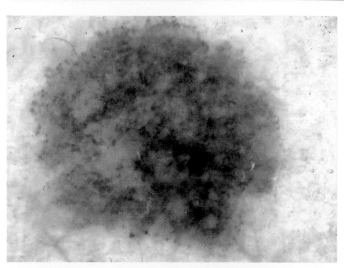

**Figure 36.28** This equivocal lesion with a non-uniform network and a reticular disorganized pattern was histologically read as a high-grade dysplastic nevus (dysplastic nevus with severe atypia). (Courtesy of Harold S. Rabinovitz, MD).

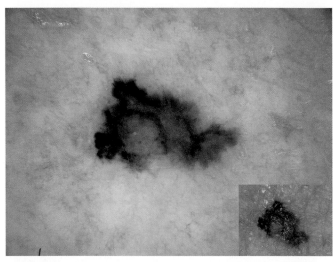

**Figure 36.26** Focal streaks are one of the melanoma-specific criteria. (Courtesy of Harold S. Rabinovitz, MD).

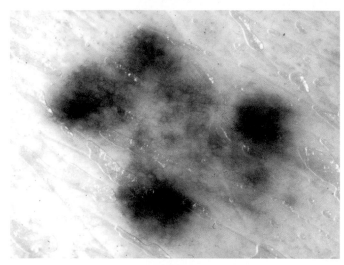

**Figure 36.29** This equivocal lesion with a reticular homogeneous disorganized pattern is characterized by a non-uniform network and an asymmetric structureless area. The histology was consistent with an atypical melanocytic nevus. (Courtesy of Harold S. Rabinovitz, MD).

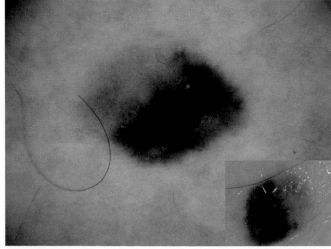

**Figure 36.27** Vessels as red dots along with other melanoma-specific criteria occasionally can be seen in melanoma. (Courtesy of Harold S. Rabinovitz, MD).

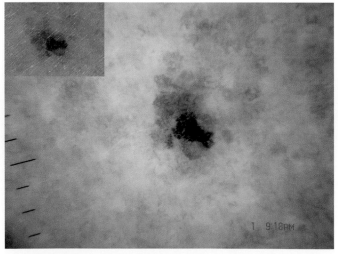

**Figure 36.30** This reticular disorganized pattern was histologically read as a high-grade dysplastic nevus/evolving melanoma in situ. Dermoscopically it was characterized by a non-uniform network with globules asymmetrically distributed. (Courtesy of Harold S. Rabinovitz, MD).

## FUTURE OUTLOOK

Dermoscopy is a valuable tool in the clinical management of skin cancer because its usage has been demonstrated to improve diagnostic accuracy and confidence levels. It is important to remember that dermoscopy is only one tool in the management of patients with suspicious skin lesions. Clinical presentation, personal and family history, and even other clinically unrelated elements must all be factored into the overall diagnostic process.

Given the continued interest in this technique, new dermoscopic structures still await to be discovered, and these findings may provide valuable clues for detecting skin cancers. Lastly, combining dermoscopy with computer-based approaches and other imaging modalities (e.g. confocal laser microscopy) has the potential to dramatically improve clinicians' ability to more accurately diagnose skin cancers in the future at an earlier point in their evolution.

## REFERENCES

1. Kittler H, Pehamberger H, Wolff K, et al. Diagnostic accuracy of dermoscopy. *Lancet Oncol*. 2002;3:159–165.
2. Pehamberger H, Binder M, Steiner A, et al. In vivo epiluminescence microscopy: improvement of early diagnosis of melanoma. *J Invest Dermatol*. 1993;100:356S–362S.
3. MacKie RM. An aid to the preoperative assessment of pigmented lesions of the skin. *Br J Dermatol*. 1971;85:232–238.
4. MacKie RM. Cutaneous microscopy in vivo as an aid to preoperative assessment of pigmented lesions of the skin. *Br J Plast Surg*. 1972;25:123–129.
5. Tripp JM, Kopf AW, Marghoob AA, et al. Management of dysplastic nevi: a survey of fellows of the American Academy of Dermatology. *J Am Acad Dermatol*. 2002;46:674–682.
6. Noor 2nd O, Nanda A, Rao BK. A dermoscopy survey to assess who is using it and why it is or is not being used. *Int J Dermatol*. 2009;48:951–952.
7. Stauffer F, Kittler H, Forstinger C, et al. The dermatoscope: a potential source of nosocomial infection? *Melanoma Res*. 2001;11:153–156.
8. Ronger S, Touzet S, Ligeron C, et al. Dermoscopic examination of nail pigmentation. *Arch Dermatol*. 2002;138:1327–1333.
9. Kelly SC, Purcell SM. Prevention of nosocomial infection during dermoscopy? *Dermatol Surg*. 2006;32:552–555.
10. Benvenuto-Andrade C, Dusza SW, Agero AL, et al. Differences between polarized light dermoscopy and immersion contact dermoscopy for the evaluation of skin lesions. *Arch Dermatol*. 2007;143:329–338.
11. Wang SQ, Dusza SW, Scope A, et al. Differences in dermoscopic images from nonpolarized dermoscope and polarized dermoscope influence the diagnostic accuracy and confidence level: a pilot study. *Dermatol Surg*. 2008;34:1389–1395.
12. Felder S, Rabinovitz H, Oliviero M, et al. Dermoscopic pattern of pigmented basal cell carcinoma, blue-white variant. *Dermatol Surg*. 2006;32:569–570.
13. Giacomel J, Zalaudek I. Dermoscopy of superficial basal cell carcinoma. *Dermatol Surg*. 2005;31:1710–1713.
14. Menzies SW, Westerhoff K, Rabinovitz H, et al. Surface microscopy of pigmented basal cell carcinoma. *Arch Dermatol*. 2000;136:1012–1016.
15. Peris K, Altobelli E, Ferrari A, et al. Interobserver agreement on dermoscopic features of pigmented basal cell carcinoma. *Dermatol Surg*. 2002;28:643–655.
16. Felder S, Rabinovitz H, Oliviero M, et al. Dermoscopic differentiation of a superficial basal cell carcinoma and squamous cell carcinoma in situ. *Dermatol Surg*. 2006;32:423–425.
17. Zalaudek I, Argenziano G, Leinweber B, et al. Dermoscopy of Bowen's disease. *Br J Dermatol*. 2004;150:1112–1116.
18. Zalaudek I, Hofmann-Wellenhof R, Argenziano G. Dermoscopy of clear-cell acanthoma differs from dermoscopy of psoriasis. *Dermatology*. 2003;207:428 author reply 9.
19. Cameron A, Rosendahl C, Tschandl P, et al. Dermatoscopy of pigmented Bowen's disease. *J Am Acad Dermatol*. 2010;62:597–604.
20. Nachbar F, Stolz W, Merkle T, et al. The ABCD rule of dermatoscopy. High prospective value in the diagnosis of doubtful melanocytic skin lesions. *J Am Acad Dermatol*. 1994;30:551–559.
21. Argenziano G, Fabbrocini G, Carli P, et al. Epiluminescence microscopy for the diagnosis of doubtful melanocytic skin lesions. Comparison of the ABCD rule of dermatoscopy and a new 7-point checklist based on pattern analysis. *Arch Dermatol*. 1998;134:1563–1570.
22. Stolz W, Riemann A, Cognetta AB, et al. ABCD rule of dermatoscopy: a new practical method for early recognition of malignant melanoma. *Eur J Dermatol*. 1994;4:521–527.
23. Henning JS, Dusza SW, Wang SQ, et al. The CASH (color, architecture, symmetry, and homogeneity) algorithm for dermoscopy. *J Am Acad Dermatol*. 2007;56:45–52.
24. Menzies SW, Ingvar C, Crotty KA, et al. Frequency and morphologic characteristics of invasive melanomas lacking specific surface microscopic features. *Arch Dermatol*. 1996;132:1178–1182.
25. Argenziano G, Soyer HP, Chimenti S, et al. Dermoscopy of pigmented skin lesions: results of a consensus meeting via the Internet. *J Am Acad Dermatol*. 2003;48:679–693.
26. Malveyh J, Braun SPP, Marghoob AA, et al., eds. *Handbook of Dermoscopy*. London: Taylor & Francis; 2006.
27. Hofmann-Wellenhof R, Blum A, Wolf IH, et al. Dermoscopic classification of atypical melanocytic nevi (Clark nevi). *Arch Dermatol*. 2001;137:1575–1580.
28. Marghoob AA, Korzenko AJ, Changchien L, et al. The beauty and the beast sign in dermoscopy. *Dermatol Surg*. 2007;33:1388–1391.
29. Kittler H, Pehamberger H, Wolff K, et al. Follow-up of melanocytic skin lesions with digital epiluminescence microscopy: patterns of modifications observed in early melanoma, atypical nevi, and common nevi. *J Am Acad Dermatol*. 2000;43:467–476.
30. Menzies SW, Gutenev A, Avramidis M, et al. Short-term digital surface microscopic monitoring of atypical or changing melanocytic lesions. *Arch Dermatol*. 2001;137:1583–1589.
31. Scope A, Dusza SW, Halpern AC, et al. The "ugly duckling" sign: agreement between observers. *Arch Dermatol*. 2008;144:58–64.
32. Grob JJ, Bonerandi JJ. The 'ugly duckling' sign: identification of the common characteristics of nevi in an individual as a basis for melanoma screening. *Arch Dermatol*. 1998;134:103–104.

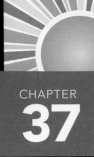

# Computer-Aided Diagnosis for Cutaneous Melanoma

*Sallyann Coleman King, Clara Curiel-Lewandowski, and Suephy C. Chen*

## Key Points

- Computer-aided diagnosis for cutaneous melanoma is a rapidly emerging but promising field of research that has the potential to help physicians to improve diagnostic accuracy for melanoma.

- The combination of rising incidence of melanomas and the need to improve diagnostic accuracy have spurred the research in this field.

- Sequential steps are involved in creating a computer-assisted analysis system. These include image acquisition, lesions segmentation, feature extraction and lesion classification.

- Current computer-assisted analysis systems use differing algorithms and specifications.

## INTRODUCTION

Early detection is critical in lowering mortality from melanoma. As incidence and mortality continue to escalate, and because definitive therapy for advanced melanoma remains elusive, clinicians strive to evolve in their ability to diagnose melanoma at earlier, surgically resectable stages. New technologies, ranging from simple techniques such as photography to more complicated computer-based ones may improve clinical acumen. Ultimately, the role of computer-based diagnostic devices should be to increase the clinician's sensitivity by enhancing the ability to detect lesions and remove them while simultaneously maintaining a high specificity and avoiding the removal of benign lesions. While there is still much work to be done, there are many promising devices which use differing computer-augmented techniques that may serve to enhance the traditional dermatologist visual examination (Table 37.1).

## COMPUTER-ENHANCED TOTAL BODY DIGITAL IMAGING (TBDI)

The use of TBDI to document and monitor patients with many potentially dysplastic nevi has been established.[1,2] Here, images capture the morphology of existing nevi with standardized lighting and body poses allowing the clinician to 'zoom in' for closer evaluation of a concerning lesion. Serial evaluation with photos allows the clinician to better determine relative change in existing nevi as well as to identify new nevi.

Several computer-based imaging systems provide high-definition photographs that can be analyzed allowing for easier tracking of atypical nevi and the appearance of new pigmented lesions. With MoleMapCD (DigitalDerm Inc, Columbia, SC), patients are sent to medical photographers for 36 high-resolution images documenting the patient's entire skin surface using standardized lighting and poses (Fig. 37.1). These images are then stored on a CD. One is given to the physician and one provided to the patients for self-skin examinations.[3] Images on the CD have embedded software which allows the clinician to enlarge and look closer at concerning nevi.

MIRROR DermaGraphix (Canfield Scientific, Fairfield, NJ) has software that enables the linking of close-up or dermoscopy images to specific points on a patient's regional body sector photos. The MIRROR DermaGraphix software is designed for image acquisition performed by, or under the supervision of, each practitioner. In this case, individual, regional, or total body digital images are obtained and downloaded into the software for storage and viewing. A CD or total body photography book can be generated and provided to the patient to enhance self-skin examination.[4]

A side-by-side comparison between total body or regional photographs and the patient skin lesions are completed by the medical provider in the office and/or the patients during self-skin examinations. This method is time-consuming and subjective to individual physician experience and style. In an attempt to automatize TBDI examination and detect changes objectively, a collaborative project between the University of Arizona and Raytheon Missile System was initiated in 2005. To date, a proof of concept has been completed by integrating sophisticated registration and change detection algorithms used in the remote sensing field to standardized TBDI images. Consecutive images can thus be objectively compared for change (Fig. 37.2). As envisioned, the proposed system will generate quantitative results in size and pigmentation that can be compared over time.

## DERMOSCOPY

Dermoscopy is being increasingly adopted as a melanoma diagnostic technique (Chapter 36). Several computer-based algorithms have recently been developed to help with dermoscopy interpretation; however, none has been shown to be superior to physician-based methods. Blum et al. created an algorithm using 64 analytic parameters evaluating 837 digital images of benign lesions and melanoma proving to have an accuracy comparable to that by dermoscopic experts.[5] Others have seen similar results.[6,7]

## Table 37.1 Comparison of Emerging Computer-Aided Melanoma Diagnostic Technologies

| Technology | Sensitivity | Specificity | Advantages | Disadvantages |
|---|---|---|---|---|
| MoleMax | N/A | N/A | Two-camera system; no oil immersion required; transparent overlay for follow-up; total body photography | No computer diagnostic analysis |
| MelaFind | 95–100% | 70–85% | Multispectral sequence of images created in < 3 s; handheld scanner | – |
| Spectrophotometric intracutaneous analysis | 83–96% | 80–87% | Diagnosis of lesions up to 2 mm; visualizes skin structure, vascular composition and reticular pigment networks; handheld scanner | – |
| SolarScan | 91% | 68% | Empirical database for comparison; session and image-level calibration; recorded on graphical map of body | Requires oil immersion |
| Confocal scanning laser microscopy (CSLM) | 98% | 98% | Histopathological evaluation at bedside with similar criteria; longer wavelengths can measure up to papillary dermis; fiber-optic imaging allows for flexible handheld devices | Poor resolution of chromatin patterns, nuclear contours and nucleoli; can only assess to depth of 300 μm; melanomas without in-situ component will likely escape detection |
| Optical coherence tomography (OCT) | N/A | N/A | High-resolution cross-sectional images resembling histopathological section of skin; higher resolution than ultrasound and greater detection depth than CSLM | Photons are scattered more than once, which can lead to image artifacts; ointment or glycerol may be needed to reduce scattering and increase detection depth; visualization of architectural changes and not single cells |
| Ultrasound technology | 99% | 99% | Cost-effective; information about inflammatory processes of skin in relationship to nerves and vessels | Tumor thickness may be overestimated due to underlying inflammatory infiltrate; melanoma metastasis cannot be separated from that of another tumor |
| Electrical bio-impedance | 92–100% | 67–80% | Complete examination lasts 7 minutes | Electrical impedance properties of human skin vary significantly with the body location, age, gender, and season |

Adapted from Patel JK, Konda S, Perez OA, et al. Newer technologies/techniques and tools in the diagnosis of melanoma. *Eur J Dermatol*. 2008;18(6):617–631.

One caveat regarding the assessment of computer-based dermoscopy is the possibility of photo selection bias of the images used for creating and testing the algorithms. A recent study[8] of three computer-program-driven diagnostic instruments found significant variability in the diagnostic accuracy of the instruments in the evaluation of suspect melanocytic lesions. While the three systems were able to accurately identify clinically obvious melanoma, they tended to incorrectly classify most seborrheic keratoses as potential malignant lesions.

Tools are also being developed to allow comparison of dermatoscopic images across time. The DermoGenius Ultra (LINOS AG, BIOCAM, Gottingen) takes and uses standardized images to quantify dermoscopic characteristics into a dermatological point score. These images and scores are compared over time to determine if significant change has occurred.[9]

## MULTISPECTRAL IMAGING (MULTISPECTRAL DIGITAL DERMOSCOPY AND COMPUTER-BASED ANALYSIS)

### Multispectral digital dermoscopy image analysis

As the wavelength of light varies, it is able to penetrate the skin to differing depths. Multispectral imaging takes sequences of images at varying wavelengths (from 400 to 1000 nm), thus supplying information about a range of depths within the lesion in vivo. The depth of penetration

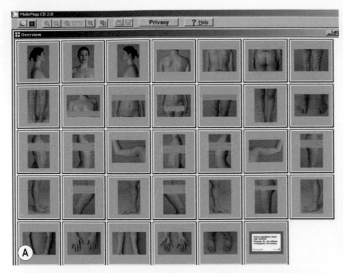

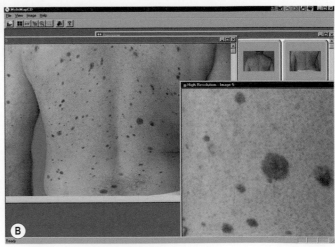

**Figure 37.1** Medical photographers use MoleMapCD to create high-resolution images documenting the patient's entire skin surface.

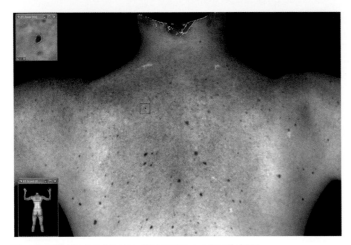

**Figure 37.2** Regional image with graphic overlay of alerts.

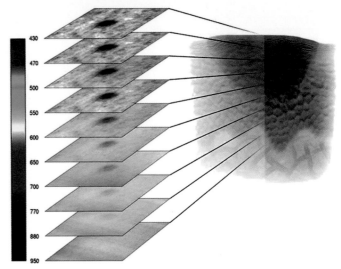

**Figure 37.3** MelaFind. Multiple depths. Light of each wavelength penetrates progressively deeper into the lesion. A digital image of each wavelength corresponding to particular levels down to 2.5 mm is obtained. The image processing algorithms can appreciate 500 characteristics of the pigmented skin lesions per each wavelength. Since there are 10 wavelengths, that means the lesion classification algorithms can choose from a universe of 5000 characteristics in arriving at the optimal group of features that separate melanomas from non-melanomas.

of light into the skin is directly related to wavelength. Information found at different depths is useful in differentiating between benign and malignant pigmented skin lesions.[10] In multispectral digital dermoscopy, a sequence of images is obtained using given bands of wavelengths (Fig. 37.3). The data obtained from differing depths are compared and analyzed by computer using a database of historical lesions. The lesion is then classified into whether biopsy is recommended (suspicious for melanoma). This technique offers the advantages of analyzing features indiscernible to the human eye, probing up to 2 mm below the surface.

The multispectral approach has been augmented through using artificial neural networks so that the diagnostic algorithm iteratively improves.

MelaFind (MelaSciences Inc, Irvington, NY) is a handheld fully automated analysis system using visible and infrared light to capture images, perform segmentation, and classify lesions against a proprietary database of melanomas and benign lesions.[11] Unlike the subjective nature of manual dermoscopy, this device is objective and does not rely on the diagnostic skills of the user.

MelaFind is composed of a handheld imaging device comprising an illuminator that shines light of 10 different specific wavelength bands ranging from 430 nm to 950 nm

(including near infra-red) controlled by narrow interference filters on a rotating wheel, a photon sensor and an image processor employing proprietary algorithms to extract specific features from the images. Each lesion generates six scores based on constrained linear classifiers. These classifiers are established to differentiate melanoma from other pigmented lesions.

The 10 digital image sequence is produced in less than 3 seconds (Fig. 37.3). The images are then analyzed for wavelet maxima, asymmetry, color variation, perimeter changes and textures changes, and the output is a binary 'biopsy' or 'no biopsy needed' recommendation. The MelaFind database of pigmented skin lesions includes in-vivo MelaFind images and corresponding histological results of approximately 9000 biopsied lesions from approximately 7000 patients. Studies demonstrated that MelaFind can achieve 95% to 100% sensitivity and 70% to 85% specificity.

Normal Skin          Superficial Spreading Melanoma (SSM)

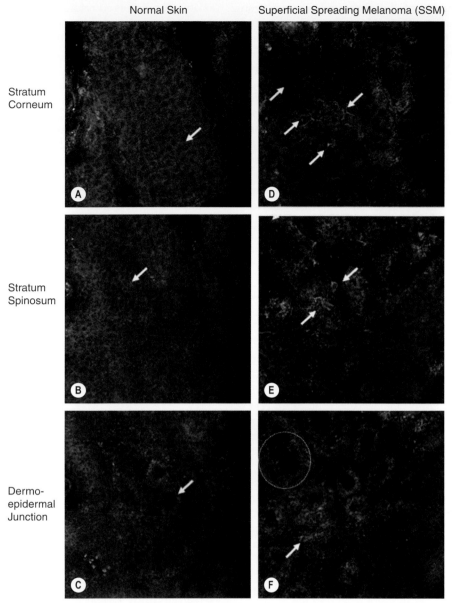

**Figure 37.4** In-vivo confocal scanning laser microscopy. Panels **A–C** show normal skin architecture with normal-appearing keratinocytes (white arrows) and dermal papillae (yellow arrows). Panels **D–F** show findings characteristics of SSM. **D)** Pigmented keratinocytes (yellow arrow) and dendritic cells with enlarged nuclei are observed (white arrows). **E)** Loss of the honeycomb structure and presence of melanocytes in pagetoid distribution. Dendritic melanocytes with enlarged nuclei (white arrows). **F)** Atypical cells (white arrows) and 'non-edged' dermal papillae (dotted circle). (Courtesy of Dr Salvador Gonzalez).

Another study matched a panel of 10 dermatoscopists against MelaFind, using 990 small pigmented lesions. This study found dermatoscopists correctly recommending biopsies with a sensitivity of 71% and a specificity of 49%. MelaFind, however, achieved a sensitivity of 98% and specificity of 44%.[12] Thus, MelaFind is promising as a sensitive adjuvant device for deciding whether or not to biopsy.

SolarScan® (Polartechnics Ltd, Sydney, Australia) has a three charge-coupled device (CCD) video camera for acquiring digital images of lesions, which is used to compare with an empirical database of more than 1800 benign and malignant lesions. The video head is coupled to the skin with oil to eliminate surface reflections. Changes in color, pattern and size are recorded along with the position of each monitored lesion on a graphical map of the patient's body. Images of a lesion from different time points can be viewed simultaneously and the corresponding analysis is displayed on four different graphs. Detection of 14 shades of dermatoscopic colors, as well as the blue-white veil structure (which is one of the best features for invasive melanoma diagnosis), is achieved with a specificity for melanoma diagnosis of 97%.[13] In a study of 2430 pigmented lesions, SolarScan was found to give a sensitivity of 91% and specificity of 68% for melanoma, which was comparable to that of experts.[14]

Spectrophotometric intracutaneous analysis (SIAscope™, Astron Clinica, Cambridge, UK) is based on the principle that individual skin components vary in their optical properties. It uses a chromophore imaging system and probes 1–2 cm² areas of skin using a handheld scanner that emits radiation ranging from 400 to 1000 nm in wavelength. Eight narrowband, spectrally filtered images are obtained, which are then calibrated and entered into computer algorithms created to assess the underlying skin microarchitecture.[15] SIAscopy yields information regarding the location, quantity and distribution of the chromophores collagen, hemoglobin and melanin in the epidermis and dermis – features that have been found to be highly specific (87%) and sensitive (96%) for melanoma.[16] This information is presented in the form of maps called SIAscans, which are then interpreted by the clinician. Moncrieff et al. found several reliable and reproducible features (presence of dermal melanin, collagen holes, and erythematous blush with blood displacement) with 83% sensitivity and 80% specificity in a dataset of 348 pigmented lesions (52 melanomas).[17]

MoleMate (Astron Clinica) is a similar device designed for primary care physicians which includes SIAscopy with a diagnostic algorithm. While this system has great potential, it requires a training program such that the user can become proficient reading the SIAscans.[18]

## CONFOCAL SCANNING LASER MICROSCOPY (CLSM) (REFLECTANCE CONFOCAL MICROSCOPY [RCM])

Confocal microscopy provides real-time in-vivo visualization of subsurface skin structures at a resolution that approaches that of light microscopy (Chapter 38).[19] The confocal microscope uses a near-infrared laser at 830 nm operating at a power of less than 20 mW. The penetration depth of imaging is 200–500 μm, allowing visualization of the epidermis and the superficial dermis (Fig. 37.4). A ×30 water-immersion objective lens provides a lateral resolution of 1–2 μm and an axial resolution of 3–5 μm. Owing to the low power of the diode laser, no tissue damage occurs (see Chapter 38).

Recently, several studies have evaluated the diagnostic accuracy of in-vivo confocal microscopy for melanocytic skin tumors,[20,21] demonstrating sensitivity superior to that of dermoscopy.[22] However, the process is technique-dependent and is somewhat tedious, requiring 5–15 minutes to evaluate a lesion.

## ELECTRICAL IMPEDANCE SPECTROSCOPY (EIS)

This method, called electronic biopsy by SciBase AB (Stockholm, Sweden), uses a probe which painlessly penetrates the stratum corneum, measuring the overall resistance in tissues at alternating currents and frequencies. Here, the device evaluates the resistance of the cells to determine whether the cells are concerning for melanoma. This product is not yet FDA approved.[23]

## CELLULAR ELECTRICAL RESISTANCE (BIO-IMPEDANCE)

Electrical resistance (bio-impedance) of lesions has been studied to assess differences in skin cancers versus benign lesions.[24] Bio-impedance levels are a function of cell shape and structure, cell membranes and the amount of water present. Based on these features, electrical impedance of cancer and benign cells are different because cancer cells typically have a different shape, size and orientation than benign cells do.[25] Bio-impedance measurements of suspicious pigmented lesions are made both over the center of the lesion as well

as on a non-involved reference skin site. Lesional and reference skin are measured at five depth levels, approximately 0.1–2 mm into the tissue, and the data are analyzed by the computer.[26] The entire process takes approximately 7 minutes to complete.

Bio-impedance has a high sensitivity of almost 100% for in-situ and thin melanomas, and can differentiate melanoma from benign nevi with 92–100% sensitivity and 67–75% specificity.[27] Spiked micro-invasive electrodes may be better for melanoma detection (92% sensitivity and 80% specificity) than the regular non-invasive probes.[28] Since electrical impedance properties of human skin vary significantly with the body location, age, gender, and season, more studies are being undertaken to better standardize results.[29]

## ULTRASOUND IMAGING

Ultrasound scanning is a safe non-invasive method that in some settings can be used to show subtle differences between nevi and melanoma. Transducers with higher-frequency wavelengths are beneficial for diagnosing skin lesions because they allow better resolution of small lesions located near the skin surface. However, higher frequency also leads to the tradeoff of decreased depth of penetration by the ultrasound waves, leaving the choice of the probe frequency dependent on the diameter and site of the lesion.[30]

High-resolution B-mode ultrasound has primarily been traditionally used to assess the depth/thickness of melanoma tumors. Reflex transmission imaging (RTI) is a form of high-resolution ultrasound that can be used in combination with white light digital photography for classification of pigmented lesions. Rallan et al. used RTI to derive sonographic parameters to differentiate melanomas from benign pigmented lesions.[31] Significant quantitative differences were noted, allowing discrimination between melanomas, seborrheic keratoses, and nevi. Using a 20-MHz ultrasound B-scan imaging system interfaced to a computer, melanoma could be distinguished from basal cell carcinoma with 100% sensitivity and 79% specificity.[32] Devices such as DermaScan C (Cortex Technology, Hadsund, Denmark) use proprietary computer software to provide skin imaging with resolution to 25 μm in depth, allowing for evaluation of the volume of skin tumors, and thus may be used as a prognostic parameter for melanoma.[33,34]

Further refinements are needed to make this technique widely applicable. Despite various frequency transducers that can probe depths greater than 1.5 cm, melanoma metastasis cannot often be separated from that of another tumor. In addition, the consistency of ultrasound results depends heavily on the skill and experience of the examiner and the anatomic site of the lesion.

## MAGNETIC RESONANCE IMAGING (MRI)

Currently, MRI is thought to be less useful in discriminating banal melanocytic lesions from those which deserve biopsy[35] but may provide some future benefit in evaluating melanoma thickness,[36] allowing better preparation for removal and treatment.

## OPTICAL COHERENCE TOMOGRAPHY

This technique uses a pulse of near-infrared, low-coherence light, splitting it and allowing half of the beam to reach the skin and half to reach the scanning reference mirror. The light on the skin penetrates to a depth of 1 mm and focuses on the papillary dermis before it backscatters and combines with the light reflected from the mirror. The system monitors for an interference signal and informs the user the position within the skin where the light was reflected.[37] The differing components of the tissue (melanin, cell membranes, etc.) reflect the light differently and provide contrast in the CT images.[38] While the resolution does not allow visualization of cell morphology, it allows characterization of the lesion architecture.[39] This is important as melanomas have been shown to have increased architectural disarray, less defined borders, and other structures not seen in normal nevi.[40] The future of this tool in the evaluation of skin lesions is uncertain as we await a better understanding of its value in melanoma diagnosis. Computer-based analysis software is being developed to enhance diagnostic accuracy. Currently, SkinDex 300 (ISIS Optronics, Mannheim, Germany) allows for a resolution of $3 \times 5$ μm.[41]

## FUTURE OUTLOOK

Until a cure for advanced-stage melanoma is found, early detection of melanoma remains the best way to improve survival for melanoma patients. While visual skin examination in dermatology is still clearly the most accessible and relied upon method of diagnosing melanoma, differentiation of suspicious lesions may frequently be difficult. This difficulty will continue to spur the development of technical advances. Many other tools are on the horizon for use, which may reduce unnecessary biopsies and provide greater accuracy in differentiating suspicious lesions for biopsy. However, the effectiveness of these devices remain dependent on the user to clinically select the appropriate lesion(s) for imaging.

## REFERENCES

1. Feit N, Dusza S, Marghoob A. Melanomas detected with the aid of total cutaneous photography. *Br J Dermatol*. 2004;150:706–714.
2. Shriner D, Wagner Jr R, Glowczwski J. Photography for the early diagnosis of malignant melanoma in patients with atypical moles. *Cutis*. 1992;50:358–362.
3. Derm D, MoleMap CD. Available from: http://www.digitalderm.com/ Accessed October 13, 2009.
4. Canfield Scientific. *Total body photography from Canfield*. Available from: http://www.canfieldsci.com/FileLibrary/BodyMap_Brochure.pdf Accessed October 13, 2009.
5. Blum A, Luedtke H, Ellwanger U, et al. Digital image analysis for diagnosis of cutaneous melanoma. Development of a highly effective computer algorithm based on analysis of 837 melanocytic lesions. *Br J Dermatol*. 2004;151(5):1029–1038.
6. Barzegari M, Ghaninezhad H, Mansoori P, et al. Computer-aided dermoscopy for diagnosis of melanoma. *BMC Dermatol*. 2005;5:8.
7. Pellacani G, Grana C, Seidenari S. Algorithmic reproduction of asymmetry and boarder cut-off parameters according to the ABCD rule for dermoscopy. *J Eur Acad Dermatol Venereol*. 2006;20:1214–1219.
8. Perrinaud A, Gaide O, French L, et al. Can automated dermoscopy image analysis instruments provide added benefit for the dermatologist? A study comparing the results of three systems. *Br J Dermatol*. 2007;157(5):926–933.
9. BIOCAM. DermoGenius Ultra. Available from: http://www.biocam.de/DermoGenius-ultra.72.0.html?&L=1. Accessed October 17, 2009.
10. Carrara M, Bono A, Bartoli C, et al. Multispectral imaging and artificial neural network: mimicking the management decision of the clinician facing pigmented skin lesions. *Phys Med Biol*. 2007;52(9):2599–2613.
11. Elbaum M, Kopf AW, Rabinowitz HS, et al. Automatic differentiation of melanoma from melanocytic nevi with multispectral digital dermoscopy: A feasibility study. *J Am Acad Dermatol*. 2001;44(1):207–218.
12. Friedman R, Gutkowicz-Krusin D, Farber M, et al. The diagnostic performance of expert dermoscopists vs a computer-vision system on small-diameter melanomas. *Arch Dermatol*. 2008;144(4):476–482.
13. Menzies SW, Gutenev A, Avramidis M, et al. Short-term digital surface microscopic monitoring of atypical or changing melanocytic lesions. *Arch Dermatol*. 2001;137:1583–1589.
14. Menzies SW, Bischof L, Talbot H, et al. The performance of SolarScan: an automated dermoscopy image analysis instrument for the diagnosis of primary melanoma. *Arch Dermatol*. 2005;141:1388–1396.
15. Goodson AG, Grossman D. Strategies for early melanoma detection: approaches to the patient with nevi. *J Am Acad Dermatol*. 2009;60:719–735.
16. Michalska M, Chodorowska G, Krasowska D. SIAscopy—a new non-invasive technique of melanoma diagnosis. *Ann Univ Mariae Curie Sklodowska [Med]*. 2004;59:421–431.
17. Moncrieff M, Cotton S, Claridge E, et al. Spectrophotometric intracutaneous analysis: a new technique for imaging pigmented skin lesions. *Br J Dermatol*. 2002;146(3):448–457.
18. Wood A, Morris H, Emery J, et al. Evaluation of the MoleMate training program for assessment of suspicious pigmented lesions in primary care. *Inform Prim Care*. 2008;16(1):41–50.
19. Meyer L, Otberg N, Sterry W, et al. In vivo confocal scanning laser microscopy; comparison of the reflectance and fluorescence mode by imaging human skin. *J Biomed Opt*. 2006;11(4):044012.
20. Gerger A, Hofmann-Wellenhof R, Samonigg H, et al. In vivo confocal laser scanning microscopy in the diagnosis of melanocytic skin tumours. *Br J Dermatol*. 2009;160(3):475–481.
21. Scope A, Benvenuto-Andrade C, Agero A, et al. In vivo reflectance confocal microscopy imaging of melanocytic skin lesions: consensus terminology glossary and illustrative images. *J Am Acad Dermatol*. 2007;57(4):644–658.
22. Langley R, Walsh N, Sutherland A, et al. The diagnostic accuracy of in vivo confocal scanning laser microscopy compared to dermoscopy of benign and malignant melanocytic lesions: a prospective study. *Dermatology*. 2007;215(4):365–372.
23. SCIBASE. Overview: SciBase electronic biopsy method. Available from: http://www.scibase.se/Templates/Article1.aspx?PageID=d2307fdd-ef31-4be2-92b9-94565b13bcc3 Accessed November 16, 2009.
24. Aberg P, Nicander I, Hansson J, et al. Skin cancer identification using multifrequency electrical impedance—a potential screening tool. *IEEE Trans Biomed Eng*. 2004;51:2097–2102.
25. Blad B, Baldetorp B. Impedance spectra of tumour tissue in comparison with normal tissue; a possible clinical application for electrical impedance tomography. *Physiol Meas*. 1996;17(Suppl 4A):A105–A115.
26. Har-Shai Y, Glickman YA, Siller G, et al. Electrical impedance scanning for melanoma diagnosis: a validation study. *Plast Reconstr Surg*. 2005;116:782–790.
27. Glickman YA, Filo O, David M, et al. Electrical impedance scanning: a new approach to skin cancer diagnosis. *Skin Res Technol*. 2003;9:262–268.
28. Aberg P, Geladi P, Nicander I, et al. Non-invasive and microinvasive electrical impedance spectra of skin cancer – a comparison between two techniques. *Skin Res Technol*. 2005;11:281–286.
29. Nicander I, Ollmar S. Electrical impedance measurements at different skin sites related to seasonal variations. *Skin Res Technol*. 2000;6:81–86.
30. Gambichler T, Moussa G, Bahrenberg K, et al. Preoperative ultrasonic assessment of thin melanocytic skin lesions using a 100-MHz ultrasound transducer: a comparative study. *Dermatol Surg*. 2007;33:818–824.
31. Rallan D, Bush NL, Bamber JC, et al. Quantitative discrimination of pigmented lesions using three-dimensional high-resolution ultrasound reflex transmission imaging. *J Invest Dermatol*. 2007;127:189–195.
32. Harland CC, Kale SG, Jackson P, et al. Differentiation of common benign pigmented skin lesions from melanoma by high-resolution ultrasound. *Br J Dermatol*. 2000;143(2):281–289.
33. Cortex Technology DermaScan C. Available from:http://www.cortex.dk/dermascan_c.htm Accessed October 18, 2009.
34. Stucker M, Wilmert M, Hoffmann K, et al. Objectivity, reproducibility and validity of 3D ultrasound in dermatology. *Bildgebung*. 1995;62(3):179–188.
35. Maurer J, Knollmann F, Schlums D, et al. Role of high-resolution magnetic resonance imaging for differentiating melanin-containing skin tumors. *Invest Radiol*. 1995;30(11):638–643.
36. Ono I, Kaneko F. Magnetic resonance imaging for diagnosing skin tumors. *Clin Dermatol*. 1995;13(4):393–399.
37. Marchesini R, Bono A, Bartoli C, et al. Optical imaging and automated melanoma detection: questions and answers. *Melanoma Res*. 2002;12(3):279–286.

**38.** Tadrous P. Methods for imaging the structure and function of living tissues and cells: optical coherence tomography. *J Pathol.* 2000;191:115–119.

**39.** Giorgi V, Stante M, Massi D, et al. Possible histopathologic correlates of dermoscopic features in pigmented melanocytic lesions identified by means of optical coherence tomography. *Exp Dermatol.* 2005;2005(14):56–59.

**40.** Gambichler T, Regeniter P, Bechara F, et al. Characterization of benign and malignant melanocytic skin lesions using optical coherence tomography in vivo. *J Am Acad Dermatol.* 2007;57(4):629–637.

**41.** ISIS Optronics. Specification of SkinDex 300. Available from: http://www.isis-optronics.de/en/skindex/produkte/content.html Accessed October 19, 2009.

# Confocal Microscopy in Skin Cancer

*Verena Ahlgrimm-Siess, Harold S. Rabinovitz, Margaret Oliviero, Rainer Hofmann-Wellenhof,*

*Ashfaq A. Marghoob, Salvador González, and Alon Scope*

## Key Points

- Reflectance confocal microscopy (RCM) enables imaging of skin lesions at cellular-level resolution either at the bedside (*in vivo*) or in freshly excised tissue (*ex vivo*).
- Like dermoscopy, in-vivo RCM acquires images in the horizontal plane (*en face*), allowing RCM investigation of tissue pathology underlying dermoscopic structures of interest.
- RCM is a promising technique for the non-invasive diagnosis of skin neoplasms as well as for monitoring surgical margins and response to non-invasive treatment.

## INTRODUCTION

The search to enhance our clinical diagnosis and to minimize unnecessary skin biopsies has led to the development of non-invasive imaging techniques. Unlike other non-invasive imaging modalities, reflectance confocal microscopy (RCM) offers imaging at cellular-level resolution. RCM imaging can be performed at the bedside – *in vivo* – or on freshly excised tissue – *ex vivo*.

In-vivo RCM enables the visualization of epidermis and upper dermis in real-time. While RCM has been applied in a variety of skin conditions, the research focus has been on diagnosis of skin neoplasms. With RCM, optical sectioning of the skin can be performed, like an 'optical biopsy'; this non-invasive approach is especially desirable for cosmetically sensitive areas such as the face. In addition, RCM enables repeated imaging of the same lesion over time, which can be used for monitoring efficacy of non-invasive treatment. The ability to visualize dynamic processes by RCM (e.g. blood flow) is of great interest for clinical as well as basic dermatological research.

Ex-vivo RCM allows immediate imaging of freshly biopsied tissue with hardly any laboratory processing. Thus, ex-vivo RCM may be used in the future to expedite surgical margin assessment (e.g. during Mohs micrographic surgery).

## HISTORY

Confocal scanning microscopy was invented in 1957 by Marvin Minsky at Harvard University.[1] However, only in the 1990s did further advances in optical and electronic technologies allow for the development of an RCM device that could image skin in real-time and that was suitable for clinical applications.[2,3]

## PRINCIPLES OF REFLECTANCE CONFOCAL MICROSCOPY

The basic principle of RCM is the use of a point source of light which is tightly focused on a specific point in the tissue. The light is reflected back by certain tissue structures due to variations of refractive indices within the skin; specifically, melanin, hydrated collagen, and keratin are highly reflective skin components which appear brighter on RCM images than the surrounding structures. Only light reflected back from the focus point is allowed to enter the RCM detector through a pinhole-sized spatial filter and be processed by the dedicated software (Fig. 38.1).

RCM uses a near-infrared, low-power laser beam (830 nm diode laser, power up to 35 mW) for imaging (Fig. 38.2A). The laser beam is scanned in a two-dimensional grid over the skin to obtain a thin horizontal optical section which is displayed as a gray scale image (500×500 µm field-of-view, Fig. 38.3). An automated stepper can be used to obtain up to 256 sequential images making a mosaic grid of 16×16 contiguous images in the horizontal plane (Fig. 38.4). By adjusting the focal length of the laser beam, a series of single images can be stacked vertically at the same point in the tissue (Fig. 38.4). A combination of both imaging settings (mosaicing and stacking) allows for collection of a cube of skin imaging data (Fig. 38.4).

To minimize motion artifacts, an adaptor ring with a disposable polymer window provided with a double-sided adhesive is fixed to the patient's skin and then coupled magnetically to the RCM probe (Fig. 38.2B,D). Water-based gel between the probe and window and crodamol oil between the window and skin are used as immersion media. Before RCM imaging, a dermoscopic image, providing a 10×10 mm field-of-view can be captured through the tissue ring with a dedicated camera attached to the RCM (Fig. 38.2C). The dermoscopic picture correlates precisely to the RCM mosaic images and can be viewed simultaneously, serving as a gross map to guide RCM imaging of sub-regions of the lesion with a high degree of accuracy (Fig. 38.3).

The RCM is equipped with a 30× water immersion objective lens, providing a 30× magnification for single images and a lateral resolution of 0.5–1 µm. The axial resolution which determines the section thickness is approximately 3–5 µm; this thickness is comparable to the thickness of histological sections. Also comparable to routine histopathology, evaluation

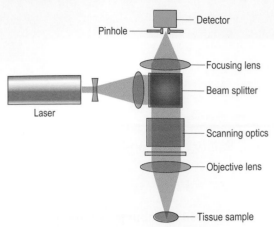

**Figure 38.1** Schematic of the pathway of light in reflectance confocal microscopy: a point within the tissue is illuminated by a point source of laser light (830 nm laser). Light that is backscattered from tissue structures that are in the focal point is collected through a small aperture (pinhole) into the detector, while light out of focus is rejected. By scanning the focal point in the horizontal plane, an image is produced that represents a thin *en face* optical section of tissue.

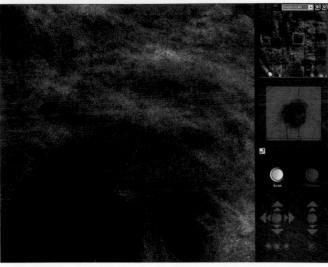

**Figure 38.3** Screenshot from the Vivascope® computer during RCM imaging. Most of the screen is taken up by a single RCM image (500 × 500 μm, displayed on the left). A mosaic (3 × 3 mm) is also seen (right upper corner); the yellow square highlighted within the mosaic corresponds to location of the single RCM image displayed on the left. The mosaic and the dermoscopic image below the mosaic may serve as gross maps for RCM imaging. Both images can be viewed as enlarged pictures by toggling them with the single RCM images. The buttons in the right lower corner are used to navigate the RCM light within the tissue along the x-, y- and z-axis and to capture RCM images and videos.

**Figure 38.2 A)** Reflectance confocal microscope equipped with a dermoscopic camera and a handheld probe (the darker blue device that resembles a drill). **B)** A metal adaptor ring (left upper corner) is attached to a disposable polymer disc (right lower corner). The metal ring provides the housing for the RCM probe. The polymer disc provides a window through which imaging is done and also provides a double-sided adhesive that sticks to the ring and secures it to the skin. **C)** A dermoscopic picture that serves as a gross map during RCM imaging is captured through the adaptor ring–polymer disc. **D)** The probe is coupled magnetically to the adaptor ring that is fixed to the skin. To reduce backscatter and distortion of light, crodamol oil is used as an immersion media between skin and the polymer window, and water-based gel is used between the polymer window and the RCM probe.

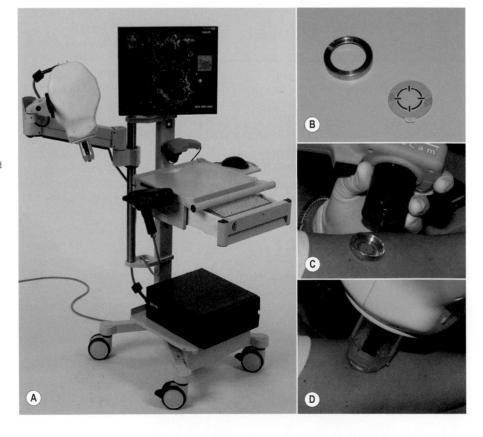

of RCM images is usually done first at 'low magnification' (e.g. 8×8 mm mosaic similar to 2× magnification in histopathology) to examine the overall lesion architecture and then at 'higher magnification' by assessing single RCM images (500×500 μm field-of-view akin to 30× magnification) to further examine architectural and cytomorphological details.

The major limitation of RCM is the limited imaging depth of approximately 250 μm, which usually correlates to the level of the papillary dermis or the upper reticular dermis. Another disadvantage is that assessment of nuclear details with RCM is significantly inferior to assessment with histopathology.

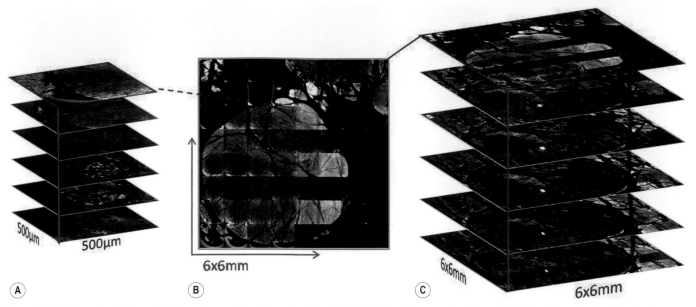

**Figure 38.4** Schematic of different RCM imaging modes. **(A)** a vertical stack of single 500×500 μm *en face* images is obtained; there is an automatic stepper that moves the focal plane deeper into the tissue (along the z-axis) at increments of ≥1 μm, while acquiring single images at the same point (x–y plane) in the tissue. **(B)** up to 256 contiguous single 500×500 μm images are captured in the horizontal plane (x–y plane) and are stitched together, forming a mosaic of up to 8×8 mm. **(C)** sequential mosaics are captured at different imaging depths (incremental steps along the z-axis) at the same area in the tissue (x–y plane), providing a cube of images of the skin.

## NORMAL SKIN

RCM imaging should follow a standardized protocol to enable accurate and reproducible image analysis. For this purpose, mosaic images of the suprabasal epidermis, the dermal–epidermal junction (DEJ) and the superficial dermis should be routinely acquired. Single images and RCM movies are taken in areas of special interest.

With RCM, the normal skin surface is seen as bright, large 'wrinkled'-appearing sheets of stratum corneum separated by dark furrows which correlate to the skin folds (Fig. 38.5A). Occasionally, single corneocytes, which appear as large, polygonal-shaped, anucleated cells, can be seen within the sheets. Below the stratum corneum, the granular cells are visualized, displaying bright grainy structures within the cytoplasm. Spinous cells resemble granular cells but are smaller and with a cytoplasm which is less bright and less grainy than that of granular cells. The cytoplasm and intercellular connections (e.g. desmosomes) of granular and spinous cells appear bright whereas the nuclei appear as central dark oval to round structures. The overall RCM appearance of the spinous and granular layers has been called 'honeycomb pattern' (Table 38.1), with bright lines of the honeycomb correlating to cytoplasm of keratinocytes and their intercellular connections and the dark holes correlating to the nuclei. In normal skin, the nuclei are regular in size and the lines show a fairly uniform thickness and reflectivity (Fig. 38.5B). In patients with darker skin color, pigmented keratinocytes can be seen at suprabasal layers. Suprabasal pigmented keratinocytes appear bright on RCM and their nuclei are obscured by the bright melanin. Thus, aggregated, bright polygonal keratinocytes laid back-to-back are observed, forming the so-called 'cobblestone pattern' (Table 38.1) instead of the honeycomb pattern.

At an average depth of 100 μm below the skin surface, a single layer of basal cells is visualized. Basal cells harbor a higher amount of melanin than do other epidermal layers.[3,4] In an undulating DEJ, basal keratinocytes will appear as disk-like bright cell aggregates when RCM sections at the suprapapillary plates, and as bright rings surrounding dark dermal papillae ('edged papillae'; Table 38.1) when RCM sections deeper, at the level of the dermal papillae (Fig. 38.5C). In a flattened DEJ, as seen in sun-damaged skin, basal keratinocytes will appear as aggregates or sheets of bright cells directly above the dermis; bright rings will not be seen. Within the dermal papillae, blood flow in capillary loops can be observed. Below the DEJ, a network of fibers and bundles can be seen within the papillary and superficial reticular dermis correlating to dermal collagen (Fig. 38.5D). In addition, hair follicles present as round to ovoid structures characterized by smaller keratinocytes at the periphery and larger, flat keratinocytes towards the center, and displaying a central dark ostium that contains a refractile hair shaft. Sweat gland openings appear as bright centrally hollow structures that spiral through the epidermis. The appearance of normal skin will vary according to the patient's age and skin color, the anatomic site being imaged, and the degree of sun damage present.[5,6]

## NON-MELANOMA SKIN CANCERS

Non-melanoma skin cancer (NMSC) tends to occur on a background of significantly photodamaged skin. Patients can have numerous basal cell carcinomas (BCCs) or squamous cell carcinomas (SCCs) concomitantly, and those need to be distinguished from the background solar lentigines, lichen planus-like keratoses, and seborrheic keratoses. Dermoscopy has limited utility when it comes to the diagnosis of pink, erythematous, non-pigmented

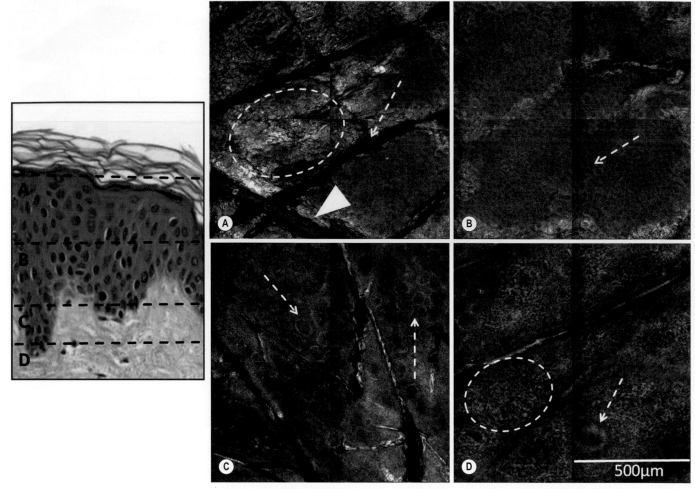

**Figure 38.5** Horizontal RCM sections (1×1 mm) of normal skin at various imaging depths, as indicated on the vertically cut histological image. **A)** Polygonal skin islands are separated by dark furrows (arrow); the furrows correlate to skin surface folds (dermatoglyphics). The stratum corneum presents as a 'wrinkled'-appearing bright reflecting sheet (circle). A refractile long cylindrical tube correlating to a hair shaft is observed (arrowhead). **B)** Regular honeycomb pattern of the granular and spinous layers seen with RCM. Dark holes of regular size, correlating to nuclei of keratinocytes (arrow) and bright lines with uniform thickness and reflectivity, correlating to cytoplasm of keratinocytes and intercellular connections, are seen. **C)** Dark, round to oval dermal papillae surrounded by a slightly brighter rim of pigmented basal keratinocytes and melanocytes ('edged papillae') are observed at the DEJ (arrows). **D)** Within the papillary dermis a web-like pattern of bright collagen fibers is seen (circle). The bright, centrally hollow structure (arrow) is a sweat duct; spiraling of the epidermal portion of the sweat duct (acrosyringium) through the epidermis can be seen when sequential images are obtained along the z-axis.

## Table 38.1 Key RCM Features of Normal Skin by Anatomic Level

| RCM Feature | Definition |
| --- | --- |
| **Superficial epidermal layers (granular-spinous layers)** | |
| Honeycomb pattern | Normal pattern of the granular-spinous layers formed by bright polygonal outlines of keratinocytes (cytoplasm and intercellular connections) with dark central nuclei |
| Cobblestone pattern | Normal pattern of basal keratinocytes at the supra-papillary plates and a variant of the normal pattern of the granular-spinous layers in darkly pigmented skin; bright round cells without a visible nucleus (pigmented keratinocytes) are closely set, separated by a less refractive polygonal outline |
| **Dermal–epidermal junction** | |
| Edged papillae | Dermal papillae demarcated by a rim of bright cells (pigmented basal keratinocytes and melanocytes) |
| **Superficial dermis** | |
| Collagen | Bright fibrillar structures that appear finely reticulated, forming a web-like pattern, or as thicker bundles |

skin lesions. RCM has been emerging as a promising imaging tool that can help diagnose with specificity solitary pink lesions.[7]

## Reflectance confocal microscopy of actinic keratosis and squamous cell carcinoma

Actinic keratoses (AK) are characterized on histopathology by crowding, jumbling and atypia of nuclei of keratinocytes and dyskeratotic keratinocytes in the lower part of the epidermis; there is typically alternating ortho- and parakeratosis (with sparing of the corneal layer above infundibula). In addition, solar elastosis is invariably observed in the dermis. SCC in situ (Bowen's disease) shows on histopathology atypia of keratinocytes that involves the full thickness of the epidermis, invasive SCC is characterized by aggregates of atypical keratinocytes that extend into the reticular dermis.

With RCM, AK and SCC show an irregular and thickened stratum corneum (Fig. 38.6B and Fig. 38.7B) which correlate to the ortho- and parakeratosis seen on histopathology. [8,9] Focally, dark nuclei are visualized on RCM within the stratum corneum, correlating with parakeratosis on histopathology. The stratum granulosum and spinosum display on RCM pleomorphism of keratinocytes – the cells are irregularly crowded, and vary in size and shape; the findings sum up to an irregular honeycomb pattern with lines that vary in width and level of brightness, and with

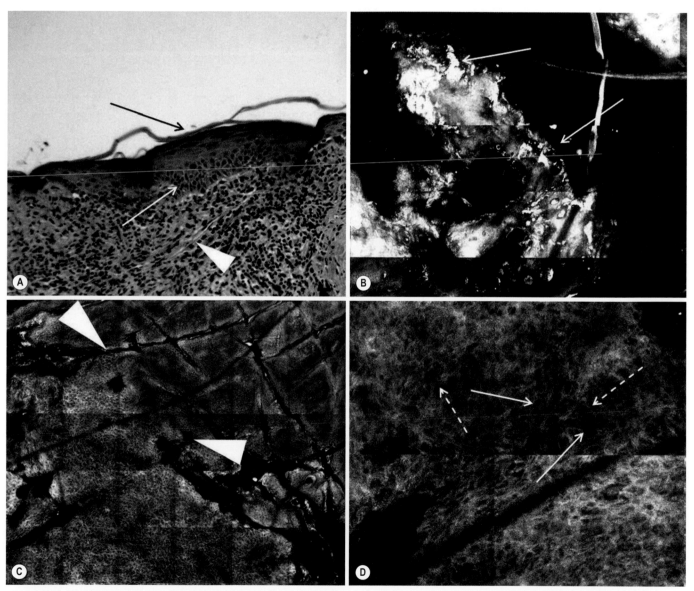

**Figure 38.6** RCM features and histopathological correlates of an actinic keratosis. **A)** On histopathology, there is orthokeratosis (black arrow), crowding of atypical keratinocytes at the lower part of the epidermis (white arrow), and a dense lichenoid infiltrate of lymphocytes and solar elastosis (arrowhead) in the underlying dermis. **B)** On RCM at the stratum corneum level (low magnification, 2.5 × 2 mm field-of-view), irregularly shaped and heterogeneously bright reflecting sheets of different sizes and shapes (arrows) are observed, correlating to the scale observed clinically and to orthokeratosis seen on histopathology. **C)** At the spinous and granular layers, the transition (arrowheads) from irregular (lower left) to regular (upper right) honeycomb patterns is seen at low magnification (3 × 2.5 mm field-of-view). **D)** An irregular honeycomb pattern is seen on higher magnification (approximately 500 × 500 µm field-of-view) at the spinous layer; the irregular honeycomb consists of lines varying in width and brightness (dashed arrows) and holes varying in size and shape (arrows) correlating on histopathology to abnormal keratinocytes whose nuclei are jumbled and vary in size and shape.

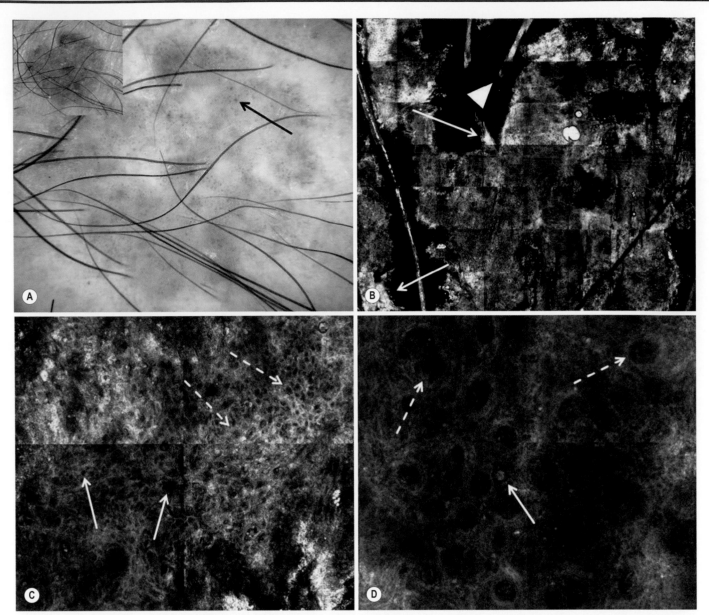

**Figure 38.7** Clinical, dermoscopic and RCM images of Bowen's disease (SCC in situ). **A)** Clinically, a red scaly plaque measuring 15 mm in diameter is seen (insert). An ill-defined pink structureless lesion with diffuse dotted vessels (arrow) is observed on dermoscopy. **B)** On RCM at the level of the stratum corneum, irregularly shaped and heterogeneously bright sheets with loss of the normal skin folds are seen at low magnification (3.5 × 4 mm field-of-view). The brighter foci (arrows) correlate to the scale seen clinically. Hair shafts (arrowhead) are also seen. **C)** An irregular honeycomb pattern is seen at the level of the spinous layer (1 × 1 mm field-of-view) with variability in the width and brightness of the lines (dashed arrows) and size and shape of the holes (arrows). In foci, large holes, representing abnormally large nuclei of keratinocytes, are seen. **D)** At the DEJ, increased density of dermal papillae having different sizes and shapes (dashed arrows) and harboring dilated blood vessels are visualized (1 × 1 mm field-of-view). In addition, a single large, round, bright non-nucleated cell is seen (arrow) at the basal layer of the epidermis, probably correlating to a dyskeratotic keratinocyte.

dark nuclei that vary in size or that are obscured (Table 38.2, Fig. 38.6C,D and Fig. 38.7C). Within the papillary dermis, abnormal bundles are seen that are wider than normal collagen bundles and that appear clumped (Fig. 38.8), correlating with solar elastosis on histopathology. Small bright stellate dots, correlating to inflammatory cells, may also be detected within the dermis.

A recent study showed high interobserver agreement on the RCM diagnosis of AK. Key RCM features were pleomorphism of keratinocytes and loss of the regular stratification of the epidermal layers whereby a clear differentiation between granular, spinous and basal layer was no longer possible. These key RCM parameters yielded a high sen-

sitivity (100%) and specificity (91.2%) for the diagnosis of AK.[10] A sensitivity and specificity of 93.34% and 88.34%, respectively, were reported for the discrimination of AK from contralateral sun-damaged skin.[11]

On RCM, SCC shows similar, albeit more pronounced, findings compared to AK.[12] Bright, round cells within the granular and spinous layers, whose nuclei are often obscured, are more frequently observed in SCC, correlating to dyskeratotic cells seen on histopathology. The honeycomb pattern is focally lost in the spinous and granular layers ('disarranged' pattern, Table 38.2). Dilated, round blood vessels (Table 38.2) running perpendicular to the horizontal confocal plane of imaging, in a looped or tortuous course, are observed

## Table 38.2 Key RCM Features of Non-Melanoma Skin Cancers

| RCM Feature | Definition |
| --- | --- |
| **Actinic keratosis and squamous cell carcinoma** | |
| Irregular honeycomb pattern | Abnormal pattern of the granular-spinous layers formed by bright cellular outlines which vary in size and shapes and in the thickness and brightness of the lines |
| Disarranged pattern | Focal or diffuse loss of the normal patterns of the granular-spinous layers (honeycomb or cobblestone) |
| Round blood vessels | Dilated blood vessels within the dermal papillae that run perpendicular to the horizontal confocal plane of imaging |
| **Basal cell carcinoma** | |
| Streaming | Basal or spinous keratinocytes that appear to be focally elongated and distorted into alignment along the same axis |
| Tumor islands | Round to oval, cord-like or lobulated structures at the level of DEJ or superficial dermis that can be either darker than the surrounding epidermis or dermis ('dark silhouettes') or bright structures, well demarcated by a surrounding dark cleft |
| Linear blood vessels | Branching and tortuous dilated blood vessels in the superficial dermis that run parallel to the horizontal (en face) confocal plane of imaging |

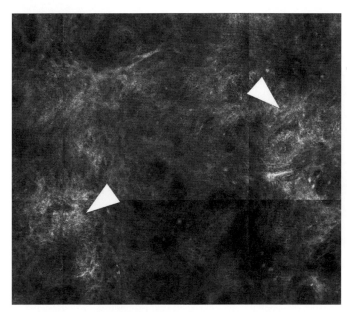

**Figure 38.8** Dermal RCM features of the Bowen's disease shown in Figure 38.7. Abnormally clumped bundles that are wider than usual (arrowheads) are seen within the papillary dermis (1×1 mm field-of-view), correlating with solar elastosis. The small bright stellate dots dispersed between the collagen bundles are inflammatory cells.

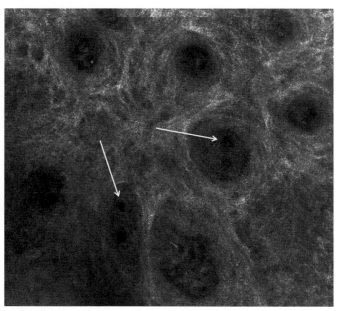

**Figure 38.9** Vascular RCM features of the Bowen's disease shown in Figure 38.7. At the level of the superficial dermis (500 × 500 μm field-of-view), dilated round blood vessels running perpendicular to the RCM plane of imaging are detected within dermal papillae. Most dermal papillae display two dark holes; one is the ascending and the other the descending portion of the capillary loop. These blood vessels would be visualized as dotted vessels on dermoscopy.

within dermal papillae in most cases of SCC and less often in AK; these vessels may be also visualized as glomerular or dotted vessels on dermoscopy (Fig. 38.7A,D and Fig. 38.9).

At present, RCM does not allow differentiation with high specificity between AK, SCC in situ, and invasive SCC. It does, however, allow differentiation from other disease entities that occur on sun-damaged skin, such as BCC, solar lentigo, lichen planus-like keratosis, and melanoma.

## Basal cell carcinoma

González et al. first described RCM features of BCC in 2002.[13] The most striking feature of BCC with RCM is the presence of tumor islands (Table 38.2) sharply demarcated

from the surrounding dermis by dark cleft-like spaces. Bright tumor islands are typically seen in pigmented BCCs (Fig. 38.10 and Fig. 38.11A). The presence of tumor islands as hyporeflective areas ('dark silhouettes') that are darker than the surrounding dermis or basal epidermis is mostly seen in non-pigmented BCCs (Fig. 38.11B). The tumor islands seen on RCM correlate on histopathology with aggregates of basaloid cells with peripheral palisading of nuclei and clefting. The bright and the darker tumor islands can also be seen in the same BCC, reflecting the degree of pigmentation within the neoplastic aggregates.

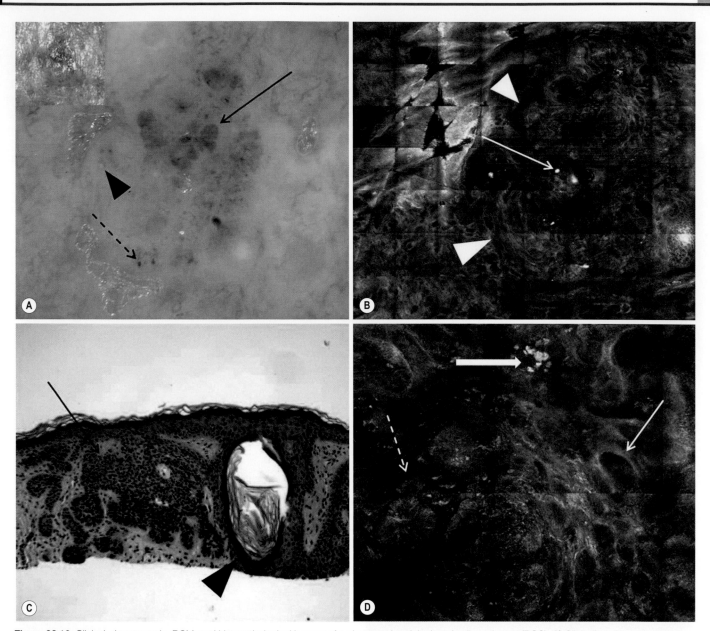

**Figure 38.10** Clinical, dermoscopic, RCM, and histopathological images of a pigmented nodular basal cell carcinoma (BCC). **A)** Clinically, a 3-mm tan papule is seen (insert). With dermoscopy, focal aggregates of brown ovoid structures (arrow) as well as grey dots (dashed arrow) are observed. In addition, subtle milia-like cysts are detected (arrowhead). **B)** On RCM, a large oval structure, sharply demarcated from the surrounding skin (arrowheads), is visualized at the DEJ/upper dermis at low magnification (3.5×4 mm field-of-view), correlating to the clinically observed tan papule. Small, highly reflective structures (arrow), correlating to the dermoscopically recognized milia-like cysts, are seen within the tumor island. **C)** Histopathology shows dermal aggregates of basaloid cells with peripheral palisading of nuclei (arrow). A dilated follicular infundibulum is additionally seen (arrowhead) amidst the neoplastic aggregates, possibly accounting for the finding of milia-like cysts on dermoscopy. **D)** At high magnification RCM (1×1mm field-of-view), reflective round to oval structures (dashed arrow) are seen in the dermis; these are bright tumor islands that correlate to pigmented basaloid aggregates. In addition, dark, oval to round structures are seen in the dermis (arrow) with RCM; these are also tumor islands, termed 'dark silhouettes', that correlate with non-pigmented basaloid aggregates in BCC. A focal aggregate of round to triangular non-nucleated cells (thick arrow), correlating to melanophages, is also seen.

Bright dendritic structures and/or dendritic cells can be seen within refractile tumor islands and represent melanocytes or Langerhans cells in pigmented BCC[14] (Fig. 38.11A). Interestingly, when viewed by RCM at the en face plane, basal or spinous keratinocytes above tumor islands in BCC appear to be focally elongated and distorted into alignment along an axis ('streaming') (Fig. 38.12 and Table 38.2). The papillary dermis displays dense bright collagen bundles between the tumor islands (Fig. 38.13) correlating to the fibrotic stroma associated with BCC. Dilated and tortuous linear blood vessels (Table 38.2) that run parallel to the horizontal plane of RCM imaging are also typically observed within the stroma (Fig. 38.14B). These vessels correlate with the arborizing or fine branching vessels seen on dermoscopy (Fig. 38.14A). In pigmented BCC, round to triangular plump-bright cells with indistinct nucleus may be observed on RCM singly or in aggregates within the stroma (Fig. 38.15C, D); these correlate with melanophages on histopathology.[15]

The reliability of RCM criteria of BCCs was subsequently validated in a multicenter study with 152 cases; the presence of four or more criteria resulted in a sensitivity of 82.9% and

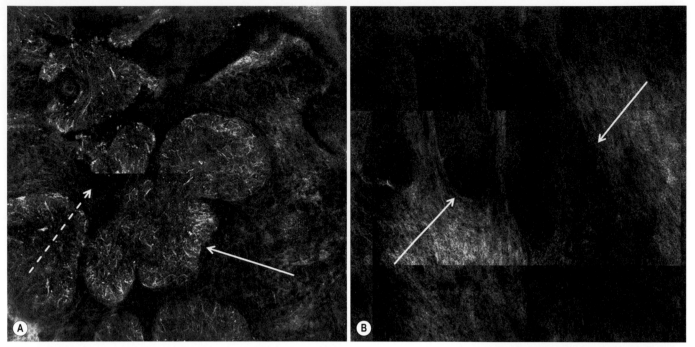

**Figure 38.11** RCM image (1×1mm field-of-view) of bright tumor islands and dark silhouettes seen in basal cell carcinoma (BCC). **A)** On RCM, the bright tumor islands of BCC harbor numerous bright dendritic structures (arrow). These are dendrites of melanocytes in pigmented basaloid aggregates of BCC. Dark cleft-like spaces are also observed surrounding the tumor islands (dashed arrow). **B)** Hyporeflective tumor islands appear as 'dark silhouettes' (arrows) within the bright collagen of the tumor stroma; these correlate with non-pigmented basaloid aggregates of BCC.

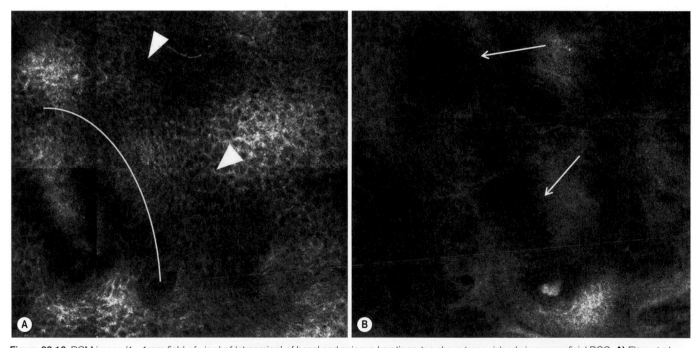

**Figure 38.12** RCM image (1 × 1mm field-of-view) of 'streaming' of basal and spinous keratinocytes above tumor islands in a superficial BCC. **A)** Elongated nuclei of keratinocytes (arrowheads) are observed oriented along the same axis (curved line) above tumor islands, creating a distortion in the honeycomb pattern. **B)** Dark tumor islands ('dark silhouettes', arrows) are observed within the dermis at a deeper section of the area shown in part A.

a specificity of 95.7%, with little variability across study site and BCC subtype.[16] However, the number of infiltrative BCCs included in the study was small, and the detection of this BCC subtype still remains challenging with RCM; the small cords and strands of neoplastic cells are difficult to detect within the bright dermal collagen. In addition, the limited depth of RCM imaging does not allow detection of more deeply infiltrating BCC.

## MELANOCYTIC NEOPLASMS

RCM is a useful tool for the evaluation of melanocytic lesions since melanin is highly reflective and provides strong contrast in RCM images. RCM enables rapid recognition of pigmented skin lesion as melanocytic or as non-melanocytic. In addition, the findings in RCM images allow differentiation of most nevi from melanoma. As the basis

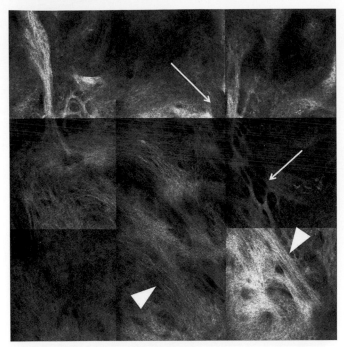

Figure 38.13 RCM image (1.5×1.5 mm field-of-view) of the fibrotic stroma associated with basal cell carcinoma. Densely packed, elongated, bright collagen bundles (arrowheads) are observed at the level of the superficial dermis. Hyporeflective, round to oval tumor islands ('dark silhouettes', arrows) are embedded in the fibrotic stroma.

for RCM evaluation of melanocytic lesions, a recent publication has provided a consensus set of RCM terms,[17] considering previously described RCM terms of melanocytic and non-melanocytic skin lesions.[18,19] Most of the terms used to evaluate melanocytic lesions showed high interobserver agreement among experts.[20]

In addition, because RCM and dermoscopy both image lesions *en face*, RCM has been helpful in elucidating the direct tissue correlates of dermoscopic structures such as streaks or blue-white structures for which indirect correlation with vertically sectioned histopathology is difficult (see Chapter 36).[21,22] Dermoscopic and histologic correlates of RCM features have been described for nevi and melanoma.[23] The value of RCM for the diagnosis of clinically and dermoscopically equivocal melanocytic neoplasms is the subject of ongoing investigation.

## RCM of melanocytic nevi

The RCM features of melanocytic nevi were first described by Langley at al.[24] Nevi typically display round to oval, bright, monomorphic melanocytes and a regular epidermal architecture. According to their dermoscopic and histopathologic appearance, different nevus types may show variable findings with RCM.[25]

In junctional nevi, melanocytes are distributed singly and in nests mostly at the tips and sides of the rete ridges. With RCM, dark, round dermal papillae surrounded by a rim of monomorphous refractive cells ('edged papillae', Table 38.3), corresponding to melanocytes and pigmented basal keratinocytes, are observed at the level of the DEJ (Fig. 38.16B,C). Small junctional dense nests of melanocytes are observed on RCM within the interpapillary spaces or protruding into the dermal papillae with connection to the basal layer of the epidermis (Fig. 38.16D and Table 38.3). The dermal papillae usually show little variability in size and shape. When viewing a mosaic image of nevi (akin to low magnification) at the DEJ level, the edged papillae, homogeneously distributed throughout the lesion, result in a regular ringed pattern, which correlates with typical pigment network seen on dermoscopy[26] (Fig. 38.16A,B).

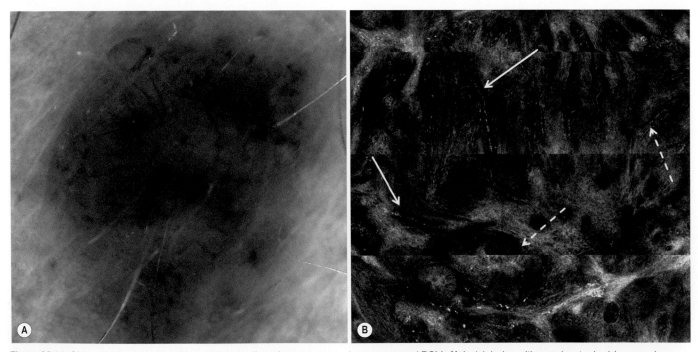

Figure 38.14 Characteristic vascular features of basal cell carcinoma seen on dermoscopy and RCM. A) A pink lesion with prominent arborizing vessels (arrows) and focal gray-blue ovoid structures as well as gray dots/granules is seen on dermoscopy. B) With RCM (1.5 × 1.5mm field-of-view), branching linear blood vessels (arrows) that run horizontally to the RCM plane of imaging are visualized adjacent to reflective, round to oval and trabecular tumor islands (dashed arrows). The blood flow is best observed during real-time imaging.

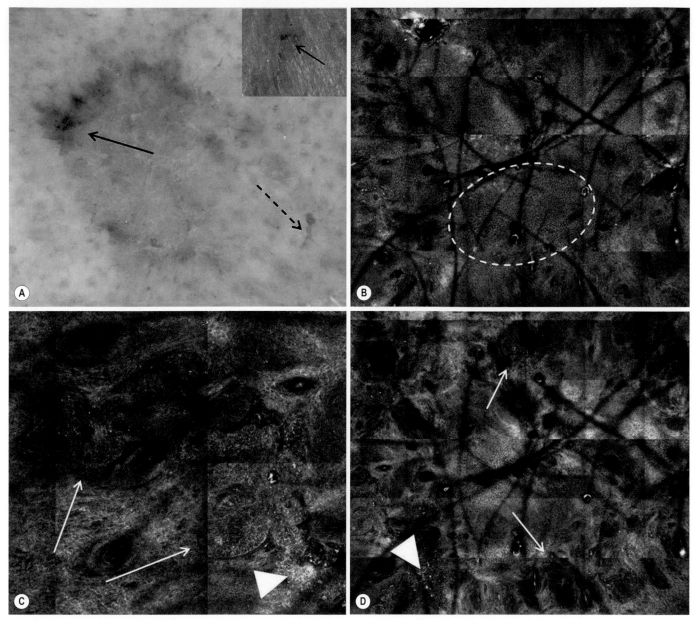

**Figure 38.15** Clinical, dermoscopic and RCM images of a pigmented superficial basal cell carcinoma (BCC) displaying only subtle clinical and dermoscopic features suggestive of BCC. **A)** A 3-mm pink to tan, flat-topped papule (arrow) with a central depression is seen clinically (insert). With dermoscopy, a structureless pink-brown center as well as peripheral tan globular structures (dashed arrow) and blotches (arrow), interpreted as leaf-like structures, are observed. **B)** On RCM, a regular honeycomb pattern (circle) is displayed at granular–spinous layers at low magnification (3 × 3mm field-of-view). **C)** Tumor strands of heterogeneous reflectivity (arrows) surrounded by dark cleft-like spaces are visualized at the level of the superficial dermis. Single bright, round to triangular non-nucleated cells (arrowhead), correlating to melanophages, are focally seen within the tumor stroma. **D)** At the level of the superficial dermis, tumor islands of variable reflectivity are observed embedded in the bright tumor stroma in a rim-like distribution (arrows) at low magnification (3 × 3 mm field-of-view); these tumor islands correlate with the leaf-like structures seen on dermoscopy. Focal aggregates of bright, round to triangular non-nucleated cells (arrowhead), correlating to melanophages, are focally seen.

In compound and dermal nevi, histopathology shows large nests of melanocytes within the dermis, with or without concomitant junctional nests. On RCM, compact aggregates of cells (also called 'dense nests'), which are round to oval in shape and show uniform brightness, are observed[27] (Fig. 38.17 and Fig. 38.18). Distinct cellular outlines of melanocytes are not always detectable within individual nests (Fig. 38.17C,D). The larger nests of melanocytes seen with RCM correlate to pigment globules seen with dermoscopy (Fig. 38.17A,B and Fig. 38.18A,B). Nevi may show on RCM at the DEJ level elongated, tubular melanocytic nests that expand the interpapillary spaces ('junctional thickening';

Table 38.3, Fig. 38.19 and Fig. 38.20). These tubular nests are composed of bright aggregates of melanocytes along the rete ridges whose individual outlines are mostly indistinct; these correlate on histopathology with confluent junctional nests of melanocytes. When viewed on mosaic RCM image at the DEJ level, junctional thickening would appear as a meshed pattern; this correlates on dermoscopy with thickened network (so-called atypical network) (Fig 38.21A,C).

Spitz nevi, some Clark nevi (Fig. 38.21), and, uncommonly, congenital nevi can present conflicting RCM criteria that may sway the observer to the diagnosis of melanoma.

## Table 38.3 Key RCM Features of Melanocytic Lesions

| RCM Feature | Definition | Favors Melanoma or Nevus? |
|---|---|---|
| **Superficial epidermal layers (granular-spinous layers)** | | |
| Disarranged pattern | Focal or diffuse loss of the normal patterns of the granular-spinous layers (honeycomb or cobblestone). Often seen in conjunction with pagetoid spread of cells | Melanoma > nevi |
| Pagetoid spread of cells | Presence of bright round or dendritic nucleated cells (melanocytes*) at suprabasal layers of the epidermis | Melanoma > nevi |
| **Dermal–epidermal junction** | | |
| Edged papillae | Dermal papillae demarcated by a rim of bright cells (pigmented basal keratinocytes and melanocytes) | Nevi > melanoma |
| Non-edged papillae | Dermal papillae without a demarcating bright rim at the DEJ | Melanoma > nevi |
| Dense nests | Compact, round to oval cell aggregates of variable reflectance in which outline of individual cells is often indiscernible<br>Junctional – the nests are connected with the basal layer of the epidermis and bulge into the dermal papillae<br>Dermal – the nests are located in the dermis without connection with the basal layer of the epidermis | Nevi > melanoma |
| Junctional thickening | Enlargement of the interpapillary spaces (i.e. rete ridges) by bright cell aggregates. Outline of individual cells is often indiscernible | Nevi > melanoma |
| Sheet-like distribution of cells | Round or dendritic nucleated cells (melanocytes) that are not aggregated in nests but closely distributed at the transition of the epidermis and dermis (DEJ) that shows loss of dermal papillae | Melanoma > nevi |
| **Superficial dermis** | | |
| Sparse (also called 'loose') nests | Aggregates of melanocytes with uneven brightness and cellular discohesion showing isolated nucleated cells at the periphery | Melanoma > nevi |
| Cerebriform nests | Confluent aggregates of low-reflecting cells in the dermis separated by a darker rim, resulting in a multilobate appearance | Melanoma |

* Dendritic cells at the spinous layer of the epidermis occasionally prove to be Langerhans cells and not melanocytes. At present, this is a morphologic pitfall of RCM.

Concerning RCM findings that can be seen in these nevi include melanocytes at suprabasal layers of the epidermis (i.e. in pagetoid pattern); large solitary melanocytes at the basal layer; dermal papillae that lack a sharp demarcation (known as 'non-edged papillae', Table 38.3); and melanocytic nests that vary in size, brightness and cohesiveness (including 'sparse nests', Table 38.3). Of note, these nevi are often also equivocal for clinical and dermoscopic diagnosis. In these nevi, RCM examination cannot rule out the possibility of melanoma. Thus, excisional biopsy and histopathological analysis are judicious in such concerning melanocytic lesions.

## Melanoma

In melanoma, an abnormal epidermal pattern is usually observed; the honeycomb pattern is not visualized, either focally or throughout the lesion ('disarranged honeycomb pattern') (Table 38.3 and Fig. 38.22C). Instead, nucleated cells and dendritic processes may be seen at suprabasal layers of the epidermis (i.e. in pagetoid pattern) (Fig. 38.22B,C).

Melanocytes disposed in pagetoid pattern may be shaped as round, triangular, spindle or dendritic nucleated cells;[28] melanocytes of different shapes, size and brightness observed concomitantly suggest cellular pleomorphism (Fig. 38.23A). Clusters of melanocytes in pagetoid pattern may be detected in addition to solitary melanocytes in pagetoid pattern. At the DEJ level, an abnormal architecture is also seen with RCM. Non-edged dermal papillae (Table 38.3) variable in size and shape may be observed; non-edged papillae are often separated by widened interpapillary spaces that may contain large reflecting nucleated cells (atypical melanocytes) (Fig. 38.23B). While junctional thickenings (on high-magnification RCM) and meshed pattern (on RCM mosaic images) can be seen at the DEJ in nevi and in some melanomas, their pattern is different. In nevi, the meshed pattern would appear more regular, while in melanoma, the junctional thickenings which make the lines of the mesh would vary in thickness and in brightness (Fig. 38.23B). In addition, large melanocytes as solitary units can be observed in melanoma at the basal layer of the epidermis (Fig. 38.23B). Foci with loss of the dermal papillae, replaced

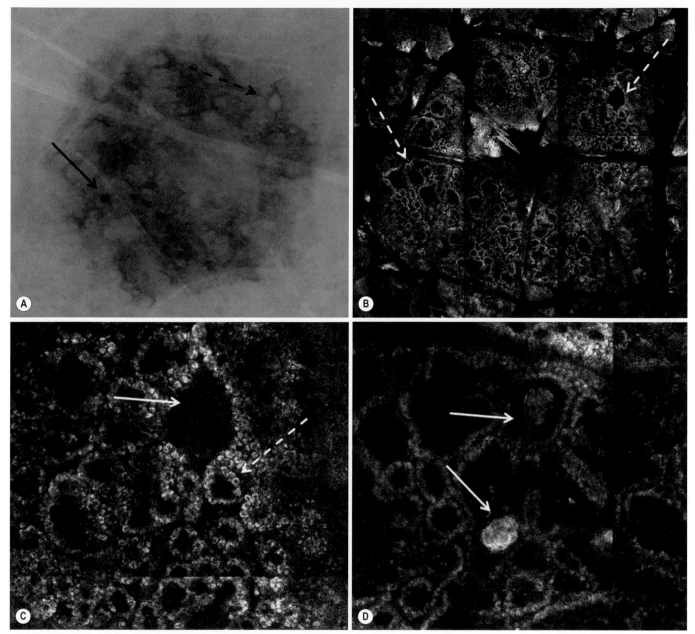

**Figure 38.16** Dermoscopic and RCM images of a junctional nevus. **A)** Dermoscopy shows a pigment network (dashed arrow) and focal small brown globules (arrow). **B)** On RCM mosaic, a ringed pattern (arrows) composed of edged dermal papillae is observed at the DEJ (2 × 2 mm field-of-view). **C)** At higher magnification (500 × 500 μm field-of-view), edged papillae are seen composed of dark, round to oval dermal papillae (arrow) surrounded by a rim of monomorphous bright cells (basal keratinocytes and melanocytes, dashed arrow). Round blood vessels traversing dermal papillae are detected during real-time imaging. **D)** A deeper section of the DEJ displays small junctional dense nests (arrows) that protrude into the papillary dermis. (B,C&D, Courtesy of Harold S. Rabinovitz, MD).

by sheets of atypical melanocytes seen on RCM (Table 38.3 and Fig 38.24D), indicate a crowded proliferation of solitary melanocytes and flattening of the DEJ on histopathology.

The cell clusters seen on RCM at the level of the superficial dermis, may appear at least focally as sparse or cerebriform aggregates[27] (Fig. 38.25B,C and Table 38.3). The variable size, shape and brightness and uneven distribution of melanocytic nests seen in melanoma on RCM mosaics (Fig. 38.25A) correlate on dermoscopy with the presence of irregular globules and dots. The finding on RCM of cell clusters or solitary bright nucleated cells in the dermis in a melanoma, suggest the presence of an invasive melanoma. Dermal aggregates of plump bright cells without visible nuclei (correlating with melanophages) as well as bright

dermal clusters of melanocytes are seen in areas showing blue-white structures on dermoscopy.[22]

The above-mentioned RCM features are well established for superficial spreading melanoma. In nodular melanoma, cerebriform dermal nests are more commonly seen, while melanocytes in pagetoid pattern or a disarranged honeycomb pattern of the epidermis are uncommon.[29] In lentigo maligna melanoma, a descent of atypical melanocytes along adnexal structures, flattening of the DEJ with cord-like rete ridges, aggregates of atypical melanocytes surrounding adnexal openings, and sheets of atypical melanocytes at basal and suprabasal layers are typically observed[30] (Fig. 38.26 and Table 38.3). RCM can also be particularly valuable in the evaluation of

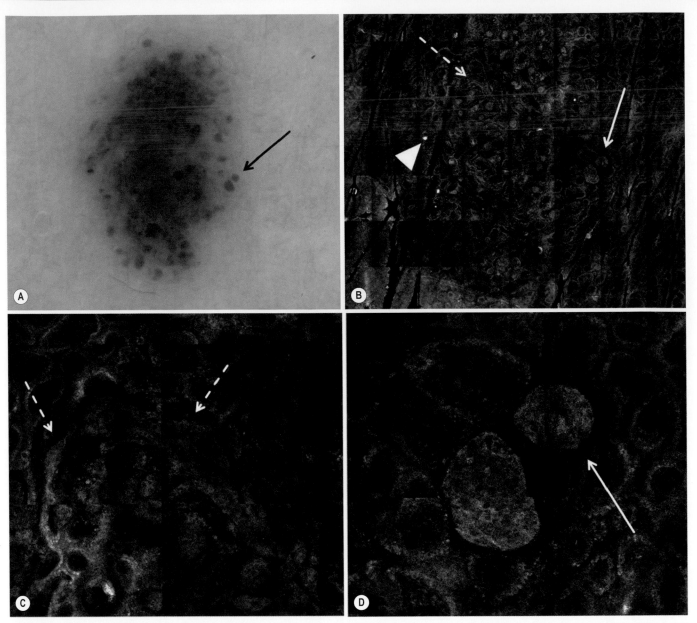

**Figure 38.17** Dermoscopic and RCM images of a compound nevus. **A)** Dermoscopy shows light to dark brown aggregated globules (arrow). **B)** On RCM, bright round structures (arrows) and elongated, tubular structures (dashed arrow), correlating to melanocytic nests, are seen at the DEJ on low magnification (3 × 4mm field-of-view). **C)** At higher magnification (1 × 1mm field-of-view), the tubular structures observed at the DEJ are junctional thickenings (dashed arrows ) that widen and bridge the rete ridges. **D)** Round to oval dense nests are seen within the dermal papillae on RCM (1 × 1mm field-of-view); these are dermal nests. (B,C&D, Courtesy of Harold S. Rabinovitz, MD).

lightly pigmented or amelanotic melanomas that often lack diagnostic features on clinical and dermoscopic examination.[31]

Pellacani et al. defined six RCM criteria for the diagnosis of melanoma based on multivariate analysis; two major criteria (non-edged papillae, atypical cells at the DEJ) and four minor criteria (roundish pagetoid cells, pagetoid cells widespread throughout the lesion, cerebriform clusters and isolated nucleated cells within dermal papillae) contribute to a scoring algorithm (each major criterion 2 points, each minor criterion 1 point). A score ≥3 signifies the diagnosis of MM with a sensitivity of 97.3% and a specificity of 72.3%.[32] A two-step algorithm for the diagnosis of melanoma

by RCM has been recently proposed.[33] In the first step, the lesion is identified by RCM as melanocytic or non-melanocytic. In the second step, the lesion is diagnosed with RCM based on Pellacani's scoring system as nevus versus melanoma. By using this algorithm, unnecessary biopsies may be reduced by more than 50% without missing a melanoma.

Limitations of RCM in the assessment of melanocytic skin lesions include the lack of nuclear staining, the limited depth of imaging, and the difficulty in distinguishing dendritic melanocytes in pagetoid pattern from Langerhans cells that may occasionally simulate pagetoid spread.

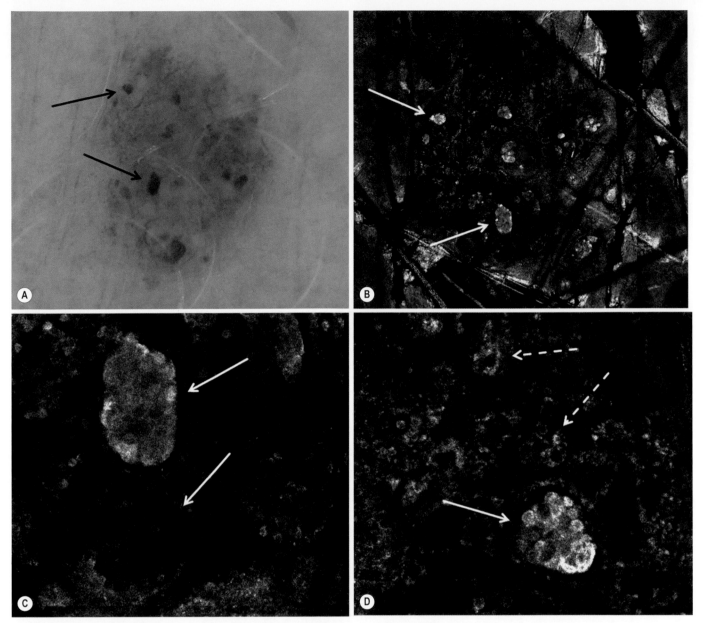

**Figure 38.18** Dermoscopic and RCM images of a compound nevus. **A)** Dermoscopy shows a lesion with a tan homogeneous area, few scattered light to dark brown, large, angulated ('cobblestone') globules (arrows) and faint peripheral reticulation. **B)** RCM mosaic (2 × 2 mm field-of-view) at the DEJ level shows large, round to oval reflective nests (arrows) which correlate with the dermoscopically identified globules and a subtle ringed pattern ('edged papillae') which correlates with the faint reticulation seen on dermoscopy. **C)** At higher magnification (500 × 500 µm field-of-view), dense nests of variable reflectivity (arrow) are observed within dermal papillae. **D)** Higher-magnification RCM (500 × 500 µm field-of-view) at the DEJ level shows a rim of bright basal cells (melanocytes and pigmented basal keratinocytes, 'edged papillae') around dermal papillae (dashed arrows). Some of the dermal papillae also harbor intradermal, dense nests in which individual brighter melanocytes may be visualized (arrow). (B,C&D, Courtesy of Harold S. Rabinovitz, MD).

## RCM IN MARGIN MAPPING AND MONITORING OF TREATMENT OF SKIN CANCER

An important area of research lies in the use of RCM for margins evaluation during microscopic-guided surgery (e.g. Mohs surgery). In previous studies, contrast agents which led to compaction of chromatin, such as acetic acid, were used to improve imaging contrast. However, micronodular and infiltrative BCCs were not consistently identified within the background of bright dermal collagen and the detection of SCCs was hindered by the bright appearance of the epidermis. The recent introduction of fluorescence confocal microscopy, using fluorophores such as acridine orange as contrast agents, may overcome these drawbacks; an overall sensitivity and specificity of 96.6% and 89.2%, respectively, was reported for the ex-vivo detection of BCCs, across all subtypes, in tissue specimens from Mohs surgery.[34]

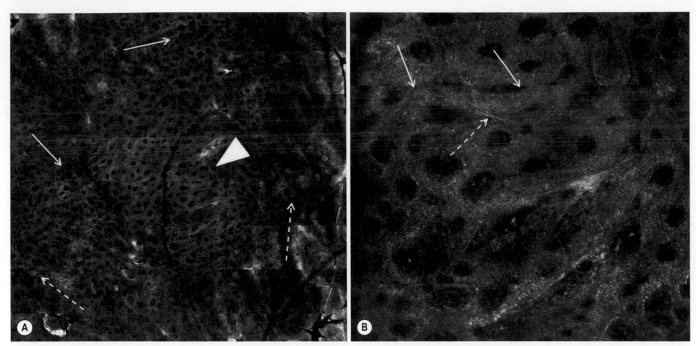

**Figure 38.19** RCM figures of a biopsy-proven congenital nevus. **A)** On RCM mosaic (4 × 4 mm field-of-view) at the DEJ level, there is a central meshed pattern (arrowhead), peripheral ringed pattern (arrows) and peripheral round reflective nests (dashed arrows). **B)** At higher magnification (1 × 1 mm field-of-view), the central area with the meshed pattern on the mosaic image shows thickenings of the interpapillary areas (i.e. the rete ridges) harboring tubular reflecting structures ('junctional thickenings', arrows), correlating to elongated junctional melanocytic nests (arrows). Few dendritic processes of melanocytes can be appreciated within the junctional nests (dashed arrow). (Courtesy of Harold S. Rabinovitz, MD).

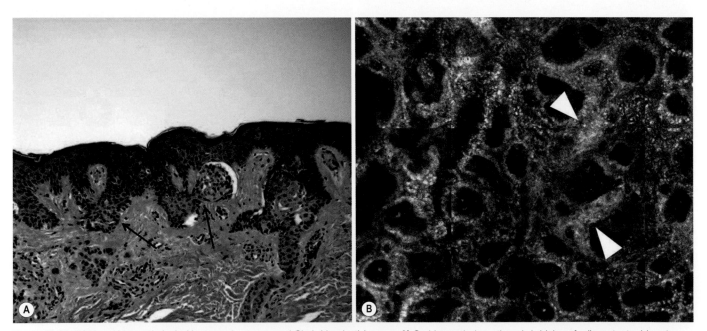

**Figure 38.20** RCM and histopathological images of a compound Clark (dysplastic) nevus. **A)** On histopathology, there is bridging of adjacent rete ridges by confluence of junctional melanocytic nests (arrows) (H&E, magnification 100 ×). **B)** These confluent junctional nests correlate on RCM at the DEJ level (1 × 1 mm field-of-view) with oval to tubular, reflective melanocytic nests in a widened interpapillary area ('junctional thickening', arrowheads).

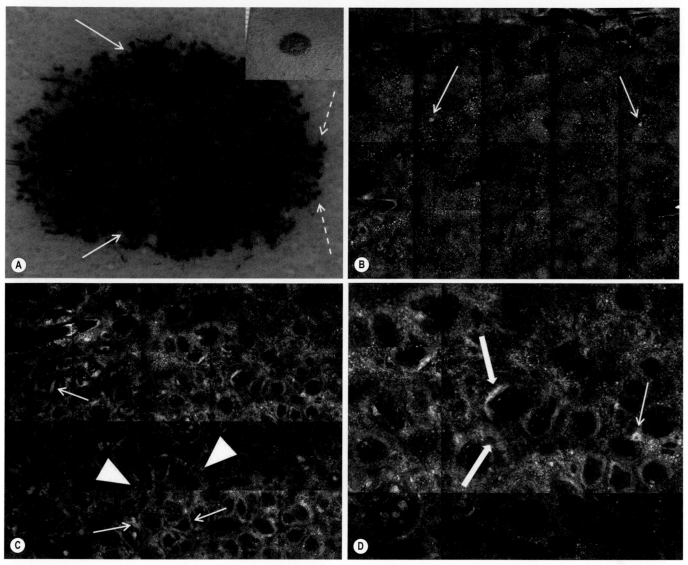

**Figure 38.21** Images of a compound Clark (dysplastic) nevus with some features raising concern for melanoma on both dermoscopy and RCM. **A)** Clinically (inset), a 4 × 5 mm dark brown, flat-topped papule is seen. With dermoscopy, a dark brown atypical pigment network (arrows) and focal pseudopods at the lesion's periphery (dashed arrows) are observed. **B)** On RCM mosaic (2 × 2.5 mm field-of-view), few bright cells (arrows) are seen at the level of the spinous layer, raising the possibility of melanocytes in pagetoid pattern. **C)** On RCM mosaic (2 × 2.5 mm field-of-view) at the DEJ level, a meshed pattern (arrowheads) is seen composed of non-edged papillae and bright tubular structures ('junctional thickening', arrows); these tubular structures correlate with confluent melanocytic nests on histopathology. **D)** Non-edged papillae are visualized on higher-magnification RCM (approximately 1 × 1 mm field-of-view) at the DEJ level. Widened interpapillary spaces harboring bright tubular structures of variable reflectivity ('junctional thickening', thick arrows), are observed. Single large, bright nucleated cells are detected (arrow); these cells represent solitary atypical melanocytes. According to Pellacani's RCM method for melanoma diagnosis, the lesion will get a score of 5 (non edged papillae – 2; atypical melanocytes at DEJ – 2; cells in pagetoid pattern – 1), denoting suspicion for melanoma. (B, C and D, Courtesy of Harold S. Rabinovitz, MD).

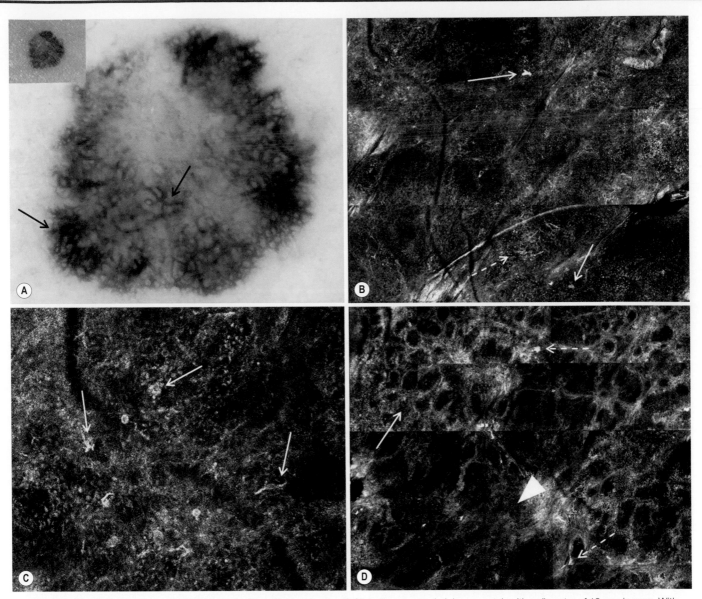

**Figure 38.22** Clinical, dermoscopic and RCM images of a melanoma in situ. **A)** Clinically, a tan to dark brown patch with a diameter of 10 mm is seen. With dermoscopy, a dark brown atypical network (arrows) is observed. **B)** On RCM mosaic (2.5 × 2.5 mm field-of-view), large bright cells are visualized within the upper epidermis (arrows). In addition, areas displaying bright dendritic processes are noted (dashed arrow). **C)** Large, bright nucleated cells of variable size and shape are detected at level of the spinous layer at higher magnification RCM (500 × 500 μm field-of-view), denoting melanocytes in pagetoid pattern displaying pleomorphism. The normal honeycomb pattern is not seen ('disarranged pattern'). **D)** On RCM mosaic (2.5 × 2.5 mm field-of-view) at the DEJ level, a meshed pattern is observed (arrow) with some variability in the width and brightness of the lines of the meshwork. Focally, the meshed pattern is not detected (arrowhead); there is absence of dermal papillae in this focus, suggesting a flattened DEJ. Single bright cells (dashed arrows) stand out both within the meshwork and in the focus that lacks the meshed pattern, suggesting focal predominance of solitary melanocytes at the DEJ. (B, C, D, Courtesy of Harold S. Rabinovitz, MD).

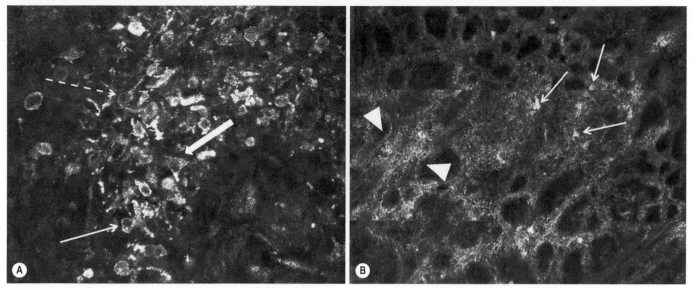

**Figure 38.23 A)** RCM image (500 × 500 µm field-of-view) displaying pleomorphism of melanocytes in a melanoma. Round, triangular, dendritic and spindle-shaped nucleated cells of variable size and reflectivity are seen at the suprabasal levels of the epidermis (arrows). There is a disarranged pattern, with loss of the normal honeycomb pattern. **B)** RCM image (1 × 1 mm field-of-view) of a melanoma at the DEJ level displays non-edged papillae with variable reflectivity and with widening of the interpapillary spaces (arrowheads). Multiple bright nucleated and dendritic cells of variable size and shape (arrows), correlating to pleomorphic melanocytes, are seen. (Courtesy of Harold S. Rabinovitz, MD).

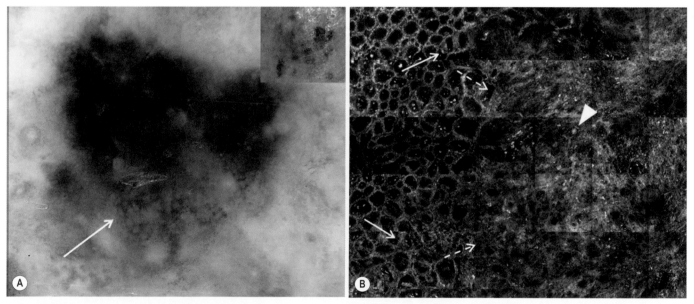

**Figure 38.24** Clinical, dermoscopic, histopathological and RCM figures of a melanoma. **A)** Clinically, a 1.5 cm in diameter, irregularly shaped patch, with color variegation ranging from tan to dark brown is seen (inset). Dermoscopy of the darker pole of the lesion displays asymmetry in distribution of colors (tan, dark brown, blue-gray), and asymmetry in the distribution of dermoscopic structures – network, dots, and granularity (regression area, arrow). **B)** RCM mosaic (2.5 × 3 mm field-of-view) at the DEJ level shows an area with almost complete absence of dermal papillae (dashed arrows), alongside an area displaying a meshed pattern (arrows). Multiple bright cells, correlating to melanocytes as solitary units (arrowhead) and small nests are seen in the area with loss of dermal papillae.

*(Continued)*

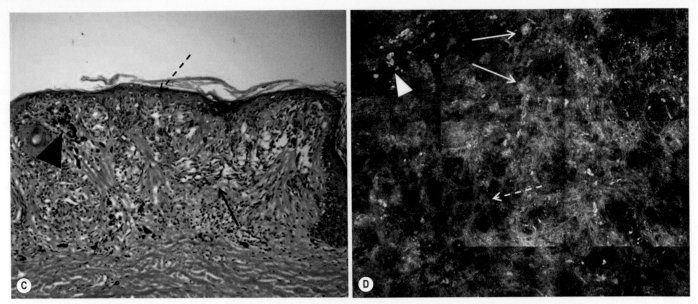

**Figure 38.24—cont'd C)** On histopathology (H&E, magnification 100×), nests that vary in size and tendency to confluence are seen at the DEJ (arrow), as well as solitary melanocytes at and above the DEJ (dashed arrow). Focal aggregates of melanophages are detected within the papillary dermis (arrowhead), correlating with the granularity seen on dermoscopy. **D)** On higher-magnification RCM (approximately 1.5 × 1.5 mm field-of-view), almost complete loss of the dermal papillae is focally observed at the DEJ; only few dermal papillae (round dark structures) are focally seen (dashed arrow). Bright solitary nucleated cells and small nests (arrows) are visualized at the DEJ. Aggregates of bright, round to triangular non-nucleated cells (arrowhead), correlating to melanophages, are detected in the superficial dermis.

**Figure 38.25** RCM images of a melanoma.
**A)** On RCM mosaic (2.5 × 2.5 mm field-of-view), multiple round, oval and tubular structures of variable reflectivity (arrowheads) are seen at the suprabasal epidermal levels; these correlate with nests of atypical melanocytes. Some of the nests are surrounded by dark cleft-like spaces. The majority of the nests appear as 'dense clusters' that are homogenous in brightness and in which individual melanocytes are mostly unapparent; however, 'sparse nests', which are discohesive aggregates of atypical melanocytes, are also seen (arrow). **B)** On high-magnification RCM (500 × 500 µm field-of-view) of the upper epidermis, sparse nests appear as aggregates of nucleated cells of variable reflectivity, in which the individual cells are discernible. **C)** High-magnification RCM (500 × 500 µm field-of-view) at the level of the superficial dermis shows 'cerebriform nests'. Cerebriform nests are confluent aggregates of low reflecting cells (melanocytes) in the dermis that are separated by a darker rim, resulting in a multilobate appearance.

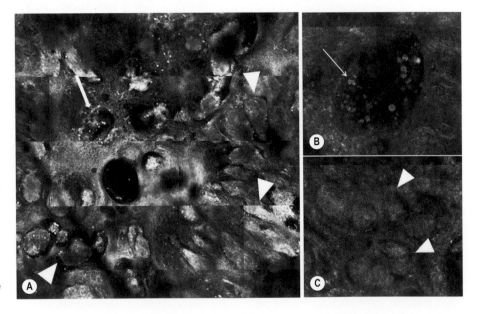

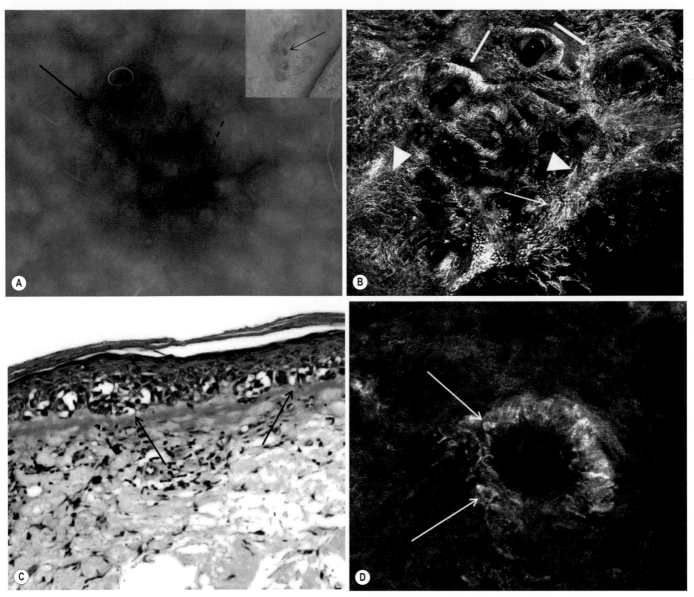

**Figure 38.26** Clinical, dermoscopic, histopathological and RCM images of a melanoma in situ (lentigo maligna) on the right cheek. **A)** Clinically (inset), a 2 × 3 cm tan macule with focal dark brown areas is seen. With dermoscopy, asymmetrically pigmented follicular openings (arrow) and early rhomboidal structures (dashed arrow) are visualized. **B)** On RCM (approximately 2 × 2mm field-of-view), bright dendritic cells and dendritic processes (arrowheads) form sheets and tubular structures at the basal layer. Small melanocytic nests are focally detected (arrow). Some of the sheets and tubular structures of dendritic cells and dendritic processes are located around adnexal structures (thick arrows). **C)** On histopathology, atypical melanocytes are seen as crowded single cells and small nests (arrows) along a flattened DEJ (H&E, magnification 100×). **D)** At high-magnification RCM (500 × 500 μm field-of-view), bright, pleomorphic nucleated and dendritic cells infiltrate the adnexal epithelium (arrows); imaging deeper into the tissue can show the extension of atypical melanocytes down adnexal structures.

## FUTURE OUTLOOK

To be broadly implemented, RCM needs to be smaller, cheaper and user-friendly. In addition, the black and white contrast imaging and limited penetration depth are barriers to adoption of RCM technology. The use of multi-wavelength RCM may allow incorporation of wavelengths that penetrate deeper as well as wavelengths that penetrate more superficially but with higher resolution.

However, at present this technique does require expertise and experience in image interpretation, while image acquisition is fairly straightforward. The inherent potential of RCM for tele-dermatologic application and automated image analyzing can address the end-user interpretation challenges. Finally, in the future, a multimodal imaging concept combining RCM with other non-invasive imaging tools (like spectroscopy) may be applied to improve non-invasive imaging.

## REFERENCES

1. Minsky M. *Microscopy apparatus*. U.S. Patent No. 3013467, 7 Nov.1957.
2. Rajadhyaksha M, Grossmann M, Esterowiz D, et al. In vivo confocal scanning laser microscopy of human skin: melanin provides strong contrast. *J Invest Dermatol*. 1995;104:946–952.
3. Rajadhyaksha M, González S, Zavislan JM, et al. In vivo confocal scanning laser microscopy of human skin II: Advances in instrumentation and comparison with histology. *J Invest Dermatol*. 1999;113:293–303.
4. Yamashita T, Kuwahara T, Gonzáez S, et al. Non-invasive visualization of melanin and melanocytes by reflectance-mode confocal microscopy. *J Invest Dermatol*. 2005;124:235–240.
5. Huzaira M, Rius F, Rajadhyaksha M, et al. Topographic variations in normal skin, as viewed by in vivo reflectance confocal microscopy. *J Invest Dermatol*. 2001;116:846–852.
6. Sauermann K, Clemann S, Jaspers S, et al. Age related changes of human skin investigated with histometric measurements by confocal laser scanning microscopy in vivo. *Skin Res Technol*. 2002;8:52–56.
7. Braga JC, Scope A, Klaz I, et al. The significance of reflectance confocal microscopy in the assessment of solitary pink skin lesions. *J Am Acad Dermatol*. 2009;61(2):230–241.
8. Aghassi D, Anderson RR, González S. Confocal laser microscopic imaging of actinic keratoses in vivo: a preliminary report. *J Am Acad Dermatol*. 2000;43:42–48.
9. Ulrich M, Maltusch A, Röwert-Huber J, et al. Actinic keratoses: non-invasive diagnosis for field cancerisation. *Br J Dermatol*. 2007;156(suppl 3):13–17.
10. Ulrich M, Maltusch A, Rius-Diaz F, et al. Clinical applicability of in vivo reflectance confocal microscopy for the diagnosis of actinic keratoses. *Dermatol Surg*. 2008;34:610–619.
11. Horn M, Gerger A, Ahlgrimm-Siess V, et al. Discrimination of actinic keratoses from normal skin with reflectance mode confocal microscopy. *Dermatol Surg*. 2008;34:620–625.
12. Rishpon A, Kim N, Scope A, et al. Reflectance confocal microscopy criteria of squamous cell carcinoma and actinic keratoses. *Arch Dermatol*. 2009;145(7):766–772.
13. González S, Tannous Z. Real-time, in vivo confocal reflectance microscopy of basal cell carcinoma. *J Am Acad Dermatol*. 2002;47:869–874.
14. Segura S, Puig S, Carrera C, et al. Dendritic cells in pigmented basal cell carcinoma. *Arch Dermatol*. 2007;143(7):883–886.
15. Charles CA, Marghoob AA, Busam KJ, et al. Melanoma or pigmented basal cell carcinoma: a clinical-pathologic correlation with dermoscopy, in vivo confocal scanning laser microscopy, and routine histology. *Skin Res Technol*. 2002;8:282–287.
16. Nori S, Rius-Díaz F, Cuevas J, et al. Sensitivity and specificity of reflectance-mode confocal microscopy for in vivo diagnosis of basal cell carcinoma: a multicenter study. *J Am Acad Dermatol*. 2004;51:923–930.
17. Scope A, Benvenuto-Andrade C, Agero AL, et al. In vivo reflectance confocal microscopy imaging of melanocytic skin lesions: consensus terminology glossary and illustrative images. *J Am Acad Dermatol*. 2007;57(4):644–658.
18. Pellacani G, Ardigo A, Bassoli S, et al. Glossary. In: Gonzalez S, Gill M, Halpern AC, eds. *Reflectance Confocal Microscopy of Cutaneous Tumors. An Atlas of Clinical, Dermoscopic and Histopathological Correlations*. London: Informa Healthcare; 2008:253–256.
19. Pellacani G, Guitera P, Longo C, et al. The impact of in vivo reflectance confocal microscopy for the diagnostic accuracy of melanoma and equivocal melanocytic lesions. *J Invest Dermatol*. 2007;127:2759–2765.
20. Pellacani G, Vinceti M, Bassoli S, et al. Reflectance confocal microscopy and features of melanocytic lesions: an internet-based study of the reproducibility of terminology. *Arch Dermatol*. 2009;145(10):1137–1143.
21. Scope A, Gill M, Benveuto-Andrade C, et al. Correlation of dermoscopy with in vivo reflectance confocal microscopy of streaks in melanocytic lesions. *Arch Dermatol*. 2007;143(6):727–734.
22. Pellacani G, Bassoli S, Longo C, et al. Diving into the blue: in vivo microscopic characterization of the dermoscopic blue hue. *J Am Acad Dermatol*. 2007;57(1):96–104.
23. Pellacani G, Longo C, Malvehy J, et al. In vivo confocal microscopic and histopathologic correlations of dermoscopic features in 202 melanocytic lesions. *Arch Dermatol*. 2008;144(12):1597–1608.
24. Langley RGB, Rajadhyaksha M, Dwyer PJ, et al. Confocal scanning laser microscopy of benign and malignant melanocytic lesions in vivo. *J Am Acad Dermatol*. 2001;45:365–376.
25. Ahlgrimm-Siess V, Massone C, Koller S, et al. In vivo confocal scanning laser microscopy of common naevi with globular, homogeneous and reticular pattern in dermoscopy. *Br J Dermatol*. 2008;158(5):1000–1007.
26. Pellacani G, Cesinaro AM, Longo C, et al. Microscopic in vivo description of cellular architecture of dermoscopic pigment network in nevi and melanomas. *Arch Dermatol*. 2005;141:147–154.
27. Pellacani G, Cesinaro AM, Seidenari S. In vivo assessment of melanocytic nests in nevi and melanomas by reflectance confocal microscopy. *Mod Pathol*. 2005;18:469–474.
28. Pellacani G, Cesinaro AM, Seidenari S. Reflectance-mode confocal microscopy for the in vivo characterization of pagetoid melanocytosis in melanomas and nevi. *J Invest Dermatol*. 2005;125:532–537.
29. Segura S, Pellacani G, Puig S, et al. In vivo microscopic features of nodular melanomas. *Arch Dermatol*. 2008;144(10):1311–1320.
30. Ahlgrimm-Siess V, Massone C, Scope A, et al. Reflectance confocal microscopy of facial lentigo maligna and lentigo maligna melanoma: a preliminary study. *Br J Dermatol*. 2009;161(6):1307–1316.
31. Guitera P, Pellacani G, Longo C, et al. In vivo reflectance confocal microscopy enhances secondary evaluation of melanocytic lesions. *J Invest Dermatol*. 2009;129(1):131–138.
32. Pellacani G, Cesinaro AM, Seidenari S. Reflectance-mode confocal microscopy of pigmented skin lesions – improvement in melanoma diagnostic specificity. *J Am Acad Dermatol*. 2005;53:979–985.
33. Segura S, Puig S, Carrera C, et al. Development of a two-step method for the diagnosis of melanoma by reflectance confocal microscopy. *J Am Acad Dermatol*. 2009;61:216–229.
34. Karen JK, Gareau DS, Dusza SW, et al. Detection of basal cell carcinomas in Mohs excisions with fluorescence confocal mosaicing microscopy. *Br J Dermatol*. 2009;160:1242–1250.

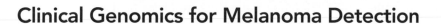

# Clinical Genomics for Melanoma Detection

*William Wachsman*

## Key Points

- Recent findings provide proof-of-principle that adhesive tape stripping of pigmented lesions suspicious for melanoma, coupled with epidermal genetic information retrieval (EGIR) and gene expression profiling, can be used to discern melanoma from nevi and solar lentigines.

- Genes differentially expressed between melanoma and nevi, as identified through these EGIR-harvested specimens, are biologically relevant to disease biology.

- Class prediction modeling of these EGIR-based genomic data produced a multigene classifier that is highly accurate for detection of melanoma.

- Further development of a non-invasive assay is underway to validate this approach for routine clinical use.

## INTRODUCTION

The Human Genome Project (HGP), begun in 1990, ostensibly culminated in 2003 with the sequencing of a complete human genome.[1] The project also provided the research community with substantially more: a physical and genetic map of the human genome, including the locations of more than 3.7 million single nucleotide polymorphisms (SNPs); identification of more than 15,000 human genes; and the basis for a myriad of tools for genomic investigation.[2] This research established a framework for attacking the molecular pathogenesis of human disease, which is now coming to fruition in terms of clinical applications. In addition to enabling development of novel, targeted therapeutics, the genomic technologies spawned by the HGP will impact the ability to: predict the likelihood that a patient will develop a specific disease, detect the presence of a disease, perform molecular disease diagnosis, characterize disease prognosis, and direct treatment management.

Melanoma, the most lethal skin cancer, has become one of the primary focal points of genomic research. Epidemiology studies have established that melanoma has a genetic predisposition, that chronic sun exposure is a significant risk factor for melanoma development, and that patients diagnosed with melanoma are at substantially higher risk for developing an additional primary. This knowledge has increased the vigilance of practitioners and dermatopathologists for the presence of melanoma. However, the application of genomics at a clinical level has the potential to greatly impact how patients are evaluated for melanoma

susceptibility (Chapter 30), early detection, diagnosis, and management by means of targeted treatment of advanced disease (Chapter 55). This chapter will focus on the evolving application of genomics for the early detection of melanoma.

## CURRENT MELANOMA DETECTION

Numerous studies have shown that early detection of melanoma is key to disease survival. This observation has placed tremendous pressure on the clinician to discern lesions suspicious for melanoma from those that are benign. The key means for melanoma detection rely upon visual examination of skin lesions and a variety of optical technologies, such as dermoscopy, to further assess the likelihood that a lesion harbors malignant melanocytes. In addition, newer optical methods for melanoma detection, including confocal microscopy and automated image analysis, are now emerging from the research setting.

Because of the highly variable visual and/or optical appearance of melanoma (in particular atypical nevi), many skin lesions are found to confound detection. These factors have substantially lowered the threshold to remove any lesion deemed in the least bit suspicious for melanoma. Yet the vast majority of these lesions considered suspicious for melanoma are found to be negative upon histopathologic analysis. In fact, various studies have shown that the ratio of melanoma to biopsies of suspicious lesions ranges from 1 in 3–5 when the assessment is performed by pigmented lesion experts, to 1 in 12–20 for non-expert practitioners, to 1 in 75–100 for primary care physicians.[3-5] Therefore, the availability of a non-invasive clinical test that significantly improves the specificity of melanoma detection, without sacrificing sensitivity, could potentially eliminate many unneeded skin biopsies.

## EPIDERMAL GENETIC INFORMATION RETRIEVAL (EGIR)

A diagnostic method using tape stripping was recently developed that enables the assay of RNA from cells overlying a pigmented lesion for the purpose of melanoma detection. The core technology to perform this assay is termed epidermal genetic information retrieval (EGIR™) (DermTech International, Inc., La Jolla, CA). EGIR was first implemented by Morhenn et al. for the purpose of discerning allergic from irritant skin reactions and later for analysis of psoriatic gene expression by means of a quantitative reverse transcription polymerase chain reaction (qPCR) assay for specific cytokine mRNA.[6,7] Subsequent work showed that EGIR-harvested RNA was also suitable for microarray-based gene expression profiling.[8] This work demonstrated that RNA present in EGIR-harvested stratum corneum samples contain messages expressed by cells found deeper in the epidermis. Therefore, it was hypothesized that mRNA produced by melanomas and nevi could by sampled by EGIR and then analyzed in order to characterize these skin lesions.

## EGIR GENOMIC CHARACTERIZATION OF MELANOMA, NEVI, AND NORMAL SKIN

A study employing tape stripping was performed whereby four adhesive tape disks were sequentially applied to skin overlying a pigmented lesion which was deemed suspicious for melanoma (Fig. 39.1). Lesions as small as 6 mm in diameter were sampled. In addition, any lesion that was observed to be bleeding, weeping, or ulcerated was excluded, thereby eliminating many lesions that most would consider to be at highest risk for melanoma. After stripping the skin surface, a lesional biopsy was performed. Each biopsy specimen was reviewed by two independent dermatopathologists by means of routinely available histopathology methods.

For this study, 20 melanoma specimens (9 in situ and 11 invasive) and 62 nevi (54 dyplastic, 4 lentiginous, and 4 congenital) were analyzed. Control tape-stripped specimens were also obtained from non-lesional skin from 17 subjects, all at greater than 10 cm from the suspicious skin lesion. Using EGIR, the RNA from the four tape disks was isolated and pooled, yielding an average of 1 ng, and then amplified to produce at least 5 µg of cDNA product. The amplified material was profiled for gene expression on the U133 Plus2.0 Affymetrix GeneChip that targets approximately 47,000 unique transcripts. Analysis of the resulting data identified 317 genes (p < 0.01, false discovery rate [FDR] < 0.05) that are differentially expressed between melanomas, nevi, and normal control specimens. These 317 differentially expressed genes were further assessed by hierarchical clustering (Fig. 39.2). As seen in the resulting 'heatmap', all of the melanoma specimens group closely together on the right site of the specimen dendogram. In addition, the appearance of the control specimen data from uninvolved skin is very similar to that of nevi. Lastly, there appear to be several different groupings of data from nevi, suggesting the existence of different classes of benign pigmented lesions. Taken together, these findings established proof-of-principle that the EGIR technology, when applied to samples of skin garnered by tape stripping, could distinguish melanoma from nevi and normal skin.[9]

Further analysis of the data from these EGIR-harvested specimens identified 89 genes differentially expressed between melanoma and nevi (p < 0.01, FDR < 0.05).[9] Bioinformatic interrogation of these differentially expressed genes revealed the presence of four major functional categories: hair and skin biology, cellular development, cell growth and proliferation, and cancer biology. Surprisingly, 9 of the 89 genes are expressed in melanocytes and melanoma and known to be involved in melanocyte development

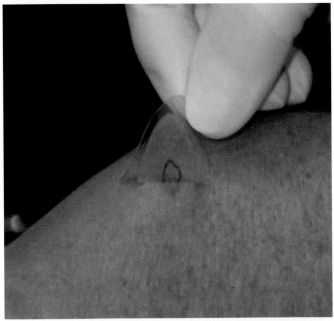

**Figure 39.1** Adhesive tape stripping of pigmented lesions for epidermal genetic information retrieval (EGIR). Shown is an adhesive disk after application to a pigmented skin lesion. The translucent coating on the tape disk is cellular material from stratum corneum. The procedure involves prepping the skin locus overlying the pigmented lesion by wiping gently with an alcohol pad and then letting the area air-dry. The adhesive disk is then applied, the lesion boundary (if smaller than the 17 mm diameter disk) demarcated, and then the surface of the disk is rubbed evenly. The disk is removed and the process is repeated to generate a total of four adhesive disks from which RNA is extracted for assay. RNA is isolated from only the area of tape overlying the lesion and that material from all four tapes is pooled for assay.

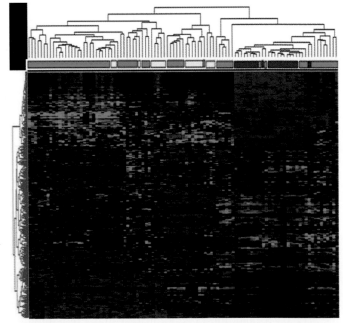

**Figure 39.2** Expression profiling of EGIR-harvested specimens differentiates melanoma from nevi and normal skin. The 'heatmap' diagram shows the results of hierarchical clustering analysis of the 317 genes differentially expressed between EGIR-harvested specimens of in-situ and invasive melanoma (■ n=20), nevi (■ n=62), and normal skin ( n=17) (p < 0.01, FDR < 0.05). Each of the 317 genes is demarcated on the dendrogram to the left of the heatmap, and the 99 samples are demarcated in the dendrogram at the top of the heatmap. Within the heatmap, an increased level of gene expression, with respect to the mean, is shown in red, a decreased level is shown in green, and no significant change in expression in black. (Adapted from a presentation by William Wachsman MD PhD at the Society for Investigative Dermatology meeting in 2007.)

| Table 39.1 Genes Expressed in Melanocytes and Melanoma Present in EGIR-Harvested Specimens | | |
|---|---|---|
| **Gene ID** | **Gene Name** | **p-Value** |
| TYRP1 | tyrosinase-related protein 1 | 1.22E-09 |
| Melan-A | melan-A | 3.13E-06 |
| KIT | Kit | 3.13E-06 |
| MYO5A | myosin 5A | 4.22E-06 |
| ENDRB | endothelin receptor type B | 5.67E-06 |
| DCT | dopachrome tautomerase | 9.35E-06 |
| TYR | tyrosinase | 4.47E-05 |
| SILV | silver homologue | 7.86E-05 |
| MLPH | melanophilin | 0.000233 |

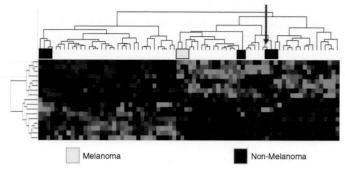

☐ Melanoma     ■ Non-Melanoma

**Figure 39.3** Analysis of EGIR-harvested specimens enables melanoma detection. Shown in heatmap format are the results from the training dataset for 37 melanoma specimens and 37 nevi, when assessed by the TreeNet algorithm for the expression of 17 genes in the classifier. Of note is that one benign specimen, initially thought to be a dyplastic nevus (denoted by the arrow) but called positive by TreeNet analysis, was found to contain invasive melanoma upon re-review of serial sectioned biopsy material.

and proliferation as well as melanoma biology and pathogenesis (Table 39.1). In that the EGIR-based tape stripping rarely samples deeper than stratum corneum,[5] it is unclear why genes expressed in melanocytes and melanoma are detected by this method. It was theorized that the pagetoid spread of the malignant melanocyte makes it accessible for sampling. However, the number of such cells would be expected to be a relatively small percentage of the total specimen and, as such, should not generate a very robust signal. Alternatively, the malignant melanocyte might either directly affect surrounding keratinocytes that become stratum corneum, possibly by the direct transfer of the melanoma RNA into adjacent cells, or indirectly induce the production of these RNA species by means of cell-to-cell interactions.

## GENOMIC DETECTION OF MELANOMA

On the basis of these findings, subsequent work focused on the development of a class prediction model that would discern melanoma from non-melanoma lesions using the EGIR technology. To accomplish this goal, RNA from a total of 202 pigmented skin lesions deemed suspicious for melanoma was harvested and extracted using the EGIR method. As in the earlier investigation, lesions that were bleeding, ulcerated, or weeping were excluded from study. Following tape stripping, the skin lesion was biopsied and each specimen was examined by two dermatopathologists. To move forward into the assay queue, a specimen was required to be called either a melanoma or nevus by both reviewers. Following gene expression profiling by means of Affymetrix GeneChip assay, the data were normalized and randomly split into two separate datasets – one for training the class prediction model, the other for testing the model. Data generated from 37 melanomas and 37 nevi composed the training set: these included both in situ and invasive superficial spreading melanoma, lentigo maligna and lentigo maligna melanoma as well as dyplastic and lentiginous nevi.

Using a supervised approach to data analysis, in which specimens of melanoma were assessed in comparison to those of nevi, 422 differentially expressed genes were identified. This cohort of differentially expressed genes was then subjected to class prediction modeling using a stochastic gradient boosting algorithm (TreeNet™, Salford Systems, San Diego, CA) resulting in discovery of a 17-gene classifier.[10] Upon testing with the independent dataset, generated from 39 in-situ and invasive melanomas and 89 nevi, this multi-gene classifier was found to be 100% sensitive and 88% specific for distinguishing specimens of melanoma from nevi. The test dataset analysis using the 17-gene classifier was found to have an area under the curve (AUC) for the receiver operator characteristic (ROC) of >0.95, confirming that it is highly robust. By comparison, the application of this classifier to a variety of EGIR-harvested negative controls, including 73 non-lesional skin specimens and 22 histopathology-confirmed solar lentigines, showed that these contained no melanoma. That this classifier was capable of predicting all of the 10 specimens of lentigo maligna and lentigo maligna melanoma as positive for melanoma and all 22 solar lentigines as negative is noteworthy because these lesions can sometimes be difficult to distinguish from each other by standard histopathologic review by even expert dermatopathologists.

This high level of assay sensitivity and specificity exhibited by the 17-gene classifier raised questions about the nature of the 13 benign specimens deemed melanoma by the assay. Therefore, each of these 13 false-positive specimens was serially sectioned and re-reviewed for pathology. One of the 13, denoted by the heatmap shown in Figure 39.3, was found to contain a focus of invasive superficial spreading melanoma.[10] It is unclear whether the remaining 12 lesions are true false-positives or lesions exhibiting molecular changes indicative of melanoma that occur in advance of any change in tissue morphology. Further testing is needed to determine whether this 17-gene genomic classifier could be more accurate than histopathology for identification of melanoma.

## FURTHER DEVELOPMENT

Several other steps need to be taken in order to develop this non-invasive EGIR-based genomic assay into an FDA-approved in-vitro diagnostic multivariate index assay

(IVDMIA) for clinical detection of melanoma. A more ergonomic device is being developed that will supplant the adhesive tape disks used in the discovery studies. This collection device, shown in Figure 39.4, should reduce the time needed for specimen collection and facilitate handling and shipping. This device contains a 4 mm by 90 mm loop of adhesive tape that, in preliminary work, has been shown to collect an adequate amount of material for assay. Second, the current microarray-based assay will likely be shifted to another assay platform that is more amenable to a high-throughput format and comparatively lower in cost to perform in the clinical setting. Initial work has shown that off-the-shelf reagents for qPCR, targeting each of the 17 genes as well as gene targets that will serve as internal controls, can successfully be used. Of the first 20 EGIR-harvested samples tested, 10 of 10 melanoma specimens were correctly called positive and 9 of 10 nevi were correctly called negative – effectively recapitulating the microarray-based assay accuracy (Fig. 39.5).

Finally, it is planned that this melanoma IVDMIA will be validated within the context of an international, multi-institution study in which it is anticipated that more than 5000 EGIR-harvested specimens – all from suspicious pigmented lesions – will be collected, assayed, and analyzed. This number of specimens is expected to yield at least 200 in-situ and invasive melanomas. Each lesion will be biopsied and reviewed for pathology by at least

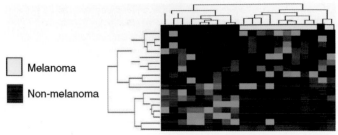

Melanoma

Non-melanoma

**Figure 39.5** Implementation of the EGIR-based genomic melanoma detection assay on a qPCR platform. Expression of each of the 17 genes in the classifier (demarcated in the dendrogram to the left of the heatmap) was measured by quantitative reverse transcriptase polymerase chain reaction (qPCR) assay using SYBR-green labeled probes. Preliminary results are shown from 10 specimens each of melanoma (in situ and invasive) and nevi (demarcated in the dendrogram above the heatmap). Resulting data were normalized to the expression of the β-actin gene in each sample.

three independent dermatopathologists. Investigators performing the assays and dermatopathologists performing specimen review will be blinded to the results of their counterparts, which at the conclusion of the study will be correlated and statistically evaluated for assay sensitivity, specificity, and ROC AUC.

The test results will be reported back to the requesting physician as a risk score (Table 39.2 and Fig. 39.6) that indicates whether a suspicious lesion is likely to contain melanoma. A preliminary version of this scoring system for melanoma IVDMIA was established from the EGIR-based microarray data and histopathology results generated with in-situ and invasive melanoma specimens, nevi, and solar lentigines. As shown, all 77 lesions found to contain either in-situ or invasive melanoma generated IVDMIA risk scores between 3 and 5, with all but one having a score of 4 or 5. In contrast, 88% of the benign lesions exhibited risk scores ranging from 0 to 2, including all of the solar lentigines. The IVDMIA score will provide a practitioner with adjunctive information to assess the risk of a lesion containing melanoma. This test is not meant to replace a biopsy or provide a diagnosis, but should help to better guide whether a lesion should undergo excisional biopsy. The final sensitivity and specificity of the IVDMIA test will be determined through the validation study. If these results are similar to those found through the preliminary studies, the test may improve the ability to better define and select suspicious pigmented lesions in need of excision.

## FUTURE OUTLOOK

The melanoma IVDMIA risk score has the potential to shift the paradigm for melanoma detection for both in-situ and invasive lesions because of its objective and simultaneous assessment of multiple disease biomarkers. The first-generation IVDMIA will likely be performed in a CLIA-certified clinical reference laboratory with a turnaround time of 3–5 days. With the rapid advances in genomic technology, it is possible that subsequent generations of IVDMIA might even be performed on a point-of-care device.

As this type of assay is formulated on genomic data, it also has the potential of providing insights about clinical aspects of melanoma that cannot be attained through visual inspection of a lesion, even when optical enhancement techniques are used.

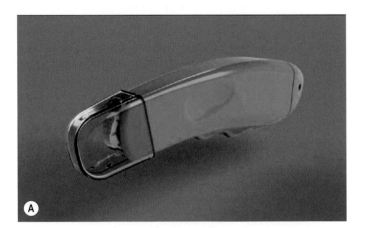

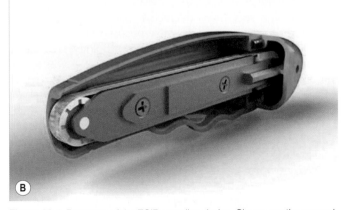

**Figure 39.4** Prototype of the EGIR sampling device. Shown are the capped exterior and cut-away views of the unit that is intended to be for single-use sample collection. Upon application to the skin surface, when an adequate amount of downward pressure is applied to the tape head, the adhesive tape is engaged to move in a unidirectional manner.

## Table 39.2 Development of an IVDMIA Score for Melanoma Risk Assessment

| Score | Total Lesions* | # Nevi (%) | # Solar Lentigines (%) | # Melanoma in situ (%) | # Invasive Melanomas (%) |
|---|---|---|---|---|---|
| 0 | 95 | 82 (86) | 13 (14) | 0 (0) | 0 (0) |
| 1 | 31 | 24 (77) | 7 (23) | 0 (0) | 0 (0) |
| 2 | 4 | 2 (50) | 2 (50) | 0 (0) | 0 (0) |
| 3 | 8 | 7 (88) | 0 (0) | 0 (0) | 1 (12) |
| 4 | 22 | 6 (27) | 0 (0) | 10 (46) | 6 (27) |
| 5 | 64 | 4 (6) | 0 (0) | 21 (33) | 39 (61) |

Specimen composition: 125 nevi, 22 solar lentigines, 77 melanomas

*Total Lesions = nevi + solar lentigines + melanomas at each score

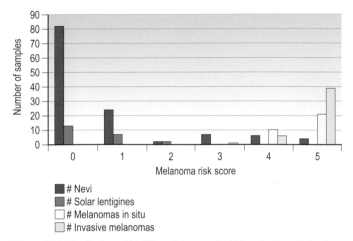

- # Nevi
- # Solar lentigines
- # Melanomas in situ
- # Invasive melanomas

**Figure 39.6** Distribution of MelDTect risk score by histopathology. Following assay of EGIR-harvested melanoma, nevi, and solar lentigines for expression of the 17 genes that compose the MelDTect classifier, the data for each specimen were assessed by the TreeNet algorithm. Based on the TreeNet outcome, each specimen was assigned a score indicative of the risk of containing melanoma (see Table 39.2).

Some of the issues that this non-invasive genomic approach, enabled by EGIR, has the potential to address include:

- Is there a field effect from melanoma that can be detected in stratum corneum? Preliminary data from EGIR sampling show that a signal indicative of melanoma can be detected at least 4 mm beyond the bounds of the pigmented lesion.

- Can EGIR be used to better gauge melanoma prognosis? Re-analysis of the microarray data, generated from only the invasive melanoma specimens, could be performed to identify a prognostic biomarker. This could potentially be used to direct the need for (or even supplant) a sentinel node biopsy.

- Can the IVDMIA detect amelanotic melanoma? Current work has just begun to collect non-pigmented lesions for EGIR-based analysis.

- Are the molecular pathways identified by expression profiling of EGIR specimens of melanoma potential targets for treatment intervention? Further bioinformatics analyses of the microarray data from melanoma may be able to identify molecular pathways for targeted treatment.

- Can an individual's susceptibility for melanoma be characterized by a biomarker generated from EGIR sampling of normal-appearing skin? Such a finding may make current DNA-based markers of melanoma susceptibility more robust.

- Can genital lesions be evaluated by IVDMIA? These lesions can be problematic to biopsy and EGIR could potentially provide a non-invasive means for their assessment.

It is anticipated that over the next few years each of these questions will be addressed to better determine the scope and efficacy of the EGIR technology in the diagnosis of melanoma.

## ACKNOWLEDGEMENTS

I am grateful for data and insights provided by DermTech International, Inc., and especially wish to thank Dr. Sherman Chang, Director of Molecular Biology at DermTech for his contributions for this chapter. In addition, I want to thank Cheryl Peters and Jennifer Larson of DermTech for their assistance with figures for this chapter.

## REFERENCES

**1.** Lander ES, Linton LM, Birren B, et al. Initial sequencing and analysis of the human genome. *Nature*. 2001;409:860–921.
**2.** Collins FS, Morgan M, Patrinos A. The Human Genome Project: lessons from large-scale biology. *Science*. 2003;300:286–290.
**3.** Tran KT, Wright NA, Cockerell CJ. Biopsy of the pigmented lesion – when and how. *J Am Acad Dermatol*. 2008;59:852–871.
**4.** Osborne JE, Chave TA, Hutchinson PE. Comparison of diagnostic accuracy for cutaneous malignant melanoma between general dermatology, plastic surgery and pigmented lesion clinics. *Br J Dermatol*. 2003;148:252–258.
**5.** Soares TF, Laman SD, Yiannias JA, et al. Factors leading to the biopsy of 1547 pigmented lesions at Mayo Clinic, Scottsdale, Arizona, in 2005. *Int J Dermatol*. 2009;48:1053–1056.
**6.** Morhenn VB, Chang EY, Rheins LA. A noninvasive method for quantifying and distinguishing inflammatory skin reactions. *J Am Acad Dermatol*. 1999;41:687–692.
**7.** Benson NR, Papenfuss J, Wong R, et al. An analysis of select pathogenic messages in lesional and non-lesional psoriatic skin using non-invasive tape harvesting. *J Invest Dermatol*. 2006;126:2234–2241.
**8.** Wong R, Tran V, Morhenn V, et al. Use of RT-PCR and DNA microarrays to characterize RNA recovered by non-invasive tape harvesting of normal and inflamed skin. *J Invest Dermatol*. 2004;123:159–167.
**9.** Wachsman W, Zapala M, Udall D, et al. Differentiation of melanoma from dysplastic nevi in suspicious pigmented skin lesions by non-invasive tape stripping. *J Invest Dermatol*. 2007;127:S145.
**10.** Wachsman W, Palmer T, Walls L, et al. *Non-invasive genomic detection of melanoma*. Manuscript submitted. 2010

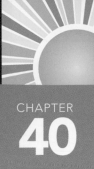

CHAPTER
## 40

# Biopsy Techniques

*Joseph F. Sobanko, Justin J. Leitenberger, Neil A. Swanson, and Ken K. Lee*

---

### Key Points

- Proper biopsy is critical in the diagnosis and management of skin cancers.

- Melanocytic lesions should be removed with an excisional biopsy where possible in order to obtain the most accurate diagnosis and prognostic factors although there is no evidence that an incisional biopsy adversely affects prognosis.

- Non-melanocytic lesions can be removed with a shave biopsy or other incisional techniques.

---

## INTRODUCTION

The biopsy is a critical start to the diagnosis of skin cancer. It is 'the process of removing tissue from patients for diagnostic examination'.[1] Fortunately, the accessibility of the skin simplifies the biopsy process relative to other organ systems. Experienced clinicians can often identify skin cancers during physical examination using both visual and tactile clues. Nevertheless, a properly performed biopsy is paramount to the diagnosis and eventual management of the skin cancer. The numerous biopsy techniques available to a clinician include: excisional, incisional, shave, saucerization and punch. Each of these modalities serves a different purpose and clinicians who manage skin cancers should understand and master all of them. Correctly biopsying pigmented lesions illustrates this importance, as there may be significant ramifications beyond the initial diagnosis of melanoma. Factors such as depth of invasion, ulceration, microsatellitosis, angiolymphatic invasion, and mitotic index can impact prognosis and proper management. The decision to implement additional prognostic and therapeutic techniques such as sentinel lymph node biopsy and systemic adjuvant therapies is often determined by the results from the initial biopsy. Therefore, procurement of an adequate specimen for presentation to the dermatopathologist is critical to assure a correct and complete diagnosis. Conversely, aesthetic outcomes should be considered since many suspicious lesions are in fact determined to be benign. This chapter reviews the decision-making process and discusses in detail the biopsy techniques and rationales for their use.

## DECISION-MAKING PROCESS

There are many different types of skin cancers which are frequently divided into two categories: melanoma and non-melanoma skin cancers. This division stems from the relative difficulty and controversy surrounding the histologic diagnosis of melanoma. The controversy arises as similar-appearing melanocytes, the pigment-forming cells of the skin, can be found in a benign nevus, atypical or dysplastic nevus, and invasive melanoma. Since the prognosis and management of melanoma is based primarily on the Breslow depth of invasion, an adequate deep margin is necessary in the diagnosis. Thus, a proper initial biopsy is critical to correctly diagnose and characterize melanoma. This type of information is best obtained in the initial biopsy. There is more flexibility in the type of biopsy technique chosen for diagnosis of non-melanoma skin cancers, with respect to important factors such as location, appearance, and the size of the lesion.

## Types of biopsies

An **excisional biopsy** refers to *en toto* removal of a suspicious lesion. This is performed with a margin (as defined below) of clinically normal tissue. It is the preferred method of removing a pigmented lesion for histologic interpretation.

An **incisional biopsy** is used to sample only a part of a suspicious lesion for histologic evaluation. It is an appropriate method to biopsy a suspicious non-melanoma skin cancer.

**Shave biopsy** refers to a shallow removal of a lesion at a depth confined to the dermis. It can be performed by a scalpel, a Dermablade®, a razor blade, or scissors.

A **saucerization** is a biopsy which occurs through viable dermis into subcutaneous fat. It is performed by angling a scalpel at approximately 45 degrees to the skin and removing a disc of tissue, including all or part of the suspicious lesion, well into the subcutaneous fat.

**Punch biopsy** refers to the use of a sharp circular instrument to remove tissue well into the subcutaneous fat. It is usually sutured.

**Fusiform ellipse** allows for full-thickness removal of the suspicious lesion, as well as a margin of surrounding skin. It is sutured.

The **margin** removed is defined as the area of normal-appearing tissue surrounding the lesion to be removed and has two components. The *peripheral margin* is the area of normal skin extending radially from the clinically suspicious lesion while the *deep margin* is the depth to which skin and subcutaneous tissue is entered and removed during the biopsy.

## Equipment

The equipment needed for biopsies need not be elaborate but should be of good quality. The equipment should be properly maintained and sterilized prior to each use.

Following is a list of commonly used equipment (Figs 40.1 and 40.2):

- Scalpel – #15 blade is the most often used
- Needle holder – Webster or Halsey
- Forceps – Adson type with teeth
- Scissors – Iris and Metzenbaum
- Skin hook – single or double prong
- Dermablade or Gillette blue blade
- Punch – 2, 3, 4, 5, 6, 8 mm
- Suture material
- Aluminum chloride – 35%
- Electrocautery
- Gauze
- Cotton-tipped applicator.

When performing a biopsy, a tray should be prepared with all the equipment that is needed for that particular

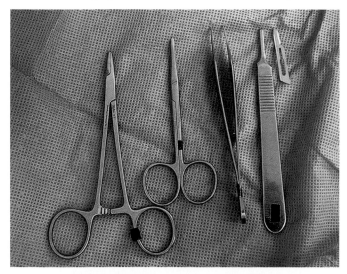

**Figure 40.1** Biopsy equipment. Some of the commonly used equipment, listed from left to right. (a) Webster needle holder, (b) small Metzenbaum scissors, (c) Adson forceps with teeth, (d) scalpel handle and #15 blade.

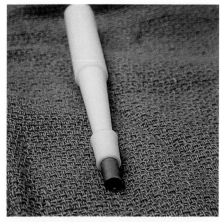

**Figure 40.2** Punch biopsy. Disposable punch device. These range from 1.5 to 10 mm. Most commonly used sizes are 2, 3, 4, 6, and 8 mm.

procedure. *On or near the tray should be the formalin-containing specimen bottle(s) with the patient's identifying information* (Fig. 40.3). This cannot be overemphasized, as there have been unfortunate cases of mislabeled specimen bottles and/or lost specimens that were left on the tray intended for subsequent transfer. Sterile surgical gloves are generally not necessary for biopsies, with the exception of excisional and incisional biopsies needing buried absorbable sutures to close the biopsied site.

## Anesthesia

Lidocaine 1% mixed with epinephrine (adrenaline) at 1:100,000 is typically used for local anesthesia. The onset of action is almost immediate with local injection and the duration of action is 1–2 hours,[2] thus making lidocaine 1% with epinephrine ideal for short biopsy procedures. However, it is optimal to wait 7–10 minutes following local infiltration to optimize the full vasoconstrictive effects of the epinephrine. Lidocaine and epinephrine mix can be obtained as a premixed formula or can be freshly mixed on a daily basis. Premixed lidocaine with epinephrine contains preservatives and has a low pH of 3.3–5.5. This low pH causes an increased amount of pain upon injection. Freshly mixed solution is desirable as it has a more neutral pH of 6.5–6.8, thus minimizing the pain from local infiltration. Sodium bicarbonate can be mixed to buffer stock (premixed) lidocaine by the addition of $1\,cm^3$ $NaHCO_3$ to every $10\,cm^3$ of lidocaine to neutralize the pH and decrease the pain of injection.[3]

Patients may describe a history of heart palpitations and tremors with local anesthesia, leading them to report this as an allergy. Very few patients are truly allergic to lidocaine and most often these symptoms are due to the systemic adrenergic effects of epinephrine. The history should be carefully assessed and the epinephrine diluted or eliminated accordingly. The most frequent side effect encountered is a vasovagal reaction manifested by hypotension and bradycardia. Amide anesthetics do not cross-react with other drugs and true allergic reactions are extremely rare. If a true allergy to lidocaine (in the amide family of anesthetics) is documented, an anesthetic from the ester family, such as procaine, can be used. It is more likely to have an allergy

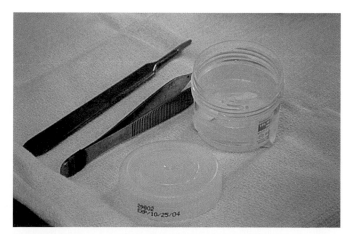

**Figure 40.3** Biopsy tray. A labeled specimen bottle should always be set out prior to the biopsy.

to the ester family anesthetics, however, as these can cross-react with para-amino benzoic acid, sulfonamides, and thiazides. Lastly, diphenhydramine solution (12.5–25 mg/kg) or normal saline can be used as local anesthesia for smaller lesions.[4] When the medical history is unclear, an evaluation by an allergist to determine a safe local anesthetic is critical.

The local anesthetic is injected intradermally using a 30-gauge needle (Fig. 40.4). Rapid needle insertion through the skin and slower infiltration of anesthetic agent causes less discomfort. Furthermore, it often eases anxiety to prepare the patient by discussing the technique prior to injection. In children and very anxious adults, a topical anesthetic cream can be applied 30 minutes to 2 hours prior to injection to reduce the pain of needle insertion and injection pain.[5]

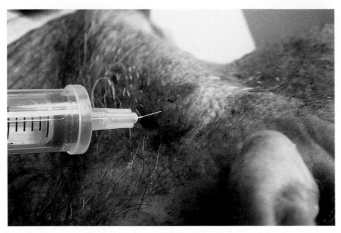

**Figure 40.4** Anesthesia injection. 1% lidocaine with epinephrine is most commonly used for local anesthesia. A 30-gauge needle is used to infiltrate slowly into the dermis.

## Contraindications to biopsy

There are no absolute contraindications to a skin biopsy. The main relative contraindication is the potential for bleeding. Many patients requiring skin biopsies are older and use anticoagulants. While there may be an elevated risk of postoperative bleeding, the use of warfarin or aspirin is not contraindicated. Extra measures such as electrocoagulation and pressure dressings may be needed for enhanced hemostasis in select cases. In patients on chemotherapy or with diseases that affect platelets, it is best if the platelet count is above 10,000 per microliter.

## BIOPSY TECHNIQUES – ILLUSTRATED

**Punch biopsy:** Trephines (handheld punches) are available in sizes that range from 1.5 mm to 10 mm and may be used for excisional or incisional biopsies. A proper punch biopsy size must be chosen in order to obtain an adequate tissue sample. Determination of trephine size is guided by whether an incisional or excisional biopsy is indicated (Table 40.1). For an excisional biopsy, the punch should be 1.0 to 1.5 mm greater in diameter than the lesion. For an incisional biopsy, a 2–4 mm punch is commonly used. After adequate anesthesia, traction is placed across the skin tension lines, converting a circular region into an elliptical shape (Fig. 40.5A–E). When traction is released, the resultant elliptical defect allows for an easier and aesthetically superior closure. The punch is rotated back and forth on the skin with constant pressure through the full thickness of the dermis. A characteristic 'give' is felt when the subcutaneous fat is reached. The specimen should be carefully grasped only on one edge so as to minimize crush artifact on histologic examination. The base of the specimen is cut at the level of the subcutaneous fat. Hemostasis is

| Table 40.1 Biopsy Selections for Neoplastic Skin Lesions | | | | |
|---|---|---|---|---|
| **Type of Biopsy** | **Indications** | **Anatomic Locations** | **Pigmented Lesion Use** | **Method of Healing** |
| Shave | Suspect non-melanoma skin cancer (BCC, SCC) | All | No | Second intention |
| Punch (incisional) | Large pigmented lesions (when excisional biopsy cannot be performed) | Cosmetically sensitive locations | Yes[†] | Simple interrupted, vertical mattress sutures |
| Punch (excisional) | Small pigmented lesions (to be removed en toto) Rare neoplasms* | All | Yes | Simple interrupted, vertical mattress sutures |
| Fusiform ellipse | Pigmented lesions (with surgical margin for diagnosis and treatment) | Aligned along relaxed skin tension lines | Yes | Linear layered closure |
| Saucerization | Pigmented lesions | Upper back, shoulders, upper arms, and anterior chest; occasionally, lower extremities and ears | Yes | Second intention |

*Lesions where the differential diagnosis includes amelanotic melanoma, atypical fibroxanthoma, dermatofibrosarcoma protuberans, Merkel cell carcinoma or other rare neoplasms of the skin should be biopsied with an incisional punch or any excisional biopsy (ellipse or excisional punch), based on the size and anatomic location, to evaluate the deep margins.

†Used when pre-test probability of suspicious lesion is low to moderate. Lesions with a high pre-test probability for melanoma should be excised.

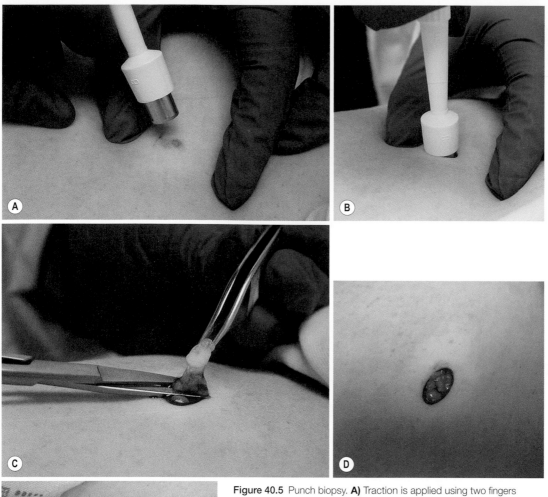

**Figure 40.5** Punch biopsy. **A)** Traction is applied using two fingers perpendicular to the relaxed skin tension lines, providing a rigid surface for the cutting edge of the punch device. **B)** The punch is then pushed through skin while applying a circular back-and-forth motion. **C)** The specimen is gently grasped on one edge and transected at the level of the subcutaneous fat. **D)** The resultant defect is elliptical because the circular biopsy was done under traction. This allows for an easier linear closure. **E)** After closure with cuticular sutures.

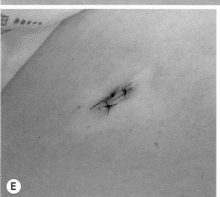

usually achieved with pressure and suture closure. Rarely, electrocauterization may be needed. Punch biopsies, with rare exception, are closed with simple interrupted or vertical mattress stitches for wound edge eversion to obtain the best cosmetic result.

**Shave biopsy:** A shave biopsy is used to remove the superficial component of a lesion raised above the level of the surrounding skin. The level at which the shave is performed is either at that of the surrounding skin or slightly deeper. The intent is usually not to remove the entire neoplasm but rather to obtain a representative sample for histopathologic examination. Accurate sampling and cosmetic outcome are two factors considered when performing a shave biopsy, as many biopsied lesions are

benign. The infiltration of anesthesia in the mid-dermis will provide a rigid plane and squeezing the surrounding skin will provide an elevated plane for shave biopsy. Using a #15 blade scalpel, Dermablade, or razor blade, a shallow horizontal incision is made through the lesion at the level of the surrounding skin or slightly below. Forceps can also be used for gentle countertraction (Fig. 40.6A,B). A Dermablade or a razor blade also allows for a precise shave biopsy. The blade is flexed to match the size of the lesion and is slid back and forth through the lesion until the entire lesion is removed (Fig. 40.7). Hemostasis is obtained with aluminum chloride 35%. The resultant scar is circular and approximates the size of the initial lesion. There may be a subtle indentation if the incision was made in a deeper plane.

**437**

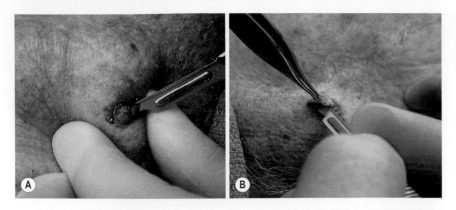

**Figure 40.6** Shave biopsy. A #15 blade scalpel is used to shave the raised component of the suspected cancer. The surrounding skin is squeezed together to provide an elevated and rigid plane (**A**) or forceps are used for countertraction (**B**).

**Saucerization:** A saucerization provides an excisional specimen for the dermatopathologist. This technique is easy to perform, time efficient, and often preferred by patients and physicians in areas of the body where it is difficult to create an elegant scar. These areas include the upper back,

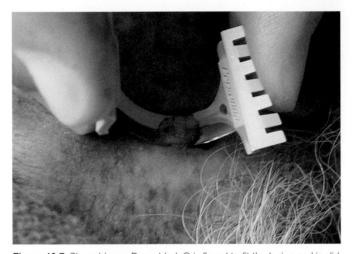

**Figure 40.7** Shave biopsy. Dermablade® is flexed to fit the lesion and is slid side to side through the lesion.

shoulders, upper arms, and anterior chest, where scars often spread and/or become hypertrophic. Occasionally, saucerizations are also used to biopsy lesions on the lower extremities and ears. The key is to perform true saucerization, i.e. a biopsy into subcutaneous fat. With saucerization, a smaller, rounder, and more cosmetically acceptable scar will replace a longer, linear spread excisional scar while providing adequate tissue for histologic interpretation. A #15 blade scalpel is placed approximately 45 degrees to the skin surface. The incision is made around a 1–2 mm peripheral margin of the lesion, then angled tangentially deeper through the dermis to the level of the subcutaneous fat. This generates a disc- or saucer-shaped piece of tissue that contains the entire lesion (Fig. 40.8A,B). The defect then heals by secondary intent without the need for sutures.

**Fusiform ellipse:** The fusiform elliptical excision is the cornerstone of cutaneous surgery. It is easy to perform, gives excellent cosmetic results, and provides tissue of sufficient depth to aid in an accurate diagnosis by the dermatopathologist.[6] In designing the ellipse, the long axis should generally be oriented along the relaxed skin tension lines and the draining lymphatics for that site. The length is approximately three times the width but this will vary depending on the adjacent skin laxity. The ideal

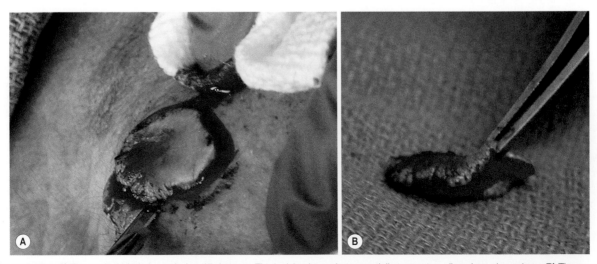

**Figure 40.8** Saucerization. **A)** The scalpel blade is angled at 45 degrees. The incision is made tangentially to create a disc-shaped specimen **B)** The specimen is removed at the level of the fat.

angle of the apices is 30 degrees in order to minimize puckering of redundant skin. The #15 scalpel blade is angled perpendicular to the skin surface and the incision is carried through the skin into the subcutaneous fat. The specimen is removed in its entirety maintaining a flat-bottomed surface (Fig. 40.9A–C).

The fusiform ellipse is usually closed in linear layered fashion. The defect is undermined at the level of the subcutaneous fat to alleviate tension and to promote wound eversion. After adequate hemostasis is achieved, the wound is carefully re-approximated using absorbable buried dermal interrupted sutures. The needle insertion should begin at the deep aspect, allowing the knot to lie deeply, decreasing the chances of a spitting suture. The superficial or cuticular layer is generally closed with a non-absorbable monofilament suture (Fig. 40.10A–E).

## DIAGNOSIS OF MELANOMA

When examining a patient with one or several suspicious pigmented lesions, the question often arises, 'Do I need to perform a biopsy, and if so, which technique do I choose?' A clinician must weigh the given risks of a particular lesion with the patient or family concern (in the case of children) for scarring, inherent in all biopsy procedures.[7]

There are several tools available to help decide whether or not to biopsy a particular pigmented lesion. These include dermoscopy, precise photography, 'mole mapping' by computer, and other tools in developmental stages (see Chapter 37). As clinicians we develop expertise to determine which group of patients and which particular lesions are concerns for the development of melanoma. If our suspicion is moderate or high, we will routinely remove the pigmented lesion and submit it for histologic analysis by a dermatopathologist. This is both reassuring to the patient as well as the clinician, and frequently may lead to a diagnosis of melanoma in its earlier, less advanced stage.

The excisional biopsy is the preferred method of removing a clinically suspicious pigmented lesion. It provides the dermatopathologist with the most adequate tissue sampling to correctly diagnose a melanoma. If present, the maximum depth of invasion of the melanoma (Breslow level) can be measured as well as other histologic criteria

of importance, which helps define the extent of further necessary surgery.

When performing an excisional biopsy, the clinician should first examine the lymph nodes in the suspected draining basin(s) from the lesion in question. If the lesion turns out to be a melanoma, inflammation from the biopsy procedure can result in a false positive 'dermatopathic' node. A Wood's light is helpful to assess the complete margin, sometimes extending beyond the obvious clinical appearance of the lesion. A 1.0–1.5 mm margin is marked around the lesion and removed at the level of the subcutaneous fat.[8,9] When possible, the biopsy is aligned along relaxed skin tension lines and along the draining lymphatics from that site. The former allows for an easier and more cosmetically acceptable procedure if the lesion is a melanoma and requires re-excision. The latter allows for a more accurate sentinel lymph node biopsy if indicated.

The excisional biopsy can be performed with either a punch or a fusiform (elliptical) excision. Choosing a punch 1.0–1.5 mm greater in diameter than the lesion to be biopsied assures a full-thickness removal of the entire lesion that is easy and quick to perform with a cosmetically acceptable scar. If the lesion is larger and/or in a cosmetically sensitive area such as the head and neck, a fusiform (elliptical) excision with full-thickness closure provides adequate tissue for the pathologist and an excellent cosmetic result if the pigmented lesion is benign.

A saucerization biopsy can also be used to provide an excisional specimen for the dermatopathologist. Again, the key is to make sure this is a true saucerization, i.e. a biopsy into fatty tissue. Because of their tendency to heal with hypertrophic or spread scars, the torso and extremities are often best biopsied by saucerization. Superficial shave biopsies should not be used for pigmented lesions, especially if one is attempting to rule out melanoma. The transection of the specimen base will lead to an uninterpretable Breslow level.

An incisional biopsy can be used to diagnose melanoma in a worrisome pigmented lesion. However, because it does not sample the entire lesion in question, incisional biopsies may lead to an inaccurate diagnosis or an inaccurate calculation of the Breslow depth. Incisional biopsies can be performed on very large lesions and/or in cosmetically

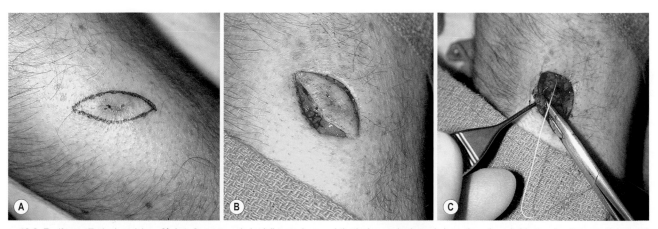

**Figure 40.9** Fusiform elliptical excision. **A)** A 1–2 mm margin is delineated around the lesion and oriented along the relaxed skin tension lines and/or direction of lymphatic drainage. **B)** Incision is made through the dermis into the fat. **C)** Defect is ready for layered closure.

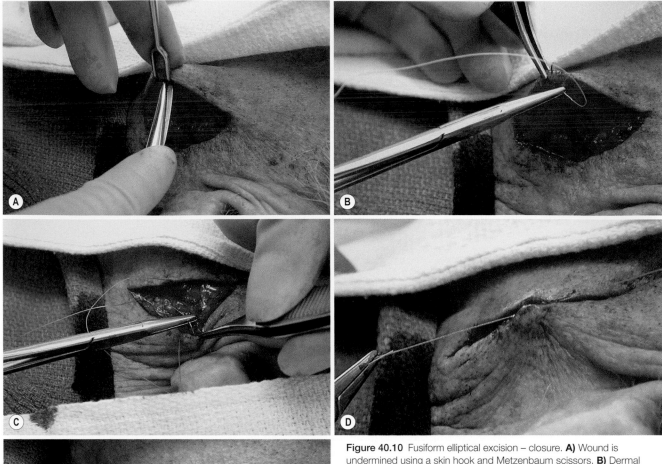

**Figure 40.10** Fusiform elliptical excision – closure. **A)** Wound is undermined using a skin hook and Metzenbaum scissors. **B)** Dermal suture is inserted from the deep aspect of the wound, then **C)** passed superficial to deep on the other side and **D)** knotted to create an everted wound. **E)** Final appearance.

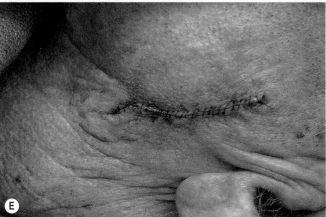

sensitive regions (Fig. 40.11A,B). The darkest pigmented and/or raised area of the lesion should be biopsied. This can be performed using a punch biopsy, small fusiform ellipse, or a saucerization down to the level of the subcutaneous fat. When performed, the incisional biopsy specimen should be cut and processed along the longitudinal axis to maximize the cross-section area available histologically for the dermatopathologist.

Although most clinicians feel that an incisional biopsy does not 'spread' tumor or influence survival,[10] there still exists a theoretical risk that cutting through the tumor may lead to local spread of the melanoma. Implantation and seeding of malignant cells with certain surgical procedures is a phenomenon known to occur with other neoplasms such as breast and colon cancer.[11-13] Most studies indicate that performing an incisional biopsy does not influence prognosis in patients with melanoma.[14-18] Nor does it appear that

incisional biopsies of melanoma influence recurrence or mortality when compared to their excisional counterpart.[19] Few studies have suggested otherwise.[20,21]

Most recently, it has been demonstrated that an incisional biopsy that leaves behind >50% of the initial clinical lesion may in fact result in false microstaging and significantly underestimate the depth of the tumor and lead to understaging. In a study of melanoma patients diagnosed by subtotal incisional biopsy, more than 20% required upstaging, with almost half of those patients then becoming eligible for sentinel node biopsy by AJCC criteria.[22] Inaccurate Breslow depth estimation from incisional punch biopsies of melanomas has been demonstrated elsewhere.[23,24] Lesions suspected to be melanoma in situ are of particular relevance as up to 25% of cases are ultimately determined to contain an invasive component upon further review.[25] Because histologic evaluation of the entire lesion depth and periphery

**Figure 40.11** Incisional biopsy. **A)** A large and ill-defined pigmented lesion on the cheek with variegate pigmentation. Punch biopsies can be taken from the darker areas, or **B)** an incisional ellipse is made through the most suspicious area. The lines demonstrate the axis of sectioning in order to maximize the cross-section seen by the dermatopathologist.

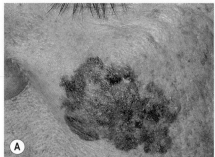
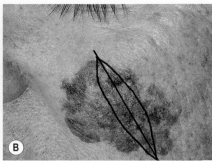

are so vitally important to staging and treatment, it must be advised to perform an excisional biopsy where possible on a lesion suspicious for melanoma.

## DIAGNOSIS OF NON-MELANOMA SKIN CANCER

The two most prevalent non-melanoma skin cancers (NMSC) are basal cell carcinoma (BCC) and squamous cell carcinoma (SCC). Incidence of these cancers number 1 million and 250,000 per year, respectively, in the United States.[26] It is thus imperative, given their high incidence, that the astute clinician recognize them clinically and obtain a biopsy for correct diagnosis.

Morphologically, NMSC can be exophytic, macular, or ulcerated. They can be pinpoint in size or consume large parts of a face, trunk, or extremity. These differences impact the choice of biopsy. An excisional biopsy is rarely needed for NMSCs.

An exophytic lesion such as a nodular BCC, or a hyperkeratotic SCC can be biopsied using the shave technique. Near-complete removal of the surface component usually results in an adequate tissue sample for an accurate diagnosis. One must be cautious, however, of lesions that have a significant hyperkeratotic component (e.g. cutaneous horn). A shave through only the hyperkeratotic component may not remove the full epidermis, necessary to distinguish SCC from an actinic keratosis. Occasionally, amelanotic melanoma can present as a skin-colored papule or nodule. If there is any concern that a lesion is something other than a clinically routine BCC or SCC, a deeper biopsy should be considered.

BCC can present as different histologic subtypes. Sclerosing (morpheaform) and infiltrative types of BCC typically have a significant component that is below the level of the skin surface which can be clinically subtle or inapparent (subclinical extension). When there is minimal or no raised component, a deeper biopsy is indicated and a punch biopsy usually results in an accurate diagnosis. Sometimes, however, multiple punch biopsies may need to be performed on the same lesion, especially when the cancer is recurrent and is adjacent to or part of a prior surgical scar.

Many different malignant and non-malignant skin conditions can present as an ulcer. Due to the dense inflammation invariably present in the ulcer bed, the biopsy should be taken from the wound edges in order to obtain proper diagnosis. As most ulcers are not cancerous, all longstanding ulcers without obvious cause should raise the concern of possible malignancy.

## POST-BIOPSY CARE

Biopsy sites that heal by secondary intent need to be cleaned daily with soap and water. They should heal under moist conditions and therefore need to be covered with an ointment and non-adherent bandage. Sutured wounds need less daily care but should be kept clean. Fusiform excisions closed with a layered closure should have a pressure bandage placed for 24 hours postoperatively. Postoperative pain is usually managed effectively with acetaminophen. Non-steroidal anti-inflammatories and aspirin are not recommended, as these can increase the risk for postoperative bleeding.

## SUMMARY

Incisional biopsies are appropriate for non-melanoma skin cancers and can be performed in limited circumstances for pigmented lesions, but should be done so with caution as sampling error may lead to missed diagnosis or inaccurate histologic criterion, such as depth. Excisional biopsies should be considered for pigmented lesions and should extend to the subcutaneous fat by means of a punch biopsy, a fusiform ellipse, or a saucerization. The clinician must also consider the cosmetic result, although not at the expense of a proper diagnosis.

## FUTURE OUTLOOK

Choosing the appropriate biopsy technique for a suspicious cutaneous lesion will continue to remain critical in establishing a correct and complete diagnosis, and, in turn, will influence the extent of further necessary surgery and/or other adjuvant therapy.

## REFERENCES

**1.** *Stedman's Medical Dictionary*. 24th ed. Baltimore: Williams & Wilkins; 1982.
**2.** Norris Jr RL. Local anesthetics. *Emerg Med Clin North Am*. 1992;10(4):707–718.
**3.** Stewart JH, Cole GW, Klein JA. Neutralized lidocaine with epinephrine for local anesthesia. *J Dermatol Surg Oncol*. 1989;15(10):1081–1083.

4. Dire DJ, Hogan DE. Double-blinded comparison of diphenhydramine versus lidocaine as a local anesthetic. *Ann Emerg Med*. 1993;22(9):1419–1422.

5. Raveh T, Weinberg A, Sibirsky O, et al. Efficacy of the topical anesthetic cream, EMLA, in alleviating both needle insertion and injection pain. *Ann Plast Surg*. 1995;35(6):576.

6. Swanson NA. *Atlas of Cutaneous Surgery*. Boston: Little Brown; 1987:20.

7. Swanson NA, Lee KK, Gorman A, et al. Biopsy techniques-diagnosis of melanoma. *Dermatol Clin*. 2002;20:677–680.

8. Brown MD, Johnson TM, Swanson NA. Changing trends in melanoma treatment and the expanding role of the dermatologist. *Dermatol Clin*. 1991;9:657–667.

9. Holmstrom H. Surgical management of primary melanoma. *Semin Surg Oncol*. 1992;8:366–369.

10. Penneys NS. Excision of melanoma after initial biopsy. *J Am Acad Dermatol*. 1985;13:995–998.

11. Schaeff B, Paolucci V, Thomopoulos J. Port site recurrences after laparoscopic surgery. A review. *Dig Surg*. 1998;15:124–134.

12. Harter LP, Curtis JS, Ponto G, et al. Malignant seeding of the needle track during stereotaxic core needle breast biopsy. *Radiology*. 1992;185:713–714.

13. Basha G, Ectors N, Penninckx F, et al. Tumour cell implantation after colonoscopy with biopsies in a patient with rectal cancer: report of a case. *Dis Colon Rectum*. 1997;40:1508–1510.

14. Eldh J. Excisional biopsy and delayed wide excision versus primary wide excision of malignant melanoma. *Scand J Plast Reconstr Surg*. 1979;13:341–345.

15. Drzewiecki KT, Ladefoged C, Christensen HE. Biopsy and prognosis for cutaneous malignant melanomas in clinical stage I. *Scand J Plast Reconstr Surg*. 1980;14:141–144.

16. Lederman JS, Sober AJ. Does wide excision as the initial diagnostic procedure improve prognosis in patients with cutaneous melanoma? *J Dermatol Surg Oncol*. 1986;12:697–699.

17. Epstein E, Bragg K, Linden G. Biopsy and prognosis of malignant melanoma. *JAMA*. 1969;208:1369–1371.

18. Martin RCG, Scoggins CR, Ross MI, et al. Is incisional biopsy of melanoma harmful? *Am J Surg*. 2005;190:927–932.

19. Bong JL, Herd RM, Hunter JAA. Incisional biopsy and melanoma prognosis. *J Am Acad Dermatol*. 2002;46:690–694.

20. Rampen FHJ, Van Houten WA, Hop WC. Incisional procedures and prognosis in malignant melanoma. *Clin Exp Dermatol*. 1980;5:313–320.

21. Austin JR, Byers RM, Brown WD, et al. Influence of biopsy on the prognosis of cutaneous melanoma of the head and neck. *Head Neck*. 1996;18:107–117.

22. Karimipour DJ, Schwartz JL, Wang TS, et al. Microstaging accuracy after subtotal incisional biopsy of cutaneous melanoma. *J Am Acad Dermatol*. 2003;48:420–424.

23. Ng PC, Barzilai DA, Ismail SA, et al. Evaluating invasive cutaneous melanoma: is the initial biopsy representative of the final depth? *J Am Acad Dermatol*. 2003;48:420–424.

24. Lorusso GD, Sarma DP, Sarwar SF. Punch biopsies of melanoma: a diagnostic peril. *Dermatol Online J*. 2005;11(1):7.

25. Dawn ME, Dawn AG, Miller SJ. Mohs surgery for the treatment of melanoma in situ. *Dermatol Surg*. 2007;33:395–402.

26. Miller DL, Weinstock MA. Nonmelanoma skin cancer in the United States: incidence. *J Am Acad Dermatol*. 1994;30(5 Pt 1):774–778.

# Curettage and Electrodesiccation

*Samuel F. Almquist, Oliver J. Wisco, and J. Michael Wentzell*

## Key Points

- Curettage and electrodesiccation (CE) is an expedient method of treating many non-melanoma skin cancers (NMSC).
- Cure rates and cosmetic outcome for CE of NMSC are site- and lesion-dependent.
- The most important aspect of CE is choosing the correct lesion to treat.
- Careful incorporation of proper lesion selection and good technique make CE a valuable therapeutic technique in the treatment of uncomplicated NMSC.

## INTRODUCTION

Curettage and electrodesiccation (CE) is a technique available to dermatologists to destroy benign entities and non-melanoma skin cancer (NMSC). The use of CE for the treatment of NMSC has been both praised and criticized, revealing its advantages and limitations. In order to appropriately employ CE to treat NMSC, it is essential to learn the basis for selecting CE, the proper technique, the likely cure rates for given lesions, and the expected cosmetic result, in order to provide patients with the best outcome.

Formerly the dermatologists' treatment of choice for many skin cancers, CE is now only one method in an increasing therapeutic armamentarium. To utilize CE most judiciously, it is valuable to examine this technique in depth and to come to some thoughtful conclusions about its use for patients with skin cancer.

## HISTORY

Electrodesiccation of skin lesion was first established in 1911 by William Clark, who noted superficial tissue drying (desiccation) when he applied a high voltage, low current to the skin, through a monoterminal electrode. Clark reported the treatment of a variety of skin lesions, including some basal cell carcinomas, with electrodesiccation alone.[1] The technique of electrodesiccation became available to the office practitioner through the development of instrumentation such as the original Hyfrecator units produced by the Birtcher Corporation.

The literature surrounding the original implementation of curettage is quite sparse. Use of the dermal curette was first reported in 1870 by Dr. Henry Piffard.[2] Several years later, Dr. Edward Wigglesworth used the dermal curette to treat a variety of skin lesions, including psoriasis and syphilitic condylomata.[3] In 1902, Dr. George Fox introduced the Fox model curette, which remains the most popular curette today.[4] As dermatology evolved in the 1950s and 1960s, an increasing number of epithelial tumors were primarily treated by CE or by curettage alone. At this time, many dermatologists received little training in surgery and most large lesions were handled either through excision by general surgeons or plastic surgeons, or by radiation therapy. As dermatologists explored avenues for office-based treatment of cutaneous tumors, the technique of CE was embraced as an efficient method for the removal of benign lesions and NMSC.

## DESCRIPTION OF PROCEDURE/THERAPY

### Electrosurgery principles

The use of electrosurgery requires understanding the principles of electricity and waveforms. The five principles of electricity are current, resistance, voltage, work, and power (Table 41.1). These principles determine the functionality of an electrosurgery unit. Waveform refers to the shape of an electromagnetic field generated from a high-frequency alternating current. The waveform factors to consider are whether it is damped or undamped and whether it is continuous or discontinuous (Fig. 41.1).

Combining the five electricity principles and the type of waveform, in addition to whether the electrosurgery unit is monoterminal (no grounding pad used, the current is randomly dispersed to the environment) or biterminal (grounding pad used, the current flows from one electrode to the other), determines the type of destruction that the electrosurgery unit creates in the tissue (Fig. 41.2). Electrodesiccation is typically performed using a monoterminal unit with high voltage, low amperage, and a discontinuous and damped waveform. The procedure invokes a superficial level of destruction with minimal damage to the deeper structures. It is performed by gliding the electrodesiccator tip gently along the surface of the tissue until a thin char is achieved.[5-7]

### The curette

Curettes come in both disposable and non-disposable forms. Clinicians who choose to use the non-disposable forms typically use a combination of standard round and oval head Fox curettes or oval Cannon curettes with or without a delicate angle (Fig. 41.3). The standard Fox round head curette has a rectangular handle with a tapered cylindrical extension to the head, which is round with a thicker dull side and

| Principle | Definition | Units | Pearls/Application |
|---|---|---|---|
| Current | Flows of electrons through a conductor per second. Density = current/conductor cross-sectional area | Amperes | The thinner the electrosurgical tip, the greater the current density, resulting in greater tissue destruction |
| Direct | Electron flow is in one direction | | Used in iontophoresis and electrolysis |
| Alternating | Electron flow is constantly alternating direction; with high frequencies there is no cellular depolarization resulting in the generation of heat | | Frequencies of 500–2000 Hz generate heat with no/minimal neuromuscular depolarization |
| Resistance | A conductor's ability to impede the passage of an electric current. Directly proportional to the length of the substance. Inversely proportional to the cross-sectional area | Ohms | Muscle: low resistance. Fat: high resistance. Skin: high when dry, low when wet |
| Voltage | Electrical force that induces electron flow. Current flows from high to low electron concentration. Volts = current × resistance | Volts | Little heat is created with low resistance |
| Work | Current flow over a distance due to voltage difference. Work = force × distance | Joules | Tissue resistance to current results in heat generation |
| Power | Rate of heat generated due to tissue resistance to the passage of current created by a voltage potential. Power = current × voltage | Watts (joules/s) | Power increases are greater with increased current rather than voltage |

**Table 41.1 Electricity Principles**

a thin sharp side. The Fox oval curette has the same handle, but the head is oval with its longest axis along the length of the curette.[4] The Cannon angled oval curette has a more delicate (thinner) handle and the head is tilted at a slight angle to facilitate curettage.

The disposable curettes that are typically used are similar to the commonly used non-disposable curettes (Fig. 41.4). The benefit of the disposable curette is that new curettes are consistently sharp, while the non-disposable curettes lose the precision of their edge over time and require sharpening. However, many experienced practitioners will argue that the non-disposable curettes give a more precise feel compared to the disposable curettes when curetting the tissue in order to delineate the margins of the tumor. Curettes are labeled by size from 0 to 8, based on the approximate diameter of the longest axis in millimeters (mm). There are some specialty sizes and the size of a 'given size' curette may vary from vendor to vendor and should be checked.

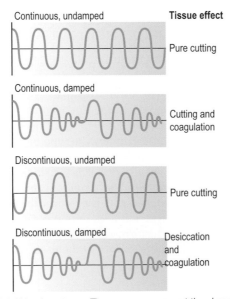

Figure 41.1 Waveform types. These waves represent the shape of the electromagnetic field created by high-frequency alternating current. The waveform dictates the effect of the current applied to tissue. A continuous, undampened sine wave is employed in electrosection and is purely cutting with minimal hemostasis. The continuous dampened waveform is advantageous as it uses uninterrupted waveforms resulting in cutting with the benefit of tissue heating resulting in coagulation. The last two waveforms are discontinuous, resulting in decreased tissue heating, allowing a surgeon to cut with less heat transferred to the tissue. (Adapted from Robinson et al., *Surgery of the Skin*, 2005 with permission from Mosby Publishing Company.)

## Preoperative management

Preoperative evaluation for CE takes into account the same considerations as for excisional removal. Risk for bleeding, keloidal scarring, and implanted cardiac devices are the main concerns. However, the risk for developing a postoperative wound infection is not a significant concern in the immunocompetent patient because of the superficial nature of the procedure. Avoid using an alcohol cleanser or ethyl chloride anesthesia, and flowing oxygen should be turned off. Smoke evacuators should also be used, but the procedure can be performed under clean, non-sterile, technique. Last, during the procedure, patients should remove all metal jewelry and should not make any contact with metal objects on the treatment table. A typical setup for CE is illustrated in Figure 41.5.

## Electrodesiccation and curettage technique

The premise behind CE is that by using a curette, the clinician can distinguish precisely between disease (tumor) and normal dermis. Most nodular and superficial basal cell carcinomas (BCC) and some squamous cell carcinomas (SCC) have a less cohesive texture than normal epidermis

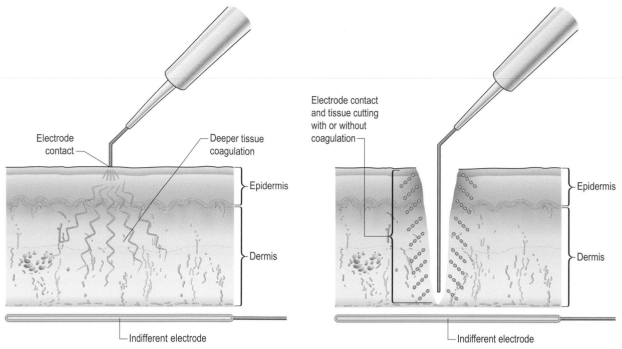

**Figure 41.2** Electrosurgery. This figure demonstrates the differences between electrosection, electrofulguration, electrodesiccation, and electrocoagulation, including electrode tip placement, and the result of the current on the tissue. (Adapted from Robinson et al., Surgery of the Skin, 2005 with permission from Mosby Publishing Company.)

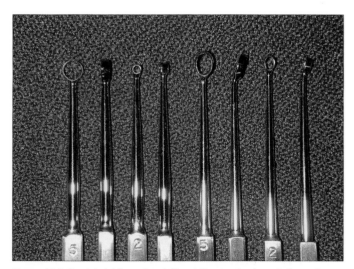

**Figure 41.3** Fox (straight) curettes (left) and Cannon (oval, angled) curettes (right).

and dermis and are thus delineated from healthy tissue by curettage.[8]

A large or medium curette is used to remove the bulk of the tumor and residual foci are removed and the defect sculpted with a fine curette. Most authors who are proponents of CE recommend vigorous and precise curettage prior to electrodesiccation. The lesion has been fully removed when a flat, off-white dermis with regularly spaced hair follicles, pinpoint bleeding and no intervening epidermal tissue is seen.

Two curettage techniques may be employed and these methods have been reviewed in detail.[9] In the pen technique, the curette is held like a pencil in the dominant hand and the lesion is stabilized with the non-dominant hand.

Most clinicians use this technique. In the potato peeler technique, which has been encouraged for larger tumors, the curette is held in the distal interdigital joint of the index finger, middle finger, ring finger and pinky. Using the thumb to brace against the tissue, the lesion is then peeled from the dermis. It is essential that the area to be treated is braced firmly to provide a taut surface for the curette. With either method, curettage is performed vigorously until all tumor is removed by tactile feel and until a firm dermis with pinpoint bleeding is observed (Fig. 41.6).[9]

A great deal has been written about the feel of curetting a skin cancer. In their 2000 review of CE, Sheridan and Dawber note that 'this feel is both undeniably and readily learnt'.[10] On the other hand, Salasche has demonstrated that even in highly experienced hands, tumor is left behind by curettage in 12–30% of facial BCC.[11] The 'feel' is far more reliable on the trunk and proximal extremities where the dermis is thick and taut, and the recurrence rate for NMSC following CE is much lower at these locations. 'Feel' is at its weakest on the eyelid, medial cheek and eyelid, which 'float' during the curettage procedure, and on the nose where BCC extending into the follicles is beyond the feel of the curette.[11]

Some authors believe that electrodesiccation (Fig. 41.7) and subsequent curettage of the char effects a higher cure rate,[10] but the data to support this assertion are weak. Likewise it is not clear that performing three cycles of CE is statistically more effective than one. It is clear that those who have reported the highest cure rates always destroy a substantial peripheral margin around the initial curettage. This is accomplished most readily by electrodesiccation and then curettage of a rim of 2 mm, to as much as 8 mm of tissue around the initial defect.[12,13]

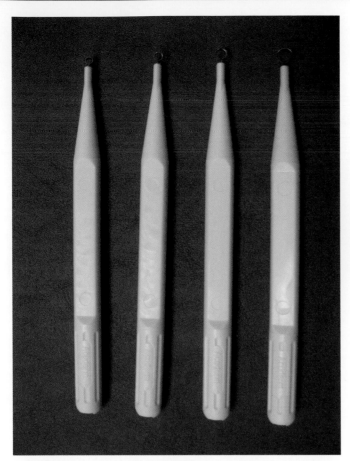

**Figure 41.4** Disposable curettes, sizes 2–5.

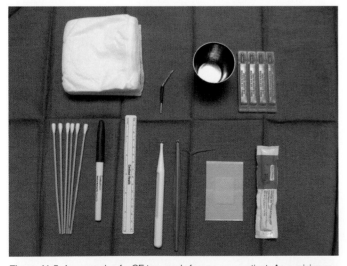

**Figure 41.5** An example of a CE tray ready for use on a patient. As a minimum, one should have the desired curette(s), 4 × 4 gauze, and the electrodesiccator present.

## Postoperative care

Immediately after the procedure, the wounds are covered with petrolatum and a non-stick bandage for the next 24 hours. Homecare consists of gently cleansing the wound daily with soap and water and covering the wound with petrolatum and a non-adherent bandage. No scheduled follow-up for the wound is needed other than re-evaluation at routine skin examinations.

## Cosmesis

In 1963, Sweet wrote that the cosmetic results from curettage and electrodesiccation were 'so astoundingly good that I think they would justify this form of treatment even if the recurrence rate were far higher'.[14] Subsequent authors who have promoted the technique of CE or curettage alone have extolled the cosmetic virtues of curettage over surgical excision. With regard to curettage alone, Reymann noted that 'it must be emphasized that after treatment solely with curettage, the cicatrices are much more satisfactory than those resulting from any other type of therapy'.[15] In contrast, Epstein noted in 1977 that 'surgical excision produces cosmetic results clearly superior to CE' and that 'the dermatology profession should stop trying to justify the second-rate cosmetic results obtainable by CE and abandon the technique in treating BCC'.[16] To date, there have been no blinded studies of the cosmetic outcome of CE versus excision.

Clearly, the cosmetic result following both CE and excision is site-dependent. On the trunk and extremities, CE often leads to a flat, white macule or patch (Fig. 41.8), but may lead to a raised or depressed oval scar, or occasionally a longstanding keloidal scar. Even if the eventual result is satisfactory, often CE sites remain pink and elevated for a period of months before improving. Surgical excision at these sites frequently leads to a fine line but can produce either a spread scar or a keloidal scar (Fig. 41.9). On the face, CE may heal with a fine white patch or macule. However, despite many claims to the contrary, healed CE sites on the face are often depressed, sometimes markedly so, often retract free margins as they heal, and can produce a firm rope-like scar due to wound contraction. It is important to note that a skillfully performed surgical excision on the face often leads to a scar that is almost imperceptible even on close inspection, while CE can never do this. In general it is the authors' feeling that excision or Mohs surgery followed by proper repair more often leads to a better aesthetic scar than does CE, particularly on the face.

## Cure rates

The discrepancy in reported cure rates has been significant.[12-34] The argument against 'feeling' for clear margins by surgeons who feel comfortable with their CE skills has been challenged in several studies. In 1983, Salasche performed three passes of CE to treat BCC and then excised the lesions with 1 mm margins to look for residual histologic cancer in nasal and non-nasal lesions. Residual BCC was found in 12% of non-nasal lesions and in 30% of nasal and paranasal lesions.[11] In 1984, Suhge d'Aubermont and Bennett attained similar findings by demonstrating residual BCC in 46.6% of head lesions versus only 8.3% of trunk lesions.[28] In 1971, Crissey's review of the 13 previous studies found an average cure rate of 92.6%. Crissey also summarized unsuitable locations and tumors for CE, including lesions involving cartilage, sclerosing BCCs, eyelid and vermilion lesions, nasal lesions >1 cm, and 'large cutaneous carcinomas'.[32] Dubin and Kopf in the 1970s and 1980s found that over a 15-year period, the 5-year recurrence rate of BCC was 26% for CE compared to the gold standard of excision which was 9.6%.[33]

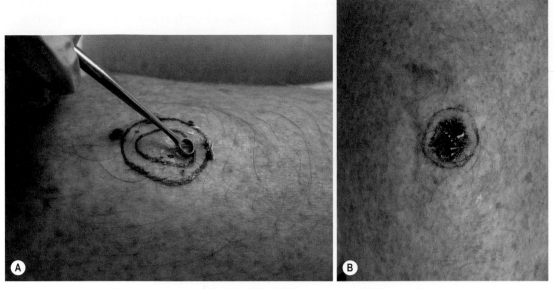

**Figure 41.6** Curettage of a squamous cell carcinoma in situ on the right thigh. **A)** Prior to curetage with the curette in place using the pen technique. **B)** Residual defect after curettage. Note the shining dermis, pinpoint bleeding, and the lack of subcutaneous tissue involvement.

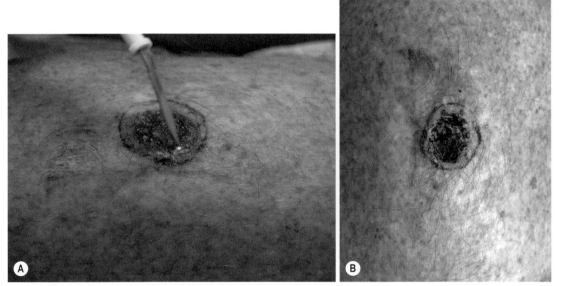

**Figure 41.7** Electrodesiccation after curettage of a squamous cell carcinoma in situ on the right thigh. **A)** Electrodesiccation technique of linear application of the hyfrecator tip to the lesion. **B)** Defect after electrodesiccation.

Silverman et al., using 30 years of data from New York University patients, performed what has since become the standard regarding the treatment of BCC with CE in 1991.[34] They identified sites of low, moderate, and high risk of recurrence following CE of a primary BCC. Low-risk locations were the neck, trunk, and extremities, with a 5-year recurrence rate of 8.6%. The scalp, forehead, and temples were designated moderate risk, at 12.9% recurrence rate. Lastly, the nose, eyelids, chin, jaw, and ear were termed high-risk locations to perform CE as there was a 17.5% risk of recurrence.[34] They were also the first to note that the size of the lesion treated by CE will affect a surgeon's recurrence rate. With the growing popularity of Mohs surgery, it is this author's opinion that the high-risk sites and many of the moderate-risk sites should not be treated with CE as first-line therapy as there is significantly increased risk of recurrence and the cosmetic outcome, which will be addressed later, is less acceptable than can be achieved with other methods.

Recurrences of NMSC pose a management dilemma and it is of utmost importance that the practicing surgeon realize the consequences of a recurrence. NMSC recurring after CE should not be retreated by CE. The following two factors significantly interfere with the effectiveness of CE for recurrent NMSC: scar tissue (prevents adequate curettage) and the potential for multifocal recurrences. NMSC recurrent after CE should be treated by Mohs micrographic surgery.[35]

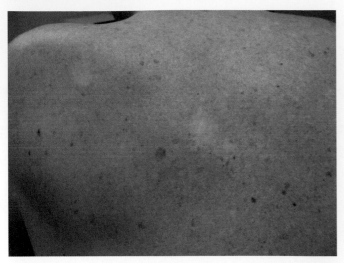

**Figure 41.8** Typical white flat smooth CE scars on the back after 1 year of maturation.

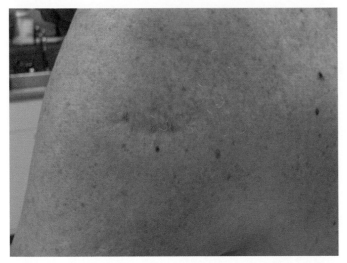

**Figure 41.9** Spread excision scar 1 year postoperatively on the left posterior shoulder

## INDICATIONS AND CONTRAINDICATIONS

### Indications

It is important to incorporate many factors in developing a formula to select the most appropriate therapy for NMSC. CE is an expedient and suitable form of treatment for selected NMSC and can be widely utilized within a set of defined guidelines.

All biopsies to diagnose NMSC should be superficial or mid-dermal shave biopsies, in order to avoid disturbing the underlying deep dermis. Caution should be taken in the setting of a superficial biopsy where the specimen has significant inflammation at the base or there is a mucinous stroma extending to the base of a BCC. The problem lies in the fact that the histopathology of NMSC is heterogeneous in a given lesion. Jones et al. found that 40% of his biopsied lesions were heterogeneous and that 13% of tumors classified as nodular had a component of infiltrative tumor.[31] Curettage biopsy specimens are inherently less reliable than saucerization biopsy specimens due to fragmentation and crush artifact. Punch biopsies, which penetrate through to the subcutis and simulate deep tumor extension, make subsequent CE difficult. If a punch biopsy has been performed prior to surgical treatment, it is reasonable to avoid CE.

In considering when to treat a given lesion by CE, it is crucial to make an assessment of lesion depth, the size, the character and thickness of the underlying dermis, and the lack or abundance of deeply seated hair follicles. Histology that supports the use of CE as primary treatment includes nodular and/or superficial basal cell carcinoma, hypertrophic actinic keratoses, and in-situ squamous carcinomas without deep follicular involvement in select locations. Infiltrative and micronodular BCC are not amenable to curettage, nor are deeply invasive SCC, and should be treated by excision or Mohs micrographic surgery.[10]

The highest cure rates are seen in those lesions less than 1 cm in diameter. Lesions greater than 2 cm in diameter should generally be treated with surgery. Relatively broad and superficial lesions which are located in areas with thick dermis (particularly the trunk and extremities) are well suited to CE. On the trunk and extremities, superficial lesions tend to just wipe off of the thick underlying dermis and are also in general quite well defined on clinical examination. At such sites, the procedure of CE is also much less invasive than a surgical excision, requires minimal wound care effort, and leads to a very high cure rate. However, in many older patients, CE on the extremities often results in a wound extending to the subcutis due to the atrophy of the skin from aging. Caution should also be taken if there is evidence of deep follicular extension on pretreatment punch biopsy. These NMSCs should be treated by excisional means.

### Contraindications

CE is relatively contraindicated in patients who readily form keloids and in patients with unshielded implanted electro-stimulative devices (cardiac, auditory, central nervous system [CNS]). Prior to undertaking CE in a patient with an implanted electro-stimulative device, the treating physician should discuss the procedure with the specialist monitoring that device. While most cardiac pacemakers are adequately shielded against electrical interference by CE, some defibrillators, cochlear implants, and CNS implants can be more vulnerable to interference. In all cases, adverse events can be minimized by using only short bursts (<5 seconds), using the lowest settings possible, grounding away from the device, and avoiding electrodesiccation near the device (preferably more than 10 inches away).[36]

When a procedure must be performed in patients that develop keloids, the judgement on whether an excisional scar or a CE scar would afford the better outcome is controversial. Making the smallest scar with the least amount of tension possible is the best option and should be accomplished by whatever means possible. One of the benefits of CE is that it provides a scar with little tension. However, because it is an open wound, the healing process is prolonged.

## FUTURE OUTLOOK

Newer treatments are heralding a paradigm shift in therapy for NMSC. In experienced hands, Mohs surgery affords the highest cure rates for NMSC with maximal tissue sparing and less scarring relative to older techniques of CE and en-bloc resection. CE is also yielding ground to photodynamic therapy and imiquimod therapy. However, CE remains a valuable, cost-effective tool for the treatment of properly selected NMSC cancers.

For years to come, CE will remain a workhorse when appropriately selected. However, the era may have already passed for the dominance of CE as the most utilized treatment for NMSC. Recurrences from the use of CE for deeper NMSCs are now commonly seen and future recurrences from inappropriate use of CE should be prevented. As dermatology continues to refine and improve upon its surgical skills, the treatment of NMSC will continue to evolve. It will be important to continue to utilize older techniques where valuable. However, it will be equally important to define and recognize the limitations of our older therapies and move forward by incorporating new available treatment modalities.

## REFERENCES

1. Clark WM. Oscillatory desiccation in the treatment of accessible malignant growths and minor surgical conditions. *J Adv Ther.* 1911;29:169–183.
2. Piffard HG. Histological contribution. *Am J Syph Derm.* 1870;1:217.
3. Wigglesworth E. The curette in dermal therapeutics. *Boston Med Surg J.* 1876;94:143.
4. Fox GH. *Photographic Atlas of the Diseases of the Skin in Four Volumes.* New York: Kettles Publishing Co; 1905:19.
5. Massarweh NN, Cosgriff N, Slakey DP. Electrosurgery: history, principles, and current and future uses. *J Am Coll Surg.* 2006;202(3):520–530.
6. Pollack SV. Electrosurgery. In: Bolognia JL, Jorizzo JL, Rapini RP, eds. *Dermatology.* Edinburgh: Mosby; 2003:2197–2203.
7. Soon SL, Washington CV. Electrosurgery, electrocoagulation, electrofulguration, electrodesiccation, electrosection, electrocautery. In: Robinson JK, Hanke CW, Sengelmann RD, et al., eds. *Surgery of the Skin, Procedural Dermatology.* Philadelphia: Mosby; 2005:177–190.
8. Sturm HM, Leider M. An editorial on curettage. *J Dermatol Surg Oncol.* 1979;5:532–533.
9. Adam JE. The technic of curettage surgery. *J Am Acad Dermatol.* 1986;15:697–702.
10. Sheridan AT, Dawber RPR. Curettage, electrosurgery and skin cancer. *Australas J Dermatol.* 2000;41:19–30.
11. Salasche SJ. Curettage and electrodesiccation in the treatment of midfacial basal cell epithelioma. *J Am Acad Dermatol.* 1983;8:496–503.
12. Knox JM, Lyles TW, Shapiro EM, et al. Curettage and electrodesiccation in the treatment of skin cancer. *Arch Dermatol.* 1960;82:197–203.
13. Whelan CS, Deckers PJ. Electrocoagulation and curettage for carcinoma involving the skin of the face, nose, eyelids and ears. *Cancer.* 1973;31:159–164.
14. Sweet RD. The treatment of basal cell carcinoma by curettage. *Br J Dermatol.* 1963;75:137–148.
15. Reymann F. Treatment of basal cell carcinoma of the skin with curettage. A follow-up study. *Arch Dermatol.* 1973;108:528–531.
16. Epstein E. Curettage-electrodesiccation vs surgical excision. *Arch Dermatol.* 1977;113:1729.
17. Knox JM, Freeman RG, Duncan WC, et al. Treatment of skin cancer. *South Med J.* 1967;60:241–246.
18. Williamson GS, Jackson R. The treatment of basal cell carcinoma by electrodesiccation and curettage. *Can Med J.* 1962;86:855.
19. Williamson GS, Jackson R. Treatment of squamous cell carcinoma of the skin by electrodesiccation and curettage. *Can Med J.* 1964;90:408–413.
20. Popkin GL. Curettage and electrodesiccation. *NY State J Med.* 1968;68:866–868.
21. Honeycutt WM, Jansen GT. Treatment of squamous cell carcinoma of the skin. *Arch Dermatol.* 1973;108:670–672.
22. Chernosky ME. Squamous cell and basal cell carcinomas: preliminary study of 3817 primary skin cancers. *South Med J.* 1978;71:802–803.
23. Reymann F. Treatment of basal cell carcinoma of the skin with curettage. *Arch Dermatol.* 1971;103:623–627.
24. Reymann F. Multiple basal cell carcinomas of the skin. Treatment with curettage. *Arch Dermatol.* 1975;111:877–879.
25. McDaniel WE. Surgical therapy for basal cell epitheliomas by curettage only. *Arch Dermatol.* 1978;114:1491–1492.
26. McDaniel WE. Therapy for basal cell epitheliomas by curettage only. Further study. *Arch Dermatol.* 1983;119:901–903.
27. Reymann F. 15 years' experience with treatment of basal cell carcinomas of the skin with curettage. *Acta Dermatol.* 1985;120:56–59.
28. Suhge d'Aubermont PC, Bennett PG. Failure of curettage and electrodesiccation for removal of basal cell carcinoma. *Arch Dermatol.* 1984;120:1456–1460.
29. Spencer JM, Tannenbaum A, Sloan L, et al. Does inflammation contribute to the eradication of basal cell carcinoma following curettage and electrodesiccation? *Dermatol Surg.* 1997;25:183–185.
30. Wagner RF, Cottel WI. Multifocal recurrent basal cell carcinoma following primary treatment by electrodesiccation and curettage. *J Am Acad Dermatol.* 1987;17:1047–1049.
31. Jones MS, Maloney ME, Billingsly EM. The heterogeneous nature of in vivo basal cell carcinoma. *Dermatol Surg.* 1998;24:881–884.
32. Crissey JT. Curettage and electrodesiccation as a method of treatment for epitheliomas of the skin. *J Surg Oncol.* 1971;3:287–290.
33. Dubin N, Kopf A. Multivariate risk scores for recurrences of cutaneous basal cell carcinomas. *J Am Acad Dermatol.* 1984;11:373–377.
34. Silverman MK, Kopf AW, Grin CM, et al. Recurrence rates of treated basal cell carcinoma. Part 2: Curettage-electrodesiccation. *J Dermatol Surg Oncol.* 1991;17:720–726.
35. Rowe DE, Carroll RJ, Day Jr CL. Mohs surgery is the treatment of choice for recurrent (previously treated) basal cell carcinoma. *J Dermatol Surg Oncol.* 1989;15(4):424–431.
36. Yu SS, Tope WD, Grekin RC. Cardiac devices and electromagnetic interference revisited: new radiofrequency technologies and implications for dermatologic surgery. *Dermatol Surg.* 2005;31:932–940.

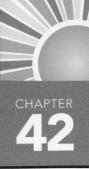

# Cryosurgery

*Paola Pasquali*

## Key Points

- Comparable cure rates to other procedures.
- Cryogen: liquid nitrogen.
- Fast freeze, slow thaw.
- Excellent cosmetic results.
- Combination treatments provide enhanced results.

## INTRODUCTION

Once a premalignant or malignant skin lesion is diagnosed, the physician decides among the multiple surgical and non-surgical treatment options having comparable cure rates for the appropriate course of action for the patient's needs.[1-5] Cryosurgery stands among the ablative methods that have stood the severe test of time, with advantages and disadvantages like any other therapeutic approach, with newer applications and scientific supportive data in dermatology as well as other specialties and with recent and exciting research in basic sciences that place cryosurgery in a new and strong position in comparison with other procedures.

This minimally invasive surgical technique has always excelled in its relatively simple application, versatility, and low cost. The speed of performing the procedure sharply contrasts with the long healing time. The high sensitivity of the melanocyte to cold, which is useful when treating lentigo maligna, can reduce the final cosmetic results whenever the depth of freezing extends to the melanocytes.

Cryosurgery is most beneficial when the surgeon is confronted with a patient with numerous lesions, with superficial tumors, patients with complex medical comorbidities, older and/or bedridden patients receiving anticoagulation treatments or having bloodborne infections.

## HISTORY

Most of the scientific support for cryosurgery began in the early 1960s, when experimental studies showed some of the mechanisms involved in cell and tissue death after freezing. Pioneering work by Douglas Torre and Setrag Zacarian opened the way for treating malignancies. Their innovations facilitated the technique and made cryogen delivery more effective. Torre's first reliable liquid nitrogen system was soon followed by a small handheld device engineered by Michael Bryne and Setrag Zacarian.

Today, cryosurgical equipment is available worldwide, the techniques have been improved, numerous long-term cure rates provide scientific support, and combination treatments based on immunological studies are opening a whole new field in the area of immunocryosurgery.

## BASIC PRINCIPLES

Cryoablation is the destruction of tissue by freezing. It has long been recognized as a powerful tool in the treatment of many tumors, including breast, prostate, kidney, bone, liver and skin. Heat flows from a warm object to a cold one. When subzero temperatures are applied to living tissue, heat extraction results, causing damage and eventual cell death.

The molecular basis of cryosurgical cell destruction[6] can be summarized as follows (Table 42.1):

1. *Direct injury.* With the initial freezing, water crystallizes outside the cells, causing a hyperosmotic environment and subsequent intracellular water movement out of the cell. Internal dehydration causes membrane and organelle damage. Further freezing makes water crystallize inside the cells and leads to eventual cell bursting. With thawing, ice crystals reorganize, forming larger crystals and inducing further cell destruction. Further thawing moves water from the outside to inside the cells.

   Additional mechanical damage occurs, such as cytoskeleton disorganization due to the weakening of membrane proteins bonds of the cell scaffold; metabolic failure because of the ionic changes and decreasing pH causing denaturalization/inactivation of proteins and enzymes; and lipid alterations by peroxidation, leading to membrane fluidity and permeability alterations.

   Most of the direct injury damage is mechanical and occurs during the freezing period. Cell death is by necrosis and mainly at the center of the lesion.[6]

2. *Vascular injury.* There is delayed, intense vasoconstriction which decreases blood flow. When the tissue thaws, the frozen area becomes congested due to vascular endothelial changes which increase permeability of capillary walls and cause platelet aggregation and microthrombi, leading finally to vascular stasis. With thawing, circulation returns with compensatory vasodilation, tissue hyperperfusion, free radical formation, and further peroxidation of the membrane lipids. Loss of blood supply through progressive microcirculatory failure occurs about 1 hour after freezing during the thawing period and causes cell death from ischemia.[7]

**Table 42.1 Molecular Basis of Cryosurgical Injury**

| | Mechanism | Time of Cycle | Location |
|---|---|---|---|
| Direct injury | Extra- and intracellular ice crystal formation + coagulation necrosis | Freezing phase | Center of the cryoinjury |
| Vascular injury | Microcirculatory failure + ischemic necrosis | Thawing phase | Periphery of the cryoinjury |
| Apoptosis | Cell death by apoptosis | Up to 8 hours after rewarming | Periphery of the cryoinjury |
| Immunological* | T-cell response mediated by dendritic cells | Late event | Whole body |

*Animal studies.

3. *Apoptosis* or gene-regulated cell death. Apoptotic cells are found at the periphery of the necrotic central area, where the temperature was not sufficient to kill cells by direct necrosis.[8,9] Apoptosis increases progressively 2–8 hours after freezing.[9,10]

4. The *immunologic effect* caused by cryoablation has long been observed. The first reports showed a reduction of metastatic disease after cryoablation of the primary tumor.[11,12] Murine models demonstrated that cryoablation of tumor tissue can result in inhibition of secondary and metastatic tumor growth,[13] which was attributed to a cytokine response induced by cryoablation.

Dendritic cells (DC) are crucial antigen-presenting cells (APC) that initiate primary T-cell response[14] if they receive stimulatory signals. If APCs do not receive stimulatory signals, they do not mature while taking up the antigen and tolerance is induced rather than immunity. Two indirect strategies to accomplish activation of the immune response are: (1) by expression of co-stimulatory molecules on tumors which can induce T-cell-mediated rejection of a variety of tumors and (2) by blocking inhibitory receptors.

Den Brok et al.[15,16] have shown in murine models that tumor debris remaining in the body after in-situ tumor cryoablation is an in-vivo tumor antigen source for the immune system. These necrotic tumor cells and debris enhance migration of DCs from the tumor site to the draining lymph nodes. The immunity induced is T-cell mediated with DCs playing a key role in the initiation of this immune response. Since patients with ablative treatments can develop systemic recurrences, simple ablation is not sufficient to induce proper immune response. Theoretically, additional immune activation stimuli by blocking inhibitor receptors like CTLA-4 or by depleting regulatory T cells given simultaneously with cryosurgery constitutes an in-situ DC vaccine.

With the concept of creating an 'in-situ' vaccine by synergistically combining cryoablation and immunomodulation, several clinical studies have been done combining topical immunomodulators with cryotherapy.[17] Imiquimod is an immunomodulatory drug that activates immune cells through the Toll-like receptor 7 (TLR-7). As a TLR-7 agonist, it stimulates immature plasmacytoid DCs (see Chapter 44). While B16/ovalbumin mice receiving either imiquimod or cryosurgery alone had only partial protection from tumor development,[18] mice that received both treatments were protected even from subsequent challenges. Clinical application of immunocryosurgery for lentigo maligna[19] and basal cell carcinomas (BCCs)[20] is an emerging field of treatment.

In a recent prospective study,[5] 18% of the patients treated with cryosurgery developed a new non-melanoma skin cancer (NMSC) in comparison with 36–50% of the patients who received other treatments. This result suggests an immunity induced by cryosurgery. Only carefully conducted randomized studies investigating recurrence rates of different treatment modalities will clarify this observation.

The amount of tissue to be frozen should include the tumor and a margin of safety comparable to the amount that would be excised in a surgical procedure. Freezing with liquid nitrogen (LN) using the appropriate delivery systems will achieve rapid cell-killing temperatures. The cooling rate should be fast in order to produce destructive intracellular ice and faster creation of a cryosurgical lesion.[1,21] This is called the fast-freeze. Slow thawing is a prime destructive factor due to recrystallization with larger and more damaging crystals, free radical formation, and peroxidation. This whole process is called the freeze–thaw cycle. One of the multiple effects of this cycle is the cellular breakdown which increases thermal conductivity. A second freeze–thaw cycle is then more damaging than the first one, increasing the extent of necrosis up to 80% of the previous volume.[22] This is the reason why cancers are treated with at least two freezing cycles.

## EQUIPMENT

Cryogen and delivery units are the two key instruments.

The ideal cryogen in dermatology for treating premalignant and malignant lesions of the skin is liquid nitrogen (LN). It combines safety in handling, low cost, and easy availability as it can be obtained from most welding supply companies. Most important is the low temperature (−195.8°C) of LN, which cools by a change of phase, i.e. by going from liquid to gas.

Destruction of malignant cells requires temperatures of −40°C to −60°C. Higher temperatures will damage but will not destroy the target cells. When the initial temperature of the cryogen is −195.8°C, as in LN, one can be assured that the temperature reached at the bottom and lateral margins of the tumor will be in the correct range. When treating premalignant or malignant lesions, cryogens and delivery systems that do not achieve this temperature range should be not be used, which includes cotton-tip applicators or metal dipped in LN. The delivery system for LN is commercially available handheld cryosurgical devices from Brymill Corporation (CRY-AC®, CRY-AC®-3 and Cry-Ac®Tracker®), Wallace or Premier, among others (Fig. 42.1).

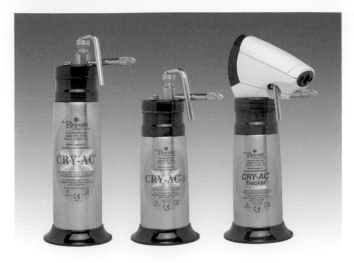

Figure 42.1 Handheld cryosurgical devices from Brymill Corporation Cryosurgical. (Image courtesy of Brymill Cryogenic Systems, Ellington, CT.)

LN is stored in containers available in 5, 10, 20, 30 and 50 liter capacity (Figs 42.2 and 42.3). The intermediate sizes (20–30 L) tend to be more practical because they hold enough LN to last 1 or 2 months (depending on the use), sparing the operator the need to do frequent refills (necessary in smaller dewars), and they are more manageable than large containers.

For treatment of lesions near the eye, non-conducting eyeshields should be used.

Thermocoupling devices are monitors that measure temperature through needles placed beneath the tumor.

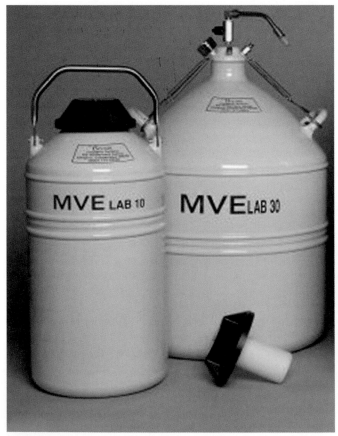

Figure 42.2 Dewar for liquid nitrogen.

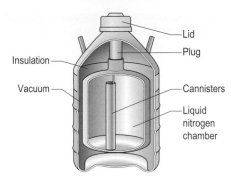

Figure 42.3 Inside a dewar.

Such placement could be selectively guided by echosonography. Thermocouples are not often used by those very experienced in the technique.

## TECHNIQUES

Since the goal is complete ablation of the target tissue, cryosurgeons have to keep in mind the following concepts:

- The freeze–thaw cycle, its repetition and the interval between cycles. Complete thawing is required from one cycle to another.
- The final freezing temperature on the target lesion. There is a difference in cold sensitivity between different cells. Connective tissue, cartilage and bone are very resistant; cancer cells are more resistant than normal cells. Preservation of the supportive framework (fibroblasts and collagen fibers), even though it is devitalized, is important, as large blood vessels and bone remain intact and are important for wound healing.
- Isotherms explain the spread of the ice ball (Fig. 42.4). The final ice ball should include the −50°C isotherm. The 5 mm treated margins correspond to a 4–5 mm frozen depth since freezing advances in a spherical manner. This total volume is comparable to the amount of tissue removed if surgical excision was chosen. Cell death at the center of the lesion is assured. Care should be taken with the margins.

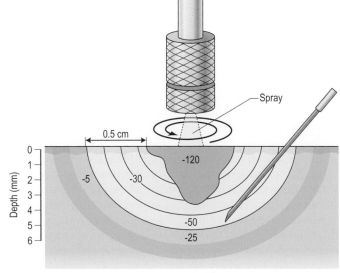

Figure 42.4 Development of isotherms in the cryosurgical site.

**Figure 42.5** Different freezing methods: **A)** spray; **B)** cone; **C)** chamber; **D)** probe.

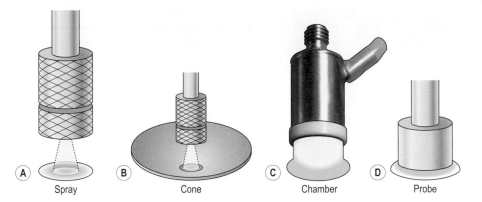

A) Spray   B) Cone   C) Chamber   D) Probe

Four different ways of delivering the cryogen are possible (Fig. 42.5):

- *Open spray* delivers LN through attachments at the open end of the unit. The spray nozzle should be positioned at 1–1.5 cm above the target and the stream is delivered perpendicular to the skin. These spraying tips or nozzles come with different apertures: A (larger), B, C, D and E (0.04, 0.031, 0.022, 0.016 and 0.013 inch/opening). Larger apertures deliver more LN in a shorter period of time and in a more 'expansive' manner. The bigger the nozzle, the larger amount of cryogen delivered and the more widespread will be the final frozen area. Smaller tips release less LN per unit of time; therefore, they take longer to deliver the same amount of LN and the application is more circumscribed. Smaller nozzles allow more delicate work and are ideal for treating small, well-defined lesions. The E tips come with a back vent that allows the most precise and streamlined spray. Larger nozzles freeze faster and are reserved for large malignancies. The B and C sizes are suitable for most treatments and are the most commonly used. Some systems clog while the spraying is done: this occurs when LN is not 'clean'. Under normal circumstances, they should not do so. Luer-lock adapters are available for attaching needles, therefore increasing the availability in spraying tip diameters. The spray or open technique is probably the more versatile way to freeze. It allows treatment of lesions of any size, and, when applied for sufficient time, the final freezing depth can be comparable to the one achieved with other cryosurgical techniques. It is the method of choice for the treatment of premalignant lesions, such as actinic keratosis, and malignant lesions, such as superficial BCCs and Bowen's disease. It is the first choice for cryosurgical treatment when a tumor has irregular surfaces, for large tumoral masses in palliative treatments, and for those lesions where previous curettage is not an option.

- *Confined-spray* or *cones* are a variant of the open-spray technique. The application of LN is circumscribed by a cone or an orifice on a plastic plate. This helps spare lateral tissue while concentrating the spray at the orifice, with greater penetration. Also, it reduces inadvertent spraying/splashing into orifices (ear, eyes, and nose). The insulated material of the cone avoids sticking to the surface, which would cause further unwanted freezing due to material conductance. A lexan cryoplate with conical openings of 3, 5, 8 and 10 mm is available to localize freezing while protecting the surrounding tissue. They need to be applied with some pressure to avoid lateral 'leaking', and are an excellent choice for small malignant tumors as a suitable orifice is fitted around the tumor. For a constant freezing time, confined spraying freezes more rapidly than open spray.

- *Chamber* or *closed-cone* are metal cylinders (available in 6, 10, 15, 18 and 31 mm diameter) with an open rubber-covered base which is firmly applied to the target tissue (Fig. 42.6). The other end has the attachment and a wide opening that allows large amounts of LN into the chamber at a constant flow. A releasing vent on a side reduces internal pressure. In a short period of time, chambers attain very deep freezing. They are powerful and destructive and their use should be reserved for thick malignancies.

- *Closed system or probes.* Available in different shapes, cryoprobes are metal (usually copper), sometimes covered with Teflon to reduce sticking, and are used for contact cryosurgery (Fig. 42.7). They have a conduit line that keeps LN circulating from the unit into the probe and out of it at a constant rate. This system keeps the probe at constant low temperatures throughout the procedure, thus delivering freezing directly into the tissue. They should be chosen to fit the size and shape of the lesion and are preferably applied over flat surfaces. For irregular surfaces, conductance will not be even because there is

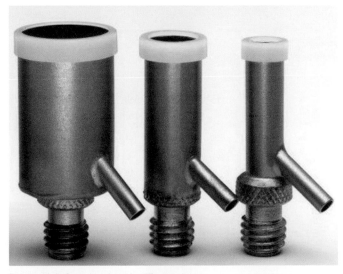

**Figure 42.6** Cryochambers in different sizes.

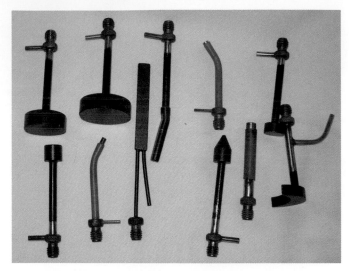

**Figure 42.7** Different types of probes.

air interposed between the probe and lesion (interphase) that makes less efficient cooling (Fig. 42.8). If the surface is irregular, then curettage to remove the uneven surface prior to freezing is helpful. Another tip is to use an aqueous gel between the probe and the lesion (Fig. 42.9). The water in the gel is a better conductant than air and optimizes freezing. If curettage were impossible, spray technique might be a better choice. Probes are ideal for malignancies and for vascular tumors. Since blood warms the lesion, probes have to be applied with pressure to make the vascular tumor bloodless.

Malleable adapters and extensions can be used in the probes, chambers and spraying tips to facilitate application in inaccessible areas. The advantages/disadvantages of each technique are summarized in Table 42.2.

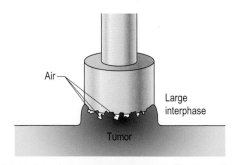

**Figure 42.8** Interphase between probe and tumor. The larger the interphase, the worse the heat transfer.

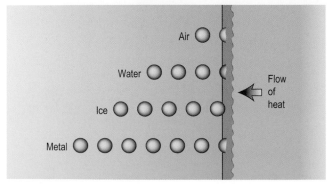

**Figure 42.9** Differences in conductivity.

## CONSIDERATIONS AND APPLICATIONS

### General considerations

Adequate treatment requires knowledge of the diagnosis, histopathology, and anatomical location in order to make comprehensive consideration of all the treatment options. Patients have to be carefully chosen to provide the best oncological and cosmetic results. Clinical diagnosis can be further confirmed by cytology, dermatoscopy or other means, but the final diagnosis will be by a skin biopsy. Dermatoscopy can be helpful in diagnosing the lesion and in following the patient for possible recurrences (Figs 42.10 and 42.11).

High-resolution ultrasonography (20 MHz) can help determine the tumor depth and lateral margins.[23] In a study by Vaillant et al.,[24] 112 BCCs were visualized by echosonography before and after cryosurgery, and the depth and lateral margins were determined. The mean echosonographic depth of the tumors was 2.42 mm. The image was typically an anechoic oval lesion and the majority of tumors had small echoic images inside them. Some cases of recurrence were diagnosed by echosonography before clinical and histological confirmation. In this series, recurrences were seen in tumors larger than 30 mm, and previously treated tumors. Echosonographically, recurrent tumors had a mean depth greater than 3 mm and lateral extension more evident by echo than by clinical examination.

Preoperative treatment is minimal. Patients should be informed of the postoperative effects, sign consent forms, and receive postoperative care instructions. For those patients with extensive actinic damage (*field cancerization*), previous treatments with antimitotic agents like 5-fluorouracil (5-FU)[25] (0.5–5%), immunomodulators (imiquimod), and keratolytics (salicylic acid, alpha-hydroxy acids, and urea) reduce surface keratin, thus improving freezing. Preoperative treatment may eliminate many lesions, reduce the size of the larger ones, and have a synergistic effect with cryosurgery (as in 5-FU and imiquimod). Adjunctive therapies have synergistic effects with cryosurgery. The comprehensive oncologic approach should target the primary lesion (premalignant or malignant) and its surroundings (Figs 42.12 and 42.13).

An oral analgesic medication before a deep freezing procedure can diminish postoperative pain.

Since freezing or certain hemostatic substances (aluminum chloride) might blur the margins, it is wise to delineate the area to be treated prior to freezing.

### Clinical considerations

- *Age.* Although there are no age limits, older patients often receive cryosurgery rather than other treatment methods because of reduced pre-surgical requirements.
- *Previous medical conditions.* It is an ideal option for patients with bleeding disorders, under anticoagulant medications; bloodborne infections; infected lesions; and patients who are bedridden or have limited mobility.
- *Anesthesia.* Most procedures can be done with local anesthesia. For actinic keratosis treatment and other cryosurgery procedures with one cycle,

## Table 42.2 Advantages/Disadvantages of Different Cryosurgery Techniques

| | Advantages | Disadvantages |
|---|---|---|
| Spray or open technique | Can be used in benign, premalignant and malignant lesions | |
| | Size: can be used in any size | If lesion is too small, there could be lateral overfreezing |
| | Excellent choice in bulky/irregular surface lesions | Care should be taken to assure depth of penetration |
| | First choice when previous curettage for debulking is not an option | Care should be taken to assure depth of penetration |
| | First choice for premalignant lesions and lesions where depth of freezing is not a concern | Care should be taken for possible 'false' freezing fronts |
| Confined spray or cones/plates | Can be used in benign, premalignant and malignant lesions | Care should be taken to firmly apply it to the skin to avoid lateral 'spilling' of LN |
| | Confines the spray to a certain diameter given by the cone/plate orifice | Cannot be used if lesion is larger than the available cone |
| | Excellent option for spraying elevated/irregular surface lesions | |
| | By concentrating the spray in one lesion, it can freeze more deeply | Care should be taken when freezing superficial lesions |
| Probe or close technique | For malignant lesions where depth of freezing and final temperature are a concern | Requires appropriate size and shape of probes/Need to have a complete set of probes |
| | Ideal for well-defined tumors | Should be avoided when surface is too irregular due to inappropriate contact with the lesion |
| | Ideal in areas where operator can 'feel' with the fingertip the advancing freezing front (as in earlobes) | Care with attached probes to avoid accidental breaking of the frozen tissue |
| | Ideal for lesions in oral cavity, in nostrils, in earlobes | |
| | Ideal for malignant lesions over bony prominences | |
| Chamber technique | For well-defined malignancies where depth of freezing and final temperature are a concern | Should not be used in premalignant lesions due to deep extent of freezing and necrosis |
| | Ideal for lesions over bony prominences | Requires perfect match between the lesion and the chamber |
| | Can be used in bulky, irregular lesions, as long as they fit into the chamber | |
| | Due to the highly destructive capacity, ideal for metastatic skin lesion | Requires highly experienced operator |

anesthesia is optional. Cryosurgery is an excellent option in patients allergic to anesthetics and those with needle phobias. No general anesthesia is required.

■ An *operative suite* is not required. The procedure can be done in most settings.

■ Patients with *multiple lesions* are excellent candidates, as it is faster and less traumatic than other forms of surgery. Since cryosurgery does not involve 'cutting', it may be offered to patients who fear surgery.

■ *Location.* For a one cycle freezing, healing time increases as one moves away from the face (e.g. face, 7–10 days; trunk, 2–3 weeks; legs, up to 2 months).

For deeper freezing procedures of malignancies, lower extremities should be avoided because the postoperative period can be extremely long. Tumors over cartilage and bone, eyelids, periocular and auricular are particularly suitable for cryosurgery (Figs 42.14 and 42.15).

## Clinical applications

For *actinic keratosis (AK)*, 5–10 seconds of freezing with a 1 mm margin is sufficient (Figs 42.16 and 42.17). Thicker/hyperkeratotic lesions will require further freezing since keratin is a poor cold conductant. One cycle is sufficient. For numerous lesions and/or field cancerization, previous

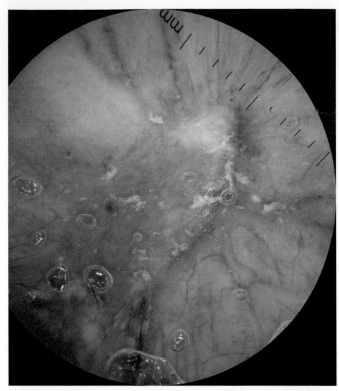

**Figure 42.10** Dermatoscopic evaluation before treatment of a BCC.

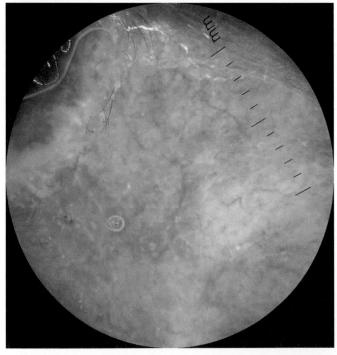

**Figure 42.11** Dermatoscopic control 2 years post cryosurgery.

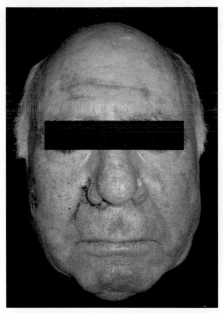

**Figure 42.12** Field cancerization before 5-FU treatment and cryosurgery of BCC.

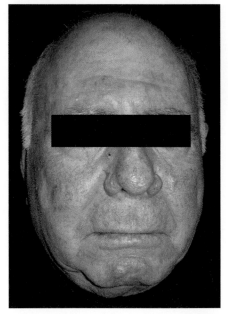

**Figure 42.13** Six months after 5-FU plus cryosurgery treatment.

treatment with 5% 5-FU or imiquimod will clear the area, clearing numerous lesions, exposing new ones and leaving only the large and thicker ones for cryosurgery. Spraying is the indicated technique.

*Basal cell carcinomas (BCCs)*[26] require 60–120 seconds of freezing (Figs 42.18–42.20). For superficial BCC, one cycle may be sufficient. A double freeze cycle is needed for the rest. Debulking reduces tumor thickness and allows freezing to

reach lower areas of the initial tumor. Combination treatment of curettage/coagulation followed by cryosurgery allows acquisition of a specimen for pathologic examination, better elucidation of the margins of the tumor, and leaves a bloodless area for treatment, with excellent results.[5,27] Cryosurgery is preferred for lesions less than 2 cm in diameter but larger lesions can also be treated. Morpheaform, ill-defined and recurrent BCC should be treated with Mohs surgery.

*Well-differentiated small-diameter squamous cell carcinoma (SCC), SCC in situ* (Bowen's disease) and keratoacanthomas respond well to cryosurgical treatment. With the diagnosis confirmed by pathology and in the absence of lymphadenopathy, treatment can be performed. For SCC, triple cycles

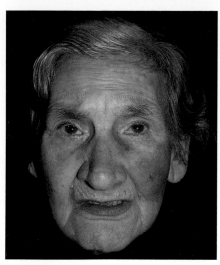

**Figure 42.23** Postoperative and post-imiquimod results at 6 months.

Carefully written instructions with expected symptoms should be given to the patient to set expectations.

Superficial freezing will require washing the area with water and soap and applying an antibiotic ointment.

- *Pain*. Some patients may require analgesic medication in the 24 hours after the procedure. During freezing, cold sensation is felt, and during immediate thawing, erythema and urtication are observed. With superficial treatment, a burning feeling can last for 5–10 minutes. Deeper freezing can be followed by a more intense burning/painful sensation that can last up to 30 minutes. After the lesion has stopped oozing, the presence of pain might be an indication of infection. Oral anesthesia is usually sufficient.
- *Edema* will be related to freezing depth/time, modality of treatment (larger for chamber followed by probe and spray), skin type (lighter skins tend to have more edema), age (in older patients tends to be more obvious due to tissue looseness) and lesion location (more for periorbital, forehead, mandibular and ear). This edema does not respond to steroids. It is non-painful even in severe cases. The edema lasts for 5–7 days and is more obvious in the morning due to the effect of gravity.
- Postoperatively, there will be *vesicle/bulla formation* which will be dependent on modality, time of freeze, and skin type. The bulla content is usually clear fluid but can be hemorrhagic if a biopsy was done in conjunction with the cryosurgical treatment, if the tumor was ulcerated, or if curettage was performed. Hemostasis prior to performing cryosurgery reduces the chance of a hemorrhagic vesicle or bulla, and bleeding if the bulla breaks. Deeper freezing will produce more edema and larger bullae. When too large, bullae can be evacuated, reducing distress and improving recovery. The exudate can be substantial, and requires frequent replacement of gauze dressings. The amount of exudate will decrease in the next few days, and a crust forms. Very rarely, the removal of a bulla or a crust can lead to hemorrhage due to the presence of an underlying persistent vascular supply. Hemostasis can be achieved by manual pressure. Sometimes a pressure dressing is required and in extreme cases electrocoagulation or ligation of the vessels is needed.
- Eschar formation is related to reduced oozing. It can be accompanied by infection. Removal of the crust is recommended.

For large procedures, weekly evaluations are recommended.

## COMPLICATIONS (Table 42.5)

Among the complications are pyogenic granuloma formation at the cryosurgical site and, very rarely, flu-like symptoms.

| Table 42.3 Premalignant and Malignant Lesions where Cryosurgery can be Used | | | | |
|---|---|---|---|---|
| **Lesion** | **Technique** | **Margins (mm)** | **Cycles** | **Freeze time (s)** |
| Actinic keratosis /0 | S | 1 | 1 | 5–10; up to 20 |
| Superficial basal cell carcinomas | S, CS | 4–5 | 1–2 | 60–120 |
| Nodular basal cell carcinomas | S, CS, P, Ch | 4–5 | 2* | 60–120 |
| Squamous cell carcinomas | S, CS, P, Ch | > 5 | 2–3 | 60–120 |
| Keratoacanthomas | S, CS, P (if flatten); Ch | 4–5 | 2 | 60–120 |
| Bowen's disease | S | 4–5 | 2 | 60–120 |
| Vascular tumors: Kaposi sarcomas | P | 4–5 | 1–2 | 60–120 |
| Lentigo maligna | S (Usually too large for CS, P) | 4–5 | 1–2 | 60–120 |
| Metastatic tumors of the skin/ Palliative treatments | S, Ch (Usually too large for CS, P) Fractional and/or segmental cryosurgery for large lesions | >5 | 2+ | >60 |

S, spray; CS, confined spray; Ch, chamber; P, probe.

* The time between both cycles should be at least 1 minute; halo thaw time of at least 30 seconds. Complete thaw can take from 1 to 5 minutes.

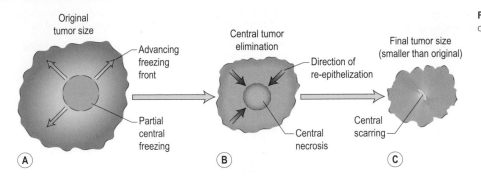

**Figure 42.24** Almeida Gonçalves' fractional cryosurgery.

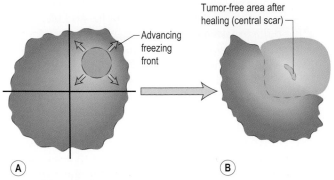

**Figure 42.25** Zacarian's segmental cryosurgery.

### Table 42.4 Indications and Contraindications of Cryosurgery

| Indications | Contraindications* |
|---|---|
| All ages; particularly suitable for older/bedridden and mobility-impaired | Patient unable to accept possible pigmentary changes (A) |
| Medical conditions such as bloodborne infections/anticoagulant medication/needle phobia/anesthesia intolerance | Cold intolerance and other cold-triggered conditions (R) |
| Well-defined tumors | Ill-defined tumors (A) |
| Tumors with diameter less than 2 cm; for larger tumors, consider fractional or segmental cryosurgery | Morpheaform or sclerodermiform BCC (A) Recurrent tumors (A) |
| Tumors over cartilage/bone | When diagnosis is not clear (A) |
| Any body area Avoid in legs due to slow wound healing | Lower legs with vascular compromise have impaired healing |
| Multiple lesions | |
| For palliative treatments | |

(A), absolute; (R), relative.

### Short-term reactions

*Nitrogen gas insufflation* is a rare occurrence but possible whenever a biopsy is followed by cryosurgery with spray technique. When previous curettage has been performed, probe technique is recommended.

*Syncope* may occur immediately after procedures, especially in nervous/fearful patients and whenever pain is involved. Patients should be placed in a supine or Trendelenburg position for recovery.

*Local infection* is not frequent but is possible whenever proper cleaning of the treated area has not been followed in the eschar period. For older patients, it is best to have close follow-up and to have a nurse or a trained family member do the local wound care.

### Long-term reactions

Most long-term expected side effects are related to depth/time of freezing. For superficial procedures, there are no side effects. Since melanocytes are extremely sensitive to cold, with cell death at −4°C to −7°C, treatment of skin cancers requiring temperatures in the range of −40°C to −60°C will result in *hypopigmentation*. It is important to differentiate between the hypopigmentation due to melanocyte destruction versus healing within severely damaged and dyschromic skin, where the newly formed skin tends to look lighter in comparison with the surrounding untreated skin.

### Table 42.5 Side Effects and Complications of Cryosurgery

| Short-term side effects |
|---|
| ***Expected*** |
| • Edema and swelling<br>• Vesicle or bulla formation<br>• Exudation<br>• Tissue sloughing<br>• Eschar formation |
| ***Occasional not expected*** |
| • LN insufflation (incorrect technique)<br>• Inadvertent burn (caused by released LN gas from vent)<br>• Syncope (in nervous patients) |
| ***Long-term side effects*** |
| • Infection (after 2–3 weeks; if proper cleaning of treated area has not been done)<br>• Hypopigmentation (in deep cryosurgery)** Can be permanent.<br>• Hyperpigmentation<br>• Pseudoepitheliomatous hyperplasia<br>• Milia<br>• Occasional scar retraction/Notching of ear or nasal ali*<br>• Alopecia* (occasional)<br>• Atrophic/depressed scar* |

* Can be permanent.

*Hyperpigmentation* can also occur, especially in darker skins and at the periphery of the lesions. This can resolve spontaneously.

*Pseudoepitheliomatous hyperplasia* is a common finding that is sometimes confused with tumor persistence or recurrence. It tends to be a linear, reddish, elevated scar in the center of the healing area. No treatment is required and local injection with corticosteroids is not recommended as tissue depression may result. It resolves spontaneously over a few months. Persistence over time (over 6–9 months) indicates the presence of a hypertrophic scar which can be left to naturally involute or injected with local steroids if it is cosmetically unacceptable to the patient.

*Alopecia* has been described.

## FUTURE OUTLOOK

Cryosurgery is a potent ablative tool that will further benefit from the newest technology. Thermocouple needles have been gradually replaced by the operators' experience; the use of non-invasive methods for in-vivo imaging, like high-resolution echosonography, confocal microscopy and optical coherence tomography,[29] will give more precise tumor margins and will be helpful in evaluating the extent of the area to be treated. Immunocryotherapy is a promising field for the treatment of tumors with an approach that will result in tumor destruction as well as inducing antitumor immunity that could protect against tumor recurrence or metastasis.

## REFERENCES

1. Zacarian SA. Cryosurgery of cutaneous carcinomas. An 18-year study of 3,022 patients with 4,228 carcinomas. *J Am Acad Dermatol.* 1983;9:947–956.
2. Graham GF, Clark LC. Statistical analysis in cryosurgery of skin cancer. In: Breitbart E, Dachow-Siwiec E, eds. *Clinics in Dermatology. Advances in Cryosurgery.* New York: Elsevier Science; 1990:101–107.
3. Nordin P. Curettage-cryosurgery for non-melanoma skin cancer of the external ear: excellent 5-year results. *Br J Dermatol.* 1999;140:291–293.
4. Kuflik EG. Cryosurgery for skin cancer: 30 year experience and cure rates. *Dermatol Surg.* 2004;30:297–300.
5. Lindemalm-Lundstam B, Dalenbäck J. Prospective follow-up after curettage-cryosurgery for scalp and face skin cancers. *Br J Dermatol.* 2009;161(3):568–576.
6. Baust JG, Gage AA. The molecular basis of cryosurgery. *BJU Int.* 2005;95(9):1187–1191.
7. Gage AA, Baust JG. Mechanisms of tissue injury in cryosurgery. *Cryobiology.* 1998;37:171–186.
8. Hollister WR, Mathew AJ, Baust JG, et al. Effects of freezing on cell viability and mechanisms of cell death in a human prostate cancer cell line. *Mol Urol.* 1998;2:13–18.
9. Gage AA, Baust JM, Baust JG. Experimental cryosurgery investigations in vivo. *Cryobiology.* 2009;59:229–243.
10. Forest V, Peoc'h M, Campos L, et al. Effects of cryotherapy or chemotherapy on apoptosis in a non-small-cell lung cancer xenografted into SCID mice. *Cryobiology.* 2005;50:29–37.
11. Gage AA. Cryosurgery for oral and pharyngeal carcinoma. *Am J Surg.* 1969;118:669–672.
12. Soanes WA, Ablin RJ, Gonder MJ. Remission of metastatic lesions following cryosurgery in prostatic cancer: immunologic considerations. *J Urol.* 1970;104:154–159.
13. Joosten JJA, van Muijen JNP, Wobbes T, et al. In vivo destruction of tumor tissue by cryoablation can induce inhibition of secondary tumor growth: an experimental study. *Cryobiology.* 2001;42(1):49–58.
14. Adams S, O'Neil DW, Bhardwaj N. Recent advances in dendritic cell biology. *J Clin Immunol.* 2005;25(3):177–188.
15. den Brok MH, Sutmuller RP, Nierkens S, et al. Efficient loading of dendritic cells following cryo and radiofrequency ablation in combination with immune modulation induces anti-tumour immunity. *Br J Cancer.* 2006;95(7):896–905.
16. den Brok MH, Sutmuller RP, Nierkens S, et al. Synergy between in situ cryoablation and TLR9 stimulation results in a highly effective in vivo dendritic cell vaccine. *Cancer Res.* 2006;66(14):7285–7292.
17. Goel R, Anderson K, Slaton J, et al. Adjuvant approaches to enhance cryosurgery. *J Biomech Eng.* 2009;131(7):074003.
18. Redondo P, del Olmo J, López-Díaz A, et al. Imiquimod enhances the systemic immunity attained by local cryosurgery destruction of melanoma lesions. *J Invest Dermatol.* 2007;127(7):1673–1680.
19. Bassukas ID, Gamvroulia C, Zioga A, et al. Cryosurgery during topical imiquimod: a successful combination modality for lentigo maligna. *Int J Dermatol.* 2008;47(5):519–521.
20. Gaitanis G, Nomikos K, Vava E, et al. Immunocryosurgery for basal cell carcinoma: results of a pilot, prospective, open-label study of cryosurgery during continued imiquimod application.. *J Eur Acad Dermatol Venereol.* 2009;23(12):1427–1431.
21. Bischof JC, Cristof K, Rubinsky B. A morphological study of the cooling rate response of normal and neoplastic human liver tissue: Cryosurgical implications. *Cryobiology.* 1993;30:482–492.
22. Gage AA, Baust JG. Cryosurgery for tumors. *J Am Coll Surg.* 2007;205(2):342–356.
23. Pesić Z, Mijailović D, Milosavljević M. Ultrasonography and surgical treatment of facial skin neoplasms. *Srp Arh Celok Lek.* 2002;130(5–6):165–167.
24. Vaillant L, Grognard C, Machet L, et al. Imaginerie ultrasonore haute résolution : utilité pour le traitement des carcinomas basocellulaires para cryochirurgie. *Ann Dermatol Venereol.* 1998;125:500–504.
25. Jorizzo J, Weiss J, Furst K, et al. Effect of a 1-week treatment with 0.5% topical fluorouracil on occurrence of actinic keratosis after cryosurgery. A randomized, vehicle-controlled trial. *Arch Dermatol.* 2004;140:813–816.
26. Telfel NR, Colver GB, Morton CA. Guidelines for the management of basal cell carcinoma. *Br J Dermatol.* 2008;159:35–48.
27. Nordin P, Stenquist B. Five-year results of curettage-cryosurgery for 100 consecutive auricular nonmelanoma skin cancers. *J Laryngol Otol.* 2002;116:893–898.
28. Gonçalves JC. Fractional cryosurgery for skin cancer. *Dermatol Surg.* 2009;35(11):1788–1796.
29. Mogensen M, Thrane L, Jørgensen TM, et al. OCT imaging of skin cancer and other dermatological diseases. *J Biophotonics.* 2009;2(6–7):442–451.

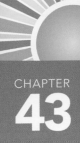
# Topical Treatment of Skin Cancer

*Victoria Williams, Theodore Rosen, Roger I. Ceilley, James Q. del Rosso, and Eggert Stockfleth*

### Key Points

- DNA analogs are effective in treating actinic keratoses.

- Immune response modifiers are effective in treating actinic keratoses, squamous cell carcinoma and basal cell carcinoma through immunomodulation.

- Inhibition of cyclo-oxygenase enzymes is effective in ablating actinic keratoses.

- Other compounds are being evaluated for their therapeutic effects as topical chemotherapeutic agents against skin cancer.

- Topical chemotherapy combined with physical modalities may be the most effective approach by combining the benefits of field and lesional therapy.

## INTRODUCTION

Cancer chemotherapy ideally produces selective destruction of the malignant or abnormal cells with minimal or no toxicity to normal cells. The application of topical chemotherapy for the treatment of actinic keratoses (AKs) and non-melanoma skin cancers (NMSCs) attempts to achieve this without the associated risks of systemic chemotherapy and is gaining increased recognition. Over the past decade, there have been many exciting new topical therapeutic modalities as well as modifications of existing treatments which represent significant advances.

AKs represent the initial manifestation of abnormal keratinocyte proliferation with the potential of progression to invasive squamous cell carcinoma (SCC). When present in limited numbers, traditional lesion-targeted AK therapies such as cryotherapy and curettage may be appropriate. However, contemporary research supports the idea of 'field cancerization', indicating that each visible lesion may be surrounded by a zone of photodamage where subclinical AKs can be present 10-fold more frequently than visible AKs.[1] Thus, topical treatment offers the opportunity to treat visible AKs while simultaneously preventing the progression of subclinical lesions. Additionally, topical chemotherapeutic agents offer the potential advantage of selectively eliminating various types of abnormal epithelial and even dermal cells with minimal toxicity to normal skin cells.

Factors to consider in choosing a topical chemotherapy agent for treating skin cancer include expected intensity of local reaction, absorption, potential for systemic side effects, efficacy, application frequency and treatment duration, potential for allergic contact dermatitis, and confounding patient factors. The confounding factors, such as the presence of an implanted pacemaker or the existence of severe thrombocytopenia, often make topical therapy an attractive option compared to surgical intervention. Nonetheless, the practitioner must readily acknowledge the single most common criticism of topical therapy, namely that it is a 'blind' procedure, unaccompanied by the inherent ability to verify diagnosis and/or check for tumor-free margins in a tissue specimen. Thus, the patient benefit must outweigh any risk when choosing to employ topical therapy as the definitive treatment of cutaneous neoplasia.

In evaluating the efficacy of topical agents, it must be understood that optimum endpoints are uncertain and that clinical studies are rarely comparable. What should be the gold standard in this regard? Should it be percentage reduction in lesions (when multiple are present, such as in AK) or absolute clearance of the treated field? If absolute clearance is selected, should this reflect clearance of initially detectable lesions only or clearance of both initial and subsequently revealed lesions? Should clinical clearance be verified by one or more test-of-cure biopsies? At what point in time should efficacy be assessed? Are long-term studies (1 year to 5 years) the most appropriate? Until the answers to these and other questions are definitively determined, the practitioner must interpret the published data in light of experience and evolving standards of care. The advantages and disadvantages of using various topical therapeutic modalities compared to surgical interventions are summarized for treating skin cancer in Table 43.1, and the current indications for specific topical chemotherapy are listed in Table 43.2.

## DNA ANALOG ANTIMETABOLITES

### 5-fluorouracil

Topical 5-fluorouracil (5-FU) is a well-established topical agent commonly used to treat patients with a large number of AKs. As an antimetabolite of uracil, 5-FU blocks the conversion of uridine monophosphate to thymidine monophosphate, impairing the synthesis of DNA and RNA, most prominently in abnormal keratinocytes. In the 1960s, cancer patients undergoing systemic treatment with 5-FU were discovered to experience an inflammatory reaction at sites of AKs followed by subsequent resolution of lesions. This observation led to the initiation of topical 5-FU for AK management. 5-FU remains a first-line treatment of AKs and has been also approved for the treatment of superficial basal cell carcinoma (sBCC).[2] The agent is neither approved nor

**Table 43.1 Summary of Advantages and Disadvantages of Topical Versus Surgical Treatments for AKs**

| | Advantages | Disadvantages |
|---|---|---|
| **Topical** | | |
| 5-fluorouracil | • Effective<br>• Can treat clinically apparent and inapparent lesions<br>• Can treat multiple lesions<br>• Minimal scarring risk | • Potential skin irritation<br>• Requires high patient compliance<br>• Risk for potentially severe inflammatory reaction<br>• Skin may require 1 to 2 months to heal |
| Imiquimod | • Effective<br>• Can be used on multiple lesions<br>• Minimal scarring risk<br>• Induces an individual's own immune system<br>• Can treat clinically apparent and inapparent lesions | • Potential skin irritation<br>• Dispensed in small packets<br>• Requires high patient compliance<br>• May rarely cause systemic symptoms |
| Diclofenac | • Can treat multiple lesions<br>• Efficacious after long treatment course<br>• Can treat clinically apparent and inapparent lesions<br>• Minimally irritating<br>• No scarring | • Requires lengthy treatment time<br>• Requires high patient compliance |
| Photodynamic therapy | • Effective<br>• Can be used on multiple lesions<br>• Patient compliance not required | • Requires two steps<br>• Stinging and burning can occur during treatment<br>• Cost and inconvenience of extra office visits<br>• Cost of light equipment<br>• Problems with reimbursement |
| Retinoids | • Can treat multiple lesions<br>• Can treat clinically apparent and inapparent lesions<br>• Can be used to augment other therapy | • Requires lengthy treatment time<br>• May cause mild to moderate inflammation<br>• Efficacy not well supported<br>• Works better as an adjunct, with minimal efficacy as a monotherapy |
| Colchicine | • Treats multiple lesions at once<br>• Short treatment course<br>• No systemic side effects<br>• Localized effect | • May cause severe inflammation<br>• Off-label usage with limited evidence of efficacy |
| **Surgical** | | |
| Cryotherapy | • Very effective<br>• Quick<br>• Few side effects<br>• Well tolerated<br>• High patient compliance | • Pain during procedure<br>• Possible residual hyper- or hypopigmentation<br>• Scarring<br>• Difficult to treat multiple lesions |
| Excision | • High success rate<br>• Can achieve a definitive diagnosis with pathology<br>• Enables removal of an entire lesion | • Scarring<br>• Limited to patients with solitary lesions<br>• Some can have delayed healing |

recommended for the treatment of nodular or other morphologic forms of invasive basal cell carcinoma.

Topical 5-FU preferentially interacts with rapidly proliferating keratinocytes, creating an intense inflammatory reaction leading to cell death with relative sparing of surrounding normal skin. Visible actinic lesions are targeted, as well as subclinical AKs in surrounding areas of photodamaged skin.[1] As a result, topical 5-FU therapy reduces the rate of local recurrence and subsequent development of primary malignancy compared with lesion-directed therapies that treat only clinically visible lesions.[1]

The standard treatment regimen for AKs is twice-daily application of 1–5% 5-FU cream or solution to the involved areas for 2–4 weeks or until a significant inflammatory reaction is achieved, at which point treatment is discontinued (Fig. 43.1). No difference in efficacy has been found between the 1%, 2% and 5% preparations.[3] More recently, a 0.5% microsphere cream formulation was approved by the United States Food and Drug Administration (FDA) for once-daily

treatment of AKs of the face and anterior scalp. Studies have shown an overall 89% reduction of AKs and a complete clearance rate of 48% in patients receiving once-daily application of the 0.5% microsphere cream for 4 weeks (Fig. 43.2).[4]

A single-blind, randomized, split-face study compared the efficacy of 5-FU 0.5% microsphere cream and 5-FU 5% cream, each being applied once daily for 4 weeks. Both agents achieved a complete lesion clearance rate of 43% at 4 weeks post-therapy.[5] Although both formulations can induce varying levels of inflammation, most patients preferred the 0.5% cream due to the convenience of once-daily dosing (compared to the recommended twice-daily application of the 5% cream), and a perception of less irritation. A recent comparative study suggested the 0.5% cream is equally efficacious to the 5% but may be more cost-effective, safer and better tolerated.[6]

Askew et al. conducted a systematic review of randomized controlled trials to determine the effectiveness of 5-FU treatment for AKs.[7] An average of 49% of patients

**Table 43.2 Summary of Indications for Topical Chemotherapy for Skin Cancers**

| Skin Lesion | 5% 5-FU | 0.5–2% 5-FU | Imiq 5% | Resiq | Diclofenac | PDT | Retinoids | Bexarotene | Colchicine | NM | T4 |
|---|---|---|---|---|---|---|---|---|---|---|---|
| AKs | ✚ | ✚ | ✚ | 🗑 | ✚ | ✚ | 🗑 | | 🗑 | | 🗑 |
| SBCC | ✚ | | ✚ | | | ☀ | 🗑 | | | | 🗑 |
| NBCC | | | 🗑 | | | 🗑 | 🗑 | | | | |
| IBCC | | | 🗑 | | | | | | | | |
| SCCIS | 🗑 | | ☀ | | | ☀ | 🗑 | | | | |
| BP | 🗑 | | ☀ | | | | | | | | |
| CIN/ VIN | | | 🗑 | | | | 🗑 | | | | |
| ISCC | | | 🗑 | | | | | | | | |
| CTCL | | | 🗑 | | | 🗑 | 🗑 | ✚ | | ✚ | |
| KS | | | 🗑 | | | | ✚ | | | | |
| LMM | | | 🗑 | | | | | | | | |
| EMPD | | | 🗑 | | | | | | | | |
| OL | | | | | | | 🗑 | | | | |
| VN | | | 🗑 | | | | | | | | |

✚ FDA-approved treatment indication.

☀ Off-label usage well supported by clinical studies.

🗑 Off-label usage supported by limited evidence.

5-FU, 5-fluorouracil; Imiq, imiquimod; Resiq, resiquimod; PDT, photodynamic therapy (ALA or MAL); NM, nitrogen mustard; T4, T4 endonuclease; AKs, actinic keratoses; SBCC, superficial basal cell carcinoma; NBCC, nodular basal cell carcinoma; IBCC, invasive basal cell carcinoma; SCCIS, squamous cell carcinoma in situ; BP, Bowen's disease of the penis; CIN, cervical intraepithelial neoplasm; VIN, vulvar intraepithelial neoplasm; ISCC, invasive squamous cell carcinoma; CTCL, cutaneous T-cell lymphoma; KS, Kaposi sarcoma; LMM, lentigo maligna melanoma; EMPD, extramammary Paget's disease; OL, oral leukoplakia; VN, vascular neoplasms including hemangiomas, pyoderma gangrenosum.

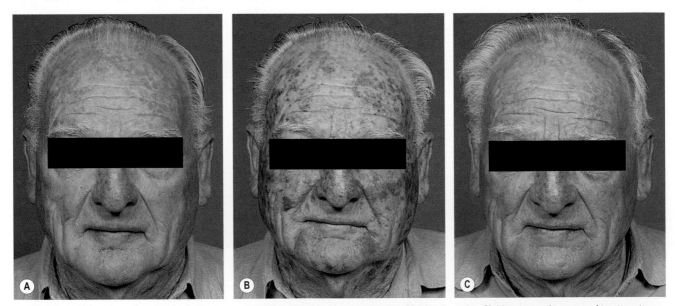

**Figure 43.1** Male with multiple actinic keratoses treated with 5% 5-FU b.i.d. **A)** Pre-treatment. **B)** After 2 weeks. **C)** After 1-month course of treatment.

treated with 5% 5-FU and 35% treated with 0.5% 5-FU achieved complete clearance. Both formulations led to an approximately 80% reduction in lesion counts. However, over 60% of patients required re-treatment after 1 year for recurrences. 5-FU is quite effective for AKs on the head and neck region but treatment is less effective for extremity AKs and hyperkeratotic AKs.

Superficial BCC has been successfully treated with 5-FU. However, current published data only support the use of the higher-strength (5%) formulation. Application should

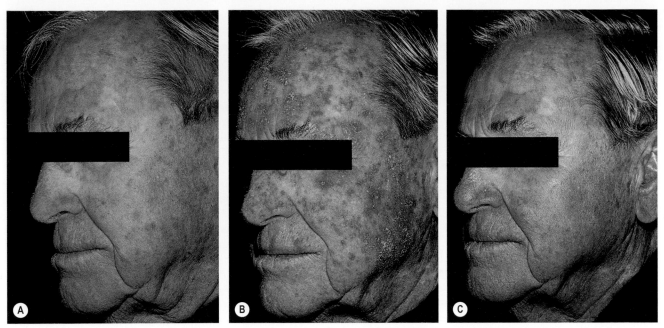

**Figure 43.2** Male with multiple actinic keratoses treated with 0.5% 5-FU q.d. **A)** Pre-treatment. **B)** After 2 weeks. **C)** Post-treatment.

be twice daily to cover the lesion plus a several-millimeter margin. The approved length of treatment is 3–6 weeks, but based on more recent studies, up to 11 weeks may be needed to completely clear lesions.[8] Gross et al. demonstrated a 90% clearance rate by histology on the basis of 3-week follow-up of 31 patients treated with twice-daily 5% 5-FU therapy.[2] More recently, a 90% cure rate for moderate-thickness BCCs was achieved by combining 5-FU with phosphatidylcholine as a transepidermal carrier.[9] Concerns have also been raised that only the superficial components of BCCs might be treated with 5-FU, leading to persistence of the deeper aspects of the tumor.

A recent systematic review compared five studies demonstrating the efficacy of topical 5-FU for the treatment of SCC in situ (SCCIS). Unfortunately, dosing schedules and lengths of treatment varied widely in these studies. A clinical clearance rate of 48–56% was achieved at 12-month follow-up after daily dosing for 1 week followed by twice-daily dosing for 3 weeks. An 85% clinical clearance rate was achieved after a more intense regimen of twice-daily dosing for 8 weeks with an average follow-up of 4.6 years.[10]

The British Association of Dermatologists' 2006 guidelines for the management of SCCIS recommended once- or twice-daily application of 5% 5-FU cream for up to 2 months, with repeat treatment cycles as needed.[11] SCCIS (Bowen's disease) of the penis can be similarly treated with 5% 5-FU twice daily for 4–5 weeks; accompanying inflammation may however limit tolerability and therefore impair patient compliance with an adequate treatment regimen. Increased efficacy has been achieved for SCCIS when administered under occlusion, or with the concurrent use of dinitrochlorobenzene, iontophoresis, or erbium:YAG laser.[11–13]

The usual treatment for extramammary Paget's disease is radical local excision. While there is very limited data proposing that topical 5-FU can substitute for surgical intervention, the agent can be utilized, via short-term pre-operative application, to expose clinically invisible foci of this often multifocal disorder.[14] This maneuver may help to better ensure adequate surgical excision.

The treatment of choice for keratoacanthomas is surgical extirpation. In selected cases, however, topical 5-FU may be of benefit. The agent can be used as an adjunct to laser ablation or as a primary intervention in the specific subtype: keratoacanthoma centrifugum marginatum. A small, clinically classic keratoacanthoma in a low-risk anatomic area may also be managed with topical 5-FU. In this situation, a therapeutic trial should be limited to 3 weeks.[15]

In all cases of SCC and BCC treated with 5-FU, careful follow-up is needed to ensure cure. Inadequate treatment may resolve only the superficial component and render the diagnosis of recurrence more difficult. Due to the small sample size of most studies and relative lack of long-term follow-up, Love et al. concluded that its use should be limited to small areas of SCCIS in low-risk areas (trunk, extremities and neck) or multiple areas of superficial BCCs in difficult-to-treat areas.[10] 5-FU may also be used in patients unable to tolerate other treatment.

The most common limitation of 5-FU therapy is the development of intense local inflammation associated with pain, erythema, erosion, ulceration and crusting. To help increase compliance, some practitioners have tried weekly pulsed dosing for longer durations. This method causes less local irritation but has not proven to be reliably effective at resolving AK lesions.[16] An inflammatory response appears to be necessary for efficacy in 5-FU treatment, and patients with the most intense reactions often achieve the best clinical responses.[17]

A high level of compliance is required to achieve a successful treatment outcome with 5-FU therapy. Patients need to be forewarned about the expected inflammatory reaction. Upon completion of the course of topical 5-FU therapy, mid-potency topical corticosteroids can be applied to the zone of inflammation to help hasten healing. Patients should be instructed to avoid application of 5-FU on mucous membranes, as well as on uninvolved periorbital, intertriginous, and genital areas, to avoid significant inflammation in these sensitive regions.

Systemic reactions related to topical application of 5-FU appear to be rare. Less than 10% of a dose of 5-FU 5% cream applied topically to intact skin is reported to be absorbed systemically.[18] Urinary excretion of 5-FU after application of 5-FU 0.5% microsponge cream was one-fortieth of that observed with 5-FU 5% cream despite only a one-tenth difference in drug concentration.[19] Systemic absorption of 5-FU may be significantly increased in patients with dihydropyrimidine dehydrogenase (DPD) deficiency because of an impaired ability to metabolize 5-FU. These patients are at risk of severe toxicity and the use of 5-FU is contraindicated in those with known DPD deficiency.[19] Routine testing for this deficiency, however, is not standard of care.

## TOPICAL IMIDAZOQUINOLONES

Imiquimod is a synthetic imidazoquinolone that functions as an immune response modulator with antiviral and antitumor activity for the treatment of skin cancer (see Chapter 44). Imiquimod's activity is mediated through Toll-like receptor (TLR) 7 and 8 signaling, resulting in secretion of pro-inflammatory cytokines (including interferons alpha and gamma, TNF alpha, IL-1, IL-6, IL-8, IL-10 and IL-12) that stimulate a localized cellular immune response against abnormal epithelial cells.[20]

## Imiquimod

Imiquimod was originally approved as a 5% cream for the treatment of external genital warts and has subsequently been approved for the treatment of non-hypertrophic AKs on the face and scalp and superficial BCCs.[20] In the United States, the 5% imiquimod preparation is approved for AKs in a regimen of twice-weekly application for 16 weeks. However, imiquimod is also typically used for treating AKs with once-daily application two to three times per week for 4 weeks, followed by a second 4-week treatment cycle if lesions have not resolved. While increased frequency of dosing has been shown to achieve a superior response, this is accompanied by increased adverse effects. Gebauer et al. found that application of 5% imiquimod more than three times a week was not well tolerated and led to a 33% clinical study withdrawal rate.[21]

In a retrospective review of 5% imiquimod topical therapy for AKs, Gaspari et al. reported overall complete clearance rates ranging from 45% to 57% and a median AK reduction rate of about 80%.[20] A systematic review of 1293 AK patients largely confirmed this, with 50% of patients treated for 12–16 weeks with imiquimod achieving complete clinical clearance.[22] In a head-to-head comparison with topical 5-FU and liquid nitrogen cryosurgery for the treatment of AKs, topical imiquimod demonstrated superior cosmetic outcomes and higher long-term complete clinical clearance rates at 12-month follow-up (73% imiquimod versus 33% 5-FU and 4% cryosurgery).[23] The use of imiquimod *in combination* with other AK treatment modalities (such as cryosurgery, 5-FU and photodynamic therapy) is evolving.

Because of the long treatment course and counter-intuitive regimen typically required for 5% imiquimod monotherapy

in the management AKs, other formulations have recently been studied.[24,25] A 3.75% formulation is likely optimum, and is utilized as daily application in a 6-week total regimen (2 weeks therapy, 2 weeks rest period, 2 weeks therapy). The 3.75% imiquimod formulation affords comparable clinical efficacy to the 5% cream, with reduced risk of unacceptable local skin reactions, a shorter course of therapy, and an intuitive (daily) application schedule (Fig. 43.3).

Numerous clinical trials and studies have demonstrated the safety and efficacy of imiquimod for the treatment of superficial BCCs. BCCs are typically treated with once-daily application, five times a week for a total of 6 weeks, with a minimum of 3 months follow-up (Fig. 43.4). A systematic review of 515 patients with superficial BCC treated with imiquimod at least daily, 5–7 days a week for 6–12 weeks, demonstrated an overall histologically confirmed clearance rate of 81% at 6 or 12 weeks.[10] A phase III study investigated the long-term efficacy of treatment: after application of imiquimod five times a week for 6 weeks to superficial BCC less than 2 cm, cure rates at 1- and 2-year follow-up were 90.4% and 82%.[26] Gollnick et al. demonstrated that after 6 weeks' application of 5% imiquimod for 5 days a week, a post-treatment clearance rate of 90.3% after 12 weeks and a sustained clearance rate of 80.9% after 5 years could be achieved. All recurrences occurred within 12 months, suggesting that assessment of initial response may be valuable for predicting the long-term outcome of patients treated with imiquimod for sBCCs.[27]

Several studies indicate that imiquimod may also be effective for nodular BCCs. However, effective treatment requires higher dosages and lower clearance rates are achieved compared to procedural modalities.[10,20,28] The largest study of 167 patients (including only low-risk BCCs: less than 2 cm in size, greater than 1 cm from the eyes, nose, mouth, ears, or hairline and excluding infiltrating morpheic and micronodular histologic patterns) found a 76% histologic clearance rate at 6 weeks after daily imiquimod for 12 weeks compared with a 42% histologic clearance rate for twice-daily imiquimod, 3 days a week for 6 weeks.[28] In a more recent report, an initial clearance rate of 78% was achieved. However, 17% of these patients subsequently had histologic evidence of residual disease, which raised concern that an excisional biopsy may be needed to confirm complete clearance of nodular BCCs, thereby defeating the purpose of topical therapy.[27] Debulking the tumor with curettage prior to imiquimod therapy enhances the cure rate.

There is growing evidence that imiquimod may be useful in the treatment of infiltrative BCC, SCCIS, and, to a lesser degree, invasive SCC. Vidal et al. demonstrated a sustained 5-year clearance rate of 60% for infiltrative BCC after imiquimod therapy.[29] To date, five studies have investigated the use of imiquimod for SCCIS. Clearance rates ranging from 73% to 88% have been achieved after daily application (or every-other-day dosing with genital lesions) for 9–16 weeks.[30-34] Tumors confined to the trunk or upper extremities had higher clearance rates compared with large facial and lower leg lesions.[31,34] Pooled analysis of randomized controlled trials, uncontrolled and cohort studies, demonstrated mean clearance rates of 51%, 70% and 48% for vulvar intraepithelial neoplasia, penile intraepithelial neoplasia

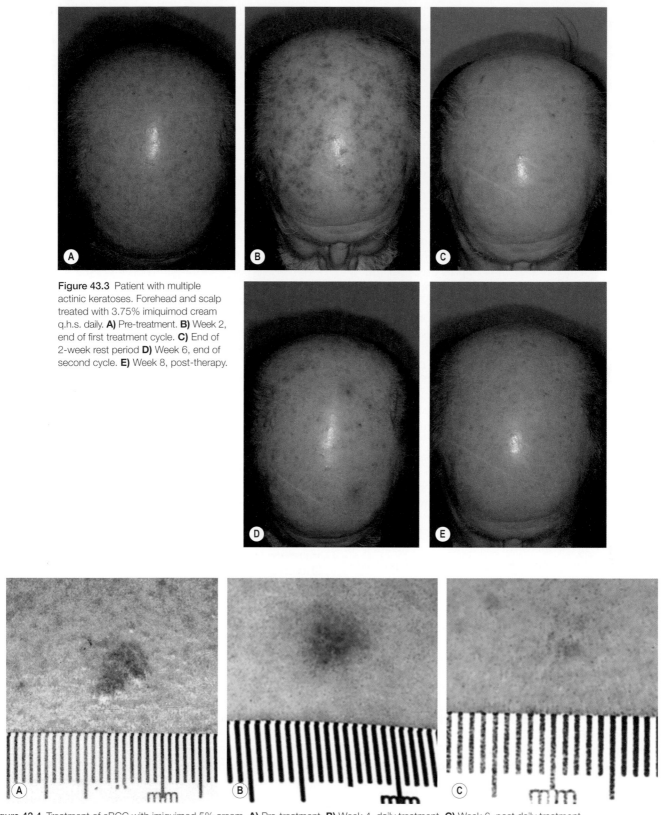

**Figure 43.3** Patient with multiple actinic keratoses. Forehead and scalp treated with 3.75% imiquimod cream q.h.s. daily. **A)** Pre-treatment. **B)** Week 2, end of first treatment cycle. **C)** End of 2-week rest period **D)** Week 6, end of second cycle. **E)** Week 8, post-therapy.

**Figure 43.4** Treatment of sBCC with imiquimod 5% cream. **A)** Pre-treatment. **B)** Week 4, daily treatment. **C)** Week 6, post daily treatment.

and anal intraepithelial neoplasia, respectively.[35] One study attempted treatment of invasive SCC with imiquimod 5 days per week for 12 weeks and achieved a 71% histological clearance rate at 28-month follow-up.[31] Scattered case reports also document the efficacy of imiquimod for invasive SCC.

Due to limited evidence of sustained 5-year clearance rates, recent systematic reviews cautioned against the use of imiquimod monotherapy in the treatment of non-superficial BCC or invasive SCC. Studies suggest limiting this approach for treating these lesions to tumors less than 2 cm in diameter, located in low-risk anatomic locations, and in patients who cannot tolerate or who refuse other well-established treatments.[10,36] A recent retrospective study revealed significantly lower clearance rates in patients with high-risk mixed aggressive BCC, nodular BCC, and SCCIS. Significant cutaneous or systemic comorbidities were also reported as risk factors for a worse prognosis.[37]

Several reports support the use of imiquimod for the treatment of rapidly appearing, multiple BCCs in basal cell nevus syndrome (BCNS), xeroderma pigmentosa (XP) or in immunosuppressed transplant patients.[3] However, the use of imiquimod as ongoing or intermittent topical prophylaxis to prevent NMSC associated with the high-risk conditions noted above has not yet become a widely accepted practice.

Imiquimod has been used in the treatment of lentigo maligna melanoma. A comprehensive post-hoc review of five studies found complete histologic clearance in 67–100% of patients treated with 5% imiquimod daily for 6–13 weeks, with one trial demonstrating no relapses at 1-year follow-up.[38] Currently, it is suggested that imiquimod only be used in a very narrow scope for lentigo maligna melanoma, such as treatment of post-excision recurrences or for adjunct management of poor surgical candidates or inoperable tumors.[39]

Imiquimod's ability to induce local release of interferon-alpha led to the investigation of its use as a treatment for Kaposi sarcoma (KS). In an open-label trial, 17 patients with classic KS were treated with imiquimod under occlusion three times a week for 24 weeks. Two complete responses and six partial responses were reported.[40] Imiquimod may therefore serve as a viable treatment option for cutaneous KS in patients who are unsuitable for more aggressive therapy.

Imiquimod has also been reported to successfully treat other forms of cutaneous malignancies, including patch stage cutaneous T-cell lymphoma (CTCL) and extramammary Paget's disease.[41,42] Based on in-vitro evidence of anti-angiogenic properties, imiquimod has also been used to treat vascular neoplasms, including hemangiomas of infancy, pyogenic granulomas and congenital port-wine stains.[43,44] The optimum dosing regimen is unknown for all of the aforementioned conditions, and sufficient long-term follow-up is also lacking.

A recent multicenter, placebo-controlled safety and efficacy study performed by the Skin Care in Organ-transplant Patients, Europe (SCOPE) research network enrolled 43 patients in six European transplant centers. Among patients randomized to imiquimod, the histologically confirmed complete clearance rate was 62%, compared to a complete clearance rate of 0% in the vehicle group.[45] In order to exclude graft rejections induced through the Th1 immune response of the immune response modifier (IRM) imiquimod, all patients were monitored for changes in hematology and serum chemistry. In all studies published to date with imiquimod in organ transplant recipients (OTR), no adverse effect of the IRM on the function of the graft has been observed.

Patients should be informed about common local application site reactions with imiquimod therapy, which are largely secondary to the inflammatory response, including erythema, crusting, flaking, erosion and ulceration, edema, and oozing or weeping.[22] If these develop in excess, treatment can be suspended for a few days without an apparent decrease in efficacy.[3] However, local inflammation appears to correlate with success, so patients should be informed that some degree of inflammation is desirable to achieve the best results.[46] Rivers et al. demonstrated that 4-week rest periods between 4-week treatment cycles for AKs decreased local skin reactions without decreasing overall efficacy of 5% topical imiquimod.[47]

The effects of imiquimod are generally localized to the skin, with minimal systemic absorption. Systemic side effects can include flu-like symptoms, experienced by fewer than 10% of patients.[20] Overall cosmetic results are favorable, with rare reports of mild residual hyperpigmentation or hypopigmentation.[36,48]

## Resiquimod

Resiquimod is another imidazoquinolamine which has currently only completed phase II studies for the treatment of AKs. Similar to imiquimod, it is a TLR-7 and TLR-8 agonist; however, it is purported to be 10 to 100 times more potent and has the ability to stimulate a greater spectrum of inflammatory cytokines.[49] Limited studies indicate that resiquimod 0.01% gel can be used three times a week for 4 weeks to face and scalp AKs to achieve a 77% overall clearance rate.[50] After a single 4-week treatment course, resiquimod achieves a clearance rate comparable to the rate imiquimod attains after two courses of treatment. However, resiquimod concentrations of 0.03% and higher lead to severe local erythema, inflammation, and increased systemic side effects that are not well tolerated.[50] Further investigation is needed to determine if resiquimod can offer a greater risk-to-benefit profile for the treatment of advanced NMSCs. Sotirimod is an additional drug in this class which might have clinical utility.

## CYCLOOXYGENASE (COX) ENZYME INHIBITORS

### Diclofenac

Diclofenac is a COX-2-selective non-steroidal anti-inflammatory drug (NSAID) that is approved for the treatment of AKs as a 3% topical gel in 2.5% hyaluronic acid. Through inhibition of arachidonic acid mediators, diclofenac is hypothesized to induce apoptosis, alter cell proliferation, and inhibit cell angiogenesis, leading to diminished carcinogenesis within keratinocytes.[51] Recently, increased levels of COX-2 have been implicated in the process of UV-induced carcinogenesis, supporting the use of diclofenac for chemoprevention of NMSCs.[52]

Long-term clearance of AKs after use of topical diclofenac has been evaluated. In a study of patients with at least five AKs involving the face, forehead or scalp, treated with diclofenac sodium 3% gel twice daily for 90 days, target AK lesions and cumulative AK lesions decreased by 95% and 77% at 1-year follow-up. Complete target and cumulative clearance of AKs at 1 year was achieved in 79% and 30% of patients, respectively. AK reductions of at least 75% were noted in 70% of patients at 1 year of follow-up.[51]

A review of randomized placebo-controlled and open-label studies demonstrated an overall 60–80% clearance rate for AKs treated with topical diclofenac for an average of approximately 110 days.[51] The most common treatment regimen included application of the gel twice daily to AK lesions for at least 3 months. Optimal treatment effect was reported to occur up to 4 weeks after the last application.[51]

Diclofenac gel applied twice daily for 4 months has led to complete clinical clearance of AKs in solid organ transplant patients. Another study demonstrated that 41% of such patients cleared. Although over half had recurrence of AK in the treatment area within a year, none of the treated cohort developed invasive SCC.[53]

The use of diclofenac 3% gel in organ transplant recipients (OTRs) was also recently evaluated in a small, open-label study in six OTRs (three kidney, one liver and two heart transplant patients) with histories of multiple NMSCs and extensive AKs. Diclofenac 3% gel, used twice daily for 16 weeks, showed a 50% complete clearance rate and 83% partial response rate (≥75% lesion reduction), with generally mild local adverse events at the site of application.[54]

Topical 3% diclofenac sodium in 2.5% hyaluronic acid is easily applied and well tolerated. The most common adverse events reported with use of topical diclofenac for AKs are mild to moderate, reversible, local tolerability reactions occurring at the application site (Fig. 43.5). These include pruritus, erythema, and dryness of the skin. Although 70–80% of patients experience some degree of local irritation and erythema at sites of diclofenac sodium 3% gel application, the extent and severity of reaction are relatively mild and tolerable in most patients and significantly less than the application site reactions characteristic of topical 5-fluorouracil, topical imiquimod, or cryosurgery.[55] No severe or systemic reactions occurred that were found to be related to topical diclofenac therapy. Anti-diclofenac antibodies were not identified in any patients.

Systemic bioavailability of diclofenac was demonstrated to be considerably lower after topical application than after systemic administration and the drug demonstrated a good safety profile. The use of diclofenac should be avoided in patients with NSAID hypersensitivity, aspirin intolerance, or bleeding diatheses.[8] There is currently no evidence to support the use of topical diclofenac for the treatment of BCCs, SCCs, or other primary cutaneous malignancies.

## PHOTODYNAMIC THERAPY

Photodynamic therapy (PDT) is a non-invasive and precisely directed treatment that involves activation of a photosensitizing agent by visible light, creating cytotoxic oxygen species and free radicals, which selectively destroy rapidly proliferating cells.[56] Currently there are two photosensitizers in use for PDT: 5-aminolevulinic acid (ALA) and methylaminolevulinate (MAL). PDT is an advantageous treatment for preinvasive and malignant skin lesions (AKs, BCC, SCC) when size, site, or number of lesions limits the efficacy or acceptability of more conventional therapies (see Chapter 45).

Adverse effects of both ALA-PDT and MAL-PDT include marked erythema, edema, crusting, vesiculation, or erosion of lesions in the 24–48 hours after light treatment. However, these reactions are desirable to achieve resolution of neoplastic lesions, which occurs over 7–10 days (Fig. 43.6).

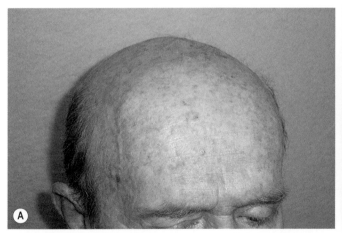
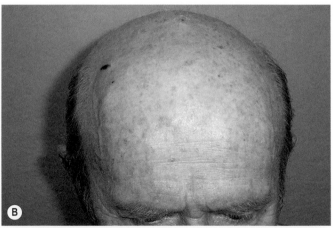
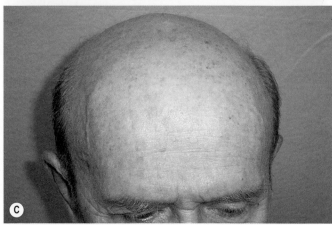

**Figure 43.5** Male with multiple actinic keratoses on the scalp treated with topical diclofenac 3% gel b.i.d. **A)** Pre-treatment. **B)** After 30 days. **C)** After 90-day course of treatment. (Images courtesy of Dr Christopher Nelson.)

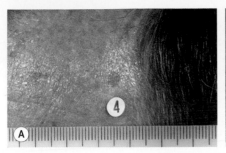
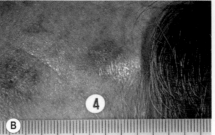
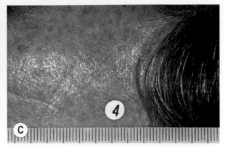

**Figure 43.6** Treatment of actinic keratoses on forehead with topical ALA-PDT. **A)** Pre-treatment. **B)** 1 week post-treatment. **C)** 6 weeks post-treatment. (Courtesy of Donald Tillman, D.O.).

Residual dyschromia, both hyperpigmentation and hypopigmentation, has been reported following PDT sessions.[57] Rarely, patients can experience a severe phototoxic reaction consisting of excessive burning, vesicle formation, crusting, and peeling.[56] Compared with other topical therapies, PDT has the disadvantage of requiring timed office visits, leading to increased personal expense and inconvenience. However, this is offset by shorter treatment courses and local adverse events being limited to a few days. Physician control of treatment eliminates any risk of patient non-compliance or abuse of the topical modality.

## RETINOIDS

Retinoids are a group of naturally occurring and synthetic derivatives of vitamin A that can modulate proliferation and differentiation of keratinocytes through interaction with nuclear retinoic acid receptors. They have been used to treat various cutaneous neoplasms, with proposed mechanisms of action including suppression of tumor growth, promotion of cell maturation, and induction of apoptosis.[58] An early study revealed that vitamin A-deficient rats developed multiple areas of squamous metaplasia, prompting investigation of the possible chemoprotective effects of retinoids against skin cancer.[59]

Oral retinoids have a long history of use as chemoprophylactics to reduce the development of AKs, BCCs and SCCs in high-risk patients with solid organ transplants, XP, BCNS, or history of prolonged exposure to PUVA.[60] Although oral retinoids have proven to be effective chemoprotective agents in these conditions, patients develop significant dose-limiting mucocutaneous and systemic side effects.[60] Topical retinoids have therefore been proposed as an alternative, more localized form of treatment for NMSCs to avoid these systemic adverse effects.

Multiple studies support the use of topical retinoids, both to treat and prevent recurrence of AKs. Various formulations, concentrations, and dosing schedules have been studied. In 1975, Bollag and Ott reported complete clearance of AKs on the forearms and hands in 55% of subjects treated with 0.1% tretinoin twice daily for 3 weeks.[61] Moglia et al. demonstrated 46% complete regression and 44% partial regression of AKs after twice-daily treatment with the retinoid fenretinide for 3 months.[62] Topical treatment with isotretinoin has produced similar results.[63] Efficacy appears to be dose-responsive, with a greater reduction of AKs after twice-daily application of 0.1% tretinoin versus 0.05% tretinoin for 15 months.[64]

Recent studies support the use of retinoids for more advanced NMSCs. When applied daily for 24 weeks to superficial or nodular BCCs, tazarotene 0.1% gel achieved a greater than 50% regression in 70.8% of tumors. After 12 weeks, biopsies confirmed that lesions showed reduced proliferation along with apoptosis of tumor cells.[65] A small pilot study of 15 patients with SCCIS on the extremities, trunk, and head revealed that daily application of 0.1% tazarotene resulted in complete resolution of lesions after 3–5 months.[66] Additionally, there is evidence that retinoids may act synergistically with other topical chemotherapies to treat NMSCs when individual therapies are ineffective.[67–69]

In 1999, the FDA approved 0.1% alitretinoin (9-cis-retinoic acid) for the treatment of cutaneous lesions of AIDS-related KS.[70] In a phase I–II trial, 37% of treated lesions compared with 11% of untreated lesions showed clinically significant responses after 0.1% alitretinoin was applied for up to 16 weeks.[70] In another phase III trial by Bodsworth et al., KS patients were treated with either alitretinoin 0.1% gel or vehicle twice daily for 12 weeks. Alitretinon patients achieved an overall response rate of 37% versus 7% for vehicle.[71] Topical treatment up to four times daily was well tolerated in all studies, with only mild associated dermal irritation.

Topical retinoids have also been studied as a treatment option for refractory CTCL lesions. In a pilot study of 20 patients with refractory T1-stage MF lesions, daily application of 0.1% tazarotene gel for 6 months achieved a 58% overall response rate.[72]

In contrast to systemic retinoid treatment, topical therapy is generally well tolerated with minimal side effects, which may include local irritation, pruritus, burning, dryness, erythema, and desquamation. Local reactions peak at 4 weeks and increase with drug concentration and frequency of application. Most topical retinoids are available in a cream or gel with no significant differences in efficacy between formulations. All retinoids are theoretically teratogenic and are not recommended for use during pregnancy.[60]

### Bexarotene

Bexarotene is a synthetic retinoid analog that can be differentiated from other retinoids by its selectivity for the biologically distinct retinoid X receptor. In 1999, oral bexarotene received FDA approval for the treatment of advanced refractory CTCL.[73] For patients who could not tolerate the systemic side effects of oral retinoids, topical bexarotene 1% gel was approved for the treatment of refractory IA and

IB cutaneous CTCL lesions. Bexarotene is thought to have activity against CTCL through its ability to produce dose-dependent apoptosis of CTCL lines and peripheral T cells in patients with Sézary syndrome.[73]

A recent phase III clinical trial of 50 patients with refractory stage IA–IIA CTCL skin lesions demonstrated a 54% overall response with topical 1% bexarotene gel applied every other day and escalated at 1-week intervals up to four times daily for 16 weeks.[74] An average relapse-free interval has been reported as ranging from 11 weeks to up to 5 years with maintenance therapy.[75] Topical bexarotene appears to be more effective for thicker lesions and in patients who have recieved no previous therapy for CTCL.[73]

Bexarotene 1% gel is easily applied and well tolerated. Adverse effects are generally mild and limited to local application site reactions, including irritation, pruritus, pain, and vesiculobullous rash. Up to 19% of patients develop severe dose-related reactions, including facial edema, neuralgia, skin necrosis, and ulceration. As with other retinoids, there is a potential for teratogenicity, and use during pregnancy is not recommended.

## COLCHICINE

Colchicine is an alkaloid plant extract that has potent anti-mitotic activity. It is best known as an anti-inflammatory agent that can arrest the chemotactic and phagocytic abilities of leukocytes for the treatment of acute gout. Studies also indicate that topical colchicine is an effective treatment for AKs. Grimarte et al. demonstrated complete clearance of AKs in 7 out of 10 patients at 60-day follow-up. Treatment included twice-daily application of 1% colchicine cream to forehead AKs for a total of 10 days.[76] Akar et al. reported an approximately 76% reduction in AKs after twice-daily application of either 0.5% or 1% colchicine cream for up to 10 days. There was no significant difference in the total clearing of AKs between the 0.5% and 1% creams.[77]

Topical colchicine induces a potent inflammatory effect after 3 days of treatment that intensifies until treatment is stopped. Inflammation is localized to AKs, with sparing of surrounding normal skin. Lesions that develop a strong inflammatory response appear to have the best cosmetic outcomes. No systemic side effects or evidence of systemic absorption have been reported. Because of significant associated inflammation, treatment of AKs should be limited to twice-daily application for up to 10 days.[76] Further studies are needed to characterize the benefit of topical colchicine over other similar topical chemotherapeutic agents. A commercially available formulation has not been released.

## NITROGEN MUSTARD

Nitrogen mustard (methchlorethamine hydrochloride) is an alkylating agent with an unclear mechanism of action. It reacts with DNA, resulting in the donation of alkyl groups and the disruption of DNA synthesis, halting cell growth. As a topical agent, it may also stimulate immune function and interact with the epidermal T cell/Langerhans cell axis.[78] Topical nitrogen mustard is a well-established treatment for early T1-stage CTCL.

Nitrogen mustard can be used in concentrations of 10–40 mg/dL, compounded with either an aqueous or ointment-based preparation. The agent can be applied daily to the entire skin surface, sparing the face, skin folds, and genital areas. Treatment should begin with broad application as the associated inflammatory reaction may unmask areas of skin not previously involved. Application can then be focused to affected areas after several weeks. Treatment should continue daily until complete skin clearance is achieved; a variable length of maintenance therapy will follow. Remissions may take up to 6–12 months.

In a retrospective study, Kim et al. reported a complete response rate of 50% and an overall response rate of 83% for 203 CTCL patients treated with daily nitrogen mustard.[78] Median time to achieve a complete response was 12 months and median time to relapse was 12 months.

Patients with T1 disease responded better and had better survival outcomes compared to those with T2 disease (overall complete response of 93% versus 72%). Freedom-from-progression rates at 5 and 10 years were 92% and 85%, respectively, for T1 disease, and 83% for T2 at both 5 and 10 years. Once a complete response was achieved, frequency of application was decreased from daily to several times a week for a period of up to 2–3 months. A more prolonged maintenance therapy appeared to add no benefit to outcomes; after cessation of maintenance therapy, CTCL relapsed at the same rate as in those not receiving maintenance therapy. Results were similar in patients treated with ointment versus aqueous preparations.[78] Long-term survival rates are similar to those achieved with more aggressive treatment with total skin electron beam therapy, but nitrogen mustard is generally more convenient and cost-effective for patients.

The most common adverse effects are irritant and true allergic contact dermatitis, occurring more often with aqueous formulations. A 7–10-day patch test can be conducted before initiation of therapy, to screen for hypersensitivity. When significant hypersensitivity is present, patients can undergo a topical desensitization program. Mild irritant reactions can be treated with low-potency topical corticosteroids or a decrease in application frequency. Patients who develop brisk local reactions often benefit from a more rapid clearance of lesions. Secondary cutaneous malignancies have been reported with prolonged therapy and in patients previously treated with total skin electron beam or long-term PUVA therapy.[78] Topical nitrogen mustard is not systemically absorbed and no systemic side effects have been observed. Overall, nitrogen mustard is safe and well tolerated, even in the pediatric setting.[78]

## EMERGING THERAPIES

### Ingenol mebutate

Ingenol mebutate (ingenol-3-angelate, formerly PEP005) is a diterpene ester that is currently being evaluated for topical field directed treatment of AKs.[79] Produced from the sap of the *Euphorbia peplus* plant, it has long been used as a 'home remedy' for AKs and other skin conditions in Australia.[80] Preclinical studies have uncovered two mechanisms of activity against keratinocyte proliferation. First, application induces rapid primary necrosis of local cells through disruption of mitochondria and plasma membranes. Then, residual tumor cells are eradicated through production of tumor-specific antibodies leading to neutrophil and antibody dependent cellular cytotoxicity.[79,81]

Ingenol mebutate is formulated in a gel base with isopropyl alcohol. Phase IIA studies indicate that the most effective dosing regimen is application of 0.05% ingenol mebutate gel to cutaneous AKs lesions once daily for 2 days.[82,83] Phase IIA and IIB studies confirm that two or three doses of 0.05% ingenol mebutate are significantly more effective than vehicle at clearing non-facial AKs (clearance rates ranged from 54% to 71%).[82,83] Ingenol mebutate potentially offers the advantage of effective clearance rates in a significantly shorter treatment period compared with other topical chemotherapies for AKs, including application of imiquimod for up to 16 weeks, 5-FU for up to 4 weeks, and diclofenac for up to 90 days.[4–7,20,22,23,49]

Ingenol mebutate induces localized necrosis and a subsequent inflammatory response, which causes dose-related transient local skin reactions consisting of erythema, scabbing, crusting, scaling, flaking and dryness. Reactions may be quite brisk and typically peak by day 3–8 and resolve by day 15–30. Most often, there is no evidence of residual scarring. Initial studies have revealed no systemic absorption. In preliminary studies, the drug has been well received by patients for its tolerability, ease of use and cosmetic results.[82,83]

## T4 endonuclease

T4 endonuclease V is a bacterial DNA repair enzyme that has demonstrated the ability to repair UV light-induced cyclobutane pyrimidine dimers which contribute to the pathogenesis of actinic keratosis and other NMSCs. T4 endonuclease has been formulated into a liposomally delivered topical medication that can enter the nucleus of keratinocytes and interact with damaged DNA. Initial studies in patients with xeroderma pigmentosa (XP) show a significant reduction in the development of new AKs after 12 months of treatment compared to a vehicle alone.[84] In clinical trials using XP patients, topical application of T4 endonuclease reduced the incidence of AKs by more than 68% and BCCs by more than 30%.[85] No adverse side effects have been noted to date. T4 endonuclease has only completed phase I and II trials for FDA approval and is not commercially available at this time. Ongoing studies are investigating whether the photoprotective effects in XP patients can be applied to other populations at risk for NMSC.[85]

## Perillyl alcohol

Perillyl alcohol (POH) is a naturally occurring hydroxylated monocyclic monoterpene that is produced as an essential oil extract from various plants.[86] In preclinical studies, POH has been shown to inhibit multiple steps of tumorigenesis in murine models of UVB-induced SCC and melanoma.[87,88] POH is postulated to induce selective apoptosis of tumor cells[89] and inhibit UVB-induced activator protein-1, which plays a key role in tumor promotion and/or progression.[90] Phase I and IIA studies have indicated that topical POH cream is well tolerated with mild local side effects that do not differ significantly from those of placebo.[91]

A phase IIA study found that application of 0.76% POH cream twice daily for 3 months to moderate/severely sun-damaged forearms achieved a significant reduction in nuclear chromatin abnormality based on karyometric analysis, possibly representing a beneficial chemopreventative effect. However, histopathologic examination did not reveal a significant change in the sun-damaged skin areas post-treatment.[86] Further studies will be needed to address the potential of POH as a therapeutic or chemoprotective agent.

## DL-alpha-tocopherol

DL-alpha-tocopherol is a biologically active form of vitamin E, a well-known epidermal antioxidant shown to be depleted in UV-radiated skin.[92] Formulated in a 12.5% cream base, DL-alpha-tocopherol has been shown to prevent skin cancer in mice and reduce UVB-induced immunosuppression.[93] However, a randomized placebo-controlled trial found that after 6 months of daily application to dorsal forearm AKs, DL-alpha-tocopherol did not significantly decrease the level of AKs compared to placebo. Of the biomarkers for tumorigenesis tested (p53, proliferating cell nuclear antigen and polyamines), only the concentration of polyamines were significantly decreased following application, indicating a possible inhibition of keratinocyte carcinogenesis.[94] The clinical utility of topical DL-alpha-tocopherol remains to be determined.

## DFMO

A newer compound being evaluated for its chemopreventative qualities is 2-(difluoromethyl)-dl-ornithine, an irreversible inhibitor of the rate-limiting step of polyamine synthesis, ornithine decarboxylase.[95,96] Polyamines are upregulated during the promotion phase of skin carcinogenesis models, and by inhibiting polyamine synthesis, DFMO is thought to attenuate this critical step in tumor formation.[97,98] A randomized placebo-controlled trial showed that 10% DFMO ointment applied to one forearm with moderate to severe AKs for 6 months achieved a 23.5% reduction in the number of AKs compared with placebo.[99] Another study found that following topical DFMO application, the local levels of p53 expression were reduced by 22%, indicating a possible decrease in local cellular DNA damage.[100] However, a recent phase III study indicated that oral DFMO taken for up to 5 years did not result in a significantly decreased rate of onset of skin cancers.[98] Further clinical studies are needed to elucidate the safety and efficacy of topical DFMO as a therapeutic or chemopreventative agent for NMSC.

## Calcipotriol

Recent research has demonstrated that vitamin D has potent immunomodulatory, antiproliferative, and prodifferentiative actions. These effects on the skin are exerted via the vitamin $D_3$ receptor (VDR) in keratinocytes.[101,102] Seckin et al.[103] reported in a pilot study that topical calcipotriol was effective in treating

AK. They noted greater than a 25–50% decrease in total AKs after 12 weeks of treatment. Further studies are needed, but the possibility of a well-tolerated therapeutic agent with possible skin cancer preventative benefits is intriguing.[104] Topical calcipotriol may also be useful as an adjuvant for MAL-PDT when applied prior to the PDT. Cicarma et al.[105] showed that calcipotriol pre-treatment improved MAL-PDT in human squamous cell carcinoma A431 cells.

## HEAD-TO-HEAD TRIALS OF TOPICAL CHEMOTHERAPY

Effective, well-designed head-to-head trials comparing various topical chemotherapeutic options would be helpful in optimizing therapy by lesion type and anatomic site. However, there are few of these in the literature.

A cumulative meta-analysis included 10 studies comparing the efficacy of topical agents imiquimod and 5-FU. The average efficacy rate was 52% (n = 6 studies, 145 subjects) for 5-FU and 70% (n = 4 studies, 393 subjects) for imiquimod. This analysis suggests that imiquimod has higher efficacy than 5-FU for AK lesions located on the face and scalp.[106]

A study in AK patients comparing imiquimod, 5-FU and cryosurgery showed, respectively, 85%, 96% and 68% initial clinical clearance and 73%, 67% and 32% histological clearance in patients treated. However, the recurrence rate was significantly lower for imiquimod after 12 months than for the other treatments, where the sustained clearance rate of initially cleared individual lesions was 73%, 54% and 28% for imiquimod, 5-FU and cryosurgery, respectively. Also the 12-month sustained clearance for the total treatment field was 73%, 33% and 4% of patients, respectively, for imiquimod, 5-FU and cryosurgery. Imiquimod treatment of AK resulted in superior sustained clearance in a 12 months follow-up period, having a superior cosmetic outcome compared with cryosurgery and 5-FU.[23]

Two studies comparing PDT with cryosurgery show different results, one showing a higher clearance rate for cryosurgery (69% PDT vs 75% cryosurgery)[107] and one showing a lower clearance rate for cryosurgery (91% PDT vs 68% cryosurgery).[108] Another study found similar response rates for PDT and cryosurgery (69–89% vs 68–86%, respectively). PDT was associated with better cosmetic results than cryosurgery and subjects in the intra-individual comparison significantly preferred PDT.[109] A right/left comparison of AK treatment on the back of the hands by PDT and 5-FU showed a similar response to both therapies, clearing 73% and 70%, respectively. Responses remained similar at 6 months.[110]

## COMBINATION THERAPY

Using topical chemotherapy agents for skin cancer has the advantage of potentially treating subclinical lesions and, with some of the agents, providing an immunologic induction for a longer-lasting clearance but may not be as effective for treating larger lesions. Surgical approaches have the advantage of effectively ablating larger individual lesions but have limited effect on an area with diffuse damage. Combining the two types of approach may be more than additive in enhancing treatment of skin cancer. Combination therapy may be either sequential or concurrent.

Several trials have shown a synergistic effect of combining imiquimod and physical modalities for the treatment of BCC and AKs. A study of 57 patients with BCC treated with curettage followed by 6 weeks of imiquimod showed no reoccurrences at 1 year, with excellent cosmetic results.[111] Another study of 101 BCCs treated with curettage followed by the application of imiquimod 5% cream resulted in clearance rates of 96% at an average 36 months follow-up.[112] In the treatment of nodular BCC, studies indicate that combining topical imiquimod with a surgical procedure can reduce risk of recurrence and improve the ultimate cosmetic result compared to curettage with electrodessication or surgical excision alone.[113] A recent study of 3.75% imiquimod following cryosurgery in 247 subjects demonstrated significantly improved clearance of AKs over cryosurgery alone.[114]

Cryosurgery followed 15 days later with use of diclofenac sodium 3% gel twice daily for 90 days proved to be superior to cryosurgery alone for multiple AKs involving the forehead, face, scalp, or hands (n = 521).[115] Complete target and cumulative lesion clearance was noted in 64% and 46%, respectively, of patients treated with cryosurgery followed by topical diclofenac, and in 32% and 21%, respectively, of patients treated with cryosurgery alone.

For hyperkeratotic AKs of the extremities, the combination therapy approach of spot treatment with liquid nitrogen cryotherapy or application of trichloroacetic acid (TCA) 35% solution, prior to initiating or after completing a course of topical 5-FU therapy, enhances results. Longer duration of therapy or combining 5-FU with other treatments may be beneficial for more persistent lesions. Success has been reported with liquid nitrogen cryotherapy, gentle curettage, or combined application of trichloroacetic acid solution, tretinoin cream, lactic acid moisturizer or topical diclofenac sodium prior to initiating or after completing a course of topical 5-FU therapy.[8,67] Bercovich et al. reported that tretinion 0.05% at bedtime given concurrently with 5-FU 5% cream twice daily for 12–28 days was significantly more effective than 5-FU alone for upper extremity AKs.[68]

PDT has also been effectively combined with other therapies. In a split-face study, two short-contact ALA-PDT treatments followed by standard 5% imiquimod therapy for 16 weeks resulted in nearly 90% median lesion reduction at 1 year, compared to 74.5% median lesion reduction following ALA-PDT monotherapy.[116]

## FUTURE OUTLOOK

Until the last decade, the only therapies for actinic keratoses and non-melanoma skin cancers had been ablative or topical 5-FU. Now, topical agents working via new specific mechanisms have been found to be effective, such as topical imiquimod (an immune modulator enhancing antigen recognition and targeted immunologic response), diclofenac (a COX inhibitor) and PDT (utilizing a combination of a topical protoporphyrin and light).

In a very short time, topical treatment options have progressed from a limited menu and very few mechanisms of disease treatment to multiple options utilizing varied treatment mechanisms. This may be only the tip of the topical therapeutic iceberg for cutaneous cancer. The use of an endpoint of sustained clearance will become increasingly important. Rigorous head-to-head studies and better evaluation of combination therapies will help determine future optimal topical chemotherapy treatment regimens for skin cancer.

## REFERENCES

1. Vatve M, Ortonne JP, Birch-Machin MA, et al. Management of field change in actinic keratosis. Br J Dermatol. 2007;157(suppl 2):21–24.
2. Gross K, Kircik L, Kricorian G. 5% 5-fluorouracil cream for the treatment of small superficial basal cell carcinoma: efficacy, tolerability, cosmetic outcome, and patient satisfaction. Dermatol Surg. 2007;33:433–440.
3. Barrera MV, Herrera E. Topical chemotherapy for actinic keratosis and nonmelanoma skin cancer: current options and future perspectives. Actas Dermosifiliogr. 2007;98:556–562.
4. Weiss J, Menter A, Hevia O, et al. Effective treatment of actinic keratosis with 0.5% fluorouracil cream for 1, 2, or 4 weeks. Cutis. 2002;70(suppl 2):22–29.
5. Loven K, Stein L, Furst K, et al. Evaluation of the efficacy and tolerability of 0.5% fluorouracil cream and 5% fluorouracil cream applied to each side of the face in patients with actinic keratosis. Clin Ther. 2002;24:990–1000.
6. Jorizzo JL, Carney PS, Ko WT, et al. Fluorouracil 5% and 0.5% creams for the treatment of actinic keratosis: equivalent efficacy with a lower concentration and more convenient dosing schedule. Cutis. 2004;74(suppl 6):18–23.
7. Askew DA, Mickan SM, Soyer HP, et al. Effectiveness of 5-fluorouracil treatment for actinic keratosis – a systematic review of randomized controlled trials. Int J Dermatol. 2009;48:453–463.
8. McGillis ST, Fein H. Topical treatment strategies for non-melanoma skin cancer and precursor lesions. Semin Cutan Med Surg. 2004;23:174–183.
9. Romadgosa R, Saap L, Givens M, et al. A pilot study to evaluate the treatment of basal cell carcinoma with 5-fluorouracil using phosphatidyl choline as a trans-epidermal carrier. Dermatol Surg. 2003;26:338–340.
10. Love WE, Bernhard JD, Bordeaux JS. Topical imiquimod or fluorouracil therapy for basal and squamous cell carcinoma: a systematic review. Arch Dermatol. 2009;145:1431–1438.
11. Cox NH, Eedy DJ, Morton CA, Therapy Guidelines and Audit Subcommittee, British Association of Dermatologists. Guidelines for management of Bowen's disease: 2006 update. Br J Dermatol. 2007;156:11–21.
12. Welch ML, Grabski WJ, McCollough ML, et al. 5-Fluorouracil iontophoretic therapy for Bowen's disease. J Am Acad Dermatol. 1997;36:956–958.
13. Wang KH, Fang JY, Hu CH, et al. Erbium:YAG laser pretreatment accelerates the response of Bowen's disease treated by topical 5-fluorouracil. Dermatol Surg. 2004;30:441–445.
14. Eliezri YD, Silvers DN, Horan DB. Role of pre-operative topical 5-fluorouracil in preparation for Mohs micrographic surgery of extramammary Paget's disease. J Am Acad Dermatol. 1987;17:497–505.
15. Gray RJ, Meland NB. Topical 5-fluorouracil as primary therapy for keratoacanthoma. Ann Plast Surg. 2000;44:82–85.
16. Jury CS, Ramraka-Jones VS, Gudi V, et al. A randomized trial of topical 5% 5-fluorouracil (Efudex cream) in the treatment of actinic keratoses comparing daily with weekly treatment. Br J Dermatol. 2005;153:808–810.
17. Sachs DL, Kang S, Hammerberg C, et al. Topical fluorouracil for actinic keratoses and photoaging: a clinical and molecular analysis. Arch Dermatol. 2009;145:659–666.
18. Dillaha CJ, Jansen GT, Honeycutt WM, et al. Further studies with topical 5-fluorouracil. Arch Dermatol. 1965;92:410–417.
19. Levy S, Furst K. A pharmacokinetic evaluation of 0.5% or 5% fluorouracil topical cream in patients with actinic keratosis. Clin Ther. 2001;23:908–920.
20. Gaspari AA, Tyring SK, Rosen T. Beyond a decade of 5% imiquimod topical therapy. J Drugs Dermatol. 2009;8:467–474.
21. Gebauer K, Shumack S, Cowen PS. Effect of dosing frequency on the safety and efficacy of imiquimod 5% cream for treatment of actinic keratosis on the forearms and hands: a phase II, randomized placebo-controlled trial. Br J Dermatol. 2009;161:897–903.
22. Hadley G, Derry S, Moore RA. Imiquimod for actinic keratosis: systematic review and meta-analysis. J Invest Dermatol. 2006;126:1251–1255.
23. Krawtchenko N, Roewert-Huber J, Ulrich M, et al. A randomized study of topical 5% imiquimod vs. topical 5-fluorouracil vs. cryosurgery in immunocompetent patients with actinic keratosis: a comparison of clinical and histological outcome including 1-year follow-up. Br J Dermatol. 2007;157(suppl 2):34–40.
24. Hanke CW, Beer KR, Stockfleth E, et al. Imiquimod 2.5% and 3.75% for the treatment of actinic keratoses: results of two placebo-controlled studies of daily application to the face and balding scalp for two 3-week cycles. J Am Acad Dermatol. 2010;62:573–581.
25. Swanson N, Abramovits W, Berman B, et al. Imiquimod 2.5% and 3.75% for the treatment of actinic keratoses: results of two placebo-controlled studies of daily application to the face and balding scalp for two 2-week cycles. J Am Acad Dermatol. 2010;62:582–590.
26. Quirk C, Gebauer K, Owens M, et al. Two-year interim results from a 5-year study evaluating clinical recurrence of superficial basal cell carcinoma after treatment with imiquimod 5% cream daily for 6 weeks. Australas J Dermatol. 2006;47:258–265.
27. Gollnick H, Barona CG, Frank RG, et al. Recurrence rate of superficial basal cell carcinoma following treatment with imiquimod 5% cream: conclusion of a 5-year long-term follow-up study in Europe. Eur J Dermatol. 2008;18:677–682.
28. Shumack S, Robinson J, Kossard S, et al. Efficacy of topical 5% imiquimod cream for the treatment of nodular basal cell carcinoma: comparison of dosing regimens. Arch Dermatol. 2002;138:1165–1171.
29. Vidal D, Matías-Guiu X, Alomar A. Fifty-five basal cell carcinomas treated with topical imiquimod: outcome at 5-year follow-up. Arch Dermatol. 2007;143:266–268.
30. Patel GK, Goodwin R, Chawla M, et al. Imiquimod 5% cream monotherapy for cutaneous squamous cell carcinoma in situ (Bowen's disease): a randomized, double-blind, placebo-controlled trial. J Am Acad Dermatol. 2006;54:1025–1032.
31. Peris K, Micantonio T, Fargnoli MC, et al. Imiquimod 5% cream in the treatment of Bowen's disease and invasive squamous cell carcinoma. J Am Acad Dermatol. 2006;55:324–327.
32. Mandekou-Lefaki I, Delli F, Koussidou-Eremondi T, et al. Imiquimod 5% cream: a new treatment for Bowen's disease. Int J Tissue React. 2005;27:31–38.
33. Mackenzie-Wood A, Kossard S, de Launey J, et al. Imiquimod 5% cream in the treatment of Bowen's disease. J Am Acad Dermatol. 2001;44:462–470.
34. Rosen T, Harting M, Gibson M. Treatment of Bowen's disease with topical 5% imiquimod cream: retrospective study. Dermatol Surg. 2007;33:427–432.
35. Mahto M, Nathan M, O'Mahony C. More than a decade on: review of the use of imiquimod in lower anogenital intraepithelial neoplasia. Int J STD AIDS. 2010;21:8–16.
36. Bath-Hextall F, Perkins W, Bong J, et al. Interventions for basal cell carcinoma of the skin. Cochrane Database Syst Rev. 2007;(1):CD003412.
37. Alessi SS, Sanches JA, de Oliveira WR, et al. Treatment of cutaneous tumors with topical 5% imiquimod cream. Clinics (Sao Paulo). 2009;64:961–966.
38. Wagstaff AJ, Perry CM. Topical imiquimod: a review of its use in the management of anogenital warts, actinic keratoses, basal cell carcinoma and other skin lesions. Drugs. 2007;67:2187–2210.
39. Junkins-Hopkins JM. Imiquimod use in the treatment of lentigo maligna. J Am Acad Dermatol. 2009;61:865–867.
40. Célestin Schartz NE, Chevret S, Paz C, et al. Imiquimod 5% cream for treatment of HIV-negative Kaposi's sarcoma skin lesions: a phase I to II, open-label trial in 17 patients. J Am Acad Dermatol. 2008;58:585–591.
41. Martínez-González MC, Verea-Hernando MM, Yebra-Pimentel MT, et al. Imiquimod in mycosis fungoides. Eur J Dermatol. 2008;18:148–152.
42. Badgwell C, Rosen T. Treatment of limited extent extramammary Paget's disease with 5% imiquimod cream. Dermatol Online J. 2006;12(1):22.
43. Martinez MI, Sanchez-Carpintero I, North PE, et al. Infantile hemangioma: clinical resolution with 5% imiquimod cream. Arch Dermatol. 2002;138:881–884; discussion 884.
44. Ezzell TI, Fromowitz JS, Ramos-Caro FA. Recurrent pyogenic granuloma treated with topical imiquimod. J Am Acad Dermatol. 2006;54(suppl 5):S244–S245.
45. Ulrich C, Bichel J, Euvrard S, et al. Topical immunomodulation under systemic immunosuppression: results of a multicentre, randomized, placebo-controlled safety and efficacy study of imiquimod 5% cream for the treatment of actinic keratoses in kidney, heart, and liver transplant patients. Br J Dermatol. 2007;157(suppl 2):25–31.
46. Neville JA, Welch E, Leffell DJ. Management of nonmelanoma skin cancer in 2007. Nat Clin Pract Oncol. 2007;4:462–469.
47. Rivers JK, Rosoph L, Provost N, et al. Open-label study to assess the safety and efficacy of imiquimod 5% cream applied once daily three times per week in cycles for treatment of actinic keratoses on the head. J Cutan Med Surg. 2008;12:97–101.
48. Sriprakash K, Godbolt A. Vitiligo-like depigmentation induced by imiquimod treatment of superficial basal cell carcinoma. Australas J Dermatol. 2009;50:211–213.
49. Jones T. Resiquimod (3M). Curr Opin Investig Drugs. 2003;4:214–218.

50. Szeimies RM, Bichel J, Ortonne JP, et al. A phase II dose-ranging study of topical resiquimod to treat actinic keratosis. *Br J Dermatol.* 2008;159:205–210.

51. Merck HF. Topical diclofenac in the treatment of actinic keratoses. *Int J Dermatol.* 2007;46:12–18.

52. Rundhaug JE, Fischer SM. Cyclo-oxygenase-2 plays a critical role in UV-induced skin carcinogenesis. *Photochem Photobiol.* 2008;84:322–329.

53. Ulrich C, Johannsen A, Rowert-Huber J, et al. Results of a randomized, placebo-controlled safety and efficacy study of topical diclofenac 3% gel in organ transplant patients with multiple actinic keratoses. *Eur J Dermatol.* 2010;20:482–488.

54. Ulrich C, Hackethal M, Ulrich M, et al. Treatment of multiple actinic keratoses with topical diclofenac 3% gel in organ transplant recipients: a series of six cases. *Br J Dermatol.* 2007;156(suppl 3):40–42.

55. Smith SR, Morhenn VB, Piacquadio DJ. Bilateral comparison of the efficacy and tolerability of 3% diclofenac sodium gel and 5% 5-fluorouracil cream in the treatment of actinic keratosis of the face and scalp. *J Drugs Dermatol.* 2006;5:156–159.

56. Choudhary S, Nouri K, Elsaie ML. Photodynamic therapy in dermatology: a review. *Lasers Med Sci.* 2009;24:971–980.

57. MacCormack MA. Photodynamic therapy in dermatology: an update on applications and outcomes. *Semin Cutan Med Surg.* 2008;27:52–62.

58. Merino R, Hurlé JM. The molecular basis of retinoid action in tumors. *Trends Mol Med.* 2003;9:509–511.

59. Wolbach SB, Howe PR. Tissue changes following deprivation of fat-soluble A vitamin. *J Exp Med.* 1925;42:753–777.

60. Pooja K, Koo JY. A review of the chemopreventative and chemotherapeutic effects of topical and oral retinoids for both cutaneous and internal neoplasms. *J Drugs Dermatol.* 2005;4:432–446.

61. Bollag W, Ott F. Vitamin A acid in benign and malignant epithelial tumors of the skin. *Acta Derm Venereol Suppl (Stockh).* 1975;74:163–166.

62. Moglia D, Fornelli F, Baliva G, et al. Effects of topical treatment with fenretinide (4-HPR) and plasma vitamin A levels in patients with actinic keratoses. *Cancer Lett.* 1996;110:87–91.

63. Alirezai M, Dupuy P, Amblard P, et al. Clinical evaluation of topical isotretinoin in the treatment of actinic keratoses. *J Am Acad Dermatol.* 1994;30:447–451.

64. Thorne EG. Long-term clinical experience with a topical retinoid. *Br J Dermatol.* 1993;127(suppl):31–36.

65. Bianchi L, Orlandi A, Campione E, et al. Topical treatment of basal cell carcinoma with tazarotene: a clinicopathological study on a large series of cases. *Br J Dermatol.* 2004;151:148–156.

66. Bardazzi F, Bianchi F, Parente G, et al. A pilot study on the use of topical tazarotene to treat squamous cell carcinoma in situ. *J Am Acad Dermatol.* 2005;52:1102–1104.

67. Robinson TA, Kligman AM. Treatment of solar keratoses of the extremities with retinoic acid and 5-fluorouracil. *Br J Dermatol.* 1975;92:703.

68. Bercovich L. Topical chemotherapy of actinic keratosis of the upper extremity with tretinoin and 5-fluorouracil: a double blind controlled study. *Br J Dermatol.* 1987;116:549–552.

69. Modi G, Jacobs A, Orengo IF, et al. Combination therapy with imiquimod, 5-fluorouracil, and tazarotene in the treatment of extensive radiation-induced Bowen's disease of the hands. *Dermatol Surg.* 2009;35:1–7.

70. Duvic M, Friedman-Kien AE, Looney DJ, et al. Topical treatment of cutaneous lesions of acquired immunodeficiency syndrome-related Kaposi sarcoma using alitretinoin gel: results of phase 1 and 2 trials. *Arch Dermatol.* 2000;136:1461–1469.

71. Bodsworth NJ, Bloch M, Bower M, et al. International Panretin Gel KS Study Group. Phase III vehicle-controlled, multi-centered study of topical alitretinoin gel 0.1% in cutaneous AIDS-related Kaposi's sarcoma. *Am J Clin Dermatol.* 2001;2:77–87.

72. Apisarnthanarax N, Talpur R, Ward S, et al. Tazarotene 0.1% gel for refractory mycosis fungoides lesions: an open-label pilot study. *J Am Acad Dermatol.* 2004;50:600–607.

73. Abbott RA, Whittaker SJ, Morris SL, et al. Bexarotene therapy for mycosis fungoides and Sézary syndrome. *Br J Dermatol.* 2009;160:1299–1307.

74. Heald P, Mehlmauer M, Martin AG, et al. Worldwide Bexarotene Study Group. Topical bexarotene therapy for patients with refractory or persistent early-stage cutaneous T-cell lymphoma: results of the phase III clinical trial. *J Am Acad Dermatol.* 2003;49:801–815.

75. Breneman D, Duvic M, Kuzel T, et al. Phase 1 and 2 trial of bexarotene gel for skin-directed treatment of patients with cutaneous T-cell lymphoma. *Arch Dermatol.* 2002;138:325–332.

76. Grimarte M, Etienne A, Fathi M, et al. Topical colchicine therapy for actinic keratoses. *Dermatology.* 2000;200:346–348.

77. Akar A, Bulent Tastan H, Erbil H, et al. Efficacy and safety assessment of 0.5% and 1% colchicine cream in the treatment of actinic keratoses. *J Dermatol Treat.* 2001;12:199–203.

78. Kim YH, Martinez G, Varghese A, et al. Topical nitrogen mustard in the management of mycosis fungoides: update of the Stanford experience. *Arch Dermatol.* 2003;139:165–173.

79. Ogbourne SM, Suhrbier A, Jones B, et al. Antitumor activity of 3-ingenyl angelate: plasma membrane and mitochondrial disruption and necrotic cell death. *Cancer Res.* 2004;64:2833–2839.

80. Green AC, Beardmore GL. Home treatment of skin cancer and solar keratoses. *Aust J Dermatol.* 1988;29:127–130.

81. Challacombe JM, Suhrbier A, Parson PG, et al. Neutrophils are a key component of the antitumor efficacy of topical chemotherapy with ingenol-3-angelate. *J Immunol.* 2006;177:8123–8132.

82. Siller G, Gebauer K, Welbrun P. PEP005 (ingenol mebutate) gel, a novel agent for the treatment of actinic keratoses: results of a randomized, double-blind, vehicle-controlled, multicentre, phase IIa study. *Australas J Dermatol.* 2009;50:16–22.

83. Anderson L, Schmieder GJ, Werschler P, et al. Randomized double-dummy, vehicle-controlled study of ingenol mebutate gel 0.025% and 0.05% for actinic keratosis. *J Am Acad Dermatol.* 2009;60:934–943.

84. Yarosh D, Klein J, O'Connor A, et al. Effect of topically applied T4 endonuclease V in liposomes on skin cancer in xeroderma pigmentosum: a randomized study. Xeroderma Pigmentosum Study Group. *Lancet.* 2001;357:926–929.

85. Cafardi JA, Elmets CA. T4 endonuclease V: review and application to dermatology. *Expert Opin Biol Ther.* 2008;8(6):829–838.

86. Strattin SP, Alberts DS, Einspahr JG, et al. A Phase 2a study of topical perillyl alcohol cream for chemoprevention of skin cancer. *Cancer Prev Res.* 2010;3(2):160–169.

87. Barthelman M, Chen W, Gensler HL, et al. Inhibitory effects of perillyl alcohol on UVB-induced murine skin cancer and AP-1 transactivation. *Cancer Res.* 1998;58:711–716.

88. Lluria-Prevatt M, Morreale J, Gregus J, et al. Effects of perillyl alcohol on melanoma in the TPras mouse model. *Cancer Epidemiol Biomarkers Prev.* 2002;11:573–579.

89. Mills JJ, Chari RS, Boyer IJ, et al. Induction of apoptosis in liver tumors by the monoterpene perillyl alcohol. *Cancer Res.* 1995;55:979–983.

90. Cooper SJ, MacGowan J, Ranger-Moore J, et al. Expression of dominant negative c-jun inhibits ultraviolet B-induced squamous cell carcinoma number and size in an SKH-1 hairless mouse model. *Mol Cancer Res.* 2003;1:848–854.

91. Stratton S, Saboda K, Myrdal PB, et al. Phase 1 study of topical perillyl alcohol cream for chemoprevention of skin cancer. *Nutr Cancer.* 2008;60:325–330.

92. Rhie G, Shin MH, Seo JY, et al. Aging and photoaging-dependent changes of enzymatic and nonenzymatic antioxidants in the epidermis and dermis of human skin in vivo. *J Invest Dermatol.* 2001;117:1212–1217.

93. Gensler HL, Aickin M, Peng Y-M, et al. Importance of the form of topical vitamin E for prevention of photocarcinogenesis. *Nutr Cancer.* 1996;26:183–191.

94. Foote JA, Ranger-Moore JR, Einspahr JG, et al. Chemoprevention of human actinic keratoses by topical DL-alpha-tocopherol. *Cancer Prev Res (Phila Pa).* 2009;2(4):394–400.

95. McCann PP, Bitonti AJ, Pegg AE. Inhibition of polyamine metabolism and the consequent effects on cell proliferation. In: Wattenberg L, ed. *Cancer Chemoprevention.* Boca Raton, FL: CRC Press; 1992:531–539.

96. Pegg AE. Polyamine metabolism and its importance in neoplastic growth and a target for chemotherapy. *Cancer Res.* 1988;48:759–774.

97. Einspahr JG, Stratton SP, Bowden GT, et al. Chemoprevention of human skin cancer. *Crit Rev Oncol Hematol.* 2002;41:269–285.

98. Bailey HH, Kim K, Verma AK, et al. A randomized, double-blind, placebo-controlled phase 3 skin cancer prevention study of alpha-difluorromethylornithine in subjects with previous history of skin cancer. *Cancer Prev Res.* 2010;3(1):35–47.

99. Alberts DS, Dorr RT, Einspahr JG, et al. Chemoprevention of human actinic keratoses by topical 2-(diflurormethyl)-dl-ornithine. *Cancer Epidemiol Biomarkers Prev.* 2000;9:1281–1286.

100. Einspahr JG, Nelson MA, Saboda K, et al. Modulation of biologic endpoints by topical difluoromethylornithine (DFMO), in subjects at high-risk for nonmelanoma skin cancer. *Clin Cancer Res.* 2002;8:149–155.

101. Reichrath J, Rafi L, Rech M, et al. Analysis of the vitamin D system in cutaneous squamous cell carcinomas. *J Cutan Pathol.* 2004;31(3):224–231.

102. Lu J, Goldstein KM, Chen P, et al. Transcriptional profiling of keratinocytes reveals a vitamin D-regulated epidermal differentiation network. *J Invest Dermatol.* 2005;124(4):778–785.

103. Seckin D, Cerman AA, Yildiz A, et al. Can topical calcipotriol be a treatment alternative in actinic keratoses? A preliminary report. *J Drugs Dermatol.* 2009;8(5):451–454.

104. Dixon KM, Deo SS, Wong G, et al. Skin cancer prevention: a possible role of 1,25 dihydroxyvitamin D3 and its analogs. *J Steroid Biochem Mol Biol.* 2005;97(1–2):137–143.

105. Cicarma E, Tuorkey M, Juzeniene A, et al. Calcitriol treatment improves methyl aminolaevulinate-based photodynamic therapy in human squamous cell carcinoma A431 cells. *Br J Dermatol.* 2009;161(2):413–418.

106. Gupta AK, Davey V, Mcphail H. Evaluation of the effectiveness of imiquimod and 5-fluorouracil for the treatment of actinic keratosis: critical review and meta-analysis of efficacy studies. *J Cutan Med Surg.* 2005;9(5):209–214.

107. Szeimies RM, Karrer S, Radakovic-Fijan S, et al. Photodynamic therapy using topical methyl 5-aminolevulinate compared with cryotherapy for actinic keratosis: a prospective, randomized study. *J Am Acad Dermatol.* 2002;47(2):258–262.

108. Freeman M, Vinciullo C, Francis D, et al. A comparison of photodynamic therapy using topical methyl aminolevulinate (Metvix) with single cycle cryotherapy in patients with actinic keratosis: a prospective, randomized study. *J Dermatolog Treat.* 2003;14:99–106.

109. Morton C, Campbell S, Gupta G, et al. AKtion Investigators. Intraindividual, right-left comparison of topical methyl aminolaevulinate-photodynamic therapy and cryotherapy in subjects with actinic keratoses: a multicentre, randomized controlled study. *Br J Dermatol.* 2006;155(5):1029–1036.

110. Kurwa HA, Yong-Gee SA, Seed PT, et al. A randomized paired comparison of photodynamic therapy and topical 5-fluorouracil in the treatment of actinic keratoses. *J Am Acad Dermatol.* 1999;41(3 Pt 1):414–418.

111. Rigel DS, Torres AM, Ely H. Imiquimod 5% cream following curettage without electrodesiccation for basal cell carcinoma: preliminary report. *Drugs Dermatol.* 2008;7(1 suppl 1):s15–s16.

112. Tillman Jr DK, Carroll MT. A 36-month clinical experience of the effectiveness of curettage and imiquimod 5% cream in the treatment of basal cell carcinoma. *J Drugs Dermatol.* 2008;7(1 suppl 1):s7–s14.

113. Berman B. Scientific rationale: combining imiquimod and surgical treatments for basal cell carcinomas. *J Drugs Dermatol.* 2008;7(1 suppl 1):s3–s6.

114. Jorrizo JL, Markowitz O, Lebwohl MG, et al. A randomized, double-blinded, placebo-controlled, multicenter efficacy and safety study of 3.75% imiquimod cream following cryosurgery for the treatment of actinic keratoses. *J Drugs Dermatol.* 2010; 9:1101–1108.

115. Berlin JS, Rigel DS. Diclofenac sodium 3% gel in the treatment of actinic keratosis post cryosurgery. *J Drugs Dermatol.* 2008;7:669–673.

116. Shaffleburg M. Treatment of actinic keratoses with sequential use of photodynamic therapy and imiquimod 5% cream. *J Drugs Dermatol.* 2009;8:35–39.

# Immune Response Modulators in the Treatment of Skin Cancer

Brian Berman, Martha Viera, Sadegh Amini, and Whitney Valins

## Key Points

- Interferons (IFNs) have antiproliferative, antiangiogenic and immunomodulatory properties that can be used to treat skin cancer, including malignant melanoma, Kaposi sarcoma (KS), basal cell carcinoma (BCC) and cutaneous T-cell lymphoma (CTCL).

- An immune response modifier stimulates both innate and acquired immune responses, including induction of IFNs, interleukin (IL)-12, and tumor necrosis factor-$\alpha$ (TNF-$\alpha$).

- A topical immune response modifier (imiquimod) is now being used for the treatment of actinic keratoses (AKs), superficial basal cell carcinoma (sBCC) and lentigo maligna (LM).

- IL-2 is being used in clinical trials as an adjuvant therapy for metastatic melanoma and advanced CTCL.

- Other immune-related medical agents are being investigated for their potential efficacy in skin cancer therapy.

## INTRODUCTION

The immune system possesses multiple effective mechanisms responsible for the surveillance, detection and elimination of cancer cells (Table 44.1). The importance of this role is appreciated in vivo by the generation of de-novo skin cancer after long-term immunosuppression following transplantation. Immunosuppression in these patients is associated with a dramatically increased risk of malignancy, most frequently non-Hodgkin lymphoma and skin cancer. Approximately 40% of transplant recipients develop premalignant skin lesions and non-melanoma skin cancer (NMSC) within the first 5 years of suppressive therapy.[1] On the other hand, cancer does not present only in immunocompromised patients, implying that tumor cells can evade the immune surveillance system. The possible mechanisms implicated in tumoral evasion of the immune system are listed in Table 44.2.[2-6]

Although surgery is the cornerstone of therapy for melanoma and NMSC, immunotherapy has also been used with success in controlling the growth and metastatic spread of tumors, particularly in patients with multiple or extensive lesions, critical tumor locations, or with certain genodermatoses or immunosuppression conditions.

This chapter focuses on the use of immune modulators in the therapy of skin cancer. Currently, therapeutic interventions to enhance tumor antigenicity or to increase the patient's immune response against cancer cells include recombinant cytokines, immune modulators, vaccination with tumor antigens, T-cell-based immunotherapy, and gene therapy. The role of retinoids, which have been suggested to possess immunomodulatory activities in the prophylaxis and treatment of cutaneous cancers, is addressed in Chapter 43.

## INTERFERONS

Interferons (IFNs) are a family of naturally occurring glycoproteins that have antiproliferative, antiviral and immunomodulatory properties. IFNs were the first immunotherapeutic modality used in the treatment of cancer. Depending upon cellular source and mode of induction, human cells produce three antigenically distinct forms of IFNs, originally described as leukocyte ($\alpha$), fibroblast ($\beta$), and immune ($\gamma$).

## Mechanism of action

In order to be active, IFN requires binding to specific receptors on the surface of target cells. The intracellular events following receptor binding leading to gene expression remain unclear.

Several mechanisms have been identified related to IFN's ability to treat skin cancer successfully (Fig. 44.1):

- Antiproliferative effects: IFNs affect all phases of the cell cycle. IFNs induce 2',5'-oligoadenylate synthetase with its products, PKR (double stranded RNA-dependent protein kinase) and MxA, through the activation of unidentified Jak kinase(s) and subsequent formation of the IFN-stimulated gene factor 3 (ISGF3) complex. Other effects include inhibition of mitosis and growth factors, downregulation of c-myc, c-fos and c-ras oncogenes, and of the p53 tumor suppressor gene. IFNs also induce or activate pro-apoptotic genes and proteins (e.g. TNF-related apoptosis-inducing ligand [TRAIL], caspases, Bak, and Bax), repress antiapoptotic genes (e.g. Bcl-2), modulate differentiation, and promote antiangiogenic activity.

- Upregulation of skin immune system: IFN-$\alpha$ and IFN-$\beta$ are generally less potent stimulators of major histocompatibility complex (MHC) antigens required for cellular immune reactions when compared with IFN-$\gamma$. IFN-$\alpha$ and IFN-$\beta$ are capable of enhancing/inducing the expression of class I and/or II MHC antigens on immunocompetent cells and tumor cells.

## Table 44.1 Antitumor Mechanisms of the Immune System

**Effector T cells:** Recognize an antigen presented in the context of class I and II major histocompatibility complex (MHC) molecules.

**Natural killer (NK) cells:** Lyse tumor cells in a non-MHC-restricted manner.

**Tumor-associated macrophages:** Stimulate CD4+ helper cells at the tumor site by expressing high levels of MHC class II antigens. Tumor killing mechanisms include secretion of cytotoxic cytokines, such as tumor necrosis factor-alpha (TNF-α), interleukin-1 (IL-1), nitric oxide, proteases and reactive oxygen intermediates.

**Co-stimulatory signals after antigen-specific stimulation:** B7-1 and B7-2 are capable of stimulating T-cell growth.

**Cytokines:**
Interleukin-2 (IL-2) activates NK cells.
Interleukin-12 (IL-12) stimulates Th1 responses, exerting a direct effect on T cells, inducing interferon-gamma (IFN-γ) production by NK cells, and augmenting the cytotoxic capacity of both NK and cytotoxic T cells.
Interferons have antiproliferative and immunomodulatory properties.

**Apoptosis** is a key factor in keratinocyte homeostasis.

## Table 44.2 Tumoral Evasion of the Immune System

### Secondary to Tumor Activity

Tumor antigens may be weakly expressed, may be recognized as 'self' antigens, or mutate.

MHC class I (or II in the case of melanoma) may not be expressed by tumor cells.

Tumor cells can secrete immune effector suppressors.

Tumor-induced immunosuppression over lymphocytes: recent studies imply that reactive oxygen species, produced by tumor-infiltrating monocyte/macrophages, may contribute to the state of lymphocyte inhibition in neoplastic tissue.[2]

Resistance of cancer cells to lysis mediated by homologous complement.[3]

Release of transforming growth factor-β1 (TGF-β1) can reduce dendritic cell (DC) migration and reduce their ability to mature into potent antigen presenting cells (APC).[4]

Expression of Fas ligand molecules on tumor cells interacting with Fas receptors on T cells, resulting in T-cell death.[5]

### Secondary to Faulty Immune System

Lack of tumor-reactive T cells.

Incomplete antigen processing.

Interleukin-10 (IL-10) may contribute to the development of skin squamous cell carcinomas after renal transplantation.[6]

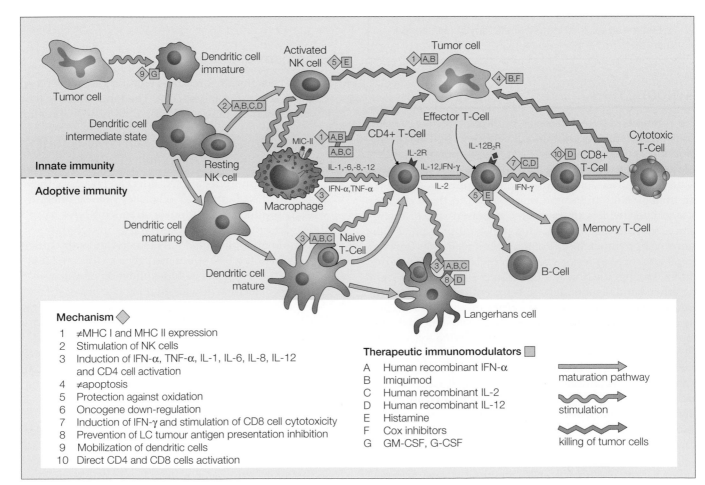

Figure 44.1 Mechanisms of action of immune response modulators in the treatment of skin cancer.

There is an increase in the number and activity of natural killer (NK) cells, macrophages and dendritic cells (DCs), following exposure to IFN, leading to an enhanced innate immune status.[7-10]

## Indications

### Malignant melanoma

Surgical excision using a 5 mm margin is the standard treatment for lentigo maligna (LM) (melanoma in situ) but currently there is evidence supporting other therapeutic modalities that can be applied in those cases where surgery is not possible.

IFN-α2b was the first immunotherapeutic agent approved for adjuvant treatment of stage IIB/III melanoma. It remains a mainstay of treatment and is the only adjuvant therapy for patients with melanomas thicker than 4 mm or with lymph node metastasis.[11] In a retrospective study, the combination of IFN-α2b and surgery led to a 48% 2-year and 36% 5-year relapse-free survival (RFS) rate in 150 patients with high-risk melanoma (stage IIC, III).[12] A randomized prospective trial did not find a significant difference between IFN-α2b-treated stage I–II melanomas and untreated controls.[13] In patients with disease limited to the skin and lymph nodes, the combination of isotretinoin and IFN-α has been reported to be only partially effective. In addition, the combination of IFN-α and chemotherapeutic regimens have failed to demonstrate efficacy over chemotherapy alone. As monotherapy for metastatic melanoma, IFN has not been shown to be efficacious, which has precluded its approval for the treatment of stage IV melanoma.[14-22]

Low-dose, adjuvant IFN-α used in stage II melanoma before sentinel node staging has been shown to prolong RFS before clinically detectable node metastases develop.[23-25] High-dose IFN has been shown to have an impact on RFS but a minor effect on overall survival (OS). In stage III melanoma, long-term adjuvant therapy (5 years) with pegylated IFN-α2b had a significant and sustained effect on RFS.[26] The efficacy was evident in sentinel-node-positive stage III patients compared with macroscopically involved stage III patients.

A high-dose IFN-α regimen incorporated an induction phase of maximally tolerated doses of IV therapy for the first 4 weeks. This is the only trial that showed prolongation of OS and RFS when compared to observation. Therefore, the induction phase may represent a critical component of this regimen, although this has not yet been tested prospectively.[11]

In a prospective, randomized study, 364 patients with melanoma stage IIB–III received either IFN-α2b five times per week for 4 weeks or the same regimen followed by subcutaneous (SC) IFN-α2b for 48 weeks. At a median follow-up of 63 months, the median RFS was 24.1 months and 27.9 months, respectively (p = 0.9) with median OS of 64.4 months and 65.3 months, respectively (p = 0.49). Patients treated with the second regimen had more hepatotoxicity, nausea/vomiting, alopecia, and neurologic toxicity.[27] An ongoing randomized trial comparing adjuvant IFN at a high dose for 1 month versus observation will provide more insight on the efficacy of this regimen in the adjuvant setting.

The identification of patients who are IFN-α sensitive is important in order to improve outcomes. Gogas et al. observed a correlation between the presence of autoimmune antibodies and improved outcomes after high-dose IFN-α treatment.[28] Other randomized trials determined that the presence of autoantibodies was not an independent predictive or prognostic factor,[29,30] but found IFN sensitivity to be higher in patients with ulcerated primary lesions.

A study assessing health-related quality of life (HRQOL) examined the effects of adjuvant pegylated IFN-α2b (PEG-IFN-α2b) on patients with stage III melanoma. At a median of 3.8 years of follow-up, RFS was reduced by 18% more in the PEG-IFN-α2b group compared with observation. Clinically, differences in social and role functioning scales and in appetite loss, fatigue, and dyspnea symptom scales were seen. The use of IFN-α2b leads to significant and sustained improvement in RFS but has negative effects on global HRQOL and selected symptoms. PEG-IFN allows patients to undergo prolonged weekly injections with the potential to improve the toxicity of IFN.[31]

Eleven biopsy-proven cases of lentigo maligna (LM) were treated three times per week with perilesional and intralesional IFN-α2b. All lesions cleared after treatment, without scarring. Controlled trials are needed to further characterize the use of IFN-α2b for LM when surgery is not an option.[32]

### Basal cell carcinoma

Although surgical modalities such as full-thickness excision and cryosurgery have high cure rates (95% and 94–99%, respectively), and acceptable associated morbidity, IFN represents an effective (70–100% cure rate) non-surgical approach to the treatment of basal cell carcinoma (BCC).[33] Buechner reported complete remission (CR) in four patients with nodular BCC (nBCC) treated with IFN-α at a low dose (1.5 million IU) three times weekly for 4 weeks.[34] A multicenter, randomized controlled trial (RCT) evaluating 172 patients with biopsy-proven BCCs reported that the optimal intralesional dose of IFN-α2b was 1.5 million IU, administered three times weekly for 3 weeks (Fig. 44.2). This IFN regimen resulted in an 86% clinical and histological CR rate compared with a 29% rate in the placebo group (P<0.0001).[35] Similar doses when used for aggressive (recurrent or morpheaform) BCC resulted in CR in only 27% of patients.[36]

In a recent study, 20 histologically proven BCC lesions were treated with intralesional IFN-α2a three times weekly for 3 weeks (1.5 × 10^6 IU for lesions <2 cm in diameter and 3.0 × 10^6 IU for lesions ≥2 cm). Eight weeks after the last injection, it was found that 55% of the lesions had clinical and histological CR, 30% had partial remission (PR), and 10% showed no response. Patients with a CR were followed up for 7 years, during which there was only one recurrence, at the fifth year.[37] Another study, by Tucker et al., using IFN-α2b to treat BCC, confirmed the long-term effectiveness of this treatment. Clinical cures were noted in 95/98 BCCs (51 nodular and 44 superficial), with a mean follow-up period of 10.5 years. The results showed 98% response rates at years 5 and 10, and a 96% response rate at year 15.[38] Although these studies show that intralesional and perilesional injections of IFN-α2b are effective in clearing

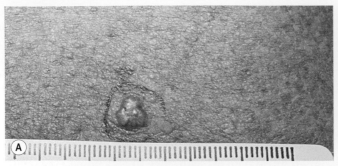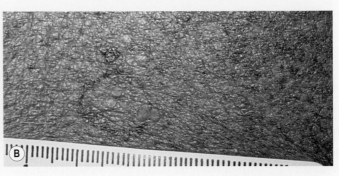

**Figure 44.2** Intralesional interferon-α2b for BCC.

BCCs with low long-term recurrence rates, it is not used as a standard treatment, due to its cost, safety profile, and the inconvenience of multiple injections.[39,40]

## Squamous cell carcinoma

Squamous cell carcinoma (SCC) of the skin constitutes 10–25% of NMSCs. The standard treatment is surgical excision or Mohs surgery; however, multiple studies have demonstrated the efficacy of intralesional IFN in the treatment of SCCs. Intralesional IFN-α2b, at a dose of 1.5 million IU, three times weekly for 3 weeks, was used in the treatment of 34 biopsy-proven SCCs, localized to sun-exposed areas. At the end of the study, 33/34 lesions revealed a histological CR.[41] Another study evaluated the efficacy and cosmetic results of intralesional recombinant IFN-α2b in 27 invasive and 7 in-situ SCCs (sizes ranging from 0.5 to 2.0 cm) at a dose of 1.5 million IU, three times weekly for 3 weeks.[42] Over 97% of the SCCs showed clinical and histological CR at 18 weeks, with a 96.2% CR rate in the 27 invasive lesions. The investigators and patients independently judged 93.9% of the cases to have a 'very good' or 'excellent' cosmetic result. In transplant-associated metastatic SCC, combination therapy with retinoids and IFN-α was used, with a 7% CR rate and a 36% PR rate.[43] IFN-α2b represents an important alternative treatment option for low-risk cases of SCC where surgery is not an option.[44]

## Keratoacanthoma

Keratoacanthomas are fast-growing, solitary, cutaneous neoplasms of unknown etiology that usually regress spontaneously. It is unclear whether or not they represent low-grade SCCs. Grob reported total resolution within 4–7 weeks with excellent cosmesis in five of six large keratoacanthomas (>2 cm in diameter) after receiving 9–20 injections with intralesional IFN-α2b.[45] Two other studies evaluated weekly doses of intralesional and perilesional IFN-α2b in a total of 11 large, rapidly growing keratoacanthomas. In a period of 7–15 weeks all lesions resolved completely, with satisfactory cosmetic results.[46,47] IFN-α is an option to treat large keratoacanthomas that cannot be surgically removed. Avoidance of scarring following surgery is one benefit of interferon, but the number of injections and patient visits may discourage its use as an alternative treatment.

## Actinic keratoses

A study evaluating intralesional IFN-α2b, 0.5 million IU three times weekly for 2–3 weeks, in the treatment of actinic keratoses (AKs) found a 93% CR following IFN-α2b injection, while no clearance was seen in the placebo group.[48] Edwards et al. examined the effects of topical IFN-α2b gel on AKs. Twenty-four subjects each treated three AKs with either topical IFN gel, 30 million IU/g, or placebo four times a day for 4 weeks. Although the results were not statistically significant, more lesions showed clinical improvement when treated with IFN.[49] The clinical usefulness of this treatment modality for AKs is quite limited because of the need for injections and multiple physician visits, which are not required by other treatments currently available.

## Cutaneous T-cell lymphoma

Cutaneous T-cell lymphoma (CTCL), including mycosis fungoides (MF) and Sézary syndrome, is a malignant proliferation of T cells with initial presentation in the skin. Most of the data on the use of IFN-α in CTCL has come from studies using recombinant IFN-α2a.

Bunn et al.[50] described an overall response rate of 55% and a CR rate of 17% among 207 patients with MF and Sézary syndrome treated with IFN-α2a. As a monotherapy, recombinant IFN-α2a is less toxic when used at low doses, and shows greater activity in patients with early-stage disease. Based on their review, the authors concluded that 3 million units administered SC three times per week is the optimal treatment for CTCL, with no apparent therapeutic differences between IFN-α2a and 2b.

The effectiveness of IFN-α has been found to be stage-dependent, with higher CR rates seen in stage I patients (50–62%) than in stage IV patients (8–16%).[51] Intralesional injection of MF lesions with IFN-α2b, at a dose of 1 million IU three times per week for 4 weeks, produced clinical and histological improvement, with 10/12 plaques obtaining CR.[52]

The effect of combining psoralen ultraviolet A (PUVA) with subcutaneous injections of IFN-α2a was evaluated in 63 CTCL patients (stage IA [n=6], IB [n=37], IIA [n=3], IIB [n=3], III [n=12], and IVA [n=2]).[53] IFN-α2a was administered at a dose of 9–12 million IU three times per week, given simultaneously with PUVA up to the minimal erythema dose. The initial treatments were administered three times a week until complete skin clearance, then once a week for 4 weeks, followed by treatments once every 2–4 weeks for an indefinite period of time. Seventy-five percent (47/63) obtained a CR, 6/63 obtained a PR, 2/63 were nonresponders and 5/63 had progressive disease. The median time to remission was 7 months; the median duration of response was 32 months, with a range of 6–57 months. CRs were obtained in all stages of disease. The combination of PUVA and IFN-α was assessed in a study involving 113 patients with all stages of MF or Sézary syndrome. A CR rate of 57% in early disease stages and 33.3% in later stages was found.[54] The combination of IFN-α and PUVA is superior to either agent alone. The combination of IFN-α and retinoic acid receptor (RAR) retinoids used in all stages of CTCL has shown an overall response rate of 60% with a CR of 11%, similar to the rates achieved with either modality when used alone.[55]

## Kaposi sarcoma

The use of IFN-α2a and IFN-α2b in the treatment of Kaposi sarcoma (KS) in patients with acquired immune deficiency syndrome (KS/AIDS) is approved by the U.S. Food and Drug Administration (FDA), but infrequently used.[56] IFN has antiviral and antiangiogenic effects, both of which are important for the survival of KS tumors.

The overall response rates with IFN-α2a and IFN-α2b were equivalent or superior to those achieved with conventional cytotoxic chemotherapy. The recommended subcutaneous doses of IFN-α2a and IFN-α2b are 36 and 30 million IU, respectively, three times per week. The average response rate of KS to high-dose IFN-α therapy has been approximately 30%. In many cases, tumor recurrence occurs within 6 months in complete responders and the response to a second treatment is not reliable. These facts led to the current recommendation of maintenance therapy as long as adverse events (AEs) are tolerated.[57]

Due to the decrease in the incidence of KS since the introduction of highly active antiretroviral therapy (HAART), it has been difficult to recruit patients for the evaluation of therapies including IFN. In addition, multiple AEs associated with IFN and the need for multiple injections has precluded its widespread use. Further research in order to better understand the mechanisms of action of IFN on KS and to determine optimal dosage is necessary.[56]

## Contraindications

Relative contraindications are cardiac arrhythmias, depression or other psychiatric disorders, leukopenia, pregnancy, and previous organ transplantation.

## Adverse events

The AEs of IFNs are dose-dependent and generally remit either during continued therapy or following dose reduction. In addition, the AEs are generally rapidly reversible upon cessation of therapy. AE management is summarized in Table 44.3.

- Anorexia.
- Influenza-like symptoms such as fever, chills, myalgias, headache and arthralgia may be controlled with acetaminophen and tend to remit with continued administration of IFN (tachyphylaxis).
- Cutaneous reactions: skin necrosis at the site of injection.

| Table 44.3 Management of the Adverse Events of Interferon | |
|---|---|
| **Adverse Event** | **Management** |
| Influenza-like symptoms | Hydration (2 L fluid daily); analgesics; antiemetics (in case of nausea and vomiting); bedtime administration of IFN |
| Cutaneous reactions | Topical antibiotics (in case of infection) and topical care with a corticosteroid-based cream can ameliorate the pain and reduce the size of the induration |
| Cardiovascular effects | Discontinue IFN; pharmacologic treatment depending on the condition (arrhythmias, hypotension, tachycardia) |
| Neurologic and psychiatric effects | Psychiatric consultation; prophylactic antidepressants in high-risk patients; initiate antidepressants in patients with symptoms of depression; assess for role of concurrent corticosteroids, β-blockers, reactive depression, brain metastases, thyroid dysfunction |
| Anorexia | Determine ideal body weight, weight history, eating habits; patient and family education; high-protein meals/supplements; multivitamins |
| Erectile dysfunction | Related pharmacologic treatment |
| Fatigue | Hydration (2 L fluid daily); assess for coexisting illnesses (anemia, electrolyte imbalance, poor nutrition, depression, hypothyroidism); improve nutrition; schedule periods of rest/activity |
| Hepatoxicity | IFN age adjustment; assess for alcohol consumption and hepatitis B |
| Hematologic toxicity | IFN dose reduction if severe |
| Hypothyroidism | Start levothyroxine; discontinue if thyroid function cannot be normalized |
| Ocular toxicity | Discontinue IFN |
| Psoriasis | Discontinue IFN; add pharmacologic therapy or phototherapy if psoriasis persists or worsens after IFN is discontinued |

- Fatal rhabdomyolysis and multiple organ failure occurred in a patient treated with high-dose IFN-α2b (20 million IU IV twice daily).[58]
- Cardiovascular effects: significant hypotension, arrhythmia or tachycardia (150 beats/min or greater) associated with IFN use can occur.
- Neurologic and psychiatric effects: spastic diplegia was reported in the treatment of infantile hemangiomas.[59] Depression and suicidal behavior have been reported in association with IFN-α therapy.
- Neutralizing antibodies can develop in patients receiving IFN-α2a and 2b. They appear to be specific to the recombinant IFN and do not neutralize natural IFN. Immune-mediated complications are infrequent, with thyroid disorders being the most common ones. The clinical spectrum of IFN-induced connective tissue disorders ranges from typical lupus erythematosus to rheumatoid arthritis. Patients with previous autoimmune phenomena should be identified.[60]
- Other AEs include gastrointestinal disturbances, erectile dysfunction, fatigue, hepatotoxicity, hematologic toxicity (leukopenia, thrombocytopenia, anemia), hypothyroidism, and ocular toxicity. Cases of exacerbated existing psoriasis and induction of de-novo psoriasis and psoriatic arthritis have been reported.[61]

PEG-IFN is a chemically modified form of recombinant human IFN. Initial data obtained in animal and phase I studies suggest that PEG-IFN injected once a week may be superior to human IFN injected three times per week. The safety of this modified form of IFN appears to be comparable to that of human IFN.[62]

## Use in pregnancy

IFNs belong to pregnancy category C and though it is unknown whether IFN is excreted in human milk, it has been shown to be excreted in mouse milk. The safety of IFN-α2b during pregnancy has not been studied formally; however, when it was administered to rhesus monkeys, it had abortifacient effects at doses equivalent to those administered to humans.[63]

## Drug interactions

IFN may cause inhibition of the cytochrome P450 enzyme system. Caution is advised when IFN is used in conjunction with potentially neurotoxic vinca alkaloids.

## IMIQUIMOD

## Introduction

Imiquimod is a potent stimulator of innate and cell-mediated immune responses with antiviral, antitumor and immunoregulatory effects, mostly through the induction of IFNs. Imiquimod 5% cream is FDA-approved for the treatment of genital and perianal warts, for non-hyperkeratotic, non-hypertrophic AKs and for sBCC, particularly in those cases where surgery is not an option.[64] Imiquimod 3.75% cream has been approved by the FDA for the treatment of AKs on the face or balding scalp.

## Mechanism of action

Imiquimod induces, in vitro and in vivo,[65] the production of cytokines, including IFN-α, TNF-α, interleukin (IL)-1, IL-2, IL-6, IL-8, and IL-12, by human peripheral blood mononuclear cells such as monocytes, macrophages, and Toll-like receptor (TLR) 7 and 8-bearing plasmacytoid DCs, where imiquimod exerts its activity in an agonistic fashion (Fig. 44.1). Through TLR, imiquimod induces nuclear factor-kappa B (NF-κB) leading to transcription of multiple genes that regulate the production of pro-inflammatory cytokines and of granulocyte colony-stimulating factor (G-CSF), granulocyte−macrophage colony-stimulating factor (GM-CSF), chemokine ligand 3 (CCL3) (macrophage inflammatory protein-1α [MIP-1α]), CCL4 (MIP-1β) and CCL2 (monocyte chemoattractant protein-1), mostly involved in the regulation of the innate immune system.[66] Imiquimod stimulates the production of IL-6, IL-8 and IFN-α by keratinocytes, resulting in a Th1-dominant response,[67-72] although antibody production by B cells, a Th2-type response, can be enhanced by imiquimod.[73] Cell-mediated immunity is stimulated by IFN-α, causing CD4 T cells to produce the IL-12 (β2) receptor. In CD4 cells, imiquimod-induced IL-12 stimulates the production of IFN-γ, which stimulates cytotoxic T cells responsible for killing virus-infected and tumor cells. Topical imiquimod has induced functional maturation of epidermal Langerhans cells in vivo and promotes their migration to regional lymph nodes.[74] Imiquimod also stimulates NK cells through the induction of 2′5′-oligoadenylate synthase, and induces perforin in cytotoxic T cells, both associated with its antitumoral effect.

Suppression of type I IFN signaling proteins is an early event leading to SCC.[75] Imiquimod increases the levels of type I IFN, improving the responsiveness to endogenous IFN-α, typically low in AKs.[76,77] The expression of FasR (CD95), a member of the tumor necrosis receptor family, has been evidenced on BCC cells after treatment with imiquimod (Fig. 44.3). Imiquimod-induced FasR-mediated apoptosis may contribute to imiquimod's efficacy in the treatment of BCC.[78] The pro-apoptotic activity of imiquimod has been attributed in part to the B-cell lymphoma/leukemia-2 (Bcl-2)-associated X (Bax) protein, independently of cell surface death receptors such as CD95, TNF receptors or TNF-related apoptosis-inducing ligand (TRAIL).[79,80] Imiquimod promotes the release of cytochrome c from the mitochondria, inducing the activation of caspases, including caspase-9 and -3, which have been linked with stress signaling, mitochondrial death pathways, and apoptosis.[81] Imiquimod's effects on the adaptive and innate immune system are summarized in Figure 44.4.

Imiquimod induces the expression of E-selectin on blood vessels in invasive SCCs after 10–14 days of treatment prior to surgical excision. E-selectin is a ligand for the skin addressin cutaneous lymphocyte antigen (CLA) which is expressed by skin resident T cells that are in charge of immunosurveillance, and is usually absent in SCCs. In addition, imiquimod has been associated with an increase in the number of infiltrating CLA+ skin homing CD8+ cytotoxic T cells and with the appearance of histological changes consistent with tumor regression, such as fibrosis surrounding SCCs. Although SCC blood vessels and dermal microvascular

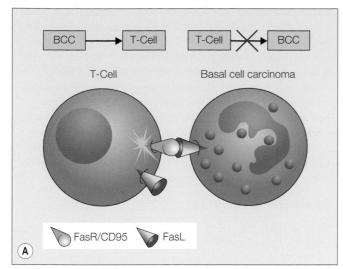
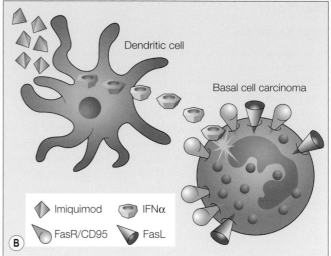

**Figure 44.3 A)** Basal cell carcinoma cells are protected by failing to express the FasR/CD95 'death receptor'. **B)** Imiquimod-induced BCC expression of FasR/CD95.

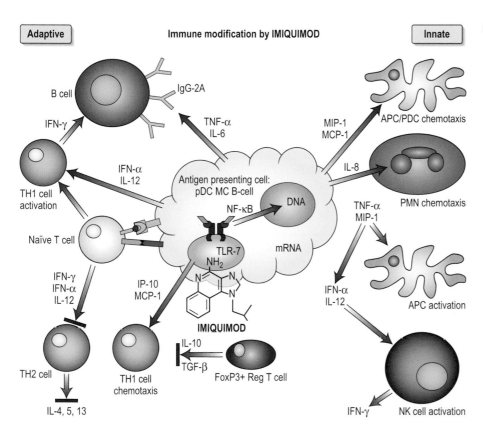

**Figure 44.4** Immune modification by imiquimod.

endothelial cells express TLR 7/8, their response to imiquimod requires the presence of antigen-presenting cells (APCs).[82]

Up to 50% of T cells infiltrating cutaneous SCCs are regulatory T cells (T reg cells) that express the transcription factor FOXP3. They are located surrounding the tumor nests and are responsible for the impairment of effector T cells that may reach the tumor. In SCCs, FOXP3+ T reg cells lack CLA and coexpress a phenotype similar to central memory T cells, usually found only in the blood or lymph nodes. Imiquimod induces a fivefold relative reduction of FOXP3+ T reg cells infiltrating SCCs, inhibits FOXP3+ T reg cells' suppressive capacity over T-cell proliferation (without reducing viability), and decreases the production of several cytokines, including IL-10 and TGF-β, in T reg cells from human skin. There is a strong correlation between high FOXP3 expression and suppression function.[82,83]

Percutaneous absorption of imiquimod is minimal, with less than 0.9% of a radiolabeled 5 mg dose being recovered in urine and feces. The site of potential metabolism and degree of protein binding, if any, is unknown.

## Indications

### Actinic keratosis

AKs are considered keratinocyte premalignant lesions with the potential to progress to SCC. Current treatments include local destruction, topical drug therapy, and photodynamic therapy. Imiquimod is a field-directed therapy with the advantage of treating multiple lesions, including subclinical AKs. Overall, CR rates achieved with imiquimod have ranged from 45% to 85%,[79,84-89] with recurrence rates of 10% and 16% within 1 year and 18 months of treatment, respectively, and approximately 20% at 24 months follow-up.[84,90]

In a multicenter non-controlled study,[91] imiquimod 5% cream was applied to 829 patients (7427 baseline AKs) three times per week for 4 weeks. After a 4-week rest period, a second 4-week course was applied in cases of remaining lesions. After the first course of treatment, a CR rate of 40.5% and an overall clearance rate of 68.9% was reported. A total of 85% of individual lesions cleared.

Several multicenter, prospective, double-blind RCTs are summarized in Table 44.4.[88,89,92-94]

Overall, thrice-weekly regimens were more effective than twice-weekly regimens. This difference appeared to be smaller than expected due to a low CR rate (40.8%) reported by one study evaluating the thrice-weekly application of imiquimod, and also due to random variation among clinical studies. Other differences between the thrice- and twice-weekly applications included the median percentage reduction in the number of AKs from baseline (>83.3% and 86%, respectively), and more local skin reactions (LSRs), more rest periods, and more treatment discontinuations due to LSRs associated with the thrice-weekly regimen.[93] The most frequent AEs reported with imiquimod included LSRs (i.e. erythema, scabbing/crusting, flaking/scaling/dryness, and erosion/ulceration) and mostly resolved 8 weeks post treatment.[88,89,93]

Forty-three post-transplant patients receiving immunosuppressive therapy within the previous 6 months applied imiquimod 5% cream or vehicle three times per week to a 100 cm² field for 16 weeks in a multicenter RCT.[95] Clinical/histological CR rates were 62.1% and 0%, respectively. The overall clearance rate of individual lesions was 73.7% and −99.1%, respectively. AEs reported with imiquimod included mild to moderate LSRs (5/29), fatigue (1/29), headache (1/29), diarrhea (1/29), nausea (1/29), rash (1/29), skin disorder (1/29), and leucopenia (1/29). No transplant rejection was reported during the study. Imiquimod was shown to be effective and well tolerated for the treatment of AKs in post-transplant immunosuppressed patients.

One or two 4-week courses of imiquimod 5% cream applied three times per week for the treatment of AKs were compared to one or two cryotherapy courses (20–40 seconds per lesion) and topical 5-fluorouracil (twice daily for 4 weeks) in an RCT.[96] A total of 85%, 68% and 96% of patients, respectively, had initial clinical clearance. However, at 12-month post-treatment evaluation, sustained clearance of initially cleared AKs was reported in 73%, 28%, and 54% of the patients, respectively (p<0.01). The histological clearance rates were 73%, 32% and 67%, respectively. Imiquimod also achieved the best cosmetic outcome (p=0.0001).

Two new concentrations of imiquimod cream (3.75% and 2.5%) were evaluated in a short-course and cyclic regimen of application in a phase III study in an attempt to optimize the use of imiquimod topically.[97] Once-daily imiquimod 3.75% for two 2-week treatment cycles, separated by a 2-week rest period, maximized tolerance while maintaining efficacy achieved with 5% imiquimod for prolonged 4 months treatment, as measured by median percent reductions in the number of AKs. The Food and Drug Administration (FDA) has recently approved imiquimod 3.75% for the treatment of clinically typical, visible or palpable AKs. This new concentration is suggested for use on large areas of skin, including the face or balding scalp, in a 6-week (2 weeks on, 2 weeks off, 2 weeks on) dosing cycle.

### Basal cell carcinoma

Several trials have documented the effectiveness of imiquimod 5% cream, an IFN-α inducer, in the treatment of sBCC or nBCC at low-risk sites. A summary of RCTs evaluating imiquimod 5% cream for the treatment of sBCC can be found in Table 44.5.[98-104] As a non-invasive treatment modality for sBCC, imiquimod may have some advantages over surgical procedures, particularly when the goal is to obtain good to excellent cosmetic outcomes.[100] The initial study of topical imiquimod 5% cream for nBCC and sBCC was a double-blind, 16-week, dose-ranging pilot RCT.[98] The histological CR rate varied depending upon the frequency of dosing, and the overall response rate was 83% (20/24) in the imiquimod-treated group and 9% (1/11) in the vehicle-treated group.

**Nodular basal cell carcinoma** Two phase II studies were performed to determine the safety and efficacy of imiquimod 5% cream for nBCC.[105] The highest response rate achieved using this modality of treatment was 76% in the twice-daily, 12-week group. The CR rates in these two studies were not as high as the CR rates seen in the studies treating sBCC with imiquimod 5% cream (Table 44.5). The efficacy levels in the treatment of nBCC does not compare with the surgical excision success rate.[36] Therefore, the candidates for this modality of treatment may be patients in whom surgery, radiotherapy or cryotherapy is not an option.

In a prospective, open-label study,[106] 19 lesions clinically diagnosed as nBCC received treatment with imiquimod 5% cream daily, three times per week on alternate days until clinical clearance of the lesion or until 12 weeks of treatment was completed. CR was obtained in 10/19 nBCCs (52.6%) in 10 patients. The most common AEs were LSRs, including erythema, erosion, ulceration, vesicle formation, and edema.

In a prospective, multicenter, open-label, randomized study,[103] 93 patients with biopsy-proven nBCC applied imiquimod 5% cream in one of four treatment regimens: twice a week without occlusion (n=21), twice a week with occlusion (n=22), three times a week without occlusion (n=24), and three times a week with occlusion (n=23) for 6 weeks. Six weeks after the end of treatment, CR rates in the thrice-weekly groups were 65% and 50% for patients with and without occlusion, respectively. CR rates in the twice-weekly groups were 50% and 57% for patients with and without occlusion, respectively. There was no significant difference in the CR rates between the groups (p=0.700). Sixty-three (70%) patients experienced at least one AE during the study. The most common AEs were LSRs, reported by 38 (42%) patients. A prospective, double-blind RCT[107] evaluated the effectiveness of imiquimod 5% cream in

## Table 44.4 Imiquimod 5% Cream for AKs: Summary of Multicenter*, Prospective, Double-Blind RCTs

| No. of Patients (no. of AKs) Location | Treatment | Outcome/Follow-up (I: Imiquimod, P: Placebo) | Adverse Events | Reference |
|---|---|---|---|---|
| 259 (855) Face or the balding scalp | OD 3×/wk for 4 wks + 4 wks rest + 3×/wk for 4 wks (in case of remaining lesions) | Complete response rate: I: 37.2% vs. P: 0.8% (p<0.0001) Overall CR rate I: 55.0% vs. P: 2.5% (p<0.0001) Overall PR rate I: 65.9% vs. P: 3.8% (p<0.0001) Individual lesion CR rate after 1 Tx I: 61.1% vs. P: 11.3% Individual lesion CR rate end of study I: 75.7% vs. P: 18.9% (p<0.001) High grade of agreement between clinical and histopathological findings Negative predictive value of investigator assessment (clinical vs. HP): 92.2% | Most common: Local skin reactions (erythema, erosion, scabbing, flaking/scaling/dryness) Most intense LSRs significantly more frequent with imiquimod than with vehicle. | Alomar et al.[92] |
| 492 (4–8 within a contiguous 25 cm² area) Face or the balding scalp | OD 3×/wk for 16 wks | CR rate I: 48.3% vs. P: 7.2% (p<0.001) PR rate I: 64.0% vs. P: 13.6% (p<0.001) F/U 8 wks: 50% of Pts had 86.6% reduction in no. of AKs vs. 14.3% (I vs. P, respectively) counted at baseline | At least 1 AE in 43.0% of Pts (I) vs. 48.2% (P) Most frequent: ASR in I: 38.8% vs. P: 7.2% (p<0.001) Most common ASR: Itching, burning, pain, tenderness | Korman et al.[93] |
| 286 (5–9 within a contiguous 25 cm² area) Face or the balding scalp | OD 3×/wk for 16 wks | CR rate I: 57.1% vs. P: 2.2% (p<0.001) PR rate I: 72.1% vs. P: 4.3% (p<0.001) Negative predictive value of investigator assessment (clinical vs. HP): 94.2% | At least 1 AE in 70.7% of Pts (I) vs. 8.8% (P) Most frequent: ASR in I: 46.3% vs. P: 11.5% Most common ASR: erythema, scabbing/crusting, flaking/scaling/dryness, erosion/ulceration Adverse events probably or possibly related to Tx: I: 51.7% vs. P: 12.9% At least one severe AE: I: 15.6% vs. P: 5% Discontinuation due to Tx: I: 4% vs. P: 3% | Szeimies et al.[89] |
| 436 (4–8 within a contiguous 25 cm² area) Face or the balding scalp | OD 2×/wk for 16 wks | CR rate I: 45.1% vs. P: 3.2% (p<0.001) PR rate I: 59.1% vs. P: 11.8% (p<0.001) F/U 8 wks: 50% of Pts had 83.3% reduction in # of AKs vs. 0% (I vs. P, respectively) counted at baseline | At least 1 AE in 77.2% of Pts (I) vs. 63.8% (P) Most frequent: ASR in I: 33% vs. P: 14.5% Most common ASR: erythema, scabbing/crusting, flaking/scaling/dryness At least one severe AE: I: 6% vs. P: 6.3% Adverse events probably or possibly related to Tx: I: 34.4% vs. P: 14.9% Discontinuation due to Tx: I: 3% vs. P: 1% | Lebwohl et al.[88] |
| 20 (at least 6 bilaterally symmetrically distributed in a 20 cm² area on the right or left side) (split face study) Face, head, or scalp | OD 2×/wk for 24 wks to one side and placebo to the other side | Marked improvement or greater I: 46.7% vs. P: 6.7% Average change in investigator assessment score I: +2.20 vs. P: −0.27 (p=0.0002) Average total lesion number score decreased I: from 1.93 to 1.47 (−0.47) vs. P: from 2.07 to 2.13 (+0.07) | AEs were minimal or non-existent Skin irritation intensity greater than mild was not reported by any Pt | Zeichner et al.[94] |

AE, adverse event; ASR, adverse skin reaction; CR, complete response; F/U, follow-up; LSR, local skin reaction; OD, once daily; PR, partial response; Pts, patients; Tx, treatment.

*Except Zeichner et al.[94] – single center.

Table 44.5 Imiquimod 5% Cream for Superficial BCC and SCC: Summary of Prospective RCTs*

| Study Design | No. of Patients (tumor), Size of TU | Treatment | Outcome/Follow-up | Adverse events | Reference |
|---|---|---|---|---|---|
| Prospective, randomized, double-blind, placebo (vehicle)-controlled study | 31 (BD) ≥1cm² to <20 cm² | OD for 16 wks | Complete clinical resolution in 9 (75%) Pts, 0 in placebo group (P<0.001). Mean change in lesion area between wk 0 and wk 28 (12 wks after stopping treatment): I: −322 mm², SD= 519 mm² P: −37 mm², SD= 114 mm² At wk 28, histological analysis confirmed that cases in the I group with clinical resolution no longer had BD 2/9 Pts had residual mild partial-thickness epidermal dysplasia In the placebo group (n=16), 10/16 Pts had persistent full-thickness epidermal dysplasia, 2/16 progressed to early invasive SCC, and 2/16 had severe epidermal dysplasia that no longer involved the full thickness of the epidermis Of those achieving clinical resolution at wk 28, no recurrence was observed at wk 52. 2/9 Pts with residual epidermal dysplasia showed no recurrences at wk 78, and further histology showed no epidermal dysplasia | 19 Pts experienced AE ranging from mild transient itching to edema with erosion and weeping | Patel GK. (JAAD 2006[76]) |
| Prospective, randomized, double-blind, vehicle-controlled study | 35 (28 sBCCs) 0.5–2.0 cm² | BID, OD, 3×/wk, 2×/wk, 1×/wk Applied 2 wks after clinical clearance or up to 16 wks | Clinical and histologic clearing: 83% (100% with BID, OD, and 3×/wk) | ASR in 92% (22/24) of treatment group. Itching, erythema, papular rash and discharge Severe reactions: erosion, induration, ulcerations (only in BID and OD groups) | Beutner et al.[98] |
| Phase II, multicenter, randomized, double-blind, vehicle-controlled, cohort study | 128 (sBCCs) 0.5–2.0 cm² | BID, OD, 5×/wk, 3×/wk, vs. vehicle for 12 wks | Clearance rates: BID: 10/10 (100%) OD: 27/31 (87.1%) 5×/wk: 21/26 (80.8%) 3×/wk: 15/29 (51.7%) Vehicle: 6/32 (18.8%) | At least 1 AE in 118/128 Pts (92.2%) Most common: ASR, including itching, pain and tenderness | Geisse JK et al.[99] |
| Two identical prospective, multicenter, randomized, double-blind, vehicle-controlled, cohort studies | 724 (sBCCs) Minimum area: 0.5 cm² and maximum diameter: 2.0 cm | OD 5×/wk, OD 7×/wk vs. vehicle for 6 wks | Clearance rates: 5×/wk: 139/185 (75%) (95% CI: 68–81%) 7×/wk: 130/179 (73%) (95% CI: 66–79%), Vehicle: 6/360 (2%) Histological clearance rate: 5×/wk: 152/185 (82%) (95% CI: 76–87%), 7×/wk: 142/179 (79%) (95% CI: 73–85%), Vehicle: 11/360 (3%). The difference between each active group and its corresponding vehicle group was statistically significant. (p<0.001) | During treatment: At least 1 AE in: 58% of Pts (5×/wk) 64% of Pts (7×/wk) 36% of Pts in the combined vehicle groups Post treatment: 33% and 31%, respectively More subjects experienced ASR in the 7× than in the 5× group (P=0.002) Most frequent: itching (16% and 26%), burning (6% and 9%), and pain (3% and 6%) in 5× and 7× respectively. Itching was significantly higher in 7× group than the 5× group (P=0.021). influenza-like symptoms, myalgia, malaise, fatigue, and fever in <3% of all pts. Severe AE in <10% of pts. | Geisse et al.[100] |

| Study design | Lesions | Dosing | Efficacy / clearance | Adverse events | Reference |
|---|---|---|---|---|---|
| Prospective, multicenter, randomized, parallel, vehicle-controlled, double-blind, phase III clinical study | 166 (sBCCs) Minimum area: 0.5 cm² and maximum diameter: 2.0 cm | OD 7×/wk for 6 wks | Post-treatment wk12, composite clearance rates: Imiquimod: 77% (95% CI 67–85%) Vehicle: 6% (95% CI 3—3%) (p<0.001) Histological clearance rates: Imiquimod: 80% (95% CI 70–87%) Vehicle: 6% (95% CI 3–13%) (p<0.001) Positive predictive value: 44% Negative predictive value: 91% | At least 1 AE in: I: 44 (52%) V: 18 (22%) (p<0.001) Most common AE :ASR in: I: 27 (32%) V: 1 (1%) (p<0.001) Most common ASR: itching, burning At least 1 SAE in: I: 8 (10%) V: 3 (4%) (p=0.211) | Schulze et al.[101] |
| Prospective, multicenter, randomized, open-label, dose-frequency | 99 (sBCCs) 0.5–2.0 cm² | BID, OD, BID 3×/wk, OD 3×/wk for 6 wks | Complete response rate: 77/99 (77.8%) Dose response gradient (intent-to-treat data): BID:3/3 (100%) OD: 29/33 (87.9%) BID 3×/wk: 22/30 (73.3%) OD 3×/wk: 23/33 (69.7%) OD application significantly correlated with the most intense erosion reaction (p=0.035) | At least 1 AE (ASR) in: BID: 3/3 (100%) OD: 22/33 (67.7%) BID 3×/wk: 16/30 (53.3%) OD 3×/wk: 17/33 (51.5%) Most common: Itching, pain, weeping. Most common: site reactions (by investigator): erythema, erosion, scabbing | Marks et al.[102] |
| Prospective, multicenter, open-label, randomized | 93 (sBCCs) 0.5–2.0 cm² | 2×/wk, 3×/wk, 2×/wk+occlusion, 3×/wk+occlusion for 6 wks | Clearance rates: 3×/wk: 20/23 (87%) 3×/wk+occ: 19/25 (76%) 2×/wk: 9/21 (43%) 2×/wk+occ: 12/24 (50%)× Significant difference between 2×/wk+occ and 3×/wk+occ (P=0.004) Clinical and histological evaluation at 6 wks post treatment: 22/66 sBCC clinically cleared, but TU remained (by histology) | At least 1 AE in 55/93 (59%) Pts. Most frequent: ASR in 30 Pts (32%). Itching, burning, and hypopigmentation Investigator assessment: most mild to moderate (erythema and induration), most frequent in 3×/wk groups Severe skin reactions seen in 3×/wk+occ > w/o occ In the 2×/wk it was the contrary: w/o occ > +occ | Sterry et al.[103] |
| Prospective, open-label, cohort study | 21 (23 BCCs), median size: 1.2 cm (0.4–1.9 cm) 19 (22 SCCs), median size: 1.1 cm (0.5–1.8 cm) 13/19 SCCs (59%) were intraepithelial | Cohort 1: OD 5×/wk, 14 days after Bx + curettage (38/45: 84%) Cohort 2: OD 5×/wk, 14 days after Bx alone (7/45) BCCs (median of 22 applications for median duration 6 wks) SCCs (median of 20 applications for median duration 6 wks) | 3–11 wks after the completion of treatment Bx showed residual tumor in 2/23 (9%) BCCs. One residual BCC received 6 additional wks of imiquimod; the other residual BCC underwent Mohs micrographic surgery 1/22 (5%) SCCs had residual tumor. The subject was treated with radiation therapy Median F/U for BCCs: 26 months. Median F/U for SCCs: 27 months. Only one subject with SCC experienced a recurrence | Most had mild to moderate skin reactions 8/21 subjects with BCCs and 3/21 with SCCs had significant skin reactions Some subjects required a rest period | Tillman et al.[104] |

* Except Tillman et al.[104]

reducing the number of Mohs stages and defect size, among other parameters. A total of 31 patients with histologically confirmed nBCC received imiquimod (n=15) or vehicle (n=16) nightly for 6 weeks under occlusion. At 4 weeks post treatment, Mohs micrographic surgery was performed at the target sites. Imiquimod 5% cream was shown to be ineffective for the reduction of the number of Mohs stages, size of the defects, and cost of the procedures and repairs. In addition, clearance rates were lower than expected in the imiquimod-treated group. The authors noted that these results were probably due to the small sample size.

### Challenging cases with multiple or large BCCs

Examples of special cases of BCCs treated with imiquimod 5% cream include a case of a large (5 × 6 cm) sBCC,[108] a patient with basal cell nevus syndrome with multiple BCCs,[109] and two patients with xeroderma pigmentosum, in whom topical imiquimod decreased the rate of new tumor formation, permitting dermatologists to 'keep up' with the surgical treatment of these new lesions.[110] Further clinical trials are required to confirm imiquimod's efficacy in larger BCCs and BCCs with aggressive growth patterns.

### Bowen's disease

A double-blind RCT[111] showing the efficacy of imiquimod 5% cream for the treatment of Bowen's disease (BD) is summarized in Table 44.5. Other studies include a phase II open-label study,[112] where 16 patients with biopsy-proven plaques of BD, with diameters ranging from 1 to 5.4 cm, received imiquimod 5% cream once daily for 16 weeks. Fourteen of 15 patients (93%) had no residual tumor histologically at 6 weeks post treatment. Six patients discontinued treatment due to LSRs, including superficial erosions and hemorrhagic crusting. No recurrences were reported after a follow-up period of 6 months. A retrospective study[113] evaluated 49 patients with BD treated with imiquimod 5% cream daily on non-genital areas and every other day on genital areas for at least 6 weeks. Eighty-six percent of the patients had clinical CR, and 4% had clinical PR. After a mean follow-up of 19 months (1–44 months) no recurrences were detected among the complete responders. In a case series,[114] four patients with a total of five BD lesions applied imiquimod 5% cream once for five consecutive nights per week until clinical clearance or until completion of 16 weeks of treatment. After 8–12 weeks of treatment, CR (complete disappearance of the lesion) was reported in 80% of the lesions, while PR (≥40% and <100% reduction in tumor size) was reported in 20% of the lesions. Post-treatment hypopigmentation in the treated areas was reported in four of five lesions. No recurrences were reported after a follow-up of 26–38 months.

Several case reports have been published illustrating the efficacy of imiquimod in treating genital and non-genital BD (Table 44.6).[115-123] The combination of imiquimod 5% cream and 5-fluorouracil (5-FU) 5% cream is an effective therapy in immunosuppressed populations. Five renal transplant patients were treated successfully with imiquimod and 5-FU for BD plaques in multiple areas, ranging in size from 1.5 to 5.0 cm, following their transplants (range: 10–18 years).[124] Imiquimod 5% cream was applied to the BD plaques and to a 1 cm rim of perilesional skin three nights a week. In addition, 5-FU 5% cream was applied every morning and on the remaining four nights of the week. Both medications were applied for 9 weeks in all patients. After 3–15 months

of follow-up, no residual lesions were reported. Figure 44.5 shows a case of BD of the face, which resolved after imiquimod once daily for 1 month.

### Invasive squamous cell carcinoma

Several case reports have shown that imiquimod 5% cream is an effective alternative for the treatment of invasive SCC, particularly in early lesions or when surgery is contraindicated.[114,125-132] In a patient with two poorly differentiated invasive SCCs,[126] imiquimod 5% cream was applied until complete clinical clearance of the lesions (19 weeks). The histopathological evaluation showed 'only a focus of dysplastic cells with no invasion' in one lesion, and 'epidermal hyperplasia with no significant cytological atypia' in another, with no evidence of invasive SCC. No recurrences after 16 months of follow-up were reported. A third lesion in the patient failed to respond to imiquimod. Since histological assessment of tumor margins are not usually performed after treatment with imiquimod, periodic clinical evaluations are warranted[125] (Fig. 44.6).

### Bowenoid papulosis

Bowenoid papulosis is a human papillomavirus (HPV)-induced condition mostly caused by the high-risk genotypes 16 and 18. Although histologically characterized by changes resembling SCC in situ and classified as such, there is low risk for progression to invasive disease.[133] Treatment with excisional surgery, electrocoagulation, cryotherapy, and 5-FU has been attempted with variable success. A 38-year-old woman with bowenoid papulosis was treated with imiquimod 5% cream on alternating days for 10 days until the skin became visibly irritated. The cream was then applied once daily for another 10 days, but washed off after 2 hours. Clinical and histological CR was noted within 8 weeks. The patient remained clinically clear for more than 18 months post treatment.[134] A 25-year-old uncircumcised male with a biopsy-proven bowenoid papulosis lesion on the glans penis received treatment with imiquimod 5% cream once every other day for 4 weeks and achieved 75% reduction in the lesion size. Four additional weeks of treatment resulted in complete clearance of the lesion. Histological evaluation at 1 month post treatment showed absence of both disease and HPV DNA.[133] Another case report described a 23-year-old male also with a biopsy-proven bowenoid papulosis lesion on the glans penis, with real-time polymerase chain reaction (RT-PCR) positive for HPV16, who obtained CR after being treated with imiquimod 5% cream every other day for 8 weeks. Evaluation at 3 months post treatment showed no recurrence of the disease.[135] A 36-year-old woman with extensive biopsy-proven bowenoid papulosis lesions in the genital and perianal regions, with HPV-16 DNA sequences detected, received treatment with imiquimod 5% cream once every other day for 4 weeks and obtained a discrete improvement. The imiquimod dose was increased to once a day for 8 weeks. At the end of the 12-week period, only 40% reduction in the lesion area was achieved. The patient refused any other treatment modality and imiquimod was continued daily for 12 more weeks, obtaining a 90% reduction in lesion size. The authors concluded that patients with limited disease respond better to imiquimod than patients with large lesions.[136]

## Table 44.6 Case Reports of Bowen's Disease Treated with Imiquimod 5% Cream

| Reference | Gender (imm. status) | Age (y) | No. of lesions | Size (cm) | Site | Treatment | Response |
|---|---|---|---|---|---|---|---|
| Schroeder & Sengelmann[115] | M | 65 | 1 | 5.2 × 3.5 | Shaft of penis | Nightly 2 cycles (11 and 13 days, 1 month apart) | 1 mo. after cycle 1: residual tumor 1 mo. after cycle 2: no evidence of tumor (clinical/histological) |
| Orengo et al.[116] | M | 41 | 1 | N/A | Glans penis | Twice daily, 3×/wk, for 12 wks | At 14 mo. post treatment: negative histological control |
| van Egmond et al.[117] | M | 62 | 1 | N/A | Perianal | 3×/wk. After 4 applications, 2 wks of rest due to LSRs. Then 4 wks | After 4 wks of treatment: CR After 3 mo.: only residual erythema + multiple Bx. showing no recurrence After 19 mo.: no recurrence |
| Thai & Sinclair[118] | M | 52 | 1 | 2 (diameter) | Penis (mid shaft) | 3×/wk for 3 wks | One mo. post treatment: CR After 6 mo. F/U: no recurrence |
| Taliaferro & Cohen[119] | M (HIV+) | 42 | 1 | 1.8 × 2 | Penis (mid shaft) | 3×/wk for 12 wks | Post treatment: clinical/histological resolution |
| Pehoushek & Smith[120] | M (HIV+) | 59 | 1 | N/A | Perianal + anal canal | 3 nights per wk + 5-FU 5% the remaining nights and all mornings, for 16 wks | 3 wks post treatment: 4 biopsies showed no residual dysplasia |
| Brannan et al.[121] | M | 75 | 1 | Within a 1 × 3 fibrotic plaque | Left lower eyelid | Twice daily every other day for 1 mo. (LSRs). Then, once daily every other day for 2 mo. Total = 3 mo. | 1 mo. post treatment: 4 Bx negative for BD 10 wks post treatment: complete resolution |
| Kossard[122] | F | 75 | 1 | 6 × 5 | Right preauricular area and cheek | Alternate nights for 6 wks | At the end of treatment: clinical CR At 8-mo. F/U: no residual lesion |
| Prabhu et al.[123] | M | 45 | 1 | 5 × 3 | Right thigh | 3×/wk for 3 mo. | At 3-mo. F/U: lesion flattened, persistent hyperpigmentation, Bx showed normal epidermis At 6-mo. F/U: Bx. negative for BD At 1-year F/U: no recurrence |

## Malignant melanoma

Imiquimod 5% cream has been suggested as a highly effective treatment for LM and may be considered in cases where surgery is not an option. Imiquimod has been found to significantly reduce the proliferation and viability of melanoma cells. In addition, imiquimod inhibits the migration and invasion of melanoma cells, even at sub-antiproliferative concentrations.

In an open-label study,[137] 30 patients with histological diagnoses of LM were treated with topical imiquimod once daily for 3 months. At 1 month post treatment, biopsies were performed on clinical and dermoscopic suspicious areas. Among the 28 patients, 26 (93%) showed clinical and histological CR. Ten patients required a rest period of more than 2 days,

because of severe LSRs that occurred from weeks 2–10, usually after seven to eight applications. Two of the patients who had CRs reported chills, malaise and headaches (considered severe AEs), leading to their early termination. Additional smaller studies[138–140] have reported similar results.

A retrospective study[141] evaluated 48 patients with biopsy-proven facial LM who applied imiquimod 5% cream to the lesion and a 2-cm margin of surrounding skin three times per week for 4 weeks, and then were instructed to increase the frequency to daily applications for a further 6 weeks if no inflammatory reaction was detected. Three months after the end of treatment, control biopsies were performed. A total of 37/40 patients (77%) had clinical and histological CR. After a follow-up ranging from 25 to 72 months (mean 48.6),

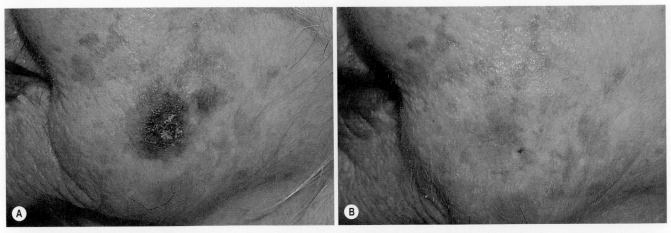

**Figure 44.5** Bowen's disease treated with imiquimod 5% cream: **A)** once daily for 1 month; **B)** 3 weeks after stopping treatment.

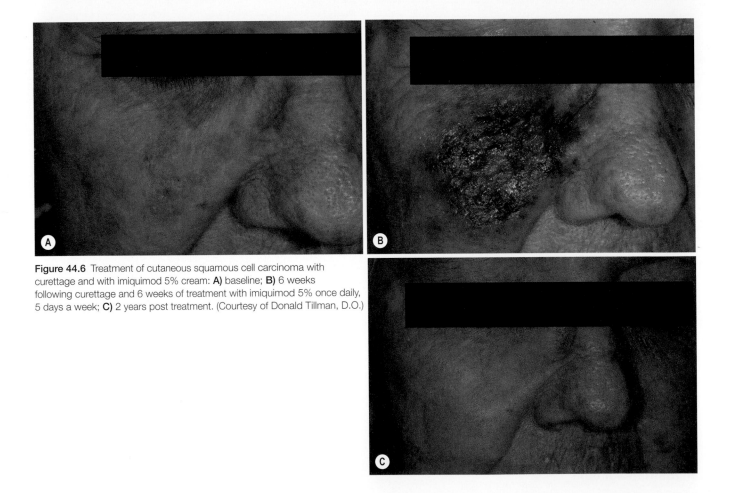

**Figure 44.6** Treatment of cutaneous squamous cell carcinoma with curettage and with imiquimod 5% cream: **A)** baseline; **B)** 6 weeks following curettage and 6 weeks of treatment with imiquimod 5% once daily, 5 days a week; **C)** 2 years post treatment. (Courtesy of Donald Tillman, D.O.)

no evidence of recurrence was reported in the imiquimod responders. In another retrospective study,[142] 40 patients with biopsy-proven LM were treated with imiquimod 5% cream five times a week for 12 weeks, and after a month, tazarotene 0.1% gel was added once nightly on weekends. Although clinical and histological clearance was obtained in 83% and 75% of patients, respectively, the authors concluded that imiquimod should be considered only as an adjuvant therapy to surgery for LM and should not be used as monotherapy.

Multiple case reports have been published in the literature showing that imiquimod 5% cream is effective in up to 93.5% (clinically) and 74.1% (histologically) for the treatment of LM,[143] for metastatic melanoma lesions unsuitable for treatment with excision or radiotherapy,[144,145] and for melanomas extending to the reticular dermis.[146] On the other hand, some reports have shown recurrences and even progression to invasive disease after treatment of LM with imiquimod 5% cream.[147-149]

## Cutaneous T-cell lymphoma

The cytokine profile expressed by clonal CD4+ tumor cells in the lesions of MF reflects an imbalance between Th1 and Th2 responses favoring Th2. Imiquimod is capable of inhibiting Th2 and stimulating Th1 responses, inducing IFN and other cytokines locally, and could be effective for the topical treatment of CTCL,[150] as IFN is effective for the systemic treatment of MF.[151] In a double-blind pilot RCT,[152] four patients with stable biopsy-proven patch or plaque stage MF were assigned to receive imiquimod 5% cream (n=3) or placebo (n=1) daily for 16 weeks, to areas measuring approximately 20 cm². The mean percentage reduction in the surface area of the lesions treated with imiquimod was 8.9%, compared with a mean percentage increase of 39.9% of the distant control areas in the same patient. There was improvement in the scaling and erythema in one patient, thickness in another, and no changes in the third patient in the imiquimod-treated group, compared to increases in the surface area, thickness and scaling in the patient receiving placebo. The authors concluded that imiquimod 5% is safe and well tolerated, and may have a therapeutic role in patch and plaque stage MF but studies are needed to further characterize this role. In an open-label pilot study,[153] six patients with stages IA–IIB MF received imiquimod 5% cream three times per week for 12 weeks. Imiquimod was well tolerated and induced a clinical CR in 50% (3/6). These three patients also had the most severe irritation on their target lesions. Histological clearance of index lesions (lesions chosen for pre- and post-treatment biopsy) correlated with significant reduction in the clinical scores for the corresponding lesions.

In a review by Martinez-González,[150] 20 cases of MF treated with imiquimod 5% cream reported in the literature were compared. The stage of the disease ranged from IA to IIB, and imiquimod was applied in varied regimens. CR was achieved by 14/20 patients (70%), PR by 3/20, and no response by 3/20 patients. The histological evaluation showed normal skin in 9/13 reports available (69%), PR in 1/13 and MF in 3/13 patients. Eight of 13 patients who showed a clinical CR also had normal skin (no MF) in their histopathological reports, while 1/13 patients had clinical CR and histological PR. The authors concluded that imiquimod could be an effective treatment modality, as monotherapy or in combination with other modalities, for the treatment of CTCL in early stages.

## Cutaneous extramammary Paget's disease

Extramammary Paget's disease (EMPD) is an infrequent epidermal malignancy with a high rate of recurrence that is associated with possible internal malignancies, and occurs most commonly in the anogenital and vulvar regions. The treatment of choice for EMPD is surgical excision, although recurrences often occur. Two cases are reported of perineal and genital EMPD treated with imiquimod 5% cream, with clinical cure occurring after 7.5–12 weeks of application of imiquimod 5% on alternating days of the week.[154] Cohen et al. describe the case of EMPD treated successfully with imiquimod 5% cream three times a week for 16 weeks. The authors also review nine cases located in the suprapubic area, scrotum, groin, penis, vulva, and buttock, which were treated with imiquimod 5% cream at least three times per week (and up to seven times per week) for 4–17 weeks. Post treatment, biopsies showed disease resolution in six of the patients for 2–14 months. The authors suggest the use of imiquimod 5% cream at least three times per week for a range of 8–16 weeks, with close follow-up.[155] One case of vulvar EMPD was treated with imiquimod 0.5% cream every other day and achieved clinical clearance at 11 weeks and biopsy-confirmed histologic remission at 27 weeks.[156] Because many cases of EMPD occur in the anogenital region, this modality of treatment offers a convenient, non-invasive therapeutic option.

## Actinic cheilitis

Actinic cheilitis can lead to invasive SCC. Therapeutic alternatives used in the treatment of this entity include superficial destructive methods, topical 5-FU, and photodynamic therapy. A retrospective review of 15 patients with a biopsy-determined diagnosis, who received topical imiquimod as a single agent three times a week for the treatment of actinic cheilitis, showed clearance of the treated area in six patients after 4 weeks of treatment and in the remaining nine patients after 6 weeks. Nine patients were followed up for at least 3 months with no evidence of recurrence.[157] In a case report, Greenberg et al. described two patients with actinic cheilitis treated with imiquimod 5% cream. In both cases, although the patients developed local severe reactions (i.e. hyperkeratotic patches and plaques, hemorrhagic crusting, edema), the actinic cheilitis resolved, with excellent cosmetic outcomes.[158]

## Major side effects

The most common AEs seen with imiquimod 5% cream are restricted to the site of application and include erythema (3%), ulceration (2%), edema (1%), excoriation (1%) and flaking (1%). Systemic AEs possibly or probably related to treatment include flu-like symptoms, fatigue, fever, headache, diarrhea and myalgia (in approximately 1–2% of patients).

## Contraindications

None known.

## Use in pregnancy

Imiquimod 5% cream belongs to pregnancy category C. It is not known whether topically applied imiquimod 5% cream is excreted in breast milk.

## Drug interactions

There are no known drug interactions with imiquimod 5% cream.

## RESIQUIMOD

Resiquimod is an imidazoquinolamine and TLR 7/8 agonist that has immunomodulatory effects comparable to imiquimod on monocytic cells, although the former is 10- to 100-times more potent than imiquimod.[159–161] Resiquimod also induces IL-1 receptor antagonist (IL-1ra), G-CSF, GM-CSF, MIP-1α, MIP-1β, and monocyte chemotactic protein (MCP-1).[70,75,161] In a phase II, dose-ranging study,[162] 132 patients with four to eight AKs in a contiguous 25 cm² area of the face or balding scalp applied resiquimod at concentrations of 0.01%, 0.03%, 0.06% or 0.1% once a day, three times a week for 4 weeks. CR rates after one course of treatment were 40.0%, 74.2%, 56.3%, and 70.6%, respectively. Patients with residual lesions received a second treatment course. Efficacy was similar with all resiquimod concentrations, but the lower two concentrations were better tolerated than the higher two concentrations.

In order to determine the direct effects of imiquimod and resiquimod on melanoma cells, a study was designed to assess cell proliferation, viability, migration and invasion in vitro.[163] In conditions devoid of TLR-7/8-bearing immune cells, imiquimod and resiquimod were found to significantly reduce the proliferation and viability of melanoma cells. In addition, both drugs inhibited the migration and invasion of melanoma cells, even at sub-antiproliferative concentrations. These effects, in addition to imiquimod's in-vivo immunomodulatory properties, may play a role in the observed clinical efficacy of imiquimod in treating LM and malignant melanoma. Further assessment of imiquimod and resiquimod as adjunctive treatments and/ or as alternatives in non-surgical melanoma patients are required.

## INTERLEUKIN-2 (IL-2)

Interleukin-2, secreted by CD4⁺ T lymphocytes after antigen recognition, has no direct effect on cancer cells. It is through stimulation of cytotoxic T lymphocytes, NK cells and macrophages that it exerts its antitumor activity (Fig. 44.1). IL-2 also induces the synthesis of specific cytokines, including tumor necrosis factor, IL-1 IL-6, and IFN-γ.

## Indications

### Cutaneous T-cell lymphoma

Seven patients with advanced stage (stage III–IVA) CTCL were treated with high-dose (20 million IU/m²/day) rIL-2, by continuous infusion, in a three-cycle 30-day induction phase, and five-cycle monthly consolidation phase. There was a CR in three patients (43%) and a PR in two patients (29%). Two of the remissions were durable (56–62 months).[164] An in-vitro study evaluating the immunologic effects of adding IL-2 to IL-12 as a model to overcome refractoriness to recombinant human IL-12 for CTCL demonstrated synergism, enhancing the levels of IFN-γ and both the NK cell activity of 15 CTCL patients, as well as the T-cell surface IL-12 receptor expression, in comparison with the effects of IL-12 or IL-2 alone.[165]

Denileukin diftitox (DD) is a fusion protein that combines the diphtheria toxin with the IL-2 receptor-binding domain, targeting cells that express the IL-2 receptor. By binding to and entering these cells, DD leads to inhibition of protein synthesis and eventually cell death.[166] DD has been approved for the treatment of CD25⁺ CTCL. It is administered IV, usually after premedication with dexamethasone, diphenhydramine and acetaminophen.[167] Interestingly, expression of CD25 is correlated with the histological stage of CTCL and with the response to DD treatment. In a prospective study involving 113 biopsy specimens from MF and Sézary syndrome patients, those with high expression of CD25 had a response rate of 78.5%, while those with low or no expression had a response rate of 20%.[168]

### Malignant melanoma

IL-2, which has been investigated in the treatment of metastatic melanoma, is the only cytokine approved for the treatment of stage IV melanoma. IL-2 in combination with histamine prolongs survival of patients with metastatic melanoma to the liver. Granulocyte–macrophage colony-stimulating factor (GM-CSF) has been used as rescue therapy in patients undergoing oncological therapy and may provide an antitumor effect that prolongs survival in clinically disease-free patients with melanoma.

## Contraindications

Patients with compromised general state, or specific cardiovascular pathology unable to tolerate the severity of IL-2 AEs.

## Side effects

Systemic high-dose IL-2 treatment is associated with severe AEs such as cardiac toxicity, thrombocytopenia, hypotension, fever and vascular leak syndrome, resembling the clinical manifestations of septic shock, in addition to respiratory toxicity.[169] Neurological and psychiatric disturbances may present as well.[170]

Others AEs include hypoalbuminemia, fever and chills, hypersensitivity reactions, nausea and vomiting, and asthenia. Elevation of liver enzymes may occur and visual acuity changes have been reported.[167] A few cases of thyrotoxicosis have been seen as well.

## OTHER THERAPIES WHICH INCLUDE IMMUNOMODULATIVE COMPONENTS

### Ingenol mebutate

Ingenol mebutate is a hydrophobic diterpene ester isolated from *Euphorbia peplus*, a plant known as milkweed, which has been reported as an effective home remedy (self-applied) in Australia for the treatment of AKs and BCCs.[171-174] Ingenol mebutate causes chemoablation by plasma membrane disruption, rapid loss of the mitochondrial membrane potential and subsequent mitochondrial swelling in dysplastic keratinocytes, followed by cell death by primary necrosis within 1 hour, and at the same time rapid induction of healing, resolution of the targeted lesions, and fast restoration of normal clinical and histological skin morphology.[171] This unique non-apoptotic mechanism of action allows ingenol mebutate to remain active even in the presence of apoptosis-resistant tumor cells.[175,176] Additional generation of tumor-specific antibodies, pro-inflammatory cytokines, and neutrophil infiltration results in antibody-dependent cellular cytotoxicity that eliminates residual cells,[177] characterizing ingenol mebutate's overall dual mechanism of action. Ongoing phase II and phase III studies are being conducted.

## Interleukin-12 (IL-12)

IL-12 stimulates Th1 responses by a direct effect on T cells, and also by induction of IFN-γ production by NK cells. IL-12 also augments the cytotoxic capacity of both NK and cytotoxic T cells. It is essential for an optimal, early response against tumors.[178] IL-12 prevents the inhibitory effects of cis-urocanic acid (cis-UCA) on tumor antigen presentation by Langerhans cells (LCs). Cis-UCA may play an important role in photocarcinogenesis by inhibiting a tumor immune response.[179]

In one study, IL-12 knockout mice were found to have an increase in the levels of cell survival kinases and an increase in UV-induced activation of NF-κB along with its downstream targets. Treatment of these mice with rIL-12 inhibited the increase in the levels of UV-induced proliferating cell nuclear factor (PCNA), cyclin D1 and NF-κB compared to untreated knockout mice. Therefore, loss of IL-12 may lead to enhanced photocarcinogenesis.[180]

A phase I dose-escalation trial with recombinant human IL-12 (rhIL-12) in patients with CTCL was conducted.[181] The study population consisted of 10 patients with the clinical and histological diagnosis of CTCL with plaques, tumors or erythrodermia (stage T1 [n=2]; stage T2 [n=3]; stage T3 [n=2]; stage T4 [n=3]). RhIL-12 was given at 50 ng/kg, 100 ng/kg, or 300 ng/kg twice a week SC. Treatment was performed for up to 24 weeks. A clinical CR was defined as complete disappearance of all measurable and evaluable lesions for at least 1 month. PR was defined as ≥50% disappearance of all CTCL skin lesions for at least 1 month. All patients with plaques had clinical improvement while receiving rhIL-12. Two of these patients who received a dose of 100 ng/kg had a CR at week 7 and 8, respectively. A previously detectable T-cell receptor rearrangement in the blood of a patient became undetectable at the time of the documented CR and remained undetectable at the conclusion of the treatment. Two other patients with plaques who received 100 ng/kg and 300 ng/kg, respectively, experienced a PR. One of three patients with Sézary syndrome completed the 24 weeks of treatment and had a documented PR. This patient started at 100 ng/kg, with dose escalation at week 4 to 300 ng/kg. Each of the two tumor-stage patients had rapidly progressive disease with numerous skin tumors at the time of initiation of rhIL-12. Both patients had progressive disease despite the treatment and both discontinued therapy. AEs were short lived (24–36 hours) and consisted of fatigue, headache, or myalgias. Two patients had transient elevations of hepatic enzymes. One patient experienced severe depression that resolved within 1 week of discontinuation of the rhIL-12. The results of this trial suggest that rhIL-12 is both efficacious and without serious AEs. In a phase II, open-label, multicenter study, rhIL-12 was administered SC twice weekly at a dose of 100 ng/kg for 2 weeks followed by 300 ng/kg thereafter to 23 patients with early CTCL (stage I–IIA), refractory to at least three other treatments. A 43% PR rate (>50% reduction in severity assessment) was seen after a median of 94 days of therapy.[182]

Intratumoral gene therapy with IL-12 has been applied through recombinant cDNA vectors and gene-modified DCs. In a phase I dose-escalation trial, plasmid IL-12 electroporation (the use of an electric charge to aid in the entry of molecules into the cell) was done in 24 patients with metastatic melanoma. The electroporation was done into the lesions on days 1, 5 and 8. Two of 19 patients with distant lesions showed complete regression of all metastases, while eight additional patients showed a PR or stabilization of disease.[183]

## FUTURE OUTLOOK

Studies assessing the effect of PPARγ on inhibition of melanoma development found ciglitazone and troglitazone to be effective.[184] Future therapies are under evaluation for the treatment of melanoma, including human antibodies (ipilimumab and tremelimumab), anti-CD137 antibody, and the TLR-9 agonist PF-3512676, and to date they have shown promising results.

Many therapies are currently under investigation, and, for some, there are already early promising data based on clinical experience. Because of the immunologic nature of most skin cancers, upcoming research that builds upon current studies will hopefully identify more effective immunomodulators that will better treat skin cancer.

## REFERENCES

1. Stockfleth E, Ulrich C, Meyer T, et al. Epithelial malignancies in organ transplant patients: clinical presentation and new methods of treatment. *Recent Results Cancer Res.* 2002;160:251–258.
2. Hellstrand C. Histamine in cancer immunotherapy: a preclinical background. *Semin Oncol.* 2002;29(3):35–40.
3. Donin N, Jurianz K, Ziporen L, et al. Complement resistance of human carcinoma cells depends on membrane regulatory proteins, protein kinases and sialic acid. *Clin Exp Immunol.* 2003;131:254–263.
4. Halliday GM, Le S. Transforming growth factor-beta produced by progressor tumor inhibits, while IL-10 produced by regressor tumor enhances, Langerhans cells migration from skin. *Int Immunol.* 2001;13:1147–1154.
5. Rabinowich H, Reichert TE, Kashii Y, et al. Lymphocyte apoptosis induced by Fas ligand-expressing ovarian carcinoma cells. Implications for altered expression of T cell receptor in tumor-associated lymphocytes. *J Clin Invest.* 1998;101:2579–2588.
6. Alamartine E, Berthoux P, Mariat C, et al. Interleukin-10 promoter polymorphisms and susceptibility to skin squamous cell carcinoma after renal transplantation. *J Invest Dermatol.* 2003;120:99–103.
7. Pestka S. Advances in cancer: interferon – achievements and potential. *N J Med.* 1987;84(1):51–56.
8. De Maeyer E, De Maeyer-Guignard J. You cannot get away from interferon. *J Interferon Res.* 1987;7(5):467–470.
9. Biron CA, Nguyen KB, Pien GC, et al. Natural killer cells in antiviral defense: function and regulation by innate cytokines. *Annu Rev Immunol.* 1999;17:189–220.
10. Theofilopoulos AN, Baccala R, Beutler B, et al. Type I interferons (alpha/beta) in immunity and autoimmunity. *Annu Rev Immunol.* 2005;23:307–336.
11. Kirkwood JM, Strawderman MH, Ernstoff MS, et al. Interferon alfa-2b adjuvant therapy of high-risk resected cutaneous melanoma: The Eastern Cooperative Oncology Group Trial EST 1684. *J Clin Oncol.* 1996;14:7–17.
12. Fluck M, Kamanabrou D, Lippold A, et al. Dose-dependent treatment benefit in high-risk melanoma patients receiving adjuvant high-dose interferon alfa-2b. *Cancer Biother Radiopharm.* 2005;20(3):280–289.
13. Creagan ET, Dalton RJ, Ahmann DL, et al. Randomized, surgical adjuvant clinical trial of recombinant interferon alfa-2a in selected patients with malignant melanoma. *J Clin Oncol.* 1995;13:2776–2783.
14. Thomson DB, Adena M, McLeod GR, et al. Interferon-alpha 2a does not improve response or survival when combined with dacarbazine in metastatic malignant melanoma: results of a multi-institutional Australian randomized trial. *Melanoma Res.* 1993;3:133–138.
15. Bajetta E, Di Leo A, Zampino MG, et al. Multicenter randomized trial of dacarbazine alone or in combination with two different doses and schedules of interferon alfa-2a in the treatment of advanced melanoma. *J Clin Oncol.* 1994;12:806–811.
16. Falkson CI, Ibrahim J, Kirkwood JM, et al. Phase III trial of dacarbazine versus dacarbazine with interferon alpha-2b versus dacarbazine with tamoxifen versus dacarbazine with interferon alpha-2b and tamoxifen in patients with metastatic malignant melanoma: an Eastern Cooperative Oncology Group Study. *J Clin Oncol.* 1998;16:1743–1751.

17. Middleton MR, Lorigan P, Owen J, et al. A randomized phase III study comparing dacarbazine, BCNU, cisplatin and tamoxifen with dacarbazine and interferon in advanced melanoma. *Br J Cancer.* 2000;82:1158–1162.
18. Young AM, Marsden J, Goodman A, et al. Prospective randomized comparison of dacarbazine (DTIC) versus DTIC plus interferon-alpha (IFN-alpha) in metastatic melanoma. *Clin Oncol (R Coll Radiol).* 2001;13:458–465.
19. Kaufmann R, Spieth K, Leiter U, et al. Temozolomide in combination with interferon-alfa versus temozolomide alone in patients with advanced metastatic melanoma: a randomized, phase III, multicenter study from the Dermatologic Cooperative Oncology Group. *J Clin Oncol.* 2005;23:9001–9007.
20. Vuoristo MS, Hahka-Kemppinen M, Parvinen LM, et al. Randomized trial of dacarbazine versus bleomycin, vincristine, lomustine and dacarbazine (BOLD) chemotherapy combined with natural or recombinant interferon-alpha in patients with advanced melanoma. *Melanoma Res.* 2005;15:291–296.
21. Bukowski RM, Tendler C, Cutler D, et al. Treating cancer with PEG Intron: pharmacokinetic profile and dosing guidelines for an improved interferon-alpha-2b formulation. *Cancer.* 2002;95:389–396.
22. Falkson CI, Falkson G, Falkson HC. Improved results with the addition of interferon alfa-2b to dacarbazine in the treatment of patients with metastatic melanoma. *J Clin Oncol.* 1991;9:1403–1408.
23. Grob JJ, Dreno B, de la Salmonière P, et al. Randomised trial of interferon alpha-2a as adjuvant therapy in resected primary melanoma thicker than 1.5 mm without clinically detectable node metastases. *Lancet.* 1998;351:1905–1910.
24. Pehamberger H, Soyer HP, Steiner A, et al. Adjuvant interferon alfa-2a treatment in resected primary stage II cutaneous melanoma. Austrian Malignant Melanoma Cooperative Group. *J Clin Oncol.* 1998;16:1425–1429.
25. Cameron DA, Cornbleet MC, Mackie RM, et al. Adjuvant interferon alpha 2b in high risk melanoma – the Scottish study. *Br J Cancer.* 2001;84:1146–1149.
26. Eggermont AM, Suciu S, Santinami M, et al. Adjuvant therapy with pegylated interferon alfa-2b versus observation alone in resected stage III melanoma: final results of EORTC 18991, a randomised phase III trial. *Lancet.* 2008;372:117–126.
27. Pectasides D, Dafni U, Bafaloukos D, et al. Randomized phase III study of 1 month versus 1 year of adjuvant high-dose interferon alfa-2b in patients with resected high-risk melanoma. *J Clin Oncol.* 2009;27(6):939–944.
28. Gogas H, Ioannovich J, Dafni U, et al. Prognostic significance of autoimmunity during treatment of melanoma with interferon. *N Engl J Med.* 2006;354:709–718.
29. Bouwhuis M, Suciu S, Kruit W, et al. Prognostic value of autoantibodies (auto-AB) in melanoma patients (pts) in the EORTC 18952 trial of adjuvant interferon (IFN) compared to observation (obs). *J Clin Oncol.* 2007;25(18S) Abstract 8507.
30. Bouwhuis M, Suciu S, Testori A, et al. Prognostic value of autoantibodies in melanoma stage III patients in the EORTC 18991 phase III randomized trial comparing adjuvant pegylated interferon a2b vs observation (abstract 5LB). *Eur J Cancer.* 2007;5:5.
31. Bottomley A, Coens C, Suciu S, et al. Adjuvant therapy with pegylated interferon alfa-2b versus observation in resected stage III melanoma: a phase III randomized controlled trial of health-related quality of life and symptoms by the European Organisation for Research and Treatment of Cancer Melanoma Group. *J Clin Oncol.* 2009;27(18):2916–2923.
32. Cornejo P, Vanaclocha F, Polimon I, et al. Intralesional interferon treatment of lentigo maligna. *Arch Dermatol.* 2000;136(3):428–430.
33. Telfer NR, Colver GB, Bowers PW. Guidelines for the management of basal cell carcinoma. British Association of Dermatologists. *Br J Dermatol.* 1999;141(3):415–423.
34. Buechner S. Intralesional interferon-alpha 2b in the treatment of basal cell carcinoma. *J Am Acad Dermatol.* 1991;24:731–734.
35. Greenway HT, Cornell RC, Tanner DJ, et al. Treatment of basal cell carcinoma with intralesional interferon. *J Am Acad Dermatol.* 1986;15:437–443.
36. Stenquist B, Wennberg AM, Gisslen H, et al. Treatment of aggressive basal cell carcinoma with intralesional interferon: evaluation of efficacy by Mohs surgery. *J Am Acad Dermatol.* 1992;27:65–69.
37. Bostanci S, Kocyigit P, Alp A, et al. Treatment of basal cell carcinoma located in the head and neck region with intralesional interferon alpha-2a: evaluation of long-term follow-up results. *Clin Drug Investig.* 2005;25(10):661–667.
38. Tucker SB, Polasek JW, Perri AJ, et al. Long-term follow-up of basal cell carcinomas treated with perilesional interferon alfa 2b as monotherapy. *J Am Acad Dermatol.* 2006;54(6):1033–1038.
39. Cornell RC, Greenway HT, Tucker SB, et al. Intralesional interferon therapy for basal cell carcinoma. *J Am Acad Dermatol.* 1990;23:694–700.
40. Chimenti S, Peris K, Di Cristofaro S, et al. Use of recombinant interferon alfa-2b in the treatment of basal cell carcinoma. *Dermatology.* 1995;190:214–217.
41. Ikic D, Padovan I, Pipic N, et al. Interferon therapy for basal cell carcinoma and squamous cell carcinoma. *Int J Clin Pharm Ther Toxicol.* 1991;29:342–346.
42. Edwards L, Berman B, Rapini RP, et al. Treatment of cutaneous squamous cell carcinoma by intralesional interferon-alpha 2b therapy. *Arch Dermatol.* 1992;128:1486–1489.
43. Kim KH, Yavel RM, Gross VL, et al. Intralesional interferon alpha-2b in the treatment of basal cell carcinoma and squamous cell carcinoma: revisited. *Dermatol Surg.* 2004;30(1):116–120.
44. Euvrard S, Kanitakis J, Claudy A. Skin cancers after organ transplantation. *N Engl J Med.* 2003;348(17):1681–1691.
45. Grob JJ, Suzini F, Richard A, et al. Large keratoacanthomas treated with intralesional interferon-alpha 2a. *J Am Acad Dermatol.* 1993;29:237–241.
46. Oh CK, Son HS, Lee JB, et al. Intralesional interferon alfa-2b treatment of keratoacanthomas. *J Am Acad Dermatol.* 2004;51(suppl 5):S177–S180. Erratum in: *J Am Acad Dermatol.* 2004;51(6):1040.
47. Somlai B, Holló P. Use of interferon-alpha (IFN-alpha) in the treatment of keratoacanthoma. *Hautarzt.* 2000;51(3):173–175.
48. Edwards L, Levine N, Weidner M, et al. Effect of intralesional interferon in actinic keratoses. *Arch Dermatol.* 1986;122:779–782.
49. Edwards L, Levine N, Smiles KA. The effect of topical interferon alpha 2b on actinic keratoses. *J Dermatol Surg Oncol.* 1990;16(5):446–449.
50. Bunn Jr PA, Hoffman SJ, Norris D, et al. Systemic therapy of cutaneous T-cell lymphomas (mycosis fungoides and the Sezary syndrome). *Ann Intern Med.* 1994;121:592–602.
51. Apisarnthanarax N, Talpur R, Duvic M. Treatment of cutaneous T-cell lymphoma: current status and future directions. *Am J Clin Dermatol.* 2002;3(3):193–215.
52. Vonderheid EC, Thompson R, Smiles KA, et al. Recombinant interferon-2b in plaque-phase mycosis fungoides – intralesional and low-dose intramuscular therapy. *Arch Dermatol.* 1987;123:757–763.
53. Chiarion-Silenu V, Bononi A, Veller Fornasa C, et al. Phase II trial of interferon-alpha 2a plus psoralen with ultraviolet light A in patients with cutaneous T-cell lymphoma. *Cancer.* 2002;95(3):596–604.
54. Anadolu RY, Birol A, Sanli H, et al. Mycosis fungoides and Sezary syndrome: therapeutic approach and outcome in 113 patients. *Int J Dermatol.* 2005;44(7):559–565.
55. Apisarnthanarax N, Talpur R, Duvic M. Treatment of cutaneous T-cell lymphoma: current status and future directions. *Am J Clin Dermatol.* 2002;3(3):193–215.
56. Krown SE. AIDS-associated Kaposi's sarcoma: is there still a role for interferon alfa? *Cytokine Growth Factor Rev.* 2007;18(5–6):395–402.
57. Krown SE. Interferon and other biological agents for the treatment of Kaposi's sarcoma. *Hem Oncol Clin N Am.* 1991;5:311–322.
58. Reinhold U, Hartl C, Hering R, et al. Fatal rhabdomyolysis and multiple organ failure associated with adjuvant high dose interferon alpha in malignant melanoma. *Lancet.* 1997;349:540–541.
59. Barlow CF. Spastic diplegia as a complication of interferon alfa-2a treatment of hemangiomas of infancy. *J Pediatr.* 1998;132:527–530.
60. Pia R, Ben-Bassat I. Immune-mediated complications during interferon therapy in hematological patients. *Acta Haematol.* 2002;107:133–144.
61. Ladoyanni E, Nambi R. Psoriasis exacerbated by interferon-alpha in a patient with chronic myeloid leukemia. *J Drugs Dermatol.* 2005;4(2):221–222.
62. Pehamberger H. Perspectives of pegylated interferon use in dermatological oncology. *Recent Results Cancer Res.* 2002;160:158–164.
63. Egberts F, Lischner S, Russo P, et al. Diagnostic and therapeutic procedures for management of melanoma during pregnancy: risk for the fetus? *J Dtsch Dermatol Ges.* 2006;4:717–720.
64. National Cancer Institute. *FDA approval for imiquimod.* < http://www.cancer.gov/cancertopics/druginfo/fda-imiquimod >; Accessed 30.10.09.
65. Dahl MV. Imiquimod: a cytokine inducer. *J Am Acad Dermatol.* 2002;47(suppl 4):S205–S208.
66. Schön M, Schön M. Imiquimod: mode of action. *Br J Dermatol.* 2007;157(suppl 2):8–13.
67. Yamamoto Y, Uede K, Otani T, et al. Different apoptotic patterns observed in tissues damaged by phenol and TCA peels. *J Dermatol Sci.* 2006;2(suppl):75–81.
68. Stuzin JM. Phenol peeling and the history of phenol peeling. *Clin Plast Surg.* 1998;25:1–19.
69. Kaminaka C, Yamamoto Y, Yonei N, et al. Phenol peels as a novel therapeutic approach for actinic keratosis and Bowen disease: prospective pilot trial with assessment of clinical, histologic, and immunohistochemical correlations. *J Am Acad Dermatol.* 2009;60(4):615–625.
70. Imbertson LM, Beaurline JM, Couture AM, et al. Cytokine induction in hairless mouse and rat skin after topical application of the immune response modifiers imiquimod and S-28463. *J Invest Dermatol.* 1998;110:734–739.
71. Wagner TL, Ahonen CL, Couture AM, et al. Modulation of TH1 and TH2 cytokine production with the immune response modifiers, R-848 and imiquimod. *Cell Immunol.* 1999;191:10–19.
72. Hemmi H, Kaisho T, Takeuchi O, et al. Small anti-viral compounds activate immune cells via the TLR7 MyD88-dependent signaling pathway. *Nat Immunol.* 2002;3:196–200.
73. Hengge UR, Ruzicka T. Topical immunomodulation in dermatology: potential of toll-like receptor agonists. *Dermatol Surg.* 2004;30(8):1101–1112.

74. Stanley MA. Imiquimod and the imidazoquinolones: mechanism of action and therapeutic potential. *Clin Exp Dermatol.* 2002;27(7):571–577.

75. Hengge UR, Benninghoff B, Ruzicka T, et al. Topical immunomodulators – progress towards treating inflammation, infection, and cancer. *Lancet Infect Dis.* 2001;1:189–198.

76. Berman B, Villa AM, Ramirez CC. Mechanisms of action of new treatment modalities for actinic keratosis. *J Drugs Dermatol.* 2006;5(2):167–173.

77. Kono T, Kondo S, Pastore S, et al. Effects of a novel topical immunomodulator, imiquimod, on keratinocyte cytokine gene expression. *Lymphokine Cytokine Res.* 1994;13:71–76.

78. Naylor MF, Boyd A, Smith DW, et al. High sun protection factor sunscreens in the suppression of actinic neoplasia. *Arch Dermatol.* 1995;131(2):170–175.

79. Schön M, Bong AB, Drewniok C, et al. Tumor-selective induction of apoptosis and the small-molecule immune response modifier imiquimod. *J Natl Cancer Inst.* 2003;95(15):1138–1149.

80. Schön MP, Wienrich BG, Drewniok C, et al. Death receptor-independent apoptosis in malignant melanoma induced by the small-molecule immune response modifier imiquimod. *J Invest Dermatol.* 2004;122(5):1266–1276.

81. Cryns V, Yuan J. Proteases to die for. *Genes Dev.* 1998;12(11):1551–1570.

82. Clark RA, Huang SJ, Murphy GF, et al. Human squamous cell carcinomas evade the immune response by down-regulation of vascular E-selectin and recruitment of regulatory T cells. *J Exp Med.* 2008;205(10):2221–2234.

83. Huang SJ, Hijnen D, Murphy GF, et al. Imiquimod enhances IFN-gamma production and effector function of T cells infiltrating human squamous cell carcinomas of the skin. *J Invest Dermatol.* 2009;129(11):2676–2685.

84. Tyring S, Conant M, Marini M, et al. Imiquimod; an international update on therapeutic uses in dermatology. *Int J Dermatol.* 2002;41(11):810–816.

85. Ooi T, Barnetson RS, Zhuang L, et al. Imiquimod-induced regression of actinic keratosis is associated with infiltration by T lymphocytes and dendritic cells: a randomized controlled trial. *Br J Dermatol.* 2006;154(1):72–78.

86. Stockfleth E, Meyer T, Benninghoff B, et al. A randomized, double-blind, vehicle-controlled study to assess 5% imiquimod cream for the treatment of multiple actinic keratoses. *Arch Dermatol.* 2002;138(11):1498–1502.

87. Salasche SJ, Levine N, Morrison L. Cycle therapy of actinic keratoses of the face and scalp with 5% topical imiquimod cream: an open-label trial. *J Am Acad Dermatol.* 2002;47(4):571–577.

88. Lebwohl M, Dinehart S, Whiting D, et al. Imiquimod 5% cream for the treatment of actinic keratosis: results from two phase III, randomized, double-blind, parallel group, vehicle-controlled trials. *J Am Acad Dermatol.* 2004;50(5):714–721.

89. Szeimies RM, Gerritsen MJ, Gupta G, et al. Imiquimod 5% cream for the treatment of actinic keratosis: results from a phase III, randomized, double-blind, vehicle-controlled, clinical trial with histology. *J Am Acad Dermatol.* 2004;51(4):547–555.

90. Gupta AK, Davey V, Mcphail H. Evaluation of the effectiveness of imiquimod and 5-fluorouracil for the treatment of actinic keratosis: critical review and meta-analysis of efficacy studies. *J Cutan Med Surg.* 2005;9(5):209–214.

91. Stockfleth E, Sterry W, Carey-Yard M, et al. Multicentre, open-label study using imiquimod 5% cream in one or two 4-week courses of treatment for multiple actinic keratoses on the head. *Br J Dermatol.* 2007;157(suppl 2):41–46.

92. Alomar A, Bichel J, McRae S. Vehicle-controlled, randomized, double-blind study to assess safety and efficacy of imiquimod 5% cream applied once daily 3 days per week in one or two courses of treatment of actinic keratoses on the head. *Br J Dermatol.* 2007;157(1):133–141.

93. Korman N, Moy R, Ling M, et al. Dosing with 5% imiquimod cream 3 times per week for the treatment of actinic keratosis: results of two phase 3, randomized, double-blind, parallel-group, vehicle-controlled trials. *Arch Dermatol.* 2005;141(4):467–473.

94. Zeichner JA, Stern DW, Uliasz A, et al. Placebo-controlled, double-blind, randomized pilot study of imiquimod 5% cream applied once per week for 6 months for the treatment of actinic keratoses. *J Am Acad Dermatol.* 2009;60(1):59–62.

95. Ulrich C, Bichel J, Euvrard S, et al. Topical immunomodulation under systemic immunosuppression: results of a multicentre, randomized, placebo-controlled safety and efficacy study of imiquimod 5% cream for the treatment of actinic keratoses in kidney, heart, and liver transplant patients. *Br J Dermatol.* 2007;157(suppl 2):25–31.

96. Krawtchenko N, Roewert-Huber J, Ulrich M, et al. A randomised study of topical 5% imiquimod vs. topical 5-fluorouracil vs. cryosurgery in immunocompetent patients with actinic keratosis: a comparison of clinical and histological outcomes including 1-year follow-up. *Br J Dermatol.* 2007;157(suppl 2):34–40.

97. Swanson N, Rosen T, Berman B, et al. *Optimizing imiquimod for treating actinic keratosis of the full face or balding scalp: imiquimod 2.5% and 3.75% applied daily for two 2-week or 3-week cycles.* Poster presented at the 12th World Congress on Cancers of the Skin; May 3-6, Tel-Aviv, Israel; 2009.

98. Beutner KR, Geisse JK, Helman D, et al. Therapeutic response of basal cell carcinoma to the immune response modifier imiquimod 5% cream. *J Am Acad Dermatol.* 1999;41(6):1002–1007.

99. Geisse JK, Rich P, Pandya A, et al. Imiquimod 5% cream for the treatment of superficial basal cell carcinoma: a double-blind, randomized, vehicle-controlled study. *J Am Acad Dermatol.* 2002;47(3):390–398.

100. Geisse J, Caro I, Lindholm J, et al. Imiquimod 5% cream for the treatment of superficial basal cell carcinoma: results from two phase III, randomized, vehicle-controlled studies. *J Am Acad Dermatol.* 2004;50(5):722–733.

101. Schulze HJ, Cribier B, Requena L, et al. Imiquimod 5% cream for the treatment of superficial basal cell carcinoma: results from a randomized vehicle-controlled phase III study in Europe. *Br J Dermatol.* 2005;152(5):939–947.

102. Marks R, Gebauer K, Shumack S, et al. Australasian Multicentre Trial Group. Imiquimod 5% cream in the treatment of superficial basal cell carcinoma: results of a multicenter 6-week dose-response trial. *J Am Acad Dermatol.* 2001;44(5):807–813.

103. Sterry W, Ruzicka T, Herrera E, et al. Imiquimod 5% cream for the treatment of superficial and nodular basal cell carcinoma: randomized studies comparing low-frequency dosing with and without occlusion. *Br J Dermatol.* 2002;147(6):1227–1236.

104. Tillman Jr DK, Carroll MT. Topical imiquimod therapy for basal and squamous cell carcinomas: a clinical experience. *Cutis.* 2007;79(3):241–248.

105. Shumack S, Robinson J, Kossard S, et al. Efficacy of topical 5% imiquimod cream for the treatment of nodular basal cell carcinoma: comparison of dosing regimens. *Arch Dermatol.* 2002;138(9):1165–1171.

106. Peris K, Campione E, Micantonio T, et al. Imiquimod treatment of superficial and nodular basal cell carcinoma: 12-week open-label trial. *Dermatol Surg.* 2005;31(3):318–323.

107. Butler DF, Parekh PK, Lenis A. Imiquimod 5% cream as adjunctive therapy for primary, solitary, nodular nasal basal cell carcinomas before Mohs micrographic surgery: a randomized, double blind, vehicle-controlled study. *Dermatol Surg.* 2009;35(1):24–29.

108. Chen TM, Rosen T, Orengo I. Treatment of a large superficial basal cell carcinoma with 5% imiquimod: a case report and review of the literature. *Dermatol Surg.* 2002;28(4):344–346.

109. Kagy MK, Amonette R. The use of imiquimod 5% cream for the treatment of superficial basal cell carcinomas in a basal cell nevus syndrome patient. *Dermatol Surg.* 2000;26(6):577–578.

110. Weisberg NK, Varghese M. Therapeutic response of a brother and sister with xeroderma pigmentosum to imiquimod 5% cream. *Dermatol Surg.* 2002;28(6):518–523.

111. Patel GK, Goodwin R, Chawla M, et al. Imiquimod 5% cream monotherapy for cutaneous squamous cell carcinoma in situ (Bowen's disease): a randomized, double-blind, placebo-controlled trial. *J Am Acad Dermatol.* 2006;54(6):1025–1032.

112. Mackenzie-Wood A, Kossard S, de Launey J, et al. Imiquimod 5% cream in the treatment of Bowen's disease. *J Am Acad Dermatol.* 2001;44(3):462–470.

113. Rosen T, Harting M, Gibson M. Treatment of Bowen's disease with topical 5% imiquimod cream: retrospective study. *Dermatol Surg.* 2007;33(4):427–431.

114. Peris K, Micantonio T, Fargnoli MC, et al. Imiquimod 5% cream in the treatment of Bowen's disease and invasive squamous cell carcinoma. *J Am Acad Dermatol.* 2006;55(2):324–327.

115. Schroeder TL, Sengelmann RD. Squamous cell carcinoma in situ of the penis successfully treated with imiquimod 5% cream. *J Am Acad Dermatol.* 2002;46(4):545–548.

116. Orengo I, Rosen T, Guill CK. Treatment of squamous cell carcinoma in situ of the penis with 5% imiquimod cream: a case report. *J Am Acad Dermatol.* 2002;47(suppl 4):S225–S228.

117. van Egmond S, Hoedemaker C, Sinclair R. Successful treatment of perianal Bowen's disease with imiquimod. *Int J Dermatol.* 2007;46(3):318–319.

118. Thai KE, Sinclair RD. Treatment of Bowen's disease of the penis with imiquimod. *J Am Acad Dermatol.* 2002;46(3):470–471.

119. Taliaferro SJ, Cohen GF. Bowen's disease of the penis treated with topical imiquimod 5% cream. *J Drugs Dermatol.* 2008;7(5):483–485.

120. Pehoushek J, Smith KJ. Imiquimod and 5% fluorouracil therapy for anal and perianal squamous cell carcinoma in situ in an HIV-1-positive man. *Arch Dermatol.* 2001;137(1):14–16.

121. Brannan PA, Anderson HK, Kersten RC, et al. Bowen disease of the eyelid successfully treated with imiquimod. *Ophthal Plast Reconstr Surg.* 2005;21(4):321–322.

122. Kossard S. Treatment of large facial Bowen's disease: case report. *Clin Exp Dermatol.* 2003;28(suppl 1):13–15.

123. Prabhu S, Rao R, Sripathi H, et al. Successful use of imiquimod 5% cream in Bowen's disease. *Indian J Dermatol Venereol Leprol.* 2007;73(6):423–425.

124. Smith KJ, Germain M, Skelton H. Squamous cell carcinoma in situ (Bowen's disease) in renal transplant patients treated with 5% imiquimod and 5% 5-fluorouracil therapy. *Dermatol Surg.* 2001;27(6):561–564.

125. Murua AA, González LC, García-Río I, et al. Coexisting perianal squamous cell carcinoma, Bowen's disease, and condylomata acuminata treated with topical imiquimod 5%. *Int J Dermatol*. 2008;47(12):1334–1336.

126. Konstantopoulou M, Lord MG, Macfarlane AW. Treatment of invasive squamous cell carcinoma with 5-percent imiquimod cream. *Dermatol Online J*. 2006;12(3):10.

127. Nouri K, O'Connell C, Rivas MP. Imiquimod for the treatment of Bowen's disease and invasive squamous cell carcinoma. *J Drugs Dermatol*. 2003;2(6):669–673.

128. Martin-Garcia RF. Imiquimod: an effective alternative for the treatment of invasive cutaneous squamous cell carcinoma. *Dermatol Surg*. 2005;31(3):371–374.

129. Oster-Schmidt C. Two cases of squamous cell carcinoma treated with topical imiquimod 5%. *J Eur Acad Dermatol Venereol*. 2004;18(1):93–95.

130. Hengge UR, Schaller J. Successful treatment of invasive squamous cell carcinoma using topical imiquimod. *Arch Dermatol*. 2004;140:404–406.

131. Flórez Á, Feal C, de la Torre C, et al. Invasive squamous cell carcinoma treated with imiquimod 5% cream. *Acta Derm Venereol*. 2004;84:227–228.

132. Oster-Schmidt C, Dirschka T. Therapy of cutaneous cell carcinoma in two retirement home residents. *J Dtsch Dermatol*. 2005;3(9):705–708.

133. Goorney BP, Polori R. A case of Bowenoid papulosis of the penis successfully treated with topical imiquimod cream 5%. *Int J STD AIDS*. 2004;15(12):833–835.

134. Petrow W, Gerdsen R, Uerlich M, et al. Successful topical immunotherapy of bowenoid papulosis with imiquimod. *Br J Dermatol*. 2001;145(6):1022–1023.

135. Matuszewski M, Michajłowski I, Michajłowski J, et al. Topical treatment of bowenoid papulosis of the penis with imiquimod. *J Eur Acad Dermatol Venereol*. 2009;23(8):978–979.

136. Ricart JM, Cordoba J, Hernandez M, et al. Extensive genital bowenoid papulosis responding to imiquimod. *J Eur Acad Dermatol Venereol*. 2007;21(1):113–115.

137. Naylor MF, Crowson N, Kuwahara R, et al. Treatment of lentigo maligna with topical imiquimod. *Br J Dermatol*. 2003;149(suppl 66):66–70.

138. Powell AM, Russell-Jones R, Barlow RJ. Topical imiquimod immunotherapy in the management of lentigo maligna. *Clin Exp Dermatol*. 2004;29(1):15–21.

139. Fleming CJ, Bryden AM, Evans A, et al. A pilot study of treatment of lentigo maligna with 5% imiquimod cream. *Br J Dermatol*. 2004;151(2):485–488.

140. Wolf IH, Cerroni L, Kodama K, et al. Treatment of lentigo maligna (melanoma in situ) with the immune response modifier imiquimod. *Arch Dermatol*. 2005;141(4):510–514.

141. Powell AM, Robson AM, Russell-Jones R, et al. Imiquimod and lentigo maligna: a search for prognostic features in a clinicopathological study with long-term follow-up. *Br J Dermatol*. 2009;160(5):994–998.

142. Cotter MA, McKenna JK, Bowen GM. Treatment of lentigo maligna with imiquimod before staged excision. *Dermatol Surg*. 2008;34(2):147–151.

143. Missall TA, Fosko SW. The use of imiquimod to minimize the surgical defect when excising invasive malignant melanoma surrounded by extensive melanoma in situ, lentiginous type. *Dermatol Surg*. 2009;35(5):868–874.

144. Steinmann A, Funk JO, Schuler G, et al. Topical imiquimod treatment of a cutaneous melanoma metastasis. *J Am Acad Dermatol*. 2000;43(3):555–556.

145. Wolf IH, Smolle J, Binder B, et al. Topical imiquimod in the treatment of metastatic melanoma to skin. *Arch Dermatol*. 2003;139(3):273–276.

146. Turza K, Dengel LT, Harris RC, et al. Effectiveness of imiquimod limited to dermal melanoma metastases, with simultaneous resistance of subcutaneous metastasis. *J Cutan Pathol*. 2010;37(1):94–8.

147. van Meurs T, van Doorn R, Kirtschig G. Recurrence of lentigo maligna after initial complete response to treatment with 5% imiquimod cream. *Dermatol Surg*. 2007;33(5):623–626.

148. Woodmansee CS, McCall MW. Recurrence of lentigo maligna and development of invasive melanoma after treatment of lentigo maligna with imiquimod. *Dermatol Surg*. 2009;35(8):1286–1289.

149. Fisher GH, Lang PG. Treatment of melanoma in situ on sun-damaged skin with topical 5% imiquimod cream complicated by the development of invasive disease. *Arch Dermatol*. 2003;139(7):945–947.

150. Martínez-González MC, Verea-Hernando MM, Yebra-Pimentel MT, et al. Imiquimod in mycosis fungoides. *Eur J Dermatol*. 2008;18(2):148–152.

151. Olsen EA, Bunn PA. Interferon in the treatment of cutaneous T-cell lymphoma. *Hematol Oncol Clin North Am*. 1995;9(5):1089–1107.

152. Chong A, Loo WJ, Banney L, et al. Imiquimod 5% cream in the treatment of mycosis fungoides – a pilot study. *J Dermatolog Treat*. 2004;15(2):118–119.

153. Deeths MJ, Chapman JT, Dellavalle RP, et al. Treatment of patch and plaque stage mycosis fungoides with imiquimod 5% cream. *J Am Acad Dermatol*. 2005;52(2):275–280.

154. Zampogna JC, Flowers FP, Roth WI, et al. Treatment of primary limited cutaneous extramammary Paget's disease with topical imiquimod monotherapy: two case reports. *J Am Acad Dermatol*. 2002;47(suppl 4):S229–S235.

155. Cohen PR, Schulze KE, Tschen JA, et al. Treatment of extramammary Paget disease with topical imiquimod cream: case report and literature review. *South Med J*. 2006;99(4):396–402.

156. Hatch KD, Davis JR. Complete resolution of Paget disease of the vulva with imiquimod cream. *J Low Genit Tract Dis*. 2008;12(2):90–94.

157. Smith KJ, Germain M, Yeager J, et al. Topical 5% imiquimod for the therapy of actinic cheilitis. *J Am Acad Dermatol*. 2002;47(4):497–501.

158. Greenberg HL, Cohen JL, Rosen T, et al. Severe reaction to 5% imiquimod cream with excellent clinical and cosmetic outcomes. *J Drugs Dermatol*. 2007;6(4):452–458.

159. Testerman TL, Gerster JF, Imbertson LM, et al. Cytokine induction by the immunomodulators imiquimod and S-27609. *J Leukoc Biol*. 1995;58:365–372.

160. Tomai MA, Gibson SJ, Imbertson LM, et al. Immunomodulating and antiviral activities of the imidazoquinoline S-28463. *Antiviral Res*. 1995;28:253–264.

161. Jones T. Resiquimod 3M. *Curr Opin Investig Drugs*. 2003;4:214–218.

162. Szeimies RM, Bichel J, Ortonne JP, et al. A phase II dose-ranging study of topical resiquimod to treat actinic keratosis. *Br J Dermatol*. 2008;159(1):205–210.

163. Berman B, Li J, Huo R. Effects of imiquimod and resiquimod on melanoma cells in vitro. (Poster P602) 67th Annual Meeting of the American Academy of Dermatology. San Francisco, CA. March 2009 *J Am Acad Dermatol*. 2009;60(3):AB11.

164. Baccard M, Marolleau JP, Rybojad M. Middle-term evolution of patients with advanced cutaneous T-cell lymphoma treated with high dose recombinant interleukin-2. *Arch Dermatol*. 1997;133:656.

165. Zaki MH, Wysocka M, Everetts SE, et al. Synergistic enhancement of cell-mediated immunity by interleukin-12 plus interleukin-2: basis for therapy of cutaneous T-cell lymphoma. *J Invest Dermatol*. 2002;118(2):366–371.

166. Kaminetzky D, Hymes KB. Denileukin diftitox for the treatment of cutaneous T-cell lymphoma. *Biologics*. 2008;2(4):717–724.

167. Scheinfeld N. A brief primer on treatments of cutaneous T cell lymphoma, newly approved or late in development. *J Drugs Dermatol*. 2007;6(7):757–760.

168. Talpur R, Jones DM, Alencar AJ, et al. CD25 expression is correlated with histological grade and response to denileukin diftitox in cutaneous T-cell lymphoma. *J Invest Dermatol*. 2006;126(3):575–583.

169. Atkins M. Interleukin-2: clinical applications. *Semin Oncol*. 2002;29(7):12–17.

170. Helgurea G, Morrison SL, Penichet ML. Antibody-cytokine fusion proteins: harnessing the combined power of cytokines and antibodies for cancer therapy. *Clin Immunol*. 2002;105(3):233–246.

171. Ogbourne SM, Suhrbier A, Jones B, et al. Antitumor activity of 3-ingenyl angelate: plasma membrane and mitochondrial disruption and necrotic cell death. *Cancer Res*. 2004;64(8):2833–2839.

172. Siller G, Gebauer K, Welburn P, et al. PEP005 (ingenol mebutate) gel, a novel agent for the treatment of actinic keratosis: results of a randomized, double-blind, vehicle-controlled, multicentre, phase IIa study. *Australas J Dermatol*. 2009;50(1):16–22.

173. Weedon D, Chick J. Home treatment of basal cell carcinoma. *Med J Aust*. 1976;1:928.

174. Green AC, Beardmore GL. Home treatment of skin cancer and solar keratoses. *Australas J Dermatol*. 1988;29:127–130.

175. Ivanov VN, Bhoumik A, Ronai Z. Death receptors and melanoma resistance to apoptosis. *Oncogene*. 2003;22:3152–3161.

176. Johnstone RW, Ruefli AA, Lowe SW. Apoptosis: a link between cancer genetics and chemotherapy. *Cell*. 2002;108:153–164.

177. Challacombe JM, Suhrbier A, Parsons PG, et al. Neutrophils are a key component of the antitumor efficacy of topical chemotherapy with ingenol-3-angelate. *J Immunol*. 2006;177(11):8123–8132.

178. Grufman P, Karre K. Innate and adaptive immunity to tumors: IL-12 is required for optimal responses. *Eur J Immunol*. 2000;30(4):1088–1093.

179. Beissert S, Ruhlemann D, Mohammad T, et al. IL-12 prevents the inhibitory effects of cis-urocanic acid on tumor antigen presentation by Langerhans cells: implications for photocarcinogenesis. *J Immunol*. 2001;167(11):6232–6238.

180. Meeran SM, Katiyar N, Singh T, et al. Loss of endogenous interleukin-12 activates survival signals in ultraviolet-exposed mouse skin and skin tumors. *Neoplasia*. 2009;11(9):846–855.

181. Rook AH, Wood GS, Yoo EK, et al. Interleukin-12 therapy of cutaneous T-cell lymphoma induces lesion regression and cytotoxic T-cell responses. *Blood*. 1999;94(3):902–908.

182. Duvic M, Sherman ML, Wood GS, et al. A phase II open-label study of recombinant human interleukin-12 in patients with stage IA, IB, or IIA mycosis fungoides. *J Am Acad Dermatol*. 2006;55(5):807–813.

183. Daud AI, DeConti RC, Andrews S, et al. Phase I trial of interleukin-12 plasmid electroporation in patients with metastatic melanoma. *J Clin Oncol*. 2008;26(36):5896–5903.

184. Botton T, Puissant A, Bahadoran P, et al. In vitro and in vivo anti-melanoma effects of ciglitazone. *J Invest Dermatol*. 2009;129(5):1208–1218.

# Photodynamic Therapy in Skin Cancer

CHAPTER 45

*Colin A. Morton*

## Key Points

- Photodynamic therapy (PDT) is a selective non-invasive therapy for non-hyperkeratotic actinic keratoses, in-situ squamous cell carcinoma, and superficial and thin nodular basal cell carcinomas.

- PDT offers particular advantages for large and multiple lesions and those in sites where standard therapies have limitations.

- Field therapy with PDT has potential as a preventive therapy for non-melanoma skin cancer.

- Superiority of cosmetic outcome following PDT is often observed over conventional therapies.

- PDT appears to be safe, with repeat treatments possible. Stinging/pain during treatment can be controlled, if required, by analgesia or local anesthesia.

## INTRODUCTION

Photodynamic therapy (PDT) is a non-invasive therapy with proven efficacy in non-melanoma skin cancer (NMSC). PDT involves the activation of a photosensitizing drug by visible light to produce activated oxygen species within target cells, resulting in their destruction.[1] Initially, systemic administration of photosensitizers was required, adding complexity to the procedure and resulting in the complication of generalized photosensitivity that could last several weeks. Subsequently, the use of the topically active agent 5-aminolevulinic acid (5-ALA), a precursor of the endogenous photosensitizer protoporphyrin IX (PpIX), was described, permitting simplification of the treatment process.[2]

Evidence-based guidelines indicate that topical PDT is effective in actinic keratoses (AK), Bowen's disease (squamous cell carcinoma in situ), superficial basal cell carcinomas (BCC) and thin nodular BCC (Table 45.1).[3] Additional evidence exists indicating the potential of topical PDT in treating localized plaques of cutaneous T-cell lymphoma, for epidermal dysplasias in organ transplant recipients (OTR), and as adjunctive therapy in extramammary Paget's disease.[4] The recent publication of studies of long-term response rates of topical PDT in NMSC, as well as evaluation of its potential use in field cancerization and as a preventive therapy for cutaneous malignancy, has stimulated increased interest in this therapy.

Topical PDT has, to date, been approved by regulatory authorities in over 30 countries worldwide, for use in at least one NMSC indication. Two photosensitizing agents are licensed: a formulation of 5-ALA, Levulan® (DUSA Pharmaceuticals, Wilmington, MA, USA), for AK, and an esterified formulation, methyl aminolevulinate (MAL), Metvix®/Metvixia® (Galderma, Paris, France), for AK, Bowen's disease, and superficial and nodular BCCs. Additional formulations are under development.

Topical PDT offers the potential of a practical, non-surgical, outpatient/office therapy in dermatology (Table 45.2). PDT may prove advantageous where size, site or numbers of lesions limit the efficacy and/or acceptability of conventional therapies.[4] Topical PDT studies consistently report a superiority of cosmetic outcome with minimal or no scarring when compared to other standard therapies including cryotherapy and surgery.

In addition to providing a novel therapy, fluorescence emitted by ALA-induced PpIX can be utilized to provide additional information about cutaneous lesions. This permits the delineation of surface tumor margins or recurrent disease where clinical margins are difficult to define and can aid diagnosis of cancer.[5] Refinement of this technique is still required, but offers an additional advantage of using the PDT process for treating skin cancer. Surface tumor delineation can be visualized even using a simple Woods UV lamp prior to illuminating lesions with the PDT lamp.

## HISTORY

The term 'photodynamic therapy' was first used over 100 years ago by von Tappeiner following experiments using eosin and a combination of natural and artificial light in the treatment of skin cancer in 1903.[6] He realized the requirement for oxygen, describing the phenomenon as an oxygen-dependent photosensitization. The subsequent observation of selective localization of porphyrins to tumors and the demonstration of a photodynamic action involving hematoporphyrin in tumors raised interest in PDT. However, large doses of the crude photosensitizer were required and the consequent phototoxicity limited development. Partial purification produced hematoporphyrin derivative (HpD) and re-ignited interest in this modality, and PDT using HpD in human cancer was reported in 1967. The first trial was performed in 1978 in 25 patients with a variety of malignancies, including SCC and BCC. Kennedy et al.[2] reported in 1990 the use of the topically active agent, 5-ALA, which has been the focus of much research activity during the past two decades.

**Table 45.1 Advantages and Disadvantages of Topical Photodynamic Therapy**

| Advantages | Disadvantages |
|---|---|
| • Relatively selective treatment<br>• Minimal or no scarring<br>• Functional preservation of tissue<br>• Treats field disease<br>• Non-invasive<br>• Multiple lesions may be treated simultaneously<br>• Large lesions can be effectively treated<br>• 'Difficult' anatomical sites for conventional therapy are usually suitable for PDT<br>• Reduced adverse events compared with standard therapies<br>• Safe – 25 years' experience suggests very low potential for carcinogenicity<br>• Repeated treatments possible<br>• Does not limit subsequent salvage therapies when used for palliation<br>• Supervised outpatient therapy ensures compliance<br>• No generalized photosensitivity<br>• Good healing rate, with ulceration very rare | • Prickling/burning/stinging sensations during and immediately following treatment are common<br>• Local anesthesia/analgesia required for a minority of patients<br>• Local erythema and edema following treatment<br>• No histological confirmation of diagnosis nor of clearance<br>• Treatment time-consuming and requires practice space and staff<br>• Initial high cost relative to certain standard therapies (offset by reduced adverse events)<br>• Recurrence rates vary – concern that deep disease may be left untreated rendering difficult salvage therapy at certain body sites<br>• Hypo- and hyperpigmentation post therapy common, but temporary<br>• Hair loss in hirsute sites observed, but much less than following radiotherapy |

**Table 45.2 Indications and Contraindications to Topical PDT for Skin Cancer**

| Indications with Strong Evidence of Efficacy | Indications with Anecdotal Experience of Efficacy | Contraindications to PDT |
|---|---|---|
| • Thin and moderate thickness AKs (face/scalp and acral)<br>• Bowen's disease<br>• Superficial BCC<br>• Nodular BCC<br>• Epidermal dysplasia in organ transplant recipients | • Local patch/plaque cutaneous T-cell lymphoma<br>• Erythroplasia of Queyrat<br>• Extramammary Paget's<br>• Vaginal intraepithelial neoplasia<br>• Actinic cheilitis<br>• Skin cancer prevention | • Malignant melanoma<br>• Invasive squamous cell carcinoma<br>• Hyperkeratotic AK<br>• Morpheaform BCC<br>• Porphyria |

## OVERVIEW

The photodynamic reaction concerns the activation of photosensitizers in target tissue following absorption of light of an appropriate wavelength. For skin tumors, the topical route of application of 5-ALA permits an additional method of tumor selectivity, with selective uptake through altered epidermis. 5-ALA is a precursor in the heme biosynthesis pathway of protoporphyrin IX (PpIX), an endogenous photosensitizer not normally present within tissue in therapeutically useful concentrations.[1,7] Exogenous administration of 5-ALA can increase the intracellular concentration of PpIX (Fig. 45.1), as 5-ALA is the first precursor of heme after the feedback control point and the conversion of PpIX to heme is relatively slow. Local application of 5-ALA is possible due to its increased passage, when in aqueous solution, through an abnormal epidermis, thus restricting the photosensitization primarily to the tumor/dysplastic cells. Proliferating, relatively iron-deficient tumor cells preferentially accumulate PpIX as iron is required for the final conversion of PpIX into heme. This tissue selectivity in 5-ALA photodynamic therapy can be demonstrated by the detection of PpIX-induced fluorescence. There is a

relatively greater specificity with the methyl ester of 5-ALA (MAL) in comparison with 5-ALA due to increased lipophilicity, with a ratio of 9:1 compared with 2:1 for BCC compared with normal skin.

Szeimies et al. demonstrated a homogenous distribution of PpIX fluorescence of nodular and superficial (but not morpheic) BCC, including tumor lobules in deep dermis, 12 hours after 10% ALA application.[8] Roberts et al. reported that PpIX distribution in BCC was most intense in those regions of tumor immediately adjacent to the dermis following application of 20% 5-ALA for 4 hours to Bowen's disease and superficial BCC.[9]

As 5-ALA is hydrophilic, to facilitate penetration, most studies report the use of a 20% concentration in an oil-in-water emulsion. Further enhancement of efficacy has been attempted using the penetration enhancer dimethylsulfoxide, and the iron chelators desferrioxamine and ethylenediaminetetra-acetic acid disodium. As MAL is more lipophilic, Peng et al. found that MAL penetrated to a 2 mm depth in BCC, contrasting with more limited penetration with ALA.[10,11] However, using similar protocols, ALA is reported to result in higher PpIX levels than MAL, but with less selectivity for the diseased compared with healthy tissue and in AK.[12] A randomized double-blind study compared ALA and MAL for the treatment of extensive scalp AK.[13] MAL was applied for 3 hours, but ALA for 5 hours. No significant difference in mean lesion count reduction was observed 1 month after treatment, although pain was more intense on the ALA side. Direct comparison of these agents remains limited, but the current literature, while indicating both to be effective, indicates reduced specificity with high efficacy in superficial lesions with ALA, but greater lesion specificity and tissue penetration with MAL. This supports the impressive clearance rates for MAL-PDT in nodular BCC as well as with superficial lesions.[4]

## Mechanism of action

The rationale for PDT is based on the cytotoxic action of products generated by excited photosensitizers.[1] When a photosensitizer absorbs light of the appropriate

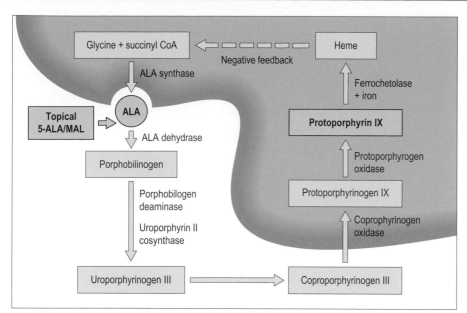

**Figure 45.1** The heme cycle in ALA/MAL-PDT. Regulation of heme synthesis – the accumulation within the mitochondria of protoporphyrin IX (PpIX) – is central to ALA- and MAL-PDT. Cellular uptake mechanisms differ between ALA and MAL, but exogenous administration acts to temporarily promote the accumulation of PpIX.

wavelength, it is converted from a stable ground state to a short-lived singlet state that may undergo conversion to a longer-lived excited triplet state. This is the photo-active species responsible for the generation of cytotoxic products. This may either directly react with substrate by hydrogen atom or electron transfer to form radicals (type I reaction), or the triplet state can transfer its energy to oxygen directly to produce singlet oxygen. Singlet oxygen is highly reactive in biological systems (type II reaction), causing photo-oxidation and cell death (Fig. 45.2). The complete process, with excitation of photosensitizer, transfer of energy through intersystem crossings, to excitation of oxygen from its triplet state and the subsequent quenching of singlet oxygen through cytotoxic mechanisms, takes place in a time scale of microseconds.

The effect of PDT on cells depends on the concentration and localization of the sensitizer and its efficiency in that environment, the light dose reaching the cell, and the oxygen supply. As the diffusion distance of singlet oxygen in cells is estimated to be only 0.1 mm, cell damage is likely to be close to the site of its generation. For lipophilic photosensitizers, including protoporphyrin IX, inhibition of mitochondrial enzymes may be the key event in PDT cell death.

The predominant mechanism of action of PDT is presumed to be direct tumor cell kill. Immunologic effects such as the elimination of small foci of cancer cells that

have escaped PDT-induced cytotoxicity may also contribute to the success of PDT, although the importance of this remains undetermined. Tumor-sensitized immune cells and the anti-tumor activity of inflammatory cells probably both contribute to this immune response.

Light of appropriate wavelength for activation of the photosensitizer is required in the target tissue. While 635 nm light may penetrate up to 6 mm (compared with 1–2 mm for light at 400–500 nm), the therapeutically effective maximum depth of PDT will depend on sufficient light dose being delivered to tissue that also has sufficient photosensitizer to achieve a photodynamic reaction. The therapeutically effective depth of PDT in the skin is therefore likely to be less, at 1–3 mm at 635 nm, depending on the tissue.[1] 5-ALA-induced photosensitivity has a porphyrin-like spectrum with maximum excitation at 410 nm and additional smaller peaks at 510, 545, 580 and 635 nm (Fig. 45.3). Using shorter wavelength light could thus achieve more efficient activation of PpIX, but at the expense of depth of therapeutic effect. In Europe, most clinical applications of PDT have used red light around 630–635 nm to achieve adequate penetration, although in the US, blue light that activates the 410 nm peak is commonly used when treating thin/moderate thickness AKs.

Several light sources have been used in clinical PDT studies for cutaneous applications, including lasers, xenon arc/discharge lamps, incandescent filament lamps, and

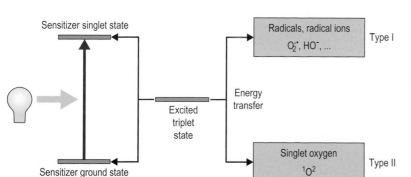

**Figure 45.2** The photodynamic reaction. The photosensitizer in the excited triplet state can react directly with substrate/solvent by hydrogen atom or electron transfer (type I reaction), which, after interaction with oxygen, produces oxygenated products. Alternatively, the sensitizer can directly transfer its energy to oxygen to form singlet oxygen (type II reaction)

**499**

**Figure 45.3** Protoporphyrin absorption spectrum – demonstrating maximum excitation at 410 nm, with further peaks at 510, 545, 580 and 635 nm

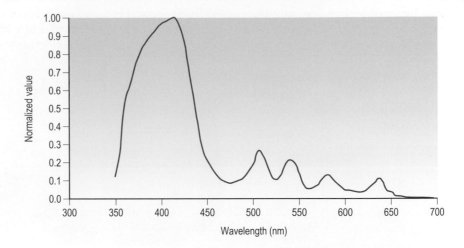

solid-state light-emitting diodes (LEDs). Coherent light is not required for PDT. The development of energy-efficient LED sources has facilitated the development of large-area, yet portable, red-light sources that have become the most frequently used lights in clinical practice.

For superficial disease such as non-hyperkeratotic AK, short wavelength blue light is a more efficient wavelength to use. This is near the maximum absorption wavelength of PpIX at 410 nm and may reduce the stinging/pain of PDT. In a randomized comparison of green with red light in Bowen's disease, however, green light was significantly inferior, suggesting deeper light penetration with longer wavelength red light is necessary to treat the entire thickness of disease (including skin appendages) in Bowen's disease.[14]

Fractionation (discontinuous illumination) may improve tumor responsiveness by permitting tissue re-oxygenation during 'dark' periods. Recent studies support superiority of the fractionation approach over conventional single illuminations in BCC, but not in Bowen's disease, although direct comparison with approved protocols is required.[15,16] MAL-PDT is approved on the basis of a double treatment 1 week apart. This 'long-interval' fractionation is presumed to target residual disease before re-epithelialization and re-growth occur.

Recent studies have suggested that pulsed light therapy may be useful in topical PDT, including a randomized trial comparing a variable pulse light with LED-PDT in AK.[17] Efficacy was equivalent, while pain was significantly less, with the pulsed light source. However, a study performed in healthy human skin in vivo following microdermabrasion and acetone scrub showed that two pulsed light sources previously reported in PDT, the pulse dye laser (PDL) and a broadband flashlamp filtered intense pulsed light (IPL), produced evidence of minimal activation of photosensitizer, with a dramatically smaller photodynamic reaction than seen with a conventional continuous wave broadband source.[18]

Current interest is focusing on developing small, potentially disposable, organic LED light devices that can be worn by patients, hence achieving 'ambulatory PDT'.[19] Initial studies are promising, with reduced pain over conventional therapy.

Ambient light as the source for ALA-PDT for AK has also been explored with a randomized ambient light-controlled

study using 5-ALA demonstrating no significant effect on lesion ablation.[20] However, a randomized right/left intra-patient comparison of conventional MAL-PDT delivered with an LED device versus daylight (for 2.5 hours) for the treatment of AK of face and scalp, showed an equivalent reduction in AK and significantly less pain with daylight, recently confirmed in a further study.[21,22] Although daylight exposure might achieve a therapeutically effective dose in certain circumstances, it is unlikely to offer a consistent, practical approach to the delivery of PDT.

Choice of light source requires consideration of their relative efficiency for the photosensitizer used and for the indications proposed. If clinical practice is limited to AK, then blue light remains a good option, while red LED devices increase the therapeutic range of office PDT.

## Therapeutic effect

Dosimetry in PDT can presently be defined only in terms of explicit parameters, including the administered photosensitizer dose, the drug–light interval, and the wavelength/band, irradiance ($mW/cm^2$) and fluence ($J/cm^2$) of light. Total effective fluence, taking into account incident spectral irradiance, optical transmission through tissue, and absorption by photosensitizer, has been proposed as a method for more accurate dosimetry but light dosage can only be estimated from the energy fluence in practice.[23] Comparison of dosimetry between studies is thus prevented as a significant proportion of incident light may be of relatively ineffective wavelengths.

### TOPICAL PDT THERAPY

Figure 45.4 demonstrates the sequence of preparation that a patient would receive for MAL-PDT for extensive AKs. Removal of overlying crust and scales with gauze soaked in saline, forceps, or by gentle curettage is often performed, although in PDT of thin/moderate AK, such preparation is possibly of limited importance. For nodular BCC, the need for lesion preparation is probably more important. A debulking curettage, avoiding the edge of the lesion, facilitates effective therapy. This is unlike typical curettage as this gentle debulking is without the need for local anesthesia, and by sparing the edges and base of the lesion, probably preserves the superior cosmesis that is consistently seen after PDT. A thin layer of photosensitizer is applied, typically of a thickness of only 1 mm, including a margin of 5–10 mm around the visible borders of lesions. An occlusive dressing to retain cream should then be applied. The patient is free to leave, returning 3 hours later (4–6 hours if standard ALA-PDT with red light) for removal of excess cream and optional check of surface fluorescence with an ultraviolet Wood's lamp (Fig. 45.5) (e.g. UVL-56, Upland CA, USA) – helpful in confirming PpIX generation at least in superficial parts of the lesion.

5-ALA for AKs involves mixing the powder together with the vehicle solution, then gently dabbing the mixed solution onto lesions, allowing them to dry, then re-applying.

Patients leave the office without the need for occlusion of lesions, but with advice to minimize light exposure and not to wash the treatment site. At 14–18 hours later, blue light is delivered via the Blu-U for 1000 seconds to provide a 10 J/cm$^2$ light dose. Recent studies have shown that shorter application times can be effective for AK treatment.

There is the option for either pre-treatment application of a topical anesthetic, applied following removal of excess 5-ALA 30–45 minutes prior to illumination, or provision during illumination of local injected anesthesia, e.g. 1–2% lidocaine. Analgesia prior to treatment is advocated by some practitioners while others recommend a fan or cool air system to minimize sensations of prickling/burning/stinging experienced during illumination with typical treatment times of 15 minutes.

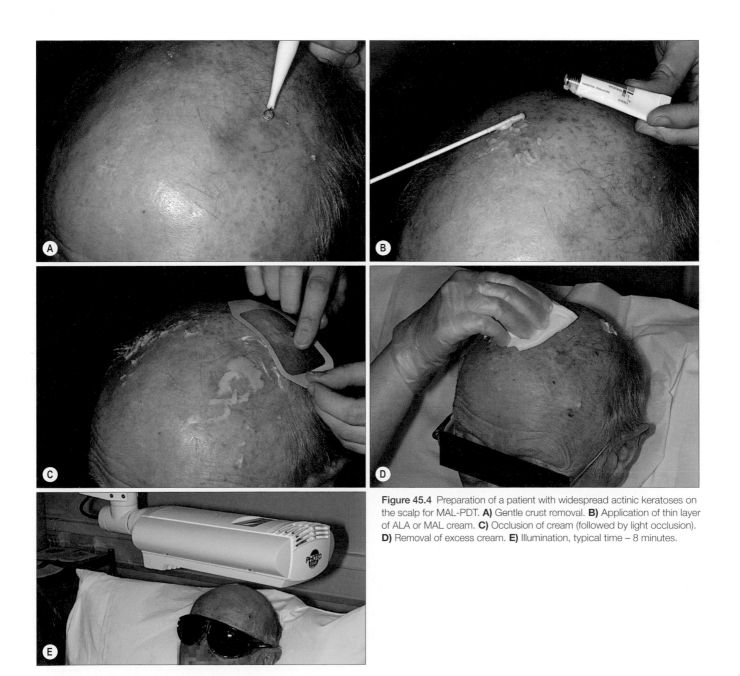

**Figure 45.4** Preparation of a patient with widespread actinic keratoses on the scalp for MAL-PDT. **A)** Gentle crust removal. **B)** Application of thin layer of ALA or MAL cream. **C)** Occlusion of cream (followed by light occlusion). **D)** Removal of excess cream. **E)** Illumination, typical time – 8 minutes.

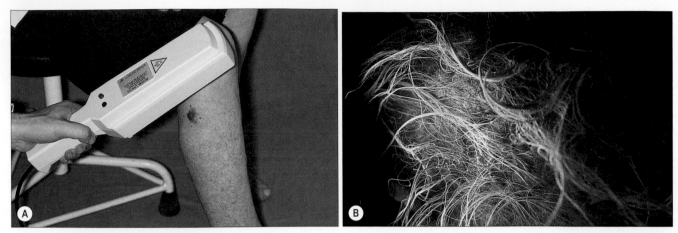

**Figure 45.5 A)** Wood's light illumination of lesion. **B)** Intense surface fluorescence in BCCs on scalp that were difficult to delineate clinically, but clearly outlined using the Wood's lamp.

The treatment site should then be protected from ambient light for up to 24–48 hours. When MAL-PDT is used for Bowen's disease or BCC, the treatment is repeated after 1 week. For 5-ALA- and MAL-PDT for AK, it is common to assess outcome after 6–12 weeks, before determining the need for repeat treatment.

## INDICATIONS

### Actinic keratoses

Topical PDT with MAL and 5-ALA have been approved only for non-hyperkeratotic AKs of the face and scalp (Fig. 45.6). ALA-PDT applied for 14–18 hours clears 75% increasing to 89% of AKs after one or two treatments, respectively.[24] Sustainability of the response of AK to ALA-PDT was reported in a study of patients each with multiple thin or moderate thickness AKs which achieved a peak target lesion clearance of 86% reducing to 78% at 12 months.[25] Recent reports of a new ALA formulation, where the prodrug is incorporated into a self-adhesive patch, observe high efficacy (82–89%) following a single treatment in mild/moderate thickness AK with no prior lesion preparation required, potentially simplifying the PDT procedure.[26]

MAL-PDT using broad-spectrum red light sources cleared 69% increasing to 89–91% of predominantly thin and moderate thickness AK of the face or scalp after a single and repeat treatments, 7 days apart.[4] In comparison, clearance rates of 68% and 75% were recorded for cryotherapy in two of these studies, and cosmetic outcome was inferior with cryotherapy. Two studies demonstrated clearance of 83% and 86% of thin/moderate AK, respectively, following the use of red LED MAL-PDT, repeated at 7 days.[27,28] Recent studies using the narrowband red LED light sources have shown that a single treatment with MAL-PDT, repeated only if required at 3 months, was as effective as the standard two treatments separated by 7 days, leading to a change in licence in several countries and saving many patients the need for a second treatment.[29] In a large randomized intra-individual study of 1501 face/scalp AKs in 119 patients, MAL-PDT was compared with double free–thaw cryotherapy, repeating treatments at 3 months if required.[30] After the initial cycle of treatments, PDT resulted in a significantly higher cure rate than cryotherapy (87% vs. 76%), but with equivalent outcome after all non-responders were retreated (89% vs. 86%). Overall subject preference significantly favoured PDT.

Acral AKs may be the poorer-responding hyperkeratotic AK, but PDT may still be a useful therapy for non-facial/head AK. A randomized intra-individual study comparing topical MAL-PDT with cryotherapy saw 78% of lesions clearing with PDT against 88% with cryotherapy

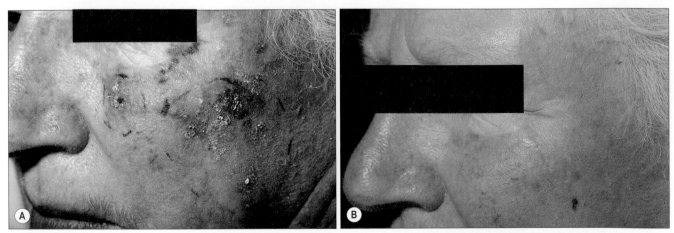

**Figure 45.6** Extensive facial actinic keratoses: **A)** pre-PDT; **B)** following ALA-PDT.

at 6 months.[31] The inferior efficacy was offset by superior cosmesis and patient preference for PDT. Given the poor healing that can occur post cryotherapy, it is perhaps an option to undertake PDT to clear as many lesions as possible, then use cryotherapy/curettage for non-responding lesions.

Although 5-ALA should be applied for 14–18 hours before light illumination, it has become common practice to apply it for much shorter times. Comparison of 3-hour with 14–18-hour 5-ALA application demonstrated equivalent efficacy of 90% at 8 months.[32] Several open studies of 'short-contact' (0.5–3-hour application) ALA-PDT achieved lesion clearance rates of 50–98% after single sessions using blue, IPL or PDL sources.[4] A similar study to compare standard 3-hour incubation with MAL versus 1-hour, demonstrated that 1-hour incubation achieved inferior rates of clearance (thin AK: 78% lesion clearance vs. 96%; moderate thickness: 74% vs. 87%) but possibly sufficiently high to permit wider use of short-incubation MAL-PDT.[33]

## Bowen's disease (squamous cell carcinoma in situ)

Topical PDT clears 86–93% of Bowen's lesions following one or two treatments (Fig. 45.7).[4] Topical MAL-PDT is now approved in many countries for Bowen's disease. Although ALA-PDT has also been demonstrated to be effective, it is not licensed for Bowen's. A randomized comparison study showed non-formulary ALA-PDT to be superior to topical 5-fluorouracil (5-FU), with initial clearance rates of 88% and 67%, respectively, and 12-month sustained clearance rates of 82% and 48%, respectively.[34] An earlier comparison of ALA-PDT with cryotherapy in Bowen's disease observed superior clearance with a single treatment (75% vs. 50%) with ulceration observed only with cryotherapy.[35] As 75% of lesions occur on the lower leg of typically elderly patients, where cryotherapy is a relative contraindication, PDT offers a highly effective alternative first-line therapy for Bowen's disease.

PDT using red light has been shown to be superior to green light, encouraging more PDT practitioners to use red light when treating Bowen's disease. In a study of 40 large (20–55 mm) lesions, an initial clearance rate after one to three treatments of 88% fell to 78% by 12 months. In the same study, 10 patients, each with three or more patches of Bowen's disease, achieved an overall clearance rate with PDT of 89% after 12 months.[36]

MAL-PDT has recently been compared with clinicians' choice of cryotherapy or 5-FU in a multicenter randomized controlled trial of 225 patients with 275 lesions.[37] Three months after last treatment, clearance rates were similar following MAL-PDT (86%), cryotherapy (82%), and 5-FU (83%). PDT gave superior cosmetic results compared with cryotherapy and 5-FU. After 24 months of follow-up, 68% of lesions remained clear following PDT, 60% after cryotherapy, and 59% after 5-FU.

Topical ALA-PDT has been observed to offer therapeutic benefit in erythroplasia of Queyrat. MAL-PDT cleared residual erythroplasia following Mohs surgery for penile SCC. Paoli et al. observed that administration of PDT (ALA/MAL) to 10 patients with penile intraepithelial neoplasia resulted in initial clearance in 7 patients, but later recurrence in 4.[38] There was sustained clearance in the remaining patients over 46 months, including clearance of HPV-DNA.

There remains limited data on the efficacy of topical PDT for primary cutaneous invasive SCC. Clearance rates for superficial lesions of 54–100% have been observed following ALA-PDT, but with recurrence rates ranging from 0% to 69%.[4] In a recent study of MAL-PDT for in-situ, microinvasive, and invasive SCC, 3-month clearance rates of 88%, 80%, and 45% were observed, with results at 24 months of 71%, 58%, and 26%, respectively.[39] Current evidence supports the potential of topical PDT for in-situ and microinvasive SCC, but in view of its metastatic potential, topical PDT should not be used for the treatment of invasive SCC.

## Basal cell carcinoma

Topical PDT can effectively clear superficial BCC (Figs 45.8 and 45.9), with efficacy for nodular lesions appearing more dependent on protocol. MAL-PDT has been licensed in many countries for the treatment of superficial and nodular BCC, with therapy-specific guidelines recommending it especially for primary superficial BCC at low-risk sites and small low-risk nodular lesions.[40]

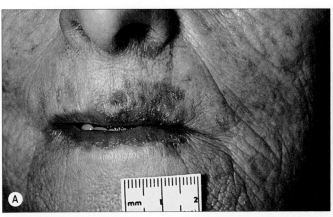
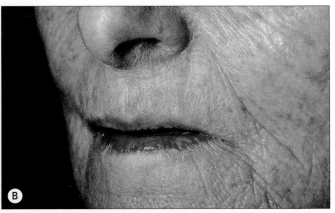

Figure 45.7 Bowen's disease on the upper and lower lip: **A)** pre-PDT; **B)** the same site 12 months following a single treatment with ALA-PDT.

Initial experience with non-formulary ALA demonstrated efficacy, with a weighted clearance rate of 87% in one review of 12 studies for superficial BCC, compared with 53% for nodular lesions.[41] A number of studies of ALA-PDT for nodular BCC employed prior debulking curettage,[4] although a recent study failed to show a significant advantage of curettage followed by PDT compared with conventional surgery for nodular BCC up to 2 cm in diameter, with clearance rates of 72% and 100%, respectively, of treatment sites reviewed at 1 year.[42]

Experiments to increase efficacy of ALA-PDT in BCC include the use of a novel iron chelator, CP94, to temporarily increase the accumulation of the photosensitizer in tumours.[43]

A 5-year follow-up study has compared cryotherapy with MAL-PDT using a broadband red light for the treatment of superficial BCC. The 3-month complete clinical response rates were similar for PDT (97%) and cryo-therapy (95%). Cosmetic outcome was superior following PDT. The complete lesion response rate at 5 years was 75% in the MAL-PDT group versus 74% in the cryotherapy group.[44]

In another recent study, comparing MAL-PDT with surgery for superficial BCC, PDT cleared 92%, surgery 99%, at 3 months, with the only recurrences by 12 months being in the PDT group – 9%.[45]

A randomized study compared double MAL-PDT using a broadband red light with treatments 7 days apart (and repeated at 3 months if required) with standard surgical excision, in patients with small nodular BCC.[46] Clinical clearance rates at 3 months were similar, 98% for surgery versus 91% following MAL-PDT, with 12-month response rates of 96% versus 83%, respectively. A 5-year follow-up of this study has revealed a significantly higher estimated sustained lesion response rate for surgery at 96% compared with 76% for MAL-PDT. Cosmetic evaluation showed significantly better results for MAL-PDT. These results imply that while surgery remains the gold standard for the treatment of nodular BCC, MAL-PDT is effective for treatment of these lesions and exhibits a more favourable cosmetic outcome. To date, there has been only one small randomized study directly comparing ALA-PDT with MAL-PDT in BCC, with no difference in lesional response observed.[47]

## Cutaneous T-cell lymphoma

Selective uptake of photosensitizers into lymphocytes after topical PDT, with inhibition of T cells has been demonstrated in topical PDT of cutaneous T-cell lymphoma (CTCL). Several case reports and small series support the efficacy of repetitive treatments with ALA and MAL-PDT

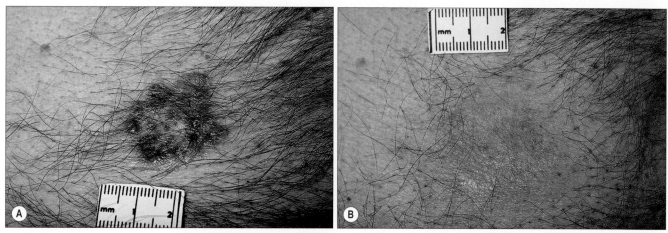

**Figure 45.8** Superficial BCC on lower leg: **A)** pre-PDT; **B)** 12 months post ALA-PDT.

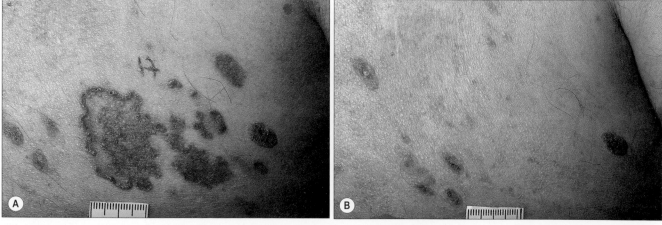

**Figure 45.9** Large superficial BCC: **A)** pre-PDT; **B)** 60 months following ALA-PDT (2 cm ruler just visible).

for localized plaque-stage CTCL, but single treatments appear less likely to be successful.[4]

## Applications for topical PDT beyond NMSC

Topical PDT can be beneficial in anal and vulval intraepithelial neoplasia, and as an adjunctive therapy for extramammary Paget's disease. However, further studies are required to determine how useful PDT is compared with conventional therapies in these indications.

PDT should not be considered an option for the treatment of melanoma, where reduced penetration of light into pigmented lesions reduces the potential for achieving a response with PDT with currently used photosensitizers. Eight cutaneous metastases of melanoma failed to clear after topical ALA-PDT with only superficial tumor necrosis achieved in those amelanotic tumors and no response with melanotic metastases.[48]

## PDT in organ transplant recipients (OTR)

OTR often develop large and multiple NMSC – the impact of PDT in this patient group has also been evaluated. ALA-PDT and MAL-PDT have both been shown to be effective in clearing AK/BD in OTR. Although initial clinical response rates appear similar to those in immunocompetent patients, it has been noted that recurrence rates were higher in OTR patients during a 48-week follow-up.[4] This lends support to the importance of the role of immune response factors in the mechanism of action of PDT. Data comparing PDT with other therapies in OTR are limited, although MAL-PDT has been shown to be superior in efficacy to topical 5-FU, even after 6 months, for the treatment of epidermal dysplasia in OTR.[4]

## Skin cancer prevention

Repeated PDT treatments have delayed the appearance of UV-induced skin cancer in several in-vivo studies.[4] A recent open intra-patient randomized study of 27 renal OTR reported a significant delay in development of new lesions at sites treated with MAL-PDT.[49] By 12 months, 62% of treated areas were free from new lesions compared with 35% of control areas. In a further study of topical PDT in 81 OTR, MAL-PDT was administered twice, 1 week apart, then at 3, 9 and 15 months.[50] The occurrence of new lesions was reduced compared with control sites during the initial months of the study, but lost by 27 months, suggesting additional treatments after 15 months might be required. However, so far, studies have failed to clearly demonstrate avoidance of squamous cell carcinoma in this important 45.1 patient group, and further study is required.

The mechanism by which PDT might delay/prevent skin cancer is unknown. There may be some contribution from the treatment of subclinical disease. In addition to biological response modifier activity, PDT may also cause selective destruction of keratinocytes bearing mutated *p53* induced by UV exposure.

There is currently considerable interest in devising protocols that can clear multiple widespread actinic keratoses using field therapy with PDT, with the expectation that this will provide additional information of the preventive potential of PDT.

## ADVERSE EFFECTS

No generalized photosensitivity reactions have been observed following topical PDT. Localized photosensitivity can remain for up to 48 hours, ALA degrading with a half-life of about 24 hours, and MAL-induced PpIX clearing from normal skin within 24–48 hours. Light protection at treatment sites is therefore advised for up to 48 hours.

Pain or discomfort, often described as 'burning,' 'stinging' or 'prickling' restricted to the illuminated area, is commonly experienced during PDT. It usually peaks within minutes of commencing light exposure and probably reflects nerve stimulation and/or tissue damage by reactive oxygen species, possibly aggravated by hyperthermia. This discomfort can occasionally persist for hours, and rarely for a few days, at a reduced intensity. Most patients will tolerate ALA-PDT without anesthesia/analgesia. The face and scalp may be more susceptible to pain and large and/or ulcerated lesions are more likely to be painful. Strategies to reduce pain include supportive nursing during treatment, explaining the mechanism of PDT, prior topical/injected local anesthetic, premedication with benzodiazepine, and cooling fans or spraying water on lesions during therapy. Nerve blocks have been employed by some practitioners treating large areas of skin.

Immediately following treatment, erythema and edema are common, with erosion, crust formation and healing over 2–6 weeks, but ulceration is very rare. Swelling can be locally marked, giving rise to occasional observations of an urticated reaction at the treatment site. Careful counseling is advised in treating large areas of the skin in patients who have never received PDT.

Hyper- or hypopigmentation can occasionally be seen in treated areas and usually resolves within 6 months. Permanent hair loss has been observed following PDT, but is much less than that observed following radiotherapy.

PDT has the potential of promoting genotoxic effects, including induction of DNA strand breaks, chromosomal aberrations and alkylation of DNA. However, porphyrin molecules also possess anti-mutagenic properties. PDT delays photocarcinogenesis in mice. Overall, evidence would indicate the risk of cancer associated with PDT to be low, but in view of the latent period for carcinogenesis, careful reporting of malignancies in sites of prior PDT is advised.

## FUTURE OUTLOOK

The potential of topical PDT is currently limited by the depth of therapeutic effect. The use of longer wavelength light with new photosensitizers and the advent of interstitial light delivery could further extend this depth. Combining iron chelators with the topical photosensitizers might be another means of extending the range of therapy.

The potential to harness the clinical benefits of fluorescence diagnosis enhances the appeal of utilizing the PDT process. Delineation of subclinical disease by fluorescence, followed by targeting of 'hot spots', could offer substantial benefit to high-risk patients, currently enduring multiple surgical excisions, sometimes with grafting.

Refining protocols remains important to identify those patients who might best benefit from local anesthesia, even nerve block, versus the majority in whom careful explanation of the therapy, including comforting explanations during treatment (talk anesthesia), is all that is required.

PDT is likely to become more simple, greatly extending its use in office dermatology. The novel self-adhesive ALA-impregnated plasters could permit home application of photosensitizer by certain patients. Routine use of daylight as the light source might be viable, at least for certain months of the year. It is more likely, however, that illumination will become better tolerated and simpler via the wider use of wearable disposable organic LED sources, with reduced discomfort due to the much lower intensities of illumination.

The multiple indications for topical PDT confirm that the modality has progressed over recent years, sitting alongside other topical field-therapies that hold the additional potential of secondary prevention.

## REFERENCES

1. Henderson BW, Dougherty TJ. How does photodynamic therapy work? *Photochem Photobiol*. 1992;55:145–157.
2. Kennedy JC, Pottier RH, Pross DC. Photodynamic therapy with endogenous protoporphyrin IX: basic principles and present clinical experience. *J Photochem Photobiol B Biol*. 1990;6:143–148.
3. Braathen LB, Szeimies RM, Basset-Seguin N, et al. Guidelines on the use of photodynamic therapy for nonmelanoma skin cancer: an international consensus. *J Am Acad Dermatol*. 2007;56:125–143.
4. Morton CA, Brown SB, Collins C, et al. Guidelines for topical photodynamic therapy: update. *Br J Dermatol*. 2008;159:1245–1266.
5. Fritsch C, Lang K, Neuse W, et al. Photodynamic diagnosis and therapy in dermatology. *Skin Pharmacol Appl Skin Physiol*. 1998;11:358–373.
6. Daniell MD, Hill JS. A history of photodynamic therapy. *Aust NZ J Surg*. 1991;61:340–348.
7. Kalka K, Merk H, Mukhtar H. Photodynamic therapy in dermatology. *J Am Acad Dermatol*. 2000;42:389–413.
8. Szeimies RM, Sassy T, Landthaler M. Penetration potency of topical applied 5-aminolaevulinic acid for photodynamic therapy of basal cell carcinoma. *Photochem Photobiol*. 1994;59:73–76.
9. Roberts DJH, Cairnduff F. Photodynamic therapy of primary skin cancer: a review. *Br J Plast Surg*. 1995;48:360–370.
10. Peng Q, Soler AM, Warloe T, et al. Selective distribution of porphyrins in thick basal cell carcinoma after topical application of methyl 5-aminolevulinate. *J Photochem Photobiol B*. 2001;62:140–145.
11. Peng Q, Warloe T, Moan J, et al. Distribution of 5-aminolevulinic acid-induced porphyrins in noduloulcerative basal cell carcinoma. *Photochem Photobiol*. 2005;62:906–913.
12. Fritsch C, Homey B, Stahl W, et al. Preferential relative porphyrin enrichment in solar keratoses upon topical application of delta-aminolevulinic acid methylester. *Photochem Photobiol*. 1998;68:218–221.
13. Moloney FJ, Collins P. Randomized, double-blind, prospective study to compare topical 5-aminolaevulinic acid methylester with topical 5-aminolaevulinic acid photodynamic therapy for extensive scalp actinic keratosis. *Br J Dermatol*. 2007;157:87–91.
14. Morton CA, Whitehurst C, Moore JV, et al. Comparison of red and green light in the treatment of Bowen's disease by photodynamic therapy. *Br J Dermatol*. 2000;143:767–772.
15. de Haas ER, Kruijt B, Sterenborg HJ, et al. Fractionated illumination significantly improves the response of superficial basal cell carcinoma to aminolevulinic acid photodynamic therapy. *J Invest Dermatol*. 2006;126:2679–2686.
16. de Haas ER, Sterenborg HJ, Neumann HA, et al. Response of Bowen disease to ALA-PDT using a single and a 2-fold illumination scheme. *Arch Dermatol*. 2007;143:264–265.
17. Babilas P, Knobler R, Hummel C, et al. Variable pulsed light is less painful than light-emitting diodes for topical photodynamic therapy of actinic keratoses: a prospective randomized controlled trial. *Br J Dermatol*. 2007;157:111–117.
18. Strasswimmer J, Grande DJ. Do pulsed lasers produce an effective photodynamic therapy response? *Lasers Surg Med*. 2006;38:22–25.
19. Attili SK, Lesar A, McNeill A, et al. An open pilot study of ambulatory photodynamic therapy using a wearable low-irradiance organic light-emitting diode light source in the treatment of nonmelanoma skin cancer. *Br J Dermatol*. 2009;161:170–173.

20. Marcus SL, Houlihan A, Lundahl S, et al. Does ambient light contribute to the therapeutic effects of topical photodynamic therapy using aminolaevulinic acid? *Lasers Surg Med*. 2007;39:201–202.
21. Wiegell SR, Haedersdal M, Philipsen PA, et al. Continuous activation of PpIX by daylight is as effective as and less painful than conventional photodynamic therapy for actinic keratoses; a randomized, controlled, single-blind study. *Br J Dermatol*. 2008;158:740–746.
22. Wiegell SR, Haedersdal M, Eriksen P, et al. Photodynamic therapy of actinic keratoses with 8% and 16% methyl aminolaevulinate and home-based daylight exposure: a double-blinded randomized clinical trial. *Br J Dermatol*. 2009;160:1308–1314.
23. Moseley H. Total effective fluence: a useful concept in photodynamic therapy. *Lasers Med Sci*. 1996;11:139–143.
24. Piacquadio DJ, Chen DM, Farber HF, et al. Photodynamic therapy with aminolevulinic acid topical solution and visible blue light in the treatment of multiple actinic keratoses of the face and scalp: investigator-blinded, phase 3, multicenter trials. *Arch Dermatol*. 2004;140:41–46.
25. Tschen EH, Wong DS, Pariser DM, et al. The Phase IV ALA-PDT Actinic Keratosis Study Group. Photodynamic therapy using aminolaevulinic acid for patients with nonhyperkeratotic actinic keratoses of the face and scalp: phase IV multicentre clinical trial with 12-month follow up. *Br J Dermatol*. 2006;155:1262–1269.
26. Hauschild A, Stockfleth E, Popp G, et al. Optimization of photodynamic therapy with a novel self-adhesive 5-aminolevulinic acid patch: results of two randomized controlled phase III studies. *Br J Dermatol*. 2009;160:1066–1074.
27. Szeimies RM, Matheson RT, Davis SA, et al. Topical methyl aminolevulinate photodynamic therapy using red light-emitting diode light for multiple actinic keratoses: a randomized study. *Dermatol Surg*. 2009;35:586–592.
28. Pariser D, Loss R, Jarratt M, et al. Topical methyl aminolevulinate photodynamic therapy using red light-emitting diode light for treatment of multiple actinic keratoses: a randomized, double-blind, placebo-controlled study. *J Am Acad Dermatol*. 2008;59:569–576.
29. Tarstedt M, Rosdahl I, Berne B, et al. A randomized multicenter study to compare two treatment regimens of topical methyl aminolevulinate (Metvix®)-PDT in actinic keratosis of the face and scalp. *Acta Derm Venereol*. 2005;85:424–428.
30. Morton C, Campbell S, Gupta G, et al. Intraindividual, right-left comparison of topical methyl aminolaevulinate-photodynamic therapy and cryotherapy in subjects with actinic keratoses: a multicentre, randomized controlled study. *Br J Dermatol*. 2006;155:1029–1036.
31. Kaufmann R, Spelman L, Weightman W, et al. Multicentre intraindividual randomized trial of topical methyl aminolaevulate-photodynamic therapy vs. cryotherapy for multiple actinic keratoses on the extremities. *Br J Dermatol*. 2008;158:994–999.
32. Alexiades-Armenakas MR, Geronemus RG. Laser-mediated photodynamic therapy of actinic keratoses. *Arch Dermatol*. 2003;139:1313–1320.
33. Braathen LR, Paredes BE, Saksela O, et al. Short incubation with methyl aminolevulinate for photodynamic therapy of actinic keratoses. *J Eur Acad Dermatol Venereol*. 2008;23:550–555.
34. Salim A, Leman JA, McColl JH, et al. Randomized comparison trial of photodynamic therapy with topical 5-fluorouracil in Bowen's disease. *Br J Dermatol*. 2003;148:539–543.
35. Morton CA, Whitehurst C, Moseley H, et al. Comparison of photodynamic therapy with cryotherapy in the treatment of Bowen's disease. *Br J Dermatol*. 1996;135:766–771.
36. Morton CA, Whitehurst C, McColl JH, et al. Photodynamic therapy for large or multiple patches of Bowen's disease and basal cell carcinoma. *Arch Dermatol*. 2001;137:319–324.
37. Morton CA, Horn M, Leman J, et al. Comparison of topical methyl aminolevulinate photodynamic therapy with cryotherapy or fluorouracil for treatment of squamous cell carcinoma in situ: results of a multicenter randomized trial. *Arch Dermatol*. 2006;142:729–735.
38. Paoli J, Ternesten Bratel A, Lowhagen G-B, et al. Penile intraepithelial neoplasia: results of photodynamic therapy. *Acta Derm Venereol*. 2006;86:418–421.
39. Calzavara-Pinton PG, Venturini M, Sala R, et al. Methyl aminolaevulinate-based photodynamic therapy of Bowen's disease and squamous cell carcinoma. *Br J Dermatol*. 2008;159:137–144.
40. Telfer NR, Colver GB, Morton CA. Guidelines for the management of basal cell carcinoma. *Br J Dermatol*. 2008;159:35–48.
41. Peng Q, Warloe T, Berg K, et al. 5-Aminolevulinic acid-based photodynamic therapy. Clinical research and future challenges. *Cancer*. 1997;79:2282–2308.
42. Berroeta L, Clark C, Dawe RS, et al. A randomized study of minimal curettage followed by topical photodynamic therapy compared with surgical excision for low risk nodular BCC. *Br J Dermatol*. 2007;157:401–403.
43. Campbell SM, Morton CA, Alyahya R. Clinical investigation of the novel iron-chelating agent, CP94, to enhance topical photodynamic therapy of nodular basal cell carcinoma. *Br J Dermatol*. 2008;159:387–393.

**44.** Basset-Séguin N, Ibbotson SH, Emtestam L, et al. Topical methyl aminolaevulinate photodynamic therapy versus cryotherapy for superficial basal cell carcinoma: a 5 year randomized trial. *Eur J Dermatol.* 2008;18:547–553.

**45.** Szeimies RM, Ibbotson S, Murrell DF. A clinical study comparing methyl aminolevulinate photodynamic therapy and surgery in small superficial basal cell carcinoma (8-20mm) with a 12 month follow-up. *J Eur Acad Dermatol Venereol.* 2008;22:1302–1311.

**46.** Rhodes LE, de Rie MA, Leifsdottir R, et al. Five-year follow-up of a randomized prospective trial of topical methyl aminolevulinate-photodynamic therapy versus surgery for nodular basal cell carcinoma. *Arch Dermatol.* 2007;143:1131–1136.

**47.** Kuijpers D, Thissen MR, Thissen CA, Neumann MH. Similar effectiveness of methyl aminolevulinate and 5-aminolevulinate in topical photodynamic therapy for nodular basal cell carcinoma. *J Drugs Dermatol.* 2006;5:642–645.

**48.** Wolf P, Reiger E, Kerl H. Topical photodynamic therapy with endogenous porphyrins after application of 5-aminolevulinic acid. An alternative treatment modality for solar keratoses, superficial squamous cell carcinomas, and basal cell carcinomas? *J Am Acad Dermatol* 1993;28(1):17–21.

**49.** Wulf HC, Pavel S, Stender I, et al. Topical photodynamic therapy for prevention of new skin lesions in renal transplant recipients. *Acta Derm Venereol.* 2006;86:25–28.

**50.** Wennberg AM, Stenquist B, Stockfleth E, et al. Photodynamic therapy with methyl aminolevulinate for prevention of new skin lesions in transplant recipients: a randomized study. *Transplantation.* 2008;86:423–429.

CHAPTER

# 46 Surgical Excision for Non-Melanoma Skin Cancer

*Sherrif F. Ibrahim and Marc D. Brown*

---

### Key Points

- Non-melanoma skin cancer (NMSC) is the most common type of cancer and has multiple management options.

- Surgical excision remains an efficient, effective, and safe method for the treatment of these tumors, particularly with thorough perioperative planning.

- Excision has advantages over destructive treatment modalities because it allows for histologic evaluation of margins and tumor characteristics that may influence further management.

- Various patient and tumor qualities support surgical excision as an appropriate approach to treating NMSC with consistently acceptable cure rates.

- Certain situations argue against treating NMSC with standard excisional techniques.

---

## INTRODUCTION

Non-melanoma skin cancers (NMSC) are the most common among all human malignancies, with their incidence approaching that of all other cancers combined.[1,2] Fortunately, mortality from these tumors is low, but their management cost to the medical system is quite high.[3,4] In the US, NMSC ranks fifth among all types of cancer in healthcare expenditures,[4] while in Australia it ranks first.[5]

Because of their contiguous growth pattern and low metastatic potential, these tumors are well suited for standard surgical excision, which can be performed under local anesthesia in an office-based setting with relatively low associated risk and cost and high cure rates. Prior to performing these procedures, the surgeon must be familiar with several factors that influence their execution in order to optimize cure rates while minimizing destruction of uninvolved tissue

## PERIOPERATIVE MANAGEMENT

Multiple patient- and tumor-associated features must be evaluated while planning surgical excisions for NMSC. A thorough history and physical examination is of paramount importance and should be performed prior to any surgical procedure in order to avoid potential adverse events. Medication allergies should be discussed, as well as complete review of all medications that the patient is currently taking and the patient's medical diagnoses. Factors such as age, general state of health, and anxiety level will directly

influence how well a given patient will be able to tolerate a procedure under local anesthesia, and, in certain cases, general anesthesia or conscious sedation may be more appropriate. Patients should be cognizant of what to expect throughout the procedure as well as in the postoperative period, including activity restrictions and the need to return to the office for suture removal if necessary. Although surgical excisions are considered extremely safe procedures, with infection and bleeding as the most common adverse events,[6] the potential for serious undesirable complications does exist.

## Minimizing infectious complications

Medical conditions such as diabetes mellitus, acquired immune deficiency syndrome (AIDS), organ transplantation, cancer, chronic disease, and nutritional deficiency are all associated with some degree of immunosuppression and can potentially increase the risk for infection.[7,8] Antiseptic handwashing with either scrub and water or alcohol-based products can significantly reduce the incidence of infection and should be employed prior to every procedure.[8] Likewise, a variety of preoperative antiseptic skin preparations are available and should be used to disinfect the skin of the patient. The skin should be cleansed in enlarging concentric circles, beginning at the site of excision and extending beyond the area to be covered by sterile drapes.[8] Patients should be instructed to bathe the evening before or the morning of their procedure, as this has also been shown to reduce the rate of infection.[9] Interestingly, preoperative shaving of hair has been linked to higher wound infection rates, presumably by causing small cuts or scratches in the skin, thus providing portals of entry for infection.[10] If hair is to be removed prior to surgery (e.g. on the scalp or on the chest of a man), scissors should be used as opposed to a razor. Additionally, infections at sites distant to the operative location increase the risk for postoperative wound infections, and should be addressed prior to excisional surgery.[8]

The use of prophylactic antibiotics in dermatologic surgery has been an evolving issue, most recently reviewed in the advisory statement published by the American Academy of Dermatology (AAD).[11–14] Bacteremia has been documented to occur during cutaneous surgery at rates ranging from 0.7% to 7%.[15,16] This value is similar to the rate of spontaneous bacteremia in healthy adults, and far less than the rates of bacteremia that occur with activities of daily living such as mastication, brushing teeth, or defecation. The American Heart Association (AHA) has published guidelines for the prevention of bacterial endocarditis and recommends antibiotic prophylaxis for procedures causing bacteremia greater than 10% of the time,[14,17] making antibiotic prophylaxis unnecessary for cutaneous surgery unless mucosal skin is involved, the operative site is inflamed or infected, or in high-risk patients. In these situations, antibiotics should be administered as a single dose 1 hour prior to surgery.

Antibiotic prophylaxis may also be considered in certain patients with prosthetic devices.[18] In high-risk patients or in high-risk locations such as nasal mucosa or the perineum, preoperative antibiotics may be considered. The use of antibiotics, however, should be balanced with their potential side effects, including the emergence of resistant strains of bacteria, severe allergic reactions, cost, and serious interactions with medications such as warfarin. Ultimately, the decision to administer prophylactic antibiotics should be made on a case-by-case basis, with definite indications for use being few in number.

Inevitably, despite proper precautions, wound infections will occur and typically present within the first week after surgery with pain, erythema, warmth, and purulent drainage. Sutures should be removed to allow drainage and cultures should be collected for correct identification of the causative organism and selection of appropriate antibiotics. First-generation cephalosporins are generally accepted as first-line empiric treatment until culture and sensitivity results are obtained.[8]

## Minimizing bleeding complications

Although the risk of postoperative bleeding is low, it remains the most common complication of dermatologic surgery, and steps taken beforehand can help further reduce this risk. Of note, over-the-counter dietary supplements can also impact proper coagulation and are often overlooked in history-taking by physicians and medication lists provided by patients.[19] The indication for anticoagulation is an important factor in determining whether it should be discontinued. It may be prudent to check the international normalized ratio (INR) level prior to surgery to confirm that it is not beyond the therapeutic range; however, a recent study of perioperative bleeding in patients taking warfarin demonstrated that patients who were taking warfarin and experienced a moderate-to-severe bleeding complication had INR levels less than 2.6 (well within the therapeutic range) at the time of surgery.[20] Hurst and colleagues have provided a set of recommendations regarding perioperative management of anticoagulants including: 1) primary preventative aspirin should be discontinued 10–14 days prior to surgery and restarted 1 week afterwards; 2) medically necessary warfarin and aspirin should be continued with an INR value measured within 1 week of the procedure; 3) NSAIDs should be stopped 3 days prior to surgery with resumption after 1 week. The authors recommend continuation of clopidogrel. However, no studies have investigated its use or the use of combination anticoagulant therapy.[21]

Despite meticulous intraoperative hemostasis, both immediate and delayed bleeding will occur, typically within the first 48 hours after surgery. Postoperative bleeding can often be controlled by patient-applied pressure and ice; however, patients with signs and symptoms concerning for hematoma formation should be evaluated as soon as possible and managed appropriately.

## Pacemakers and defibrillators

Electrosurgical instruments are often used for hemostasis during skin surgery and may interfere with the proper function of pacemakers and implantable cardioverter-defibrillators (ICD). Interference may lead to inappropriate triggering of pulses, inhibition of proper triggering, or alteration of the programming of the device. Despite recent advances in the circuitry of pacemakers and ICDs, recommendations published in 1998 for patients with cardiac devices undergoing dermatologic procedures[22] were not changed significantly from suggested guidelines posed in 1975.[23]

When possible, in patients with implantable cardiac devices who are in need of surgery, thermal cautery is the safest alternative as no electric current is passed through the patient. Other suggested precautions include the use of short (<5 second) bursts of current for electrocautery, minimal use of power, and avoiding usage of electric current in the immediate vicinity of a cardiac device.[24,25] When in any doubt, consultation with a cardiologist should be obtained. Cardiac crash carts and staff trained in advanced cardiac life support should also be present in any dermatologic surgical facility.

## PLANNING AN EXCISION

Preferably, a diagnostic biopsy has been performed prior to excisional procedures, as these results along with patient and tumor characteristics contribute directly to the decision to proceed with a given course of management. The ideal treatment option considers not only long-term recurrence risk, but also risks associated with the procedure itself, comorbidities, as well as patient needs and expectations.

Most commonly, lesions are excised with a fusiform ellipse (Fig. 46.1) with a long axis oriented along relaxed skin tension lines (lines of Langer), or variations thereof (Fig. 46.2). The length-to-width ratio should be between 3:1 and 4:1 and the angles formed at the ends should approximate 30° to avoid producing standing cones (dog-ears) at the poles. Once the tumor has been excised, the wound edges are undermined to reduce tension across the wound and to enable eversion of the edges. The defect is then closed primarily. Typically, dissolving deep sutures are placed to close dead space and remove tension from the wound. Cutaneous sutures are then placed to finely approximate wound edges and provide additional eversion for optimal wound healing and cosmesis.

Alternate approaches include crescenteric closures in areas such as the preauricular cheek or near the nasolabial fold where the relaxed skin tension lines are curved. When suturing such an excision, the side with greater curvature will have tissue redundancy. Crescentic excisions are best closed using the rule of halves to equally distribute the excess tissue along the length of the defect (Fig. 46.3). In areas where the relaxed skin tension lines lie in opposite directions at the edges of the ellipse or on convex surfaces, an S-shaped or curvilinear approach may be used.

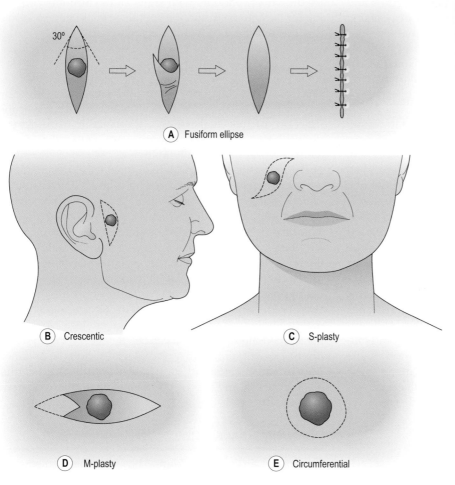

**Figure 46.1** Excision shapes. **A)** Fusiform ellipse. Note that the angle formed by the ends approximates a 30° angle. This results in optimal apposition of the wound edges and minimizes the possibility of redundancies at the ends. **B)** Crescentic. **C)** S-plasty. **D)** M-plasty. **E)** Circumferential.

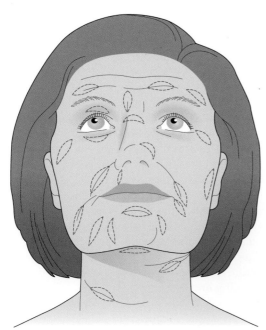

**Figure 46.2** Excision orientation incorporating relaxed skin tension lines (lines of Langer).

M-plasty is a technique used to decrease the length of a scar when encroaching upon vital anatomic structures (see Fig. 46.1). In instances where the relaxed skin tension lines cannot be adequately determined, lesions can be excised circumferentially.

In certain situations, such as for large tumors or in areas of minimal tissue movement such as the scalp or pretibial region, primary closure may not be possible. In such cases, circumferential excision can be planned with subsequent purse-string closure or healing by secondary intention.

## CLINICAL, SURGICAL, AND HISTOLOGIC MARGINS

Surgical excision of NMSC requires a margin of healthy skin because the true margin of a tumor is felt to extend subclinically to some degree. The term 'margin' can be interpreted in several ways. Clinical margin refers to the gross edges of a tumor – those which are clinically ascertained by visual and tactile inspection under bright surgical lighting with magnification when appropriate. Surgical margin is defined as the distance of normal-appearing skin (i.e. uninvolved by tumor) measured outward from the clinical margin. Based on these definitions, a tumor can be categorized as well-defined – when the clinical margin is easily determined – or ill-defined – when the clinical margin is not readily apparent (e.g. with diffuse actinic damage, sclerotic lesions, or surrounding erythema). Lastly, histologic margin refers to the measurements made by the pathologist from the deep edge of the tumor to the base of the specimen and from the lateral borders of the tumor to the lateral edges of the specimen when examining the excised tumor.

It is common for pathologists to remark that a given tumor extends 'close to the margin' and the definition

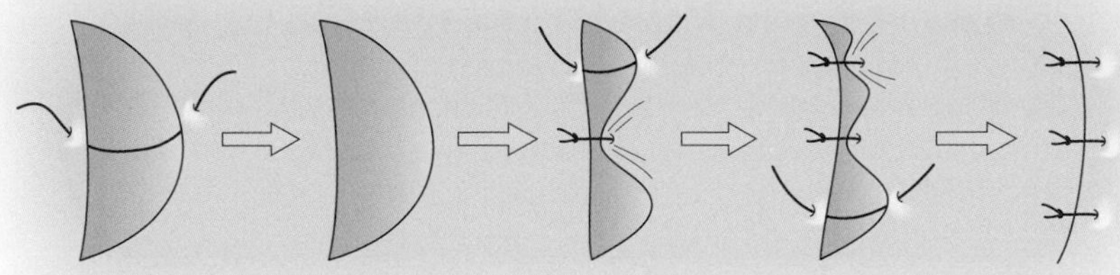

**Figure 46.3** Closing by following the rule of halves.

of this assessment varies between pathologists from a distance of a few cells to as much as 5 mm, making it necessary for the surgeon to familiarize themselves with the pathologist generating the postoperative report.[26,27] This is of importance because excisional specimens are almost always examined using vertical ('bread-loaf') sectioning, where the large majority of surgical margin is not visually inspected by the pathologist, making false-negative clear margins possible.[28] A histologic margin of only a few cells may prompt the surgeon to re-excise the lesion, whereas several millimeters may be sufficient for a cure. Of note, it is generally accepted that fixation of tissue results in an approximately 25% reduction in size when postoperative lesions are compared to preoperative measurements, and this should also be taken into account when interpreting histologic margins.[29]

## Surgical margins for NMSC

The aim of treatment of NMSC by surgical excision is to completely remove the tumor while minimizing the destruction of normal skin. When planning excisions of NMSC that lie in anatomic locations other than the head and neck, it is often possible to take larger surgical margins with minimal effect on outcome; however, the vast majority of these tumors occur on the head and neck, where excess skin is not available and tissue preservation is of utmost importance. Furthermore, vital structures of the face may limit the distance that a margin can extend in one or more direction from the tumor. The surgeon should be familiar with the circumstances in which smaller margins may be allowable, or when alternative approaches such as Mohs micrographic surgery (MMS) may be more appropriate. When extirpating tumors on the head and neck, differences in surgical margins as small as 1 mm can have profound effects on the success rate of excision and careful planning beforehand can ensure the highest chance for cure as well as determine those tumors better suited for alternative management approaches.

Well-designed, prospective, qualitative studies examining surgical margins for NMSC are few in number. Currently, recommendations for margins range from 2 to 10 mm for basal cell carcinoma (BCC) and up to 15 mm for squamous cell carcinoma (SCC).[29]

### Surgical margins for basal cell carcinoma

Despite a widely published 'standard' excision margin of 4 mm, review of the literature reveals that there is no single answer for optimal margin when excising a BCC and that several factors must be taken into account when deciding upon how large a surgical margin will completely remove the tumor an acceptable percentage of the time, particularly for tumors on the head and neck. Studies which fail to subdivide individual cases along these lines are difficult to interpret and provide less practical information when planning a surgical excision. Features that unequivocally must be considered (as they have been demonstrated to have direct relationship to recurrence rates and/or histologic margin) include: 1) tumor appearance (well-defined or ill-defined); 2) tumor diameter; 3) histologic subtype; 4) anatomic location; and 5) previous treatments[30] (Table 46.1). Each of these parameters is discussed below.

**Tumor appearance** Ill-defined tumors are generally poor candidates for surgical excision. If an adequate assessment of clinical margin is not possible, surgical margins cannot be measured accurately and this will have a direct outcome on cure rate. In these cases, it may be more appropriate to refer the patient for MMS, or to use curettage to help delineate the clinical margins prior to planning the excision.[31] Because tumor cells are less cohesive than normal skin, curetting the lesion results in an erosion that can act as a surrogate for clinical margin. Johnson and colleagues reported that aggressive curettage prior to surgical excision with a 2 mm margin from the edge of the curetted erosion leads to a 98% histologic cure rate.[32] A more recent study

| Table 46.1 Factors for and Against Standard Surgical Excision for NMSC |
|---|
| **Factors supporting standard surgical excision for NMSC** |
| • Well-defined tumors<br>• Tumor diameter <2 cm<br>• Non-aggressive histologic subtype (superficial, nodular BCCs; well-differentiated SCCs)<br>• Low- and intermediate-risk anatomic location<br>• Primary tumors |
| **Factors against standard surgical excision for NMSC** |
| • Ill-defined tumors<br>• Tumor diameter >2 cm<br>• Aggressive histologic subtype (infiltrative, morpheaform, micronodular BCCs; poorly differentiated SCCs)<br>• Intermediate- and high-risk anatomic location<br>• Recurrent tumors |

looked at periocular BCCs and noted that when tumors are well defined, a 2 mm margin is sufficient for histologic clearance in 78% of cases.[33]

**Tumor size** It has been well documented that subclinical extension extends in parallel with increasing diameter of BCCs.[34] However, the degree of subclinical spread becomes unpredictable when tumor diameter exceeds 2 cm, necessitating MMS, large surgical margins, or rapid examination of complete tumor margins with frozen sections prior to reconstruction.[30] A direct study on the implications of tumor diameter on surgical margins necessary for histologic clearance examined primary, well-defined BCCs that were being treated by MMS that were inked with concentric markings at 2 mm intervals beyond the clinical margin.[35] For BCCs less than 2 cm in diameter, a 2 mm margin would have resulted in a histologic cure for 75% of lesions, whereas 4 mm would have resulted in a cure rate of 98%. However, those tumors greater than 2 cm required significantly larger and unpredictable surgical margins to be cleared.

Tumor diameter is correlated with 5-year recurrence rates after surgical excision: for tumors <0.6 cm, 0.6–0.9 cm, and >1.0 cm, recurrence rates were 3.2%, 8.0%, and 9.0%, respectively.[36,37] An additional study demonstrated that for BCCs <1 cm in diameter, a 5 mm surgical margin resulted in a 95% cure rate, whereas a 1.2 cm margin was needed for those tumors >2 cm.[38]

**Histologic subtype** The majority of dermatopathologists classify BCCs into different histologic subtypes that can have implications as to the biologic behavior of a tumor. It is generally accepted that these types in order of increasing aggressiveness are: superficial, nodular, nodulocystic, micronodular, morpheaform, and infiltrating.[30] The corollary is that more aggressive BCCs should be treated with larger surgical margins or should be referred for MMS. In a series of 1039 consecutively treated BCCs, those tumors of increasing aggressiveness resulted in a significantly higher rate of positive histologic margins, suggesting wider subclinical extension of these tumors.[39] Lang and Maize reviewed a series of BCCs treated with MMS and calculated that the degree of this extension was 0.86 cm for aggressive histologic subtypes versus 0.66 cm for non-aggressive tumors.[40] This difference was even greater in the study by Salasche and Amonette, which demonstrated subclinical extensions of 0.21 cm and 0.72 cm for non-morpheaform versus morpheaform BCCs, respectively.[41]

Breuninger and Dietz reported a statistically significant difference in surgical margins needed to achieve a 95% cure rate between aggressive (infiltrating and morpheaform) and non-aggressive (superficial and nodular) subtypes of BCCs of 0.9 cm versus 0.6 cm.[38] In this same study, when aggressive subtypes were stratified by preoperative tumor diameter, the average margin needed for tumors <1 cm in diameter was 0.65 cm, increasing to 1.3 cm for tumors >2 cm in diameter. In a case–control study, Hendrix and Parlette demonstrated that the average margin needed to clear nodular versus infiltrative BCC was 0.47 cm versus 0.72 cm, respectively.[42]

Collectively, these studies and others[43] indicate that aggressive subtypes of BCC demonstrate increased subclinical spread and may be more appropriately managed with MMS or with larger (> 1 cm) surgical margins when possible.

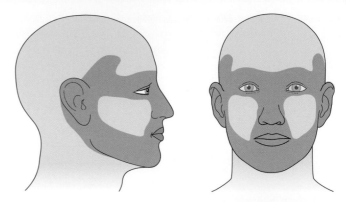

**Figure 46.4** H-zone of the face (purple) which denotes areas of higher risk for recurrence of BCC and SCC.

**Anatomic location** Certain anatomic locations of BCCs are associated with lower histologic clearance and higher rates of recurrence, designating them as high-risk locations (Fig. 46.4). Several studies have independently determined that high-risk areas include the H-zone of the face, hands, feet, and genitalia.[30,34,37,44,45] Swanson further subdivided anatomic locations as high risk (central, periorbital, perioral, mandible, preauricular, postauricular, ears, temples), intermediate risk (cheeks, forehead, scalp, neck), and low risk (trunk and extremities).[46] Kimyai-Asadi and colleagues demonstrated a positive histologic margin as high as 24% for BCCs on the face excised with margins of <4 mm despite tumors being well defined.[47] Additional studies of primary BCC excisions determined that incomplete excision was associated with location of the tumor in high-risk areas.[43,48,49]

**Tumor treatment history** Recurrent tumors have been shown in multiple studies to have greater subclinical extension and higher rates of additional recurrences when treated with either re-excision or MMS, often requiring >1.0 cm for histologic clearance.[36,41,42,46,47,50] When available, MMS should be the treatment of choice for recurrent BCC, as clinical margins are unpredictable, particularly when located anywhere on the face.[51]

### Surgical margins for squamous cell carcinoma

Excisions have the benefit of removing the entire lesion, allowing thorough histologic analysis. Aspects of the tumor such as depth of invasion, histologic grade, and involvement of structures such as nerves and muscle may lead to additional staging or adjuvant treatment for high-risk tumors.[52] The role of sentinel lymph node biopsy for these tumors is currently under investigation.[53] As with BCC, tumor appearance, size, histologic subtype, location, and treatment status can be used to adequately estimate surgical margins. An additional parameter that applies to SCC is vertical depth of invasion.[30] The clinical endpoints in the study of SCCs often include the rate of metastasis in addition to rates of recurrence and positive histologic margins.[54] It is important to note, however, that these features are averaged across large populations and cross-sectional studies, and that even lesions of SCC that are considered low risk have been shown to metastasize.[55] For this reason, all patients with a history of SCC should be followed longitudinally.

**Tumor size** In a study of 141 consecutively treated SCCs, a surgical margin of 4 mm was sufficient to clear 95% of tumors that were <2 cm, as compared to 6 mm that was needed to achieve this cure rate for tumors >2 cm.[56] Rowe and colleagues calculated an overall local recurrence rate for SCCs <2 cm of 7.4%, which increased to 15.2% for tumors >2 cm.[57]

**Histologic subtype** SCC is commonly subdivided into histologic subtypes that impact tumor behavior. Unlike BCC, however, these characteristics have a direct impact on survival. SCC histologic evaluation describes degree of differentiation as opposed to growth pattern, and the degree of differentiation is inversely related to the surgical margin required for histologic clearance. Local recurrences approach 30% for those SCCs that are poorly differentiated.[57] Brodland and Zitelli correlated Broder's grades of SCC with surgical margins, revealing that those tumors that were poorly differentiated required 0.6 mm for histologic clearance in 95% of cases.[56] Tumors that are poorly differentiated should be referred for MMS or undergo wide local excision.[58]

**Anatomic location** Beyond location in the H-zone of the face, SCCs occurring on the lip and ear have received particular attention as high-risk tumors requiring greater than 4 mm margins.[34,54,57,58] More recently, periocular SCC has also been designated as high risk, given the higher rate of perineural invasion of these tumors.[59]

**Depth of invasion** As SCC invades deeper within tissue, the surgical margins needed to clear the tumor also increase.[30,56] This becomes a difficult issue, however, as this feature is only apparent after the tumor is subjected to postoperative analysis. Deeper invasion is correlated with tumor size, location, and histologic grade. With deeper invasion, the risk for perineural invasion also increases, further contributing to a higher risk of metastatic spread.

## INCOMPLETE EXCISION AND TUMOR RECURRENCE

Despite extensive preoperative assessment and appropriate selection of tumors for surgical excision, recurrences will occur. The presence of NMSC at a histological margin, however, does not necessarily translate into recurrence. Likewise, NMSC has been shown in multiple studies to recur despite negative histologic margins.[50,55] Furthermore, metastases of both BCC and SCC have been reported even with clear histologic margins.[60] Recurrence may be manifested by a sensation of pruritus or tingling, ulceration, crusting, or papules/swelling in the surgically treated area.[61]

Tumor recurrences can pose significant management challenges, and dermatologic surgeons should have a low threshold for treatment of these lesions with MMS or wide excision. Reports of tumor recurrence after an excision with positive margins vary, with average reported rates ranging from 30% to 40%.[5,62–64] In a study of incompletely excised BCCs, 75% were re-excised to reveal residual tumor in 54% of cases.[65]

While certain reports indicate that re-excision is not necessary for all tumors, other studies have further investigated this situation and support a second procedure to eradicate residual tumor. Robinson and Fisher collected data over a 20-year span and determined that observation was contraindicated in male patients over age 65, BCCs of aggressive histology on the nose, cheek, or perioral areas, and tumors reconstructed with a flap or graft, as these parameters contributed to a delayed (>5 year) recurrence and significantly more extensive surgery.[61] Furthermore, Boulinguez et al. demonstrated that tumors previously documented as non-aggressive subtypes often recurred as a more aggressive variant, suggesting that unless there are extenuating circumstances, all tumors with positive histologic margins should be re-excised.[66] It is difficult, however, to determine if these tumors are true recurrences or second primary lesions.[67,68] In certain settings, such as with elderly or disabled patients with low-risk BCCs, watchful waiting may be justifiable. For higher-risk BCCs and all SCCs, however, re-excision is recommended. Recurrent BCCs that undergo additional surgical excision have a 5-year recurrence rate of 17.4%; however, when treated with MMS, this figure is reduced to 5.4%.[57]

## FUTURE OUTLOOK

Surgical excision is the mainstay of therapy for a large percentage of NMSC and will remain so for the immediate future. The National Comprehensive Cancer Network has established guidelines for excision of NMSC[52,69] but there needs to be better-defined recommendations which take into account important tumor and patient characteristics. Regardless of the management approach, thorough knowledge of the patient's medical history and tumor characteristics, careful planning, and early management of complications will continue to be essential to achieving desirable outcomes.

## REFERENCES

1. Geller AC, Annas GD. Epidemiology of melanoma and nonmelanoma skin cancer. *Semin Oncol Nurs.* 2003;19:2–11.
2. ACS. *How many people get basal and squamous cell skin cancers?* Available at: http://www.cancer.org/docroot/CRI/content/CRI_2_2_1X_How_many_people_get_nonmelanoma_skin_cancer_51.asp?sitearea=.
3. John Chen G, Yelverton CB, Polisetty SS, et al. Treatment patterns and cost of nonmelanoma skin cancer management. *Dermatol Surg.* 2006;32:1266–1271.
4. Housman TS, Feldman SR, Williford PM, et al. Skin cancer is among the most costly of all cancers to treat for the Medicare population. *J Am Acad Dermatol.* 2003;48:425–429.
5. Pua VSC, Huilgol S, Hill D. Evaluation of the treatment of non-melanoma skin cancers by surgical excision. *Australas J Dermatol.* 2009;50:171–175.
6. Chan BCY, Patel DC. Perioperative management and the associated rate of adverse events in dermatological procedures performed by dermatologists in New Zealand. *Australas J Dermatol.* 2009;50:23–28.
7. Maragh SLH, Brown MD. Prospective evaluation of surgical site infection rate among patients with Mohs micrographic surgery without the use of prophylactic antibiotics. *J Am Acad Dermatol.* 2008;59:275–278.
8. Hurst EA, Grekin RC, Yu SS, et al. Infectious complications and antibiotic use in dermatologic surgery. *Semin Cutan Med Surg.* 2007;26:47–53.
9. Seal LA, Paul-Cheadle D. A systems approach to preoperative surgical patient skin preparation. *Am J Infect Control.* 2004;32:57–62.
10. Mangram AJ, Horan TC, Pearson ML, et al. Guideline for prevention of surgical site infection, 1999. Centers for Disease Control and Prevention (CDC) Hospital Infection Control Practices Advisory Committee. *Am J Infect Control.* 1999;27:97–132 quiz 133–134 discussion 96.
11. Affleck AG, Birnie AJ, Gee TM, et al. Antibiotic prophylaxis in patients with valvular heart defects undergoing dermatological surgery remains a confusing issue despite apparently clear guidelines. *Clin Exp Dermatol.* 2005;30:487–489.
12. Hirschmann JV. Antimicrobial prophylaxis in dermatologic surgery. *Cutis.* 2007;79:43–51.
13. Moorhead C, Torres A. I PREVENT bacterial resistance. An update on the use of antibiotics in dermatologic surgery. *Dermatol Surg.* 2009;35:1532–1538.

14. Wright TI, Baddour LM, Berbari EF, et al. Antibiotic prophylaxis in dermatologic surgery: advisory statement 2008. *J Am Acad Dermatol.* 2008;59:464–473.

15. Carmichael AJ, Flanagan PG, Holt PJ, et al. The occurrence of bacteraemia with skin surgery. *Br J Dermatol.* 1996;134:120–122.

16. Halpern AC, Leyden JJ, Dzubow LM, et al. The incidence of bacteremia in skin surgery of the head and neck. *J Am Acad Dermatol.* 1988;19:112–116.

17. Dajani AS, Taubert KA, Wilson W, et al. Prevention of bacterial endocarditis: recommendations by the American Heart Association. *Clin Infect Dis.* 1997;25:1448–1458.

18. American Dental Association; American Academy of Orthopedic Surgeons. Antibiotic prophylaxis for dental patients with total joint replacements. *J Am Dent Assoc.* 2003;134:895–899.

19. Dinehart SM, Henry L. Dietary supplements: altered coagulation and effects on bruising. *Dermatol Surg.* 2005;31:819–826 discussion 826.

20. Blasdale C, Lawrence CM. Perioperative international normalized ratio level is a poor predictor of postoperative bleeding complications in dermatological surgery patients taking warfarin. *Br J Dermatol.* 2008;158:522–526.

21. Hurst EA, Yu SS, Grekin RC, et al. Bleeding complications in dermatologic surgery. *Semin Cutan Med Surg.* 2007;26:189–195.

22. LeVasseur JG, Kennard CD, Finley EM, et al. Dermatologic electrosurgery in patients with implantable cardioverter-defibrillators and pacemakers. *Dermatol Surg.* 1998;24:233–240.

23. Krull EA, Pickard SD, Hall JC. Effects of electrosurgery on cardiac pacemakers. *J Dermatol Surg.* 1975;1:43–45.

24. Yu SS, Tope WD, Grekin RC. Cardiac devices and electromagnetic interference revisited: new radiofrequency technologies and implications for dermatologic surgery. *Dermatol Surg.* 2005;31:932–940.

25. Matzke TJ, Christenson LJ, Christenson SD, et al. Pacemakers and implantable cardiac defibrillators in dermatologic surgery. *Dermatol Surg.* 2006;32:1155–1162 discussion 1162.

26. Bennett RG. The meaning and significance of tissue margins. *Adv Dermatol.* 1989;4:343–355 discussion 356–357.

27. Abide JM, Nahai F, Bennett RG. The meaning of surgical margins. *Plast Reconstr Surg.* 1984;73:492–497.

28. Lane JE, Kent DE. Surgical margins in the treatment of nonmelanoma skin cancer and mohs micrographic surgery. *Curr Surg.* 2005;62:518–526.

29. Thomas DJ, King AR, Peat BG. Excision margins for nonmelanotic skin cancer. *Plast Reconstr Surg.* 2003;112:57–63.

30. Huang CC, Boyce SM. Surgical margins of excision for basal cell carcinoma and squamous cell carcinoma. *Semin Cutan Med Surg.* 2004;23:167–173.

31. Connelly T, Dixon A. Delineating curettage as an adjunct to excision of basal cell carcinoma: results in 334 cases. *Plast Reconstr Surg.* 2009;123:59e–60e.

32. Johnson TM, Tromovitch TA, Swanson NA. Combined curettage and excision: a treatment method for primary basal cell carcinoma. *J Am Acad Dermatol.* 1991;24:613–617.

33. Chadha V, Wright M. Small margin excision of periocular basal cell carcinomas. *Br J Ophthalmol.* 2009;93:803–806.

34. Rieger KE, Linos E, Egbert BM, et al. Recurrence rates associated with incompletely excised low-risk nonmelanoma skin cancer. *J Cutan Pathol.* 2009; July 14 [Epub ahead of print].

35. Wolf DJ, Zitelli JA. Surgical margins for basal cell carcinoma. *Arch Dermatol.* 1987;123:340–344.

36. Silverman MK, Kopf AW, Bart RS, et al. Recurrence rates of treated basal cell carcinomas. Part 3: Surgical excision. *J Dermatol Surg Oncol.* 1992;18:471–476.

37. Silverman MK, Kopf AW, Grin CM, et al. Recurrence rates of treated basal cell carcinomas. Part 2: Curettage-electrodesiccation. *J Dermatol Surg Oncol.* 1991;17:720–726.

38. Breuninger H, Dietz K. Prediction of subclinical tumor infiltration in basal cell carcinoma. *J Dermatol Surg Oncol.* 1991;17:574–578.

39. Sexton M, Jones DB, Maloney ME. Histologic pattern analysis of basal cell carcinoma. Study of a series of 1039 consecutive neoplasms. *J Am Acad Dermatol.* 1990;23:1118–1126.

40. Lang PG, Maize JC. Histologic evolution of recurrent basal cell carcinoma and treatment implications. *J Am Acad Dermatol.* 1986;14:186–196.

41. Salasche SJ, Amonette RA. Morpheaform basal-cell epitheliomas. A study of subclinical extensions in a series of 51 cases. *J Dermatol Surg Oncol.* 1981;7:387–394.

42. Hendrix JD, Parlette HL. Duplicitous growth of infiltrative basal cell carcinoma: analysis of clinically undetected tumor extent in a paired case-control study. *Dermatol Surg.* 1996;22:535–539.

43. Su SY, Giorlando F, Ek EW, et al. Incomplete excision of basal cell carcinoma: a prospective trial. *Plast Reconstr Surg.* 2007;120:1240–1248.

44. Newman JC, Leffell DJ. Correlation of embryonic fusion planes with the anatomical distribution of basal cell carcinoma. *Dermatol Surg.* 2007;33:957–964 discussion 965.

45. Swanson NA, Grekin RC, Baker SR. Mohs surgery: techniques, indications, and applications in head and neck surgery. *Head Neck Surg.* 1983;6:683–692.

46. Swanson NA. Mohs surgery. Technique, indications, applications, and the future. *Arch Dermatol.* 1983;119:761–773.

47. Kimyai-Asadi A, Alam M, Goldberg LH, et al. Efficacy of narrow-margin excision of well-demarcated primary facial basal cell carcinomas. *J Am Acad Dermatol.* 2005;53:464–468.

48. Farhi D, Dupin N, Palangié A, et al. Incomplete excision of basal cell carcinoma: rate and associated factors among 362 consecutive cases. *Dermatol Surg.* 2007;33:1207–1214.

49. Bogdanov-Berezovsky A, Cohen AD, Glesinger R, et al. Risk factors for incomplete excision of squamous cell carcinomas. *J Dermatolog Treat.* 2005;16:341–344.

50. Koplin L, Zarem HA. Recurrent basal cell carcinoma. A review concerning the incidence, behavior, and management of recurrent basal cell carcinoma, with emphasis on the incompletely excised lesion. *Plast Reconstr Surg.* 1980;65:656–664.

51. Mosterd K, Krekels GA, Nieman FH, et al. Surgical excision versus Mohs' micrographic surgery for primary and recurrent basal-cell carcinoma of the face: a prospective randomised controlled trial with 5-years' follow-up. *Lancet Oncol.* 2008;9:1149–1156.

52. Miller SJ, Alam M, Andersen J, et al. Basal cell and squamous cell skin cancers. *J Natl Compr Canc Netw.* 2007;5:506–529.

53. Sahn RE, Lang PG. Sentinel lymph node biopsy for high-risk nonmelanoma skin cancers. *Dermatol Surg.* 2007;33:786–792 discussion 792–793.

54. Johnson TM, Rowe DE, Nelson BR, et al. Squamous cell carcinoma of the skin (excluding lip and oral mucosa). *J Am Acad Dermatol.* 1992;26:467–484.

55. Weinberg AS, Ogle CA, Shim EK. Metastatic cutaneous squamous cell carcinoma: an update. *Dermatol Surg.* 2007;33:885–899.

56. Brodland DG, Zitelli JA. Surgical margins for excision of primary cutaneous squamous cell carcinoma. *J Am Acad Dermatol.* 1992;27:241–248.

57. Rowe DE, Carroll RJ, Day CL. Prognostic factors for local recurrence, metastasis, and survival rates in squamous cell carcinoma of the skin, ear, and lip. Implications for treatment modality selection. *J Am Acad Dermatol.* 1992;26:976–990.

58. Petter G, Haustein UF. Histologic subtyping and malignancy assessment of cutaneous squamous cell carcinoma. *Dermatol Surg.* 2000;26:521–530.

59. Thosani MK, Schneck G, Jones EC. Periocular squamous cell carcinoma. *Dermatol Surg.* 2008;34:585–599.

60. Talmi YP, Horowitz Z, Wolf M, et al. Delayed metastases in skin cancer of the head and neck: the case of the "known primary". *Ann Plast Surg.* 1999;42:289–292.

61. Robinson JK, Fisher SG. Recurrent basal cell carcinoma after incomplete resection. *Arch Dermatol.* 2000;136:1318–1324.

62. Dellon AL, DeSilva S, Connolly M, et al. Prediction of recurrence in incompletely excised basal cell carcinoma. *Plast Reconstr Surg.* 1985;75:860–871.

63. Richmond JD, Davie RM. The significance of incomplete excision in patients with basal cell carcinoma. *Br J Plast Surg.* 1987;40:63–67.

64. Walker P, Hill D. Surgical treatment of basal cell carcinomas using standard postoperative histological assessment. *Australas J Dermatol.* 2006;47:1–12.

65. Griffiths RW. Audit of histologically incompletely excised basal cell carcinomas: recommendations for management by re-excision. *Br J Plast Surg.* 1999;52:24–28.

66. Boulinguez S, Grison-Tabone C, Lamant L, et al. Histological evolution of recurrent basal cell carcinoma and therapeutic implications for incompletely excised lesions. *Br J Dermatol.* 2004;151(3):623–636.

67. Griffiths RW, Suvarna SK, Stone J. Basal cell carcinoma histological clearance margins: an analysis of 1539 conventionally excised tumours. Wider still and deeper? *J Plast Reconstr Aesthet Surg.* 2007;60:41–47.

68. Metze K, Bedin V, Adam RL, et al. 'Recurrent' basal cell carcinomas may represent new primary neoplasias: differences between aggressive and nonaggressive histologic subtypes. *J Plast Reconstr Aesthet Surg.* 2007;60:451–453.

69. Guidelines of care for cutaneous squamous cell carcinoma. Committee on Guidelines of Care. Task Force on Cutaneous Squamous Cell Carcinoma. *J Am Acad Dermatol.* 1993;28:628–631.

# Mohs Surgery

CHAPTER 47

*Edward Upjohn and R. Stan Taylor*

## Key Points

- Mohs micrographic surgery (MMS) involves the extirpation of tumor and correct processing of tissue with frozen section histology to ensure that 100% of the margin is examined and has the advantage of sparing normal tissue.

- MMS has the highest cure rate for both primary and recurrent basal and squamous cell carcinomas.

- MMS is a useful technique for the management of some melanomas and less common malignancies.

- Defects resulting from MMS are either allowed to heal by secondary intention, repaired by the Mohs surgeon or referred to another reconstructive surgeon for closure.

## INTRODUCTION

Dr. Frederick Mohs pioneered the technique of micrographically mapped and margin controlled surgery and in honor of his discovery the name Mohs Micrographic Surgery (MMS) was applied to this procedure. MMS is now considered the treatment of choice for many skin cancers, especially where 100% margin examination is required and tissue sparing is sought.[1,2] MMS fulfils the two major requirements for skin cancer treatment: complete removal of the tumor and minimal damage to adjacent normal tissue and structures.

Many studies including large multicenter designs have demonstrated the safety and efficacy of MMS for the treatment of cancers of the skin.[3-5] MMS has the lowest recurrence rate for the treatment of both primary and recurrent or previously incompletely treated basal cell carcinomas and squamous cell carcinomas of the skin. These results have made MMS the treatment of choice for primary skin cancers found in functionally and cosmetically sensitive sites and for the treatment of recurrent tumors.

Central to the success of MMS is the role of the Mohs surgeon, who identifies the tumor and its clinical margin, excises the tumor and carefully maps its orientation, and finally examines the margin using a microscope to ensure the tumor is completely excised before reconstruction is undertaken. This process is described in detail below.

## DESCRIPTION OF PROCEDURE

Originally, MMS was performed by fixing tissue in situ prior to its excision. This required the application of zinc chloride paste, a painful and cumbersome procedure. The paste was applied to the tumor and allowed to fix the tissue (usually overnight) and then the fixed tissue was excised, processed and mounted on a slide, and finally examined by the treating surgeon. This in-situ tissue fixation was replaced with the 'fresh tissue' technique whereby tumor and a small margin of normal skin is excised, the margin is flattened and then rapidly frozen and processed so that the three-dimensional margin becomes a two-dimensional plane. The tissue is cut in a cryostat, mounted on one or more glass slides, stained and then examined by the surgeon. Positive margins are marked on the operative map and more tissue is then removed from the site where tumor is present and the processing and examination is repeated until a clear margin is obtained. These steps are illustrated in Figure 47.1. There are variations in how individual surgeons may perform MMS but the fundamental steps are the same regardless of individual technique.

First, the tumor is visually identified and the clinical margins delineated on the patient prior to injecting local anesthesia. Second, the clinically obvious tumor is debulked using either a scalpel or a curette, which facilitates removal of a specimen of uniform thickness at the base of the debulked area; thus, flattening of the initial margin of the specimen can be achieved during processing.[6] Next the initial margin specimen is excised around and underneath the area of debulking. Margin specimens are typically excised to include 1–2 mm margins but may be larger depending on the tumor type or whether it is a primary or recurrent lesion. The incisions used to harvest the specimens from the margin are often beveled, resulting in a bowl-shaped specimen, which also facilitates flattening of the tissue during processing. Beveled incisions are not always necessary and some Mohs surgeons no longer bevel their incisions.[7]

Before the specimen is removed, orienting marks are made on the specimen and the corresponding site on the patient. These marks can be applied with ink or may take the form of shallow, short nicks made with a scalpel bridging from the specimen to the adjacent rim of remaining tissue. Aligning the marks on the margin specimen with the marks at the edge of the patient's defect allows orientation of positive margins later in the process.

Typically, four marks are made on the specimen and patient's defect, one each at the 12, 3, 6 and 9 o'clock positions. If nicks are used, then the nicks on the margin specimen are commonly marked, with different colored tissue ink. Analysis of a single specimen with four evenly placed marks of different colors provides clear direction when correlating microscopic findings with their location on the patient. Unfortunately, to clear larger tumors it is not

515

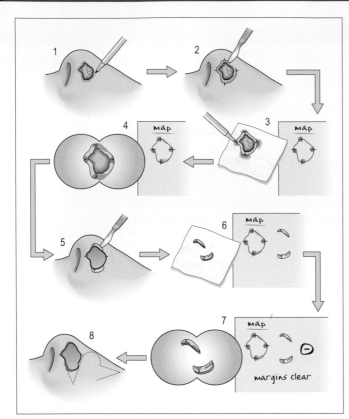

**Figure 47.1** MMS technique. (1) First step. Careful physical examination under bright lighting with delineation and marking of tumor margins. (2) Second step. Excision of tumor. (3) Third step. Inking of tissue with tissue dye. A map of the tissue with color coding is made. (4) Fourth step. Microscopic examination of prepared slides and identification of residual tumor. Corresponding marks are made on the map. (5–7) Repeat steps 2, 3 and 4 until histologically tumor-free margins are obtained. (8) Reconstruction of defect.

be visualized microscopically, but critical evaluation of each microscopic section by the surgeon is required to achieve this goal. Each section is examined to ensure 100% of the epidermis is present. Epidermal 'drop out' may occur due to incorrect flattening and mounting of the specimen or separation of the epidermis from the dermis during sectioning on the microtome. Visualization of continuous ink edges is also essential. Once all epidermal and inked edges are visualized, then the histology bordered by these edges is evaluated. Assuming that 100% of the epidermis and deep margin can be visualized, then the next goal is to find the 'absence of tumor', which by implication means the tumor has been completely excised. If tumor is visible, then the positive margin is carefully located in relation to the inked nicks and corresponding sites marked on the map. With the positive margins marked on the map, it is used to direct the excision of additional specimens to include the positive margins. The process is repeated until a negative margin is confirmed. The resulting defect may be repaired by the Mohs surgeon, allowed to heal by secondary intention, or the patient may be referred to another surgical colleague for reconstruction.

## The use of special stains

While the majority of basal and squamous cell carcinomas are examined with H&E or toluidine blue stains, for the examination of certain tumors additional stains can be helpful. These include oil-red-O for the staining of sebaceous carcinoma and immunohistochemical stains for other tumors such as melanoma, dermatofibrosarcoma protuberans (DFSP), and certain aggressive squamous cell carcinomas. It is desirable that these special stains be easy and quick to perform so as to minimize any additional waiting time between stages. Ideally they should also be specific for the tumor of interest and not stain normal cells or tissue which may confuse the Mohs surgeon reading the slide. Immunohistochemistry stains involve the use of a monoclonal antibody to detect a specific antigen in the tissue. In most situations, a secondary antibody that is specific for the primary antibody is then added to bind to the now tissue-bounded primary antibody. This secondary antibody is conjugated with an enzyme which subsequently catalyzes a chromogen to develop the stain, highlighting those cells or the structures in the tissue that have the specific antigen.[8] Immunohistochemistry staining traditionally takes around 90 minutes to perform, although newer techniques claim to reduce this to as short as 19 minutes.[9] Tissue sections should be thin enough to avoid excessive background staining, which may cause difficulty with interpretation of the histologic findings, and, therefore, 4 μm sections are recommended. Positive and negative controls are also required for the interpretation of immunostains. Immunostains are expensive and may have a short shelf-life, but in busy MMS units, with appropriately trained staff, their use can be cost-effective. A summary of the stains that are helpful for different tumors is included in Table 47.1. In general, the use of immunostains is reserved for those less commonly treated tumors that are difficult to identify on routine H&E stains. However, in certain subtypes of squamous cell carcinoma and basal cell carcinoma, their use is also desirable – for example, in the identification of perineural invasion of

possible to process a single large margin specimen and either the single specimen must be cut into multiple specimens or multiple specimens are harvested directly from the patient. In order to confirm that the entire margin has been evaluated and to piece the microscopic findings together, all edges of these specimens must be defined by an epidermis or be inked. Technicians processing these specimens look for the epidermis or inked vertical edges of the specimens when cutting the tissue in order to provide the surgeon with a histologic section that incorporates all edges and the intervening histology. The surgeon orients findings to the inked edges when evaluating sections at the microscope. Next, a map is carefully drawn by the surgeon to indicate the orientation of the margin specimen to local anatomic landmarks and the location of ink markings or the nicks along with their corresponding ink color. Tissue is then taken to the Mohs laboratory where it is flattened, mounted in tissue medium, frozen and processed using a microtome/cryostat into 6-μm-thick sections (thickness can vary with personal preference and staining requirements). The sections are placed on a glass slide and stained with hematoxylin and eosin (H&E) or toluidine blue; they are then cover slipped and examined by the Mohs surgeon.

If care has been taken to harvest, mark, map, cut and stain the margin specimens, then 100% of the margin can

**Table 47.1 Tumors and the Special Stains that may be Useful in their Treatment**

| Tumor | Stain | Characteristics |
|---|---|---|
| Melanoma | MART-1 | • A melanocyte differentiation antigen<br>• Most sensitive for melanoma and melanoma in situ<br>• Also known as Melan-A |
| | HMB-45 | • Recognizes a melanosome-associated glycoprotein, found in immature and neoplastic melanocytes<br>• Not as sensitive as other stains |
| | S100 | • Most sensitive stain for melanoma but not specific, also stains dendritic cells such as nerve and Langerhans cells<br>• Useful for desmoplastic melanoma |
| | Micro-ophthalmic transcription factor (MITF) | • Tyrosinase gene transcription factor<br>• Nuclear staining |
| Extramammary Paget's disease (EMPD) | Cytokeratin 7 | Paget's cells stain for low molecular weight keratin<br>Regarded as the most reliable stain for EMPD[78] |
| Dermatofibrosarcoma protuberans (DFSP) | CD34 | Selectively expressed by DFSP<br>Staining may be variable in individual tumors |
| Squamous cell carcinoma (SCC) | Pan-cytokeratin AE1/AE3 | Broad-spectrum anticytokeratin (high molecular weight keratin) |
| Basal cell carcinoma (BCC) | Ber-EP4 | Recognizes an epithelial glycoprotein antigen found in benign and malignant tissues<br>Stains BCC but not keratinocytes or SCC, generally absent from hair follicles (except the base) |
| Sebaceous carcinoma | Oil-red-O | Avid for lipid found in sebocytes |
| | Cam 5.2 | Low molecular weight keratin stain<br>Positive in 72% of sebaceous carcinomas but negative in benign sebaceous neoplasms[8] |
| | Cytokeratin AE1/AE3 | Stains 100% of sebaceous carcinomas (but also BCC and SCC) |
| Atypical fibroxanthoma (AFX) | CD10 | Stains AFX strongly and diffusely<br>Useful for poorly differentiated tumors with follicular extension |

these tumors, as well as the identification of squamous cell carcinoma showing single cell infiltration.[10]

## GENERAL INDICATIONS AND CONTRAINDICATIONS

### Indications

The indications for MMS have evolved over the years as the technique has become more widely adopted and even actively sought out by patients. Traditionally it had been reserved for recurrent tumors or primary tumors at high risk of incomplete excision or recurrence, such as those in periocular, nasal or auricular sites, those of an aggressive histological subtype and those that are large (e.g. >2cm in diameter). In more recent years, it has become common for the technique to be applied to all tumors on the head and neck and for larger tumors at other sites. Current recommendations state that immunosuppressed patients, such as solid organ transplant recipients with an increased lifetime risk of large skin tumor burdens, should be offered MMS, and these recommendations do not specify tumor site or size.[11] Patients are today aware of the technique from sources such as the internet and will often request it. MMS can be safely performed on patients of a wide range of age. Almost all areas of the body can be treated with MMS.

Individual surgeons must counsel their patients about the risks and benefits of the various treatment options available including MMS and come to a mutual decision based on available evidence and likely benefit for the patient. These issues are explored in further detail at the end of this chapter under the heading of 'Controversies'.

### Contraindications

As MMS is performed under local anesthesia, patients should be able to tolerate a medical procedure while conscious. Anxiolytics can be used during MMS but this may initiate other problems such as an inability for the patient to consent to a particular surgical closure after taking an anxiolytic. The fresh tissue technique is not able to easily process bone, so tumors with bony involvement should be referred for other treatment modalities. Superficial skin cancers such as Bowen's disease and superficial basal cell carcinoma may be amenable to less invasive treatment with topical imiquimod or photodynamic therapy. While treatments such as this may be appropriate for some tumors, careful follow-up of these patients is required in the light of case reports of invasive tumor recurring at the sites of previously treated squamous cell carcinoma in situ.[12] Superficial skin cancers are therefore an indication for MMS, especially where their margins may be clinically indistinct. For certain tumor presentations, the treatment algorithm is evolving and with this evolution the role or timing of MMS may change. An example is the treatment of DFSP with neoadjuvant imatinib prior to MMS.[13]

The cost of MMS in terms of patient and medical personnel's time, hospital or clinic resources, and money paid either by private insurance companies, public insurance or by self-funded patients should be considered, especially where MMS is a 'scarce' resource. The cost of the procedure must be balanced against the cost of the alternative and the cost of recurrence if the alternative treatment is less efficacious in clearing the tumor.

For very large tumors, the window of opportunity for using MMS may have passed and instead the patient should be referred to a surgical oncologist for tumor resection or for radiotherapy. On occasion, the Mohs surgeon may be asked to assist surgical oncologists in resecting larger tumors by clearing the peripheral margins but leaving deep margins for the surgical oncologist to resect. This may be helpful for tumors that are very deeply invasive into structures such as cartilage, muscle or bone, which may make MMS impractical for clearing the deep margin. By defining the peripheral extent of the tumor with MMS the surgical oncologist can focus on ensuring the deep margin is adequately resected.

## MMS FOR SKIN CANCER TREATMENT

### Basal cell and squamous cell carcinomas

The most evidence for the efficacy of MMS exists for the treatment of basal cell carcinoma (BCC – see Chapter 11) and squamous cell carcinoma (SCC – see Chapter 12). There are a growing number of treatment options for BCC and SCC, including surgical and non-surgical options. The choice of treatment is guided by many factors, including: the location of the tumor, the age and co-morbidities of the patient, the patient's preference, and of course the cure and failure rate of a particular treatment and the consequences of failed therapy. Whilst a small-diameter recurrent BCC on the back following treatment with curettage and electrodesiccation may be easily managed, a recurrent BCC in the nasofacial sulcus following curettage may be deeply invading and destructive. The definitive removal of such a recurrent facial BCC may be a far more complicated procedure than if it had been definitively managed in the first place. A proportion of previously incompletely excised BCC recur and when they recur they may exhibit more aggressive histology than at the time of their initial excision. In one study, 8 of 33 (24%) recurrent BCC became histologically more aggressive.[14] Standard excision of BCC is routinely associated with an incomplete excision rate of around 10% and risk factors for incomplete excision include periocular or nasal location and multifocal or infiltrative histological subtypes.[15]

MMS has the best documented and highest cure rate of all treatment modalities for BCC and SCC. In a review of the Australian Mohs database – a prospective, multicenter study that included 3370 patients in Australia treated with MMS for BCC – there was a 5-year recurrence rate of 1.4% for primary (previously untreated) BCC and 4% for previously treated and recurrent BCC.[3] The same group reported their 5-year follow-up for SCC treated with MMS and recurrence occurred in 15 of 381 patients (3.9%) at 5 years. The recurrence rate was 2.6% in patients with primary SCC and 5.9% in patients with previously recurrent SCC.[16]

## Melanoma

MMS is being increasingly utilized for melanoma management.[17] Controversy exists about the indications for MMS for melanoma and invasive melanoma in particular. This has continued with the increasing use of sentinel lymph node biopsy (SLNB) for invasive melanoma. SLNB is usually performed at the time of definitive and wide local excision (WLE) of the primary tumor and this can create a challenge for the scheduling of MMS. If MMS is performed some time before SLNB, then this may theoretically interfere with lymphatic drainage and therefore interfere with the correct identification of the sentinel lymph node.

There are particular sites, however, where MMS may provide advantages for tissue conservation in the treatment of melanoma and where it is unlikely to disrupt lymphatic drainage; an example of such a site is the nail apparatus. Brodland reviewed 14 patients treated for melanoma and melanoma in situ of the nail with MMS. He found a 79% disease-free survival which compared favorably to historical controls and had the advantage of sparing amputation, thus preserving the important function of the digit.[18] This article did not describe patients undergoing SLNB; however, theoretically there should be no difficulty in doing SLNB after performing resection of the primary nail melanoma with MMS.

### Melanoma in situ

Melanoma in situ is confined to the epidermis and by definition has no metastatic potential. Lentigo maligna, superficial spreading melanoma, and acral lentiginous melanoma may all be in situ. The ability to examine 100% of the surgical margin is of great theoretical benefit in these tumors as standard bread-loaf or vertical sections may miss the insidious spread that these tumors can exhibit. Lentigo maligna in particular is commonly found on the sun-damaged head and neck with indistinct clinical and histological margins. Sentinel lymph node biopsy is not indicated in the management of melanoma in situ. However, melanoma in situ may harbour a 'hidden' invasive component. Hill and Gramp found 32% of 66 lentigo malignas showed evidence of invasion after complete surgical excision. The majority of these (76%) were less than 1 mm in thickness.[19] For this reason it is essential that any melanoma in situ that is treated with MMS is debulked by an en-bloc removal and that this debulked specimen be submitted for paraffin-embedded permanent sectioning so that invasion can be detected and accurately measured.

Traditionally, 5 mm margins have been recommended for the WLE of melanoma in situ but this has been challenged, in particular for tumors of larger diameter. For example, in a study of head and neck lentigo malignas, margins greater than 5 mm were required to clear tumors in 22% of cases.[20] Standard 5 mm margins also may encroach on cosmetically and structurally sensitive areas such as eyelids and periocular structures. In this situation, a narrower margin that will still completely excise a tumor is highly desirable.

Various techniques have been described to achieve 100% margin control for the treatment of melanoma.[21] These include standard MMS, MMS with immunohistochemistry, and staged excision with permanent paraffin sections using a 'square technique'.[22,23] The major disadvantages of permanent sections using the square technique is the time required to process specimens, the loss of tissue conservation as a result of the geometric configuration of the defect, and the fact that the role of surgeon and pathologist may be separated, which can introduce discordance in the identification of residual tumor location.

The definition of a positive margin is key to the utility of MMS for melanoma in situ. Bricca et al. gave the criteria for diagnosing a positive margin (Table 47.2), and according to this group, isolated atypical melanocytes and melanocytic hyperplasia are commonly seen in sun-damaged skin and are not excised.[24] The key to the utility of MMS for melanoma in situ is the ability to confidently determine when margins are positive or negative on frozen section histology. Published figures for the sensitivity and specificity of frozen section histology range widely, from 59% sensitive and 81% specific for the detection of single melanocyte atypia[25] to 100% sensitivity and 90% specificity when frozen section was compared to paraffin section for the detection of melanoma.[26]

Immunostains are a valuable tool for the Mohs surgeon to aid in the diagnosis of positive margins in melanoma in situ, but some studies suggest that caution is needed when interpreting immunostained sections. In particular, the increased density of MART-1-positive melanocytes in sun-damaged skin has been discussed in the literature.[10] The conclusion of one group is that in normal sun-damaged skin there is an average density of 15–20 melanocytes per high-powered field, up to nine melanocytes may be confluent and melanocytes can extend into follicular structures.[27]

Single melanocyte atypia is a controversial facet of melanoma management. Firstly, the identification of atypia of a single melanocyte is more challenging, and some would argue impossible, with frozen section histology when compared with paraffin histology.[25] Secondly, the significance of such atypia when present is controversial. Should it be used as a marker for a positive margin resulting in a subsequent stage being taken? Or is it a more common finding in the epidermis of sun-damaged individuals and therefore a function of actinic damage and not a useful identifier of melanoma in situ? One method for ascertaining the presence of single melanocyte atypia in a timely manner may be the use of microwave-assisted rapid preparation of permanent paraffin sections. This method allows permanent paraffin sections to be produced in 2 hours and these slides were found to be comparable to standard conventional paraffin processed slides for the assessment of normal and abnormal melanocytes.[28]

Evidence for the efficacy of MMS for melanoma in situ is encouraging; Bricca et al. report a 0.3% recurrence rate after a mean of 58 months follow-up in their series of melanomas in situ treated with MMS.[24] This compares favorably to a British review with a recurrence rate of 20% after 42 months follow-up following standard WLE.[29] This same British study reported an initial incomplete excision rate of 9% when standard excision was performed for melanoma in situ. The use of MMS could therefore potentially avoid incomplete initial excisions in 9% of all melanoma in situ cases and also significantly reduce the recurrence rate of these tumors.

One technique for the management of melanomas in situ using MMS is outlined below and illustrated in Figures 47.2–47.8:

- The extent of the tumor (Fig. 47.2) is assessed with both natural and Wood's light examination.
- The clinical margin, as defined by the Wood's lamp, is marked, as is the first Mohs stage margin. The Mohs margin is marked 5 mm beyond the clinical margin (Fig. 47.3).

| Table 47.2 Identifying positive margins for melanoma in situ with MMS* |
| --- |
| **Criteria for the Identification of Positive Margins in Melanoma in situ** |
| • Nests of at least three atypical melanocytes<br>• Melanocytes above the dermoepidermal junction, or<br>• 'Non-uniform' contiguous hyperplasia of melanoyctes along the basement membrane |
| **Other Histologic Findings Raising Suspicion and Requiring Careful Interpretation** |
| • Extension of confluent, atypical melanocytes down adnexal structures<br>• Excessive number of melanophages<br>• Brisk inflammatory response, and<br>• Presence of dermal scarring |

Data from Bricca GM, Brodland DG, Ren D, et al. Cutaneous head and neck melanoma treated with Mohs micrographic surgery. *J Am Acad Dermatol.* 2005; 52(1): 92-100.

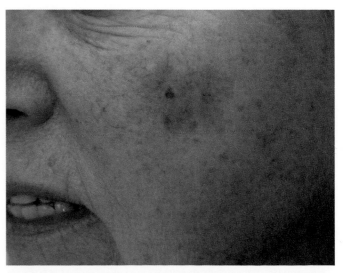

**Figure 47.2** A patient with a biopsy-proven Stage 1A melanoma of the left cheek.

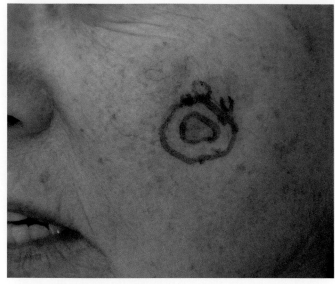

**Figure 47.3** The tumor outlined (inner circle) and the 5 mm margin (outer circle) after careful clinical examination and Wood's lamp examination.

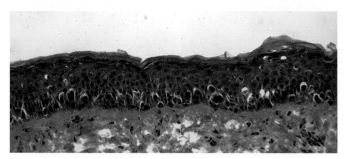

**Figure 47.4** Photomicrograph of the first stage H&E staining from the patient in Figure 47.2, showing nesting of melanocytes, large atypical melanocytes, increased melanocyte density, and pagetoid spread of melanocytes.

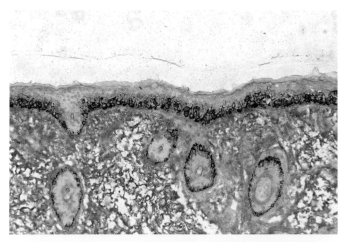

**Figure 47.5** Photomicrograph of the first stage MART-1 immunostaining from the patient in Figure 47.2, showing increased melanocyte density, nesting of melanocytes, and involvement of adnexal structures

- The tumor is excised to the deep dermis or subcutaneous fat along the clinical margin and sent for paraffin histological examination to check for invasive melanoma.
- The 5 mm Mohs margin is excised and processed by frozen section using the Mohs technique with H&E and MART-1 immunostains.

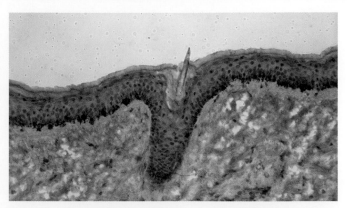

**Figure 47.6** Photomicrograph of the final stage MART-1 immunostaining from the patient in Figure 47.2, showing normal melanocyte density and no pagetoid spread of melanocytes.

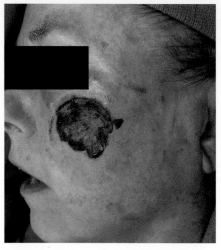

**Figure 47.7** The defect after four stages of MMS. (Reproduced by permission of James Thornton M.D.)

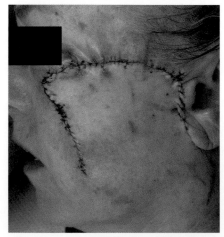

**Figure 47.8** The reconstruction. (Reproduced by permission of James Thornton M.D.)

- Positive margins (either on H&E or MART-1 stained slides) are re-excised on subsequent stages and examined again with H&E and MART-1 until clear margins are obtained.

If MMS is used for melanoma or melanoma in situ, it is essential that rigorous protocols are adhered to (especially for the successful use of immunostains) and that follow-up is instigated and records kept of any recurrence so that the true efficacy of MMS for this tumor can be properly assessed.

## Dermatofibrosarcoma protuberans

Dermatofibrosarcoma protuberans (DFSP) is a spindle cell tumor of the dermis (see Chapter 15). DFSP commonly presents as a growing nodule or plaque on the trunk, often with 'multiple protuberances'.[30] Metastases are very rare and often represent a fibrosarcomatous transformation. DFSP frequently recurs locally following WLE, with rates ranging from less than 10% to greater than 20%.[31-33] Given this high local recurrence rate, thought to be due to a propensity for subclinical extension, MMS is an excellent option for tumor clearance. Aggressive debulking of tumors and wider initial margins for the first stage (10–20 mm) are often indicated, especially for large or previously recurrent tumors. The use of CD34 immunostains may be helpful in the removal of this tumor. CD34 stains the spindle fibroblasts of the tumor and is especially helpful when operating at the peripheral extensions of the tumor so that tumor cells are more easily distinguished from the normal connective tissue. Much lower recurrence rates are reported for DFSP treated with MMS than with standard WLE, with rates of 1.6% (n=64, follow-up 5–96 months) and 0% (n=39, follow-up 1–155 months) for MMS compared to 20% (n=489, follow-up 1–360 months) for WLE.[34-36] Because of the subclinical extension and the requirement for wide margins, the ratio of defect size post MMS to lesion size is large for DFSP. In a review of 39 patients with DFSP treated at their institution with MMS, Thomas et al. found their ratio of defect area to lesional area was 7.7.[36] However, the final size of the defect is postulated to be smaller post MMS than post WLE; Hancox et al. using modified MMS (where MMS is performed but permanent paraffin sections are obtained instead of frozen sections) calculated that their defect to lesion size ratio was 5.1 (smaller than Thomas's) and that standard 3 cm margins would have produced a defect to lesion ratio of 7.[34]

Preoperative magnetic resonance imaging (MRI) may be indicated for larger tumors. This is of particular importance when tumors may be impinging upon viscera. For example, large DFSP located in the shoulder region can be in proximity to or invade into the lung apex. Situations like this require special considerations and coordination of specialty care. On MRI scans, the DFSP is hyperintense on T2 sequences.[37] A recent development in the treatment of DFSP, particularly for larger tumors, is the neoadjuvant use of imatinib.[13] Imatinib is an oral chemotherapeutic agent that inhibits the PDGFβ receptor tyrosine kinase which is overactivated in DFSP. Han et al. described four patients with DFSP who received imatinib for 3–7 months prior to undergoing MMS. Clinical tumor size was reduced on average by 36.9% and all four patients were free of recurrence at 1.5–4 years follow-up.

## Atypical fibroxanthoma

Atypical fibroxanthoma (AFX – see Chapter 13) is a spindle cell tumor typically occurring on the sun-exposed head and neck of older patients. The histology comprises an admixture of spindle cells, histiocyte-like cells, xanthomatous cells and multinucleate giant cells. Necrosis, vascular and perineural invasion are not considered features of AFX,[38] and if seen during MMS, their presence should prompt a reconsideration of the diagnosis to that of another spindle cell tumor such as spindled cell SCC.

Treatment is by surgical excision, radiotherapy is contraindicated and metastases are rare.[39] AFX treated with MMS appears to have a lower recurrence rate than with WLE. Davis et al. had no recurrences of AFX in 19 patients after an average follow-up of 29.6 months.[40] In contrast, Fretzin and Helwig reported a 9% recurrence rate in 101 patients treated with WLE with a longer follow-up of 4.1 years.[41] A review of 91 patients with 93 tumors treated at the Mayo Clinic by Ang et al. showed no recurrence in those patients treated with MMS, but two recurrences in the 23 patients treated with WLE.[42] Traditionally, radiotherapy has not been recommended as a therapy; however, Ang described its successful use as adjuvant therapy post MMS in a patient who developed multiple primary AFX.

## Malignant fibrous histiocytoma

Malignant fibrous histiocytoma (MFH) is an aggressive soft tissue sarcoma. In contrast to AFX which is found on the head and neck, MFH is more common on the extremities (60% occur in the lower extremities), retroperitoneum and internal viscera. AFX tumor cells are located in the superficial layers of the skin while MFH cells tend to occur in the deeper layers of the skin or subcutaneous tissues. MFHs arising from skeletal muscle or deep fascia require preoperative imaging and are usually not candidates for MMS. Smaller, more superficial tumors are the ones that have been amenable to MMS. There are five clinicopathologic subtypes of MFH: pleomorphic, myxoid, giant cell, inflammatory, and angiomatoid.[39] The largest series of patients treated with MMS was published 20 years ago.[43] Brown and Swanson reported 22 cases (which included 5 cases of AFX) with a mean follow-up of 3 years. Recurrence was noted in 9% but it is not clear whether these were AFX or MFH. In contrast, a much higher recurrence rate was noted in a large series of 196 cases treated with WLE, with tumors recurring in 44% of cases.[44] Unlike AFX, MFH can more commonly metastasize, usually to lung and lymph nodes. Size and depth of tumor are reported risk factors.[44] As with DFSP, initial first stage margins using MMS are wider for MFH (around 5–10 mm) than other tumors such as BCC or SCC.

## Microcystic adnexal carcinoma

Microcystic adnexal carcinoma (MAC) is a locally aggressive adnexal tumor which often has marked subclinical extension and a high risk of local recurrence. It is slow growing but locally aggressive. Mortality due to MAC is difficult to assess from the literature. MAC is often misdiagnosed on initial biopsy, particularly if this was a shallow shave, and it may therefore be confused with morpheic BCC, syringoma or desmoplastic trichoepithelioma. It is thus possible that a patient referred for MMS with a 'morpheic BCC' in fact has a MAC and a surgeon should therefore be ready to reconsider this diagnosis based on histologic findings at the time of surgery. MAC is common on the head and neck, in particular in the nasolabial and periorbital regions. Given high recurrence rates with standard excision of up to 30–40%, MMS is the recommended treatment option.[45,46] MAC is a radio-resistant tumor and may even be associated with prior irradiation. Radiotherapy is therefore not recommended as a treatment. It can be a locally destructive tumor but metastasis and mortality are considered exceptional.[47] In the largest follow-up series of MAC treated with MMS, 44 patients with 44 tumors were treated with MMS and included in an Australian database over a 9-year period. Ninety percent of these were located on the head and neck and 31% were recurrent tumors; 17.5% of tumors demonstrated perineural invasion and 85% of these were recurrent. Twenty patients completed 5 years of follow-up post MMS and there was a single documented recurrence, giving a 5% recurrence rate.[48] Other reviews have documented higher recurrence post MMS. The Geisinger group had an overall marginal recurrence rate of 12%; however, in those tumors that had been previously treated, recurrence rates were much higher at 33% (2 of 6 recurrent tumors treated with MMS recurring at follow-up).[36] Similar to DFSP, MACs treated with MMS have a large ratio of defect to lesion size; in the Geisinger review, this ratio was 6.2. Pre-surgical assessment should include close questioning to elucidate possible neurotropic involvement, which may be indicated by pain, burning or paresthesia.

## Merkel cell carcinoma

Merkel cell carcinoma is a rare carcinoma of neuroendocrine origin (see Chapter 17). It is commonly found on the head and neck of sun-damaged adults and has a propensity to metastasize to loco-regional lymph nodes. While MMS is typically used to gain clear surgical margins, the metastatic potential of Merkel cell carcinoma must be appreciated and an opinion sought from a radiation oncologist about the suitability of loco-regional radiotherapy post surgical clearance, especially as this tumor is highly radiosensitive.[49] SLNB has also been described for Merkel cell carcinoma and if this becomes more widespread it could be expected to have an effect on the logistics and timing of MMS in a similar way to the treatment of invasive melanomas.[50] MMS would seem to be an appropriate surgical therapy for Merkel cell carcinoma but whether cure rates for smaller tumors are higher with MMS than with WLE remains to be seen.

## Extramammary Paget's disease

Extramammary Paget's disease (EMPD – see Chapter 14) is an adenocarcinoma that is intraepidermal (but may become invasive) and is considered either primary to the skin (probably derived from intraepidermal sweat ducts) or secondary to an underlying malignancy, usually of the genitourinary or gastrointestinal tract. It is typically located on the genitals or elsewhere on the perineum of either males or females and is named for its clinical similarity to Paget's disease of the nipple.[51]

EMPD requires careful evaluation to determine whether it is primary or secondary to an underlying malignancy.

For EMPD of the perineum, this requires imaging of the genitourinary tract with cystoscopy and the gastrointestinal tract with colonoscopy. If an underlying internal malignancy is not found, then the EMPD is considered primary to the skin. The intraepidermal nature of EMPD, the fact that it commonly has microscopic extension beyond its clinical margins and that cutaneous EMPD is located in functionally and cosmetically sensitive areas makes MMS an appealing treatment option. Recurrence rates following MMS are significantly lower than for standard excision or other therapies. A Korean study found a lower recurrence rate of EMPD with MMS than with WLE, where 2 of 11 cases (18.2%) recurred after MMS compared with 8 recurrences of 22 (36.4%) after WLE.[52] Techniques that may aid in the treatment of EMPD with MMS include photodynamic diagnosis (where the tendency for EMPD to fluoresce after the application of ALA and irradiation with UV light is utilized), preoperative mapping biopsies and the use of cytokeratin-7 immunostains on Mohs stages.[53]

## Sebaceous carcinoma

Sebaceous carcinoma is an uncommon and aggressive tumor typically occurring on the eyelids. It may be extraocular as well, but the extraocular variant accounts for only 25% of cases. In some series, sebaceous carcinoma accounts for up to 25% of referred eyelid malignancies.[54] Clinically, it is a painless yellow papule, nodule or plaque. It can locally invade and damage the underlying structures of the orbit. Loco-regional lymph node metastases occur in 17–28% of cases.[55] In addition to spreading via direct extension, sebaceous carcinoma may exhibit pagetoid spread.[56] Special stains can be very helpful when using MMS to treat sebaceous carcinoma, in particular the use of oil-red-O stain, which highlights sebum-containing cells. A diagnosis of sebaceous carcinoma should prompt consideration of whether the patient may have Muir–Torre syndrome, a familial cancer syndrome with greatly increased incidence of sebaceous tumors, including sebaceous carcinoma.

Due to the risk of pagetoid spread in ocular sebaceous carcinoma, it is recommended that bulbar and palpebral conjunctival biopsies be performed of the involved eye at the time of MMS. These biopsies are processed in the Mohs laboratory with care being taken not to let the fragile tissue desiccate or be crushed during handling. If conjunctival biopsies are positive, as with advanced stage disease, then it becomes difficult to clear the tumor with a conservative approach and exenteration of the orbital contents is often considered the best option for cure. Consultation with ocular surgical colleagues is an important part of care for these patients.

## Angiosarcoma

Angiosarcoma is a rare, aggressive tumor with a 5-year survival rate of 12% (see Chapter 15).[57] The utility of MMS for the treatment of this tumor is not established and the literature contains only a few case reports of its use.[58,59] It may be considered for very small tumors, but, unfortunately, angiosarcoma is often an insidious and late-presenting tumor, at which time it may be unresectable. Careful examination using the recently described 'head tilt' maneuver may reveal a tumor's true extent and this can be confirmed with mapping biopsies.[60]

## Granular cell tumor

Granular cell tumors are unusual neoplasms that typically are found on the head and neck. About 60% of tumors are found on the skin and the remaining 40% are found on the tongue. The characteristic cell is large, located in the dermis and full of granules. The majority are considered benign, but malignant granular cell tumors are also described. On immunohistochemistry they are S100-positive.[61] MMS has been recommended for granular cell tumors that are clinically behaving as malignant.[62] Others have recommended that MMS be used for granular cell tumors that are in cosmetically or functionally sensitive sites.[63]

## Hidradenoma

Hidradenoma is a rare tumor of sweat glands that typically occurs on the head and neck or limbs, usually as a solitary solid or cystic nodule. Hidradenoma may be skin colored, erythematous or blue. Histologically they are circumscribed tumors with round eosinophilic cells clustered with clear cells, often with a small eccentric nucleus; duct-like structures are present. They may appear atypical with pleomorphic nuclei and giant cells. Atypical subtypes may be at higher risk of local recurrence or even have malignant potential.[47] For large or recurrent hidradenomas, MMS may be the treatment of choice.[61]

## THERAPUETIC CONTROVERSIES

Recently, the cost-effectiveness of MMS has been questioned following the publication of a randomized controlled trial of MMS and standard surgical excision for BCC of the face in The Netherlands. Primary outcome measure was the recurrence of tumor. The authors found slightly fewer recurrences after MMS than after standard excision in the treatment of primary and recurrent facial BCC, but the difference was not significant. Eighteen percent of primary and 32% of recurrent BCC were incompletely excised after the first excision in the standard excision group.[64] The authors did conclude that MMS had the advantage of avoiding large defects and obtaining better cosmetic outcomes for primary aggressive and all recurrent facial BCCs. The cost of MMS was significantly higher than standard excision for both primary and recurrent tumors.

This study provoked a wave of correspondence both supporting and rejecting the authors' conclusions. The initial margin taken in both MMS and standard excision patients was 3 mm which is larger than the usual initial margin for MMS and may well account for the lack of difference in aesthetic outcomes between MMS and standard excision patients for non-aggressive primary BCC. Comments that MMS is more time-consuming than standard excision are not necessarily correct. In an efficient practice it is possible to clear a tumor in a single stage and repair the defect in under an hour. Obviously, more complicated tumors will require more stages, but even so the time taken may still be comparable to standard excision, particularly if excision is incomplete and needs to be repeated.

A lack of clear, understandable and 'real world' follow-up data bedevils any attempt to compare different therapies for skin cancers. Many quoted cure rates are from studies that utilized different follow-up methodologies. The opportunity cost and emotional cost of incomplete excisions of tumors using standard excision is difficult to quantify and is to a large extent intangible. Even in tertiary referral centers with experienced surgeons, the incomplete excision rate for previously untreated primary BCC is as high as 11.2%. For recurrent BCC the rate of incomplete excision jumps to 26.8%.[65] It is probably only the fact that BCC is considered 'non-life-threatening' that these high initial 'treatment failure' rates are tolerated by the medical community and patients.

A recent study has confirmed the tissue-sparing nature of MMS for the treatment of BCC.[66] In this randomized controlled study a comparison was made between standard excision of BCC with 4 mm margins and MMS with initial 2 mm margins. The median area of the surgical defects in the MMS group was 116.6 mm², versus 187.7 mm² in the control group. In the Smeets study[64] there was no significant difference in defect size between single-stage MMS defects and standard surgical defects for both primary and recurrent BCC, but defect size was not a primary outcome measure in that study.

## SAFETY

MMS is a very safe procedure and is routinely carried out in the office setting. Like all surgical procedures, however, it is associated with risks. Much has been published recently about the cessation of anticoagulants prior to dermatologic surgery and MMS.[67–69] The consensus is that the risk associated with bleeding post dermatologic surgery and MMS in patients who take anticoagulants is much less than the risk of thromboembolic events that may occur if this anticoagulation is ceased.[70] Exceptional cases in which cessation of long-term anticoagulation or antiplatelet therapy should be considered are those in which large defects result from MMS, placing patients at greater risk of postoperative bleeding, and when hemorrhage would compromise optimal outcome of the post-MMS repair procedure. Switching these patients to short-acting anticoagulation therapy may be most appropriate.

Lidocaine toxicity must be avoided during MMS. Careful record-keeping of the quantity and timing of local anesthetic administered to the patient is critical, especially where tumors are large and may require multiple stages to clear. Lidocaine toxicity may manifest as talkativeness, perioral paresthesia, tinnitus, vomiting, tremors, seizures, and ultimately cardiopulmonary arrest. The maximum lidocaine dose in adults is 5 mg/kg for straight lidocaine and 7 mg/kg for lidocaine mixed with epinephrine (adrenaline).[71]

Postoperative infection rates in cutaneous surgery are generally low but the published rates of wound infection do vary widely, from 1.9% to 8.6%.[72,73] To ensure that infection rates are as low as possible, the use of alcohol-based hand rubs,[74] good hemostasis and excellent aseptic technique are required. Recently updated guidelines for the use of prophylactic antibiotics prior to cutaneous surgery, based on the most recent American Heart Association, American Dental Association, and American Academy of Orthopedic Surgeons guidelines, have been published.[75]

The correct preoperative diagnosis is key to the safe and effective use of MMS. For example, plaque-like syringomas may mimic large morpheic BCC or MAC, and large MMS defects being created unnecessarily for this benign tumor are not acceptable. Some Mohs surgeons have their own dermatopathologist review the slides of all patients referred to them for MMS. Butler et al. reviewed 3345 cases and in 2.2% of cases the diagnosis was revised, resulting in a change of management plan in 61% of those cases.[76]

Occasionally, during the course of performing MMS, tumors will be encountered which are unresectable, but this may not be apparent until after many stages have been performed. In this situation, it is important to map positive margins as accurately as possible, preferably with the aid of clinical photographs, so that further surgery or adjuvant radiotherapy can be targeted accurately. Examples where this may occur include perineural invasion that involves the trigeminal nerve and tracks back through the trigeminal foramen; this situation may require neurosurgery or stereotactic radiotherapy to treat the trigeminal nerve. Digital photography combined with graphics software used in most office settings allows surgeons to note on images of Mohs defects the location of positive margins. Using e-mail, these images are easily accessible to consultants and other members of the treatment team.

Two cases of cerebral air emboli have been described following MMS for tumors of the scalp.[77] While MMS is commonly performed on scalp tumors and this complication is rare, it is important to recognize that air embolism may occur via the non-collapsing veins of the head and neck such as the epiploic veins and the emissary veins which then drain to the dural venous sinuses. Therefore, for patients with large scalp tumors, especially those that may possibly involve the underlying bone, careful patient positioning is required to limit negative pressure gradients that can facilitate such air emboli. This should include the time when the patient is undergoing surgery and also whilst he or she is waiting between stages.

## FUTURE OUTLOOK

With more trained Mohs surgeons operating now than at any time in the past, the future of MMS would appear certain. MMS is also becoming more widely known outside of its country of origin (the US). Like all therapies, the use of MMS must be justified by robust evidence, and as with all surgical techniques, outcomes are dependent on the meticulous execution and attention to detail. Even the smallest Mohs practice is a team effort, with at least a Mohs surgeon, a histotechnologist and a nurse needing to work together and communicate effectively for the benefit of their patient. The acquisition, maintenance and enhancement of skills required for MMS will continue to be of paramount importance to the Mohs surgeon in order to provide optimal care for his or her patients.

## REFERENCES

1. Brodland DG, Amonette R, Hanke CW, et al. The history and evolution of Mohs micrographic surgery. *Dermatol Surg.* 2000;26(4):303–307.
2. Randle HW, Roenigk RK, Brodland DG. Giant basal cell carcinoma (T3). Who is at risk? *Cancer.* 1993;72(5):1624–1630.
3. Leibovitch I, Huilgol SC, Selva D, et al. Basal cell carcinoma treated with Mohs surgery in Australia II. Outcome at 5-year follow-up. *J Am Acad Dermatol.* 2005;53(3):452–457.
4. Rowe DE, Carroll RJ, Day Jr CL. Long-term recurrence rates in previously untreated (primary) basal cell carcinoma: implications for patient follow-up. *J Dermatol Surg Oncol.* 1989;15(3):315–328.
5. Rowe DE, Carroll RJ, Day Jr CL. Prognostic factors for local recurrence, metastasis, and survival rates in squamous cell carcinoma of the skin, ear, and lip. Implications for treatment modality selection. *J Am Acad Dermatol.* 1992;26(6):976–990.
6. Ratner D, Bagiella E. The efficacy of curettage in delineating margins of basal cell carcinoma before Mohs micrographic surgery. *Dermatol Surg.* 2003;29(9):899–903.
7. Weber PJ, Moody BR, Dryden RM, et al. Mohs surgery and processing: novel optimizations and enhancements. *Dermatol Surg.* 2000;26(10):909–914.
8. Thosani MK, Marghoob A, Chen CS. Current progress of immunostains in Mohs micrographic surgery: a review. *Dermatol Surg.* 2008;34(12):1621–1636.
9. Cherpelis BS, Moore R, Ladd S, et al. Comparison of MART-1 frozen sections to permanent sections using a rapid 19-minute protocol. *Dermatol Surg.* 2009;35(2):207–213.
10. Stranahan D, Cherpelis BS, Glass LF, et al. Immunohistochemical stains in Mohs surgery: a review. *Dermatol Surg.* 2009;35(7):1023–1034.
11. Berg D, Otley CC. Skin cancer in organ transplant recipients: epidemiology, pathogenesis, and management. *J Am Acad Dermatol.* 2002;47(1):1–17 quiz 18–20.
12. Goh MS. Invasive squamous cell carcinoma after treatment of carcinoma in situ with 5% imiquimod cream. *Australas J Dermatol.* 2006;47(3):186–188.
13. Han A, Chen EH, Niedt G, et al. Neoadjuvant imatinib therapy for dermatofibrosarcoma protuberans. *Arch Dermatol.* 2009;145(7):792–796.
14. Boulinguez S, Grison-Tabone C, Lamant L, et al. Histological evolution of recurrent basal cell carcinoma and therapeutic implications for incompletely excised lesions. *Br J Dermatol.* 2004;151(3):623–626.
15. Farhi D, Dupin N, Palangie A, et al. Incomplete excision of basal cell carcinoma: rate and associated factors among 362 consecutive cases. *Dermatol Surg.* 2007;33(10):1207–1214.
16. Leibovitch I, Huilgol SC, Selva D, et al. Cutaneous squamous cell carcinoma treated with Mohs micrographic surgery in Australia I. Experience over 10 years. *J Am Acad Dermatol.* 2005;53(2):253–260.
17. MacKie RM, Hauschild A, Eggermont AM. Epidemiology of invasive cutaneous melanoma. *Ann Oncol.* 2009;20(suppl 6):vi1–vi7.
18. Brodland DG. The treatment of nail apparatus melanoma with Mohs micrographic surgery. *Dermatol Surg.* 2001;27(3):269–273.
19. Hill DC, Gramp AA. Surgical treatment of lentigo maligna and lentigo maligna melanoma. *Australas J Dermatol.* 1999;40(1):25–30.
20. Huilgol SC, Selva D, Chen C, et al. Surgical margins for lentigo maligna and lentigo maligna melanoma: the technique of mapped serial excision. *Arch Dermatol.* 2004;140(9):1087–1092.
21. Dawn ME, Dawn AG, Miller SJ. Mohs surgery for the treatment of melanoma in situ: a review. *Dermatol Surg.* 2007;33(4):395–402.
22. Johnson TM, Headington JT, Baker SR, et al. Usefulness of the staged excision for lentigo maligna and lentigo maligna melanoma: the "square" procedure. *J Am Acad Dermatol.* 1997;37(5 Pt 1):758–764.
23. Demirci H, Johnson TM, Frueh BR, et al. Management of periocular cutaneous melanoma with a staged excision technique and permanent sections: the square procedure. *Ophthalmology.* 2008;115(12):2295–2300.e3.
24. Bricca GM, Brodland DG, Ren D, et al. Cutaneous head and neck melanoma treated with Mohs micrographic surgery. *J Am Acad Dermatol.* 2005;52(1):92–100.
25. Barlow RJ, White CR, Swanson NA. Mohs' micrographic surgery using frozen sections alone may be unsuitable for detecting single atypical melanocytes at the margins of melanoma in situ. *Br J Dermatol.* 2002;146(2):290–294.
26. Zitelli JA, Moy RL, Abell E. The reliability of frozen sections in the evaluation of surgical margins for melanoma. *J Am Acad Dermatol.* 1991;24(1):102–106.
27. Hendi A, Brodland DG, Zitelli JA. Melanocytes in long-standing sun-exposed skin: quantitative analysis using the MART-1 immunostain. *Arch Dermatol.* 2006;142(7):871–876.
28. Mallipeddi R, Stark J, Xie XJ, et al. A novel 2-hour method for rapid preparation of permanent paraffin sections when treating melanoma in situ with mohs micrographic surgery. *Dermatol Surg.* 2008;34(11):1520–1526.
29. Osborne JE, Hutchinson PE. A follow-up study to investigate the efficacy of initial treatment of lentigo maligna with surgical excision. *Br J Plast Surg.* 2002;55(8):611–615.

30. Rapini RP. *Practical Dermatopathology*. Philadelphia: Elsevier Mosby; 2005.

31. Chang CK, Jacobs IA, Salti GI. Outcomes of surgery for dermatofibrosarcoma protuberans. *Eur J Surg Oncol*. 2004;30(3):341–345.

32. Gloster Jr HM. Dermatofibrosarcoma protuberans. *J Am Acad Dermatol*. 1996;35(3 Pt 1):355–374 quiz 375–376.

33. Lindner NJ, Scarborough MT, Powell GJ, et al. Revision surgery in dermatofibrosarcoma protuberans of the trunk and extremities. *Eur J Surg Oncol*. 1999;25(4):392–397.

34. Hancox JG, Kelley B, Greenway Jr HT. Treatment of dermatofibroma sarcoma protuberans using modified Mohs micrographic surgery: no recurrences and smaller defects. *Dermatol Surg*. 2008;34(6):780–784.

35. Gloster Jr HM, Harris KR, Roenigk RK. A comparison between Mohs micrographic surgery and wide surgical excision for the treatment of dermatofibrosarcoma protuberans. *J Am Acad Dermatol*. 1996;35(1):82–87.

36. Thomas CJ, Wood GC, Marks VJ. Mohs micrographic surgery in the treatment of rare aggressive cutaneous tumors: the Geisinger experience. *Dermatol Surg*. 2007;33(3):333–339.

37. Bergin P, Rezaei S, Lau Q, et al. Dermatofibrosarcoma protuberans, magnetic resonance imaging and pathological correlation. *Australas Radiol*. 2007;51 Spec No: B64–B66.

38. McKee PH, Calonje E, Granter SR. Connective tissue tumors. In: McKee PH, Calonje E, Granter SR, eds. *Pathology of the Skin with Clinical Correlations*. Philadelphia: Elsevier Mosby; 2005:1757–1760.

39. Calonje E, MacKie RM. Soft-tissue tumours and tumour-like conditions. In: Burns T, Breathnach SM, Cox N, et al., eds. *Rook's Textbook of Dermatology*. Oxford: Blackwell; 2004:53.1–53.47.

40. Davis JL, Randle HW, Zalla MJ, et al. A comparison of Mohs micrographic surgery and wide excision for the treatment of atypical fibroxanthoma. *Dermatol Surg*. 1997;23(2):105–110.

41. Fretzin DF, Helwig EB. Atypical fibroxanthoma of the skin. A clinicopathologic study of 140 cases. *Cancer*. 1973;31(6):1541–1552.

42. Ang GC, Roenigk RK, Otley CC, et al. More than 2 decades of treating atypical fibroxanthoma at Mayo Clinic: what have we learned from 91 patients? *Dermatol Surg*. 2009;35(5):765–772.

43. Brown MD, Swanson NA. Treatment of malignant fibrous histiocytoma and atypical fibrous xanthomas with micrographic surgery. *J Dermatol Surg Oncol*. 1989;15(12):1287–1292.

44. Weiss SW, Enzinger FM. Malignant fibrous histiocytoma: an analysis of 200 cases. *Cancer*. 1978;41(6):2250–2266.

45. LeBoit PE, Sexton M. Microcystic adnexal carcinoma of the skin. A reappraisal of the differentiation and differential diagnosis of an underrecognized neoplasm. *J Am Acad Dermatol*. 1993;29(4):609–618.

46. Burns MK, Chen SP, Goldberg LH. Microcystic adnexal carcinoma. Ten cases treated by Mohs micrographic surgery. *J Dermatol Surg Oncol*. 1994;20(7):429–434.

47. Brenn T, McKee PH. Tumors of the sweat glands. In: McKee PH, Calonje E, Granter SR, eds. *Pathology of the Skin with Clinical Correlations*. Philadelphia: Elsevier Mosby; 2005:1632–1635.

48. Leibovitch I, Huilgol SC, Selva D, et al. Microcystic adnexal carcinoma: treatment with Mohs micrographic surgery. *J Am Acad Dermatol*. 2005;52(2):295–300.

49. Veness MJ. Merkel cell carcinoma (primary cutaneous neuroendocrine carcinoma): an overview on management. *Australas J Dermatol*. 2006;47(3):160–165.

50. Mehrany K, Otley CC, Weenig RH, et al. A meta-analysis of the prognostic significance of sentinel lymph node status in Merkel cell carcinoma. *Dermatol Surg*. 2002;28(2):113–117 discussion 117.

51. McKee PH, Calonje E, Granter SR. Cutaneous metastases and Paget's disease of the skin. In: McKee PH, Calonje E, Granter SR, eds. *Pathology of the Skin with Clinical Correlations*. Philadelphia: Elsevier Mosby; 2005:1514–1518.

52. Lee KY, Roh MR, Chung WG, et al. Comparison of Mohs micrographic surgery and wide excision for extramammary Paget's disease: Korean experience. *Dermatol Surg*. 2009;35(1):34–40.

53. O'Connor WJ, Lim KK, Zalla MJ, et al. Comparison of Mohs micrographic surgery and wide excision for extramammary Paget's disease. *Dermatol Surg*. 2003;29(7):723–727.

54. Lazar AJF, McKee PH. Tumors and related lesions of the sebaceous glands. In: McKee PH, Calonje E, Granter SR, eds. *Pathology of the Skin with Clinical Correlations*. Philadelphia: Elsevier Mosby; 2005:1579–1586.

55. Ratz JL, Luu-Duong S, Kulwin DR. Sebaceous carcinoma of the eyelid treated with Mohs' surgery. *J Am Acad Dermatol*. 1986;14(4):668–673.

56. Berlin AL, Amin SP, Goldberg DJ. Extraocular sebaceous carcinoma treated with Mohs micrographic surgery: report of a case and review of literature. *Dermatol Surg*. 2008;34(2):254–257.

57. Holden CA, Spittle MF, Jones EW. Angiosarcoma of the face and scalp, prognosis and treatment. *Cancer*. 1987;59(5):1046–1057.

58. Goldberg DJ, Kim YA. Angiosarcoma of the scalp treated with Mohs micrographic surgery. *J Dermatol Surg Oncol*. 1993;19(2):156–158.

59. Muscarella VA. Angiosarcoma treated by Mohs micrographic surgery. *J Dermatol Surg Oncol*. 1993;19(12):1132–1133.

60. Asgari MM, Cockerell CJ, Weitzul S. The head-tilt maneuver: a clinical aid in recognizing head and neck angiosarcomas. *Arch Dermatol*. 2007;143(1):75–77.

61. Chilukuri S, Peterson SR, Goldberg LH. Granular cell tumor of the heel treated with Mohs technique. *Dermatol Surg*. 2004;30(7):1046–1049.

62. Dzubow LM, Kramer EM. Treatment of a large, ulcerating, granular-cell tumor by microscopically controlled excision. *J Dermatol Surg Oncol*. 1985;11(4):392–395.

63. Gardner ES, Goldberg LH. Granular cell tumor treated with Mohs micrographic surgery: report of a case and review of the literature. *Dermatol Surg*. 2001;27(8):772–774.

64. Smeets NW, Krekels GA, Ostertag JU, et al. Surgical excision vs Mohs' micrographic surgery for basal-cell carcinoma of the face: randomised controlled trial. *Lancet*. 2004;364(9447):1766–1772.

65. Su SY, Giorlando F, Ek EW, et al. Incomplete excision of basal cell carcinoma: a prospective trial. *Plast Reconstr Surg*. 2007;120(5):1240–1248.

66. Muller FM, Dawe RS, Moseley H, et al. Randomized comparison of Mohs micrographic surgery and surgical excision for small nodular basal cell carcinoma: tissue-sparing outcome. *Dermatol Surg*. 2009;35(9):1349–1354.

67. Lewis KG, Dufresne Jr RG. A meta-analysis of complications attributed to anticoagulation among patients following cutaneous surgery. *Dermatol Surg*. 2008;34(2):160–164 discussion 164–165.

68. Hurst EA, Yu SS, Grekin RC, et al. Bleeding complications in dermatologic surgery. *Semin Cutan Med Surg*. 2007;26(1):40–46.

69. Alcalay J, Alkalay R. Controversies in perioperative management of blood thinners in dermatologic surgery: continue or discontinue? *Dermatol Surg*. 2004;30(8):1091–1094 discussion 1094.

70. Otley CC. Continuation of medically necessary aspirin and warfarin during cutaneous surgery. *Mayo Clin Proc*. 2003;78(11):1392–1396.

71. Soriano TT, Lask GP, Dinehart SM. Anesthesia and analgesia. In: Robinson JK, Hanke CW, Sengelmann RD, et al., eds. *Surgery of the Skin*. Philadeplphia: Elsevier; 2005:39–58.

72. Rogues AM, Lasheras A, Amici JM, et al. Infection control practices and infectious complications in dermatological surgery. *J Hosp Infect*. 2007;65(3):258–263.

73. Heal C, Buettner P, Browning S. Risk factors for wound infection after minor surgery in general practice. *Med J Aust*. 2006;185(5):255–258.

74. Widmer AF, Rotter M, Voss A, et al. Surgical hand preparation: state-of-the-art. *J Hosp Infect*. 2010;74(2):112–122.

75. Wright TI, Baddour LM, Berbari EF, et al. Antibiotic prophylaxis in dermatologic surgery: advisory statement 2008. *J Am Acad Dermatol*. 2008;59(3):464–473.

76. Butler ST, Youker SR, Mandrell J, et al. The importance of reviewing pathology specimens before Mohs surgery. *Dermatol Surg*. 2009;35(3):407–412.

77. Goldman G, Altmayer S, Sambandan P, et al. Development of cerebral air emboli during Mohs micrographic surgery. *Dermatol Surg*. 2009;35(9):1414–1421.

78. Smith KJ, Tuur S, Corvette D, et al. Cytokeratin 7 staining in mammary and extramammary Paget's disease. *Mod Pathol*. 1997;10(11):1069–1074.

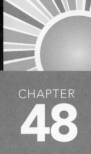

# Treatment of Disseminated Non-Melanoma Skin Cancers

*Kathryn A. Gold and Merrill S. Kies*

---

## Key Points

- Basal cell carcinomas only rarely disseminate widely.
- Squamous cell carcinoma of the skin has a variable risk of distant metastasis up to 16%.
- Platinum-based combination therapy is used to treat both metastatic basal and squamous cell carcinoma; data from randomized trials are lacking.
- Merkel cell carcinoma is an aggressive malignancy of the skin which frequently metastasizes. It is treated in a similar manner to small cell carcinoma of the lung, with platinum–etoposide combination regimens.
- Targeted agents are being tested in these rare tumors, and this represents a promising area of research.

## INTRODUCTION

Melanoma is a well-recognized and potentially invasive primary skin cancer, with comprehensive discussion in this textbook. However, other forms of skin cancer, particularly Merkel cell carcinoma, adnexal cancers and a percentage of squamous cell carcinomas, may also be regionally invasive or metastasize widely and become life-threatening. In the United States, over 2,000,000 cases of non-melanoma skin cancer are diagnosed yearly, and the incidence is increasing.[1,2] Physicians are encountering larger numbers of patients with these tumors who also have metastatic disease. Management may be particularly difficult because reports of systemic therapy have tended to be anecdotal, clinical trials devoted to metastatic skin malignancies are few and not widely available, and the medical literature devoted to this topic is limited. This chapter reviews published data and provides an outline of the systemic approach to treatment of advanced non-melanoma skin cancers as practiced at MD Anderson.

## DISSEMINATED BASAL CELL CARCINOMA

Basal cell carcinoma is the most common cancer worldwide, accounting for 75% of all non-melanoma skin cancers,[3] and for the majority of cases is effectively treated by surgical resection (see Chapter 11). A minority of patients may require radiotherapy in addition to surgery, or may be candidates for primary treatment with radiotherapy, depending upon the precise site and extent of tumor. Disseminated metastases are rare, with few case reports in the literature.[4] With clinical or radiographic evidence for distant metastases, biopsy is required to firmly establish the diagnosis, and to rule out other metastatic cancers, before proceeding with chemotherapy. Even biopsy evidence may sometimes be difficult to interpret, as poorly differentiated malignancies may appear 'basaloid' but not truly represent metastatic basal cell carcinoma of the skin. Distant metastases occur most often in association with primary cancers of the head and neck area, and have been recognized a median of 9 years following the original diagnosis.[5] Phase II clinical trials of chemotherapy and newer targeted agents are not reported in this rare disease. Nonetheless, there are reports of cisplatin-based regimens that have been shown to induce antitumor responses, but an effect on overall survival is not yet possible to conclude.[6] Molecular abnormalities often seen in basal cell carcinoma include *p53* mutation and activation, and alterations of the hedgehog signaling pathway.[7,8]

Activation of the hedgehog pathway is seen in both sporadic and familial cases, and has therefore been a target of therapeutic trials. In an intriguing recent report, Von Hoff et al. observed striking albeit brief responses of basal cell carcinoma to the hedgehog inhibitor GDC-0449 in a phase I trial. Eighteen of 33 patients with locally advanced or metastatic basal cell carcinoma had some measure of objective response (Fig. 48.1).[9] Currently, a multicenter, single-arm phase II trial of this agent is in progress.

Patients with objective clinical and radiographic signs of multiple and progressive metastases are generally not amenable to salvage surgical resection, and are candidates for chemotherapy. Most often a platin and taxane-based regimen, incorporating cis- or carboplatin and paclitaxel or docetaxel are used as these combinations have activity in a wide spectrum of epithelial cancers and toxicities are predictable. Patients are generally treated with two cycles of therapy and then formally assessed for response including CT or CT-PET imaging to assess the relative benefit before a decision to continue the program or not is made. An attractive alternative would be recommendation for entry to a clinical trial, as indicated above, or more often a phase I study.

## DISSEMINATED SQUAMOUS CELL CARCINOMA

Squamous cell carcinoma is the second most common human cancer, after basal cell carcinoma; it is frequently encountered by dermatologists and effectively managed with surgical resection in the vast majority of cases (Chapter 12). Over 100,000 cases are diagnosed yearly in the United States. The natural history tends to be more

**Figure 48.1** Demonstration of responses of advanced basal cell carcinoma following treatment with an experimental hedgehog inhibitor. (From Von Hoff DD, LoRusso PM, Rudin CM, et al. Inhibition of the hedgehog pathway in advanced basal-cell carcinoma. *N Engl J Med.* 2009;361(12):1164-1172.)

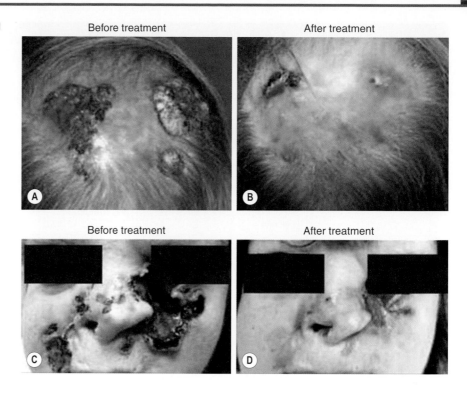

aggressive than that of basal cell carcinoma, with regional tumor invasion, and nodal and distant metastases affecting a significant minority of patients. The observed risk of developing distant metastatic disease is not clearly established and there is a broad range reported in the literature, from 0.05% to 16%,[3] dependent upon the clinical and pathologic presentation. Increasing tumor bulk, depth of invasion, poorly differentiated or variant histology, perineural spread, and involved surgical margins predict for tumor recurrence and disease-specific mortality.[10] Moreover, squamous cell carcinomas arising in a burn site, or from severely injured or chronically diseased skin from excessive sun exposure or other reasons, have a higher rate of metastasis approaching 40% at 5 years.[11] Patients chronically immunosuppressed after transplant procedures or known to have chronic lymphocytic leukemia are at high risk of developing squamous cell carcinoma, and more often have aggressive courses with increased risk of regional and distant metastases.[3]

Phase II clinical trials for advanced cutaneous squamous cell carcinoma have been infrequently reported in the literature and studies have been limited by slow accrual. However, there has been an emerging literature to guide the choice of therapy. Of some note, there has been a tendency to enroll patients with either locally advanced or distant metastatic disease, and so variability in patient selection for uncontrolled studies may make comparison of results hazardous. Generally, locally advanced disease appears to be more sensitive to chemotherapy than distant metastatic disease. Tumor response rates may also be higher for disease in sites not previously irradiated and in patients with favorable performance status, Eastern Cooperative Oncology Group (ECOG) 0 or 1. A majority of the trials discussed here enrolled patients both with locally advanced disease and with distant metastases.

There have been anecdotal reports and underpowered studies with small numbers showing moderate to high response rates with cisplatin-based combination therapy. Effects upon overall survival have not been clearly demonstrated. Denic[12] reported the use of cisplatin and bleomycin in the pre-operative setting for patients with locally advanced disease, observing partial tumor responses in 80% of patients. Surgical pathology showed no complete pathologic responses and all patients were reported to be rendered free of disease after surgery, though long-term follow-up was not available. Cisplatin has been administered with doxorubicin[13] and with fluorouracil and bleomycin[14] in small series, with observations of tumor responses in 87% and 84% of patients, respectively. Long-term survival data are not available. The combination of carboplatin (AUC 5 to 6) and paclitaxel (175–200 mg/m$^2$) is more commonly used today in the setting of widely metastatic non-curable disease. Table 48.1 summarizes reported phase II studies.[12-18]

Given the higher rates of squamous cell carcinoma in patients with chronic immune suppression, immunomodulating therapy has been attempted in this disease. Immunotherapy to modify the immune suppression is now feasible with a range of new agents that deserve evaluation. In an innovative trial, Lippman and colleagues studied a combination of interferon-α-2a and 13-*cis*-retinoic acid and observed responses in 68% of 28 patients with advanced, inoperable squamous cell carcinoma. Responses were greater in locally advanced albeit inoperable disease (93%) than in patients with distant metastases (25%).[16] Side effects of the drug regimen were significant – fatigue, flu-like symptoms, and dry skin – prompting dose modulation in 18 patients.[16]

A similar regimen was tested as adjuvant therapy following surgical resection of aggressive lesions in a randomized,

**Table 48.1 Selected Phase II Studies in Advanced Cutaneous Squamous Cell Carcinoma**

| Study | Regimen | Patients Enrolled | Response Rate | Comments |
|---|---|---|---|---|
| Guthrie et al., 1985[13] | Cisplatin 75 mg/m² IV and doxorubicin 50 mg/m² IV every 3 weeks | Locally advanced | 87% | |
| Sadek et al., 1990[14] | Cisplatin 100 mg/m² IV, 5-FU 650 mg/m²/day IV × 5 days, and bleomycin 15 mg IV bolus, then 16 mg/m²/day IV × 5 days every 3 to 4 weeks | Locally advanced | 84% | Pre-operative study |
| Khansur & Kennedy, 1991[15] | Cisplatin 100 mg/m² IV and 5-FU 1 g/m²/day × 4 days every 3 weeks | Locally advanced and metastatic | 86% | |
| Lippman et al., 1992[16] | 13cRA 1 mg/kg PO daily and IFN-α 3 million units SQ daily | Locally advanced and metastatic | 68% | Response rates higher in patients with locally advanced disease (93%) than in patients with metastatic disease (25%) |
| Denic, 1999[12] | Cisplatin 20 mg/m² IV daily × 4 days and bleomycin 20 mg IV daily × 4 days every 3 weeks | Locally advanced | 80% | Pre-operative study |
| Shin et al., 2002[17] | Cisplatin 20 mg/m² IV weekly, 13cRA 1 mg/kg PO daily, and IFN-α 5 million units SQ 3 times weekly | Locally advanced and metastatic | 34% | Most patients had metastatic disease; response rate was significantly higher for patients with locally advanced disease (67%) |
| Weber et al., 2009[18] | Gefitinib 250 mg PO daily, increasing to 500 mg PO daily if well tolerated | Locally advanced | 68% | Pre-operative study; patients had to be eligible for definitive local therapy |

Abbreviations: 13cRA, 13-*cis*-retinoic acid; PO, orally; IV, intravenous; SQ, subcutaneously; IFN-α, interferon-α2a; 5-FU, 5-fluorouracil.

controlled phase II trial, though no differences in either recurrence or second primary tumors were observed.[19] Shin et al.[17] combined chemotherapy with immune modulation in a phase II study. Interferon-alfa, 13-*cis*-retinoic acid, and cisplatin were administered to 39 patients with advanced squamous skin cancer, with regional or distant metastatic disease not considered potentially curable with local therapy. The partial response rate was 34%, and median overall survival was 14.6 months.[17]

Targeted therapies have the potential to exploit tumor cell dependent metabolic pathways and have been tested in this disease. The epidermal growth factor receptor (EGFR) is frequently overexpressed in these tumors,[20] prompting study of EGFR inhibition. Please see Figure 48.2 for a schematic representation of the EGFR pathway. The small molecule tyrosine kinase inhibitor (TKI) gefitinib has been studied at 250 mg/m² as induction therapy in a group of patients with locally advanced cutaneous squamous cell carcinoma.[18] Responses were observed in 68% of patients, some quite striking (Fig. 48.3). Correlative EGFR studies showed tumor surface overexpression, by immunohistochemistry, in 45%. Mutations were not seen. However, preliminary analyses do not reveal a correlation of EGFR with response. Toxicities were tolerable and predictable, with grade 3 facial folliculitis and/or diarrhea affecting 25% of patients.[18] A similar study of gefitinib in patients with recurrent or metastatic squamous cell carcinoma not amenable to surgery showed modest activity.[21]

As metabolism of this family of tyrosine kinase inhibitors may be affected by tobacco use, William and colleagues have initiated an innovative study of erlotinib, again in the pre-operative setting, with dosage adjustments related to previous tobacco consumption and patient tolerance. Correlative biomarker studies are to be obtained and there will be a determination of the potential for a dose–response effect. In our anecdotal experience, we are observing tumor responses with this strategy which indicate that dose intensity is important.

Cetuximab is a human–murine chimeric antibody directed against the external domain of the EGFR, and has been shown to enhance the treatment efficacy of radiotherapy[22] and cytotoxic chemotherapy[23] in squamous cancer of the head and neck. Jalili et al. have reported an impressive case study of cetuximab combined with celecoxib, a COX-2 inhibitor, in a patient with cutaneous squamous cell carcinoma with induction of a substantial response.[24] Phase II studies of cetuximab-based therapy are anticipated.

Dasatinib, a small molecule SRC inhibitor, is also now under study for both chronically immunosuppressed patients and non-immunocompromised. Phase I targeted therapy trials offer a broad range of systemic treatment strategies for new drugs, as single agents are administered in combination with other targeting principles, or with traditional cytotoxic chemotherapy. This may lead to the observation of active agents or regimens which would then become candidates for more extensive phase II testing.

**Figure 48.2** Schematic representation of the EGFR pathway. (From Ciardiello F, Tortora G. EGFR antagonists in cancer treatment. *N Engl J Med.* 2008;358(11):1160-1174.)

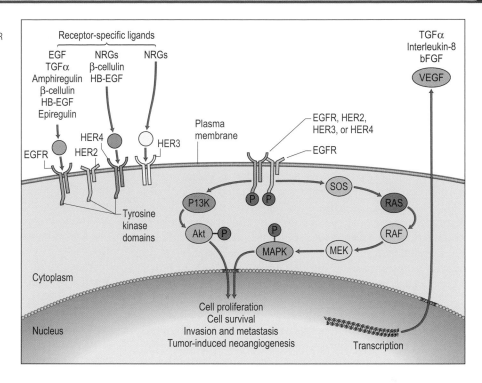

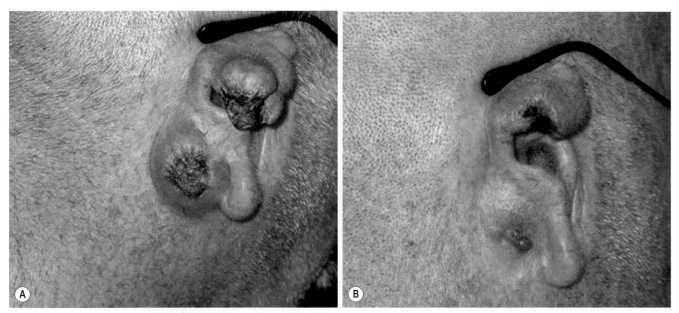

**Figure 48.3** Excellent response of a locally advanced squamous cell carcinoma following 7 weeks of treatment with gefitinib. (Courtesy of Randal S. Weber, MD.)

There is clearly a need for continued study of advanced squamous cancer, with attention directed to treatment efficacy and tolerance. The effects of experimental drug strategies on survival are uncertain. Targeted therapies offer the potential of treatment efficacy with fewer side effects, and merit further investigation. Importantly, we must also perform correlative scientific inquiries as tumors are often accessible for biopsies before and after therapy, to assess molecular biomarkers which may provide signals for improved patient selection to identify potential therapeutic targets.

## DISSEMINATED MERKEL CELL CARCINOMA

Merkel cell carcinoma (MCC) is a rare and potentially highly malignant neuroendocrine skin cancer (see Chapter 17). MCC arises in the dermis, and tumor cells possess histologic and ultrastructural features typical of small cell lung cancer (SCLC), but with distinctive characteristics such as staining with CK20 and the absence of reactivity to thyroid transcription factor. Recent molecular studies have demonstrated a polyomavirus that appears to be a causative factor,[25] presently designated as MCPyV. Most often occurring in the head and neck region, the incidence increases after age 50. There also is increased risk in persons with fair skin, and with chronic immune suppression, especially AIDS. This year in the United States, approximately 1500 new cases will be diagnosed, and, like many skin cancers, the incidence is increasing.[26] Distant metastatic disease occurs in 20% to 50% of patients,[27] and the 2-year mortality rate is 25–30%.

MCC is not often suspected at diagnosis, although rapidly progressive, erythematous lesions in immune-deficient patients should elicit concern. Regional lymph node involvement is common and, if positive, is associated with increased risk for systemic recurrence: 60% in patients with positive sentinel node biopsy versus 20% in those with negative nodal sampling.[28] The American Joint Committee on Cancer is expected soon to publish a widely acceptable staging system[29] on the basis of findings from the National Cancer Center Database.

The primary treatment is most often surgical excision, with postoperative radiotherapy for all but small tumors less than 0.5 cm with no signs of regional or nodal metastases. Although recognized as sensitive to chemotherapy, combined treatment programs with induction or adjuvant chemotherapy have not yet become established as the standard of care. Despite the lack of level I data, the National Comprehensive Center Network (NCCN) supports consideration of systemic chemotherapy as a component of treatment for patients at high risk of systemic recurrence, with 'large' primary cancers or demonstrated regional nodal disease. However, 'adjuvant chemotherapy is not routinely recommended as adequate trials to evaluate usefulness have not been done' (National Comprehensive Center Network Guidelines. Version 1.2010. 6/07/2010), and the NCCN recommends participation in a clinical trial if feasible.

In the setting of recurrent or advanced disease, treatment strategies tend to parallel those for small cell lung cancer (SCLC), another neuroendocrine tumor. The most frequently used regimens are similar to those used to treat SCLC, such as either cisplatin or carboplatin with etoposide.[30] High response rates have also been described with a combination of cyclophosphamide, doxorubicin, and vincristine.[30,31] These regimens have considerable activity, with response rates in the range of 40% to 70%,[31] but effects on overall survival are not clear, with the median probably being less than 1 year. Camptothecins such as topotecan also have activity and may be used in the palliative setting as single agents.[30] Phase II chemotherapy trials have not been conducted.

The discovery of the Merkel cell polyomavirus (MCPyV) as a potential causative factor is prompting increasing study of the molecular biology of MCC, in part with a goal of developing novel targeted therapy. Creation of a tissue microarray, identification of the transcriptone, and further molecular pathology studies may be fruitful. Vaccine development for MCPyV will require more careful immunological studies in the human, and may benefit from establishing a small-animal model for preclinical studies. Given the immunosuppression that is associated with this neoplasm, immunomodulator therapy is also reasonable to explore.

## ADNEXAL CARCINOMAS

Skin adnexal neoplasms represent a diverse group of relatively rare benign and malignant tumors that demonstrate features reflecting adnexal structures of the skin (see Chapter 13). Table 48.2 offers a classification of both benign and malignant lesions, most often surgically excised as primary therapy.[32,33] Adenocarcinomas of the sweat glands, unspecified, and sebaceous cell carcinomas have the potential to metastasize widely. Microcystic adnexal carcinoma may be quite slow-growing and locally aggressive, but distant metastases are rare.[34] In contrast, Dasgupta et al.[35] recently reported a large series of 1349 sebaceous cell carcinoma patients, from the NCI Surveillance, Epidemiology and End Results (SEER) database. The median age at diagnosis was 73 years, with 82% of patients white, 54% male, the most frequent primary site the eyelid, and with cause of death attributed to cancer in 31% of patients.

For patients with advanced or metastatic disease there have been anecdotal reports of tumor responses to regimens containing cisplatin, fluorouracil, etoposide, or methotrexate.[34,36] Eccrine carcinomas may express hormonal receptors and Her 2/neu, similar to receptor-positive breast cancers. There have been scattered reports of tumor activity for tamoxifen in estrogen receptor positive tumors[37,38,39] and trastuzumab has been administered to a patient with HER2/neu positive disease.[40] Unfortunately, organized trials of hormonal therapy have yet to be conducted in this rare disease.

## FUTURE OUTLOOK

Current treatment recommendations for these tumors are generally based upon small case series or personal experience. The accumulation of clinical trial data, the identification of treatment selection factors, and prospective serum and tumor tissue banking for correlative scientific study will contribute to improved therapies.

| Table 48.2 Selected Malignant Neoplasms of the Skin Adnexa[32,33] | |
|---|---|
| **Tissue of Origin** | **Tumor** |
| Hair or hair follicle | Trichilemmal carcinoma<br>Trichoblastic carcinoma<br>Malignant proliferating trichilemmal cyst<br>Pilomatrix carcinoma |
| Sebaceous glands | Sebaceous carcinoma<br>Basal cell carcinoma with sebaceous differentiation |
| Sweat gland (mixed origin) | Malignant mixed tumor of the skin |
| Sweat gland (eccrine) | Porocarcinoma<br>Hidradenocarcinoma<br>Spiradenocarcinoma<br>Microcystic adnexal carcinoma<br>Adenoid cystic carcinoma |
| Sweat gland (apocrine) | Syringocystadenocarcinoma<br>Apocrine carcinoma |

Clinical trials are needed to better define the appropriate approaches to patients with disseminated non-melanoma skin cancer. However, due to the rarity of disseminated disease in these neoplasms, even large cancer centers likely may not see sufficient numbers of patients to generate sequential clinical trials leading to comparative phase III studies. For this reason, multicenter or international trials are reasonable to consider as our understanding of the biology of these skin cancers improves.

## REFERENCES

1. Jemal A, Siegel R, Ward E, et al. Cancer Statistics, 2008. *CA Cancer J Clin*. 2008;58(2):71–96.
2. Rogers HW, Weinstock MA, Harris AR, et al. Incidence estimate of nonmelanoma skin cancer in the United States, 2006. *Arch Dermatol*. 2010;146(3):283–287.
3. Thomas VD, Aasi SZ, Wilson LD, et al. Cancer of the skin. In: DeVita VT, Lawrence TS, Rosenberg SA, eds. *Cancer: Principles and Practice of Oncology*. 8th ed.Philadelphia, PA: Lippincott Williams & Wilkins; 2008.
4. Pena T, LoRusso PM, Ruckdeschel JC, et al. Pulmonary metastasis of basal cell carcinoma: a rare manifestation of a common disease with variable clinical course. *J Thorac Oncol*. 2009;4(8):1026–1027.
5. Walling HW, Fosko SW, Geraminejad PA, et al. Aggressive basal cell carcinoma: presentation, pathogenesis, and management. *Cancer Metastasis Rev*. 2004;23(3–4):389–402.
6. Pfeiffer P, Hansen O, Rose C. Systemic cytotoxic therapy of basal cell carcinoma: a review of the literature. *Eur J Cancer*. 1990;26(1):73–77.
7. Epstein EH. Basal cell carcinomas: attack of the hedgehog. *Nat Rev Cancer*. 2008;8(10):743–754.
8. Ziegler A, Leffell DJ, Kunala S, et al. Mutation hotspots due to sunlight in the p53 gene of nonmelanoma skin cancers. *PNAS*. 1993;90(9):4216–4220.
9. Von Hoff DD, LoRusso PM, Rudin CM, et al. Inhibition of the hedgehog pathway in advanced basal-cell carcinoma. *N Engl J Med*. 2009;361(12):1164–1172.
10. Clayman GL, Lee JJ, Holsinger FC, et al. Mortality risk from squamous cell skin cancer. *J Clin Oncol*. 2005;23(4):759–765.
11. Alam M, Ratner D. Cutaneous squamous-cell carcinoma. *N Engl J Med*. 2001;344(13):975–983.
12. Denic S. Preoperative treatment of advanced skin carcinoma with cisplatin and bleomycin. *Am J Clin Oncol*. 1999;22(1):32–34.
13. Guthrie TH, McEleveen LJ, Porubsky ES, et al. Cisplatin and doxorubicin: an effective chemotherapy in the treatment of advanced basal cell and squamous carcinoma of the skin. *Cancer*. 1985;55(8):1629–1632.
14. Sadek H, Azli N, Wendling JL, et al. Treatment of advanced squamous cell carcinoma of the skin with cisplatin, 5-fluorouracil, and bleomycin. *Cancer*. 1990;66(8):1692–1696.
15. Khansur T, Kennedy A. Cisplatin and 5-fluorouracil for advanced locoregional and metastatic squamous cell carcinoma of the skin. *Cancer*. 1991;67(8):2030–2032.
16. Lippman SM, Parkinson DR, Itri LM, et al. 13-cis-retinoic acid and interferon α-2a: effective combination therapy for advanced squamous cell carcinoma of the skin. *J Natl Cancer Inst*. 1992;84(4):235–241.
17. Shin DM, Glisson BS, Khuri FR, et al. Phase II and biologic study of interferon alfa, retinoic acid, and cisplatin in advanced squamous skin cancer. *J Clin Oncol*. 2002;20(2):364–370.
18. Weber RS, Lustig RA, El-Naggar A, et al. Gefitinib for advanced cutaneous squamous cell carcinoma of head and neck: phase II trial. *J Clin Oncol*. 2009;27(15S):6054.
19. Brewster AM, Lee JJ, Clayman GL, et al. Randomized trial of adjuvant 13-cis-retinoic acid and interferon alfa for patients with aggressive skin squamous cell carcinoma. *J Clin Oncol*. 2007;25(15):1974–1978.
20. Maubec E, Duvillard P, Velasco V, et al. Immunohistochemical analysis of EGFR and HER-2 in patients with metastatic squamous cell carcinoma of the skin. *Anticancer Res*. 2005;25(2B):1205–1210.
21. Glisson BS, Kim ES, Kies MS, et al. Phase II study of gefitinib in patients with metastatic/recurrent squamous cell carcinoma of the skin. *J Clin Oncol*. 2006;24(18S):5531.
22. Bonner JA, Harari PM, Giralt J, et al. Radiotherapy plus cetuximab for squamous cell carcinoma of the head and neck. *N Engl J Med*. 2006;354(6):567–578.
23. Vermorken JB, Mesia R, Rivera F, et al. Platinum-based chemotherapy plus cetuximab in head and neck cancer. *N Engl J Med*. 2008;359(11):1116–1127.
24. Jalili A, Pinc A, Pieczkowski C, et al. Combination of an EGFR blocker and a COX-2 inhibitor for the treatment of advanced cutaneous squamous cell carcinoma. *J Dtsch Dermatol Ges*. 2008;6(12):1066–1069.
25. Feng H, Shuda M, Chang Y, et al. Clonal integration of a polyomavirus in human Merkel cell carcinoma. *Science*. 2008;319(5866):1096–1100.
26. Zhan FQ, Packianathan VS, Zeitouni NC. Merkel cell carcinoma: a review of current advances. *J Natl Compr Canc Netw*. 2009;7(3):333–339.
27. Voog E, Biron P, Martin J-P, et al. Chemotherapy for patients with locally advanced or metastatic Merkel cell carcinoma. *Cancer*. 1999;85(12):2589–2595.
28. Gupta SG, Wang LC, Penas PF, et al. Sentinel lymph node biopsy for evaluation and treatment of patients with Merkel cell carcinoma: the Dana-Farber experience and meta-analysis of the literature. *Arch Dermatol*. 2006;142(6):685–690.
29. Rockville Merkel Cell Carcinoma Group. Merkel cell carcinoma: recent progress and current priorities on etiology, pathogenesis, and clinical management. *J Clin Oncol*. 2009;27(24):4021–4026.
30. Miller SJ, Alam M, Andersen J, et al. Merkel cell carcinoma: clinical practice guidelines in oncology. *J Natl Compr Canc Netw*. 2009;7(3):322–332.
31. Tai PT, Yu E, Winquist E, et al. Chemotherapy in neuroendocrine/Merkel cell carcinoma of the skin: case series and review of 204 cases. *J Clin Oncol*. 2000;18(12):2493–2499.
32. Alsaad KO, Obaidat NA, Ghazarian D. Skin adnexal neoplasms - part 1: an approach to tumours of the pilosebaceous unit. *J Clin Pathol*. 2007;60(2):129–144.
33. Obaidat NA, Alsaad KO, Ghazarian D. Skin adnexal neoplasms - part 2: an approach to tumours of cutaneous sweat glands. *J Clin Pathol*. 2007;60(2):145–159.
34. Wetter R, Goldstein GD. Microcystic adnexal carcinoma: a diagnostic and therapeutic challenge. *Dermatol Ther*. 2008;21(6):452–458.
35. Dasgupta T, Wilson LD, Yu JB. A retrospective review of 1349 cases of sebaceous carcinoma. *Cancer*. 2009;115(1):158–165.
36. Meyer TK, Rhee JS, Smith MM, et al. External auditory canal eccrine spiradenocarcinoma: a case report and review of literature. *Head Neck*. 2003;25(6):505–510.
37. Sridhar KS, Benedetto P, Otrakji CL, et al. Response of eccrine adenocarcinoma to tamoxifen. *Cancer* 1989;64:366.
38. Schroder U, Dries V, Klussmann JP, et al. Successful adjuvant tamoxifen therapy for estrogen receptor-positive metastasizing sweat gland adenocarcinoma: need for a clinical trial? *Ann Otol Rhinol Laryngol*. 2004;113(3 Pt 1):242.
39. Daniel SJ, Nader R, Kost K, et al. Facial sweat gland carcinoma metastasizing to neck nodes: a diagnostic and therapeutic challenge. *Arch Otolaryngol Head Neck Surg*. 2001;127:1495.
40. Nash JW, Barrett TL, Kies M, et al. Metastatic hidradenocarcinoma with demonstration of Her-2/neu gene amplification by fluorescence in situ hybridization: potential treatment implications. *J Cutan Pathol*. 2007;34(1):49–54.

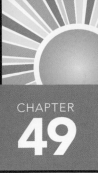

# Surgical Excision of Melanoma

*Robert H.I. Andtbacka*

---

## Key Points

- Surgical excision is the cornerstone for the initial management of primary melanoma.

- The major focus of surgical excision for melanoma is to remove the primary tumor and any local disease.

- The initial treatment for melanoma should include excision with 5 mm margins (for in-situ lesions), 1 cm margins (for tumors 0.01–1.00 mm of invasion), 1–2 cm margins (for tumors 1.01–2.00 mm of invasion), 2 cm margins for tumors greater than 2 mm invasion and depth to fascia with consideration for sentinel lymph node biopsy if appropriate criteria are met.

- Closure techniques are varied as a function of excision size and anatomic sites.

---

## INTRODUCTION

Surgical excision remains the main treatment modality for patients with primary cutaneous melanoma. The main goal of surgical excision is to remove all melanoma tumor cells at the primary melanoma site in order to provide the best oncological outcome that minimizes the risk of local recurrence. The surgical excision should also be carried out in such a manner as to minimize functional impairment and cosmetic disfigurement. The appropriate width of surgical resection has been a longstanding controversy. Traditionally, many institutions have promoted wide local excisions of melanomas with margins of 3 to 5 cm. Most of these recommendations were not based on scientific data but rather on anecdotal evidence that patients treated with wider excisions experienced lower likelihood of recurrence at the resection site. Well-conducted randomized clinical trials have now resolved many of these excision margin controversies, and this chapter will highlight the current recommendations for excision of primary cutaneous melanoma.

## HISTORY

William Norris in 1857 first reported on the need for a wide excision of primary melanoma with surrounding normal tissue after he observed a local recurrence of melanoma with extensive tumor dissemination after an initial excision with minimal margins.[1,2] In 1907, W. Sampson Handley observed histological evidence of 'centripetal lymphatic spread' in an autopsy of a patient with a locally advanced melanoma.[3] Based on this somewhat minimal information, he recommended an even more aggressive excision with 2 inches (5 cm) of normal skin surrounding the primary melanoma with concomitant excision of the underlying subcutaneous tissue down to the muscle fascia and a regional lymph node dissection. These findings formed the basis for a recommendation of extensive margin resection of primary melanoma over the following 60 years. The recommendation was based on the belief that undertreatment of the patient with a narrow excision increased the risk of local recurrence and distant metastatic spread. It was not until the 1970s that the need for such an extensive margin excision was questioned.

In 1977 Breslow and Macht[4] investigated the incidence of local recurrence in 62 patients with melanomas of 0.76 mm or less in thickness treated with 0.1 cm to 5.5 cm excision margins. Of the 62 patients, 20 underwent excisions with margins of 1.0 cm or less. None of the 62 patients developed a local recurrence or metastatic disease. This study and other studies established that local recurrence and metastatic disease rates were primarily governed by the melanoma thickness and biology of disease, and less by the margins of excision. The Breslow thickness subsequently became an important stratification criterion for randomized clinical trials evaluating different excision margins.

## EXCISION MARGIN TRIALS

Prior to the 1970s, no randomized trials had been conducted evaluating the safety of narrow margin excisions. Based on the findings of Breslow and Macht,[4] several large randomized clinical trials have been conducted evaluating the safety of narrow margin excision. These trials have tested the following paradigms: 1) local failure is a function of both biology of the primary tumor and extent of excision; 2) narrow (1 cm) margins are safe in thin melanomas with a low risk of recurrence; 3) wider excisions lower the risk of local and/or regional recurrences in thicker and/or ulcerated melanomas; 4) increased rates of local/regional failure may or may not have an impact on survival.

To date, five large prospective randomized clinical trials, published in 11 reports, have evaluated the excision margins and the impact of these on the risk of local recurrence and survival (Table 49.1).[5-16] All of these randomized clinical trials were multicenter and four were multinational. In all of them, the surgical excision margins was measured clinically and no specific correlation between clinical margins and histological margins was given. Two of the trials compared 1 to 3 cm excision margins (World Health Organization [WHO] Melanoma Program Trial No. 10,[5-7] and the United Kingdom Melanoma Study Group Trial[16]),

| Randomized Surgical Trial | N | Tumor Thickness (mm) | Surgical Excision (cm) | | Median Follow-up (Years) |
|---|---|---|---|---|---|
| | | | Narrow | Wide | |
| WHO Melanoma Group Trial No. 10[5–7] | 612 | ≤2 | 1 | ≥3 | 15 |
| French Group of Research on Malignant Melanoma Trial[8,9] | 337 | <2.1 | 2 | 5 | 16 |
| Swedish Melanoma Trial Group[10,11] | 989 | >0.8, ≤2 | 2 | 5 | 11 (survival) 8 (recurrence) |
| Intergroup Melanoma Surgical Trial[12–15] | 468 | 1–4 | 2 | 4 | 10 |
| UK Melanoma Study Group[16] | 900 | ≥2 | 1 | 3 | 5 |

Table 49.1 Prospective Randomized Trials Assessing Surgical Excision Margins for Primary Cutaneous Melanoma

one compared 2 to 4 cm excision margins (the Intergroup Melanoma Surgical Trial[12–15]) and two compared 2 to 5 cm margins (the French Cooperative Group Trial[8,9] and the Swedish Melanoma Group Trial[10,11]).

## The French Cooperative Group Trial (melanomas ≤ 2mm, margins 2 vs 5 cm)

The French Cooperative Group Trial, conducted by the French Group of Research on Malignant Melanoma, was initiated in 1981 and randomized 337 patients with cutaneous melanomas ≤2 mm (in the later publication this was referred to as <2.1 mm) in Breslow thickness on the trunk, limbs, head and neck to either 2 cm or 5 cm excision margins. Patients with melanomas on the fingers, toes and nails were excluded from the study. The results of the study were reported initially in 1993 in abstract format[8] and published in 2003.[9] After a median follow-up of 16 years (192 months), 55 (16.8%) patients developed recurrent disease; 22 (13.6%) of these underwent a 2 cm excision and 33 (20%) underwent a 5 cm excision. This difference was not statistically significant, P=0.22. The majority of recurrences were in regional lymph nodes and distant sites, whereas the local recurrence rate was very low in both of the randomized groups. A total of five patients developed a local recurrence, one (0.6%) in the 2-cm group and four (2.4%) in the 5-cm group. This difference was not statistically different. There were no significant differences in the 10-year disease-free survival rates (85% vs 83% for the 2-cm and 5-cm groups, respectively) and the 10-year overall survival rates (87% vs 86%) (Table 49.2). Based on this, the authors concluded that in patients with cutaneous melanomas ≤ 2 mm, a 2 cm excision margin is sufficient, and a traditional 5 cm margin is not necessary.

## WHO Melanoma Program Trial No. 10 (melanomas ≤2 mm, margins 1 vs 3 cm)

The WHO Melanoma Program initiated a wide-excision randomized clinical trial at the same time as the French group and between 1980 and 1985 randomized 703 patients with primary cutaneous melanomas ≤2 mm in Breslow thickness to a 1 cm or ≥3 cm radial wide excision margin (Table 49.2). An excision margin more conservative than that of the French group (2 cm vs 5 cm) was deemed safe by the WHO group, since the risk of local recurrence was presumed to

be low in patients with melanomas ≤2 mm. Patients with melanomas on the trunk or limbs were included, excluding patients with melanomas on the face, fingers, or toes.

Of the 703 randomized patients, 612 were evaluated, and the results have been reported in three publications.[5–7] The patients were stratified a priori and the results reported according to primary melanoma thickness ranges of <1 mm and 1 to 2 mm. Long-term follow-up at 4, 8 and 12 years showed no statistically significant differences in recurrence-free and overall survival rates between the 1 cm and 3 cm excision margins. In the second analysis of the trial at a mean length of follow-up of 7.5 years, four (0.6%) of the 612 patients had developed a local recurrence as a first sign of recurrent melanoma.[6] Local recurrence was defined as a cutaneous or subcutaneous nodule occurring in the surgical scar or within a radius of 1 cm or less from the scar. All four local recurrences occurred in patients with excisions of 1 cm and with primary melanomas between 1.01 and 2.0 mm. At the time of the third analysis with a median follow-up of 12 years, 11 (1.8%) of 612 patients had developed a local recurrence as a first sign of recurrent melanoma.[5] Eight of these recurrences occurred in patients with 1 cm excision margins, and five of these eight patients had primary melanomas between 1.01 and 2.0 mm in Breslow thickness.

This study indicated that the overall incidence of local recurrence was extremely low in patients with primary cutaneous melanomas with a Breslow thickness ≤2 mm. The risk of local recurrence appeared to be primarily a function of tumor thickness and possibly margin of excision. However, due to the low incidence of local recurrence, an impact of these factors on overall survival could not be detected, and based on the data the authors concluded that a 1 cm excision margin appeared safe in patients with melanomas ≤2 mm in thickness. Some clinicians, however, have been reluctant to adopt a 1 cm margin for all patients with melanomas ≤2 mm in thickness. Although the incidence of local recurrence is low in these patients, over time there is an absolute increase in the incidence, especially in patients with melanomas 1.01–2.0 mm in thickness. In the WHO study, the absolute number of local recurrences in the 1.01–2.0 mm cohort treated with a 1 cm margin increased from 2.5%[7] to 3.4%[6] in progressive follow-up reports, to an incidence of 4.2% (5 out of 119 patients) after 12 years of follow-up.[5] The incidence of local recurrence in the same cohort of patients treated with a 3 cm excision margin was 0%, 0% and 1.5%, respectively. In patients with melanomas ≤1 mm,

Table 49.2 Actuarial Rates of Overall Survival, Disease-Free Survival, and Recurrence in Prospective Randomized Trials Assessing Surgical Excision Margins for Primary Cutaneous Melanoma

| Category | French Cooperative Group Trial (≤2 mm) | | | WHO Melanoma Group Trial No. 10 (≤2 mm) | | | Swedish Melanoma Trial Group (>0.8–2 mm) | | | Intergroup Melanoma Surgical Trial (1–4 mm) | | | UK Melanoma Study Group (≥2 mm) | | |
|---|---|---|---|---|---|---|---|---|---|---|---|---|---|---|---|
| Breslow thickness | 2 cm | 5 cm | P | 1 cm | 3 cm | P | 2 cm | 5 cm | P | 2 cm | 4 cm | P | 1 cm | 3 cm | P |
| **Disease-Free Survival** | | | | | | | | | | | | | | | |
| 5-year | – | – | | – | – | | 81% | 83% | NS | 75% | 80% | NS | 51% | 56% | 0.06 |
| 10-year | 85% | 83% | NS | 82%* | 84%* | NS | 71% | 70% | NS | – | – | NS | – | – | |
| **Overall Survival** | | | | | | | | | | | | | | | |
| 5-year | 93% | 90% | NS | 97%† | 96%† | NS | 86% | 89% | NS | 76% | 82% | NS | 68% | 69% | NS |
| 10-year | 87% | 86% | NS | 90%* / 87%‡ | 90%* / 85%‡ | NS / NS | 79% | 76% | NS | 70% | 77% | 0.074 | – | – | |
| Local recurrence as first relapse | – | – | | 2.6%‡ | 1.0%‡ | NS | 0.2%* | 1.0%* | NS | 0.4% | 0.9% | NS | 3.3% | 2.9% | NS |
| Local recurrence at any time | 0.6% | 2.4% | NS | – | – | | 0.6%* | 1.0%* | NS | 2.1% | 2.6% | NS | – | – | |
| Locoregional recurrence | 8.7% | 9.1% | NS | 8.9%* | 8.5%* | NS | 19.3%* | 14.8%* | 0.06 | – | – | | 37.1% | 31.8% | 0.05 |
| Overall recurrence | 13.6% | 20% | NS | 14.4%* | 13.0%* | NS | 21%* | 19%* | NS | – | – | NS | 45.5% | 38.5% | 0.03 |

–, not reported; NS, not significant; WHO, World Health Organization; UK, United Kingdom.

†4-year follow-up.

*8-year follow-up.

‡12-year follow-up.

the incidence of local recurrence after 12 years of follow-up was 1.6% and 0.6% in patients treated with 1 and 3 cm margins of resection, respectively. Although these were not statistically different, the absolute risk of local recurrence increases over time and excision margins greater than 1 cm may be considered in patients with melanomas 1.01–2.0 mm in thickness.

## The Swedish Melanoma Group Trial (melanomas >0.8–2 mm, margins 2 vs 5 cm)

The Swedish Melanoma Trial randomized patients with primary cutaneous melanomas of the trunk and extremities to a wide excision with either a 2 cm or 5 cm margin (Tables 49.1 and 49.2). Between 1982 and 1991, a total of 989 patients with melanomas >0.8 mm but ≤2 mm were enrolled. The results from the study have been presented in two reports in 1996 and 2000.[10,11] After a median follow-up of 8 years for local recurrence and 11 years for survival, 20% of patients experienced disease recurrence and 15% of patients had died of melanoma. There was no statistical difference in recurrence rates between the two excision cohorts.

Specifically, local recurrence, defined as recurrence in the 'scar or transplant', was very rare as a first event of recurrence at 0.2% (1 out of 476 patients) in patients treated with a 2 cm excision, compared to 1% (4 out of 513 patients) in the 5 cm margin cohort. This difference was not statistically different. There was a trend for increased locoregional metastasis in patients treated with a 2 cm excision. The patients in this study did not undergo sentinel lymph node biopsy, and most of the difference in locoregional metastasis was due to regional lymph node metastasis, not local or in-transit recurrences. It is possible that this trend may have been eliminated had patients with microscopic lymph node metastases been treated with early completion lymph node dissection. The estimated 10-year overall survival was not different between the two groups, 79% for patients treated with a 2 cm margin excision compared with 76% for the 5 cm group. Hence, the authors concluded that patients with melanomas >0.8 mm and ≤2.0 mm 'can be treated with a resection margin of 2 cm as safely as with a resection margin of 5 cm'.[10] These results are similar to the ones seen in the French trial, again underscoring that in patients with primary melanomas ≤2 mm, a more conservative 2 cm margin can safely be used without apparent compromise.

## The Intergroup Melanoma Surgical Trial (melanomas 1.0–4.0 mm, margins 2 vs 4 cm)

The French Melanoma Trial, the WHO Melanoma Program Trial No. 10, and the Swedish Melanoma Trial all evaluated patients with melanomas ≤2 mm and established that a 1 to 2 cm resection margin was safe in these patients. The Intergroup Melanoma Surgical Trial was initiated in 1983 and included patients with primary melanomas 1.0–4.0 mm in thickness. A total of 740 patients were enrolled into the trial and divided into two groups – Group A: proximal extremity and trunk, and Group B: head and neck, and distal extremity (Fig. 49.1). The 468 patients in Group A were randomized to either a 2 cm or 4 cm margin of excision, whereas patients in Group B underwent a 2 cm excision.

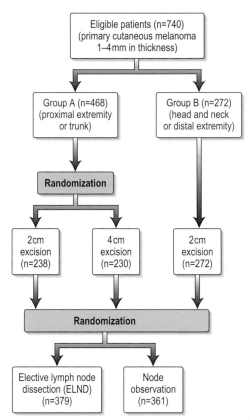

**Figure 49.1** Treatment schema for the Intergroup Melanoma Surgical Trial. Patients with 1–4 mm cutaneous melanoma of the proximal extremity and trunk (Group A) were randomized to 2 or 4 cm margins of excision. All patients from Group A and Group B were randomized to elective lymph node dissection of nodal observation.

A second randomization of elective lymph node dissection versus nodal observation was also built into the trial for both Group A and Group B patients. All patients were a priori stratified according to tumor thickness (1.0–2.0 mm, 2.1–3.0 mm, and 3.1–4.0 mm), and presence or absence of ulceration.

The initial results from this trial were reported in 1993,[14] and a long-term follow-up (median 10 years) was reported in 2001.[13] Among the 468 patients in Group A (238 randomized to 2 cm vs 230 randomized to 4 cm), there was no statistical difference in local recurrence as a first event (0.4% vs 0.9%), local recurrence at any time (2.1% vs 2.6%), in-transit metastasis (5.9% vs 5.2%), and 10-year survival (70% vs 77%; P=0.074) (Table 49.2).[13] Elective lymph node dissection did not influence survival.

The median time to local recurrence was 1.7 years, and the median survival after local recurrence was only 1 year. The extent of local excision did not influence the time to local recurrence or survival after local recurrence. In a univariate analysis, local recurrence was associated with the presence of primary tumor ulceration (1.1% no ulceration vs 6.6% with ulceration; P<0.001) and increasing tumor thickness (1.0% for 1.0–2.0, 4.6% for 2.1–3.0 mm; P<0.001, 4.1% for 3.1–4.0 mm; P=0.05). In a multivariate analysis, only primary tumor ulceration was prognostic of an increased risk of local recurrence. There was a difference in local recurrence depending on the site of primary tumor location.

Anytime local recurrence for tumor of the proximal extremity, trunk, distal extremity, and head or neck was 1.1%, 3.1%, 5.3%, and 9.4%, respectively.

Although there was no difference in recurrence and survival in patients undergoing a narrower 2 cm margin excision, there was a difference in the extent of surgery needed and hospital stay. Patients who underwent a 4 cm excision, compared to those who had a 2 cm excision, had a significantly longer stay in hospital (5.2 vs 3.0 days, respectively; $P<0.001$) and increased split-thickness skin grafting rates (46% vs 11%, respectively; $P<0.001$). Based on these findings, the authors concluded that 2 cm margins can safely be performed in patients with intermediate-thickness melanomas of 1.0–4.0 mm, and allows for surgery that is less disfiguring with less use of skin grafts. The longer hospital stay is less relevant today, since most patients undergoing a wide local excision for melanoma are treated on an outpatient basis.

## The United Kingdom Melanoma Study Group Trial (melanomas ≥2 mm, margins 1 vs 3 cm)

In a fifth large randomized trial, the United Kingdom Melanoma Study Group, the British Association of Plastic Surgeons, and the Scottish Cancer Therapy Network randomized 900 patients with melanomas ≥2 mm to 1 cm versus 3 cm excision margins.[16] Local recurrence was defined as recurrence within 2 cm of the scar or graft, and in-transit recurrence was defined as a recurrence from beyond the first 2 cm of the scar or graft to the regional nodes. All locoregional recurrences were detected clinically and confirmed by biopsy. Sentinel lymph node biopsy was not done as part of this trial.

After a median follow-up of 5 years, 15 (3.3%) out of 453 patients randomized to 1 cm excision experienced a local recurrence as a first event, compared to 13 (2.9%) out of 447 patients randomized to 3 cm (Table 49.2). This difference was not statistically significant. However, when all locoregional recurrences (local, in-transit and regional lymph nodes) were considered, patients receiving a 1 cm margin excision had a significantly higher locoregional recurrence as first event rate of 37.1% compared to 31.8% in patients receiving 3 cm margin excisions ($P=0.05$). Interestingly, the majority (85%) of locoregional first event recurrences were nodal recurrences. The overall recurrences were statistically greater in the 1 cm excision group, $P=0.03$. There was a trend ($P=0.06$) towards decreased disease-free survival in the 1 cm excision group. There were no differences in melanoma-specific survival and overall survival between patients in the two treatment groups.

It is important to note that none of the patients in this study underwent staging of the regional lymph node basin with elective lymph node dissection or sentinel lymph node biopsy. The large proportion of regional lymph node recurrence observed in this study likely would not occur in current surgical practice since most, if not all, patients would have been offered sentinel lymph node biopsy. As a result, regional lymph node involvement would have been diagnosed earlier and would have been treated with a completion lymph node dissection, hence decreasing the risk for regional lymph node recurrence. Nonetheless, the results of this analysis do suggest that there may be a benefit in performing a wider resection to decrease the risk of locoregional recurrence.

## CURRENT RECOMMENDATIONS

The five randomized clinical trials described above serve the basis for the current recommendation of margins of excision in melanoma. When proposing recommendations, it is important to evaluate the data available in the context of the goals of surgical excision: optimizing survival, local control and minimizing morbidity. Currently, several national guidelines have been developed in the US, Europe and Australia (Table 49.3).[17-23] Although these guidelines provide some consistent generalizations regarding appropriate margins of excision, they do offer slightly different advice.

## Melanoma in situ

For melanoma in situ, the margin recommendation of 0.5 to 1 cm is based on consensus. Although these lesions are noninvasive, an inadequate surgical resection may result in a local invasive recurrence with the potential for metastasis. In most in-situ melanoma, an excision incorporating 0.5 to 1 cm of normal skin around the melanoma and a layer of subcutaneous tissue is sufficient. However, in some in-situ

| Breslow Thickness | US (2009)*[17] | Australia (2008)[18] | German (2008)[19] | Dutch (2005)[20] | Swiss (2005)[21] | UK (2002)[22,23] |
|---|---|---|---|---|---|---|
| In situ | 0.5 cm | 0.5 cm | 0.5 cm | 0.5 cm | 0.5 cm | 0.2–0.5 cm |
| 0.01–1.00 mm | 1 cm | 1 cm | 1 cm | 1 cm | 1 cm | 1 cm |
| 1.01–2.00 mm | 1–2 cm | 1–2 cm | 1 cm | 1 cm | 1 cm | 1–2 cm |
| 2.0–4.00 mm | 2 cm | 1–2 cm[†] | 2 cm | 2 cm | 2 cm | 2–3 cm |
| >4.00 mm | 2 cm | 2 cm | 2 cm | 2 cm | 2 cm | 2–3 cm |

Table 49.3 National Guidelines for Excision Margins for Primary Cutaneous Melanoma

*'Margins may be modified to accommodate individual anatomic or functional considerations.'

[†]'Caution be exercised for melanomas 2 to 4 mm thick, because evidence concerning optimal excision margins is unclear. Where possible, it may be desirable to take a wider margin (2 cm) for these tumors depending on tumor site and surgeon/patient preference.'

melanoma, such as lentigo maligna melanoma, a greater margin may be required to obtain a histologically negative excision. These lesions may also require a more extensive closure with skin grafts and flaps.

## Melanomas ≤1 mm thick

Three of the randomized clinical trials included patients with melanomas ≤1.0 mm in thickness (French study, 159 patients; Swedish study, 244 patients; and WHO study, 359 patients). Of these, only 185 patients in the WHO study were treated with 1 cm margins of excision. In the WHO study, there was no difference in the locoregional recurrence and overall survival between patients treated with 1 cm and 3 cm margins. Hence, based on these data, a 1 cm margin of normal skin and subcutaneous tissue around the primary melanoma or melanoma biopsy site is widely accepted as sufficient. Most of these lesions can be closed primarily by undermining the surrounding tissue. In rare instances, such as on distal extremities, the face and scalp, wound reconstruction with flaps and skin graft may be necessary.

## Melanomas 1–2 mm thick

Four of the randomized clinical trials included patients who had melanomas between 1.01 and 2.0 mm (French study, WHO study, Swedish study, and the Intergroup study). None of the studies revealed a survival difference between patients treated with narrow (1 or 2 cm) or wide (3, 4 or 5 cm) margin excision. Based on this, a 1 to 2 cm margin of excision is recommended for patients with 1.01–2.0 mm thick melanomas. To date, a direct comparison between a 1 cm and 2 cm margin has not been conducted in this group of patients. However, in the WHO study, the 12-year rate of local recurrence as a first sign of recurrence in patients with 1.01–2.0 mm melanomas undergoing a 1 cm excision was 4.2% compared to 1.5% in patients having a 3 cm excision. Although not statistically significant, this difference suggests a trend towards an increased local recurrence rate in patients treated with a 1 cm excision.

In the Intergroup study, the local recurrence rate in patients with 1.01–2.0 mm thick melanomas treated with 2 cm excision was 0.6%. For this reason, a 2 cm margin is recommended in these patients if anatomically feasible and primary closure can be achieved. However, in areas that are anatomically restrictive, such as distal extremities, the face and scalp, where a 2 cm margin may require extensive reconstruction with a skin graft or flap closure, a margin less than 2 cm but at least 1 cm can be considered.

## Melanomas 2–4 mm thick

Two randomized clinical trials have evaluated patients with melanomas between 2 and 4 mm thick. In the Intergroup trial, 190 patients had melanomas in this thickness range, and in the United Kingdom Melanoma Study Group trial, 660 patients fell into this category. There was no statistical difference in overall or disease-free survival between the narrow (1 or 2 cm) margin of resection and the wide (3 or 4 cm) margin of resection in either study. However, in the United Kingdom Melanoma Study Group trial, a 3 cm margin of resection demonstrated an improved locoregional recurrence-free survival compared to 1 cm. Although a 3 cm margin may be superior to a 1 cm margin based on the United Kingdom Melanoma Study Group trial, a 4 cm margin was not shown to be superior to a 2 cm margin in the Intergroup trial. Hence, logically, a 3 cm margin cannot be superior to a 2 cm margin. For this reason, excision margins of 2 cm are recommended for patients with melanomas 2–4 mm in thickness, since there are no data to suggest that an excision margin greater than 2 cm is superior.

## Melanomas >4 mm thick

Only the United Kingdom Melanoma Study Group trial included patients with melanomas greater than 4 mm in thickness. In this trial, 243 patients had melanomas >4 mm in thickness, and the rate of locoregional recurrence was significantly greater (56% greater for 5 mm melanomas and 82% greater for 6 mm melanomas) in patients treated with 1 cm margins compared to those treated with a 3 cm margin. Based on this improved locoregional recurrence-free survival in patients treated with a 3 cm margin of resection, the authors recommended that a 3 cm margin be used in patients with melanomas >4 mm in thickness. However, the general acceptance of this recommendation has been met with reluctance for the following reasons: 1) no overall survival benefit has been demonstrated; 2) the locoregional recurrence rate would likely be lower with the routine use of sentinel lymph node biopsy in these patients; 3) most of the recurrences were regional lymph node recurrences, and the statistical difference in locoregional recurrence is lost when nodal recurrence is taken out of the analysis; 4) 3 cm margins are associated with a greater morbidity, and increased use of skin grafts and complex reconstructions.

In a retrospective study of 278 patients with melanomas >4 mm in thickness treated at M.D. Anderson Cancer Center and the Lakeland Regional Cancer Center, no statistical difference in local recurrence rates or survival was observed in patients treated with margins ≤2 cm compared to >2 cm.[24] Local recurrence appeared to be a function of primary tumor factors such as ulceration rather than margins of excision. In a multivariate analysis, overall survival was affected by nodal status, tumor ulceration, and thickness greater than 6 mm, but not by margin width or local recurrence. Although this study was retrospective, it included a large set of patients (n=278) in this high-risk group with a 27-month follow-up. Current recommendations for patients with melanomas >4 mm in thickness call for an excision margin of at least 2 cm. A margin greater than 2 cm in this population is not clearly indicated until more data become available from an ongoing Swedish melanoma trial evaluating 2 cm versus 4 cm margins of resection in 936 patients with melanomas greater than 2 mm in thickness.

## SPECIAL EXCISIONAL CONSIDERATIONS

### Head and neck melanoma

When providing specific guidelines on margins of excision, it is essential to ensure that the patient populations the guidelines address have been evaluated in clinical trials. Of the five randomized clinical trials, only the French Cooperative Group trial enrolled patients with melanomas on the face, head and neck.[9] In this study, only 16 patients had melanomas on the head and neck (10 underwent a 2 cm margin excision and 6 underwent a 5 cm excision). Based on this small number of patients, little guidance is available for the clinician on the appropriate margins of resection in these melanomas. Melanomas on the head and neck and face are different to melanomas on the trunk and extremities, and it is unclear whether the recommendations for the trunk and extremities can be extrapolated to the head and neck and face. In the Intergroup Melanoma Surgical Trial, the 272 patients in Group B with primary melanomas of the head and neck and distal extremity who underwent a non-randomized 2 cm margin excision had a higher rate of local recurrence, with 10 (3.7%) patients having a first local recurrence and 17 (6.2%) having an anytime local recurrence. Of these, the 64 patients with melanomas of the head and neck had the highest rate of local recurrence at 9.4%, with a local recurrence rate of 16.2% in patients with ulcerated primaries. The anatomic constraints and cosmetic consequences of a wider excision in the head and neck and face regions often make it difficult to ensure 2 cm margins. Based on the findings in the Intergroup study, the higher local recurrence rates in patients with melanomas of the head and neck and face are concerning and require further evaluation. Until these data are available, resection margins similar to those for the trunk and extremity should be followed.

## EXCISION OF HISTOLOGIC VARIANTS

### Desmoplastic melanoma

Desmoplastic melanoma is a relatively uncommon fibrosing variant of melanoma, constituting 2% to 4% of all melanomas.[25,26] Most desmoplastic melanomas are amelanotic and can be mistaken for a scar/keloid, fibroma or basal cell carcinoma. Desmoplastic melanomas are slightly more common in men and occur primarily in sun-damaged skin in the head and neck region. Compared to other cutaneous melanomas, pure desmoplastic melanomas tend to have a higher rate of local recurrence and a lower rate of lymph node metastases.[27] Many desmoplastic melanomas exhibit histological evidence of perineural invasion, and this neurotropism has been associated with an increased risk of local recurrence.[28] Traditionally, desmoplastic melanoma has been classified as a locally very aggressive melanoma, with local recurrence rates of 39% to 52%.[29,30] However, with wide excision margins and careful margin assessment by experienced dermatopathologists, the local recurrence rate can decrease to 4% to 7%.[31,32] Patients excised with margins <1 cm have a higher risk of local recurrence, and margins of at least 2 cm appear appropriate to decrease the risk of local recurrence, especially in desmoplastic melanomas with neurotropism.[28]

### Lentigo maligna (melanoma)

Lentigo maligna, also known as Hutchinson's melanotic freckle, most commonly occurs in sun-exposed areas such as the face and head and neck of elderly persons. It may also occur on other sites of high sunlight exposure such as the extremities and in younger individuals, although this is less common. Lentigo maligna refers to a pure in-situ type of melanoma and lentigo maligna melanoma is used to designate an invasive component associated with lentigo maligna. The lifetime risk of invasive melanoma arising in lentigo maligna is estimated at 5%.[33]

Lentigo maligna and lentigo maligna melanoma often pose a surgical challenge since they can be quite large and occur in anatomically restrictive areas such as the face and the scalp, where obtaining surgically negative margins has the potential of being cosmetically disfiguring. Reconstruction after surgical resection in these areas often requires skin graft and elaborate flap closures. Lentigo maligna and lentigo maligna melanoma can exhibit an extensive radial growth phase and clinically it may be difficult to determine the extent of the lesions. A Wood's lamp can be used to more accurately determine the gross macroscopic extent of the lesion, allowing for better preoperative planning of the reconstruction.

Despite such maneuvers, the microscopic extent of disease can be underestimated. Historically, intraoperative frozen section using standard histological staining techniques to determine margin status has not been very accurate. Newer techniques with rapid immunohistochemical staining of frozen sections with Melan-A (MART-1) have shown promise in assessing margins of resection intraoperatively.[34-36] If accurate intraoperative margin assessment is not available, lentigo maligna and lentigo maligna melanomas should be resected in a staged fashion. The surgical defect can be covered with a moist dressing or DuoDERM during the 1 to 3 days it takes to perform a formal permanent histological evaluation of the margins. Definitive surgical reconstruction of the surgical defect should not be done until negative surgical margins have been obtained.

## Excision of atypical melanocytic lesions

Occasionally, it may be very difficult to establish the precise histological diagnosis for pigmented lesions. Even with specialized immunohistochemical stains and expert analysis by qualified dermatopathologists, it may be very difficult to determine the malignant potential of some pigmented lesions. For example, in young individuals, Spitz nevi may pose a particularly difficult problem. These lesions are often quite thick and it may be difficult to differentiate between a deep penetrating nevus, a Spitz nevus, a malignant Spitz nevus, and a spitzoid melanoma. If a firm diagnosis cannot be made, these lesions are classified as melanocytic lesions of unknown malignant potential. In order to differentiate between Spitz nevi and spitzoid melanoma, many institutions now routinely use comparative genomic hybridization (CGH) to evaluate chromosomal changes in the melanocytic cells.[37] CGH evaluates changes in DNA copy number. Nevi rarely exhibit DNA copy number changes and Sptiz nevi exhibit a consistent and unique deletion at q11 whereas spitzoid melanomas may have DNA copy number changes characteristic of other cutaneous melanomas.

In patients with melanocytic lesions of unknown malignant potential and where diagnostic uncertainty exists, it is prudent to treat patients according to the lesion in the differential diagnosis that carries the worst prognosis.

Depending on the measured thickness of the melanocytic lesion, a wide excision with a 1 to 2 cm margin and primary closure carries a relatively low morbidity compared to the risk of inadequately excising a melanoma. In certain patients, evaluation of lymph nodes with sentinel lymph node biopsy should also be considered, especially if there are CGH changes suggestive of melanoma transformation.

## TECHNIQUES FOR WOUND CLOSURE OF RESECTED MELANOMAS

### Routine wound closure

The majority of patients diagnosed with primary cutaneous melanoma can be treated with a wide local excision and primary wound closure. Wide local excisions with margins of 2 cm or less can often be accomplished on an outpatient basis with local anesthesia with or without intravenous sedation. Patients who also undergo a concomitant sentinel lymph node evaluation can also be treated in an outpatient setting with regional or general anesthesia.

From a technical perspective, the margin of resection is first measured out with a ruler as a radius from the edge of an intact primary melanoma or the edge of a previous biopsy site (Fig. 49.2). The markings are then extended in an elliptical or fusiform fashion to achieve a full-thickness closure. The long axis of the wide local excision should be three to four times its width to promote a tension-free closure.

Many surgeons often use an ellipse with a length two to three times the width to lessen the cosmetic impact of the wide local excision. The long axis of the wide local excision should be oriented to make maximal use of laxity in the tissue to achieve a full-thickness tension-free primary closure. The long axis should also be oriented towards the draining lymph node basin wherever possible so that draining lymphatic vessels from the primary melanoma site are incorporated with the excision (Fig. 49.3). Some surgeons prefer to offset the wide local excision, such that two-thirds of the fusiform is directed towards the draining lymph node basin, allowing for increased incorporation of draining lymphatic vessels (Fig. 49.3B). Once the wide local excision has been marked out, the excision includes removal of skin and underlying subcutaneous tissue down to the underlying muscle fascia. There is no evidence that removal of the muscular fascia provides any benefit or detriment to local control or survival.[38,39]

The wide local excision should be marked for orientation before being removed from the excision bed, to ensure proper assessment of histologic margins. Advancement flaps are often required to allow primary closure of the surgical defect. This is accomplished by detaching skin and subcutaneous tissue from the muscular fascia in a loose connective tissue plane. The advancement flaps in the most central part of the incision need to be mobilized the most, since this is the part of the incision with the greatest amount of tension. The mobilized flaps are then stretched over the surgical defect and closed primarily in a layered fashion. Absorbable intradermal interrupted sutures are used for the deeper layer and the skin is closed with a

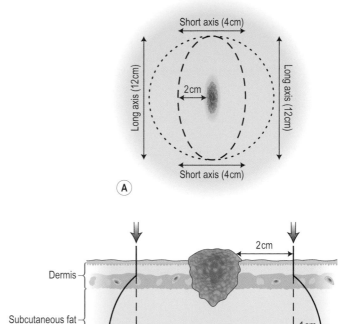

(A)

(B)

Figure 49.2 A) Schematic showing 2 cm margins of wide local excision of melanoma. The margins are measured as a radius from the outer (lateral) edge of an intact primary melanoma or prior biopsy site. To assure a tension-free primary closure, the long axis of excision should be at least three to four times the width of excision. After the wide excision is performed, skin flaps are raised in a plane above the deep muscle fascia to ensure a tension-free closure. B) The melanoma wide excision is extended down to the deep muscle fascia. Skin flaps are developed in a plane just above or just below the fascia. The mobilization of flaps is at least 1 cm as shown. Many times, the mobilization has to be greater than the width of the excisions, especially in the center of the excision, to ensure a tension-free closure. The wound is closed in a layered fashion; the subcutaneous tissue and deep dermis is joined first with interrupted sutures, after which the skin is approximated with interrupted sutures, skin staples or a subcuticular suture.

running absorbable subcuticular suture, with skin staples, or with interrupted nylon sutures, depending on the closure tension and the anticipated wound stress and range of motion. Depending on the size and anatomical location of the wide local excision, a closed suction drain may be beneficial to decrease the size of a seroma (Fig. 49.3B).

Primary wound closure with local advancement is almost always preferable over closure with a skin graft which is more costly, has an increased surgical morbidity and is often cosmetically more disfiguring. However, in some anatomical locations, such as the scalp and distal extremities, primary closure is not always possible and a split-thickness or full-thickness skin graft or a rotation flap closure may be necessary. In cosmetically sensitive areas, such as the face, rotation flaps may also offer a cosmetically more satisfying alternative. It is essential for the surgeon to provide the patient with an accurate understanding of the expected postoperative physical appearance following excision of the melanoma. Patient dissatisfaction with the cosmetic outcome of the wide local excision is more often

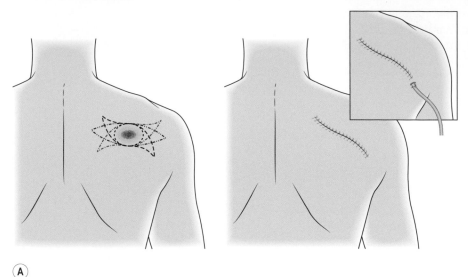

**Figure 49.3 A)** Examples of wide local excision on the right upper back. A 2 cm margin is measured out from the edge of the melanoma biopsy site. Various options for direction of the wide local excision are shown. The preferred direction of the wide local excision is towards the draining lymph node basin. A complete full-thickness closure is shown with or without a suction drain. **B)** A 2 cm margin wide local excision of the left thigh is shown. The long axis of the wide local excision should be oriented towards the draining lymph node basin in the left groin. This will promote incorporation of afferent lymphatic channels from the primary melanoma site in the wide local excision. The center of the wide local excision may be offset so that two-thirds of the excision is directed towards the draining lymph node basin, promoting incorporation of a greater proportion of afferent lymphatic channels.

Ⓐ

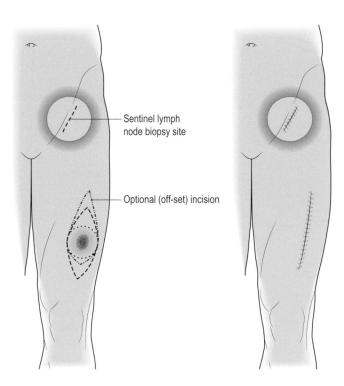

Sentinel lymph node biopsy site

Optional (off-set) incision

Ⓑ

associated with the degree of soft tissue depression rather than the length of the wound.[40] An informed preoperative discussion of these issues and a review of the potential lethality of inadequately treated primary melanoma often alleviate the negative psychological impact of surgical treatment of the melanoma.

## External ear helix melanoma

Thin primary melanomas of the external ear located on the outer helix can often be managed with a wedge excision and primary closure (Fig. 49.4). For patients who wear glasses, a special effort should be made to preserve the upper part of the ear when performing the wedge resection. Patients with intermediate-thickness and thick melanomas requiring a 2 cm margin of resection often require more extensive

reconstruction of the ear and in some patients a complete auriculectomy with reconstruction with a prosthetic ear device often provides an excellent functional and cosmetic outcome.

## Melanoma of digits

Amputation of a single toe rarely results in a significant functional impairment, and melanomas arising from the skin or nail bed of toes can be managed by amputation at the metatarsal-phalangeal joint. This can often be accomplished with a disarticulation of the joint with soft tissue coverage of the joint with a plantar and/or dorsal soft tissue flap. The metatarsal head of the great toe provides stability during ambulation and should be preserved if at all possible.

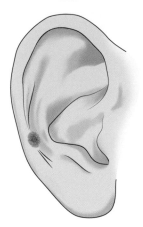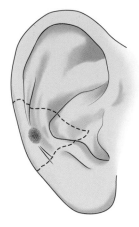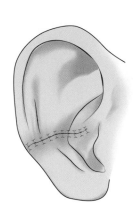

**Figure 49.4** Technique for wide local excision of a melanoma of the outer helix of the ear. A full-thickness external ear helix wedge resection with cartilage is performed, The apex of the wedge is located at the external auditory canal to allow full mobilization of the ear and decreased wound tension.

Complete amputation of fingers or a thumb often results in more functional impairment compared to amputation of toes. For this reason, when treating melanomas of the distal phalanx, especially the nail bed, the amputation should preserve as much as possible of the finger. In these melanomas, if the melanoma does not extend to the interphalangeal joint, the digit is preferentially amputated just proximal to the distal interphalangeal joint of the finger and just proximal to the interphalangeal joint of the thumb (Fig. 49.5). Total finger amputation or amputation to include the metacarpal bone (e.g. ray amputation) is not indicated in melanomas of the distal phalanx, since excision of bone does not offer any oncologic benefit unless the bone is involved with tumor. Mohs surgery is sometimes considered for distal digit lesions.[41]

## Melanomas of the webspace

Melanomas arising in the webspace between fingers and in the webspace next to the great toe require special consideration. Traditionally, ray amputations (partial removal of the metacarpal bone) have been performed for these lesions (Fig. 49.6B). However, en-bloc removal of the digits with partial removal of the metacarpal bone does not provide an oncologic benefit and the functional impairment of a ray

amputation can be significant. Soft tissue dissection alone is usually possible in the webspace and the wound defect can be covered with a full-thickness skin graft or a local rotation flap (Fig. 49.6A).

## Melanomas of the breast

Melanomas arising on the breast do not require more radical excisions such as a formal mastectomy. These cancers should be treated in accordance with the above-mentioned guidelines, and most wide local excisions can be performed without significant distortion of the contour of the breast. The nipple–areola complex should only be removed if the primary melanoma directly involves or is located immediately adjacent to the complex. It the complex is removed, the nipple–areola complex can be reconstructed.

## MOHS SURGERY IN MELANOMA

Mohs micrographic surgery was first introduced by general surgeon Frederic Mohs in 1950 as a means to histologically map the extent of melanoma and to resect the melanoma with a minimal margin.[42] This technique initially required in-situ fixation of the tissue before surgical excision. However, most Mohs surgeons performing the technique now use post-excision fixation of the tissue. In Mohs surgery, the location of residual tumor at the margin of resection is graphically mapped out and repeat sections are taken until the involved margins are clear of tumor (Chapter 47). This allows for maximum sparing of normal tissue adjacent to the primary tumor. This can be of cosmetic benefit in sensitive areas such as the face.

Mohs surgery in the treatment of melanoma has primarily been used in patients with melanoma in situ and thin invasive melanomas. The risk of local recurrence in these melanomas is quite low and the local recurrence rates reported with Mohs surgery appear comparable to rates reported with standard surgical wide local excisions.[43,44] However, to date, no direct comparison has been made between Mohs surgery and standard surgical excision for melanoma. For this reason, until more direct comparisons are available, Mohs surgery for melanoma should be limited to patients with melanoma in situ or minimally invasive melanomas in anatomically sensitive areas such as the face and digits where preservation of adjacent normal tissue is preferred for cosmetic and functional reasons.

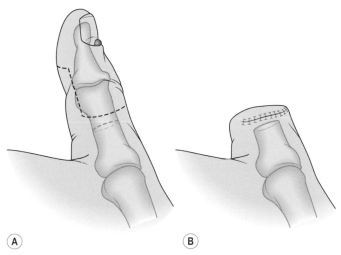

(A)  (B)

**Figure 49.5** Amputation of the thumb for a subungual melanoma. **A)** The thumb is amputated just proximal to the interphalangeal joint. A skin flap on the volar side of the thumb is created to cover the stump. **B)** The wound is closed in a layered fashion with absorbable interrupted sutures for the deep layer and non-absorbable interrupted sutures for the skin.

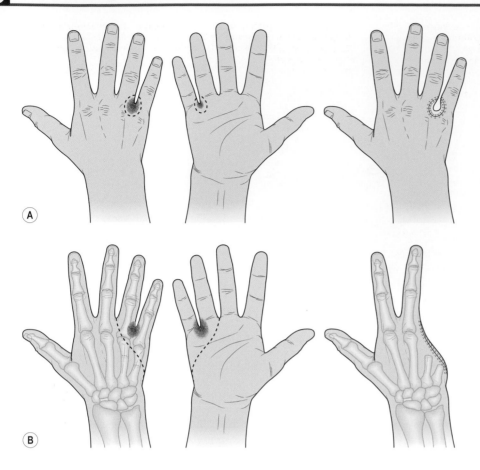

**Figure 49.6 A)** Melanomas of the webspace on the hand can often be resected with negative margins followed by reconstruction of the soft tissue defect with a full-thickness skin graft or rotational flap. **B)** For melanomas of the 4th webspace, a ray amputation with partial amputation of the 4th and 5th metacarpal bones can be performed. However, there is no oncologic benefit to removing the bone and the functional deficit is substantial with the ray amputation. For this reason, a wide local excision of the soft tissue with a full-thickness skin graft reconstruction (as shown in panel A) is preferred.

## FUTURE OUTLOOK

The use of immune response modifiers as an adjunct for surgical treatment of melanoma is being evaluated both preoperatively and postoperatively. Topical therapy may result in a reduction in the size of large tumors, which may require a less extensive surgical operation, which may be of value for tumors located in cosmetically sensitive areas. The use of imiquimod following resection of lentigo maligna may also be of benefit as an adjunctive treatment by inducing the destruction of any residual melanoma cells that were not resected.

The development of instrumentation to non-invasively visualize tumor margins will lead to more narrow surgical margins being taken for cancer removal. Enhancements to newer techniques such as in-vivo confocal microscopy will better allow for the real-time high-resolution imaging of live tissue without the need for tissue fixation and processing. A number of diagnostic features with this type of imaging have been elucidated for melanoma to assess margins. Although the sensitivity and specificity of these criteria have not been determined, approaches of this sort may enable cutaneous surgeons in the future to preoperatively define tumor borders with greater accuracy and consequently enable the further reduction of surgical margins and local recurrence rates.

## REFERENCES

**1.** Davis NC, McLeod GR, eds. *From Hunter to Handley (1787-1907): A Retrospective on Management Approaches to Melanoma.* 3rd ed.St. Louis: Quality Medical Publishing; 1998.

**2.** Norris W. *Eight cases of melanosis with pathological and therapeutical remarks of that disease.* London: Longman, Brown, Green, Longman, and Robert; 1857.

**3.** Handley WS. The pathology of melanotic growths in relation to their operative treatment. *Lancet.* 1907;1:927–933.

**4.** Breslow A, Macht SD. Optimal size of resection margin for thin cutaneous melanoma. *Surg Gynecol Obstet.* 1977;145:691–692.

**5.** Cascinelli N. Margin of resection in the management of primary melanoma. *Semin Surg Oncol.* 1998;14:272–275.

**6.** Veronesi U, Cascinelli N. Narrow excision (1-cm margin). A safe procedure for thin cutaneous melanoma. *Arch Surg.* 1991;126:438–441.

**7.** Veronesi U, Cascinelli N, Adamus J, et al. Thin stage I primary cutaneous malignant melanoma. Comparison of excision with margins of 1 or 3 cm. *N Engl J Med.* 1988;318:1159–1162.

**8.** Banzet P, Thomas A, Vuillemin E. Wide versus narrow surgical excision in thin (equal to or less than 2mm) stage I primary cutaneous malignant melanoma: long term results of a French multicentric prospective randomized trial on 319 patients. *Proc Am Assoc Clin Oncol.* 1993;12:387.

**9.** Khayat D, Rixe O, Martin G, et al. Surgical margins in cutaneous melanoma (2 cm versus 5 cm for lesions measuring less than 2.1-mm thick). *Cancer.* 2003;97:1941–1946.

**10.** Cohn-Cedermark G, Rutqvist LE, Andersson R, et al. Long term results of a randomized study by the Swedish Melanoma Study Group on 2-cm versus 5-cm resection margins for patients with cutaneous melanoma with a tumor thickness of 0.8-2.0 mm. *Cancer.* 2000;89:1495–1501.

**11.** Ringborg U, Andersson R, Eldh J, et al. Resection margins of 2 versus 5 cm for cutaneous malignant melanoma with a tumor thickness of 0.8 to 2.0 mm: randomized study by the Swedish Melanoma Study Group. *Cancer.* 1996;77:1809–1814.

**12.** Balch CM, Soong S, Ross MI, et al. Long-term results of a multi-institutional randomized trial comparing prognostic factors and surgical results for intermediate thickness melanomas (1.0 to 4.0 mm). Intergroup Melanoma Surgical Trial. *Ann Surg Oncol.* 2000;7:87–97.

**13.** Balch CM, Soong SJ, Smith T, et al. Long-term results of a prospective surgical trial comparing 2 cm vs. 4 cm excision margins for 740 patients with 1-4 mm melanomas. *Ann Surg Oncol.* 2001;8:101–108.

**14.** Balch CM, Urist MM, Karakousis CP, et al. Efficacy of 2-cm surgical margins for intermediate-thickness melanomas (1 to 4 mm). Results of a multi-institutional randomized surgical trial. *Ann Surg.* 1993;218:262–267; discussion 7–9.

15. Karakousis CP, Balch CM, Urist MM, et al. Local recurrence in malignant melanoma: long-term results of the multiinstitutional randomized surgical trial. *Ann Surg Oncol.* 1996;3:446–452.

16. Thomas JM, Newton-Bishop J, A'Hern R, et al. Excision margins in high-risk malignant melanoma. *N Engl J Med.* 2004;350:757–766.

17. *NCCN Clinical Practice Guidelines in Oncology: Melanoma.* National Comprehensive Cancer Network; 2010 V.2.2010. www.nccn.org

18. Australian Cancer Network Melanoma Guidelines Revision Working Party. In: *Clinical Practice Guidelines for the Management of Melanoma in Australia and New Zealand.* Wellington, New Zealand: The Cancer Council Australia, Australian Cancer Network, Sydney and New Zealand Guidelines Group; 2008:73–77.

19. Garbe C, Terheyden P, Keilholz U, et al. Treatment of melanoma. *Dtsch Arztebl Int.* 2008;105:845–851.

20. van Everdingen JJ, van der Rhee HJ, Koning CC, et al. Guideline 'Melanoma' (3rd revision). *Ned Tijdschr Geneeskd.* 2005;149:1839–1843.

21. Dummer R, Panizzon R, Bloch PH, et al. Updated Swiss guidelines for the treatment and follow-up of cutaneous melanoma. *Dermatology.* 2005;210:39–44.

22. Roberts DL, Anstey AV, Barlow RJ, et al. U.K. guidelines for the management of cutaneous melanoma. *Br J Dermatol.* 2002;146:7–17.

23. Bishop JN, Bataille V, Gavin A, et al. The prevention, diagnosis, referral and management of melanoma of the skin: concise guidelines. *Clin Med.* 2007;7:283–290.

24. Heaton KM, Sussman JJ, Gershenwald JE, et al. Surgical margins and prognostic factors in patients with thick (>4mm) primary melanoma. *Ann Surg Oncol.* 1998;5:322–328.

25. Conley J, Lattes R, Orr W. Desmoplastic malignant melanoma (a rare variant of spindle cell melanoma). *Cancer.* 1971;28:914–936.

26. Busam KJ, Mujumdar U, Hummer AJ, et al. Cutaneous desmoplastic melanoma: reappraisal of morphologic heterogeneity and prognostic factors. *Am J Surg Pathol.* 2004;28:1518–1525.

27. Hawkins WG, Busam KJ, Ben-Porat L, et al. Desmoplastic melanoma: a pathologically and clinically distinct form of cutaneous melanoma. *Ann Surg Oncol.* 2005;12:207–213.

28. Quinn MJ, Crotty KA, Thompson JF, et al. Desmoplastic and desmoplastic neurotropic melanoma: experience with 280 patients. *Cancer.* 1998;83:1128–1135.

29. Egbert B, Kempson R, Sagebiel R. Desmoplastic malignant melanoma. A clinicohistopathologic study of 25 cases. *Cancer.* 1988;62:2033–2041.

30. Jaroszewski DE, Pockaj BA, DiCaudo DJ, et al. The clinical behavior of desmoplastic melanoma. *Am J Surg.* 2001;182:590–595.

31. Arora A, Lowe L, Su L, et al. Wide excision without radiation for desmoplastic melanoma. *Cancer.* 2005;104:1462–1467.

32. Chen JY, Hruby G, Scolyer RA, et al. Desmoplastic neurotropic melanoma: a clinicopathologic analysis of 128 cases. *Cancer.* 2008;113:2770–2778.

33. Weinstock MA, Sober AJ. The risk of progression of lentigo maligna to lentigo maligna melanoma. *Br J Dermatol.* 1987;116:303–310.

34. Cherpelis BS, Moore R, Ladd S, et al. Comparison of MART-1 frozen sections to permanent sections using a rapid 19-minute protocol. *Dermatol Surg.* 2009;35:207–213.

35. Gross EA, Andersen WK, Rogers GS. Mohs micrographic excision of lentigo maligna using Mel-5 for margin control. *Arch Dermatol.* 1999;135:15–17.

36. Zalla MJ, Lim KK, Dicaudo DJ, et al. Mohs micrographic excision of melanoma using immunostains. *Dermatol Surg.* 2000;26:771–784.

37. Bauer J, Bastian BC. Distinguishing melanocytic nevi from melanoma by DNA copy number changes: comparative genomic hybridization as a research and diagnostic tool. *Dermatol Ther.* 2006;19:40–49.

38. Kenady DE, Brown BW, McBride CM. Excision of underlying fascia with a primary malignant melanoma: effect on recurrence and survival rates. *Surgery.* 1982;92:615–618.

39. Olsen G. Removal of fascia – cause of more frequent metastases of malignant melanomas of the skin to regional lymph nodes? *Cancer.* 1964;17:1159–1164.

40. Cassileth BR, Lusk EJ, Tenaglia AN. Patients' perceptions of the cosmetic impact of melanoma resection. *Plast Reconstr Surg.* 1983;71:73–75.

41. Whalen J, Leone D. Mohs micrographic surgery for the treatment of malignant melanoma. *Clin Dermatol.* 2009;27:597–602.

42. Mohs FE. Chemosurgical treatment of melanoma; a microscopically controlled method of excision. *Arch Derm Syphilol.* 1950;62:269–279.

43. Zitelli JA, Brown CD, Hanusa BH. Surgical margins for excision of primary cutaneous melanoma. *J Am Acad Dermatol.* 1997;37:422–429.

44. Zitelli JA, Brown C, Hanusa BH. Mohs micrographic surgery for the treatment of primary cutaneous melanoma. *J Am Acad Dermatol.* 1997;37:236–245.

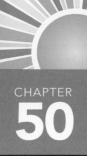

# Regional Lymph Node Surgery in Melanoma Patients

*Merrick I. Ross*

## INTRODUCTION

The regional lymph nodes that receive direct lymphatic drainage from a primary melanoma site are the most common first site(s) of metastatic disease. Lymph node involvement may be clinically occult (microscopic), as determined by sentinel lymph node biopsy (SLN), or clinically apparent (palpable). Palpable nodal involvement more commonly develops over time subsequent to the treatment of the primary cutaneous melanoma but is occasionally present at the time of primary tumor diagnosis, particularly in association with a thick and ulcerated cutaneous lesion. Patients may present with palpable disease in lymph nodes in the absence of a known concurrent primary melanoma or primary melanoma treated in their past, referred to as metastatic melanoma of unknown primary.

Surgery remains the most effective modality to treat regional lymph node involvement, whether it is microscopic or clinically apparent. A formal therapeutic lymph node dissection or lymphadenectomy is the current standard for the treatment of the involved nodal basin(s). The clinical course of disease and prognosis, however, are often

more favorable when the nodal disease is microscopic, explaining the recent increasing use of SLN biopsy in the management of primary melanoma patients presenting with clinically negative regional lymph nodes.

This chapter presents the rationale, indications, goals, techniques and postoperative issues for the two forms of regional lymph node surgery in the melanoma patient: sentinel lymph node (SLN) biopsy and formal therapeutic dissection.

## APPROACH TO CLINICALLY NEGATIVE NODAL BASINS

The vast majority of patients newly diagnosed with melanoma present with disease clinically localized to the primary site (stage I and II).[1] Establishing standards of care for this large group of patients has been an important goal for clinicians challenged with the continually increasing public health problem of melanoma.

The stage I and II population is very heterogeneous in prognosis and outcome. Surgical management recommendations have evolved over the decades based on reported findings from single and multi-institutional databases and completed prospective randomized trials in an effort to consistently achieve the following goals: accurate staging and prognosis, long-term local/regional disease control, and optimizing the chance for cure. Further emphasis has been placed on accomplishing these goals in the context of minimizing treatment-related morbidities.

## SENTINEL LYMPH NODE BIOPSY (SLN)

### History and rationale

Surgical strategies for stage I and II patients have included two main components: wide excision of the primary tumor or biopsy site and regional lymph node evaluation. While recommendations for the extent of excision margins are well established and widely accepted, the approach to the clinically uninvolved regional lymph nodes has been the center of ongoing controversy. How to best manage the following clinical scenario is often called into question: A 36-year-old patient with a biopsy-proven 1.8 mm melanoma. Physical examination reveals the absence of enlarged lymph nodes in any potential regional lymph node group. The chest X-ray is normal and the patient is otherwise healthy. Traditionally, this patient would have been offered one of two options in addition to excision of the primary tumor: 1) observation of the regional lymph nodes and formal node dissection only if the patient subsequently develops clinically evident (palpable) nodal disease, an approach termed therapeutic lymph node dissection (TLND); or, 2) a formal lymph node dissection as a component of the initial surgical treatment, referred to as elective lymph node dissection (ELND). Both of these approaches have theoretical and very real disadvantages.[1]

A significant percentage of individuals, predicted by increasing primary tumor thickness, ulceration, or other unfavorable histologic features of the primary tumor, harbor clinically undetectable regional lymph node metastases, which in most patients will progress to palpable (macroscopic) nodal disease if left untreated. Once clinical nodal involvement develops, the ability to achieve long-term survival and durable regional disease control with a TLND may be compromised compared to surgical approaches targeted at treating microscopic nodal burden.[2] The rate of distant metastatic disease and relapse in the treated nodal basin is at least 50% and 15–50%, respectively, following TLND.

The practice of ELND was popularized for the sole intent of reducing these high rates of disease recurrence. Proponents of ELND suggested that removal of microscopically involved lymph nodes would prevent the development of clinically apparent lymph node disease, which in turn could, in a significant percentage of patients, eliminate a potential source of distant failure. Furthermore, a dissection performed when the lymph node involvement is microscopic would more completely eradicate regional metastases and prevent recurrence in the treated basin and the potential sequelae of pain, skin ulceration, blood vessel and nerve involvement, and advanced lymphedema that can be associated with this pattern of failure. In the majority of patients, however, microscopic nodal disease is absent at diagnosis and therefore they cannot benefit from an ELND and are subjected to the cost and morbidity of an unnecessary operation. It is therefore not surprising that overall survival advantage with ELND was not observed in prospective randomized trials that compared the outcome of stage I and II patients receiving either ELND or nodal observation.[3–6]

For these reasons, the routine practice of ELND has been appropriately challenged. A rational compromise emerged when the technique of lymphatic mapping and SLN biopsy was introduced as a minimally invasive method for determining if occult nodal metastases are present.[7] Patients with proven occult nodal disease in the SLN could then undergo an early TLND, and those without disease could be safely observed, an approach popularized as *selective lymphadenectomy*. This approach has been extensively studied worldwide.

## Scientific support for the sentinel node concept

Lymphatic mapping relies on the hypothesis that the dermal lymphatic drainage from cutaneous sites to the regional lymph node basin is an orderly and definable process and that these lymphatic drainage patterns should mimic the metastatic spread of melanoma cells in the lymphatics (Fig. 50.1). In this way, the first lymph node(s) receiving

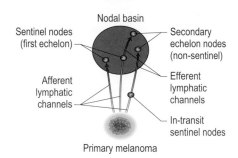

**Figure 50.1** Schematic of potential afferent lymphatic channels draining from a primary cutaneous site to sentinel (first echelon) nodes in the nodal basin. Secondary echelon nodes may be identified by pass through of the intradermally injected blue dye or radiolabeled colloid. Occasionally, a sentinel node is located between the injection site and the formal nodal basin, defined here as 'in-transit' sentinel node, but also referred to as 'interval' or 'ectopic' sentinel node.

lymphatic drainage (the sentinel nodes) are the most likely to contain metastatic disease. The successful identification, surgical removal, and careful histologic examination of these nodes should provide accurate nodal staging.

To test this hypothesis, clinical studies were performed using intradermal injections of blue lymphatic dyes (isosulfan blue or patent blue V) at the primary tumor site followed by the visual identification of the SLNs in the nodal basin. These studies established the following: 1) SLN identification rates, and 2) the accuracy of the SLN in determining the presence or absence of regional nodal metastases.

The first report published by Morton et al. in 1992 evaluated 237 patients and demonstrated an 82% SLN identification rate.[7] Subsequent studies from the M. D. Anderson and Moffitt Cancer Centers[8,9] and the Sydney Melanoma Unit[10] reported similar findings. Accuracy assessment was accomplished through the use of synchronous ELND performed at the time of the SLN biopsy. These initial studies evaluated 402 patients with successful SLN localization, 86 of whom were found to have regional node metastases (81 patients with a positive SLN and 5 additional patients with disease only in a non-SLN). This low false-negative rate of 5% supported the SLN concept.

Additional evidence that regional node metastasis is an orderly and non-random event was provided from the M. D. Anderson Cancer Center reporting on the examination of 105 lymphadenectomy specimens in patients with at least one positive SLN.[11] Investigators found that the SLN was the only node involved in 83 (79%) of the basins, with disease in additional nodes identified in 21% of the lymphadenectomy specimens. Presented in another way, 68% of all the SLNs removed from all patients with at least one involved SLN and only 1.8% of all non-SLNs were involved with metastatic disease.[11]

Tremendous interest was generated from these initial studies, and many centers subsequently adopted the selective lymphadenectomy approach for newly diagnosed intermediate- and high-risk stage I and II melanoma patients. Improvements in SLN localization techniques, insights into the biologic relevance of the SLN (discussed below), and additional findings supporting the SLN concept emerged. In a report of nearly 250 SLN-negative patients followed for over 3 years, only 10 patients (4%) developed nodal failure within the previously mapped regional basin.[12] Such failures represent a false-negative rate similar to the 5% determined by concomitant ELND. More careful histologic scrutiny of the negative SLNs from these same 10 patients revealed the presence of disease in 8. These data not only further supported the validity of the SLN concept, but also suggested that routine histologic examinations of SLNs may fail to detect clinically relevant disease.

## Technical advances

Initial SLN identification rates of 80% to 85% using blue dye injections provided a promising beginning. The use of high-resolution cutaneous lymphoscintography[13–15] and an intraoperative handheld gamma detection device to locate radiolabeled colloids that have accumulated in SLNs after being injected at the primary site have yielded higher SLN identification rates.[11,15–17] The use of a gamma probe was first described by Krag et al., who reported a 95% SLN identification rate.[17] Studies comparing combined modality techniques (radiocolloid plus blue dye) versus blue dye alone demonstrated a significant increase in SLN identification to 99% with the combined approach.[11,16]

The intraoperative use of the gamma probe provides a method of detection that is independent of and more sensitive than visualization of blue-stained nodes and can locate SLNs that might otherwise be undetected. The number of SLNs identified was greater when both modalities were employed compared to blue dye alone (1.74 versus 1.31, respectively).[11] This more complete removal of SLNs may further reduce the already low false-negative rate. Figure 50.2 summarizes the components necessary for successful identification and removal of an SLN.

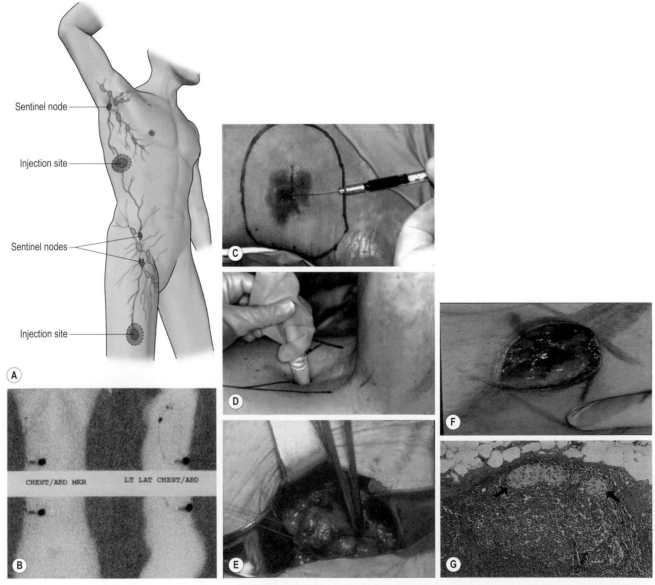

**Figure 50.2** Lymphatic mapping and sentinel lymph node (SLN) concept and technique. **A)** The SLN concept is illustrated demonstrating potential afferent drainage patterns from primary tumor sites to the first draining nodes (sentinel node) in the regional basins. **B)** Lymphoscintigraphy is an important component of the procedure which identifies nodal basin(s) at risk for primary melanomas arising in ambiguous lymphatic drainage sites and the number of sentinel nodes in the basin. Here, lymphatic drainage from the low back is to the axilla rather than the closer inguinal basin. **C)** Injection of isosulfan blue intradermally around biopsy site. **D)** Transcutaneous localization of SLN using gamma detection probe. **E, F)** Exploration of nodal basin and visualization of SLN. **G)** Histologic detection of occult metastases in subcapsular sinus.

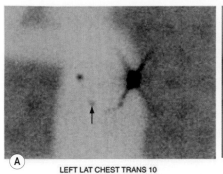
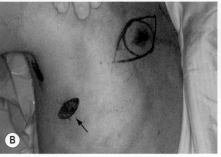
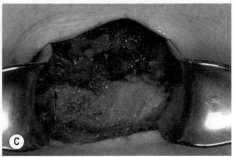

LEFT LAT CHEST TRANS 10

**Figure 50.3** In-transit sentinel node. **A)** Lymphoscintigraphy shows lymphatic drainage pattern from injection site over left upper back to the ipsilateral axilla and an in-transit sentinel node (arrow) over the scapular spine. **B)** Intraoperative photograph showing the primary site over the upper back and sentinel node biopsy sites in the axilla and in-transit region (arrow). **C)** Close-up view of exposed in-transit node (arrow) with blue afferent channel.

These techniques can also aid in the localization of SLNs that may exist outside and/or proximal to the formal nodal basin; referred to as interval, in-transit, or ectopic SLNs[18-22] (Fig. 50.3). According to published studies, the frequency of such SLN locations is in the range of 5% to 10% of patients, and the frequency of involvement with microscopic disease is the same as that of SLNs harvested from formal basins.[22] The failure to identify these nodes risks under-staging some patients and leaving behind potential sources of clinical recurrences.

## SLN biologic and prognostic significance

Studies have demonstrated that the incidence of SLN metastases correlates directly with increasing tumor thickness[11,23-26] (Table 50.1). SLN involvement is also associated with a variety of other known primary tumor factors predictive of overall survival, including ulceration, lymphatic invasion, mitotic rate, Clark level, anatomic site, and host factors such as age.[25-28] In a multivariate analysis, the two variables that independently best predicted SLN involvement were tumor thickness and the presence of ulceration.[26] This analysis uncovered a unique interaction between tumor thickness and ulceration in that the presence of ulceration within a specific tumor thickness stage worsened the prognosis of patients equivalent to those in the next-higher thickness group without ulceration.[29] A similar relationship between thickness and ulceration in terms of predicting the incidence of SLN metastases exists, as shown in Table 50.1.[26]

These observations support the hypothesis that the prognostic value of tumor thickness and ulceration is largely dependent on the fact that these two same factors predict SLN metastases, and in this way offers convincing evidence that SLN involvement is a biologically important event.

Further supporting this conclusion are findings from survival analyses of large numbers of stage I and II patients managed in prospective selective lymphadenectomy programs. Consistently, these reports revealed that the SLN-positive patients experienced a significantly lower survival compared to SLN-negative patients (Fig. 50.4), and that the histologic status of the SLN was the most powerful independent predictor of overall survival in the clinically node-negative melanoma patients when analyses were carried out including previously described primary tumor prognostic factors[30] (Table 50.2). Several similar analyses have since been published from large single institutional as well as multi-centered experiences corroborating these findings.[31-33]

While the patients with a negative SLN as a whole enjoy an excellent survival, a negative SLN is not a perfect prognostic factor. Five-year melanoma-specific survival rates are generally 90% for the SLN-negative patients, with recurrence and death occurring secondary to the following reasons: a false-negative SLN or pure hematogenous pattern of metastases. Predictors of relapse and death in the SLN-negative group include increasing tumor thickness and primary tumor ulceration. The development of clinical nodal disease in a nodal basin previously determined to be

### Table 50.1 Incidence of SLN Metastases According to Primary Tumor Factors

| Tumor Thickness (mm) | Total No. of Patients (N) | All (%) | Positive SLN | |
| --- | --- | --- | --- | --- |
| | | | Non-Ulcerated (%) | Ulcerated (%) |
| ≤1.00 | 326 | 4.2 | 3.9 | 12.5 |
| 1.01–2.00 | 490 | 11.4 | 10.8 | 21.2 |
| 2.01–4.00 | 310 | 28.5 | 23.1 | 37.0 |
| ≥4.01 | 190 | 45.5 | 31.2 | 55.4 |
| Total | 1316 | 17.4 | 11.9 | 37.0 |

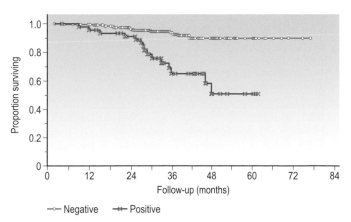

**Figure 50.4** Melanoma-specific survival of stage I and II patients according to SLN status.

### Table 50.2 Prognostic Factors Influencing Disease-Specific Survival in Stage I and II Patients Undergoing SIN Biopsy

| Prognostic Factor | Univariate | Multiple Covariate Hazard Ratio | P Value |
|---|---|---|---|
| Age | NS | – | NS |
| Sex | NS | – | NS |
| Axial location | 0.03 | – | NS |
| Tumor thickness | <0.0001 | 1.1 | 0.04 |
| Clark level >III | 0.001 | 2.3 | 0.01 |
| Ulceration | <0.0001 | 3.3 | <0.0001 |
| SLN status | <0.0001 | 6.5 | <0.0001 |

without microscopic involvement defines a false-negative event and occurs in approximately 3–5% of these patients. Theoretically, three explanations exist for these events: 1) the main SLN was not properly identified during the SLN procedure, leaving behind a microscopically involved lymph node; 2) the original SLN procedure was accurate, but microscopic in-transit disease was present at the onset that had not yet traveled to the nodal basin; 3) the correct SLN was removed and microscopic disease was present but undetected by the histologic examination either as a result of a very small burden of disease or within a portion of the node that was not sampled.

## Rationale for SLN biopsy

The original motivation to study SLN biopsy was to establish an effective method of preventing the development of clinically palpable regional disease in the stage I and II melanoma patients. Many have questioned its therapeutic role. Results of recent clinical trials demonstrated survival benefits[5,6] and improved regional disease control afforded by SLN dissection in patients with microscopic nodal involvement, and improved survival with the use of adjuvant interferon in node-positive patients.[34] These studies provided additional motivation to incorporate SLN biopsy in the management of stage I and II patients.

## Does early node dissection impart a survival benefit?

The potential for improved survival with early node dissection was the goal for the routine application of ELND as part of the initial management of newly diagnosed stage I and II patients. The question of survival impact with the use of ELND relative to nodal observation and therapeutic dissection for those patients who develop clinically detectable nodal disease has been evaluated in four prospective randomized trials. The first two trials, one from the Mayo Clinic[3] and one from the World Health Organization,[4] performed in the 1970s and prior to knowledge concerning primary tumor prognostic factors, demonstrated no survival advantage. Accordingly, ELND was strongly contested and

largely abandoned. These trials were subsequently criticized because the study populations were at low risk for occult nodal disease and therefore unlikely to benefit from the surgical treatment being tested.

Two additional ELND trials were performed targeting the higher-risk clinically node-negative patients.[5,6] Trends for improved survival following ELND were observed in both trials. However, these differences were not statistically significant. While many concluded that early treatment of nodal metastases had little impact on disease progression, others suggested that these trials were underpowered because only the 20% of patients harboring nodal disease could potentially benefit from the procedure.[1] Long-term results published in 1998 from the WHO ELND Trial, which included patients with trunk primaries >1.5 mm, demonstrated that patients with microscopic nodal disease in the ELND treatment arm experienced improved overall survival compared to patients who developed clinical adenopathy after randomization to excision alone.[5] Results published in 2000 from the Intergroup ELND Trial in which patients with melanomas 1 to 4 mm in thickness were studied, demonstrated that prospectively stratified subgroups (1 to 2 mm and all non-ulcerated primaries) derived a survival benefit with ELND.[6]

While overall survival rates for the entire study cohorts in both trials were not statistically different (confirming that not all patients can benefit from ELND), these studies do suggest that specific subsets of patients (most notably those with microscopic nodal disease and possibly additional patients with nodal disease undetected by routine histologic techniques) can benefit from earlier dissections. These data offer evidence-based credence to the theoretical concerns of delaying the lymphadenectomy until palpable nodal disease develops and supports the selective lymphadenectomy approach.

The survival impact of the selective lymphadenectomy strategy, using SLN biopsy as an alternative to ELND, was formally studied in a prospective randomized multi-centered international trial comparing the outcomes of nodal observation after wide excision to SLN biopsy and completion dissection for patients with microscopic nodal involvement. The design and primary and secondary endpoints of the Multicenter Selective Lymphadenectomy Trial-1 (MSLT-1) are presented in Figure 50.5. The results of the third interim analysis of the MSLT-1 were recently published in the New

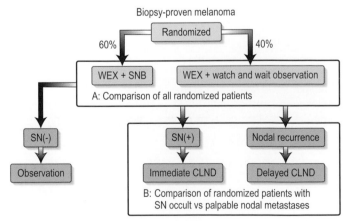

**Figure 50.5** Treatment algorithm for recently completed Multicenter Selective Lymphadenectomy Trial-1 (MSLT-1).

England Journal of Medicine.[32] Data were available for 1269 patients. In the biopsy group, the presence of metastases in the SLN was the most important prognostic factor. The 5-year melanoma-specific survival rate was 72.3±4.6% among patients with tumor-positive SLNs and 90.2±1.3% among those with tumor-negative SLNs (P<0.001), confirming the previously reported observations from several other groups. The melanoma-specific death rate at 5 years was similar in the two groups (13.8% in the observation group and 12.5% in the biopsy group), as was the melanoma-specific survival rate at 3 years (90.1±1.4% and 93.2±0.9%, respectively) and 5 years (86.6±1.6% and 87.1±1.3%, respectively). The incidence of SLN micrometastases was 16%, while the rate of relapse in regional nodes in the observation group was 15.6%. The mean number of tumor-involved nodes at lymphadenectomy was 1.4 in the biopsy group and 3.3 in the observation group (P<0.001). A pronounced overall survival advantage was observed when the analysis was performed including only the node-positive patients. Compared to the patients who underwent a therapeutic (delayed) dissection for clinical nodal failure after being randomized to nodal observation, the SLN-positive patients who underwent immediate lymphadenectomy enjoyed a 20% improved 5-year survival rate (72.3±4.6% versus 52.4±5.9%; hazard rate for death 0.51, 95% CI 0.32–0.81; P=0.004) (Fig. 50.6).

The interim results of the MSLT-I Trial provide important insights into the value of selective lymphadenectomy compared with delayed lymphadenectomy. The lack of an overall survival difference between the two treatment arms is not surprising in that this trial suffers from the same limitations as the ELND trials: being underpowered because of the low percentage of patients (16% in this trial) who could

benefit from complete lymphadenectomy. Assuming that early lymphadenectomy for SLN-positive patients is associated with a 20% survival benefit, one would predict an overall survival advantage of no more than 3.2% compared with delayed lymphadenectomy. Nonetheless, survival differences can emerge with longer follow-up. If future events follow the patterns observed in the two ELND trials, more recurrences in the nodal observation arm may develop over time than in the SLN biopsy arm.

The results of the secondary survival analysis comparing SLN-positive patients with those who developed clinically palpable nodes following nodal observation are particularly noteworthy. The improved survival of the SLN-positive group not only corroborates the results of the WHO ELND trial but also supports the concept that, if left intact, microscopic nodal disease progresses and is associated with a worse prognosis. In some patients, therefore, increasing nodal burden can be a source of systemic dissemination; early treatment of nodal disease can favorably alter the natural history of their disease.

## Regional disease control

The most common first recurrence in primary melanoma patients initially treated with excision of the primary site alone is palpable lymph node metastases. These patients are generally treated with a TLND for attempts at cure and regional control of disease. Reported in-basin, post-dissection failure rates range from 9% to 50% depending on a variety of factors, including basin site, number and size of involved nodes, and presence of extracapsular extension.[34–37] In-basin recurrences are very difficult to treat surgically and may be the source of significant morbidity in the form of pain, severe lymphedema, venous obstruction, skin ulceration, nerve involvement, and bleeding. In-basin failures in patients treated with ELND and found to harbor microscopic disease occur in less than 10% of patients and are reported to be even lower after completion dissection in SLN-positive patients.[38,39] The potential for improved regional disease control when dissections are performed for microscopic disease further supports the use of SLN biopsy.

## Histologic examination of SLNs

The fundamental goal of SLN biopsy is to accurately stage the regional basin. This is accomplished first by the accurate identification and complete surgical removal of all the SLNs from the appropriate nodal basins at risk, and then by the careful histologic examination of these nodes. Although the definition of careful histologic examination continues to evolve, it is clear that as pathologic scrutiny becomes more extensive, it is more feasible to apply novel and sensitive techniques to one or two nodes (SLNs) rather than 20 to 30 nodes submitted following an ELND. Utilizing careful evaluation of the most likely nodes to contain metastatic disease, more accurate nodal staging is possible and is accomplished with little morbidity to the patient.

Historically, the standard approach for evaluating lymph nodes, and therefore initially applied to SLNs as well, was to bivalve a clinically negative node and stain a section from

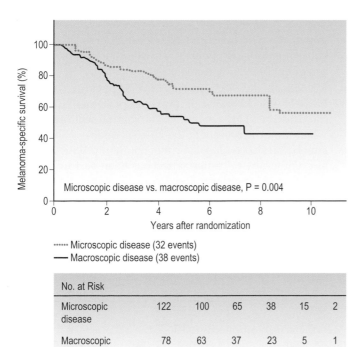

| No. at Risk | | | | | | |
|---|---|---|---|---|---|---|
| Microscopic disease | 122 | 100 | 65 | 38 | 15 | 2 |
| Macroscopic disease | 78 | 63 | 37 | 23 | 5 | 1 |

**Figure 50.6** Melanoma-specific survival curves of node-positive patients in MSLT-1. SLN-positive patients enjoyed better survival than patients randomized to receive nodal observation and underwent node dissection after developing clinically involved nodes.

each half with hematoxylin and eosin (H&E). As a result, only a small percent of the lymph node(s) were sampled and this likely explains why conventional histologic techniques underestimated the incidence of regional nodal disease in stage I and II patients. For example, the incidence of nodal failure following surgical excision alone for primary melanomas 2 to 4 mm is approximately 35–50%, while the incidence of microscopic nodal disease as determined by ELND or SLN biopsy specimens, when applying the routine pathologic technique of bivalving the nodes, is approximately 25–40%

While subsequent nodal failure may in part result from clinically occult in-transit disease, several lines of evidence support the concept that nodal disease is more often present at diagnosis than is demonstrated by conventional histology: 1) step sectioning (i.e. better sampling) improves the ability to detect microscopic disease; 2) 80% of patients who develop nodal basin failure after a negative SLN biopsy initially assessed by routine pathology are determined to be node positive following more careful analysis of the paraffin blocks;[12,40] and 3) evaluation of SLNs using the reverse transcriptase–polymerase chain reaction (PCR) to detect the presence of messenger-RNA encoding for melanoma-specific proteins (i.e. tyrosinase) as potential surrogate markers of nodal disease results in higher SLN-positive rates.[41-43]

Reports indicate that essentially all H&E positive SLNs and anywhere from 25% to 50% of H&E negative SLNs are PCR positive. While preliminary clinical correlation studies demonstrate that the PCR-positive–H&E-negative group exhibit recurrence rates intermediate between the PCR-negative and H&E-positive patients,[41-44] long-term follow-up failed to demonstrate an overall decreased survival in the PCR-positive patients compared to the PCR-negative patients in two recently published series.[44,45] As histologic techniques become more sensitive, specificity may be compromised, but the more careful and complete the evaluation of SLNs, the more likely we are to define a true and homogeneous SLN-negative subset.

Current recommendations include multiple H&E sections and immunohistology using HMB-45 and MART-1, but established standards are still in evolution.[40,46] Frozen section at the time of SLN biopsy probably reduces the sensitivity and is therefore not recommended,[47] but imprint touch cytology performed on multiple sections of the SLN at the time of the procedure can accurately detect microscopic disease in a significant percentage with occult metastases and facilitate same-day completion dissections without compromising the formal permanent histological examination.[48] For all of these reasons, PCR evaluation at present should only be considered in the setting of a clinical trial.

## Patient selection for SLN biopsy

Candidates for SLN biopsy include those with newly diagnosed primary melanoma who are clinically node-negative and predicted to be at intermediate or high risk of harboring occult nodal disease, based on primary tumor characteristics.[25,26] Specific percent risk thresholds are still in question, but tumor thickness thresholds of 1 mm have gained wide

consensus. The routine use of SLN biopsy in patients with thin (<1 mm) tumors is not cost-effective because of the overall low risk of nodal involvement in this group.[49] However, a selective approach in patients with thin melanomas based on the presence of Clark level IV and/or ulceration is rational, as these two factors were the most powerful predictors of recurrence in the patients with thin melanomas in the recent AJCC analysis.[2] Simply stated, stage IB and higher may be offered SLN biopsy.

Another primary tumor prognostic factor commonly used in the decision process in patients with thin melanomas is vertical growth phase. Specifically, an important primary tumor risk factor for SLN involvement is the presence and number of mitotic figures in the vertical growth phase as a surrogate for aggressive biology.[50,51] In a study from the University of Pennsylvania, the incidence of SLN metastases in patients with thin melanomas of at least 0.76 mm and exhibiting one or more mitotic figures per square millimeter was 12.5%.[51] Increasingly, the presence of mitotic figures is being used to identify the higher-risk subset of patients as candidates for SLN biopsy. Mitotic rate of 1 or greater per mm squared has recently been incorporated in the 2010 AJCC analysis for patients with thin melanomas (<1mm) and advances the stage designation to IB[52] and therefore is included in the factors used to recommend SLN biopsy in patients with thin melanoma.

It should be emphasized that SLN biopsy is also appropriate for patients with thick melanomas (>4 mm) even though this group is also at high risk for distant disease, as recently published experiences from more than one center demonstrates that SLN status is the single most important independent predictor of survival in the subset of patients with thick melanoma.[53-54]

Other clinical scenarios that arise where SLN biopsy may be useful are:

- in patients who develop a true local recurrence subsequent to a relatively narrow excision as prior treatment of a primary melanoma
- for patients in whom the exact tumor thickness cannot be ascertained because of improper placement in the paraffin block, resulting in tangential sectioning when tumor is present at the base secondary to a superficial shave biopsy; or when a manipulation such as cryotherapy or cauterization has been performed on the same lesion prior to the diagnosis of melanoma
- when the pathologic diagnosis of an atypical melanocytic lesion is ambiguous but may possibly include a primary melanoma >1 mm in the differential diagnosis[55]
- for patients who have already received a formal wide excision with or without a skin graft and then wish to have accurate assessment of their draining lymph node basins.

In the last-mentioned situation, the accuracy of the technique is in question because the lymphatic drainage of the remaining skin may be different than that of the skin that existed immediately adjacent to the original primary melanoma. A few small published series compared the incidence of positive SLNs in groups of patients who had already undergone a 1 cm or wider excision to patients who had intact lesions or an excision for diagnosis. The patient groups were matched in terms of primary tumor factors and the incidence of positive SLNs was similar, suggesting that SLN biopsy may still be accurate in patients who have had prior wide excisional biopsies.[56]

## Is completion dissection in patients with a positive SLN necessary?

Only 8–33% of patients with a positive SLN will be found to have additional microscopic nodal disease within non-sentinel nodes removed by a subsequent therapeutic dissection.[57–61] These data must be viewed with some concern of underestimating disease, as the pathologic techniques used to evaluate additional non-SLN(s) removed through a therapeutic lymphadenectomy procedure has been limited to bisecting lymph nodes rather than multiple step section or special histochemical stains. An international randomized trial (MSLT-2) is currently accruing patients using the basic framework design of a randomization to therapeutic node dissection versus nodal basin observation after a positive SLN biopsy. This trial will answer the following questions: 1) the incidence of nodal failure after removal of a positive SLN in the absence of a completion dissection; 2) the incidence and predictors of additional positive nodes in the same basin; and 3) the survival impact, if any, for completion dissection. Some surgeons are already inconsistently omitting the completion dissection in SLN-positive patients and others are selectively not recommending completion dissection based on published predictors of a very low incidence of non-SLN involvement.[59–61]

The largest study on the predictors of non-SLN involvement in the completion node dissection specimen included a retrospective analysis of 343 patients with a positive SLN who underwent a completion dissection.[61] Fourteen percent of patients had at least one additional lymph node involved with occult metastases. Upon multivariate analysis, the following features were independent predictors of non-SLN involvement: tumor thickness >2 mm, increasing SLN tumor burden, and the number of SLNs removed. Using these three factors, a predictive model was developed that identified four risk quartiles, ranging from 0% to 55%. The two lowest risk groups together comprise nearly half of the patients and have a risk of 0% and 4%, respectively

While such selective approaches to completion dissection are attractive, until independent validation is established, omission of a completion node dissection outside of a clinical trial should be discouraged. Therefore, completion dissection should be considered the current standard of care.

## Complications and morbidity following SLN biopsy

Complications following lymphatic mapping and SLN biopsy are relatively uncommon. Investigators from the Sunbelt Melanoma Trial reported the complication rates following SLN biopsy alone in more than 1202 trial patients and in 277 patients who required a complete lymph node dissection as part of the trial. The incidence of seroma,

lymphedema, and wound problems was 3% versus 7.9%, 0.7% versus 9.8%, and 1.7% versus 11.9%, respectively. Each significant difference favored the SLN dissection–alone arm.[62] The observation of low complication rates following SLN biopsy has also been reported by others,[63,64] as well as in the Multicenter Selective Lymphadenectomy Trial, in which an overall complication rate of 10.4% after lymphatic mapping and sentinel node biopsy (wound infection, 4.6%; wound separation, 1.2%; seroma/hematoma, 4.6%) increased to 32.7% after completion lymph node dissection.[32] Although allergic reactions, including anaphylactic reactions, have been reported on rare occasions following use of vital blue dye, they have not occurred in large melanoma populations.[65]

## Potential increased risk of in-transit metastasis – a possible 'biologic' complication?

Although the SLN biopsy technique has gained widespread acceptance for a number of reasons – accurate nodal staging, enhanced regional control, possible survival benefit, limited surgical morbidity compared to formal lymphadenectomy – some authors have suggested that SLN biopsy should not be employed outside the confines of a formal clinical investigation.[66–68] Among their concerns is that SLN biopsy may increase the risk of in-transit metastasis (ITM), thereby reducing, eliminating, or reversing any potential survival advantage associated with the SLN biopsy technique.[69,70] In considering whether ITM is promoted by regional lymph node basin intervention, a full appreciation of the biology and incidence of ITM in melanoma patients prior to the advent of SLN biopsy is helpful. The hypothesis that the SLN biopsy technique and subsequent completion lymph node dissection in SLN-positive patients may disturb lymph flow by mechanical disruption of the proximal nodal basin and lead to increased rates of ITM – if accurate – is of particular concern since SLN biopsy has been widely adopted as the standard of care for many patients with clinically localized melanoma.

The collective experience at several large academic centers does not support the hypothesis that SLN biopsy increases the risk of in-transit metastasis.[71–73] Among 1395 patients who underwent SLN biopsy at the University of Texas M. D. Anderson Cancer Center, the overall incidence of ITM as a first site of recurrence was 6.2%.[71] Compared with SLN-negative patients, SLN-positive patients had thicker tumors (median, 3.0 mm vs 1.3 mm), a higher incidence of ulceration (45% vs 12%), and a higher rate of ITM (12% vs 3.5%).[71] Among patients with primary melanomas at least 1.0 mm thick treated between 1993 and 2003 at the Sydney Melanoma Unit, rates of ITM among 1035 patients treated with wide local excision (WLE) alone and 754 patients with similar primary tumor characteristics treated with WLE plus SLN biopsy were not significantly different (6.5% and 3.7%, respectively).[72] These data have also been corroborated by another study and by the results of the MSLT-I Trial,[32,73] both of which also demonstrated no increased risk of ITM following sentinel node biopsy. Taken together, these results strongly support the proposition that the risk of in-transit melanoma metastasis depends on tumor biology and not the surgical approach to regional lymph nodes.[74]

## SLN conclusions

It is important to emphasize that the fundamental goal of SLN biopsy is to improve the disease outcome of the node positive patients. SLN biopsy is proven to accurately stage the regional lymph node basins in stage I and II melanoma patients with little morbidity and promotes the selective application of formal node dissections only for the node positive patients. The SLN-positive patients are then treated when the nodal tumor burden is microscopic (stage IIIa), optimizing the chance for long-term survival and durable regional disease control.

With the introduction of more sensitive histologic techniques, SLN biopsy offers the opportunity to more accurately stage patients and defines a more pure and homogeneous node-negative population. The node-positive patients can then receive standard adjuvant therapy or participate in prospective clinical trials assessing the value of novel adjuvant therapy regimens, while the low-risk patients can be safely spared the morbidity of additional surgery and adjuvant therapy. Until molecular studies are readily available and have the ability to accurately determine the metastatic phenotype in primary melanomas, SLN biopsy offers the opportunity to accomplish the aforementioned goals in managing stage I and II patients: optimizing the chance for cure, providing durable regional control, accurate staging, and minimizing treatment morbidity. In many western countries practicing melanoma experts routinely recommend SLN biopsy in the above mentioned clinical settings. Therefore, a recent international consensus panel concluded that SLN biopsy should be considered a standard of care practice.[75]

### REGIONAL LYMPHADENECTOMY: INDICATIONS, TECHNIQUE AND EXTENT, AND MORBIDITY

## Indications

Nodal metastases are divided into microscopic (detected at the time of sentinel lymph node biopsy) and macroscopic (disease identified by clinical evaluation). Standard treatment of melanoma patients found to have occult or clinically evident regional lymph node metastases includes complete dissection of the lymphatic basin for the purpose of regional disease control and attempts at cure.

The current version of the AJCC staging system for melanoma includes classification by the number of involved nodes – N1 (one node positive), N2 (two or three nodes positive), and N3 (four or more nodes positive) – and, therefore, staging is an important goal of a formal dissection.

While patients with advanced (palpable) regional nodal metastasis from melanoma are at relatively high risk for distant and in-basin tumor recurrence after a TLND, and therefore are candidates for postoperative systemic adjuvant therapy with high-dose interferon-alpha or a clinical trial and for the selective use of post-dissection adjuvant nodal basin irradiation,[76,77] a therapeutic node dissection in this clinical setting is still most often performed with curative intent and when performed correctly can offer the patient durable regional disease control the best opportunity for long-term survival.

Patients with advanced nodal disease but who also are found to have widespread extra-regional metastatic disease may be poor candidates for formal lymph node dissection. Surgeons must consider symptoms related to the regional nodal disease, the morbidity of the lymph node dissection, and the potential effectiveness of alternative treatment modalities, before proceeding with a regional surgical procedure that does not render the patient disease-free. In some patients with distant metastases, however, aggressive surgical intervention to address regional nodal metastasis may be justified for the purpose of palliation, particularly when there is significant morbidity related to the regional disease and the distant metastatic disease is limited in extent.

Patients who cannot medically tolerate general anesthesia are generally not considered for regional lymphadenectomy; although, from a technical standpoint, some regional lymphadenectomies can be completed under a regional block.

## Extent and technique of regional lymphadenectomy

Regional basins which may be involved and can be surgically addressed include axillary, cervical, parotid, epitrochlear, popliteal, inguinal/femoral, and iliac/obturator. Generally speaking, whether the disease to be treated is microscopic or clinically evident, the surgical approach to the lymphadenectomy is the same. However, differences may exist in terms of the extent to which the patient is evaluated for the presence of distant metastatic disease and the extent of the actual surgical procedure.

## Pre-surgical planning

Several issues should be considered when preparing a patient to undergo regional lymphadenectomy. Initial planning should begin at the time of SLN biopsy. The surgeon who performs the SLN biopsy should orient the biopsy incision so as to allow for a subsequent completion lymphadenectomy incision to be performed including excision of the biopsy scar en bloc with the lymphadenectomy specimen. This planning can be facilitated by first identifying the area of greatest focal gamma activity representing the location of the sentinel lymph node, and then drawing the incision that would be used for the completion lymphadenectomy incision in a way that would include that focus. The incision for the SLN biopsy is then made the appropriate length within the completion lymphadenectomy planned incision line.

Prior to completion lymphadenectomy, patients should undergo a chest X-ray and an age-appropriate preoperative laboratory evaluation. In terms of extensive evaluation for distant, stage IV disease, two recent studies have demonstrated that routine imaging for staging purposes in patients with only a single positive SLN is not indicated.[78,79] In contrast, in patients with multiple positive nodes or in those undergoing therapeutic lymphadenectomy for clinically detected metastases, we routinely perform a formal staging evaluation; though recognize that even in this situation the yield is low.

The standard evaluation for patients who are being considered for lymphadenectomy includes a complete blood count, blood urea nitrogen, creatinine, LDH, computed tomography (CT) of the chest, abdomen and pelvis, and magnetic resonance imaging of the brain. Recently, positron emission tomography (PET)/CT examinations have become very popular to provide total body imaging. While PET imaging is very sensitive, false-positive findings are relatively frequent, rendering its routine use controversial. Patients considered candidates for postoperative adjuvant therapy will require a similar staging evaluation prior to beginning systemic therapy. In order to avoid the need for repeat imaging studies, we will usually delay formal staging of a patient with regional nodal involvement limited to occult disease identified on SLN biopsy until after formal lymphadenectomy and just prior to beginning adjuvant therapy.

## Axillary lymphadenectomy

In order to perform a complete axillary dissection, the following anatomic landmarks have to be identified and skeletonized: the axillary vein, the ribcage at the thoracic inlet, and the latissimus dorsi, serratus anterior, and the subscapular muscles. The removal of all of the lymph node-bearing tissue is found within the confines of these structures and ensures that all three lymph node levels of axillary node-bearing areas are included in the specimen. The three levels are defined as follows: level 1, lateral to the lateral border of the pectoralis minor muscle; level 2, deep to the pectoralis minor muscle; and level 3, medial to the pectoralis minor muscle. Lymph nodes are also found superficial and superior to the axillary vein and between the pectoralis major and minor muscles (referred to as the Rotter's nodes) and can safely be removed en bloc with the above-described three levels. The important neurovascular structures, including the long thoracic nerve, thoracodorsal neurovascular bundle, medial and lateral pectoral bundles, and axillary vein, are generally spared but can be sacrificed if directly involved by tumor without significant morbidity.

## Inguinofemoral (superficial groin) and ilioinguinal (deep pelvic) lymphadenectomy

### Superficial groin (inguinofemoral) dissection

The targeted lymph node-bearing tissue within this regional basin can be found between the following landmarks: the inguinal ligament, the adductor muscles, the pubic tubercle, the spermatic cord (in males), and the sartorius muscle. The dissection removes all of the tissues within this triangle, sparing the femoral vein, artery, and nerve. Lymph nodes are also found superior to the inguinal ligament but superficial to the external oblique aponeurosis and should be included as part of the en-bloc resection, particularly in patients with a known primary on the trunk. The saphenous vein is often sacrificed as well, particularly in patients with palpable nodal disease, but can be spared in patients undergoing a dissection for a positive SLN. For patients with palpable nodal disease, most surgeons would also include a deep dissection at the same time, inclusive of the iliac and obturator nodes in the pelvis, because of the very high risk for finding synchronous microscopic disease in these nodes (see below).

## Ilioinguinal (deep pelvic) lymphadenectomy

Patients with obvious disease in the iliac and/or obturator nodes based on either palpation or CT imaging are candidates for a deep pelvic lymph node dissection. In most situations, there is proven concomitant disease in the superficial femoral nodes, but it can occur in isolation or may develop subsequent to a previous superficial femoral dissection. In the absence of clinical disease in the pelvis, a selective approach to the resection of the pelvic nodes in the same operative setting as the superficial femoral lymphadenectomy is commonplace. The indications for the inclusion of a deep dissection of the clinically uninvolved pelvic nodes along with a femoral dissection are based on published predictors for the presence of microscopic disease in the pelvic nodes, and include one of the following: palpable disease in the femoral nodes, multiple involved nodes in the femoral compartment, or a positive Cloquet's node. Cloquet's node is the highest lymph node in the femoral canal and has recently been termed the 'sentinel node' of the pelvis. In other words, if Cloquet's node is negative, the risk of disease in the pelvis is low. While some surgeons use this approach routinely, others use it only when making a decision whether or not to perform a deep dissection when a completion femoral node dissection is being performed for a positive SLN.

From a technical perspective, since most patients undergoing a pelvic lymphadenectomy will have a synchronous superficial groin dissection, the skin incision is extended vertically several centimeters over the lower quadrant of the abdomen. The external and internal oblique muscles and aponeuroses are incised to obtain a retroperitoneal approach to the iliac and obturator nodes. The pertinent pelvic nodes are found from superior to inferior from just above the bifurcation of the external and internal iliac vessels (where the ureter crosses over the common iliac vessels) to the inguinal ligament, pubic ramus, and obturator canal, respectively; and from medial to lateral from the lateral sidewall of the bladder and rectum to the pelvic sidewall, respectively. The posterior extent is to the pelvic floor deep to the obturator vessels. An en-bloc resection of these nodes can generally be accomplished without compromise to the ureter, the iliac vessels, and the obturator nerve and vessels. When the dissection is complete, there is direct communication between the deep and superficial inguinal compartments at the level of the femoral canal.

## Cervical lymphadenectomy

The cervical lymph node basins are at risk for harboring clinical or occult metastasis from primary melanomas of the head and neck region or upper trunk, and are also an occasional site for melanoma metastasis from an unknown primary site.

While radical neck dissections were historically recommended as treatment for patients with clinically evident regional melanoma metastasis, modified (also referred to as functional or comprehensive) neck dissection, including levels II, III, IV and V but sparing the spinal accessory nerve, the sternocleidomastoid muscle, and the internal jugular vein, has supplanted the more radical operation except in circumstances where there is direct tumor extension to one or more of these important anatomic structures (Figs 50.7–50.9).

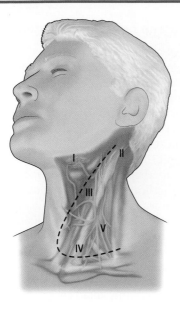

**Figure 50.7** The author's preferred cervical incision, which should be inclusive of any previous biopsy site. The incision extends along the anterior border of the sternocleidomastoid and is carried laterally out over the clavicle.

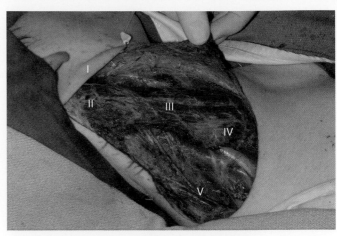

**Figure 50.8** Completed comprehensive cervical dissection.

Since patients with occult disease identified by SLN biopsy generally have a lower tumor burden than those with clinically detected disease, it is conceivable that selective neck dissection (including fewer anatomic regions than traditional comprehensive neck dissection) may achieve equivalent regional control and cure rates with lower morbidity. However, in the absence of more accurate information regarding the anatomic compartments involved in patients undergoing completion lymphadenectomy following excision of an involved SLN, we continue to advocate comprehensive neck dissections as standard surgical therapy for patients with occult regional melanoma metastasis.

## Epitrochlear dissection

### Incision and surgical technique

The incision is started several centimeters above and slightly anterior to the medial epicondyle and traverses in a slight 'hockey stick' fashion across the antecubital fossa for a distance of 4–5 cm in the joint crease. The transverse

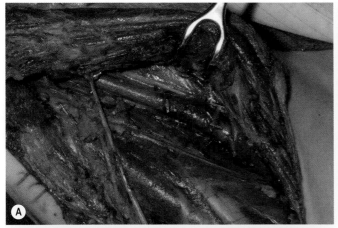

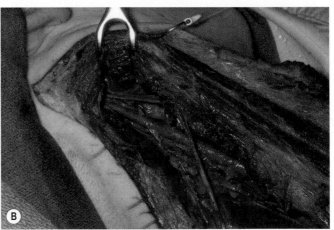

**Figure 50.9** Completed comprehensive cervical dissection demonstrating the preserved important neurovascular structures.

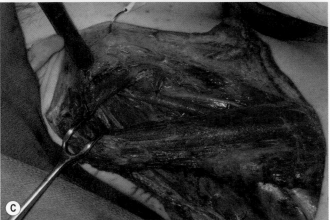

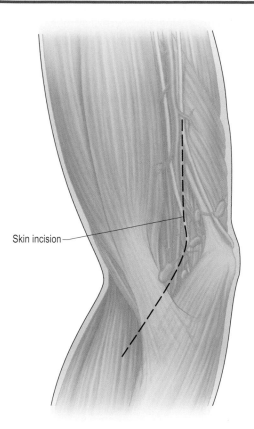

**Figure 50.10** Incision for an epitrochlear dissection, carried medially across the biceps tendon.

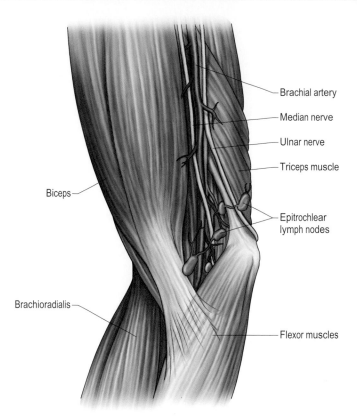

**Figure 50.11** Location of nodal specimen from an epitrochlear lymphadenectomy.

portion of the incision is carried over the tendinous portion of the biceps muscle (Fig. 50.10). Flaps are raised posteriorly to just behind the epicondyle and anterolaterally over the biceps muscle. Node-bearing tissue is then dissected off the biceps and into the fossa. The fibrofatty, node-bearing tissue between the biceps and triceps muscles is dissected, identifying the brachial artery and vein, and median and ulnar nerves. These structures are all preserved. The node-bearing tissue is then swept distally off the vessels and nerves for the remainder of the dissection to the intersection of the biceps muscle and the wrist flexors (Fig. 50.11).

## Popliteal dissection

### Incision and surgical technique

A 'lazy-S' incision from 10 cm above the joint crease on the lateral thigh (overlying biceps femoris) in a longitudinal fashion, moving transversely across the joint and ending up 10 cm distal to the joint crease longitudinally along the medial aspect of the calf (overlying gastrocnemius just medial to semimembranosus) is preferred (Fig. 50.12). Flaps are raised to incorporate a rectangle formed by imaginary extensions of the longitudinal limits of the incision. The goal of these flaps should be to expose the boundaries of the popliteal fossa which includes the biceps femoris and semitendinosus muscles. Between these muscles, the tibial and common peroneal nerves are identified, exposed and preserved. The fibrofatty, node-bearing tissue is swept from around the nerves and dissected distally while exposing the popliteal artery and vein and removing the node-bearing

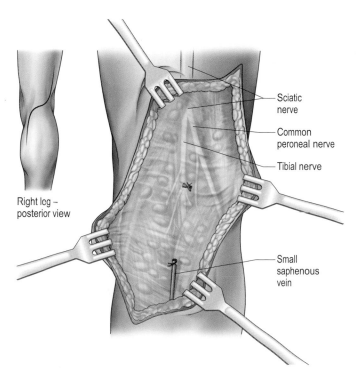

**Figure 50.12** Incision for popliteal lymphadenectomy of the right leg.

tissue from around them (it is important to address the tissue on the far side of the vessels as the only nodes in the specimen may be in this area). The inferior limit of dissection is where the vessels dive behind the gastrocnemius muscle (Fig. 50.13).

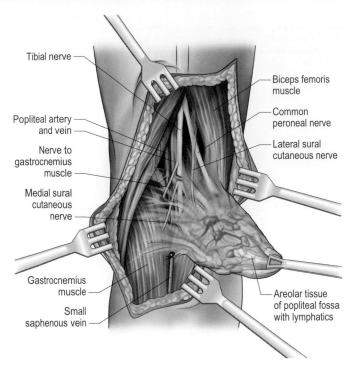

Tibial nerve

Popliteal artery
and vein

Nerve to
gastrocnemius
muscle

Medial sural
cutaneous
nerve

Gastrocnemius
muscle

Small
saphenous vein

Biceps femoris
muscle

Common
peroneal nerve

Lateral sural
cutaneous nerve

Areolar tissue
of popliteal fossa
with lymphatics

**Figure 50.13** Borders of the dissection for a popliteal dissection along with a depiction of the nodal specimen.

## Postoperative care and morbidity

An overnight stay after a node dissection is routine regardless of the basin dissected, primarily for observation for the development of a hematoma which may require re-operation and for pain control. Fortunately, early complications are rare, and pain is well controlled with oral analgesics by the first postoperative morning. Therefore, most patients who undergo axillary, epitrochlear, popliteal or neck dissection will be discharged the day following surgery. The hospital stay for patients undergoing groin dissection is usually longer because of more severe postoperative pain and issues related to early ambulation. While patients who undergo only a superficial femoral dissection are often ready for discharge on the first or second postoperative day, patients receiving a superficial and deep pelvic dissection will require longer stays.

Since closed suction drains are routinely placed at the completion of every dissection, home drain care instructions are required upon discharge. The drains remain in place until the drainage output is less than 30–40 cm$^3$ per day in order to minimize a seroma collection. A lower threshold for drain removal, around 20 cm$^3$, is required for epitrochlear and popliteal basins because of the smaller operative field.

The most common early complications following discharge include seroma, infected seromas, cellulitis, and wound edge necrosis (almost exclusively related to groin dissections). Most are easily handled in the outpatient setting with needle aspirations and oral antibiotics or sharp debridement of devitalized tissue. Recurrent seromas can be managed by a percutaneously placed small closed suction drainage catheter. Occasionally, a very extensive cellulitis may develop requiring hospitalization for intravenous antibiotic administration and open surgical drainage of infected fluid collections.

The most concerning long-term complication is extremity lymphedema. This generally develops over the ensuing months after surgery and is clearly more common and more severe as a result of a groin dissection[80-84]. The risk and severity of lymphedema are probably best predicted by a high body mass index and a postoperative infectious complication[80,81]. Following a groin dissection, while many have suggested the incidence is increased when patients undergo a deep pelvic dissection in addition to a superficial dissection, the data do not strongly support this contention[80,82-84]. Surprisingly, the incidence of arm lymphedema is very low following an axillary dissection[80,81]. Even though the extent of axillary dissection is greater than what is performed in the treatment of axillary disease for breast cancer, severe arm lymphedema, which is not infrequently encountered in patients with breast cancer, is rarely experienced after a dissection for melanoma, unless postoperative nodal basin radiation therapy is applied in the adjuvant setting in the management of very bulky disease. This unexpected finding is probably best explained by the fact that when patients receive axillary surgery for breast cancer, the chest wall lymphatics are also treated either by breast irradiation that is routinely used in the breast conservation setting or by a mastectomy. These preserved chest wall lymphatics may provide important collateral lymphatic drainage routes after a nodal dissection in patients with axillary melanoma metastases.

A cervical lymphadenectomy is very well tolerated. The risk of postoperative wound infection is very low, owing to the fact that the skin flaps are very well vascularized, and the risk of extremity lymphedema is essentially non-existent except in the setting when both an ipsilateral axillary and cervical dissection is performed for patients with disease in both basins. Unique to the cervical basin, however, are complications related to injury to specific structures in the operative field.

When performing a comprehensive left neck dissection, the thoracic duct is often encountered. While actually ligating the thoracic duct can be performed without significant morbidity, missed injuries to the main duct or small side branches can be the source of persistent chylous drainage output. When the volume of this output is large, dehydration and loss of triglycerides may occur. Fortunately, these chylous leaks can most often be managed successfully without surgical intervention, by instructing the patient to adhere to a low-fat diet. This will almost always decrease the output and facilitate closure of the leak. The use of subcutaneous injections of octreotide can also be helpful in reducing the output of chyle.

While the spinal accessory nerve can often be preserved, a comprehensive dissection involves the skeletonization of this nerve throughout its length, resulting in temporary postoperative paresis and weakness of the trapezius muscle. Early postoperative physical therapy can be valuable in managing this problem.

## Concurrent disease in more than one regional lymph node basin

Not infrequently, primary melanomas in ambiguous lymphatic drainage areas (trunk and head and neck regions) may be the source of concomitant regional spread of disease in more than one lymph node basin. The following combinations of nodal involvement occur: bilateral axillae or bilateral groin or bilateral cervical, one axilla and one groin, one axilla and one neck. The performing of more than one nodal basin dissection can be performed safely in one operative setting, sparing the patient a second general anesthetic and shortening the overall recovery time compared to two separate surgical procedures.

## FUTURE OUTLOOK

Lymphatic mapping and SLN biopsy has changed the standard of care for the patient with primary melanoma. The technique has proven to have less morbidity than the old methods of nodal staging, such as elective lymph node dissection. In addition, the ability to perform a more detailed examination of the SLN allows for a more accurate staging. This nodal staging will continue to be improved upon with the introduction of molecular assays for metastatic disease.

In the future, the possibility of 'ultra-staging' exists in that the SLN and peripheral blood will be more carefully examined to come closer to identifying patients who can most likely be surgically cured of their disease. In addition, the long-term results of ongoing clinical trials will help define which patients with a positive SLN will benefit from a completion lymph node dissection and therefore reduce the overall morbidity of surgical therapies. In this way, patients with the appropriate nodal characteristics can be spared the side effects of more radical surgery or the toxicities of adjuvant therapy. Finally, the application of specialized minimally invasive surgical technologies such as laparoscopic and robotic assistance to formal lymph node dissections, particularly in the inguinal region, is currently being evaluated to reduce the surgical morbidity in those patients who benefit from additional surgery. Hopefully, the extent of lymph node dissection as described above can be carried out using these less invasive approaches and comparison studies will demonstrate reduced morbidity without compromising regional disease control.

## REFERENCES

1. Ross MI. Surgical management of stage I and II melanoma patients: approach to the regional lymph node basin. *Semin Surg Oncol.* 1996;12:394–401.
2. Balch CM, Soong SJ, Gershenwald JE, et al. Prognostic factors analysis of 17,600 melanoma patients: validation of the American Joint Committee on Cancer melanoma staging system. *J Clin Oncol.* 2001;19:3622–3634.
3. Sim FH, Taylor WF, Pritchard DJ, et al. Lymphadenectomy in the management of stage I malignant melanoma: a prospective randomized study. *Mayo Clin Proc.* 1986;61:697–705.
4. Veronesi U, Adamus J, Bandiera DC, et al. Inefficacy of immediate node dissection in stage I melanoma of the limbs. *N Engl J Med.* 1977;297:627–630.
5. Cascinelli N, Morabito A, Santinami M, et al. Immediate or delayed dissection of regional nodes in patients with melanoma of the trunk: a randomised trial. *Lancet.* 1998;351(9105):793–796.
6. Balch CM, Soong S, Ross MI, et al. Long-term results of a multi-institutional randomized trial comparing prognostic factors and surgical results for intermediate thickness melanomas (1.0 to 4.0 mm). Intergroup Melanoma Surgical Trial. *Ann Surg Oncol.* 2000;7(2):87–97.
7. Morton D, Wen D, Wong J, et al. Technical details of intraoperative lymphatic mapping for early stage melanoma. *Arch Surg.* 1992;127:392–399.
8. Ross M, Reintgen D, Balch C. Selective lymphadenectomy: emerging role for lymphatic mapping and sentinel node biopsy in the management of early stage melanoma. *Semin Surg Oncol.* 1993;9:219–223.
9. Thompson J, McCarthy W, Bosch C, et al. Sentinel lymph node status as an indicator of the presence of metastatic melanoma in regional lymph nodes. *Melanoma Res.* 1995;5:255–260.
10. Reintgen D, Cruse C, Wells K, et al. The orderly progression of melanoma nodal metastases. *Ann Surg.* 1994;220:759–767.
11. Gershenwald JE, Tseng C-H, Thompson W, et al. Improved sentinel lymph node localization in patients with primary melanoma with the use of radiolabeled colloid. *Surgery.* 1998;124(2):203–210.
12. Gershenwald J, Colome M, Lee J, et al. Patterns of recurrence following a negative sentinel lymph node biopsy in 243 patients with stage I or II melanoma. *J Clin Oncol.* 1998;16:2253–2260.
13. Uren R, Howman-Giles R, Thompson J, et al. Lymphoscintigraphy to identify sentinel lymph nodes in patients with melanoma. *Melanoma Res.* 1994;4:395–399.
14. Berger DH, Feig BW, Podoloff D, et al. Lymphoscintigraphy as a predictor of lymphatic drainage from cutaneous melanoma. *Ann Surg Oncol.* 1997;4:247–251.
15. Albertini J, Cruse C, Rapaport D, et al. Intraoperative radiolymphoscintigraphy improves sentinel lymph node identification for patients with melanoma. *Ann Surg.* 1996;223:217–224.
16. Kapteijn BA, Nieweg OE, Liem I, et al. Localizing the sentinel node in cutaneous melanoma: gamma probe detection versus blue dye. *Ann Surg Oncol.* 1997;4:156–160.
17. Krag D, Meijer S, Weaver D, et al. Minimal-access surgery for staging of malignant melanoma. *Arch Surg.* 1995;130:654–658.
18. Thompson JF, Uren RF, Shaw HM, et al. Location of sentinel lymph nodes in patients with cutaneous melanoma: new insights into lymphatic anatomy. *J Am Coll Surg.* 1999;189(2):195–204.
19. Uren RF, Thompson JF, Howman-Giles R. Sentinel nodes. Interval nodes, lymphatic lakes, and accurate sentinel node identification. *Clin Nucl Med.* 2000;25(3):234–236.
20. Uren RF, Thompson JF, Howman-Giles R, et al. Melanoma metastases in triangular intermuscular space lymph nodes. *Ann Surg Oncol.* 1999;6(8):811.
21. Uren RF, Howman-Giles R, Thompson JF, et al. Interval nodes: the forgotten sentinel nodes in patients with melanoma. *Arch Surg.* 2000;135(10):1168–1172.
22. Sumner 3rd WE, Ross MI, Mansfield PF, et al. Implications of lymphatic drainage to unusual sentinel lymph node sites in patients with primary cutaneous melanoma. *Cancer.* 2002;95(2):354–360.
23. Thompson JF. The Sydney Melanoma Unit experience of sentinel lymphadenectomy for melanoma. *Ann Surg Oncol.* 2001;8(suppl 9):44S–47S.
24. Cascinelli N, Belli F, Santinami M, et al. Sentinel lymph node biopsy in cutaneous melanoma: the WHO Melanoma Program experience. *Ann Surg Oncol.* 2000;7(6):469–474.
25. McMasters KM, Wong SL, Edwards MJ, et al. Factors that predict the presence of sentinel lymph node metastasis in patients with melanoma. *Surgery.* 2001;130(2):151–156.
26. Rousseau Jr DL, Ross MI, Johnson MM, et al. Revised AJCC staging criteria accurately predict sentinel lymph node positivity in clinically node-negative melanoma patients. *Ann Surg Oncol.* 2003;10(5):569–574.
27. Sondak VK, Taylor JM, Sabel MS, et al. Mitotic rate and younger age are predictors of sentinel lymph node positivity: lessons learned from the generation of a probabilistic model. *Ann Surg Oncol.* 2004;11(3):247–258.
28. Thompson JF, Shaw HM. Should tumor mitotic rate and patient age as well as tumor thickness, be used to select melanoma patients for sentinel node biopsy? *Ann Surg Oncol.* 2004;11(3):233–235.
29. Balch CM, Buzaid AC, Soong SJ, et al. Final version of the American Joint Committee on Cancer staging system for cutaneous melanoma. *J Clin Oncol.* 2001;19(16):3635–3638.
30. Gershenwald JE, Thompson W, Mansfield PF, et al. Multi-institutional melanoma lymphatic mapping experience: the prognostic value of sentinel lymph node status in 612 stage I or II melanoma patients. *J Clin Oncol.* 1999;17(3):976–983.
31. Clary BM, Brady MS, Lewis JJ, et al. Sentinel lymph node biopsy in the management of patients with primary cutaneous melanoma: review of a large single-institutional experience with an emphasis on recurrence. *Ann Surg.* 2001;233(2):250–258.
32. Morton DL, Thompson JF, Cochran AJ, et al. Sentinel-node biopsy or nodal observation in melanoma. *N Engl J Med.* 2006;355(13):1307–1317.
33. Cascinelli N, Bombardieri E, Bufalino R, et al. Sentinel and nonsentinel node status in stage IB and II melanoma patients: two-step prognostic indicators of survival. *J Clin Oncol.* 2006;24(27):4464–4471.
34. Lee RJ, Gibbs JF, Proulx GM, et al. Nodal basin recurrence following lymph node dissection for melanoma: implications for adjuvant radiotherapy. *Int J Radiat Oncol Biol Phys.* 2000;46:467–474.
35. O'Brien CJ, Coates AS, Petersen-Schaefer K, et al. Experience with 998 cutaneous melanomas of the head and neck over 30 years. *Am J Surg.* 1991;162:310–314.
36. Calabro A, Singletary SE, Balch CM. Patterns of relapse in 1001 consecutive patients with melanoma nodal metastases. *Arch Surg.* 1989;124:1051–1055.
37. Ballo MT, Strom EA, Zagars GK, et al. Adjuvant irradiation for axillary metastases from malignant melanoma. *Int J Radiat Oncol Biol Phys.* 2002;52:964–972.
38. Slingluff Jr CL, Stidham KR, Ricci WM, et al. Surgical management of regional lymph nodes in patients with melanoma: experience with 4682 patients. *Ann Surg.* 1994;219:120–130.

39. Gershenwald JE, Berman RS, Porter G, et al. Regional nodal basin control is not compromised by previous sentinel lymph node biopsy in patients with melanoma. *Ann Surg Oncol.* 2000;7(3):226–231.

40. Cook MG, Green MA, Anderson B, et al. The development of optimal pathological assessment of sentinel lymph nodes for melanoma. *J Pathol.* 2003;200:314–319.

41. Wang X, Heller R, VanVoorhis N, et al. Detection of submicroscopic lymph node metastases with polymerase chain reaction in patients with malignant melanoma. *Ann Surg.* 1994;220(6):768–774.

42. Shivers SC, Wang X, Li W, et al. Molecular staging of malignant melanoma: correlation with clinical outcome. *JAMA.* 1998;280(16):1410–1415.

43. Reintgen D, Balch C, Kirkwood J, et al. Recent advances in the care of the patient with malignant melanoma. *Ann Surg.* 1997;225:1–14.

44. Kammila US, Ghoussein R, Bhattacharya S, et al. Serial follow-up and the prognostic significance of reverse transcriptase-polymerase chain reaction-staged sentinel lymph nodes from melanoma patients. *J Clin Oncol.* 2004;22:3989–3996.

45. Scoggins CR, Ross MI, Reintgen DS, et al. Prospective multi-institutional study of reverse transcription polymerase chain reaction for molecular staging of melanoma. *J Clin Oncol.* 2006;24(18):2849–2857.

46. Clark SH, Prieto VG. Processing of sentinel lymph nodes for detection of metastatic melanoma: proposal for an alternative method to serial sectioning. *Lab Invest.* 2001;14:66A.

47. Stojadinovic A, Allen PJ, Clary BM, et al. Value of frozen-section analysis of sentinel lymph nodes for primary cutaneous malignant melanoma. *Ann Surg.* 2002;235(1):92–98.

48. Soo V, Shen P, Pichardo R, et al. Intraoperative evaluation of sentinel lymph nodes for metastatic melanoma by imprint cytology. *Ann Surg Oncol.* 2007;5:1612–1617.

49. Agnese DM, Abdessalam SF, Burak WE, et al. Cost-effectiveness of sentinel lymph node biopsy in thin melanomas. *Surgery.* 2003;134:542–548.

50. Thompson JF, Shaw HM. Sentinel node metastasis from thin melanomas with vertical growth phase. *Ann Surg Oncol.* 2000;7(4):251–252.

51. Kesmodel SB, Karakousis GC, Botbyl JD, et al. Mitotic rate as a predictor of sentinel lymph node positivity in patients with thin melanomas. *Ann Surg Oncol.* 2005;12(6):1–10.

52. Balch CM, Gershenwald JE, Soong SJ, et al. Final version of the AJCC melanoma staging and classification. *J Clin Oncol.* 2009;27(36):6199–6206.

53. Gershenwald JE, Mansfield PF, Lee JE, et al. Role for lymphatic mapping and sentinel lymph node biopsy in patients with thick (> or = 4 mm) primary melanoma. *Ann Surg Oncol.* 2000;7(2):160–165.

54. Jacobs IA, Chang CK, Salti GI. Role of sentinel lymph node biopsy in patients with thick (>4 mm) primary melanoma. *Am Surg.* 2004;70(1):59–62.

55. Lohmann CM, Coit DG, Brady MS, et al. Sentinel lymph node biopsy in patients with diagnostically controversial spitzoid melanocytic tumors. *Am J Surg Pathol.* 2002;26(1):47–55.

56. Gannon CJ, Rousseau DL, Ross MI, et al. Accuracy of lymphatic mapping and sentinel node biopsy after previous wide local excision in patients with primary melanoma. *Cancer.* 2006;107(11):2647–2652.

57. Reeves ME, Delgado R, Busam KJ, et al. Prediction of nonsentinel lymph node status in melanoma. *Ann Surg Oncol.* 2003;10:27–31.

58. Shaw HM, Thompson JF. Frequency of nonsentinel lymph node metastasis in melanoma. *Ann Surg Oncol.* 2002;9:934.

59. Vylsteke RJCLM, Borgstein PJ, van Leeuwen PAM, et al. Sentinel lymph node tumor load: an independent predictor of additional lymph node involvement and survival in melanoma. *Ann Surg Oncol.* 2005;12:1–9.

60. Govindarajan A, Ghazarian DM, McCready DR, et al. Histological features of melanoma sentinel lymph node metastases associated with status of the completion lymphadenectomy and rate of subsequent relapse. *Ann Surg Oncol.* 2007;14:906–912.

61. Gershenwald JE, Andtbacka RH, Prieto VG, et al. Microscopic tumor burden in sentinel lymph nodes predicts synchronous nonsentinel lymph node involvement in patients with melanoma. *J Clin Oncol.* 2008;26(26):4296–4303.

62. Wrightson WR, Wong SL, Edwards MJ, et al. Complications associated with sentinel lymph node biopsy for melanoma. *Ann Surg Oncol.* 2003;10:676–680.

63. Guggenheim MM, Hug U, Jung FJ, et al. Morbidity and recurrence after completion lymph node dissection following sentinel lymph node biopsy in cutaneous malignant melanoma. *Ann Surg.* 2008;247:687–693.

64. Kretschmer L, Thoms KM, Peeters S, et al. Postoperative morbidity of lymph node excision for cutaneous melanoma-sentinel lymphonodectomy versus complete regional lymph node dissection. *Melanoma Res.* 2008;18:16–21.

65. Daley MD, Norman PH, Leak JA, et al. Adverse events associated with the intraoperative injection of isosulfan blue. *J Clin Anesth.* 2004;16:332–341.

66. Thomas JM, Clark MA. Sentinel lymph node biopsy: not yet standard of care for melanoma. *BMJ.* 2004;329:170.

67. Thomas JM, Clark MA. Are there guidance issues relating to sentinel node biopsy for melanoma in the UK? *Br J Plast Surg.* 2004;57:689–690.

68. Estourgie SH, Nieweg OE, Kroon BB. The sentinel node procedure in patients with melanoma. *Eur J Surg Oncol.* 2004;30:713–714.

69. Thomas JM, Clark MA. Selective lymphadenectomy in sentinel node-positive patients may increase the risk of local/in-transit recurrence in malignant melanoma. *Eur J Surg Oncol.* 2004;30:686–691.

70. Estourgie SH, Nieweg OE, Kroon BB. High incidence of in-transit metastases after sentinel node biopsy in patients with melanoma. *Br J Surg.* 2004;91:1370–1371.

71. Pawlik TM, Ross MI, Johnson MM, et al. Predictors and natural history of in-transit melanoma after sentinel lymphadenectomy. *Ann Surg Oncol.* 2005;12:587–596.

72. van Poll D, Thompson JF, Colman MH, et al. A sentinel node biopsy does not increase the incidence of in-transit metastasis in patients with primary cutaneous melanoma. *Ann Surg Oncol.* 2005;12:597–608.

73. Kang JC, Wanek LA, Essner R, et al. Sentinel lymphadenectomy does not increase the incidence of in-transit metastases in primary melanoma. *J Clin Oncol.* 2005;23:4764–4770.

74. Pawlik TM, Ross MI, Thompson JF, et al. The risk of in-transit melanoma metastasis depends on tumor biology and not the surgical approach to regional lymph nodes. *J Clin Oncol.* 2005;23:4588–4590.

75. Balch CM, Morton DL, Gershenwald JE, et al. Sentinel node biopsy and standard on care for melanoma. *J Am Acad Dermatol.* 2009;60(5):872–875.

76. Ballo MT, Strom EA, Zagars GK, et al. Adjuvant irradiation for axillary metastases from malignant melanoma. *Int J Radiat Oncol Biol Phys.* 2002;52:964–972.

77. Ballo MT, Zagars GK, Gershenwald JE, et al. A critical assessment of adjuvant radiotherapy for inguinal lymph node metastases from melanoma. *Ann Surg Oncol.* 2004;11:1079–1084.

78. Aloia TA, Gershenwald JE, Andtbacka RH, et al. Utility of computed tomography and magnetic resonance imaging staging before completion lymphadenectomy in patients with sentinel lymph node-positive melanoma. *J Clin Oncol.* 2006;24:2858–2865.

79. Miranda EP, Gertner M, Wall J, et al. Routine imaging of asymptomatic melanoma patients with metastasis to sentinel lymph nodes rarely identifies systemic disease. *Arch Surg.* 2004;139:831–836 discussion 836–837.

80. Karakousis CP. Surgical procedures and lymphedema of the upper and lower extremity. *J Surg Oncol.* 2006;93:87–91.

81. Serpell JW, Carne PW, Bailey M. Radical lymph node dissection for melanoma. *ANZ J Surg.* 2003;73:294–299.

82. Beitsch P, Balch C. Operative morbidity and risk factor assessment in melanoma patients undergoing inguinal lymph node dissection. *Am J Surg.* 1992;164:462–465 discussion 465–466.

83. Hughes TM, Thomas JM. Combined inguinal and pelvic lymph node dissection for stage III melanoma. *Br J Surg.* 1999;86:1493–1498.

84. Karakousis CP, Heiser MA, Moore RH. Lymphedema after groin dissection. *Am J Surg.* 1983;145:205–208.

# Reconstructive Surgery for Skin Cancer

*Justin M. Sacks, Kriti Mohan, and Donald Baumann*

## Key Points

- Strategies employed in skin cancer reconstruction balance the requirements of the resulting wound defect – location, dimension, functional properties and aesthetics – to achieve the goal of a well-healed durable reconstruction with minimal donor morbidity.

- Options for reconstruction of skin cancer defects range from primary closure, to skin grafts, local flaps, regional flaps and microvascular free flaps, depending on the complexity of the defect and the availability of surrounding soft tissue.

- Complex reconstructive surgeries are favored over local flaps or skin grafts when local tissue is unavailable, the wound bed is radiated, or the extirpative defect requires well-vascularized tissue coverage over critical neurovascular or bony structures.

- Timing of reconstruction is dictated by the tumor histology along with surgical pathological margins. Reconstruction can be deferred and performed in a delayed fashion if margins are not conclusively established by frozen section or if specific immunological stains are required.

- The deleterious effects of radiation therapy on wound healing must be considered in any reconstruction of a skin cancer defect.

- Multidisciplinary coordination is paramount to the success of both functional and aesthetic outcomes in the treatment of the skin cancer patient.

## INTRODUCTION

The goal of reconstructive surgery for skin cancer is to restore form and function following extirpation of the neoplasm. The partition of oncologic ablation and plastic surgery reconstruction facilitates resection of a cancer lesion independent of the steps required for restoration. Reconstructive strategies balance the characteristics of the resulting wound defect, including both the dimensions of the defect and its inherent functional properties.

Careful analysis of the surgical defect reveals the types of soft and bony tissue that are required to appropriately reconstruct the tissue defect. This analysis allows the reconstructive surgeon to formulate a logical plan that emphasizes conservative measures, such as primary closure and the use of local flaps and skin grafts. As the complexity of the defects increase, including a paucity of local structures or a wound bed with previous radiation or surgery, more complex soft tissue reconstructions such as pedicle flaps or microvascular free tissue transfer become necessary. In general, successful reconstructive surgery restores form and function with minimal donor site deformity, which enhances the patient's quality of life.

## PLANNING RECONSTRUCTIVE SURGERY FOR SKIN CANCER

The surgical margins for skin malignancies are chosen based on the risk of locoregional recurrence and the etiology of the malignancy.[1] The role of the ablative surgeon is to determine an appropriate diagnosis and attain negative surgical margins. Once negative margins have been determined by frozen section analysis or, depending on the tumor type, by final pathological analysis, the reconstructive surgeon repairs the wound defect. It is therefore critical that both the extirpation and reconstruction are performed in a timely manner that does not interfere with the ultimate goal of obtaining negative pathological margins. A soft tissue flap placed prior to achieving final pathological margins can result in a negative outcome in the management of the skin malignancy, possibly resulting in the removal of the reconstruction. In cases of cutaneous melanoma where the pathological margins are not necessarily determined at the time of surgery, a delayed reconstruction is favored.[2] In contrast, for basal cell or squamous cell carcinoma, margins of 0.5 or 1.0 cm, respectively, are accepted pathological measures of negative margins.[3]

In addition, skin grafts, local flaps, or free flaps used for the reconstruction of skin malignancies can potentially interfere with lymphatic mapping.[1] Thus, it is advantageous to perform reconstruction following lymphatic mapping versus before.

For lesions that are too large to be excised completely without immediate reconstruction, it is important to coordinate the reconstructive process with the surgical oncologist, dermatologic surgeon, or general surgeon and determine which donor sites are available to complete the reconstruction. Temporizing a partially excised wound with a biological dressing is a consideration prior to final reconstruction. It is critical to coordinate both the extirpation and the wound reconstruction taking into consideration the oncologic status of the patient.

Immediate and reliable soft tissue coverage is the primary goal of reconstruction following the excision of a skin malignancy. When reconstruction is performed immediately following extirpation, tissue planes are readily available and the soft tissue wound bed is preserved with little to no fibrotic tissue. When the reconstruction is delayed, scar tissue, fibrosis, and wound contracture can inhibit optimal reconstruction. If immediate reconstruction is not possible, the wound bed must be prepared for the eventual reconstruction with appropriate dressings, and debridement may be necessary either prior to or at the time of reconstruction.

The timing of the reconstruction is dictated by the status of the tumor and the surgical pathological margins. For example, basal cell carcinoma can potentially be reconstructed immediately if frozen tissue sections show negative margins. However, for more aggressive types of basal cell carcinoma such as morpheaform, the reconstruction must be delayed until the tumor margins are clearly determined by thorough pathological review or with Mohs surgery.[3] In addition, reconstruction must be delayed in cases of melanoma or other aggressive skin malignancies, such as Merkel cell carcinoma, when the surgeon performing the ablative resection is concerned about the margins and when the margins are not established immediately because of the need for specific immunological stains of the tissue samples. Such is often the case with advanced primary desmoplastic melanoma or large lentigo maligna melanoma of the head and neck region.[4]

However, if certain mitigating factors are evident, such as advanced age, multiple comorbidities, or the need for locoregional control with adjuvant radiotherapy, then a one-stage procedure may be warranted. If a one-stage procedure cannot be accomplished, the wound is temporized, and the final status of the pathological margins is determined. Delayed wound reconstruction, although not optimal, is at times unavoidable and required. In the case of delayed reconstruction, there is typically a greater soft tissue deficit requiring reconstruction. However, with proper wound care and planning, delayed reconstruction of soft tissue defects secondary to skin malignancy resection can be performed appropriately and with optimal success.

Surgical wounds are assessed by measuring their physical dimensions and on the basis of their location. In many instances, the wound is adjacent to critical structures, such as ocular, oral, and nasal structures. Aesthetic as well as functional parameters must also be considered. In addition, previous incisions must be taken into consideration when assessing the wound, as they may interfere with the planned reconstruction. A clinical and radiographic examination of the structural components involved is required to plan a successful reconstruction. Loss of skin, subcutaneous tissue, fascia, muscle, nerves, bone, and, often, mucosa must also be accounted for. For example, a large skin malignancy of the lip can involve structures outside and inside the oral cavity (Fig. 51.1), which would require reconstruction of all the components of the cheek, including both extraoral and intraoral components.

## SELECTION OF RECONSTRUCTIVE TECHNIQUES

The selection of appropriate reconstructive techniques is critical. The physiological status of the patient must be considered and balanced with the overall reconstructive plan. A patient unable to tolerate lengthy surgery owing to multiple comorbidities must be considered for a more conservative type of reconstruction rather than a lengthier procedure involving protracted general anesthesia or the potential for multiple surgeries.

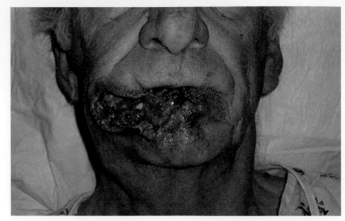

**Figure 51.1** A 68-year old man with an ulcerative squamous cell carcinoma of the lip, with intraoral extension.

The deleterious effects of radiation therapy on wound healing must be considered in any reconstruction of an acquired cancer defect. Prior radiation therapy can preclude the use of local tissue transfer for the reconstruction of a wound bed owing to its negative effects on the inherent vascularity of the local tissue.[5] Free tissue transfer of composite soft tissue constructs can potentiate wound healing in a previously irradiated bed by recruiting normal, robust vascularized tissue. In addition, if a reconstructed wound requires adjuvant radiation therapy, the vascularized tissue will help with the durability of wound healing.

Reconstruction of any skin defect is performed by primary closure, skin graft, local flaps, or microvascular free tissue transfer. The core principle of this reconstructive algorithm is to progress from simple to more complex reconstructions on the basis of the specific wound requirements. The primary goal of any surgeon should be to close a wound primarily with local tissue under physiologic tension. When primary closure is not feasible, skin grafts or local flaps of tissue can be used.

Local flaps allow the defect to be reconstructed with like tissue. These flaps typically are based on a random subdermal plexus for their blood supply. Local flaps can also be based on named blood vessels and be raised as fasciocutaneous, myocutaneous, or adipofascial flaps. These are specifically described as axial pattern flaps. Free microvascular tissue transfers can also be used, requiring the use of tissue constructs based on named vessels that are raised separately in a different part of the body and transplanted to the recipient vessels at the site of the defect. Complex reconstructive surgeries are favored over local flaps when the local tissue is unavailable, the wound bed is fibrotic or irradiated, or the patient's defect requires well-vascularized tissue over critical neurovascular or bony structures.

### Skin grafts

Skin grafts are components of tissue that contain epidermis and variable amounts of dermis. A partial-thickness skin graft uses a component of the dermis, while a full-thickness graft uses the entire portion of the dermis. Over time, a full-thickness graft contracts less than a split-thickness skin graft. In regions such as the face, a full-thickness graft is preferable because it contracts less over time, and wound bed contraction near ocular and nasal structures is not desirable.

Skin grafts become incorporated into the wound bed by inosculation or the diffusion of nutrients and oxygen across the wound–graft interface. This is followed by neovascularization 3–5 days after surgery, when the graft takes on its own blood supply. Skin grafts require a vascularized bed for ingrowth, such as granulation tissue, fascia, muscle, or periosteum. Skin grafts are excellent options for low-morbidity reconstruction; however, aesthetic outcomes are inferior to those of local or free tissue flap options in many instances.

## Local flaps

Local flaps allow surgeons to reconstruct soft tissue defects with similar tissue from an adjacent location. These random flaps represent skin and subcutaneous tissue based on a subdermal plexus vascular supply. By definition, random flaps do not have a distinct named blood supply, in contrast to axial flaps, which are based on named blood vessels (e.g. pectoralis flap or anterolateral thigh flap; Fig. 51.2). Local random flaps can be raised using various methods, including rotation-advancement, transposition, z-plasties and rhomboid flaps (Fig. 51.3). An axial pattern flap, with its named blood supply, is elevated with an arterial and venous pedicle. These flaps can be fasciocutaneous, myocutaneous, or osteocutaneous, which allows the surgeon to reconstruct a skin cancer defect using like tissue with its own intrinsic blood supply and possibly using other tissue components to obliterate dead space, contour the wound, and cover critical neurovascular structures.

## Microvascular free tissue transfer

Microvascular free tissue transfer allows tissue constructs with a named blood supply to be removed from distant regions of the body and placed into a wound defect. A vascular anastomosis is performed with the assistance of magnification, which is typically provided by a surgical microscope or loupes. The decision to use one flap over another is based on the wound defect requirements for skin, adipose tissue, fascia, muscle, and sometimes bone. The primary advantage of this type of reconstruction is to recruit tissue of like quality from a remote part of the body, allowing for reconstruction with optimal aesthetic form and function. Drawbacks of these types of reconstructions are the surgical time required, technical expertise required, and distant donor site morbidity.

## Tissue expansion

Tissue expansion of local tissue may be employed selectively to facilitate a formal delayed reconstruction. This process uses a prosthetic device to expand local and regional tissue so that it can be advanced into the wound defect in a delayed fashion. The prosthetic device can be inserted at the time of extirpation or at a second procedure. Office visits are required to inflate the expander with serial injections that are given through a remote or integrated port. Once the tissue is sufficiently expanded, it can then be advanced into the defect. This type of reconstruction takes time, and both the patient and surgeon must be patient. This method is not feasible for immediate reconstruction and has limited value in areas of previous irradiation.

## RECONSTRUCTION OF THE HEAD AND NECK

Reconstruction of the head and neck region is based on functional as well as aesthetic demands. Skin malignancies often involve ocular, nasal, and oral structures, and the appropriate planning and execution of reconstructive procedures must be performed. The ultimate goal is to preserve function, resurface vital structures such as bone, mucosa, sinuses, nerves, and vessels, and maximize the aesthetic outcomes. This can be accomplished with skin grafts, local tissue, or free microvascular transfer. Each region of the head and neck consists of unique anatomical structures and functional dynamics, which require special consideration for reconstruction.

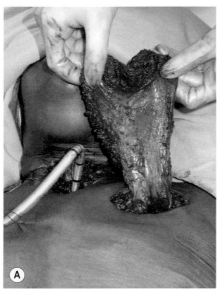 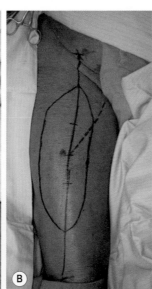 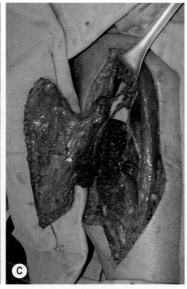

**Figure 51.2** Axial pattern flaps. **(A)** Pectoralis flap based on the pectoral vessels of the thoracoacromial vascular axis. **(B,C)** Anterolateral thigh flap (ALT) skin island design and flap elevation on the descending branch of the lateral circumflex femoral vessels.

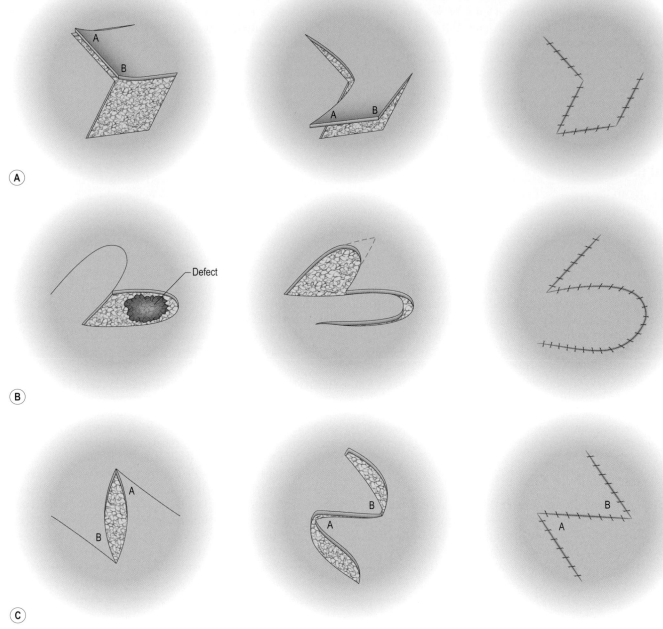

**Figure 51.3** Random flaps. **A)** Rhomboid flap. **B)** Transposition flap. **C)** Z-plasty.

## Scalp reconstruction

The scalp is a well-vascularized region composed of five layers: skin, subcutaneous tissue, galea aponeurosis, loose areolar, and pericranium. The galea aponeurosis is a dense fibrous connective tissue layer that is interspersed between the frontalis, occipitalis, and temporalis muscles. It fuses with the temporoparietal fascia at the temporal crest. To appropriately reconstruct scalp defects, the defect must be accurately assessed prior to reconstruction. This involves determining whether there is a full-thickness or partial-thickness defect. Partial-thickness defects can potentially be allowed to granulate and heal secondarily. These wounds can also be covered with split-thickness skin grafts if an appropriate vascularized wound bed, such as pericranium, is obtained or in this example without the availability of

pericranium through the use of Integra™, a dermal regeneration template (Fig. 51.4).

Primary closure of the scalp can be considered for scalp defects less than 2 cm in width with wide undermining below the galea. Further lengthening of these flaps can be accomplished by scoring the galea to increase its length, which results in several centimeters of scalp advancement. Scoring of the galea must be meticulously performed so as not to transect the subcutaneous blood vessels and compromise the flap. Local rotation flaps are optimal for small defects (<3 cm; Fig. 51.5). Defects greater than 3 cm but less than 5 cm can generally be reconstructed with rotation flaps with skin grafting of the donor site on the pericranium.

As the defects become larger, multiple local flaps can be designed based on named blood vessels in the scalp, with further skin grafting of the donor sites. Occasionally,

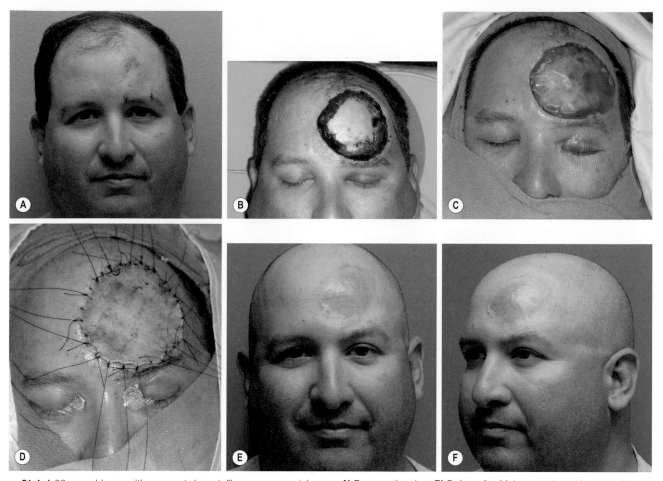

**Figure 51.4** A 36-year old man with recurrent dermatofibrosarcoma protuberans. **A)** Preoperative view. **B)** Defect after Mohs resection with exposed frontal bone devoid of periosteum. **C,D)** Reconstruction with Integra™ dermal regeneration template and split-thickness skin graft. **E,F)** Twelve-month follow-up.

skin cancers of the scalp or their oncological resection can involve bone and necessitate the removal of the outer-table or full-thickness calvaria. These reconstructions can require the use of autologous bone grafts such as split calvarial grafts or the use of prosthetic materials such as titanium mesh or methyl methacrylate in addition to microvascular free tissue transfer (Fig. 51.6). Scalp defects secondary to malignancy extirpation in the field of radiation injury can often preclude the use of local flaps and tissue expansion. In these specific instances, the use of free tissue transfer is required. Typically, these defects are reconstructed with a free muscle flap and skin graft placed over the muscle.

## Facial reconstruction

Facial reconstruction can be divided into specific regions, each with its own intrinsic anatomy and function. The face can be divided into the forehead, periorbital region, cheek, nose, lips, and neck. Each region must be considered independently, as well as collectively when defects cross facial zone boundaries. Facial defects secondary to skin cancer excision tend to be several centimeters wide. However, they can be located in aesthetically and functionally challenging regions. For instance, lesions in the lower eyelid need to be reconstructed appropriately so as not to cause ectropion of the lower eyelid (Fig. 51.7). In addition, nasal defects can be full thickness, encompassing skin, cartilage, and the internal nasal lining.

Small superficial defects of the facial skin are treated primarily with skin grafts and local flaps. Most facial defects are small and can be closed primarily after an elliptical incision. It is critical to keep the scar short and in the direction of the facial skin-lines. If the wound cannot be closed primarily, then a local tissue flap is preferable. Local flaps based on a random blood supply, such as transposition or rhomboid flaps, can be performed. Full-thickness skin grafts can be used if they match the thickness and color of the skin at the wound site. The best donor site for facial skin grafts is the region just above the clavicle, as it matches both the color and texture of the facial skin. Defects in the face larger than 4–5 cm often require large fasciocutaneous rotation flaps from the cervical and deltopectoral region (Fig. 51.8). Rarely, skin malignancies of the face require free tissue transfer reconstruction. Often these clinical situations arise when it is known the patient will require adjuvant radiation therapy, or if critical neurovascular structures are exposed (Fig. 51.9).

## Forehead reconstruction

The forehead region consists of layers similar to the scalp, which include skin, subcutaneous skin, frontalis muscle, loose areolar tissue, and pericranium.[1] The superficial temporal, supraorbital, and supratrochlear vessels provide the blood supply to the scalp. Reconstruction of this region is

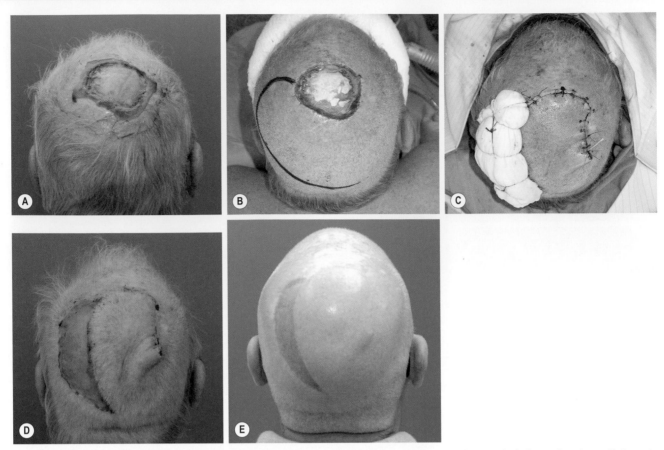

**Figure 51.5** A 68-year old man with squamous cell carcinoma of the scalp. **A)** Full-thickness resection of soft tissue, including pericranium, with the outer table preserved. **B)** The design of the rotation advancement flap was based on the right superficial temporal and occipital vessels. **C)** Flap transfer and inset. The split-thickness skin graft covers the flap donor site. **D)** Three-week follow-up. **E)** Twelve-month follow-up after completion of radiation therapy.

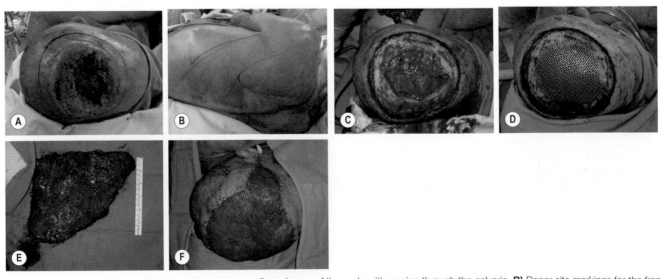

**Figure 51.6 A)** A 68-year old man with recurrent squamous cell carcinoma of the scalp with erosion through the calvaria. **B)** Donor site markings for the free latissimus dorsi muscle flap. **C)** Defect after radical debridement of bone and soft tissue. **D)** The bone defect was reconstructed with titanium mesh. **E)** The latissimus flap was transferred into the scalp defect and anastomosed to the left superficial temporal vessels. **F)** A skin graft was then placed over the muscle for skin coverage.

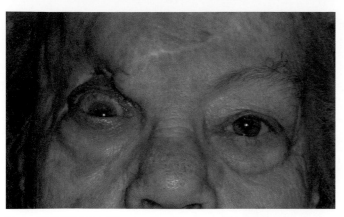

**Figure 51.7** Ectropion after resection of an upper lid tumor.

limited owing to the inelasticity of the underlying soft tissues. Defects in the forehead greater than 2 cm typically require local flaps to close. For patients with skin laxity, wide undermining leads to primary closure. Aesthetic considerations in this region are the hairline and brow line. These anatomical boundaries must be taken into consideration when performing local flap advancement. Placing full-thickness skin grafts onto vascularized muscle or pericranium is often sufficient to cover the exposed underlying structures (Fig. 51.10).

Local flaps are appropriate for forehead defects greater than 2 cm. Local flaps must be designed within natural skin tension lines, with scars being placed in natural wrinkles or in the hairline. Free flaps are appropriate when the defect is greater than one-third the size of the forehead. In these cases, thin, pliable fasciocutaneous flaps such as the radial forearm flap or the anterolateral thigh flap are

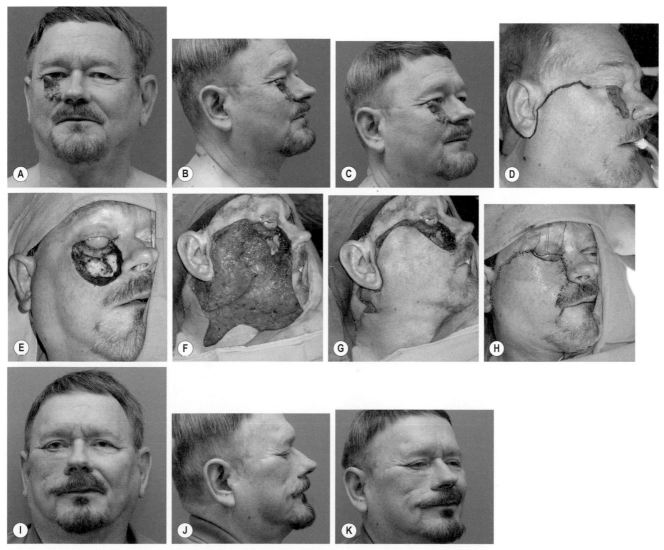

**Figure 51.8** A 58-year old man with an ulcerating basal cell carcinoma of the left lower medial eyelid. **A–C)** Preoperative view. **D)** Preoperative markings for the cervicofacial rotation advancement flap. **E)** Lower eyelid defect. **F–H)** Flap elevation, advancement, and inset. **I–K)** Twelve-month follow-up after the lower eyelid defect was reconstructed with cervicofacial rotation advancement (Mustarde flap).

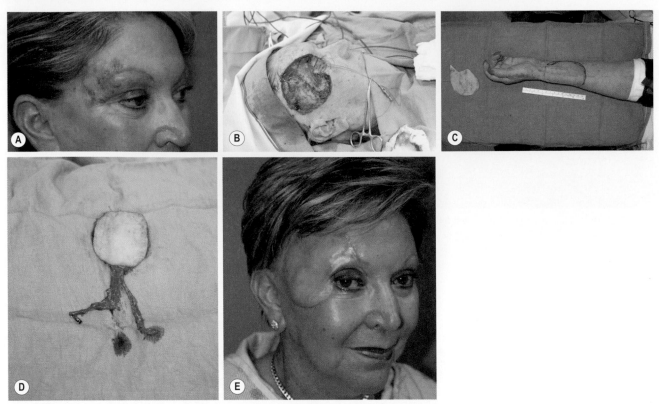

**Figure 51.9 A)** A 68-year old woman with melanoma of the right superolateral brow. **B)** Radical resection of periorbital soft tissue, including the outer lamellae upper and lower eyelid skin. The advanced stage of the disease increased the possibility of adjuvant radiation therapy. Thus, the plan for reconstruction focused on a free tissue transfer owing to the lack of available surrounding soft tissue for local flap reconstruction. In an elderly patient requiring adjuvant radiation therapy, the brow should be reconstructed with a free microvascular radial forearm flap. **C,D)** Design and harvest of a left radial forearm free flap based on the radial artery and the cephalic vein. **E)** Six-month follow-up displaying the balanced tone and position of the upper and lower eyelids and stable soft tissue resurfacing of the lateral periorbital region.

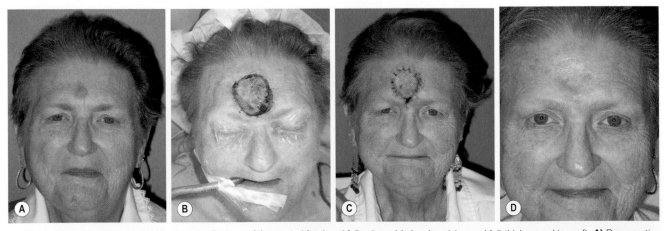

**Figure 51.10** A 78-year old woman with a basal cell tumor of the central forehead following wide local excision and full-thickness skin graft. **A)** Preoperative view. **B)** Defect after Mohs resection. **C)** Interval healing 2 weeks postoperatively. **D)** Twelve-month follow-up.

appropriate. The relatively long vascular pedicle of the radial forearm allows versatility in insetting the flap, even in central forehead defects (Fig. 51.11). Recipient blood vessels from this region in order of preference are the superficial temporal, facial, and great vessels in the neck. If the facial and neck vessels are used, vein grafting may be required.

## Nasal reconstruction

The nose consists of nine aesthetic subunits: the dorsum, sidewalls (two), tip, columella, soft triangles (two), and alae (two).[6] The adage to replace 'like with like' is critical in this anatomical region. If less than 50% of an aesthetic subunit is removed, then the defect can be reconstructed with a local

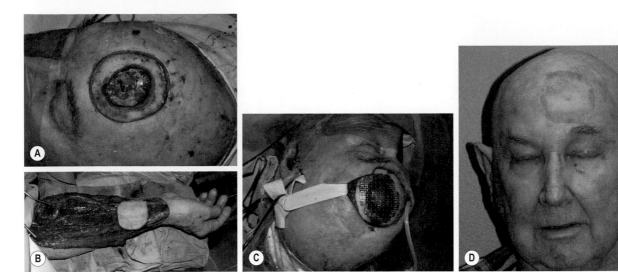

**Figure 51.11** A 74-year old man with recurrent squamous cell carcinoma of the central forehead with frontal bone invasion. The patient was previously treated with resection and skin graft reconstruction and subsequently required radiation therapy. **A)** Full-thickness defect exposing the dura covering the frontal lobe. **B)** The radial forearm flap was selected as it provides thin fasciocutaneous tissue to match that of the forehead. The microanastomosis was performed to the superficial temporal artery and vein. **C)** Central frontal cranioplasty with titanium mesh. **D)** Four-month follow-up.

flap or full-thickness skin graft, with the remainder of the subunit retained. If the defect encompasses more then 50% of the subunit, it is beneficial to reconstruct the entire subunit. Full-thickness defects of the nose consist of external skin coverage, cartilage, and the nasal lining. All three layers must be considered when reconstructing these defects.

The nasal lining can be reconstructed with local flaps obtained from the nasal mucosa. Rib or ear cartilage grafts can be used to reconstruct cartilaginous structures. The nasolabial flap, which is based on the angular artery inferiorly or the dorsal branch of the ophthalmic artery superiorly, can be used to reconstruct defects of the lower portion of the nasal elements.[7] Local flaps such as bilobed flaps (Fig. 51.12) can be used to reconstruct defects of the nasal sidewall and dorsum. The paramedian forehead flap, based on the supratrochlear artery, can be used to resurface the entire exterior nasal skin. Cartilage grafts along with either skin grafts or nasal mucosal flaps are used to reconstruct full-thickness defects of the nasal architecture (Fig. 51.13). The nasal mucosal flaps are pedicle flaps that must be inset and then divided approximately 3 to 4 weeks after inset.

## Lip reconstruction

The lips are distinct anatomical structures that are important for the articulation of speech, eating, and intimacy. The skin of the lip is made up of dry and wet vermilion. The vermiliocutaneous junction, the border between the red of the lip and normal skin, is a distinct anatomical line that must be meticulously reconstructed.[8] Asymmetries at the vermilion junction less than 1 mm will lead to visual irregularities in a reconstructed lip.

Defects that are one-third or less the width of the lower or upper lip are repaired by wedge resection and primary closure. When the defect becomes larger than one-third the width of the lip, a local flap must be considered. These local flaps are called lip switch flaps. These pedicled flaps transferred from the lower or upper lip are based on the labial branch of the facial artery. Lip switch flaps such as

the Abbe or Estlander flap are used for defects that are between one-third and two-thirds of the lip width. Defects larger than two-thirds of the lip width require bilateral rotation or advancement flaps such as the Karapandzic flap. With the Karapandzic flap, the skin and orbicularis oris are advanced medially from the cheek bilaterally into the defect. These flaps recruit larger segments of tissue from nearby adjacent cheek tissue. The Karapandzic flap is a neurovascular flap that keeps the elements of the facial nerve branches to the orbicularis oris intact. A drawback of using these flaps is that the oral aperture can be reduced, resulting in microstomia. Total lip defects can be reconstructed with a free radial forearm flap with a palmaris longus tendon graft to support the lower lip.

## Ear reconstruction

The ear is composed of skin closely applied to an underlying cartilaginous framework. Intrinsic and extrinsic muscles related to its anatomical structure are not significant obstacles when deciding upon the reconstruction of the ear following skin cancer surgery. The surface anatomy of the ear consists of the helix, antihelix, concha, tragus, and lobule. These structures must be preserved or reconstructed to keep the inherent anatomy and contour of the ear intact.

Small defects of the helical rim can be reconstructed with direct approximation after excision of a triangular wedge. If direct approximation cannot be obtained, the remaining helix with chondrocutaneous flaps can be rearranged.[9] In this instance, the remaining helical rim is dissected off the scapha and advanced. A post-auricular or tubed flap can be raised to cover large defects of the helical rim (Fig. 51.14). This is a staged procedure with division and inset performed 2–3 weeks following the initial transposition of the flap. If there is a cartilage defect of the helical rim, a graft can be taken from the contralateral ear. Larger defects of the helix with missing cartilaginous components can be reconstructed using cartilage grafts obtained from the ribs

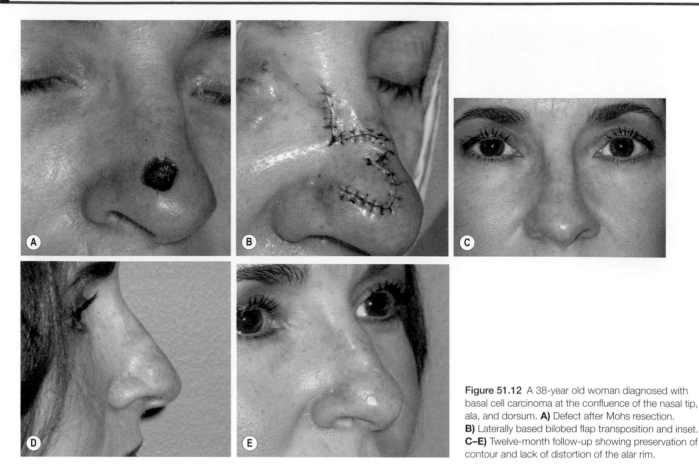

**Figure 51.12** A 38-year old woman diagnosed with basal cell carcinoma at the confluence of the nasal tip, ala, and dorsum. **A)** Defect after Mohs resection. **B)** Laterally based bilobed flap transposition and inset. **C–E)** Twelve-month follow-up showing preservation of contour and lack of distortion of the alar rim.

and covered with a pedicled temporoparietal fascia flap based on the superficial temporal artery. Rib cartilage can be sculpted to conform to the missing helical rim.

Alloplastic frameworks such as high-density polyethylene (Medpor) have been used to reconstruct auricular defects, obviating the need for donor cartilage.[10] The implants must be covered with vascularized tissue such as the temporoparietal fascial flap. Ultimately, if a total auriculectomy is performed secondary to an invasive cutaneous malignancy, the goal is to provide vascularized soft tissue coverage if the bone or skin grafting over vascularized tissue is exposed (Fig. 51.15). Alternatively, ear prosthetics can be fashioned for total auriculectomy defects, with excellent aesthetic results.

## Neck reconstruction

The neck is often a site for primary cutaneous malignancies. In addition, it is commonly the site of sentinel or completion lymph node dissections for cutaneous malignancies of the scalp and face. Often, a deltopectoral, cervicofacial, or trapezius flap (Fig. 51.16) can be elevated to these acquired neck defects. In addition, the pectoralis major flap can be transferred based on the thoracoacromial vessels to cover the acquired neck defects. If the defect exceeds the size of the local flap options, then a free flap is required. Flap options for this region include the latissimus dorsi, anterolateral thigh, and radial forearm flaps. All of these flaps can be anastomosed to the carotid and jugular systems. If the carotid artery or jugular vein is unavailable because of prior surgery or radiation, the transverse cervical vessels are routinely used as secondary donor and recipient vessels.[11]

## RECONSTRUCTION OF THE TRUNK

The trunk encompasses both the thoracic and the abdominal cavities. The chest and abdominal wall account for roughly one-third of the entire surface area of the human adult body. In this region, there is less concern for exposure of or compromise of critical anatomical structures than in the head and neck region. In the trunk, wide undermining of subcutaneous tissue down to the level of the deep investing fascia, along with local flaps, is favored for the reconstruction of cutaneous malignancies. Neoplasms that involve the full thickness of the abdominal wall or chest wall require potentially larger and vascularized pedicle and free flaps.

## Reconstruction of the thorax

The majority of skin cancers arise primarily in areas frequently exposed to the sun, and as such, the incidence of skin cancer on the chest wall is comparatively low. For instance, only 4% of squamous cell carcinomas arise on the chest and abdomen, and only 15% of basal cell carcinomas occur on the trunk.[12] Depending on the extent of the defect, particular consideration must be given to the pleural cavity, skeletal support, and soft tissue coverage. To preserve the intrathoracic negative pressure gradient, forming an airtight seal at the time of closure is crucial.[13] Skeletal stabilization with prosthetic materials is performed for resections involving either four or more rib segments or chest wall cavities greater than 6 cm in diameter to reduce the risk of paradoxical chest wall motion (flail chest).

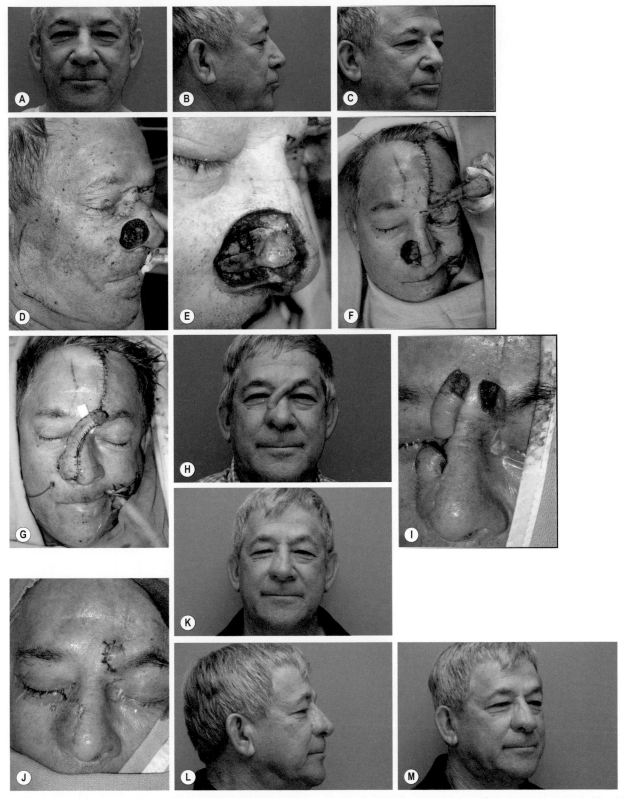

**Figure 51.13** A 66-year old man with basal cell carcinoma of the right nasal ala and sidewall. **A–C)** Preoperative view. **D)** Intraoperative defect of the skin, subcutaneous tissue, and lower lateral cartilage. **E)** Cartilage graft reconstruction with grafts harvested from conchal cartilage. **F,G)** Paramedian forehead flap elevated and transposed as an interpolated axial flap based on the supratrochlear vessels. **H)** Three weeks after surgery, the flap maintained on the distal blood supply was ready for division. **I,J)** Flap division and inset. **K–M)** Six-month follow-up showing re-establishment of the ala/sidewall contour.

The majority of thoracic defects can be repaired with local and regional musculocutaneous flaps. Muscle flap options for sternal wound coverage include the pectoralis major muscle, either as a pedicled flap based on the thoracoacromial vessels or as a turnover flap based on perforators from the internal mammary vessels, and the rectus abdominis muscle based on the superior epigastric vessels. Options for axillary coverage include the pectoralis major and latissimus dorsi flaps. The latissimus dorsi and trapezius flaps can provide coverage of the posterior thorax and paraspinous muscle flaps.

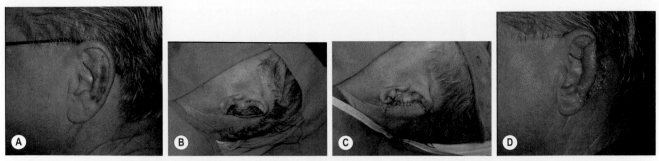

**Figure 51.14** A 59-year old man with a superficial melanoma of the left helical rim. **A)** Preoperative view. **B)** Defect of the middle third of the helical rim with loss of anterior skin and cartilage. **C)** Reconstruction with a postauricular flap based on a random circulation pattern. **D)** Early result after division of the flap base and skin graft coverage of the postauricular donor site.

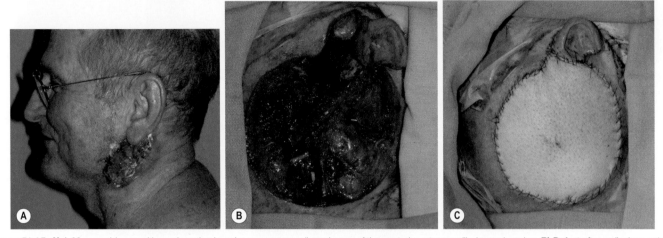

**Figure 51.15 A)** A 66-year old man with an ulcerating invasive squamous cell carcinoma of the posterior retromandibular neck region. **B)** Defect after radical resection, subtotal auriculectomy, posterior mandibulectomy, and neck dissection. **C)** Soft tissue reconstruction was achieved with a free anterolateral thigh flap (ALT).

Chest wall defects can be divided into full-thickness and partial-thickness defects. Partial-thickness defects possess an intact bony wall and thus do not require as extensive reconstruction or the use of muscle flaps, while full-thickness defects have to be reconstructed with regard to the respiratory physiology.[14] A variety of flaps, including local rotation flaps, advancement flaps, and transposition flaps, can be used. A defect that is too large for a single flap can be converted to three rhomboids, which can be closed with three smaller circumferential rhomboid flaps.[15] Another approach that has been described for the reconstruction of large defects is a pedicled flap from the abdomen, such as a pedicled transverse rectus abdominis myocutaneous (TRAM) flap or vertical rectus abdominis myocutaneous flap (VRAM). These flaps can reach up to the axilla or clavicle, and the donor site can be closed primarily.[16] A pedicle flap from either the abdomen or the back, such as a myocutaneous latissimus dorsi muscle flap, can also be used. If the skin defect is too large for the myocutaneous latissimus dorsi flap, then muscle is typically transposed and covered with a skin graft (Fig. 51.17).

## Abdominal reconstruction

Following surgery for removal of skin cancers of the abdomen, most cutaneous skin defects can be closed primarily as a result of skin laxity and subcutaneous tissue in the abdomen. Large fasciocutaneous flaps can be raised off the abdominal wall based on musculocutaneous perforators and closed in layers to obliterate dead space. If the cutaneous defect involves the abdominal wall fascia, the goal of reconstruction is to restore the integrity and continuity of the abdominal wall. Component separation, in which the layers of the abdominal wall fascia and muscle are separated to gain increased medialization of the rectus components, is often employed in situations where there is a paucity of fascia and when primary closure is required.[17] Autologous fascial grafts can be taken from the tensor fascia lata in the thigh if required. A bioprosthetic mesh in the form of an acellular dermal matrix has also been proven to be effective in reconstructing abdominal wall integrity. Pedicled flaps such as the anterolateral thigh myocutaneous flap can be used to reconstruct skin, subcutaneous, and fascial elements and obliterate dead space. Rarely is free tissue transfer required with these types of defects, but it is an option if there is a paucity of local or regional tissue.

## RECONSTRUCTION OF THE PELVIS/PERINEUM AREA

The perineal surface is distinct from other surfaces of the body both in form and function and thus may present a unique challenge in terms of reconstruction. The perineum is important for pregnancy, intercourse, bowel/bladder

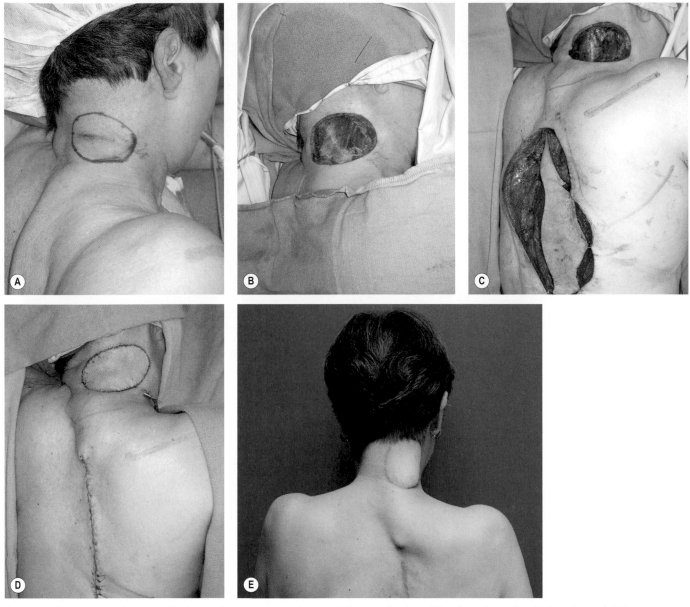

**Figure 51.16** A 55-year old woman with dermatofibrosarcoma protuberans. **A)** Preoperative view of the planned resection. **B)** Posterior neck defect. **C,D)** Trapezius flap elevation and inset. Donor site was closed primarily. **E)** Twelve-month follow-up.

motility, and hip mobility. Perineal skin and fatty tissue are also unique in that they are very sensitive to pressure and touch, and they are durable, elastic, and weight bearing. In addition, perineal skin is softly padded, pigmented, and hair bearing, which makes it impossible to match with distant tissue.[18]

Skin cancers such as Bowen's disease and invasive squamous cell carcinoma most commonly result in defects of the vulvoperineal surface, which involves loss of skin and subcutaneous tissues only.[19] For superficial defects, a split-thickness skin graft is useful, especially when there is ambiguity regarding excision margins and the risk of local recurrence is high.[20] A skin graft has a better aesthetic outcome, although it possesses an increased risk of not healing owing to fluid collection below the graft or shear.

Both partial-thickness and full-thickness skin grafts can be obtained from the suprapubic area, incorporating as much of the pubic hairline as possible to conceal the donor site. Full-thickness skin grafts can be used for larger surface area defects when there is adequate redundancy of the abdominal wall to serve as a donor site.[19] In cases of irradiated tissue, a local or regional flap can be used. For small defects that have only skin loss, a local rotational flap such as a rhomboid skin flap is useful.[21] These flaps are most effective when used in the lateral and posterior aspects of the perineal area, which have the most skin laxity. Larger defects may require regional sensate fasciocutaneous flaps or muscle flaps such as the posterior thigh flap or the pedicled gracilis muscle flap. In this case, the patient must avoid putting pressure on the area of the pedicle for several weeks.[18]

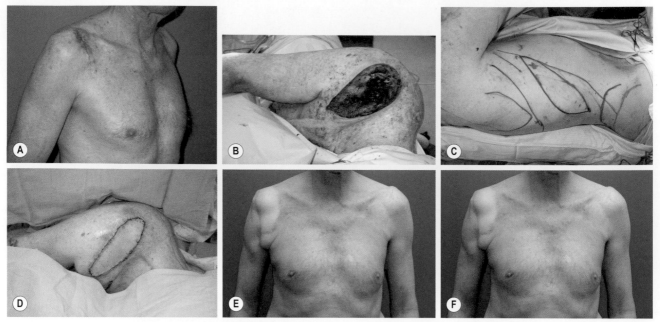

**Figure 51.17** A 57-year old man with recurrent basal cell carcinoma treated with previous resection and radiation therapy. **A)** Preoperative view. **B)** Intraoperative defect that extends to the acromion. **C)** Planned skin island incision for pedicled latissimus dorsi myocutaneous flap for soft tissue coverage and obliteration of dead space. **D)** Flap inset. **E,F)** Twelve-month follow-up showing stable soft tissue coverage and preservation of shoulder range of motion.

## RECONSTRUCTION OF THE UPPER AND LOWER EXTREMITIES

In the reconstruction of the extremities, aesthetic outcome as well as function is of primary importance. This balance often depends on the extremity in question. For instance, the distal portions of the extremities, such as the forearm and leg, are more often exposed and visible than the proximal portions of the extremities, such as the upper arm and thigh. Thus, more consideration must be given to scar formation and the ultimate aesthetic outcome in the distal portions of the extremities. With regard to the hands and feet, dexterity and sensation are more important than aesthetics.[22] In general, however, regardless of the extremity in question, preserving dexterity and ambulation take precedence over aesthetic outcomes.

When reconstructing the proximal extremities such as the thigh and arm, many patients have adequate skin laxity to allow the defects to be closed directly. This is often the case for the excision of lesions with up to a 2 cm margin.[22] If there is a risk of dehiscence or if the cancer is locally advanced, local tissue such as a rhomboid flap can be used for the reconstruction.[15] For larger defects of the anterior knee, a pedicled gastrocnemius muscle flap or a reverse anterolateral thigh flap can be used.

For defects of the proximal upper extremity, a pedicled latissimus dorsi muscle flap can be used with or without a skin paddle. Free flaps such as anterolateral thigh or lateral arm flaps based on a single perforating vessel can be useful to reconstruct medium to large skin defects if local tissue is absent. In general, local and regional flaps are preferred to skin grafts, as they provide a better match for color and texture and do not produce contour defects.[23] However, for patients with comorbidities that limit the use of anesthesia, those who are obese, or those whose dermis is atrophic, a

full-thickness or split-thickness skin graft is preferred over direct closure or flap reconstruction.[24]

Considerations in reconstructing surgical defects of the distal extremities, including the forearm and leg, differ significantly from those of the proximal extremities. Depending on the width of required excision margins, direct closure of these wounds is sometimes implausible owing to a general lack of skin laxity, thick investing fascia, the subcutaneous location of long bones, and the general tapering of the circumference of the limbs towards the more distal regions of the extremities.[2] Using a skin graft is the simplest procedure but is often associated with a poor aesthetic outcome and requires that the extremity be immobilized for many days.[15] Local flaps are a better alternative to the use of skin grafts, though the less reliable and less substantial blood flow to these areas makes local flap reconstruction more difficult and dangerous.[2]

After Ponten showed that the underlying fascia could be used to protect the vascularity of flaps on the legs,[25] local flap reconstruction has gained popularity. A fasciocutaneous flap that is commonly used to reconstruct defects on the leg is one that is advanced into the defect in a V-Y fashion, using a straight flap, curved flap, or straight flap with an oblique fascial cut.[26–28] Since the amount of advancement available with this technique is often limited in the upper two-thirds of the leg or forearm, one solution is to raise the flap as a fasciocutaneous island on a single perforating vessel.[29] One complication of this procedure, however, is that the tendons in the lower one-third of the leg and forearm limit the mobilization of the perforating vessels.

An alternative to the traditional V-Y flaps is a keystone design flap, which was initially described by Behan.[30] The keystone flap incorporates two V-Y flaps, but the flaps are oriented parallel to the defect instead of perpendicular to it, which creates greater tissue laxity. Also, the flap is usually orientated in a longitudinal manner so that the circumference of the leg or forearm does not limit its size. In one study, defects up to 6 cm in diameter could be reconstructed with the use of this flap, and, in addition, patients were ambulatory after one night of rest with elevation of the leg.[31]

In areas such as the malleoli, where tissue laxity is greatly limited, free flap reconstruction with muscle flaps plus skin grafts is recommended. With greater sophistication in perforator flap surgery, fasciocutaneous flaps based on single perforating vessels can be harvested with varying amounts of skin, subcutaneous tissue, and fascia to cover these distal defects.

## Reconstruction of defects on the hand

The most common malignant tumor of the hand is squamous cell carcinoma, followed by melanoma.[32] The three different areas of the hand that are affected by skin cancer are the nail bed, the palmar skin, and the dorsal skin. These areas have different intrinsic characteristics and also different tumor biology and thus require different reconstructive considerations. Given that the hand is crucial for dexterity and normal function, baseline functional assessment should be performed before tumor excision, and, as a general principle, digit length should be preserved as much as possible.[1] The skin of the dorsum of the hand has moderate laxity and is thin, mobile, and pliable and protects the superficial extensor tendons.

Defects up to 1–2 cm can be closed primarily and all attempts should be made to preserve the paratenon so as to minimize scarring around the tendon, thus optimizing the preservation of function. If primary closure would result in contracture, then transposition flaps can be used.[1] Defects larger than 2–3 cm can be resurfaced using skin grafts, as long as the paratenon is preserved so that the skin graft will not adhere to the underlying extensor tendons. Full-thickness skin grafts provide a better contour match than split-thickness skin grafts and result in less contracture, although a sheet graft is aesthetically acceptable if a large area is involved.[2] When the paratenon cannot be preserved, local flaps such as rotation and advancement flaps or transposition flaps (rhomboid flap) can be used.

For large defects of the dorsum of the hand, the reverse-flow pedicled radial forearm flap can be used, though it has the disadvantage of sacrificing a major vessel which supplies blood to the hand and creates a forearm donor site that typically requires a skin graft. An alternative to this may be to perform a free tissue transfer with an anterolateral thigh flap or lateral arm flap (Fig. 51.18). If the tendon requires excision, then a tendon graft may also be required to preserve tendon excursion and function.[1]

Defects of the distal cutaneous or subungual regions of the fingertips require a balance between the wide surgical excisions used for treatment and the maintenance of function by preserving the length of the digits.[2] When amputation is necessary, most cases are managed by distal interphalangeal- or middle phalangeal-level amputation. With middle phalangeal-level amputations, the insertion of the flexor digitorum superficial tendon into the base of the second phalanx is preserved to maintain finger flexion. Reconstruction then involves the use of full-thickness skin grafts or local flaps.[15] The cross-finger flap is effective for defects up to 3 cm long and 2 cm wide that are located over any of the phalanges (Fig. 51.19). These flaps are taken from the adjacent finger and are based along the mid-axial line.[1] Defects that require removing the nail plate and excising the nail bed can be resurfaced with full-thickness skin grafts.

In contrast to the dorsum of the hand, palmar skin is glabrous, thick, and receives significant sensory innervation.[2] Defects of the palm are usually resurfaced with full-thickness skin grafts, and larger defects can be reconstructed using pedicled reversed radial forearm flaps.

## Reconstructing defects on the foot

When reconstructing defects of the feet, the ambulatory status of the patient and their ability to wear shoes in the future must be considered. Planning the procedure for reconstructing the feet should also include an examination of the vascular status of the patient, as vascular insufficiency often results in poor outcomes. The main goals of foot reconstruction include preserving function, conserving the padding of

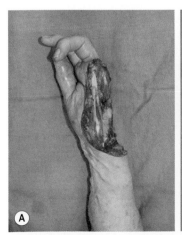
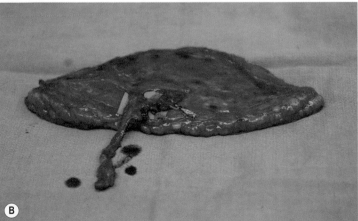
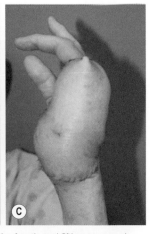

**Figure 51.18** A 64-year old woman with sarcoma of the left hand. **A)** Radical resection of the ulnar hand and wrist involving the fourth and fifth metacarpal bones and ring and small fingers. **B)** Anterolateral thigh flap (ALT) elevation on two perforating branches of the descending branch of the lateral femoral circumflex artery and vein. The flap was anastomosed to the ulnar artery and venae comitantes. **C)** Early follow-up. The patient will undergo a flap debulking procedure after a period of interim healing.

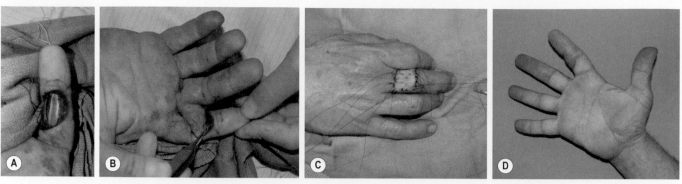

Figure 51.19 A 43-year old man who underwent resection of a squamous cell carcinoma of the right index finger. A) Full-thickness defect from the volar side of the mid phalanx to the flexor tendon. B) Cross finger flap from the dorsal proximal phalanx of the long finger. C) Skin graft coverage of the flap donor site. D) Six-month follow-up after division and inset of the cross finger flap. Full extension at the proximal and distal interphalangeal joints.

the plantar surface of the foot, and maintaining ambulation by preserving normal tendon excursion.[1]

The dorsal portion of the foot is covered by thin, mobile skin and contains superficial nerves and extensor tendons. Superficial defects can be covered with skin grafts if the paratenon is intact and preserved. Compromise of the paratenon or larger defects, however, require local flaps or fasciocutaneous free transfer (Fig. 51.20). In contrast, the plantar surface is thick and relatively immobile and consists of glabrous skin, subcutaneous fat, and neurovascular structures.[1] For non-weight-bearing areas such as the foot arch, local flaps or skin grafts can be used.[1]

Distal plantar defects can be repaired with the use of fillet flaps, which requires sacrificing a toe or advancing a V-Y flap into the defect.[1] For large defects of the heel up to 6 cm, a medial plantar flap, which is based on medial plantar vessels, can be used.[33] The donor site from where the flap is harvested is typically covered with a split-thickness skin graft. The lateral calcaneal flap can also be used to reconstruct defects on the weight-bearing aspect of the posterior heel; this is a flap based on the lateral calcaneal artery (terminal branch of the perineal artery) and innervated by the sural nerve.[1] Large defects in the mid-plantar or heel region may require a free tissue transfer.[1] In contrast to subungual and digital lesions of the hand, such lesions

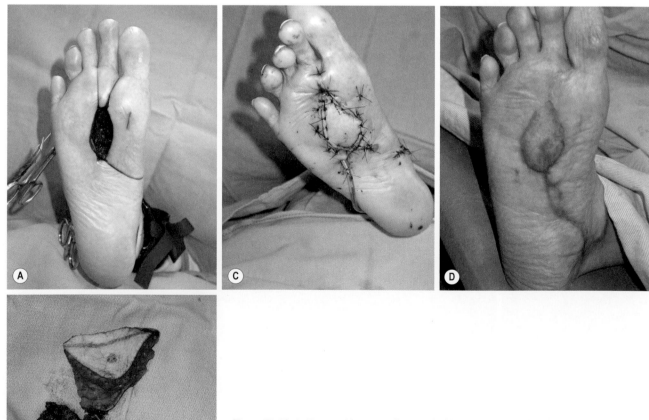

Figure 51.20 A 47-year old woman diagnosed with a melanoma of the plantar forefoot. A) Intraoperative defect. B) Anterolateral thigh flap (5 × 8 cm²) anastomosed to the posterior tibial vessels. C) Flap inset. D) Four-month follow-up.

of the foot are routinely removed by amputating the toes to the metatarsal joint,[1] since there is no benefit to preserving length and a distal stump can often contribute to postoperative morbidity.[2]

## FUTURE OUTLOOK

Reconstruction of defects created by appropriately resecting skin malignancies requires attention to both aesthetic and functional requirements. Using a systematic approach to analyzing both the defect and oncological principles, reconstruction of these defects can be accomplished routinely and safely.

The ultimate goal of reconstructive surgery of skin malignancies is a healed and durable wound with minimal patient morbidity. The wide spectrum of plastic and reconstructive procedures, which range from primary closure to skin grafting to microvascular free tissue transfer, enables optimum delivery of oncological care without compromising pathological margins. Coordinated and specialized reconstructive techniques which optimize both aesthetic and functional outcomes for the skin cancer patient is paramount to a successful outcome.

## REFERENCES

1. van Aalst JA, McCurry T, Wagner J. Reconstructive considerations in the surgical management of melanoma. *Surg Clin North Am.* 2003;83(1):187–230.
2. Moncrieff MD, Thompson JF, Quinn MJ, et al. Reconstruction after wide excision of primary cutaneous melanomas: part II—the extremities. *Lancet Oncol.* 2009;10(8):810–815.
3. Madan V, Lear JT, Szeimies RM. Non-melanoma skin cancer. *Lancet.* 2010;375(9715):673–685.
4. Moncrieff MD, Spira K, Clark JR, et al. Free flap reconstruction for melanoma of the head and neck: indications and outcomes. *J Plast Reconstr Aesthet Surg.* 2010;63(2):205–212.
5. Tibbs MK. Wound healing following radiation therapy: a review. *Radiother Oncol.* 1997;42(2):99–106.
6. Gonzalez-Ulloa M. Regional aesthetic units of the face. *Plast Reconstr Surg.* 1987;79(3):489–490.
7. Burget GC, Menick FJ. Nasal reconstruction: seeking a fourth dimension. *Plast Reconstr Surg.* 1986;78(2):145–157.
8. Burget GC, Menick FJ. Aesthetic restoration of one-half the upper lip. *Plast Reconstr Surg.* 1986;78(5):583–593.
9. Antia NH, Buch VI. Chondrocutaneous advancement flap for the marginal defect of the ear. *Plast Reconstr Surg.* 1967;39(5):472–477.
10. Wellisz T. Reconstruction of the burned external ear using a Medpor porous polyethylene pivoting helix framework. *Plast Reconstr Surg.* 1993;91(5):811–818.
11. Yu P. The transverse cervical vessels as recipient vessels for previously treated head and neck cancer patients. *Plast Reconstr Surg.* 2005;115(5):1253–1258.
12. English DR, Armstrong BK, Kricker A, et al. Demographic characteristics, pigmentary and cutaneous risk factors for squamous cell carcinoma of the skin: a case-control study. *Int J Cancer.* 1998;76(5):628–634.
13. Arnold PG, Pairolero PC. Chest-wall reconstruction: an account of 500 consecutive patients. *Plast Reconstr Surg.* 1996;98(5):804–810.
14. Arnold PG, Johnson CH. Chest wall reconstruction. *Surg Oncol Clin N Am.* 1997;6(1):91–114.
15. Ariyan S. Reconstructive surgery in melanoma patients. *Surg Oncol Clin N Am.* 1996;5(4):785–807.
16. Skoracki RJ, Chang DW. Reconstruction of the chestwall and thorax. *J Surg Oncol.* 2006;94(6):455–465.
17. Vargo D. Component separation in the management of the difficult abdominal wall. *Am J Surg.* 2004;188(6):633–637.
18. McCraw JB, Papp C, Ye Z, et al. Reconstruction of the perineum after tumor surgery. *Surg Oncol Clin N Am.* 1997;6(1):177–189.
19. Friedman J, Dinh T, Potochny J. Reconstruction of the perineum. *Semin Surg Oncol.* 2000;19(3):282–293.
20. Korlof B, Nylen B, Tillinger KG, et al. Different methods of reconstruction after vulvectomies for cancer of the vulva. *Acta Obstet Gynecol Scand.* 1975;54(5):411–415.
21. Cronje HS, Van Zyl JS. Resurfacing the vulva and vagina. *Int J Gynaecol Obstet.* 1988;27(1):113–118.
22. Moncrieff MD, Thompson JF, Quinn MJ, et al. Reconstruction after wide excision of primary cutaneous melanomas: part I—the head and neck. *Lancet Oncol.* 2009;10(7):700–708.
23. Ariyan S. General principles of reconstruction following cancer surgery. *Surg Oncol Clin N Am.* 1996;5(4):741–750.
24. Lewis JM, Zager JS, Yu D, et al. Full-thickness grafts procured from skin overlying the sentinel lymph node basin; reconstruction of primary cutaneous malignancy excision defects. *Ann Surg Oncol.* 2008;15(6):1733–1740.
25. Ponten B. The fasciocutaneous flap: its use in soft tissue defects of the lower leg. *Br J Plast Surg.* 1981;34(2):215–220.
26. Venkataramakrishnan V, Mohan D, Villafane O. Perforator based V-Y advancement flaps in the leg. *Br J Plast Surg.* 1998;51(6):431–435.
27. Dini M, Innocenti A, Russo GL, et al. The use of the V-Y fasciocutaneous island advancement flap in reconstructing postsurgical defects of the leg. *Dermatol Surg.* 2001;27(1):44–46.
28. Georgeu GA, El-Muttardi N. The horn shaped fascio-cutaneous flap usage in cutaneous malignancy of the leg. *Br J Plast Surg.* 2004;57(1):66–76.
29. Niranjan NS, Price RD, Govilkar P. Fascial feeder and perforator-based V-Y advancement flaps in the reconstruction of lower limb defects. *Br J Plast Surg.* 2000;53(8):679–689.
30. Behan FC. The keystone design perforator island flap in reconstructive surgery. *ANZ J Surg.* 2003;73(3):112–120.
31. Moncrieff MD, Bowen F, Thompson JF, et al. Keystone flap reconstruction of primary melanoma excision defects of the leg-the end of the skin graft? *Ann Surg Oncol.* 2008;15(10):2867–2873.
32. Haws MJ, Neumeister MW, Kenneaster DG, et al. Management of nonmelanoma skin tumors of the hand. *Clin Plast Surg.* 1997;24(4):779–795.
33. Koshima I, Narushima M, Mihara M, et al. Island medial plantar artery perforator flap for reconstruction of plantar defects. *Ann Plast Surg.* 2007;59(5):558–562.

# Radiation Therapy in the Treatment of Skin Cancers

*Jay S. Cooper*

## Key Points

- Radiation therapy is curative for >90% of primarily treated basal and squamous cell carcinomas of the skin; the cosmetic appearance years later is a function of the manner in which the treatment course is fractionated.

- Malignant melanomas are the least sensitive type of skin tumor; however, 25% of metastatic malignant melanomas completely regress following radiation therapy. Elective irradiation of high-risk tumor beds substantially improves locoregional control of disease.

- Kaposi sarcomas are universally responsive to radiation therapy in all clinical settings. The role and nature of radiation therapy depends on the overall health status of the patient.

- The role of and response to radiation therapy for cutaneous lymphomas depends upon the stage of the disease. Both localized and total skin electron beam radiation therapy have roles and offer benefits.

- Elective adjuvant radiation therapy decreases the local and regional risk of recurrence of resected Merkel cell carcinomas.

## INTRODUCTION

Despite decades of success, radiation therapy currently is being selected for the treatment of skin cancer less often than in the past. In part, this appropriately reflects the increasing variety of effective alternative therapies for skin cancer and a realization that radiation therapy is not the best treatment for all skin cancers. However, radiation therapy does represent an effective and potentially optimal therapy. A substantial body of information exists to suggest radiation therapy as a possible treatment in situations where it offers a better alternative than other forms of skin cancer management.

## PRINCIPLES OF RADIATION THERAPY

### Physical factors

Radiation can be produced electronically (X-rays and electrons) or obtained from the disintegration of unstable isotopes (alpha, beta and gamma rays). In dermatology, the vast majority of lesions are better suited for treatment by radiations that are produced electronically and delivered at a distance from the radiation source (teletherapy). Isotope therapy essentially is limited to implantation techniques

(brachytherapy) that result in less homogeneous dose patterns and, while a type of radiation therapy, are essentially as different from teletherapy as Mohs technique and electrodesiccation and curettage are as forms of surgery.

### Superficial-quality X-ray radiation (teletherapy)

X-rays are massless, chargeless, electromagnetic packages (photons) of energy that are generated when electrons, produced from an electrically excited filament and accelerated across an electric potential, interact with a heavy metal target. Superficial-quality X-rays cannot penetrate very far into tissue because they are attenuated rapidly by interactions with atoms in the tissues traversed. Under typical circumstances, the intensity of a superficial-quality X-ray beam (approximately 100 kVp, i.e. 100 kilovolt peak energy and 2 mm aluminum filtration, the type of radiation traditionally provided by dermatologists) decreases to approximately 80–85% (i.e. loses 15–20%, depending on field size) of its maximum deposited energy (surface dose) after traversing only 0.5 cm of tissue. It drops to 50% of its maximum intensity by 2 cm. Because most cutaneous tumors lie within a few millimeters of the skin surface, superficial-quality X-rays more than adequately penetrate such neoplasms. However, tumors that are more than 5 mm thick are better irradiated with more penetrating electrons.

### Electron beam radiation (teletherapy)

Electron beam-producing linear accelerators are now far more common than superficial-quality X-ray-producing units. To some degree, a relatively low-energy electron beam (e.g. 6 MeV [million electron volt]) and a superficial-quality X-ray (e.g. 100 kVp) penetrate tissue similarly. Because of their mass and charge, electrons can penetrate only limited distances through tissue before interacting and expending all of their energy and essentially stop. Most accelerators have the ability to produce electrons at several different energies, permitting selection of the depth of penetration that most closely matches the patient's needs; however, megavoltage electrons are more difficult to shield than are superficial X-rays.

### Field size

Because it is not possible to examine the histologic margins of an irradiated tumor, normal-appearing tissue margins need to be slightly greater than is absolutely required for surgery. For the typical, well-demarcated lesion, a margin of 0.5 to 1.0 cm is adequate. Large tumors and those with less well-defined edges may require up to 2 cm margins.

Poorly demarcated tumors are usually better treated by Mohs surgery; in the odd circumstance when radiation therapy is chosen, small circumferential punch biopsies can be used to map the tumor edge, beyond which a generous margin should be applied. Choo et al.[1] investigated the borders necessary to encompass microscopic tumor extension beyond the clinically detectable lesion in 64 consecutive patients who were selected for surgical excision with frozen-section-assisted assessment of the margins because they had features such as poorly defined edges and/or had diameters larger than 2 cm and/or had morpheaform or sclerotic patterns. In these patients, microscopic disease extended from 1 mm to 15 mm beyond the gross lesion, with a mean of 5.2 mm and larger tumors having further extension than small tumors. In this series, to have had a 95% likelihood of encompassing all disease, a margin of 10 mm beyond gross disease would have been required.

## Anatomic site

The nature of the normal tissues in various anatomic sites also influences the response to radiation. Skin that is subjected to repeated physical trauma tends to blister and/or ulcerate following radiotherapy. Consequently, there are relatively few situations in which a small basal cell carcinoma (BCC) of the arms, legs or trunk would not be better treated by an alternative modality. In contrast, mucosal surfaces tolerate radiation therapy well. Squamous cell carcinomas (SCCs) of the lip are often good candidates for treatment by radiation therapy. Some sites are ideally suited for treatment by radiation therapy. Tumors of the eyelids or at the tip of the nose tend to have a better cosmetic result when treated by a well-fractionated course of radiotherapy than by surgery.

## Biologic factors

Cellular changes in response to radiation therapy reflect both biologic processes and physical processes that determine the outcome of treatment. All tissues are less likely to be damaged or killed by the same dose of radiation when their cells are in specific phases of the cell cycle (cells in S, G1 and early G2 are less sensitive), when oxygen is less plentiful, when they have a relatively long time to repair radiation-induced damage before being damaged again, and when they have sufficient time to grow and divide between fractions of treatment. The '4Rs' of radiobiology (reassortment, reoxygenation, repair and repopulation) help explain why radiation therapy generally is most effective when a fractionated regimen is used. Regaud and Ferroux[2] long ago performed a series of experiments in radiation fractionation, examining the effect of radiation on scrotal skin and testicular function. When radiation was administered in a single fraction, there was no dose that could be delivered to a rabbit's testes that would be sufficient to cause sterility without producing unacceptable reactions in the scrotal skin as well. In contrast, when the radiation was given in a fractionated manner, it was possible to sterilize the animals without producing complications in the irradiated skin. Thus, to understand the literature, the reader must understand the precise implications of the dose-fractionation pattern employed.

For most human neoplasms, curative-intent external beam radiation therapy is delivered in one fraction per day, 180–200 cGy per fraction, 5 days per week, to total doses of 5000–7000 cGy. (Radiation is currently measured in 'Gray' or in units 1/100 as large, centiGray [cGy]. One cGy numerically equals one rad, the previous standard of dose.) However, skin tumors are among the smallest neoplasms at the time of discovery and are so superficial that it is relatively easy to protect nearby normal tissues. Consequently, one can 'get away' with a wide variety of regimens that would not be tolerated in other anatomic sites and more variations have been used for the radio therapeutic management of cutaneous tumors than could be used for tumors arising in other tissues in the body. Each of these variations has a predictable influence on the outcome of treatment (both in the short term and in the long term).

## The concept of equivalent dose

Because the total dose is not independent of the manner in which it is administered, it would be useful to have a biologic-dose-equivalent number that compared different fractionation patterns, if it could be defined accurately. It is possible to expose patches of skin to differing courses of radiation and define 'equivalent doses' by scoring the degree of acute (short-term) damage produced shortly after treatment. From such experiments, it became clear that as the total length of a treatment course increased, the greater the numerical total dose had to be, to produce an equivalent reaction.

Ellis took this concept one step further by describing a mathematical formula that related the total numerical dose, the number of fractions, and the total time of a course of treatment to a single number termed the nominal standard dose (NSD). (In the NSD equation, the influence of the number of fractions exceeds the influence of the total time. The generally cited form of the equation is $D = NSD \times N^{.24} \times T^{.11}$ where D represents the total numerical dose, N represents the number of fractions and T represents the total time in days of the course of radiation.) Orton and Ellis[3] subsequently simplified matters by publishing a set of derivative tables, written in TDF (time-dose-fractionation) units, that allow physicians to look up the equivalent acute responses based on the daily dose, number of fractions per week and total number of fractions. Unfortunately, it is now clear that the amount of damage that is evident in the acute phase of a reaction does not accurately predict what will happen in the long term.

Although the radiobiologic laws that govern the production of damage are not yet understood completely, it is now becoming apparent that damage has at least two components, termed alpha ($\alpha$) and beta ($\beta$). Some cells are killed by a single interaction ($\alpha$ killing). The number of cells killed in this manner is directly proportional to the dose-per-fraction. However, other cells merely are damaged. Such cells appear to have more than one target that needs to be destroyed for the radiation to be lethal ($\beta$ killing); the killing of such cells by radiation is proportional to the square of the dose-per-fraction.

This concept has many implications for the clinical application of radiation therapy. (The ratio of $\alpha$ to $\beta$ killing appears to be an intrinsic property of individual tissues.

For many rapidly dividing tissues, including tumors, the α/β ratio appears to be about 10. For slowly growing tissues, such as normal connective tissues, the α/β ratio is closer to 3. Because late complications are believed to occur in slowly proliferating normal tissues, late complications are made worse by larger doses per fraction. One commonly expressed form of the alpha-beta model is E = n(αd + βd²) where E is the cell kill [measured in logs], n is the number of fractions and d is the dose in Gray of a single fraction of radiation. For the current discussion, the concept predicts that for an equivalent amount of short-term damage, larger daily fractions will produce greater long-term damage, because the cells involved in long-term damage are disproportionately affected by β killing. In practice, this concept implies that two different radiation regimens may be equally effective in controlling cutaneous carcinomas (and may produce similar short-term cosmetic changes), but the one that uses the higher dose-per-fraction to reach the same total dose will inevitably lead to a poorer long-term cosmetic appearance.

## TREATMENT OF BASAL AND SQUAMOUS CELL CARCINOMAS

Basal cell and squamous cell carcinomas can be treated very effectively by several different modalities. The selection of radiotherapy for a particular BCC or SCC depends less on the likelihood of tumor control than on the anticipated cosmetic and functional results. These considerations tend to favor the use of radiation therapy for small lesions arising on or near the eyelids, nose, ears and lips in patients who are age 60 or greater. However, about 85% of all BCCs arise in the head and neck region and such lesions therefore are common.[4,5] There is rarely a reason to favor radiation therapy elsewhere in the body if the lesion can readily be excised without substantial cosmetic and/or functional consequence and the patient is a surgical candidate. Patient preference, essential anticoagulation therapy, and major medical comorbidities are examples of host-related factors that might render radiation therapy the treatment of choice. Within these constraints, radiation therapy can be used for primary therapy, treatment of post-surgical recurrences, and adjuvant therapy.

There appears to be little argument that surgery and radiotherapy are effective treatments for non-melanoma skin cancer. However, many physicians behave as if they believe that surgery conclusively has been shown to be a more effective treatment than radiation therapy; the use of radiation therapy for skin cancers has decreased to the point that a 1996 survey[6] revealed that radiation therapy was used as first-line treatment for just 8% of the BCCs treated in the UK and only 2% in The Netherlands. Yet, a recent Cochrane review concluded that 'there has been very little good quality research on the efficacy of the treatment modalities used' in the management of cutaneous BCCs.[7] In fact, the review could find only one 'suitable randomized controlled trial' of radiation therapy versus surgery. And that trial, conducted in Villejuif, France, and reported by Avril et al.[8] and subsequently by Petit et al.,[9] was far too complex to be interpreted in a simple straightforward manner as suggesting routine superiority of surgery over radiation therapy. Although 93% of lesions in that trial were 2 cm or less, surgery was not as simple as might be assumed: frozen section assessment of the tumor margins was obtained for 91% of patients and 39% required additional resection. Following histologic examination of the permanent tumor specimen, 3% patients required additional resection of residual disease, 3% required additional surgery to improve the appearance of the incision or correct an ectropion, and 1% needed salvage radiation therapy.

The radiation therapy also differs substantially from the approximately 100 kV superficial X-rays or equivalent electrons discussed throughout this chapter: 55% of tumors were treated by implantation of interstitial radioactive sources (brachytherapy); 33% were treated by 50 kV contact X-ray therapy delivered in two very large fractions of 1800 to 2000 cGy each, spaced 2 weeks apart (treatment that predictably will give poorer cosmetic results than a more fractionated, smaller individual-size fraction regimen) and only 12% were treated with more conventional 85 to 250 kV therapy of 200–400 cGy per fraction, three to four times per week, up to 6000 cGy. Results of the trial were described only as 'surgery' or 'radiotherapy' independent of the specific treatment delivered. After 24 months and 36 months, the observed differences in outcome between surgery and radiotherapy were relatively small. However, not surprisingly, after 48 months, only 69% of patients considered their cosmetic appearance 'good' following radiotherapy versus 87% after surgery; 8% of patients deemed their result poor after radiotherapy versus 2% after surgery. Moreover, surgery was not better in every anatomic location: the percentage of good cosmetic results was equal for tumors arising on the nose. Consequently, this study demonstrates better cosmetic outcome for surgery only when compared to radiotherapy done in the same manner as was used in the trial … a manner I would not recommend if optimal cosmetic outcome is important!

## Dose, time, fractionation

Skin cancers can be cured by treatment as simple as one large fraction of radiation therapy. For example, Chan et al.[10] recently reviewed the outcome of 1005 BCCs/SCCs (arising in 806 patients; 94% having a mean diameter of 3 cm or less) treated with single doses of 1800, 2000 or 2250 cGy at Nottingham University Hospital, UK, and followed for at least 10 years. The disease-free rate at 5 years was 90%; however, the necrosis-free rate at 5 years was only 84%. No significant difference in tumor recurrence was evident between 2000 and 2250 cGy (P=0.3), but skin necrosis occurred significantly more frequently following 2250 cGy (P=0.003). Consequently, fractionated doses that are considerably better tolerated by normal skin generally are preferable. As normal skin tolerance also is inversely related to the amount of skin irradiated, BCCs and SCCs often are treated according to a size-graduated scale, with larger lesions receiving larger numerical total doses delivered in smaller daily fractions. For example, Solan et al.[11] recommend 4000 cGy in 10–16 fractions for small lesions, and 4500 cGy in 15–18 fractions to 6000 cGy in 20–30 fractions for larger lesions.

## Tumor control: rates and modifiers

Silverman et al.[12] reviewed the outcome of 862 primary BCCs uniformly treated with (relatively large fractions of) 680 cGy for five fractions over 2.5 weeks between 1955 and 1982. The 5-year recurrence rate was 7.4% and larger tumor size was the only independent factor that correlated with local recurrence. Petrovich et al.[13] reported the outcome of radiotherapy in 646 patients who had carcinomas of the eyelids, pinna, or nose (72% BCC, 18% SCC, and 10% mixed). Using a size-graduated philosophy, they observed 5-, 10-, and 20-year control rates of 99%, 98%, and 98%, respectively, for 502 tumors less than 2 cm in diameter. For larger tumors between 2 and 5 cm in diameter, the 5- and 10-year control rates dropped to 92% and 79%, respectively; and for still larger tumors, 60% at 5 years and 53% at 8 years. Schulte et al.[14] reported a series of 1267 cutaneous BCCs and SCCs consecutively treated by radiation therapy with resultant local control of 95.3% at 5 years, 93.1% at 10 years, and 92.6% at 15 years. Zagrodnik et al.[15] observed a higher 5-year recurrence rate following 20–50 kilovolt soft X-ray therapy of sclerosing BCCs than of nodular BCCs (27% vs 8%, respectively), but concluded that 'radiotherapy may be the therapy of choice for patients with all BCC subtypes, depending on the individual patient's characteristics'.

There appears to be a slightly higher local recurrence rate for SCC as compared with BCC. Solan et al.[11] reported that 96% (426/444) of BCCs and 92% (144/156) of SCCs were controlled for at least 4 years after radiation therapy. Lovett et al.[16] observed that size-for-size, BCCs exhibited better control following radiotherapy: for lesions less than 1 cm, control was 97% (86/89) versus 91% (21/23); for tumors 1–5 cm, control was 87% (116/133) versus 76% (39/51); and for lesions greater than 5 cm, control was 87% (13 of 15) versus 56% (9/16), for BCC and SCC, respectively. Schulte et al.[14] observed a slightly higher 5-year recurrence rate for SCC (6.0%) than for BCC (4.2%); in part, this reflected the size of the lesions (most squamous cells were T2 whereas most basal cells were T1) and a greater likelihood of recurrence for larger SCCs (T2, 7.4% for SCC vs. 4.2% for BCC; T3, 25.9% for SCC vs. 11.4% for BCC).

The influence of specific anatomic sites as a factor for evaluating the effectiveness of radiotherapy relates more to the difficulty of applying other forms of treatment and their cosmetic implications than to the radiocurability of tumors that arise at these sites. Size for size, there appears to be no difference in response of lesions situated at different anatomic sites. Lesions near embryologic fusion planes tend to extend relatively deeply and require more penetrating therapy (radiation or other). Lesions of the eyelids often can be cured without needing to resort to complex plastic repairs. Lesions of the medial orbit can be irradiated with preservation of the functioning tear duct.

BCCs and SCCs adjacent to cartilage, once thought to be inappropriate for treatment by radiation because of the fear of subsequent chondronecrosis, are now known to be suitable for fractionated radiotherapy. Caccialanza et al.[17] recently have published their experience in treating 671 BCCs and SCCs overlying cartilage of the nose by superficial radiotherapy between 1972 and 2007. Their 5-year cure rate was 88%, cosmetic appearance was deemed 'good' or 'acceptable' in 97%, and no complications of treatment were observed. The authors concluded that radiation therapy is 'a safe, effective and non-invasive method, superior, on the basis of the literature data, to any other available therapeutic modality in the management of basal and squamous cell skin carcinomas localized over the nasal cartilages'. Similarly, Tsao et al.[18] reported a local relapse-free rate of 90% and 85% at 2 and 5 years, respectively, in 100 patients treated with radiation therapy for SCC of the skin of the nose. Silva et al.[19] reported an 87% 2-year control rate following radiation therapy of 334 lesions overlying the pinna (201 BCCs and 122 SCCs). Although the authors also reported a 5% severe complication rate, such complications were most often associated with large lesions and/or the use of large doses in each fraction. There were no severe complications associated with fractions of 300 cGy or less.

The success rate of radiotherapy also depends upon knowing when to treat a patient by alternative means. Lesions arising on skin subjected to continual trauma tend not to be treated ideally by radiotherapy. For this reason, lesions on the extremities (particularly the hands, legs and feet) usually are better treated surgically. Lesions of the trunk typically can be excised and the defect closed primarily in one session. For such patients it is unnecessarily inconvenient to attend for repetitive fractions of radiation. In addition, cosmetic considerations will not likely be as important for lesions on the trunk as on the face. This is not to say that such lesions cannot be treated by radiotherapy, merely that radiotherapy usually is not the treatment of choice.

## Cosmetic considerations

It is generally acknowledged that the cosmetic appearance of irradiated lesions shortly after treatment is excellent. Particularly for lesions of the eyelids, nose, and ears, the short-term cosmetic appearance of lesions treated by irradiation generally exceeds that attainable by surgery (Figs 52.1–52.7). More problematic is the cosmetic appearance years after treatment. Oddly, until recently there have been very few reports describing differences in cosmetic outcome based on dose fractionation. Brennan et al.[20] attempted to do precisely that by investigating the cosmetic appearance of tissues following three different dose-fractionation schemes. Patients were randomly assigned to receive three fractions of 987 cGy each (total dose 2961 cGy), seven fractions of 513 cGy each (total dose 3591 cGy), or ten fractions of 387 cGy each (total dose 3870 cGy). When measured 2 years later, there was no difference in the cure rate or cosmetic result obtained by any of these dose-fractionation schemes. Whether longer follow-up or smaller fractions of 180–200 cGy would have produced different results was not addressed. A poll of our patients[21] irradiated 10 or more years previously according to a graduated treatment scale based on the size of their lesions, found them to be very satisfied with their cosmetic result. Fifty percent rated the appearance of the irradiated region 'excellent'. The data reported by Locke

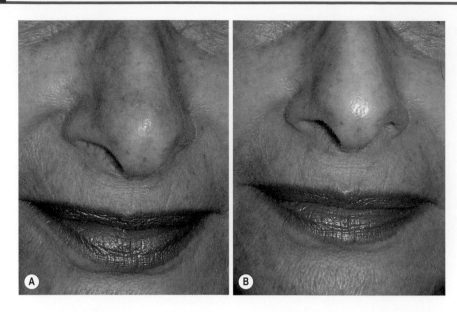

Figure 52.1 **A)** Basal cell carcinoma of the tip of the nose prior to treatment. **B)** Same patient, 10 months following 5400 cGy/18 fractions, 100 kv therapy.

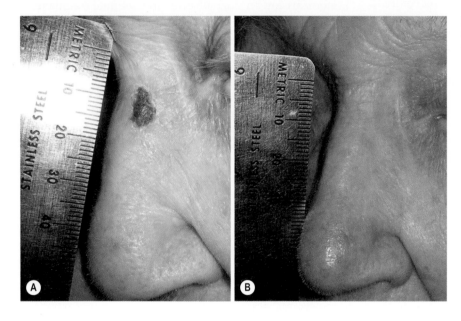

Figure 52.2 **A)** Squamous cell carcinoma of the left side of the nose. **B)** Same patient, 15 months following 5400 cGy/18 fractions, 100 kv therapy.

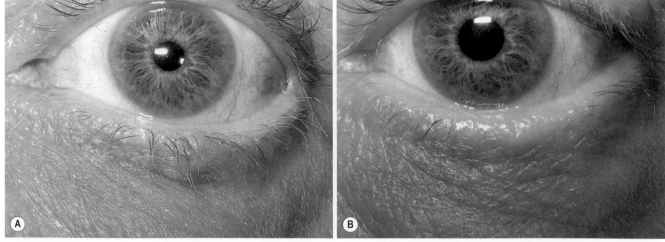

Figure 52.3 **A)** Basal cell carcinoma of the left lower eyelid prior to treatment. **B)** Same patient, 14 months following 5400 cGy/18 fractions, 100 kv therapy.

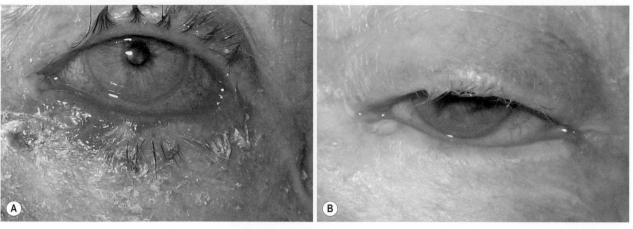

**Figure 52.4 A)** Basal cell carcinoma of the left lower eyelid prior to treatment. **B)** Same patient, 22 months following 4500 cGy/15 fractions, 100 kv therapy.

**Figure 52.5 A)** Centrally ulcerated basal cell carcinoma on posterior helix of ear. **B)** Same patient, 2 months following superficial X-ray radiotherapy. The lesion healed over completely and chondritis did not develop.

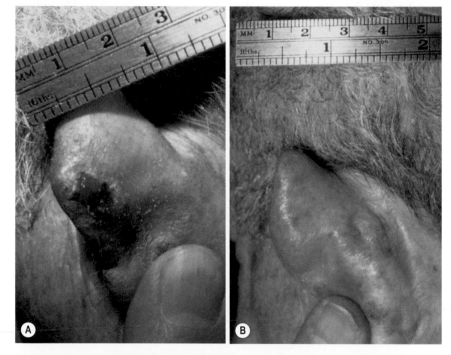

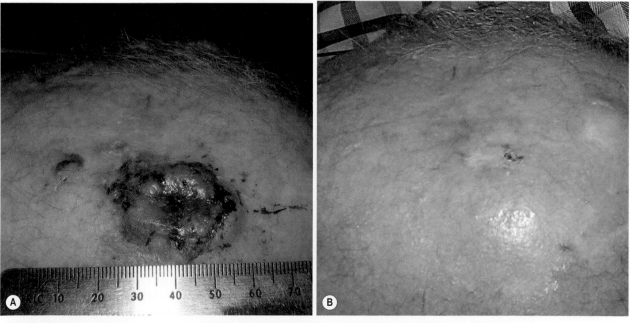

**Figure 52.6 A)** Squamous cell carcinoma of the scalp. **B)** Same patient, 3 months following 6540 cGy/35 fractions, 6 MeV therapy.

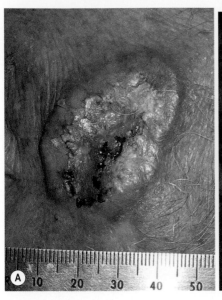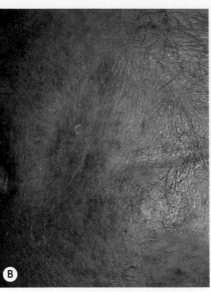

**Figure 52.7 A)** Squamous cell carcinoma of the left temple. **B)** Same patient, 24 months following 5750 cGy/22 fractions, 6 MeV therapy.

et al.[22] yielded a similar conclusion. The most common fractionation scheme they used (in 68% of their patients) delivered daily doses of no more than 300 cGy and total doses of 4001 to 6000 cGy. With these regimens, 53% of their patients had excellent cosmetic results and 94% had good or excellent results. Still more recently, Olschewski et al.[23] reported the treatment of 104 BCCs of the face and head that were predominantly (95%) treated with 300 cGy daily up to a total dose of 5700 cGy. No recurrences were observed; 87% of courses were associated with 'only low acute toxicity' and the cosmetic result was graded 'excellent' or 'good' in 94%.

## Adjuvant irradiation of high-risk cutaneous squamous cell cancers

Although there are no prospective randomized trials of adjuvant radiation therapy for resected SCCs that are believed to be at high risk for recurrence, some physicians recommend adjuvant irradiation in such circumstances, particularly when perineural invasion is seen in the surgical specimen.[24] Jambusaria-Pahlajani et al.[25] recently reviewed the Medline database and concluded that there currently is insufficient evidence to identify high-risk features that might justify adjuvant irradiation. However, they did find that involvement of larger nerves was associated with a worse prognosis. Similarly, Han and Ratner[26] reviewed the literature, confirmed the paucity of evidence-based medicine, and concluded that a multicentered, prospective, randomized trial will be needed to clarify the value of elective irradiation in patients who have perineural invasion. They also gingerly suggested that the extent of nerve involvement might be helpful in deciding appropriate candidates for treatment. In support of this concept, Galloway et al.[27] were able to correlate more evident imaging findings with decreasing prognosis; perineural spread was defined as an 'enlargement or abnormal enhancement of the nerve, obliteration of the normal fat plane surrounding the nerve, and/or erosion or enlargement of its related foramen'.

## Salvage by radiation therapy

Ríos-Buceta[28] recently reviewed the management of BCCs that had surgically involved margins and concluded that '(a)lthough no conclusive evidence is available, the studies analyzed and common sense suggest that a wait-and-see approach in patients with aggressive tumors may be risky.' Based on 13 series including 704 patients (who had surgical specimens that had involved margins) who were then simply observed, recurrence can be expected in 27% with follow-up averaging just over 31 months. However, it is not clear that unnecessarily treating the remaining 73% to cure the 27% is a good trade. Liu et al.[29] reported a retrospective analysis of BCCs that were incompletely excised. With a median follow-up of 2.7 years, the actuarial 5-year recurrence rate was 9% for the 119 patients who were irradiated versus 39% for the 67 lesions that were simply observed. However, in the latter group, if relapse occurred, 85% of the relapses were salvaged by either radiation or surgery. Consequently, the 10-year actuarial probability of local control was similar in the groups: 92% following elective treatment and 90% following salvage therapy. As further evidence that radiation therapy can eradicate basal or squamous cell carcinomas that have recurred after surgical therapy, Caccialanza et al.[30] retrospectively reviewed the outcome of salvage radiotherapy for 249 lesions that had recurred after a variety of non-radiologic treatments. The 5-year cure rate was 83.6% and 'good or acceptable' cosmetic results were observed in 92.6% of the lesions that were controlled. The retrospective review by Kwan et al.[31] suggested that radiotherapeutic salvage was more likely for post-surgically recurrent BCCs than for post-surgically recurrent SCCs.

## TREATMENT OF MALIGNANT MELANOMA

Unlike the other tumors included in this chapter, malignant melanoma is not very radioresponsive. In fact, for many years, malignant melanoma was believed to be impervious to radiation, until data demonstrated that radiotherapy palliated distressing signs and symptoms of metastatic disease in more than 50% of patients.

## High-dose-per-fraction radiotherapy for palliation

For some years there was a debate about the seemingly better response to radiation therapy packaged as larger individual fractions.[32] To clarify the situation, the Radiation Therapy Oncology Group (RTOG) conducted a prospective randomized trial[33] for metastatic malignant melanomas, comparing 800 cGy delivered four times at weekly intervals ('high-dose-per-fraction therapy') versus 250 cGy daily for 20 fractions over 26–28 days ('conventional-dose-per-fraction therapy'). The results showed no difference in response rates between the techniques, and clearly demonstrated that metastatic malignant melanomas do respond to radiation therapy and that complete response can be expected approximately 25% of the time.

## Potentially curative radiotherapy

Surgery is the treatment of choice for the vast majority of potentially curable malignant melanomas. Despite some evidence[34-36] that radiation therapy can control very thin lesions (particularly lentigo maligna and lentigo maligna melanoma), radiation therapy should be considered only in those situations where surgery is 'impossible or not reasonable'.[37]

## Elective treatment of high-risk resected melanomas

Following surgery alone, some melanomas have a high likelihood of recurring locally. For example, Lee et al.[38] reported a 30% nodal basin recurrence rate following resection of histologically involved lymph nodes and correlated some pretreatment factors with even greater risks: extracapsular extension of disease (63%), multiple nodes invaded by tumor (46% for 4–10 nodes and

63% for >10 nodes), and cervical lymph node involvement (43%). Because the efficacy of radiation therapy is inversely related to the volume of disease requiring treatment, radiation therapy has been electively applied to microscopic-sized disease in situations where a high risk for recurrence remains despite expertly done surgery (e.g. following resection of aggressive primary tumors, resection of locally recurrent disease or resection of metastases in regional lymph nodes).

Several groups[39-42] have described retrospective analyses that are highly suggestive of better control of locoregional disease by elective radiation therapy in these high-risk postoperative situations. Unfortunately, such therapy has not appeared to have a similar beneficial effect on survival. Recently, Henderson et al.[43] reported a multicenter prospective randomized trial of adjuvant radiation therapy (4800 cGy in 20 fractions) versus observation in 250 patients who were believed to be at a greater than 25% risk of local recurrence following lymphadenectomy for a regional recurrence. Regional control of disease was significantly better in the group receiving adjuvant radiation therapy; however, overall survival was not significantly different between the two groups.

## TREATMENT OF KAPOSI SARCOMA

Kaposi sarcoma (KS) occurs in four different clinical settings ('classic' KS, 'endemic' African KS, transplant-related KS [Chapter 16] and AIDS-related 'epidemic' KS [Chapter 19]), but is highly radiosensitive in all four (Figs 52.8 and 52.9). In fact, there likely is no substantial difference in the radiosensitivity of the disease between the variants and the results of treatment are remarkably consistent worldwide. For example, Stein et al.,[44] writing from Johannesburg General Hospital in South Africa, compared response to irradiation in all four groups and concluded 'Kaposi's sarcoma showed a very high response rate to radiation therapy, regardless of variant, radiation modality or schedule.' However, the benefit of radiation therapy varies; the more localized the disease, the greater the potential contribution of radiation therapy.

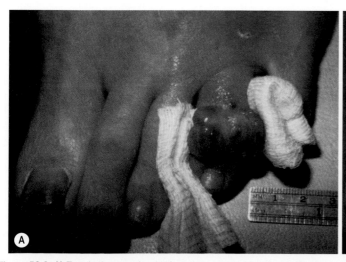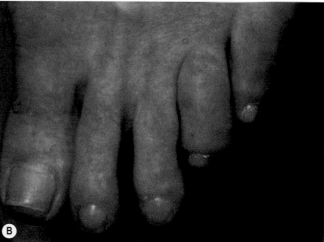

**Figure 52.8 A)** Exophytic-type classic Kaposi sarcoma of fourth toe. **B)** Same patient, 1 month following treatment. Because of the bulky nature of his tumor, the patient received cobalt therapy with bolus.

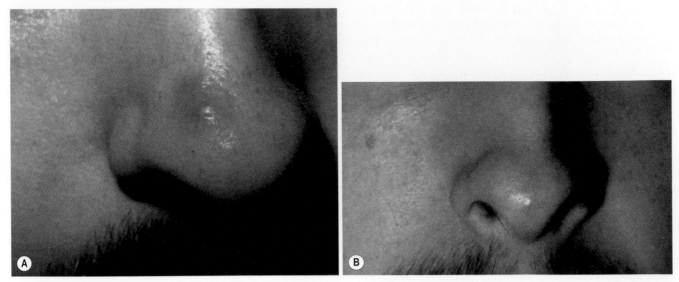

Figure 52.9 **A)** Epidemic Kaposi sarcoma of skin of nose. **B)** Same patient, 4 months following superficial X-ray treatment.

## 'Classic' KS

Because classic KS tends to be a slowly progressive disease that remains confined to the legs for many years, the highly radioresponsive nature of the lesions often renders radiation therapy the treatment of choice. Radiotherapy generally is delivered solely to involved areas of skin plus a small normal-appearing tissue border, although elective irradiation of adjacent clinically uninvolved areas has been advocated.

Fenig et al.[45] reviewed the outcome of radiation therapy in 123 Israeli patients who had classic KS. Radiotherapy produced an 88% objective (complete plus partial ) response rate and symptomatic relief in 95% of patients. Similarly, Tombolini et al.,[46] using doses ranging from 800 cGy in one fraction to 3000 cGy in ten fractions, observed a 92% objective response rate (54% complete response, 38% partial response) and complete remission of symptoms in all patients. Our own experience[47] treating 82 classic Kaposi sarcomas in New York with doses ranging from 650 cGy in one fraction to 3500 cGy in ten fractions demonstrated that more than 50% of classic KS lesions regressed completely and did not recur during a minimum follow-up of 10 years. We were also able to correlate the intensity of the treatment and the likelihood of long-term response. Doses of 2750 cGy or more delivered in ten fractions over 2 weeks, or their equivalent, were associated with significantly better long-term local control. A dose of 3000 cGy in ten fractions over 2 weeks appeared to provide an optimal balance between tumor control and rapidity of treatment. Recently, Hauerstock et al.[48] reported a retrospective review from McGill University Health Centre, Montreal, QC, of 16 patients who had classic KS that was treated by radiation therapy (most commonly by 30 Gy in 15 daily fractions). The complete response rate was 88% and all tumors responded at least partially.

## AIDS-related KS

After the initial 'epidemic' explosion, the incidence of AIDS-related KS has dramatically declined in response to highly active antiretroviral therapy (HAART). Moreover, the typically disseminated nature of epidemic KS not infrequently requires a more widespread systemic approach to the palliation of distressing lesions than radiation therapy can provide. Thus, the current role for radiation therapy is considerably diminished in the United States as compared with at the beginning of the epidemic.

Yet, there remain selected patients who can benefit from radiation therapy and the individual lesions remain as highly radiosensitive as those in classic KS. Objective response rates to radiation therapy (complete and partial response) often exceed 90% although residual benign pigmentation remains in 20–40%, the rate varying inversely with the dose delivered.

As in classic KS, there appears to be a dose–response relationship for AIDS-related KS. Stelzer and Griffin[49] conducted a landmark prospective randomized trial testing three different dose regimens in epidemic KS: 800 cGy in one fraction, 2000 cGy in ten fractions, or 4000 cGy in 20 fractions. Complete response occurred in 50% of tumors treated with 800 cGy, 79% of tumors treated with 2000 cGy, and 83% of tumors treated with 4000 cGy. In addition, in the 4000 cGy group, recurrence was less frequent, the median time to recurrence was longer, and residual purple pigmentation was less likely to be evident.

Saran and colleagues[50] also suggest that the likelihood of complete response is approximately 40% lower when comparing total doses below 2000 cGy to larger doses. However, the ideal dose for any lesion represents the likely effects of that dose viewed in terms of the patient's needs; every patient does not need the maximum tolerated dose. Singh et al.[51] could not detect a difference between 24 Gy in 12 fractions and 20 Gy in five fractions in terms of response, local control, or toxicity. Harrison et al.[52] concluded that 'a single fraction of 8 Gy is an appropriate treatment for acceptable response and normal skin pigmentation within a group of patients in whom the median life expectancy is limited'. Similarly, de Wit et al.[53] stated that 'a single dose of 800 cGy is an effective treatment for patients with a predicted survival of only a few months'.

Selection of dose should also reflect the likelihood of inducing toxicity at a given anatomic site. Belembaogo et al.[54] and Kirova et al.[55] irradiated 643 patients with doses ranging from 1000 to 3000 cGy and observed objective responses in 92% of cutaneous lesions, with 'acceptable' (7% grade I, 70% grade II, and 23% grade III) toxicity. Oral mucosal reactions were frequent after relatively low doses, prompting the authors to recommend 3000 cGy in fractionated doses for cutaneous epidemic KS (to small local fields), 2000 cGy for lesions involving eyelids, conjunctiva, and genitals, and 1500 cGy for oral lesions.

Conill et al.[56] treated 251 cutaneous lesions with doses ranging from 800 cGy in one fraction (68% of irradiated tumors) to 3000 cGy in ten fractions (27% of irradiated tumors) and concluded that radiation therapy provides 'excellent local control with minimal toxicity'. Based on their experience, Stein et al.[57] concluded that 'radiation therapy can provide good to excellent palliation with only minimal side-effects, producing a lesser impact on the hematological and immunological system than chemotherapy.'

In summary, KS is highly sensitive to radiation therapy in both its classic and AIDS-related forms. In a recent review of 1482 lesions, Caccialanza et al.[58] observed similarly high rates of local control of disease: 98.7% for classic KS (711 patients) and 91.4% for AIDS-related KS (771 patients).

## TREATMENT OF CUTANEOUS LYMPHOMAS

### T-cell lineage

The majority of cutaneous lymphomas are of T-cell lineage and mycosis fungoides accounts for the majority of these neoplasms (Chapter 21). Many forms of management should be considered (including expectant observation), but when intervention is warranted, mycosis fungoides, like most lymphomatous tumors, is very sensitive to ionizing radiation. Both plaques and tumor nodules typically regress completely following modest doses of radiation (Fig. 52.10) and radiation therapy can be used to treat discrete areas ('spot' radiation therapy) or the entire skin surface (total skin electron beam therapy, TSEB). The European Organization for Research and Treatment of Cancer (EORTC)[59] recently has published guidelines for the treatment of mycosis fungoides. While recognizing that the available evidence-based literature is limited and the grade of recommendation essentially is only C (evidence from a case series, or poor-quality cohort study, or poor-quality case–control studies), radiation therapy was recommended as a first-line therapy for all stages of mycosis fungoides.

Single fraction doses of only a few hundred cGy may be sufficient to control individual lesions; however, fractionated radiotherapy is usually chosen because of its vastly superior cosmetic result. Cotter et al.[60] reviewed the response of 191 lesions in 20 patients who received fractionated irradiation for mycosis fungoides. Complete response to treatment was noted in all lesions that received more than a numerical total of 2000 cGy. Unfortunately, local recurrence was noted, despite initial complete response, when relatively small doses were used. The in-field recurrence rate was 42% in patients receiving 1000 cGy or less, 32% in patients receiving 1001–2000 cGy, 21% in patients receiving 2001–3000 cGy, and 0% in patients receiving more than 3000 cGy. This prompted the authors to recommend tumor doses equivalent to at least 3000 cGy delivered at 200 cGy per fraction, five fractions per week, for long-term local control. And the intention of obtaining long-term control appears to be appropriate; in contrast to the relatively long survival times associated with mycosis fungoides, the authors observed that 83% of local recurrences became evident within 1 year of treatment and all were evident within 2 years.

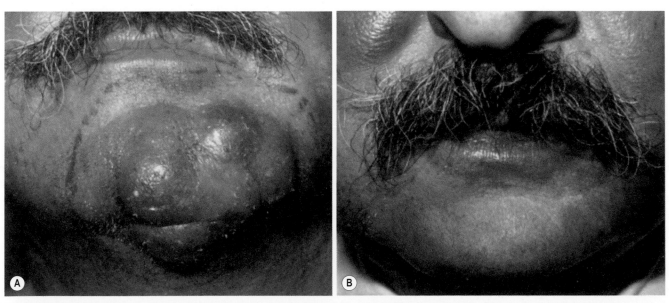

**Figure 52.10 A)** Nodular stage mycosis fungoides of the chin prior to treatment. **B)** Same patient, 1 month following electron beam treatment. Note new lesions on right cheek.

There appears to be a small subset of patients (approximately 5%) who have very limited disease ('minimal' stage IA) at presentation who are effectively treated with localized superficial radiation therapy.[61,62] Relapse of treated disease appears to be very rare, progression of disease in other anatomic sites uncommon (and, when it occurs, amenable to further therapy), and 10-year survival assured.

Unfortunately, some patients have much wider involvement of the skin at presentation, requiring irradiation of the entire skin surface. The EORTC has published consensus guidelines for total skin electron beam radiation of mycosis fungoides.[63] For patients who have previously untreated limited patches and/or plaques (more than 'minimal' disease but less than 10% of their skin surface involved, with or without clinically enlarged but histologically uninvolved lymph nodes), TSEB, using doses of 3000–3600 cGy over 8 to 10 weeks, offers the prospect of long-term progression-free survival. Approximately 95% of patients will experience complete response of disease and 50% will survive for at least 10 years free of progression of disease.

## B-cell lineage

Although level 1 evidence currently does not exist, radiation therapy appears to be the most proven effective therapy for cutaneous B-cell lymphomas. The EORTC[64] recently has published 'consensus guidelines' for the management of these diseases. For primary cutaneous marginal zone B-cell lymphoma, they recommend that patients whose disease presents as a solitary or a few scattered skin lesions are best treated with local radiotherapy (20–36 Gy) or excision. For primary cutaneous follicle center lymphoma, they recommend that for patients whose disease presents as a solitary or localized skin lesions, radiation therapy with a dose of at least 30 Gy and a margin of clinically uninvolved skin of at least 1 to 1.5 cm is the best form of treatment. For primary cutaneous diffuse large B-cell lymphoma, leg type, they comment that the complete response rate following radiation therapy is less than for the other types of cutaneous B-cell lymphomas (CR = 88% in the literature) and that extracutaneous spread occurs in approximately 30% of cases. Consequently, they recommend R-CHOP chemotherapy with or without radiation therapy, and reserve radiation therapy alone for situations in which the patient's condition would not permit R-CHOP chemotherapy.

## TREATMENT OF MERKEL CELL CARCINOMA

Merkel cell carcinomas are uncommon malignancies that originate from a neuroendocrine cell within the basal layer of the epidermis (Chapter 17). Like most neuroendocrine tumors, the cells are very sensitive to radiation therapy; however, the propensity of such cells to spread rapidly and widely, limits our ability to cure a high percentage of these tumors.

There is general agreement that surgical therapy is the most appropriate first step in their management. However, there are no prospective randomized trials evaluating the value of elective postoperative irradiation. Instead, we currently need to rely on retrospective series and meta-analyses. And, based on the available literature,

it appears that following surgery alone, local recurrence becomes evident in approximately 30% of patients and regional recurrence in nearly 40% of patients within the first year of follow-up.[65] With the addition of elective postoperative irradiation, these risks drop to 10% and 15%, respectively. Unfortunately, the addition of radiation therapy does not appear to influence the rate of distant metastasis, implying that such spread generally occurs before the patient comes for treatment. And, as a consequence, radiation therapy does not have a substantial effect on 5-year survival (approximately 50% without radiation and 57% with it).[65] As it is likely that patients who had more worrisome tumors and a worse prognosis were offered radiation therapy, the true benefit of radiation may be even greater. Furthermore, the potential adverse effects of radiation therapy are relatively modest. Because of the relative sensitivity of Merkel cell carcinomas to radiation therapy, a dose of approximately 5000 cGy delivered at 200 cGy per fraction usually is sufficient to control residual microscopic size disease.[66] When feasible, the tumor bed and draining lymphatics generally are encompassed en bloc.

Some question exists about the relative contribution of elective radiation therapy following Mohs surgery. Again, in this situation, absolute conclusions are prevented by the small database upon which they can be based. It seems reasonable, however, to assume that Mohs surgery should be more effective than non-controlled surgery in eliminating local disease. In fact, some physicians suggest that Mohs micrographic surgery is sufficiently effective at controlling local disease that elective radiation adds little. For example, Boyer et al.[67] stated that 'adjuvant radiation appears unessential to secure local control of primary MCC lesions completely excised with Mohs micrographic surgery' based on a retrospective analysis of 45 patients (treated by 11 Mohs surgeons) in which tumor-free margins and adequate follow-up were obtained. In this analysis, the local recurrence rate was 16% following Mohs and 0% following Mohs plus radiation; in-transit metastases became evident in 12% of patients treated only by Mohs versus in 0% of patients who received Mohs plus radiation therapy. Although neither of these differences reach mathematical statistical significance, it seems reasonable to conclude that this more likely reflects the small numbers at risk rather than an absence of difference. Furthermore, it seems reasonable to wonder why some patients were treated with radiation (while others were not) in this retrospective analysis.

## FUTURE OUTLOOK

Radiation therapy already provides highly effective, relatively non-toxic therapy for a variety of tumors and recent years have witnessed a move away from ablative surgery to radiation therapy (with or without chemotherapy) for tumors of the head and neck, breast, esophagus, prostate and anus. The same trends may be seen in the future for some skin cancers.

A number of radiosensitizing and radioprotective drugs that change the relative sensitivity of tumors to the adjacent normal tissues (either by making the tumors more sensitive or the normal tissues more resistant to damage) are in development or clinical trial and offer the potential of even more effective treatment. In addition, when more effective systemic therapies are developed for malignant melanomas, the value of elective irradiation of high-risk tumors beds will increase. Physicians who ignore the long, proud history of dermatologic radiation therapy and believe that radiation therapy is passé may be very surprised by the future.

## REFERENCES

1. Choo R, Woo T, Assaad D, et al. What is the microscopic tumor extent beyond clinically delineated gross tumor boundary in nonmelanoma skin cancers? *Int J Radiat Oncol Biol Phys.* 2005;62(4):1096–1099.
2. Regaud C, Ferroux R. Discordance des effets des rayons X, d'une part dans la peau, d'autre part dans le testicule par le fractionnement de la dose: diminution de l'efficacité dans la peau, maintien de l'efficacité dans le testicule. *Compt Rend Soc Biol.* 1927;97:431–434.
3. Orton CG, Ellis F. A simplification in the use of the NSD concept in practical radiotherapy. *Br J Radiol.* 1973;46:529–537.
4. Roenigk RK, Ratz JL, Bailin PL, et al. Trends in the presentation and treatment of basal cell carcinomas. *J Dermatol Surg Oncol.* 1986;12:860–865.
5. McCormack CJ, Kelly JW, Dorevitch AP. Differences in age and body site distribution of the histological subtypes of basal cell carcinoma: a possible indicator of differing causes. *Arch Dermatol.* 1997;133:593–596.
6. Thissen MR, Neumann HAM, Berretty PJM, et al. De behandeling van patienten met basalecelcarcinomen door dermatologen in Nederland. *Ned Tijdschr Geneeskd.* 1998;142:1563–1567.
7. Bath-Hextall FJ, Perkins W, Bong J, et al. Interventions for basal cell carcinoma of the skin. *Cochrane Database Syst Rev.* 2007;(1) CD003412.
8. Avril MF, Auperin A, Margulis A, et al. Basal cell carcinoma of the face: surgery or radiotherapy? Results of a randomized study. *Br J Cancer.* 1997;76:100–106.
9. Petit JY, Avril MF, Margulis A, et al. Evaluation of cosmetic results of a randomized trial comparing surgery and radiotherapy in the treatment of basal cell carcinoma of the face. *Plast Reconstr Surg.* 2000;105:2544–2551.
10. Chan S, Dhadda AS, Swindell R. Single fraction radiotherapy for small superficial carcinoma of the skin. *Clin Oncol (R Coll Radiol).* 2007;19(4):256–259.
11. Solan MJ, Brady LW, Binnick SA, et al. Skin. In: Perez CA, Brady LW, eds. Principles and Practice of Radiation Oncology. 3rd ed. Philadelphia, PA: Lippincott-Raven; 1997:723–744.
12. Silverman MK, Kopf AW, Grin CM, et al. Recurrence rates of treated basal cell carcinomas, Part 4: X-ray therapy. *J Dermatol Surg Oncol.* 1992;18(7):549–554.
13. Petrovich Z, Kuisk H, Langholz B, et al. Treatment results and patterns of failure in 646 patients with carcinoma of the eyelids, pinna, and nose. *Am J Surg.* 1987;154(4):447–450.
14. Schulte KW, Lippold A, Auras C, et al. Soft x-ray therapy for cutaneous basal cell and squamous cell carcinomas. *J Am Acad Dermatol.* 2005;53(6):993–1001.
15. Zagrodnik B, Kempf W, Seifert B, et al. Superficial radiotherapy for patients with basal cell carcinoma: recurrence rates, histologic subtypes, and expression of p53 and Bcl-2. *Cancer.* 2003;98(12):2708–2714.
16. Lovett RD, Perez CA, Shapiro SJ, et al. External irradiation of epithelial skin cancer. *Int J Radiat Oncol Biol Phys.* 1990;19(2):235–242.
17. Caccialanza M, Piccinno R, Percivalle S, et al. Radiotherapy of carcinomas of the skin overlying the cartilage of the nose: our experience in 671 lesions. *Eur Acad Dermatol Venereol.* 2009;23(9):1044–1049.
18. Tsao MN, Tsang RW, Liu FF, et al. Radiotherapy management for squamous cell carcinoma of the nasal skin: the Princess Margaret Hospital experience. *Int J Radiat Oncol Biol Phys.* 2002;52(4):973–979.
19. Silva JJ, Tsang RW, Panzarella T, et al. Results of radiotherapy for epithelial skin cancer of the pinna: the Princess Margaret Hospital experience, 1982-1993. *Int J Radiat Oncol Biol Phys.* 2000;47(2):451–459.
20. Brennan D, Young CM, Hopewell JW, et al. The effects of varied numbers of dose fractions on the tolerance of normal human skin. *Clin Radiol.* 1976;27(1):27–32.
21. Cooper JS. Patients' perceptions of their cosmetic appearance more than ten years after radiotherapy for basal cell carcinoma. *Radiat Med.* 1988;6:285–288.
22. Locke J, Karimpour S, Young G, et al. Radiotherapy for epithelial skin cancer. *Int J Radiat Oncol Biol Phys.* 2001;51(3):748–755.
23. Olschewski T, Bajor K, Lang B, et al. Radiotherapy of basal cell carcinoma of the face and head: importance of low dose per fraction on long-term outcome. *J Dtsch Dermatol Ges.* 2006;4(2):124–130.
24. Garcia-Serra A, Hinerman RW, Mendenhall WM, et al. Carcinoma of the skin with perineural invasion. *Head Neck.* 2003;25(12):1027–1033.
25. Jambusaria-Pahlajani A, Miller CJ, Quon H, et al. Surgical monotherapy versus surgery plus adjuvant radiotherapy in high-risk cutaneous squamous cell carcinoma: a systematic review of outcomes. *Dermatol Surg.* 2009;35(4):574–585.
26. Han A, Ratner D. What is the role of adjuvant radiotherapy in the treatment of cutaneous squamous cell carcinoma with perineural invasion? *Cancer.* 2007;109(6):1053–1059.
27. Galloway TJ, Morris CG, Mancuso AA, et al. Impact of radiographic findings on prognosis for skin carcinoma with clinical perineural invasion. *Cancer.* 2005;103(6):1254–1257.
28. Ríos-Buceta L. Management of basal cell carcinomas with positive margins. *Actas Dermosifiliogr.* 2007;98(10):679–687.
29. Liu FF, Maki E, Warde P, et al. A management approach to incompletely excised basal cell carcinomas of skin. *Int J Radiat Oncol Biol Phys.* 1991;20(3):423–428.
30. Caccialanza M, Piccinno R, Grammatica A. Radiotherapy of recurrent basal and squamous cell skin carcinomas: a study of 249 re-treated carcinomas in 229 patients. *Eur J Dermatol.* 2001;11(1):25–28.
31. Kwan W, Wilson D, Moravan V. Radiotherapy for locally advanced basal cell and squamous cell carcinomas of the skin. *Int J Radiat Oncol Biol Phys.* 2004;60(2):406–411.
32. Habermalz HI, Fischer JJ. Radiation therapy of malignant melanoma. *Cancer.* 1976;38:2258–2262.
33. Sause WT, Cooper JS, Rush S, et al. Fraction size in external beam radiation therapy in the treatment of melanoma. *Int J Radiat Oncol Biol Phys.* 1991;20:429–432.
34. Harwood AR, Cummings B. Radiotherapy for malignant melanoma: a re-appraisal. *Cancer Treat Rev.* 1981;8:271–282.
35. Panizzon RG. Die Roentgenweichstrahlentherapie als Alternative bei alteren Patienten. In: Burg G, Hartmann AA, Konz B, eds. *Onkologische Dermatologie. Fortschritte der dermatologischen und onkologischen dermatologie, BAND 7.* Heidelberg: Springer; 1992:263–267.
36. Harwood AR, Dancuart F, Fitzpatrick P, et al. Radiotherapy in nonlentiginous melanoma of the head and neck. *Cancer.* 1981;48:2599–2605.
37. Garbe C, Hauschild A, Volkenandt M, et al. Evidence and interdisciplinary consensus-based German guidelines: surgical treatment and radiotherapy of melanoma. *Melanoma Res.* 2008;18(1):61–67.
38. Lee RJ, Gibbs JF, Proulx GM, et al. Nodal basin recurrence following lymph node dissection for melanoma: implications for adjuvant radiotherapy. *Int J Radiat Oncol Biol Phys.* 2000;46(2):467–474.
39. Ang KK, Peters LJ, Weber RS, et al. Postoperative radiotherapy for cutaneous melanoma of the head and neck region. *Int J Radiat Oncol Biol Phys.* 1994;30(4):795–798.
40. O'Brien CJ, Petersen-Schaefer K, Stevens GN, et al. Adjuvant radiotherapy following neck dissection and parotidectomy for metastatic malignant melanoma. *Head Neck.* 1997;19(7):589–594.
41. Corry J, Smith JG, Bishop M, et al. Nodal radiation therapy for metastatic melanoma. *Int J Radiat Oncol Biol Phys.* 1999;44(5):1065–1069.
42. Cooper JS, Chang WS, Oratz R, et al. Elective radiation therapy for local-regional control of resected high-risk malignant melanomas. *Cancer J.* 2001;7:498–502.
43. Henderson MA, Burmeister B, Thompson JF, et al. *Adjuvant radiotherapy and regional lymph node field control in melanoma patients after lymphadenectomy: results of an intergroup randomized trial (ANZMTG 01.02/TROG 02.01) ASCO Meeting Abstracts 27: LBA9084.* ASCO; 2009.
44. Stein ME, Lachter J, Spencer D, et al. Variants of Kaposi's sarcoma in Southern Africa. A retrospective analysis (1980–1992). *Acta Oncol.* 1996;35(2):193–199.
45. Fenig E, Brenner B, Rakowsky E, et al. Classic Kaposi sarcoma: experience at Rabin Medical Center in Israel. *Am J Clin Oncol.* 1998;21(5):498–500.
46. Tombolini V, Osti MF, Bonanni A, et al. Radiotherapy in classic Kaposi's sarcoma (CKS): experience of the Institute of Radiology of University 'La Sapienza' of Rome. *Anticancer Res.* 1999;19:4539–4544.
47. Cooper JS. The influence of dose on the long-term control of classic (non-AIDS associated) Kaposi's sarcoma by radiotherapy. *Int J Radiat Oncol Biol Phys.* 1988;15(5):1141–1146.
48. Hauerstock D, Gerstein W, Vuong T. Results of radiation therapy for treatment of classic Kaposi sarcoma. *J Cutan Med Surg.* 2009;13(1):18–21.
49. Stelzer KJ, Griffin TW. A randomized prospective trial of radiation therapy for AIDS-associated Kaposi's sarcoma. *Int J Radiat Oncol Biol Phys.* 1993;27(5):1057–1061.
50. Saran F, Adamietz IA, Mose S, et al. The value of conventionally fractionated radiotherapy in the local treatment of HIV-related Kaposi's sarcoma. *Strahlenther Onkol.* 1995;171(10):594–599.
51. Singh NB, Lakier RH, Donde B. Hypofractionated radiation therapy in the treatment of epidemic Kaposi sarcoma—a prospective randomized trial. *Radiother Oncol.* 2008;88(2):211–216.
52. Harrison M, Harrington KJ, Tomlinson DR, et al. Response and cosmetic outcome of two fractionation regimens for AIDS-related Kaposi's sarcoma. *Radiother Oncol.* 1998;46(1):23–28.
53. de Wit R, Smit WG, Veenhof KH, et al. Palliative radiation therapy for AIDS-associated Kaposi's sarcoma by using a single fraction of 800 cGy. *Radiother Oncol.* 1990;19(2):131–136.

54. Belembaogo E, Kirova Y, Frikha H, et al. Radiotherapy of epidemic Kaposi's sarcoma: the experience of the Henri-Mondor Hospital. *Cancer Radiother*. 1998;2(1):49–52.

55. Kirova YM, Belembaogo E, Frikha H, et al. Radiotherapy in the management of epidemic Kaposi's sarcoma: a retrospective study of 643 cases. *Radiother Oncol*. 1998;46(1):19–22.

56. Conill C, Alsina M, Verger E, et al. Radiation therapy in AIDS-related cutaneous Kaposi's sarcoma. *Dermatology*. 1997;195(1):40–42.

57. Stein ME, Spencer D, Kantor A, et al. Epidemic AIDS-related Kaposi's sarcoma in southern Africa: experience at the Johannesburg General Hospital (1980–1990). *Trans R Soc Trop Med Hyg*. 1994;88(4):434–436.

58. Caccialanza M, Marca S, Piccinno R, et al. Radiotherapy of classic and human immunodeficiency virus-related Kaposi's sarcoma: results in 1482 lesions. *Eur Acad Dermatol Venereol*. 2008;22(3):297–302.

59. Trautinger F, Knobler R, Willemze R, et al. EORTC consensus recommendations for the treatment of mycosis fungoides/Sézary syndrome. *Eur J Cancer*. 2006;42(8):1014–1030.

60. Cotter GW, Baglan RJ, Wasserman TH, et al. Palliative radiation treatment of cutaneous mycosis fungoides – a dose response. *Int J Rad Oncol Biol Phys*. 1983;9:1477–1480.

61. Micaily B, Miyamoto C, Kantor G, et al. Radiotherapy for unilesional mycosis fungoides. *Int J Radiat Oncol Biol Phys*. 1998;42(2):361–364.

62. Wilson LD, Kacinski BM, Jones GW. Local superficial radiotherapy in the management of minimal stage IA cutaneous T-cell lymphoma (mycosis fungoides). *Int J Radiat Oncol Biol Phys*. 1998;40(1):109–115.

63. Jones GW, Kacinski BM, Wilson LD, et al. Total skin electron radiation in the management of mycosis fungoides: consensus of the European Organization for Research and Treatment of Cancer Cutaneous Lymphoma Project Group. *J Am Acad Dermatol*. 2002;47(3):364–370.

64. Senff NJ, Noordijk EM, Kim YH, et al. European Organization for Research and Treatment of Cancer; International Society for Cutaneous Lymphoma. European Organization for Research and Treatment of Cancer and International Society for Cutaneous Lymphoma consensus recommendations for the management of cutaneous B-cell lymphomas. *Blood*. 2008;112(5):1600–1609.

65. Lewis KG, Weinstock MA, Weaver AL, et al. Adjuvant local irradiation for Merkel cell carcinoma. *Arch Dermatol*. 2006;142(6):693–700.

66. Goessling W, McKee P, Mayer R. Merkel cell carcinoma. *J Clin Oncol*. 2002;20(2):588–598.

67. Boyer JD, Zitelli JA, Brodland DG, et al. Local control of primary Merkel cell carcinoma: review of 45 cases treated with Mohs micrographic surgery with and without adjuvant radiation. *J Am Acad Dermatol*. 2002;47(6):885–892.

# Adjuvant Therapy for Cutaneous Melanoma

*Ahmad A. Tarhini, Stergios J. Moschos, and John M. Kirkwood*

## Key Points

- Chemotherapy regimens, non-specific immunostimulants and vaccines alone have failed to show any survival benefit in the adjuvant setting.

- High-dose interferon-α2b is the only approved drug shown to improve relapse-free and overall survival in large multi-institutional randomized controlled trials in melanoma patients with high risk for relapse.

- High-dose interferon-α2b has significant side effects and financial cost, necessitating the identification of subgroups of patients who would likely benefit from treatment.

- Peginterferon alfa-2b has shown relapse-free survival benefits overall but no improvement in overall survival or distant metastasis-free survival (EORTC 18991).

- Ongoing randomized controlled trials are currently investigating standard high-dose interferon-α2b versus CTLA-4 blockade with ipilmumab (US Intergroup E1609) and ipilimumab versus placebo (EORTC 18071).

## INTRODUCTION

### General

The incidence of cutaneous melanoma is increasing at a rate greater than that of any other malignancy. Although it represents the fifth and sixth most common cancer in American men and women, respectively, melanoma affects young members of society who are in their most productive years. For this reason, the cost to society is far greater than that of many other more prevalent solid tumors such as prostatic carcinoma. Treatment of localized, early-stage disease is associated with cure rates of 90% or better. Conversely, in its disseminated form, melanoma is a devastating illness refractory to a wide range of chemotherapy agents and combinations. Melanoma has shown significant benefit from immunotherapy with the prospect for cure in the adjuvant postoperative setting and long-lasting responses that provide a hope for patients with advanced disease.

Surgery remains the cornerstone of treatment for this tumor when it is discovered at local or local-regional stages. To this, systemic therapy has been added in the adjuvant setting, i.e. when all the detectable tumor has been resected. Although adjuvant treatment can theoretically be applied at any stage, it has traditionally been applied to treat patients with American Joint Committee on Cancer (AJCC) stages II and III.

## What stages of disease are appropriately considered 'high risk' for adjuvant treatment?

Along with the search for effective treatments for melanoma over the past two decades, considerable research has been conducted to identify clinical and pathologic features that are prognostic for relapse, metastasis and overall survival (OS). These prognostic factors have been incorporated in the TNM staging system recently revised as the seventh edition of the AJCC staging system (Tables 53.1 and 53.2).[1]

Five independent prognostic factors are correlated with relapse and mortality. Breslow's tumor thickness is the single most important prognostic factor for localized melanoma and has eclipsed the importance of Clark's level of invasion for primary melanoma lesions that are ≤1.0 mm in thickness. Ulceration is the second most important prognostic factor for localized melanoma, defined as absence of intact epidermis overlying a significant portion of melanoma as evaluated in microscopic analysis. Its presence connotes a worse prognosis. In the 7th AJCC edition, the prognostic significance of the mitotic activity (histologically defined as mitoses/mm$^2$) has been recognized as an important primary tumor prognostic factor. The mitotic rate (≥1/mm$^2$) has now replaced the level of invasion as a primary criterion for defining the subcategory of T1b in addition to tumor ulceration. Regional metastases, either in the regional lymph nodes or intra-lymphatic (satellite or in-transit) metastasis, as well as the extent of lymph node tumor burden (i.e. micro- or macro-metastasis), are important predictors of outcome. The number of involved lymph nodes, defined by sentinel lymph node mapping or complete lymphadenectomy, best correlates with 10-year survival and has replaced the size of lymph nodes in the TNM staging system. In the 7th AJCC edition, there is no lower threshold of tumor burden defining the presence of regional nodal metastasis. Specifically, nodal tumor deposits less than 0.2 mm in diameter (previously used as the threshold for defining nodal metastasis) are not ignored in the staging of nodal disease, as a result of the consensus that smaller volumes of metastatic tumor are still clinically significant. Another important addition to the 7th AJCC edition is the criterion that the presence of nodal micrometastases is defined by the presence of any volume of tumor cells observed either by hematoxylin and eosin (H&E) or by immunohistochemical staining (in the 6th edition, only H&E could be used). Finally, the site of distant metastasis, the number of metastatic sites, and the serum lactate dehydrogenase (LDH) level are important prognostic factors for

### Table 53.1   AJCC Melanoma Classification System

| T Classification | Thickness | Ulceration Status |
|---|---|---|
| T1 | ≤1.0 mm | a: Without ulceration and level IV/V<br>b: With ulceration or level IV/V |
| T2 | 1.01–2.0 mm | a: Without ulceration<br>b: With ulceration |
| T3 | 2.01–4.0 mm | a: Without ulceration<br>b: With ulceration |
| T4 | >4.0 mm | a: Without ulceration<br>b: With ulceration |

| N Classification | No. of Metastatic Nodes | Nodal Metastatic Mass |
|---|---|---|
| N1 | 1 node | |
| N2 | 2–3 nodes | |
| N3 | 4 or more metastatic nodes<br>Matted nodes<br>In-transit metastasis(es)/satellite(s) with metastatic node(s) | |

| M Classification | Site | Serum LDH |
|---|---|---|
| M1a | Distant skin, subcutaneous or nodal metastases | Normal |
| M1b | Lung metastases | Normal |
| M1c | All other visceral metastases | Normal |
| | Any distant metastasis | Elevated |

T, tumor; N, node; M, metastasis; LDH, lactate dehydrogenase.

advanced-stage melanoma. These prognostic factors allow clinicians to identify patients at high risk for developing recurrence at local, regional and distant sites who would best benefit from adjuvant therapy.

The AJCC staging system divides patients into four stages depending on whether tumors are only localized to the skin (stage I and II), have regional metastases (to lymph nodes or satellite or in-transit intralymphatic sites, stage III), or have distant metastatic disease (stage IV). Subgroups are based on the interplay of the above-described prognostic factors and reflect the prognostic heterogeneity of patients with the same tumor. Traditionally, the high-risk group is described as subjects with primary deep melanomas (T4 N0 M0) or stage III disease, whereas the intermediate-risk group includes patients with melanoma thickness >1.0 mm.

## PRIOR APPROACHES

Table 53.3 lists the most important randomized controlled trials (RCTs) performed for intermediate- and high-risk cutaneous melanoma that have tested non-interferon-based

regimens in an adjuvant setting.[2-22] Chemotherapy as a single agent, in combination with other chemotherapeutic agents, hormones, or biologics, except under special settings (isolated limb perfusion), have not improved disease-free survival (DFS) or overall survival (OS) significantly in any reported prospective randomized multicenter studies to date. Single-center studies that have not utilized the current accepted rigorous standards of concurrent randomized comparators have suggested that adjuvant therapy with vindesine has benefit in stage III melanoma.[23] However, these results have not been reproduced in RCTs. Following early suggestion of benefit from small single-institution non-randomized trials, negative results were also obtained using megestrol acetate, vitamin A, and non-specific immunostimulants such as BCG, *Corynebacterium parvum*, or transfer factor.

Melanoma vaccines have been extensively investigated for more than three decades and are presented in greater detail elsewhere in this textbook (Chapter 54).[24] Morton and co-workers were among the earliest to use this approach to treat patients after surgery. Several of those vaccines that have shown some benefit in the adjuvant setting are (Table 53.3): (a) a polyvalent vaccine derived from three allogeneic melanoma cell lines which all together express more than 20 common melanoma-associated antigens studied by Morton; (b) a polyvalent, shed antigen prepared from material shed into culture medium by four melanoma cells studied by Bystryn; (c) a tumor cell vaccine derived from two cultured cell lines expressing HLA class I (HLA-A2, C3, B4) that has been recently evaluated in the cooperative groups with benefit in patients expressing these alleles and initially developed by Mitchell; and (d) vaccinia viral lysates of a single allogeneic melanoma cell line. Several large prospective RCTs of vaccination have failed to demonstrate significant benefit using vaccinia viral melanoma lysate.[17-19] Two trials showed a benefit only in subsets of patients defined by expression of a limited number of HLA alleles[16] or antibody production.[20] One small trial of vaccination with shed antigens of culture melanoma has been promising[21] but this requires further evaluation in a larger appropriately powered study.

Morton's studies of vaccination with a polyvalent vaccine, known commercially as Canvaxin®, in stage III melanoma patients was evaluated in a retrospective study. The suggestion of improvement in OS[25] was subsequently tested in a phase III RCT for resected stage III or IV melanoma, where adjuvant Canvaxin failed to improve either relapse-free or overall survival compared with BCG.[22] As more knowledge is accumulated in relation to the basic cancer biology and host immunology, and with the advent of adoptive transfer of immune cells including engineered T cells and primed matured dendritic cells, with an understanding of the constraints and obstacles to vaccination, this approach will likely achieve more meaningful immune responses and may rationally be combined with biological therapy tailored to the specific immunophenotype of the host.

## PRESENT CONCEPTS

### Interferons

In their research to explain the molecular mechanisms of viral 'interference', namely a protective effect against subsequent viral infection in cells previously infected by another

## Table 53.2 Staging Groups for Cutaneous Melanoma

| | Clinical Staging | | | Pathologic Staging | | |
|---|---|---|---|---|---|---|
| | T | N | M | T | N | M |
| 0 | Tis | N0 | M0 | Tis | N0 | M0 |
| IA | T1a | N0 | M0 | T1a | N0 | M0 |
| IB | T1b | N0 | M0 | T1b | N0 | M0 |
| | T2a | N0 | M0 | T2a | N0 | M0 |
| IIA | T2b | N0 | M0 | T2b | N0 | M0 |
| | T3a | N0 | M0 | T3a | N0 | M0 |
| IIB | T3b | N0 | M0 | T3b | N0 | M0 |
| | T4a | N0 | M0 | T4a | N0 | M0 |
| IIC | T4b | N0 | M0 | T4b | N0 | M0 |
| III | Any T | N1 N2 N3 | M0 | | | |
| IIIA | | | | T1–4a | N1a | M0 |
| | | | | T1–4a | N2a | M0 |
| IIIB | | | | T1–4a | N1a | M0 |
| | | | | T1–4a | N2a | M0 |
| | | | | T1–4a | N1b | M0 |
| | | | | T1–4a | N2b | M0 |
| | | | | T1–4a/b | N2c | M0 |
| IIIC | | | | T1–4b | N1b | M0 |
| | | | | T1–4b | N2b | M0 |
| | | | | Any T | N3 | M0 |
| IV | Any T | Any N | Any M1 | Any T | Any N | Any M1 |

is, in situ.

## Table 53.3 Most Important Randomized Controlled Trials of Adjuvant Non-IFN-Based Therapy of Cutaneous Melanoma

| Study Reference | Enrolled Patients (N) | Stage | Treatment Arms | Average Follow-up (Years) | Comments |
|---|---|---|---|---|---|
| **1. Chemotherapy** | | | | | |
| Veronesi 1982[2] | 931 | II III | DTIC BCG DTIC + BCG Observation | 5 | NS |
| Lejeune 1988[3] | 325 | I IIA IIB | DTIC Levamisole Placebo | 4 | NS |
| Fisher 1981[4] | 181 | II III | CCNU Observation | 3 | NS |
| Koops 1998[5] | 832 | II III | Isolated limb perfusion + hyperthermia Observation | 6.4 | BS |
| Meisenberg 1993[6] | 39 | III | Autologous bone marrow transplant Observation | NA | NS |

**Table 53.3 Most important Randomized Controlled Trials of Adjuvant Non-IFN-Based Therapy of Cutaneous Melanoma—cont'd**

| **2. Vitamins, Hormones** | | | | | |
|---|---|---|---|---|---|
| Meyskens 1994[7] | 248 | II III | Vitamin A Observation | 8 | NS |
| Markovic 2002[8] | 262 | IIB III | Megestrol Observation | 4.5 min | NS |
| **3. Non-Specific Immunostimulants** | | | | | |
| Czarnetzki 1993[9] | 353 | II | BCG (RIV) BCG (Pasteur) Observation | 6 | NS |
| Paterson 1984[10] | 199 | I II | BCG Observation | 4 | NS |
| Balch 1982[11] | 260 | I II | Corynebacterium parvum Observation | 2 | NS |
| Lipton 1991[12] | 262 | III | Corynebacterium parvum BCG | 4–9 | BS |
| Quirt 1991[13] | 577 | I IIA IIB III | Levamisole BCG BCG + levamisole Observation | 8 | NS |
| Spitler 1991[14] | 216 | I IIA IIB III IV | Levamisole Placebo | 10 | NS |
| Miller 1988[15] | 168 | II III | Transfer factor Observation | 2 | NS |
| **4. Vaccines** | | | | | |
| Sondak 2002[16] | 689 | IIA | Melacine with DETOX Observation | 5.6 | NS |
| Hershey 2002[17] | 700 | IIB | Vaccinia melanoma cell lysate Placebo | 8 | Trend on RFS/OS |
| Wallack 1998[18] | 250 | III | Vaccinia melanoma oncolysate Placebo | 3 | NS |
| Wallack 1995[19] | 250 | II | Virus allogeneic polyvalent melanoma cell lysate | 2.5 min | NS |
| Livingston 1994[20] | 123 | III | GM2–BCG–Cytoxan BCG alone–Cytoxan | 5 | NS |
| Bystryn 2001[21] | 38 | III | Polyvalent shed antigen Placebo | 2.5 | S |
| Morton 2007[22] | 1656 | III/IV | Allogeneic melanoma vaccine BCG | NA | NS |

DITC, dacarbazine; BCG, Bacille Calmette-Guerin; min, minimal duration of follow-up; NS, not statistically significant; S, statistically significant; NA, not available; BS, borderline significance; RFS, relapse-free survival; OS, overall survival; GM2, ganglioside GM2.

virus, Isaacs and Lindenmann discovered interferon (IFN). IFN is not a single molecule but a family of distinct proteins, many of which are structurally related and produced by most eukaryotic cell types. In the early 1970s, it became known that IFN does not only have antiviral but also antitumor activity. Its use in the clinic became possible in the early 1980s when the gene was cloned and therefore became commercially available.[26]

## Biology and proposed mechanisms of antitumor activity of type I IFNs

IFNs are classified as types I and II according to their structural and functional properties. The sole member of the type II family is IFN-γ, but there are multiple members of the type I IFN class, which is divided into IFN-α, IFN-β, IFN-ε, IFN-κ, IFN-λ and IFN-ω (Table 53.4). More distantly

**Table 53.4  The Interferon Species**

| Interferon Type | | Chromosome locus | Source | Subtypes | Receptor |
|---|---|---|---|---|---|
| I | α | 9p21 | Leukocytes | 13 | IFN-αβR |
| | β | | Fibroblasts | 1 | |
| | ε | | Brain, lung, kidney, small intestine | 1 | |
| | κ | | Keratinocytes | 1 | |
| | ω | | Leukocytes | 1 | |
| I/IL-10 | λ | 19q13 | ? | 3 | IFN-λR |
| II | γ | 12q24 | T cells, NK cells | 1 | IFN-γR |

IL, interleukin; NK, natural killer.

related molecules, such as limitin, also signal through the type I IFN receptor. In humans, excluding pseudo genes, there are 13 non-allelic IFN-α genes and a single IFN-β, IFN-ε, IFN-κ, and IFN-ω gene. In the clinic, IFN-α2 has been the most extensively evaluated agent, three subspecies of which are commercially available: IFN-α2a (Roferon-A, Roche Pharmaceuticals, Nutley, NJ), IFN-α2b (Intron A, Schering Plough, Kenilworth, NJ), and IFN-α2c (Boehringer/Ingelheim, Ingelheim, Germany). Type I IFNs interact with the same receptor and signal through distinct but related pathways to those used by IFN-γ.[27]

Type I IFNs are highly pleiotropic cytokines with potent immunoregulatory, antiproliferative, differentiation-inducing, apoptotic, and antiangiogenic properties.[28] While most cells of the body are capable of secreting IFNs, IFN-α is secreted in large amounts only by a rare type of blood cell, the plasmacytoid dendritic cell precursor, in response to infectious and other stimuli. Type I IFNs connect innate and adaptive immunity (Fig. 53.1).[29] The importance of these natural IFN-producing cells in tumor immunity is suggested by their increased migration to the primary tumor site.[30] In addition, the role of basal and/or tumor-induced production of type I IFNs in the host-mediated inhibition of tumor growth has been shown in early animal studies with antibodies specific for murine type I IFNs.[31] IFNs may indirectly affect tumor growth by inhibiting angiogenesis through several mechanisms.[32] Their direct effects on tumor cells are pleiotropic: they may induce cell cycle arrest that may be necessary for completion of differentiation,[33] or the induction of apoptosis.[34]

## Adjuvant IFN for cutaneous melanoma – phase I and II trials to optimize the route, dose, and toxicity profile

A multitude of IFN-α regimens testing a variety of forms of non-recombinant and recombinant DNA-produced IFN-α in melanoma and other cancers have been reported. Maximum tolerated daily dose depends on the schedule and route, but differs little with the IFN-α subspecies. Subcutaneous (s.c.) administration results in persistence of measurable levels of IFN-α2b after 24 hours, but peak serum

levels are relatively low, whereas intravenous (i.v.) administration leads to significantly higher peak levels in a dose-dependent fashion, and intramuscular (i.m.) administration has an intermediate pharmacokinetic profile (Fig. 53.2).[35] Cumulative increases of serum IFN-α2b levels over time may account for the better tolerance and toxicity profile of therapy administered by the i.v. as compared with the s.c. route, mandating alternate-day dosing for the s.c. administration of recombinant IFN-α. More recently, the coupling of IFN-α with polyethylene glycol (PEG) has yielded a formulation that requires administration only weekly.

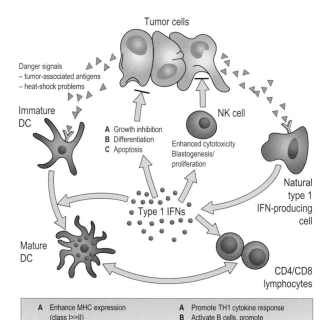

**Figure 53.1** Immunomodulatory effects of interferons. Type I interferons (IFNs) belong to a group of cytokines (such as GM-CSF, IL-12, etc.) important for immunosurveillance and provide a link between innate and adaptive immunity. NK, natural killer; DC, dendritic cell; TH, T-helper cell; MHC, major histocompatibility complex; GM-CSF, granulocyte–monocyte colony-stimulating factor; IL, interleukin.

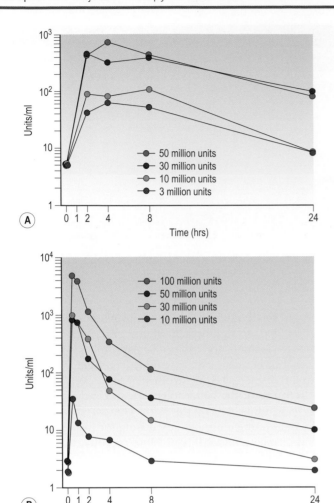

**Figure 53.2** Pharmacokinetics of IFN-α2 according to route of administration: (a) intramuscular and (b) intravenous dosage in 33 patients.[35]

A number of phase II trials of IFN-α in metastatic melanoma have attempted to identify the optimal dose and treatment duration with an acceptable toxicity and optimal response rate (Table 53.5).[36–44] The studies differ in terms of the IFN-α subspecies used, the dosing, the route of administration and the scheduling. Although the number of patients was small, meaningful regressions were reported in approximately 15% overall. Response rates varied with the burden of tumor, and were higher in patients with smaller disease, indicating that the most effective results might be seen in patients with microscopic disease (adjuvant therapy).

High-dose IFN-α2b with an intravenous induction phase is the only adjuvant therapy that has demonstrated durable effects on melanoma relapse and an impact upon survival to date. Table 53.6 shows the IFN-α regimens that have been evaluated for patients with a high risk for relapse.[45–56] The regimens are diverse in terms of IFN-α subspecies used, dosing, route of administration, and duration of therapy. The trials are summarized based on high-, intermediate-, and low-dose regimens.

High-dose IFN-α regimens are of two types: one, evaluated by the Eastern Cooperative Group (ECOG) and US Intergroup, comprises an induction phase consisting of

1 month of daily i.v. bolus IFN-α2b, followed by a prolonged (11-month) maintenance with lower doses that approach the maximum tolerable dosage given s.c.[45–47] The other is a regimen evaluated in a single trial conducted by the North Central Cancer Treatment Group (NCCTG) utilizing a high dose of IFN-α2a administered i.m. three times weekly for 12 weeks.[48]

The E1684 trial was the first RCT that showed a significant prolongation in DFS and OS in patients with deep primary tumor (>4 mm, T4 N0 M0), or the presence of regional lymph node metastases (Tx N1–3 M0, AJCC stage III).[45] In-transit, satellite, or extracapsular spread of disease was excluded and all patients had pathologic staging of regional lymph nodes before enrollment. Patients were assigned either to the treatment arm group – which received IFN-α2b 20 MU/m² i.v. 5 days per week for 4 weeks, followed by 10MU/m² s.c. 3 days per week for 48 weeks – or to the observation group. After a median follow-up time of more than 6.9 years, the estimated 5-year relapse-free survival (RFS) rate in the IFN-α2b-treated group was 37% (95% confidence interval [CI] 30–46%) versus 26% in the observation group (95% CI, 19–34%), whereas the 5-year OS in the IFN-α2b-treated group was 46% (95% CI, 39–55%) versus 37% in the observation arm (95% CI, 30–46%). Although the patients with deep primary, node-negative melanoma were underrepresented (11% of the overall accrual of patients), it appeared that the node-positive patients benefited the most from IFN-α2b therapy, the impact of which was manifested early in the first year of treatment. The results of this pivotal trial led the United States Food and Drug Administration (FDA) to approve the above regimen as the standard of care for adjuvant therapy of high-risk melanoma patients.

The substantial toxicities associated with high-dose i.v. IFN-α2b and the joint discussion of alternatives with the World Health Organization (WHO) led to the parallel evaluation of low-dose IFN-α2a and IFN-α2b (3 MU s.c. three times a week). The WHO Trial 16 of low-dose IFN-α2a versus observation was initially reported as effective,[57] but later, at maturity, no significant differences remained in RFS or OS.[51]

ECOG intergroup trial E1690 compared the benefit of the E1684 high-dose, 1-year regimen as well as the low-dose regimen of IFN-α2b at 3 million units s.c. three times a week for 2 years versus observation.[46] High risk for relapse was defined in the WHO trial as the presence of nodal disease whereas in the E1690 trial it was defined as lymph node involvement, detected clinically or pathologically at elective lymph node dissection, or deep (>4 mm) primary lesions without clinically or pathologically defined nodal disease (as in E1684). In E1690, patients were spared the need for pathologic staging of regional nodes if there was no clinical evidence of node metastasis and the primary tumor was at least 4 mm deep (T4, stage IIB). Also in E1690, 75% of patients had stage III disease, and 25% had deep primary disease without pathologically staged regional lymph node involvement – more than double the fraction of patients with this stage of disease that entered the E1684 trial. E1690 was unblinded by the external data monitoring committee before reaching the planned number of events because of the improved OS of groups in this study and the low projected likelihood that the survival results would differ

Table 53.5 Phase II Clinical Trials of IFN-α Evaluating Treatment Schedules for Metastatic Melanoma

| Study Reference | Enrolled No. Patients | IFN-α Subspecies | Dose Range (MU/m²) | Schedule | Route | Overall Response Rate | CR | PR |
|---|---|---|---|---|---|---|---|---|
| Ernstoff 1983[36] | 17 | 2b | 10–100 | qd (5 d/week, × 4 weeks) | i.v. | | | 2 |
| Creagan 1984[37] | 23 | 2a | 50 | q2d (3×/week, × 3 months) | i.m. | 20 | 1 | 5 |
| Creagan 1985[38] | 35 | 2a + cimetidine | 50 | q2d (3×/week, × 12 weeks) | i.m. | 23 | 0 | 8 |
| Creagan 1984[39] | 31 | 2a | 12 | t.i.w. × 3 months | i.m. | 23 | 3 | 4 |
| Legha 1987[40] | (a) 35 | 2a | (a) Escalating 3→36, q3d | (a) Induction × 70 d, then maintenance | i.m. | 1 | 0 | 3 |
| | (b) 31 | | (b) Fixed 18 | (b) t.i.w. | | 6 | 0 | 2 |
| Hersey 1985[41] | 20 | 2a | Escalating 15→50 | t.i.w. | i.m. | 10 | 2 | 0 |
| Neefe 1990[42] | 97 | 2a | Escalating 3→36 | 3 MU for 10 d then escalate over 10 d | s.c. | 8 | 6 | 2 |
| Dorval 1986[43] | 22 | 2b | 10 | t.i.w. | | 24 | 2 | 4 |
| Coates 1986[44] | 15 | 2a | 20 | 5 d/week, every 2 weeks | i.v. | 0 | 0 | 0 |

CR, complete remission; PR, partial remission; i.v., intravenously; i.m., intramuscularly; s.c., subcutaneously; d, day; q.d., every day; t.i.w., three times a week; MU, mega units.

**Table 53.6  Phase III Trials of Adjuvant IFN-a Therapy in Patients with Melanoma at Intermediate and High Risk for Relapse**

| Study Reference | Enrolled Patients (n=total) | Stage | Treatment Arm* | Median Follow-up at Reporting (Years) | DFS | OS |
|---|---|---|---|---|---|---|
| **High Dose** | | | | | | |
| Eastern COG-E1684 Kirkwood[45] | 287 | IIB III | IFN-α2b 20 MU/m² i.v. q.d. 5 d/week × 4 weeks then 10 MU/m² s.c. t.i.w. × 48 weeks | 6.9 | S | S |
| Eastern COG-E1690 Kirkwood[46] | 642 | IIB III | IFN-α2b 20 MU/m² i.v. q.d. 5 d/week × 4 weeks then 10 MU/m² s.c. t.i.w. × 48 weeks vs 3 MU t.i.w. for 2 years | 4.3 | NS | S |
| Eastern COG-E1694[†] Kirkwood[47] | 774 | IIB III | IFN-α2b 20 MU/m² i.v. q.d. 5 d/week × 4 weeks then 10 MU/m² s.c. t.i.w. × 48 weeks vs GMK vaccine 1 cm³ s.c. on d 1, 8, 15, 22 q12 weeks (weeks 12 to 96) | 1.3 | S | S |
| NCCTG 83-7052 Creagan[48] | 262 | IIB III | IFN-α2a 20 MU/m² i.m. q.d. for 3 months | 6.1 | NS | NS |
| **Intermediate Dose** | | | | | | |
| EORTC 18952 Eggermont[49] | 1318 | IIB III | IFN-α2b 10 MU s.c. 5 d/week × 4 weeks then 10 MU s.c. t.i.w. for 1 year vs | 4.65 | NS | NS |
| | | | IFN-α2b 10 MU s.c. 5 d/week × 4 weeks then 5 MU s.c. t.i.w. for 2 years | | –/+ | NS |
| EORTC 18991 Eggermont[50] | 1256 | III | Peg-IFN-α2b s.c. 6 µg/kg/week (8 weeks) then 3 µg/kg/week (5 years) | 3.8 | S | NS |
| **Low Dose** | | | | | | |
| WHO-16 Cascinelli[51] | 444 | III | IFN-α2a 3 MU s.c. t.i.w. for 3 years | 7.3 | NS | NS |
| AIM HIGH (UKCCCR) Hancock[52] | 674 | IIB III | IFN-α2a 3 MU s.c. t.i.w. for 2 years | 3.1 | NS | NS |
| EORTC 18871/ DKG-80 Kleeberg[53] | 830 | IIB III | IFN-α2b 1 MU s.c. alternate days, for 1 year vs | 8.2 | NS | NS |
| | | | IFN-γ 0.2 mg s.c. alternate days for 1 year vs | | NS | NS |
| | | | Iscador M◊ | | NS | NS |
| Scottish Melanoma COG Cameron[54] | 96 | II III | IFN-α2b 3 MU s.c. t.i.w. for 6 months | 6.5 | NS | NS |
| Austrian Melanoma COG Pehamberger[55] | 311 | II | IFN-α2a 3 MU s.c. q.d. for 3 weeks then 3 MU s.c. t.i.w. for 1 year | 3.4 (mean) | –/+ | NS |
| French Melanoma COG Grob[56] | 499 | II | IFN-α2a 3 MU s.c. t.i.w. for 18 months | 5 | –/+ | NS |

COG, cooperative group; WHO, World Health Organization; EORTC, European Organization for Research and Treatment of Cancer; UKCCCR, United Kingdom Committee for Cancer Research; NCCTG, North Central Cancer Treatment Group; DKG, German Cancer Society; Iscador M◊, a mistletoe extract (placebo); MU, million units; i.v., intravenously; s.c., subcutaneously; d, day; q.d., every day; t.i.w., three times a week; DFS, disease-free survival; OS, overall survival; S, statistically significant; NS, non-significant; GMK, ganglioside GM2 coupled to keyhole limpet hemocyanin (KLH).

*All clinical trials also include an observation arm, except the ECOG trial E1694.

†Statistical comparisons with the GMK vaccine

to the extent that had originally been stipulated for either treatment. Thus, at a median follow-up of 4.3 years, and in an intention-to-treat analysis, the 5-year estimated RFS rate of those treated with high-dose IFN was significantly better than that of the observation group (44% vs 35%, P 2 =0.05 log-rank test) but the 5-year OS estimates were similar for all three groups (52% high dose vs 53% low dose vs 55% observation). Subset analysis reached statistical significance for relapse-free benefit for patients with two or three positive lymph nodes, but not in other groups. The low-dose arm had no significant relapse-interval or survival benefit.

The unexpected differences between results of high-dose IFN-α2b in the E1690 trial and the E1684 trial were explained in part on the basis of the overall improvements observed between E1684 and E1690 for RFS and OS outcomes – where the patients on the observation arms of the E1690 and E1684 clinical trials differed at a significance level of $P=0.001$. When evaluated in terms of RFS, the improvement in 5-year RFS was 35% versus 26%, and 5-year OS 54% versus 37%, respectively, for observation (Fig. 53.3).

The demographic analysis of these studies reveals that the E1690 trial recruited more patients with T4N0 disease (25%) and a smaller proportion of relapsed patients than the prior E1684 trial. Of potentially greater significance, as the US FDA approved high-dose IFN for the treatment of high-risk melanoma in 1995, many of the patients assigned to the observation arm of E1690 had the opportunity to 'cross over' to receive IFN-α2b high-dose therapy as a 'salvage' regimen outside the trial when relapse occurred. This opportunity did not exist for patients in the earlier E1684 trial. Finally, the large fraction of patients who entered E1690 with deep T4 primary tumors and were not surgically staged with lymphadenectomy, presented the frequent scenario of nodal relapse in previously undissected regional nodes, coupled with the advent of a therapy for this (IFN-α2b) that was the tested agent in the E1690 trial. Post-hoc analysis of the actual crossover frequency in fact demonstrated a significant and asymmetrical delivery of IFN-α2b therapy for patients who were assigned to observation in E1690, at relapse. Thus, the use of IFN in post-protocol therapy for patients who entered the study in high numbers with deep primary melanoma and relapsed thereafter may have confounded the detection of an OS benefit without significantly affecting the DFS impact in this trial.

The subsequent E1694 trial[47] tested a vaccine that had shown a trend toward relapse-interval benefit in a single-institution phase III study at Memorial Sloan Kettering Cancer Center (MSKCC). It was undertaken to develop a therapy that would be superior to high-dose IFN-α2b treatment. This study was the first in which high-dose IFN-α2b treatment was taken as the standard of adjuvant therapy against which new options were tested. Thus, this trial also had the capacity to resolve the controversy regarding the benefit of high-dose IFN-α2b on OS which arose following the E1690 trial.[47]

The GMK vaccine consists of the purified ganglioside GM2 coupled to keyhole limpet hemocyanin (KLH) and combined with the new and more potent QS-21 adjuvant, piloted at MSKCC by Livingston.[58] This modified GM2 regimen induced more consistent high-titered IgM and IgG antibodies than the original GM2-BCG vaccine that had previously improved RFS in stage III melanoma at MSKCC. An important observation in the first trial was that patients who produced IgM anti-GM2 antibodies benefited most from the vaccine, affording an intermediate endpoint for the E1694 phase III multicenter trial.[59] It was felt to be ethically difficult to continue with an observation arm, given the well-publicized E1684 data and despite the question interjected by the subsequent E1690 results. Eligible patients for E1694 had either deep primary tumors (>4.0 mm) without clinical evidence of lymph node metastasis (T4 N0 M0, AJCC stage IIB), based on clinical or pathologic grounds, or nodal metastatic disease, after completion of lymphadenectomy (T1–4 N1–2 M0, AJCC stage III).

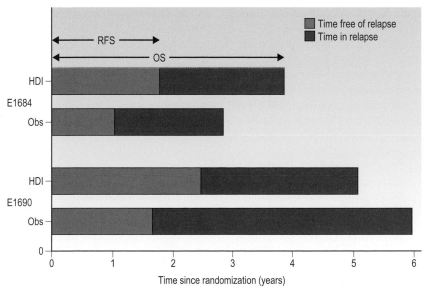

**Figure 53.3** Relapse-free (RFS) and overall survival (OS) benefits of high-dose IFN-α2b (HDI) versus observation (Obs) demonstrated in each of the ECOG trials E1684, E1690 and E1694.

This trial was unblinded after a median follow-up of 1.3 years by the external data safety and monitoring committee when the interim analysis revealed the superiority of high-dose IFN-α2b in terms of both RFS (hazard ratio [HR] 1.47 [95% CI, 1.14–1.90]) and OS (HR 1.52 [95% CI, 1.07–2.15]). These results demonstrated a 33% lower relapse and death rate for IFN-α2b, compared with the GMK vaccine. Despite the absence of an observation arm, E1694 has served as powerful confirmation of the original E1684 results.

One of the concerns in this trial is whether the GMK vaccine adversely influenced outcome, making high-dose IFN-α2b appear effective artefactually. The antibody responses induced by the GMK vaccine have been analyzed to address this question, as all vaccine recipients were serially monitored for the induction of anti-GM2 antibody responses. The results showed that patients who developed antibody response by day 29 demonstrated a trend to OS benefit (P=0.06), making it highly unlikely that the vaccine adversely influenced outcome. In addition, the vaccine arm outcome for E1694 was similar to, or slightly better than, the observation arm of the immediate preceding intergroup trial with identical entry criteria, E1690. On the other hand, an interim analysis of a phase III trial (EORTC 18961) of adjuvant GMK vaccination versus observation after resection of the primary in AJCC stage II (T3–4 N0 M0) melanoma patients was recently reported after the criteria for stopping for futility were met for the primary endpoint.[60] For OS, the results suggested a detrimental effect of the vaccine. However, this trial is still early in its follow-up and longer follow-up is important to more accurately interpret this finding.

The analysis of the three foregoing high-dose IFN-α2b studies (E1684, E1690, E1694) has been updated in a pooled analysis of survival and relapse-free outcomes to April 2001.[61] Analysis of treatment effects versus observation was based on data from 713 patients randomized to high-dose IFN-α2b (HDI) or observation in trials E1684 and E1690. The pooled analysis has firmly demonstrated that melanoma relapse has been prevented by IFN to intervals that now exceed 20 years. However, this analysis has not yielded compelling evidence of an impact upon overall survival versus observation despite the positive survival results of two independent randomized US Cooperative Group and Intergroup studies (E1684 and E1694). This may not be surprising, given that the larger of the two observation-controlled trials included in the pooled analysis (E1690) did not show an OS benefit for HDI. As discussed previously, the OS analysis of E1690 has been confounded by the routine occurrence of post-trial crossover to HDI in all but one of the 37 patients assigned to initial observation, after US FDA approval of HDI. This therapy for patients with nodal relapse during the trial was associated with an unusually prolonged post-relapse survival of those patients in the observation arm treated with HDI, which may have been responsible for this outcome variability. Patients treated with HDI in E1694 have not been included in the pooled analysis because the comparator in that trial was the GMK vaccine and not observation as was the case in E1684 and E1690.

A meta-analysis of 12 randomized trials of adjuvant IFN-α2b for high-risk melanoma has confirmed a highly significant reduction in the odds of recurrence in patients treated with IFN compared to observation. The meta-analysis included studies employing multiple IFN-α regimens, which may be categorized as high-dose, intermediate-dose, or low-dose regimens, which have been evaluated as adjuvant therapy for intermediate/high-risk (T3–4, lymph node positive) surgically resected melanoma. The analysis also demonstrated evidence of increased benefit with increasing IFN dose and a trend for improved benefit with increasing total dose. This meta-analysis did not find a statistically significant overall survival benefit for IFN-α2b.[62] However, a larger individual patient data meta-analysis of 13 randomized trials showed a significant though small impact of IFN upon overall survival, but without clarifying whether there is an optimal (high, intermediate or low) dose of IFN.[63] In this latter meta-analysis, there was statistically significant benefit for IFN for both EFS (OR=0.87, CI=0.81–0.93, p=0.00006) and OS (OR=0.9, CI=0.84–0.97, p=0.008). This survival advantage translates into an absolute benefit of about 3% (CI 1%–5%) at 5 years.

## Role of dose, route, and duration of IFN-α therapy in melanoma

Less intensive (less toxic) regimens tested as adjuvant therapy for melanoma have not previously ever demonstrated durable effects upon relapse or death versus what has been seen observed with high-dose IFN-α2b (HDI). These include the very-low-dose IFN (1 MU s.c. every other day) as tested in EORTC 18871 (melanoma stage IIB, III)[53] and low-dose interferon (3 MU s.c. three times per week) as tested in WHO Trial 16 (stage III),[51] ECOG 1690 (T4, N1),[46] UKCCR AIM-High trial (T4 N1),[52] and the Scottish trial.[54] These also include intermediate-dose interferon regimens (given s.c.) tested in EORTC 18952 (T4 N1–2)[49] and EORTC 18961 (Tx N1).[60]

The Hellenic Oncology Group conducted a randomized phase III trial (N=364) to evaluate a modification of the E1684 high-dose regimen of IFN-α2b in which the intravenous component (15 MU/m² 5 days a week) given for 4 weeks was compared with the same intravenous component followed by 11 months of modified maintenance subcutaneous therapy (10 MU/day 3 days a week).[64] The study design proposed that the 1-month treatment would be considered at least as good as the 1-year regimen if the relapse rate at 3 years from study entry were at most 15% higher in the former arm. A sample size of 152 (182 enrolled) patients per treatment arm was planned. The trial concluded that at the 5% level of significance the 3-year relapse rate of the 1-month group was not 15% higher than that of the 1-year group. There were also no significant differences in OS, DFS or severe toxicities between the arms. In interpreting this study's results, it is important to remark on a number of factors. First, the study adopted a modification of the original E1684 high-dose IFN regimen in which only three-quarters of the established dosage was used for IFN induction for 1 month (15 MU/m²) followed by a modification of the maintenance regimen in which 10 MU/dose rather than 10 MU/m²/dose was administered for the balance of 1 year. The investigational study arm of 1 month would have been termed as non-inferior if it were associated with 15% lower 3-year RFS/OS. Beyond this, in the absence of an observation control it is not certain what level of activity was achieved by either arm of this study. By comparison, a US cooperative group proposal to test equivalence of 1 month and 1 year (with a 5% threshold for declaring inferiority) was designed and abandoned when it became apparent that it would have required 3000 patients.

The Sunbelt Melanoma Trial was designed to evaluate the role of high-dose IFN-α2b or completion lymph node dissection (CLND) in patients with melanoma staged by sentinel lymph node (SLN) biopsy. Eligible patients with primary melanoma of ≥1.0 mm Breslow thickness underwent SLN biopsy. In Protocol A of this complex study, patients with a single tumor-positive lymph node after SLN biopsy and CLND were randomized to observation (N= 112) versus high-dose IFN (20 MU/m$^2$/day i.v. for 4 weeks followed by 10 MU/m$^2$ s.c. three times a week for 48 weeks; N=106). In Protocol B, patients with tumor-negative SLN by standard histopathology and immunohistochemistry underwent investigational molecular staging of the SLN by reverse transcriptase polymerase chain reaction (RT-PCR) to detect melanoma-specific mRNA (tyrosinase, MART 1, MAGE 3, gp100); patients with RT-PCR-positive SLN were randomized to observation (N=108) versus CLND (N=192) versus CLND + IFN (20 MU/m$^2$/day i.v. for 4 weeks only) (N=184). With the small numbers of subjects enrolled in the trial, this study was clearly underpowered to detect significant differences or to draw any conclusive results. Not surprisingly, in Protocol A intention-to-treat analysis, there were no significant differences in DFS or OS for patients randomized to IFN versus observation. Similarly, in Protocol B there were no significant differences in DFS or OS among patients randomized to CLND or CLND + IFN versus observation.[65]

Another question that has not clearly been answered is what the optimal duration of therapy is and whether prolonged adjuvant therapy may offer improved results. A DeCOG study of lower-dose IFN-α2a treatment using 3 MU s.c. three times per week for 5 years versus 18 months showed no difference in RFS or OS.[66] The EORTC 18952 trial tested two intermediate dosages of IFN (IDI) administered over 2 years versus 1 year and showed non-significant differences in favor of the 2-year regimen.[49] The Nordic IFN-α trial comparing an identical IDI regimen for 2 years versus 1 year showed non-significant differences in favor of the 1-year regimen.[67] More recently, the EORTC trial 18991 testing pegylated IFN-α has shown neither improved OS nor distant metastasis-free survival (DMFS) overall, although benefits upon RFS have been noted on analysis for regulatory review, which appear to be confined to the subset of patients without gross nodal disease (sentinel node positive).[50] In the subset of patients with the lowest tumor burden (N=382), IFN significantly improved RFS and DMFS, but not OS, compared with observation alone. This trial was designed to deliver 5 years of therapy, but has shown a median treatment interval of little over 1 year, so the question of whether longer therapy with this regimen achieves more significant antitumor effects cannot be answered at this time.

Two further trials have been conducted but are not yet fully mature or reported in the literature – testing the growth factor GM-CSF on the one hand, and chemobiotherapy on the other hand. The ECOG has led an intergroup trial testing the benefit of GM-CSF given for 1 year in monthly cycles of 14 days out of 28 with 250 μg s.c. per day, with a secondary randomized evaluation of peptide vaccination among patients of tissue type HLA-A2. Eligibility for this trial required either resectable nodal disease or distant solitary metastases; more than 815 patients were enrolled between 1999 and 2007, and this study has been presented to the American Society of Clinical Oncology demonstrating a lack of significant improvement in overall survival with either GM-CSF or the peptide vaccine intervention among HLA-A2 expressing patients.[67a] The SWOG designed a second adjuvant trial for patients with resectable nodal or distant metastases to test the role of chemobiotherapy given for 3 months (cisplatin, vinblastine, dacarbazine, and interleukin-2 [IL-2] with IFN-α) in comparison to high-dose IFN administered as in E1684. This intergroup trial S0008 enrolled more than 400 subjects between 2000 and 2007 and remains in follow-up.

Together, these results establish high-dose IFN-α2b as administered in E1684, E1690 and E1694 (with an intravenous induction phase and a full year of maintenance therapy) as the logical standard of care for adjuvant therapy of resected high-risk melanoma.

## Candidate biomarkers of therapeutic benefit with IFN-α

Recent studies of immunotherapy for melanoma, including high-dose IL-2 and anti-CTLA-4 antibody, have suggested a correlation of antitumor effects and autoimmune phenomena like thyroiditis, hypophysitis, enteritis, hepatitis and dermatitis.[68–81] More recently, patients who have shown a strong correlation of prolonged relapse-free and overall survival after treatment with the modified adjuvant IFN regimen (HeCOG 13A/98) have demonstrated a strong correlation with autoimmune phenomena and/or the appearance of autoantibodies in the serum.[82] Autoantibodies were detected in 52 (26%) of the group of 200 patients tested. Clinical manifestations of autoimmunity were observed in 15 patients (7%), including vitiligo-like depigmentation in 11 (5%). A total of 113 patients have relapsed and 82 have died. The median time to progression (TTP) was 27.6 months and the median survival was 58.6 months. The median TTP for the patients who did not develop clinical or serological evidence of autoimmunity was 15.9 months while it has not been reached for the 52 patients who developed autoimmunity (106 vs 7; p<0.0001). The median survival was 37.5 months for those who were negative and has not been reached for the other group (80 vs 2; p<0.001). In multivariate analysis the presence of autoimmunity was an independent favorable prognostic marker.

The two most recent ECOG-led studies E2696 and E1694 have been analyzed to better understand the prognostic value of autoimmunity induced by HDI. In E2696, patients with resectable high-risk melanoma were randomized to GM2-KLH/QS-1 (GMK) vaccine plus concurrent HDI, GMK plus sequential HDI, or GMK alone. Sera from 103 patients in E2696 and 691 patients in E1694 banked at baseline and up to three additional time points were tested by ELISA for the development of five autoantibodies. In E2696, autoantibodies were induced in 17/69 subjects (25%) receiving HDI and GMK versus 2/34 (6%) receiving GMK without HDI (2p-value=0.029). In E1694, 67/347 subjects (19.3%) who received IFN developed autoantibodies versus only 15/344 (4.4%) in the vaccine control group (2p-value <0.001). In the HDI arms, almost all induced autoantibodies were detected at ≥12 weeks after initiation of therapy. A 1-year landmark analysis of E1694 resected stage III patients showed survival advantage associated with HDI-induced autoimmunity that approaches statistical significance (HR=1.54; p=0.072) adjusting for treatment.[83]

Baseline pro-inflammatory cytokine levels were shown to predict relapse-free survival benefit with HDI in the E1694 trial.[84] The detection of serum biomarkers that are either prognostic of clinical outcome or predictive of response to IFN-α2b has been pursued using high-throughput xMAP® multiplex immunobead assay technology (Luminex Corp.). This technology was utilized to simultaneously measure the levels of 29 cytokines, chemokines, angiogenic and growth factors as well as soluble receptors in the sera of 179 patients with high-risk melanoma who have participated in the E1694, and 378 healthy age- and gender-matched controls. These banked sera that have been tested were prospectively collected in the course of the intergroup E1694 trial. The 179 melanoma patients were chosen at random from the two trial arms according to disease status (whether the subject had relapsed at < 1 year, between 1 and 3 years, or more than 5 years). Of those samples tested, 93 were derived from patients who received GMK vaccination and 86 were derived from patients treated with HDI. The clinical data from the E1694 trial were then mature to a median of 4.6 years of follow-up.

The results demonstrated that serum concentrations of IL-1α, IL-1β, IL-6, IL-8, IL-12p40, IL-13, G-CSF, MCP-1, MIP-1α, MIP-1β, IFN-α, TNF-α, EGF, VEGF, and TNFRII are significantly higher among patients with resected high-risk melanoma, when compared to healthy controls. Serum levels of immunosuppressive, angiogenic/growth stimulatory factors (VEGF, EGF, HGF) were decreased by IFN-α2b therapy significantly, while levels of anti-angiogenic IP-10 and IFN-α were elevated post treatment. Comparing patients according to relapse outcome, the pretreatment levels of pro-inflammatory cytokines IL-1α, IL-1β, IL-6 and TNF-α, and chemokines MIP-1α and MIP-1β, were significantly higher in sera of patients with longer RFS of >5 years, compared with patients who experienced shorter RFS of less than 1 year.

## INDICATIONS AND CONTRAINDICATIONS FOR IFN

High-dose IFN-α2b therapy is currently the standard of care for patients with high risk for relapse. Table 53.7 lists indications, contraindications and cautions to observe in the use of high-dose IFN-α2b therapy. Eligible patients are not restricted by age but should maintain a performance status of ECOG 0 or 1 (i.e. have normal activity, or have some symptoms but otherwise be nearly fully ambulatory) and have no significant hematologic, cardiac, hepatic or psychiatric comorbidities. Appropriate dosage adjustments need to be done for any hepatic, renal, or hematologic impairment.

High-dose IFN-α2b is associated with a number of potential adverse events ranging from flu-like symptoms

**Table 53.7  Indications, contraindications and cautions for high dose IFN- 2b therapy**

**Indications**

- ECOG performance status 0 or 1

**Contraindications**

- Pregnancy, lactation or planning to become pregnant
- Infancy
- Active autoimmune disease or history or requirement for immunosuppressive therapy
- Immunosuppression or requirement for immunosuppressive therapy (e.g. organ transplantation)
- Decompensated liver disease
- Severe functional disturbances of the kidneys
- Severe neuropsychiatric diseases (i.e. depression)
- Myelosuppression
- Life-threatening infection
- Thyroid disease if uncontrolled by conventional therapeutic measures
- Active psoriasis or a history of significant psoriasis
- Severe mental disturbances with active disease

**Cautions**

- Diabetes mellitus
- Cardiovascular disease
- Pulmonary disease
- Renal disease
- Epilepsy or other diseases of the CNS

that may interfere with daily activities and pose a threat to patients' compliance to severe (life-threatening) toxicities that mandate dose interruption or modification as well as aggressive supportive care.[85] Table 53.8 summarizes the most common toxicities and the frequency with which they have been observed in the three Cooperative Group phase III studies. It is notable that there are significant differences between the incidences and severities of toxicities reported among these three trials, demonstrating that as clinicians gained experience in recognizing and managing IFN-associated toxicities in the earlier trials (ECOG trials E1684/E1690), toxicities were more effectively managed and more patients were thus able to complete therapy in the later trial (E1694). The initial trial (E1684) was associated with toxicity attrition of 26%, the second trial (E1690) saw a 13% toxicity attrition, while in the most recent trial (E1694), toxicity accounted for attrition of only 10%. Dose delays or reductions were required in 28% to 44% of patients during induction and 36% to 52% during maintenance treatment in the three large HDI trials, with lower figures observed in the most recent trial (28% and 37%, respectively).[45–47] Education of participants in the cooperative group trials regarding the importance of providing supportive care has allowed the delivery of the full year of planned treatment in 90% of patients entering study E1694.

It is important to distinguish toxicities associated with peak dose exposure (i.e. the induction component of the E1684 regimen) from those that are associated with cumulative and continuous exposure (i.e. the maintenance phase of E1684 and the other alternate-day regimens). In fact, many patients tolerate the induction i.v. therapy phase with little difficulty, only to develop insidiously progressive

**Table 53.8 Toxicity and its Management in Patients with Melanoma Undergoing High-dose IFN-α2b Therapy**

| Adverse Event | All Grades (%)[a] | Grade 3/4 (%)[b] | Proposed Mechanism | Management |
|---|---|---|---|---|
| Myelosuppression | 92 | 26–60 | IP-10, IL-1 release | Dose reduction |
| Increased aspartate aminotransferase | 63 | 14–29 | Suppress activity of certain cytochrome P450 isoenzymes | Dose reduction |
| Fatigue | 96 | 18 | Acts as ACTH-like, DA-agonist (acute), or DA-antagonist (chronic) Via IL-1, -2, -6, and TNF-α affects HPA axis Thyroid dysfunction | Stimulants, Methylphenidate |
| Fever | 81 | 18 | | Acetaminophen, and as needed, NSAIDs |
| Myalgia | 75 | 4–17 | IL-1, IL-6, TNF-α | Tylenol[†] Demerol[‡] |
| Nausea | 66 | 5–9 | IFN-α, IL-1, 5-HT3 | Chlorpromazine[†] |
| Vomiting | 66 | 5 | | Metoclopramide[†] Ondasetron[‡] Graniserton[‡] |
| Neuropsychiatric including depression | 40 | 2–10 | Disturbance of HPA/HPG axis (IL-6 and glucocorticoids) Dysregulation of NE-/5HT3-ergic neurotransmitters | SSRI's |

IP-10, IFN-inducible protein; IL, interleukin; ACTH, adrenocorticotropic hormone; DA, dopamine; HPA, hypothalamus–pituitary–adrenal axis; HPG, hypothalamus–pituitary–gonadal axis; TNF-α, tumor necrosis factor-alpha; NE, norepinephrine; 5-HT3, serotonin; SSRI, serotonin selective reuptake inhibitors.

[a]Based on data from E1684 (n=143).

[b]Based on data from E1684 (n=143), E1690 (n=216) and E1694 (n=394).

[†]Behavioral

[‡]Pharmacologic

toxicity during the maintenance phase. However, others tolerate maintenance with little difficulty but experience acute effects of the induction regimen that require dose interruption and reduction.

The maintenance phase requires attention to the patient's complaints; some noting difficulty with the treatment at the start of each week while others have problems that mount over the week (signifying cumulative effects). Some acute effects demonstrate tachyphylaxis, and dissipate over time (fever, chills, malaise), whereas others are chronic and cumulative (anorexia, fatigue). Patients need to understand the scope and likely intensity of toxicity, and that persisting functional decrements of more than 25–33% will result in dose interruption or dose reduction until day-to-day functions have resumed a level that is at least 60% of normal. Careful follow-up of laboratory and clinical findings is critical to the successful safe delivery of this therapy. Follow-up is recommended weekly during induction therapy and monthly during maintenance (for at least 3 months) and at 3-monthly intervals to the conclusion of the year of therapy, once the patient has achieved a stable and acceptable profile.

Despite concerns regarding the toxicity of high-dose IFN-α2b, experience gained in a succession of nationwide intergroup studies has demonstrated that this regimen can be safely administered and is tolerable for the majority of patients. Close follow-up for early detection of side effects, especially the potentially life-threatening hepatic, hematologic and neurological toxicities, is mandatory.

Quality-of-life analyses have been performed. Using the Q-TWiST (quality-adjusted time without symptoms or toxicity) methodology, Cole et al. have shown that treatment with high-dose IFN-α2b results in a significant improvement in quality-adjusted time once the time with toxicity is factored out, even presuming the worst valuations of time with toxicity.[86] Kilbridge and colleagues have reported strikingly poorer valuations of time with asymptomatic relapse than might generally be presumed and rather better valuations of time with toxicity.[87] These, together, provide useful tools to portray the utility of treatment for individual patients, using indices that are specific for each individual patient.

## Alternatives to high-dose IFN-α2b therapy

Lower-dose IFN-α therapy may have a better toxicity profile, but has not been shown to improve OS significantly or RFS durably in high- or intermediate-risk melanoma. Pegylated IFN-α2b as tested in the EORTC trial 18991 has shown RFS benefits overall but neither improved OS nor DMFS.[50] The RFS benefits noted in EORTC 18991 appear to be more confined to the subset of patients without gross nodal disease (sentinel node positive), where pegylated IFN-α significantly improved RFS and DMFS, but not OS, compared with observation alone.

It is important to evaluate preliminary reports of immature data from current trials with caution to avoid interim reports of trials before they reach maturity, save where trials require interruption for outcome differences that an external data safety monitoring committee regard as compelling. There has been a tendency to report trials prematurely at interim assessments that ought to be eschewed in favor of definitive mature assessments. Trials that include patients of lower stage require longer intervals for final assessment of the benefit, and where trials conducted in very-high-risk resectable stage IIIB and IV may mature at 5 years, those including stage IIA–IIB and IIIA may require 7–10 years for maturity.

## NEXT PHASES OF DEVELOPMENT OF ADJUVANT THERAPIES

Previous clinical studies in this area have raised several critical questions that will need to be answered:

- What is the contribution of the induction phase of the high-dose E1684 IFN-β2b regimen to the overall benefit?

All trials of IFN-α with durable RFS and OS impact utilized an intravenous (i.v.) induction phase given at 20 MU/m$^2$ 5 days a week for 4 weeks (Cmax >10,000 U/mL). Based on this experience, a US Intergroup trial, E1697, was designed to evaluate the impact of a 4-week course of high-dose IFN-α2b similar to the induction phase of the HDI regimen tested in the E1684/E1690/E1694 trials. Eligibility for this trial includes patients with resected melanoma in the following categories: 1) T2b N0, 2) T3a–b N0, 3) T4a–b N0, 4) T1–4 N1a,2a (microscopic), and the control arm is observation. The E1697 intergroup trial has recently been closed for futility, and this large trial now argues that one month of IV IFN has no durable significant impact upon either relapse or survival of intermediate to high-risk patients. One year of HDI therefore remains the standard for adjuvant therapy of melanoma. Other groups are also testing the role of the i.v. induction phase of HDI, including the Italian Melanoma Intergroup (HDI induction given every 2 months for a total of 4 courses; 80 doses, N=300) and DeCOG (HDI induction given every 4 months for 1 year; 60 doses, N=800). Unfortunately, both the Hellenic and Sunbelt Melanoma Trials were underpowered to address the question related to the induction phase of the high-dose IFN, in addition to the use of a substandard regimen in the Hellenic trial.

- Is there any additional benefit from combining chemotherapy and other biologicals with IFN?

Studies of metastatic melanoma using combination chemobiotherapy (cisplatin, vinblastine and dacarbazine, CVD with IFN-α and IL-2) have shown higher response rates (44.8%, P=0.001) than IL-2 therapy alone, IL-2 plus IFN-α and IL-2 plus chemotherapy in a phase II trial.[88] Therefore, biochemotherapy has been tested both in the neoadjuvant setting in node-positive disease in small phase II studies[89,90] and in the adjuvant setting in high-risk melanoma. The current Intergroup phase III trial by SWOG (S0008) joined by ECOG and CALGB tests chemobiotherapy for 3 months versus high-dose IFN-α2b, and will be awaited with interest as it matures over the next couple of years. The results of the Intergroup E3695 study of chemobiotherapy in metastatic disease showed no survival benefit of biochemotherapy versus poly-chemotherapy alone, so the adjuvant exploration of this same regimen will be particularly interesting.[91]

- Will any subgroups with completely resected melanoma benefit from IFN-α2b more than others?

The meta-analysis of individual patient data from 13 IFN-α trials has suggested that the histological presence of primary tumor ulceration predicts increased susceptibility to IFN therapeutic effects.[63] A more recent analysis of the adjuvant trials EORTC 18952 and EORTC 18991 suggests a predictive value of primary tumor ulceration in relation to the therapeutic impact of IFN-α. In analyses for IFN impact upon RFS, DMFS and OS, there was a correlation of the presence of ulceration and outcome analyzed overall and stratified according to stage (IIB and III; N1 microscopic nodal and N2 macroscopic nodal disease). Among 2644 patients randomized into these studies, fewer than one-third (849) had ulcerated primaries, and there were 1336 non-ulcerated primaries, while for 459 the ulceration status was unknown. In the group of patients with ulcerated primary melanomas, the impact of IFN was noted to be greater than in the non-ulcerated group for RFS (test for interaction: p=0.02), DMFS (p<0.001), and OS (p<0.001). The greatest effects of therapy were noted in patients with ulceration and stages IIB/III-N1. Based on this retrospective analysis, the EORTC 18081 trial has been planned, which will compare the benefit of pegylated IFN-α2b versus observation in patients with ulcerated primaries and Breslow depth of more than 1 mm (node negative). It is noteworthy that unlike US cooperative groups, the EORTC does not require central pathology review for EORTC melanoma trials.[92] In the absence of an effect of ulceration in trials using high-dose IFN to date, one may speculate that the lower-dose regimens have an effect that occurs through a different mechanism than the high-dose regimen, where immunomodulation has been shown in the neoadjuvant setting[93] but whether this effect is an antivascular effect or not, as speculated in the past, awaits analyses of corollary side-studies performed in the context of these trials.

Sentinel lymph node biopsy, the results of which correlate with DFS and OS, and the preliminary data correlating the molecular detection of melanoma cells by RT-PCR with clinical outcome, raise the question of whether only some patient subgroups benefit from adjuvant IFN therapy. The Sunbelt Melanoma Trial, using molecular or 'ultra-staging' by RT-PCR, has failed to answer this question.[65,94]

- What is the role of adjuvant post-surgical CTLA blockade therapy utilizing ipilimumab for patients with high-risk resected melanoma compared to IFN-α2b?

Monoclonal antibodies blocking CTLA-4 and allowing prolonged T-cell activation have shown promising durable clinical activity in patients with advanced inoperable melanoma.[95] Ongoing randomized controlled trials are currently investigating standard high-dose interferon-α2b versus CTLA-4 blockade with ipilmumab (US Intergroup E1609) and ipilimumab versus placebo (EORTC 18071).

## FUTURE OUTLOOK

The obstacle of high-dose IFN-α2b toxicity may be overcome by defining patient subgroups that are likely to respond to IFN-α2b. Results from the E2690 laboratory corollary of Intergroup adjuvant trial E1690 show that: (a) in the pretreatment tumor biopsies, IFN-α2b treatment in vitro resulted in upregulation of HLA-DR and downregulation of molecule ICAM; and (b) at 1 month in patients receiving the high-dose regimen there was significant elevation of the percentage of CD4$^+$CD3$^+$ (T helper cells).[96,97]

More precise knowledge of IFN's molecular mechanism of action and novel molecular research tools, such as microarray assays[88,98–100] and proteomic spectra in serum generated by mass spectroscopy, will hopefully identify signatures of patient subpopulations with different patterns of natural history and patients in whom therapy is more predictable.[101,102]

The observations associating the induction of autoimmunity with therapeutic benefit and survival prolongation support the hypothesis that the prevention of melanoma relapse and mortality with IFN is associated with immunomodulation that may increase resistance to melanoma. IFN-α2b induction of autoimmunity may provide a useful surrogate biomarker of adjuvant therapeutic benefit. Studies of autoimmunity and its genetic determinants are currently being carried out in an NIH-funded E1697 corollary project that may help identify patients most likely to benefit from high-dose IFN-α2b. These studies may be applicable to other newer immunotherapies associated with autoimmunity, such as the anti-CTLA-4 blocking antibodies ipilimumab and tremelimumab. A predictive biomarker corollary project is also planned as part of E1609.

## REFERENCES

1. Balch CM, Buzaid AC, Soong SJ, et al. Final version of the American Joint Committee on Cancer staging system for cutaneous melanoma. *J Clin Oncol.* 2001;19(16):3635–3648.
2. Veronesi U, Adamus J, Aubert C, et al. A randomized trial of adjuvant chemotherapy and immunotherapy in cutaneous melanoma. *N Engl J Med.* 1982;307(15):913–916.
3. Lejeune FJ, Macher E, Kleeberg U, et al. An assessment of DTIC versus levamisole or placebo in the treatment of high risk stage I patients after surgical removal of a primary melanoma of the skin. A phase III adjuvant study. EORTC protocol 18761. *Eur J Cancer Clin Oncol.* 1988;24(suppl 2): S81–S90.
4. Fisher RI, Terry WD, Hodes RJ, et al. Adjuvant immunotherapy or chemotherapy for malignant melanoma. Preliminary report of the National Cancer Institute randomised clinical trial. *Surg Clin North Am.* 1981;61(6):1267–1277.
5. Koops HS, Vaglini M, Suciu S, et al. Prophylactic isolated limb perfusion for localized, high-risk limb melanoma: results of a multicenter randomized phase III trial. European Organization for Research and Treatment of Cancer Malignant Melanoma Cooperative Group Protocol 18832, the World Health Organization Melanoma Program Trial 15, and the North American Perfusion Group Southwest Oncology Group-8593. *J Clin Oncol.* 1998;16(9):2906–2912.
6. Meisenberg BR, Ross M, Vredenburgh JJ, et al. Randomized trial of high-dose chemotherapy with autologous bone marrow support as adjuvant therapy for high-risk, multi-node-positive malignant melanoma. *J Natl Cancer Inst.* 1993;85(13):1080–1085.
7. Meyskens FL, Liu PY, Tuthill RJ, et al. Randomized trial of vitamin A versus observation as adjuvant therapy in high-risk primary malignant melanoma: a Southwest Oncology Group study. *J Clin Oncol.* 1994;12(10):2060–2065.
8. Markovic S, Suman VJ, Dalton RJ, et al. Randomized, placebo-controlled, phase III surgical adjuvant clinical trial of megestrol acetate (Megace) in selected patients with malignant melanoma. *Am J Clin Oncol.* 2002;25(6):552–556.
9. Czarnetzki BM, Macher E, Suciu S, et al. Long-term adjuvant immunotherapy in stage I high risk malignant melanoma, comparing two BCG preparations versus non-treatment in a randomized multicentre study (EORTC Protocol 18781). *Eur J Cancer.* 1993;29A(9):1237–1242.
10. Paterson AH, Willans DJ, Jerry LM, et al. Adjuvant BCG immunotherapy for malignant melanoma. *Can Med Assoc J.* 1984;131(7):744–748.
11. Balch CM, Smalley RV, Bartolucci AA, et al. A randomized prospective clinical trial of adjuvant C. parvum immunotherapy in 260 patients with clinically localized melanoma (Stage I): prognostic factors analysis and preliminary results of immunotherapy. *Cancer.* 1982;49(6):1079–1084.
12. Lipton A, Harvey HA, Balch CM, et al. Corynebacterium parvum versus bacille Calmette–Guerin adjuvant immunotherapy of stage II malignant melanoma. *J Clin Oncol.* 1991;9(7):1151–1156.
13. Quirt IC, Shelley WE, Pater JL, et al. Improved survival in patients with poor-prognosis malignant melanoma treated with adjuvant levamisole: a phase III study by the National Cancer Institute of Canada Clinical Trials Group. *J Clin Oncol.* 1991;9(5):729–735.
14. Spitler LE. A randomized trial of levamisole versus placebo as adjuvant therapy in malignant melanoma. *J Clin Oncol.* 1991;9(5):735–740.
15. Miller LL, Spitler LE, Allen RE, et al. A randomized, double-blind, placebo-controlled trial of transfer factor as adjuvant therapy for malignant melanoma. *Cancer.* 1988;61(8):1543–1549.
16. Sondak VK, Liu PY, Tuthill RJ, et al. Adjuvant immunotherapy of resected, intermediate-thickness, node-negative melanoma with an allogeneic tumor vaccine: overall results of a randomized trial of the Southwest Oncology Group. *J Clin Oncol.* 2002;20(8):2058–2066.
17. Hersey P, Coates AS, McCarthy WH, et al. Adjuvant immunotherapy of patients with high-risk melanoma using vaccinia viral lysates of melanoma: results of a randomized trial. *J Clin Oncol.* 2002;20(20):4181–4190.
18. Wallack MK, Sivanandham M, Balch CM, et al. Surgical adjuvant active specific immunotherapy for patients with stage III melanoma: the final analysis of data from a phase III, randomized, double-blind, multicenter vaccinia melanoma oncolysate trial. *J Am Coll Surg.* 1998;187(1):69–77.
19. Wallack MK, Sivanandham M, Balch CM, et al. A phase III randomized, double-blind multi-institutional trial of vaccinia melanoma oncolysate-active specific immunotherapy for patients with stage II melanoma. *Cancer.* 1995;75(1):34–42.
20. Livingston PO, Wong GY, Adhuri S, et al. Improved survival in stage III melanoma patients with GM2 antibodies: a randomized trial of adjuvant vaccination with GM2 ganglioside. *J Clin Oncol.* 1994;12(5):1036–1044.
21. Bystryn JC, Zeleniuch-Jacquotte A, Oratz R, et al. Double-blind trial of a polyvalent, shed-antigen, melanoma vaccine. *Clin Cancer Res.* 2001;7(7):1882–1887.
22. Morton DL, Mozzillo N, Thompson JF, et al. An international, randomized, phase III trial of bacillus Calmette-Guerin (BCG) plus allogeneic melanoma vaccine (MCV) or placebo after complete resection of melanoma metastatic to regional or distant sites. 2007 ASCO Annual Meeting Proceedings. *J Clin Oncol.* 2007;25(18S) Abstr. 8508.
23. Retsas S, Quigley M, Pectasides D, et al. Clinical and histologic involvement of regional lymph nodes in malignant melanoma. Adjuvant vindesine improves survival. *Cancer.* 1994;73(8):2119–2130.
24. Minev BR. Melanoma vaccines. *Semin Oncol.* 2002;29(5):479–493.
25. Morton DL, Hsueh EC, Essner R, et al. Prolonged survival of patients receiving active immunotherapy with Canvaxin therapeutic polyvalent vaccine after complete resection of melanoma metastatic to regional lymph nodes. *Ann Surg.* 2002;48(9):438–448.
26. Hall S. *A Commotion in the Blood: Life, Death, and the Immune System.* New York, NY: Henry Holt; 1997.
27. Stark GR, Kerr IM, Williams BR, et al. How cells respond to interferons. *Annu Rev Biochem.* 1998;67:227–264.
28. de Veer MJ, Holko M, Frevel M, et al. Functional classification of interferon-stimulated genes identified using microarrays. *J Leukoc Biol.* 2001;69(6):912–920.
29. Belardelli F, Ferrantini M. Cytokines as a link between innate and adaptive antitumor immunity. *Trends Immunol.* 2002;23(4):201–208.
30. Zou W, Machelon V, Coulomb-L'Hermin A, et al. Stromal-derived factor-1 in human tumors recruits and alters the function of plasmacytoid precursor dendritic cells. *Nat Med.* 2001;7(12):1339–1346.
31. Gresser I, Belardelli F, Endogenous type I. interferons as a defense against tumors. *Cytokine Growth Factor Rev.* 2002;13(2):111–118.

32. McCarty MF, Bielenberg D, Donawho C, et al. Evidence for the causal role of endogenous interferon-alpha/beta in the regulation of angiogenesis, tumorigenicity, and metastasis of cutaneous neoplasms. *Clin Exp Metastasis*. 2002;19(7):609–615.

33. Grander D, Sangfelt O, Erickson S. How does interferon exert its cell growth inhibitory effect? *Eur J Haematol*. 1997;59(3):129–135.

34. Thyrell L, Erickson S, Zhivotovsky B, et al. Mechanisms of interferon-alpha induced apoptosis in malignant cells. *Oncogene*. 2002;21(8):1251–1262.

35. Kirkwood JM, Ernstoff MS, Davis CA, et al. Comparison of intramuscular and intravenous recombinant alpha-2 interferon in melanoma and other cancers. *Ann Intern Med*. 1985;103(1):32–36.

36. Ernstoff MS, Reiss M, Davis CA, et al. Intravenous (IV) recombinant alpha-2 interferon (IFNα-2) in metastatic melanoma (abstr C-222). *Proc Am Soc Clin Oncol*. 1983;2:57.

37. Creagan ET, Ahmann DL, Green SJ, et al. Phase II study of recombinant leukocyte A interferon (r-IFN-A) in disseminated malignant melanoma. *Cancer*. 1984;54:2844–2849.

38. Creagan ET, Ahmann DL, Green SJ, et al. Phase II study of recombinant leukocyte A interferon (IFN-rA) plus cimetidine in disseminated malignant melanoma. *J Clin Oncol*. 1985;3(7):977–981.

39. Creagan ET, Ahmann DL, Green SJ, et al. Phase II study of low-dose recombinant leukocyte A interferon in disseminated malignant melanoma. *J Clin Oncol*. 1984;2(9):1002–1005.

40. Legha SS, Papadopoulos NE, Plager C, et al. Clinical evaluation of recombinant interferon alfa-2a (Roferon-A) in metastatic melanoma using two different schedules. *J Clin Oncol*. 1987;5(8):1240–1246.

41. Hersey P, Hasic E, MacDonald M, et al. Effects of recombinant leukocyte interferon (rIFN-alpha A) on tumour growth and immune responses in patients with metastatic melanoma. *Br J Cancer*. 1985;51(6):815–826.

42. Neefe JR, Legha SS, Markowitz A, et al. Phase II study of recombinant alpha-interferon in malignant melanoma. *Am J Clin Oncol*. 1990;13(6):472–476.

43. Dorval T, Palangie T, Jouve M, et al. Clinical phase II trial of recombinant DNA interferon (interferon alpha 2b) in patients with metastatic malignant melanoma. *Cancer*. 1986;58(2):215–218.

44. Coates A, Rallings M, Hersey P, et al. Phase-II study of recombinant alpha 2-interferon in advanced malignant melanoma. *J Interferon Res*. 1986;6(1):1–4.

45. Kirkwood JM, Strawderman MH, Ernstoff MS, et al. Interferon alfa-2b adjuvant therapy of high-risk resected cutaneous melanoma: the Eastern Cooperative Oncology Group Trial EST 1684. *J Clin Oncol*. 1996;14(1):7–17.

46. Kirkwood JM, Ibrahim JG, Sondak VK, et al. High- and low-dose interferon alfa-2b in high-risk melanoma: first analysis of intergroup trial E1690/S9111/C9190. *J Clin Oncol*. 2000;18(12):2444–2458.

47. Kirkwood JM, Ibrahim JG, Sosman JA, et al. High-dose interferon alfa-2b significantly prolongs relapse-free and overall survival compared with the GM2-KLH/QS-21 vaccine in patients with resected stage IIB–III melanoma: results of intergroup trial E1694/S9512/C509801. *J Clin Oncol*. 2001;19(9):2370–2380.

48. Creagan ET, Dalton RJ, Ahmann DL, et al. Randomized, surgical adjuvant clinical trial of recombinant interferon alfa-2a in selected patients with malignant melanoma. *J Clin Oncol*. 1995;13(11):2776–2783.

49. Eggermont AM, Suciu S, MacKie R, et al. EORTC Melanoma Group. Post-surgery adjuvant therapy with intermediate doses of interferon alfa 2b versus observation in patients with stage IIb/III melanoma (EORTC 18952): randomised controlled trial. *Lancet*. 2005;366(9492):1189–1196.

50. Eggermont AM, Suciu S, Santinami M, et al. Adjuvant therapy with pegylated interferon alfa-2b versus observation alone in resected stage III melanoma: final results of EORTC 18991, a randomized phase III trial. *Lancet*. 2008;372(9633):117–126.

51. Cascinelli N, Belli F, MacKie RM, et al. Effect of long-term adjuvant therapy with interferon alpha-2a in patients with regional node metastases from cutaneous melanoma: a randomised trial. *Lancet*. 2001;358(9285):866–869.

52. Hancock BW, Wheatley K, Harris S, et al. AIM HIGH: Adjuvant Interferon in Melanoma (HIGH risk) – United Kingdom Coordinating Committee on Cancer Research randomized study of adjuvant low dose extended duration interferon alfa 2a in high risk resected malignant melanoma. *J Clin Oncol*. 2003;22(1):53–61.

53. Kleeberg UR, Suciu S, Brocker EB, et al. Final results of the EORTC 18871/DKG 80-1 randomised phase III trial. rIFN-alpha2b versus rIFN-gamma versus ISCADOR M versus observation after surgery in melanoma patients with either high-risk primary (thickness >3 mm) or regional lymph node metastasis. *Eur J Cancer*. 2004;40(3):390–402.

54. Cameron DA, Cornbleet MC, Mackie RM, et al. Adjuvant interferon alpha 2b in high risk melanoma – the Scottish study. *Br J Cancer*. 2001;84(9):1146–1149.

55. Pehamberger H, Soyer HP, Steiner A, et al. Adjuvant interferon alfa-2a treatment in resected primary stage II cutaneous melanoma. Austrian Malignant Melanoma Coop Group. *J Clin Oncol*. 1998;16(4):1425–1429.

56. Grob JJ, Dreno B, de la Salmoniere P, et al. Randomised trial of interferon alpha-2a as adjuvant therapy in resected primary melanoma thicker than 1.5 mm without clinically detectable node metastases. French Cooperative Group on Melanoma. *Lancet*. 1998;351(9120):1905–1910.

57. Cascinelli N, Bufalino R, Morabito A, et al. Results of adjuvant interferon study in WHO melanoma programme. *Lancet*. 1994;343(8902):913–914.

58. Helling F, Zhang S, Shang A, et al. GM2-KLH conjugate vaccine: increased immunogenicity in melanoma patients after administration with immunological adjuvant QS-21. *Cancer Res*. 1995;55(13):2783–2788.

59. Livingston PO, Wong GY, Adluri S, et al. Improved survival in stage III melanoma patients with GM2 antibodies: a randomized trial of adjuvant vaccination with GM2 ganglioside. *J Clin Oncol*. 1994;12(5):1036–1044.

60. Eggermont AM, Suciu S, Ruka W, et al. EORTC 18961: Post-operative adjuvant ganglioside GM2-KLH21 vaccination treatment vs observation in stage II (T3-T4 N0M0) melanoma: 2nd interim analysis led to an early disclosure of the results. 2008 ASCO Annual Meeting Proceedings Part I. *J Clin Oncol*. 2008;26(May 20 suppl): Abstr 9004.

61. Kirkwood JM, Manola J, Ibrahim J, et al. A pooled analysis of eastern cooperative oncology group and intergroup trials of adjuvant high-dose interferon for melanoma. *Clin Cancer Res*. 2004;10(5):1670–1677.

62. Wheatley K, Ives N, Hancock B, et al. Does adjuvant interferon-alpha for high-risk melanoma provide a worthwhile benefit? A meta-analysis of the randomised trials. *Cancer Treat Rev*. 2003;29(4):241–252.

63. Wheatley K, Ives N, Eggermont A, et al. on behalf of International Malignant Melanoma Collaborative Group. Interferon-α as adjuvant therapy for melanoma: an individual patient data meta-analysis of randomised trials. 2007 ASCO Annual Meeting Proceedings Part I. *J Clin Oncol*. 2007;25(18S) Abstr 8526.

64. Pectasides D, Dafni U, Bafaloukos D, et al. Randomized phase III study of 1 month versus 1 year of adjuvant high-dose interferon alfa-2b in patients with resected high-risk melanoma. *J Clin Oncol*. 2009;27(6):939–944.

65. McMasters KM, Ross MI, Reintgen DS, et al. Final results of the Sunbelt Melanoma Trial. *J Clin Oncol*. 2008;26(May 20 suppl): Abstr 9003.

66. Hauschild A, Volkenandt M, Tilgen W, et al. Efficacy of interferon alpha 2a in 18 versus 60 months of treatment in patients with primary melanoma of ≥1.5 mm tumor thickness: A randomized phase III DeCOG trial. *J Clin Oncol*. 2008;26(May 20 suppl): Abstr 9032.

67. Hansson J, Aamdal S, Bastholt L, et al. Results of the Nordic randomised adjuvant trial of intermediate-dose interferon alfa-2b in high-risk melanoma. *Eur J Cancer*. 2007;6(suppl 5):4.

67a. Lawson DH, Lee SJ, Tarhini AA, et al. E4697: Phase III cooperative group study of yeast-derived granulocyte macrophage colony-stimulating factor (GM-CSF) versus placebo as adjuvant treatment of patients with completely resected stage III-IV melanoma. 2010 ASCO Annual Meeting Proceedings, Vol. 28, No 15S, 46th Annual Meeting, June 4–8, 2010.

68. Atkins MB, Mier JW, Parkinson DR, et al. Hypothyroidism after treatment with interleukin-2 and lymphokine-activated killer cells. *N Engl J Med*. 1988;318(24):1557–1563.

69. Weijl NI, Van der Harst D, Brand A, et al. Hypothyroidism during immunotherapy with interleukin-2 is associated with antithyroid antibodies and response to treatment. *J Clin Oncol*. 1993;11(7):1376–1383.

70. Scalzo S, Gengaro A, Boccoli G, et al. Primary hypothyroidism associated with interleukin-2 and interferon alpha-2 therapy of melanoma and renal carcinoma. *Eur J Cancer*. 1990;26(11–12):1152–1156.

71. Krouse RS, Royal RE, Heywood G, et al. Thyroid dysfunction in 281 patients with metastatic melanoma or renal carcinoma treated with interleukin-2 alone. *J Immunother Emphasis Tumor Immunol*. 1995;18(4):272–278.

72. Phan GQ, Attia P, Steinberg SM, et al. Factors associated with response to high-dose interleukin-2 in patients with metastatic melanoma. *J Clin Oncol*. 2001;19(15):3477–3482.

73. Becker JC, Winkler B, Klingert S, et al. Antiphospholipid syndrome associated with immunotherapy for patients with melanoma. *Cancer*. 1994;73(6):1621–1624.

74. Rosenberg SA, White DE. Vitiligo in patients with melanoma: normal tissue antigens can be targets for cancer immunotherapy. *J Immunother Emphasis Tumor Immunol*. 1996;19(1):81–84.

75. Franzke A, Peest D, Probst-Kepper M, et al. Autoimmunity resulting from cytokine treatment predicts long-term survival in patients with metastatic renal cell cancer. *J Clin Oncol*. 1999;17(2):529–533.

76. Sanderson K, Scotland R, Lee P, et al. Autoimmunity in a phase I trial of a fully human anti-cytotoxic T-lymphocyte antigen-4 monoclonal antibody with multiple melanoma peptides and Montanide ISA 51 for patients with resected stages III and IV melanoma. *J Clin Oncol*. 2005;23(4):741–750.

77. Dranoff G. CTLA-4 blockade: unveiling immune regulation. *J Clin Oncol*. 2005;23(4):662–664.

78. Ribas A, Bozon VA, Lopez-Berestein G, et al. Phase 1 trial of monthly doses of the human anti-CTLA4 monoclonal antibody CP-675,206 in patients with advanced melanoma ASCO Meeting Abstracts. *J Clin Oncol*. 2005;23: Abstr 7524.

79. Phan GQ, Yang JC, Sherry RM, et al. Cancer regression and autoimmunity induced by cytotoxic T lymphocyte-associated antigen 4 blockade in patients with metastatic melanoma. *Proc Natl Acad Sci USA*. 2003;100(14):8372–8377.

**80.** Ribas A, Camacho LH, Lopez-Berestein G, et al. Antitumor activity in melanoma and anti-self responses in a phase I trial with the anti-cytotoxic T lymphocyte-associated antigen 4 monoclonal antibody CP-675,206. *J Clin Oncol.* 2005;23(35):8968–8977.

**81.** Tarhini AA, Moschos SS, Schlesselman JJ, et al. Phase II trial of combination biotherapy of high-dose interferon alfa-2b and tremelimumab for recurrent inoperable stage III or stage IV melanoma. ASCO Meeting Abstracts. *J Clin Oncol.* 2008;26(May 20 suppl): Abstr 9009.

**82.** Gogas H, Ioannovich J, Dafni U, et al. Prognostic significance of autoimmunity during treatment of melanoma with interferon. *N Engl J Med.* 2006;354:709–718.

**83.** Stuckert II JJ, Tarhini AA, Lee S, et al. Interferon alfa-induced autoimmunity and serum S100 levels as predictive and prognostic biomarkers in high-risk melanoma in the ECOG-intergroup phase II trial E2696. 2007 ASCO Annual Meeting Proceedings Part I. *J Clin Oncol.* 2007;25(18S): Abstr. 8506.

**84.** Yurkovetsky ZR, Kirkwood JM, Edington HD, et al. Multiplex analysis of serum cytokines in melanoma patients treated with interferon-alpha2b. *Clin Cancer Res.* 2007;13(8):2422–2428.

**85.** Kirkwood JM, Bender C, Agarwala S, et al. Mechanisms and management of toxicities associated with high-dose interferon alfa-2b therapy. *J Clin Oncol.* 2002;20(17):3703–3718.

**86.** Cole BF, Gelber RD, Kirkwood JM, et al. Quality-of-life-adjusted survival analysis of interferon alfa-2b adjuvant treatment of high-risk resected cutaneous melanoma: an Eastern Cooperative Oncology Group study. *J Clin Oncol.* 1996;14(10):2666–2673.

**87.** Kilbridge KL, Cole BF, Kirkwood JM, et al. Quality-of-life-adjusted survival analysis of high-dose adjuvant interferon alpha-2b for high-risk melanoma patients using intergroup clinical trial data. *J Clin Oncol.* 2002;20(5):1311–1318.

**88.** Legha SS, Ring S, Eton O, et al. Development of a biochemotherapy regimen with concurrent administration of cisplatin, vinblastine, dacarbazine, interferon alfa, and interleukin-2 for patients with metastatic melanoma. *J Clin Oncol.* 1998;16(5):1752–1759.

**89.** Buzaid AC, Colome M, Bedikian A, et al. Phase II study of neoadjuvant concurrent biochemotherapy in melanoma patients with local-regional metastases. *Melanoma Res.* 1998;8(6):549–556.

**90.** Gibbs P, Anderson C, Pearlman N, et al. A phase II study of neoadjuvant biochemotherapy for stage III melanoma. *Cancer.* 2002;94(2):470–476.

**91.** Keilholz U, Gore ME. Biochemotherapy for advanced melanoma. *Semin Oncol.* 2002;29(5):456–461.

**92.** Eggermont AM, Suciu S, Testori A, et al. EORTC Melanoma Group. Ulceration of primary melanoma and responsiveness to adjuvant interferon therapy: analysis of the adjuvant trials EORTC18952 and EORTC18991 in 2,644 patients. ASCO Meeting Abstracts 2009. *J Clin Oncol.* 2009;27(15s): Abstr 9007.

**93.** Moschos SJ, Edington HD, Land SR, et al. Neoadjuvant treatment of regional stage IIIB melanoma with high-dose interferon alfa-2b induces objective tumor regression in association with modulation of tumor infiltrating host cellular immune responses. *J Clin Oncol.* 2006;24(19):3164–3171.

**94.** McMasters KM. The Sunbelt Melanoma Trial. *Ann Surg Oncol.* 2001;8(9):41S–43S.

**95.** O'Day S, Weber J, Lebbe C, et al. Effect of ipilimumab treatment on 18-month survival: update of patients (pts) with advanced melanoma treated with 10 mg/kg ipilimumab in three phase II clinical trials. ASCO Annual Meeting, 2009. *J Clin Oncol.* 2009;27(15s): Abstr. 9033.

**96.** Motzer RJ, Rakhit A, Ginsberg M, et al. Phase I trial of 40-kD branched pegylated interferon alfa-2a for patients with advanced renal cell carcinoma. *J Clin Oncol.* 2001;19(5):1312–1319.

**97.** Kirkwood JM, Richards T, Zarour HM, et al. Immunomodulatory effects of high-dose and low-dose interferon alpha2b in patients with high-risk resected melanoma: the E2690 laboratory corollary of intergroup adjuvant trial E1690. *Cancer.* 2002;95(5):1101–1112.

**98.** Bukowski R, Ernstoff MS, Gore ME, et al. Pegylated interferon alfa-2b treatment for patients with solid tumors: a phase I/II study. *J Clin Oncol.* 2002;20(18):3841–3849.

**99.** Certa U, Seiler M, Padovan E, et al. High density oligonucleotide array analysis of interferon-alpha2a sensitivity and transcriptional response in melanoma cells. *Br J Cancer.* 2001;85(1):107–114.

**100.** de Veer MJ, Holko M, Frevel M, et al. Functional classification of interferon-stimulated genes identified using microarrays. *J Leukoc Biol.* 2001;69(6):912–920.

**101.** Barthe C, Mahon FX, Gharbi MJ, et al. Expression of interferon-alpha (IFN-alpha) receptor 2c at diagnosis is associated with cytogenetic response in IFN-alpha-treated chronic myeloid leukemia. *Blood.* 2001;97(11):3568–3573.

**102.** Petricoin EF, Ardekani AM, Hitt BA, et al. Use of proteomic patterns in serum to identify ovarian cancer. *Lancet.* 2002;359(9306):572–577.

# Vaccine Therapy for Melanoma

*Amod A. Sarnaik, Nasreen Vohra, Shari Pilon-Thomas, and Vernon K. Sondak*

## Key Points

- Vaccine therapy is promising but still an investigational treatment for melanoma.
- Vaccines can be derived from peptides, allogeneic tumor cell lines, or autologous tumor cells and have demonstrable activity in preclinical studies and phase I/II clinical trials.
- Most phase III vaccine trials have failed to show benefit; however, more appropriate patient selection may improve outcomes.
- Future strategies involving the combination of vaccine therapy with immunostimulatory cytokines or antibodies may improve outcomes.

## INTRODUCTION

Vaccination aimed at reducing the incidence of certain infectious diseases has led to vast improvements in health care. Substantial research has been directed toward the development of vaccine therapy for the treatment of cancer, and melanoma has been an attractive target. Advanced melanoma is a disease with high cancer-specific mortality and few effective treatment options. Traditional treatment modalities such as chemotherapy and radiation have limited utility in the treatment of advanced melanoma, but it has been observed, albeit in isolated cases, that immune mechanisms can slow the progression of melanoma and even cause regression of established melanoma metastases (Fig. 54.1). In addition, tumor-reactive T cells can be measured in the peripheral blood as well as within the resected tumors of melanoma patients. When recovered from patients, these T cells are able to respond to melanoma antigens derived from the same patient in vitro.[1,2]

Preclinical studies such as these have spurred interest in the development of vaccine therapy for the treatment of melanoma. In general terms, this involves the provision of antigens to patients in order to engender an anti-tumor immune response and eventual regression of disease. This chapter will review the different types of anti-melanoma vaccines that have been developed, the past successes and failures of vaccine therapy in clinical trials, as well as future directions that are being explored to improve the efficacy of vaccine therapy for melanoma.

## REQUIREMENTS FOR AN EFFECTIVE ANTI-MELANOMA VACCINE

In order for a vaccine to be effective in treating melanoma, several conditions must be satisfied. First, the vaccine must contain antigens that are sufficient to induce a specific immune response when administered to patients. Second, these target antigens must be expressed on the tumor in order for the vaccine to induce an effective anti-tumor immune response. Third, the vaccine must be safe; it must generate a long-lasting tumor-specific immune response without causing significant autoimmunity or inducing a tolerant state that could actually promote tumor growth. Finally, the vaccine must be amenable to large-scale production in a uniform fashion in order for it to be feasible to administer on a large scale. The above requirements must all be taken into consideration when designing an anti-melanoma vaccine.

## TYPES OF VACCINES

Vaccine therapy involves the exogenous administration of antigens, which are substances that induce a specific immune response. Upon ongoing or subsequent exposure to the same or similar antigens, an immune response is recalled, resulting in the destruction of tissue harboring the target antigens.

There are two general categories of anti-melanoma vaccines based on the source of antigen: defined-antigen vaccines and whole-cell vaccines. Defined-antigen vaccines contain previously isolated and characterized antigens. Most reported defined-antigen vaccines are peptide vaccines, composed of one or more purified protein fragments expressed in tumor. Other types of defined antigens include gangliosides, which are glycosphingolipids, and MUC1, a mucin-containing glycoprotein.

Vaccines may use epitopes, which are fragments of antigens that are sufficient to stimulate an immune response. These epitopes can be artificially modified to generate a stronger immune response than that observed from the 'naturally occurring' form; these are termed 'heteroclitic' epitopes. Ideally, each antigen peptide or epitope should be known to be sufficient to generate an in vitro immune response in preclinical studies.

An ideal target antigen is tumor-specific, meaning it is expressed exclusively by tumor cells and not by normal cells. This has a theoretical advantage of minimizing autoimmunity, and therefore potential toxicity, induced by

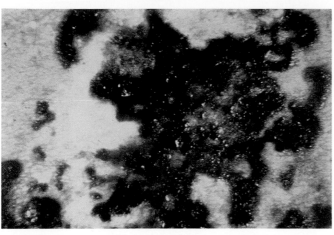

**Figure 54.1** Partial regression of primary melanoma. The white areas within this primary cutaneous melanoma are areas of tumor regression, indicating that there are defense mechanisms in humans that kill melanoma cells. Note that the skin immediately adjacent to regressing areas remains normally pigmented, indicating that the defense mechanism selectively attacks malignant cells. (Image courtesy of New York University Department of Dermatology.)

vaccine therapy. The likelihood of the vaccine generating an immune response against normal cells is relatively low, since the target antigen is not expressed on normal cells. Alternatively, antigens can be tumor-associated, meaning the antigens are expressed in tumor but are also found at lower levels and/or frequencies in normal cells. Commonly used antigens in defined-antigen vaccines are summarized in Table 54.1. Most antigens used in peptide melanoma vaccines, such as tyrosinase, gp100, and MART-1, are tumor-associated proteins mainly expressed by normal melanocytes and melanoma.

Perhaps the greatest theoretical advantages of defined-antigen vaccines include the relative ease and the standardized process involved with the manufacturing of such vaccines. The small and distinct pool of antigens contained within a given defined-antigen vaccine makes it relatively easy to adopt a reproducible production process and to establish effective quality-assurance measures. Vaccination with defined antigens rather than whole cells also facilitates immune monitoring of the response of patients to the few specific antigens contained in the vaccine. The quality and magnitude of a specific immune response to the relevant antigens can be readily assessed in the immune cells of individual patients by relatively straightforward laboratory assays. In contrast, immune monitoring can be much more difficult to accomplish with other vaccine strategies where the antigens are largely unclassified, since the targets of the immune response are unknown.

### Table 54.1 Defined Antigens Commonly Used in Melanoma Vaccines

- GM2 ganglioside
- gp100
- MART-1
- Tyrosinase
- Tyrosinase-related protein 1
- MAGE-1
- S100

Significant disadvantages of defined antigen vaccines include the requirement that relevant individual antigens must be isolated and characterized, which has proven to be a costly, labor-intensive process. Furthermore, in the case of peptide vaccines, antigenic peptides are often HLA-class restricted, which means that only patients with a certain HLA haplotype can optimally recognize and respond to certain peptides. This limits the broad application of peptide vaccines to a population, as only a subset of patients will have the HLA haplotype necessary to recognize peptide antigens contained in a given vaccine.

In addition, within a tumor, different tumor cells have been found to express unique variants of a targeted antigen, a phenomenon known as antigenic heterogeneity. These antigenic variants may not be immunogenic compared to the wild-type antigen, ultimately limiting the effectiveness of a defined-antigen vaccine. Also, a certain percentage of tumor cells in the same metastatic focus, or in a different nodule, or individual circulating tumor cells may not express the targeted antigen at all. Finally, after an initial immune response from vaccine treatment against a specific pool of tumor antigens, there is selective pressure for tumors to lose or downregulate expression of these targets, which are rarely critical to tumor cell survival, a process known as immune escape.

Following loss of tumor antigen, or downregulation of MHC class I that is required for antigen presentation, the tumor is able to successfully evade the patient's immune response. Unfortunately, the possibility of tumor escape is not limited to defined-antigen vaccines but instead is a potential problem shared by all cancer vaccine strategies. However, the fewer the antigens contained within a vaccine, the more likely this phenomenon is to occur. Therefore, tumor escape is considered to be more of a problem with defined-antigen vaccines compared to whole-cell vaccines but theoretically can be offset by increasing the number of defined antigens.

Whole-cell vaccines involve the use of tumor cells rather than isolated purified peptides. There are two types of whole-cell vaccines: allogeneic and autologous. Allogeneic whole-cell vaccines are derived from melanoma cell lines that have been generated from previous patients and are administered as irradiated intact whole cells or as cell lysates. One of the benefits of allogeneic vaccines is that their manufacturing can be standardized, as allogeneic vaccines do not require harvesting tumor and custom manufacturing for each individual patient. Unlike peptide vaccines, allogeneic vaccines contain numerous tumor antigens that do not require the laborious isolation and characterization process. Also, a higher number of antigens theoretically reduces the chance of tumor escape. Drawbacks to allogeneic vaccines include the possibility that since allogeneic vaccines are derived from unrelated tumor lines, the target tumor may not express the same antigens contained in the vaccine, rendering the vaccine ineffective. Immune monitoring can be more challenging than with peptide vaccines as the important target antigens may be uncharacterized. Also, since the tumor used to derive the vaccine is unrelated to the patient, HLA class restriction of the important tumor antigens may limit vaccine response in a broad patient population. This phenomenon has been observed in phase III clinical trials, as discussed below.

Autologous whole-cell vaccines are derived from the patient's own tumor. Compared with the other vaccine strategies, this approach has the theoretical advantage of having a relatively higher likelihood of containing the important tumor antigens for a significant immune response while avoiding the labor-intensive task of identification and purification of individual antigens. Furthermore, since autologous tumor vaccines are derived from the tumor of individual patients, the vaccines are by definition appropriately HLA-matched for optimum antigen presentation. Disadvantages include the requirement of resecting the individual patient's tumor in order to generate the vaccine. In many cases, tumor is inaccessible or the amount available is inadequate for the multiple administrations that are typically required. Also, the time it takes to resect and manufacture vaccine may result in significant tumor progression prior to the initiation of treatment. Finally, unlike the other vaccine strategies, autologous tumor vaccines require a technically challenging manufacturing process that is difficult to standardize for all patients.

In order for vaccines to stimulate a T-cell response, regardless of the type of vaccine strategy employed, the antigens from the vaccine must be taken up by 'professional' antigen-presenting cells (APC), such as dendritic cells (DC). This has led to investigations that combine DC with vaccine therapy or directly apply antigen to the DC. In preclinical tests, DC-based vaccines have been shown to induce potent primary and memory T-cell anti-tumor responses.[3–6] Clinical trials are currently underway to examine the combination of DC with multi-peptide vaccines. However, similar to autologous vaccines, DC-based vaccines are limited by the need to obtain autologous DC and to grow the cells in vitro. This process is expensive, time-consuming, and difficult to standardize for all patients.

## THE USE OF IMMUNOSTIMULATORY ADJUVANTS

Despite the great effort to develop cancer vaccines, the typical anti-cancer immune responses yielded by vaccination are relatively weak and transient in nature. Because of this, investigators have employed immunostimulatory adjuvants, substances that are administered along with vaccines to improve the immune response. Several immunostimulatory adjuvant strategies are listed in Table 54.2. Selection of an appropriate adjuvant is challenging because there have been few direct comparisons of the various adjuvants in any clinical trial. In addition, an adjuvant that is successful in augmenting the immune response with one vaccine in a given patient may not have the same effect with a different vaccine in the same patient or the same vaccine in a different patient.

A promising novel approach to augmenting response to vaccine involves encapsulating the vaccine into liposomes with immune-stimulating cytokines such as interleukin-2 (IL-2) or granulocyte–macrophage colony-stimulating factor (GM-CSF). Antigen presentation is thought to be optimal for immune activation when it occurs in the lymph node. The liposomal formulation prolongs the half-life of the cytokines and may allow the delivery of antigen to the draining lymph node where immune stimulation can be

**Table 54.2 Immunostimulatory Adjuvants Used in Melanoma Vaccine Preparations**

| Adjuvant | Description |
|---|---|
| Alum | Aluminum-containing compound empirically found to improve the immune response; typically used in vaccines for infectious disease |
| BCG | Antigens derived from *Mycobacterium bovis*; initially used as a tuberculosis vaccine |
| QS-21 | A saponin; derived from the bark of a South American tree empirically found to improve the immune response |
| DETOX (detoxified Freund's adjuvant) | Mycobacterial cell wall/endotoxin mixture |
| Liposomes | Lipid micelles that encapsulate proteins in a hydrophobic environment; used as a delivery agent to increase exposure of antigens to lymph nodes |
| Interleukin-2/GM-CSF | Proinflammatory cytokines |
| Dendritic cells | Professional antigen-presenting cells which present peptide fragments to naïve T cells |

maximized.[7] Alternatively, vaccine-incorporated DCs have been genetically modified to express CCL21, a chemokine that is important for stimulating immune cells to migrate to lymph nodes.[8] These novel concepts designed to augment immune response to vaccine therapy have been supported in preclinical studies but need to be validated in large clinical trials.

## PATIENT SELECTION FOR VACCINE THERAPY

In vitro correlative studies have indicated that anti-melanoma vaccines can result in measurable immunologic responses to tumor antigens. In isolated cases, the immunological response is associated with measurable clinical tumor regression. However, when vaccine therapy for advanced metastatic melanoma has been held to the same standards for clinical outcome as traditional chemotherapy, the results have been disappointing. Rosenberg et al.[9] reviewed the results of 440 patients with advanced metastatic cancer, mainly melanoma, treated with 541 different vaccines in clinical trials at the National Cancer Institute. Using established response criteria, the overall response rate was only 2.6%.

Most phase III trials involving vaccine therapy for advanced metastatic melanoma have been equally disappointing, as direct comparison of multiple different vaccine types to 'standard' treatments, or even to placebo, have generally not shown improved outcome. Since vaccine therapy for melanoma has not been successful in the setting of advanced metastatic melanoma, focus has shifted to treating patients with less extensive disease. Patients with a lower burden of disease tend to have a better performance status and have a theoretically improved capacity to mount an immune response to the vaccine. Furthermore,

### Table 54.3 Summary of Recent Phase III Clinical Trials Investigating Vaccine Therapy for Melanoma

| Study | Vaccine Arm | Control | Stage | n | Result |
|---|---|---|---|---|---|
| Morton et al.[15,16] | Allogeneic whole cell + BCG | BCG + placebo | Stage III resected | 1160 | Control arm exhibited superior survival (p=0.04) |
| Morton et al.[15,16] | Allogeneic whole cell + BCG | BCG + placebo | Stage IV resected | 496 | No significant difference |
| Kirkwood et al.[17] | Defined antigen GMK (GM2 ganglioside coupled to KLH+QS-21 adjuvant) | High-dose interferon-α2b | IIb/III | 774 | Control arm exhibited superior disease-free and overall survival (p=0.035) |
| Eggermont et al.[18] | Defined antigen GMK (GM2 ganglioside coupled to KLH+QS-21 adjuvant) | Observation | II | 1314 | Control arm exhibited superior overall survival (p=0.02) but identical disease-free survival |
| Sondak et al.[19] | Allogeneic whole cell lysate + DETOX | Observation | T3N0 resected | 600 | No significant difference |
| Testori et al.[22] | Autologous tumor-derived antigens complexed with heat shock proteins | Best alternative care | IV with measurable disease | 322 | No significant difference |
| Schwartzentruber et al.[23] | Defined tumor antigen gp100 + high dose IL-2 | High dose IL-2 | IV with measurable disease | 185 | Vaccine arm exhibited superior response rate (p=0.02) and progression-free survival (p=0.01) |

such patients also tend to have a shorter disease duration compared to patients with advanced metastatic disease and therefore have a theoretically lower chance for tumor immune escape through mutation.

This fact underscores the importance of appropriate patient selection when considering vaccine therapy for melanoma. It is therefore not surprising that recent vaccine trials have typically included patients with excellent performance status who undergo complete surgical resection but have a high risk for recurrence. These patients are treated with vaccine therapy in the adjuvant setting, meaning the vaccine is administered after definitive surgical resection as an additional treatment to reduce the risk of recurrence. Examples of recent phase III vaccine trials for melanoma are discussed below and are enumerated in Table 54.3.

## CLINICAL TRIALS

Canvaxin was a promising allogeneic vaccine consisting of irradiated cells from three different cell lines administered with the adjuvant bacille Calmette-Guérin (BCG). This preparation was found to be potentially beneficial in preclinical studies as well as in phase I/II clinical trials.[10–13] The vaccine appeared to have significant benefit in the post-surgical adjuvant setting when compared to historical controls, and a retrospective study found that patients who exhibited a higher response to the vaccine based upon in vitro correlative assays had improved outcomes.[14]

Canvaxin was then studied in a pair of phase III clinical trials comparing the vaccine plus the adjuvant BCG to BCG alone in resected stage III and IV melanoma patients. The studies involved completely resected melanoma patients with a relatively high risk of recurrence rather than including

patients with widely metastatic unresectable disease. While the results of the trials have not yet been published in a full format, the results were reported in abstract form after the trials were stopped early due to inadequate benefit of the vaccine at interim analysis. For the 496 stage IV patients studied, the control group actually had a trend for improved 5-year survival rate compared to the Canvaxin-treated group (44.9% vs 39.6%, p=0.24). For the 1160 stage III patients studied, the control group exhibited a statistically significantly improved 5-year survival rate compared to the Canvaxin group (59.1% vs 67.7%, p=0.04). Thus, despite the preceding non-randomized studies indicating benefit compared to historical controls, Canvaxin failed to improve patient outcome when broadly applied in phase III clinical trials and might possibly have worsened it.[15,16] This is a theme that has been repeated by a number of other anti-melanoma vaccine trials.

E1694 was a phase III clinical trial comparing the use of high-dose interferon-alfa to a vaccine known as GMK, containing the non-protein melanoma antigen ganglioside GM2 with QS21 as the immunologic adjuvant. A total of 774 eligible patients with resected stage IIB/III were included in the trial. The trial was stopped early after interim analysis revealed a significantly worse outcome for the vaccine group. Patients receiving interferon exhibited a significantly improved freedom from relapse (hazard ratio 1.47, p=0.0027), and overall survival (hazard ratio 1.52, p=0.0147). On further analysis of the GMK-treated group, those patients with higher antibody titers in response to the vaccine had a trend for improved overall survival (p=0.068).[17] An even larger phase III trial involving 1314 patients with resected stage II melanoma compared adjuvant GMK vaccination to observation. This trial was also stopped early, as, on interim analysis, patients in the observation arm exhibited a trend toward improved overall survival with no difference in disease-free survival.[18] The results of these trials have prompted questions regarding the safety of vaccine therapy (see below).

SWOG-9035 was a phase III clinical trial involving the use of Melacine, an allogeneic cell lysate derived from two melanoma-derived cell lines administered with detoxified Freund's adjuvant. The study involved patients following resection of clinically node-negative intermediate-thickness melanoma (1.5–4 mm or Clark level IV). A total of 600 eligible patients were randomized 1:1 to vaccine versus observation. The estimated 5-year relapse-free survival was 65% in the vaccine arm compared to 63% in the observation arm (p=0.83). While these results were disappointing, on subsequent analysis, a subset of patients expressing at least two of five pre-specified HLA haplotypes had a superior 5-year relapse-free survival (83% vs 59%; p=0.0002). Most of the benefit was derived in patients with two HLA haplotypes: A2 and/or C3.[19,20]

The reason for the beneficial association noted was not clear. However, this observed phenomenon is consistent with previous phase I and II trials involving Melacine that also demonstrated superior responses for treated patients with HLA-A2 and C3 haplotypes.[21] It is possible that these two haplotypes are more efficient at presenting melanoma-derived antigens. Alternatively, the two haplotypes may be closely linked to other genes which confer a better response to vaccine. These possibilities could be exploited to improve responses to the vaccine but have yet to be fully explored. In addition to selecting patients with less burden of disease, this trial indicates the potential importance of selecting patients with genetic factors that may predict an improved response to the vaccine.

A phase III clinical trial involving an autologous melanoma vaccine for the treatment of metastatic measurable disease was recently reported. Vitespen, also known as Oncophage, contains heat shock proteins complexed with antigenic peptides derived from autologous resected tumors. This trial randomized 322 stage IV melanoma patients at a 2:1 ratio to either the vaccine arm or best alternative care. There was no observed difference in overall survival between the two groups. However, of the patients randomly assigned to the vaccine group, only 62% received one or more doses of the vaccine. The main reason patients who were randomized to the vaccine group failed to receive continued vaccine therapy was due to technical difficulties associated with custom manufacturing of the vaccine. A minority of patients failed to receive the vaccine due to inability to undergo surgical resection and/or significant disease progression prior to the preparation of the vaccine.[22] While the overall results of the trial did not indicate a benefit, pre-selection of patients with sufficient tumor volume to generate ample vaccine may be a necessary prerequisite to adequately explore the potential benefit of autologous vaccination strategies.

Another prospective randomized phase III clinical trial compared high-dose IL-2 to peptide vaccination with the melanoma-associated antigen gp100 followed by high-dose IL-2.[23] The multicenter trial involved 185 patients with stage IV or locally advanced stage III disease, all of whom were pre-selected to be HLA-A2 positive. The tumor antigen

gp100 is a melanocyte-lineage protein and its dominant peptide is efficiently presented by HLA-A2. While publication of the trial is pending, results have been presented in abstract form. When compared to the control arm, the vaccine arm had a significant improvement in response rate (22.1% vs 9.7%; p=0.022), and progression-free survival (2.9 months vs 1.6 months; p=0.010), and had a trend towards an improvement in overall survival (17.6 months vs 12.8 months; p=0.096). As seen in the Melacine trial, this trial demonstrates the importance of patient selection. The study appropriately included only HLA-A2-positive patients who were likely to respond to the vaccination. However, the HLA-A2 class restriction of this gp100 peptide vaccine prevents its application to all patients.

## COULD VACCINES ACTUALLY BE HARMFUL?

Vaccine therapy, which has been enormously successful in the prevention of traditional infectious disease, has been disappointing when applied to established cancer. In fact, several clinical trials have raised the question of whether certain vaccine strategies may actually worsen patient outcome. In the trials involving Canvaxin described above, the stage IV melanoma control group had a trend for improved 5-year survival compared to the vaccine-treated group (44 months vs 39 months, p=NS). Alarmingly, the stage III melanoma control group had a statistically significant improvement in 5-year survival compared to the vaccine group (67 months vs 59 months, p=0.04). The above-described phase III study comparing the ganglioside vaccine GMK to interferon in 1314 resected stage II melanoma patients was stopped early by a safety committee due to inferior survival in the vaccine arm.[18] This finding was similar to the previous E1694 study described above involving patients with stage IIB and III melanoma where interferon alone exhibited an improved survival compared to interferon and GMK vaccine.[17] The reason for a potentially worse outcome in this study with the addition of vaccine therapy is unclear. It was noted that the survival of the patients treated in the ECOG GMK vaccine trial exhibited survival that was comparable to historical controls. Therefore the difference in outcome could be explained by the beneficial effects of interferon rather than any deleterious effects of the vaccine. However, some experts have speculated that vaccine therapy may induce an immuno-inhibitory effect that blunts the native anti-tumor immune response, but this has yet to be proven.

This controversy of potentially harmful effects generated by vaccine therapy underscores the fact that a better understanding of tumor immunology and the basic science of the immune system is required to develop more effective vaccine therapy for melanoma. Vaccine therapy alone may not be sufficient to cure cancer. Combinations of vaccines with novel forms of immunotherapy may be required to elicit a truly therapeutic immune response to melanoma.

## CURRENT VACCINE THERAPY TRIALS

Selection of patients likely to benefit from any systemic therapy has been emphasized as a critical component of any clinical trial. In line with such thinking, a global phase III double-blinded, placebo-controlled randomized trial is now underway evaluating the efficacy of a MAGE-3 vaccine. Only patients with MAGE-3-positive tumors (approximately 65% of melanoma patients) following resection of advanced regional lymph node metastases via a formal lymphadenectomy are eligible. The vaccine preparation includes the purified MAGE-3 antigen combined with a new immunologic adjuvant that is more potent than other adjuvants that have been used in previous vaccine trials. Furthermore, a favorable gene profile from the inflammatory cell population within the tumor has been identified as a potential marker for response to vaccine therapy. This gene profile has been detected in approximately 50% of the MAGE-3 population and may ultimately be used to select patients for therapy. Both the overall efficacy of the vaccine as well as the impact of this gene profile on outcome are the primary endpoints of the trial.

Recently, focus has been directed toward the combination of immunomodulatory agents with vaccine therapy. In order for vaccine-induced T-cell activation to occur, two signals are required. First, antigens must be presented in the context of MHC to stimulate the T-cell receptor. Next, T cells receive an activating signal induced by binding of ligands on APC with co-stimulatory receptors present on the T-cell membrane. To avoid autoimmunity, T cells do not receive the second signal when self antigens are presented on MHC. Tumor cells exploit this as an escape mechanism, essentially deceiving the immune system into treating them as normal self antigens.

One particular inhibitory protein found on T cells, called CTLA-4, has been extensively investigated.[24] While inhibition by CTLA-4 ostensibly limits the potential for deleterious autoimmunity under normal circumstances, this process also limits the beneficial anti-tumor immunity induced by vaccination. Antibodies that block CTLA-4 have been commercially developed with the hope of breaking immune tolerance to tumor antigens. The combination of CTLA-4 antibody treatment with vaccine therapy has yielded promising initial results in early-phase clinical trials. Interestingly, many of these trials reported a correlation between clinical benefit and the generation of autoimmune side effects, including dermatitis, vitiligo, enterocolitis, hepatitis, and hypophysitis. A recent phase III clinical trial randomized patients with unresectable, advanced melanoma to one of three groups: CTLA-4 blocking antibody, gp100 peptide vaccine, or both. The authors found a statistically significant improvement in overall survival in the groups receiving CTLA-4 blocking antibody compared to the group randomized to gp100 peptide vaccine alone. Disappointingly, there was no evidence of either improved efficacy or decreased toxicity in the group receiving both the antibody and the vaccine.[25] In addition to CTLA-4, studies involving the blockade or stimulation of other immune modulators, such as PD-1, 4-1BB, and OX-40, are under preclinical and early clinical investigation, either alone or in combination with vaccine therapy.[26] The positive results of the CTLA-4 blocking antibody phase III trial have created a renewed wave of excitement about immunotherapy in general, but how this will translate into improving the prospects for vaccine therapy remains to be seen.

## FUTURE OUTLOOK

The potential utility of vaccine therapy for the treatment of melanoma is still as tantalizing as ever. While preclinical data as well as early phase I and II clinical vaccine trials indicate a theoretical benefit, these results have not been reproduced in phase III clinical vaccine trials. It is likely that past strategies for the use of anti-melanoma vaccines have not been ideal. Rather than treating patients with advanced metastatic disease, focus has shifted towards treating patients with completely resected disease in the adjuvant setting to reduce future recurrence. Further characterization of the immune response to vaccine therapy in different patients may identify genetic markers that can be used to pre-select patients with a higher chance of clinical benefit.

In the future, vaccine therapy may have an enormous impact on melanoma care when applied to the right patients, at the right time, and with the right combination of adjuvants and immunomodulatory agents. Until this can be established in randomized controlled clinical trials, vaccine therapy for melanoma may continue to remain a promise that is unfulfilled.

## REFERENCES

1. Tran KQ, Zhou J, Durflinger KH, et al. Minimally cultured tumor-infiltrating lymphocytes display optimal characteristics for adoptive cell therapy. J Immunother. 2008;31(8):742–751.
2. Dudley ME, Yang JC, Sherry R, et al. Adoptive cell therapy for patients with metastatic melanoma: evaluation of intensive myeloablative chemoradiation preparative regimens. J Clin Oncol. 2008;26(32):5233–5239.
3. Mulé JJ. Dendritic cell-based vaccines for pancreatic cancer and melanoma. Ann N Y Acad Sci. 2009;1174:33–40.
4. Redman BG, Chang AE, Whitfield J, et al. Phase Ib trial assessing autologous, tumor-pulsed dendritic cells as a vaccine administered with or without IL-2 in patients with metastatic melanoma. J Immunother. 2008;31(6):591–598.
5. Koike N, Pilon-Thomas S, Mulé JJ. Nonmyeloablative chemotherapy followed by T-cell adoptive transfer and dendritic cell-based vaccination results in rejection of established melanoma. J Immunother. 2008;31(4):402–412.
6. Palucka K, Ueno H, Fay J, et al. Harnessing dendritic cells to generate cancer vaccines. Ann N Y Acad Sci. 2009;1174:88–98.
7. Koppenhagen FJ, Küpcü Z, Wallner G, et al. Sustained cytokine delivery for anticancer vaccination: liposomes as alternative for gene-transfected tumor cells. Clin Cancer Res. 1998;4(8):1881–1886.
8. Terando A, Roessler B, Mulé JJ. Chemokine gene modification of human dendritic cell-based tumor vaccines using a recombinant adenoviral vector. Cancer Gene Ther. 2004;11(3):165–173.
9. Rosenberg SA, Yang JC, Restifo NP. Cancer immunotherapy: moving beyond current vaccines. Nat Med. 2004;10(9):909–915.
10. Morton DL, Foshag LJ, Hoon DS, et al. Prolongation of survival in metastatic melanoma after active specific immunotherapy with a new polyvalent melanoma vaccine. Ann Surg. 1992;216(4):463–482.
11. Hsueh EC, Gupta RK, Qi K, et al. Correlation of specific immune responses with survival in melanoma patients with distant metastases receiving polyvalent melanoma cell vaccine. J Clin Oncol. 1998;16(9):2913–2920.
12. Shen P, Foshag LJ, Essner R, et al. Postoperative adjuvant therapy using a polyvalent melanoma vaccine improves overall survival of patients with primary melanoma. Proc Am Soc Clin Oncol. 1999;18S: abstr 2059.
13. Morton DL, Hsueh EC, Essner R, et al. Prolonged survival of patients receiving active immunotherapy with Canvaxin therapeutic polyvalent vaccine after complete resection of melanoma metastatic to regional lymph nodes. Ann Surg. 2002;236(4):438–448.
14. DiFronzo LA, Morton DL. Melanoma vaccines: current status of clinical trials. Adv Oncol. 2000;6:23–29.
15. Morton DL, Mozzillo N, Thompson JF, et al. An international, randomized, phase III trial of bacillus Calmette-Guerin (BCG) plus allogeneic melanoma vaccine (MCV) or placebo after complete resection

of melanoma metastatic to regional or distant sites. *J Clin Oncol.* 2007;18S: abstr 8508.

16. *CancerVax Corporation media release.* October 3, 2005. Available from: http://www.accessmylibrary.com/coms2/summary_0286-31746079_ITM.

17. Kirkwood JM, Ibrahim JG, Sosman JA, et al. High-dose interferon alfa-2b significantly prolongs relapse-free and overall survival compared with the GM2-KLH/QS-21 vaccine in patients with resected stage IIB-III melanoma: results of intergroup trial E1694/S9512/C509801. *J Clin Oncol.* 2001;19(9):2370–2380.

18. Eggermont AM, Suciu S, Ruka W, et al. EORTC 18961: Postoperative adjuvant ganglioside GM2-KLH21 vaccination treatment vs observation in stage II (T3-T4 N0M0) melanoma: 2nd interim analysis led to an early disclosure of the results. *J Clin Oncol.* 2008;26S: abstr 9004.

19. Sondak VK, Liu PY, Tuthill RJ, et al. Adjuvant immunotherapy of resected, intermediate-thickness, node-negative melanoma with an allogeneic tumor vaccine: overall results of a randomized trial of the Southwest Oncology Group. *J Clin Oncol.* 2002;20(8):2058–2066.

20. Sosman JA, Unger JM, Liu PY, et al. Southwest Oncology Group. Adjuvant immunotherapy of resected, intermediate-thickness, node-negative melanoma with an allogeneic tumor vaccine: impact of HLA class I antigen expression on outcome. *J Clin Oncol.* 2002;20(8):2067–2075.

21. Mitchell MS, Harel W, Groshen S. Association of HLA phenotype with response to active specific immunotherapy of melanoma. *J Clin Oncol.* 1992;10(7):1158–1164.

22. Testori A, Richards J, Whitman E, et al. Phase III comparison of vitespen, an autologous tumor-derived heat shock protein gp96 peptide complex vaccine, with physician's choice of treatment for stage IV melanoma: the C-100-21 Study Group. *J Clin Oncol.* 2008;26(6):955–962.

23. Schwartzentruber DJ, Lawson D, Richards J, et al. A phase III multi-institutional randomized study of immunization with the gp100:209-217(210M) peptide followed by high-dose IL-2 compared with high-dose IL-2 alone in patients with metastatic melanoma. *J Clin Oncol.* 2009;18S: abstr 9011.

24. Sarnaik AA, Weber JS. Recent advances using anti-CTLA-4 for the treatment of melanoma. *Cancer J.* 2009;15(3):169–173.

25. Hodi FS, O'Day SJ, McDermott DF, et al. Improved survival with ipilimumab in patients with metastatic melanoma. *N Engl J Med.* 2010;363(8):711–23.

26. Vohra N, Pilon-Thomas S, Weber J, et al. New approaches for optimizing melanoma vaccines. In: Agarwala SS, Sondak VK, eds. *Melanoma: Translational Research and Emerging Therapies.* New York: Informa Healthcare; 2008:143–160.

# Targeted Therapy for Melanoma

*Stergios Moschos*

---

## Key Points

- A number of targets in melanoma cells and the melanoma tumor microenvironment exist.

- Early targeted clinical studies against the oncogenic form of B-Raf (V600E) using PLX-4032 have shown promising results.

- Rational drug combinations will prevent inevitable drug resistance using single-agent therapies.

---

## INTRODUCTION

Conventional systemic chemotherapies and immunotherapies have not translated into clinically significant benefit for the treatment of melanoma and other skin cancers over the last 30 years, as summarized in a recent meta-analysis.[1] In parallel with these largely unsuccessful clinical efforts, advances in understanding the biology of melanocytes, the genetic makeup of melanoma cells as well as the role of the tumor microenvironment have provided important insights regarding the role of several molecules in melanoma development and progression, and the resistance of melanoma cells to chemotherapy, and melanoma's genetic heterogeneity. Finally, the emergence of clinical-grade compounds that potently and specifically inhibit the pathways of progression has provided us with opportunities to make a significant impact in the lives of patients with metastatic melanoma (MM).

Targeted cancer therapies ideally take into consideration the higher, or even exclusive, expression of particular molecules in cancer cells and their neighboring host cells (immune, endothelial, and stromal cells) over the other normal cells of the body. If the above conditions are present, we may expect that treatment with agents that *selectively* and *potently* inhibit the target(s) will have a high therapeutic index (Fig. 55.1). Obviously, successful use of targeted therapies is dependent upon the precise knowledge of the molecules/pathway(s) that drive the disease at a particular stage.

## TARGETS IN METASTATIC MELANOMA

As in many other cancers, melanoma development and progression may be regarded as a complex process, rather than the isolated deregulation of melanocyte proliferation, cell senescence and survival mechanisms. Melanoma cells interact closely with and depend upon their microenvironment, defined as stromal, endothelial, and immune cells (Fig. 55.2).

One of the most important recent advances in the field of melanoma has been the realization that it is a genetically heterogeneous disease, based on distinct molecular changes within different molecular pathways[2–4] that can, to a certain extent, be clinically defined.[5] This has triggered an increasing number of clinical trials in patients with MM testing molecularly targeted therapies. For example, constitutive activation of the *Ras/Raf*/MEK/ERK pathway is observed in up to 90% of melanoma patients and is most commonly mediated via mutations in *N-Ras* or *B-Raf*.[2,6] The *Ras/PI3K/Akt* cascade is another important signaling pathway that is activated in 60% of melanomas. In contrast with the *Raf/MEK/ERK* pathway, however, the activation of the *PI3K/Akt3* pathway is usually secondary to activation of upstream receptor tyrosine kinases and other epigenetic mechanisms and less attributable to mutations.[7] One of these upstream kinases is c-Kit, the stem cell factor receptor that, upon activation, triggers several other downstream events apart from PI3K activation, such as the MAPK kinase pathway. c-Kit aberrations, in the form of either mutations or gene amplifications, have been observed in up to 40% of mucosal, acral lentiginous, and chronically sun-damaged melanomas, providing opportunities for therapeutic intervention in this small subset of melanomas, as will be discussed below.

As a result of these and other deregulated signal transduction pathways, melanoma cells are able to shape their microenvironment by secreting growth factor(s) and other enzymes that stimulate lymph and blood vessel growth and/or acquire the ability to migrate, invade and metastasize. A number of angiogenic growth factors and their corresponding receptors have been shown to play an important role in melanoma, and they synergize with integrins, extracellular matrix components and matrix metalloproteinases.[8] Furthermore, melanoma cells may secrete cytokines and chemokines that create an immunosuppressive microenvironment in which immune cells either cannot enter the tumor site or are present within the tumor but are dysfunctional and fail to eradicate the tumor. Over the last decade, a number of cells and molecules expressed by either the host immune or melanoma cells have been shown to play a role in tumor-mediated immune suppression, such as the immunosuppressive T regulatory cells (CD4+CD25+FoxP3+), the cytotoxic T-lymphocyte antigen 4 (CTLA-4), and the programmed cell death-1 (PD-1) protein.[9]

Targeted therapies can be grouped based on the molecular target of interest and the presumed mechanism of action, i.e. in melanoma cell versus the cellular components of the tumor microenvironment (vascular endothelium, extracellular matrix, and immune cell compartment).

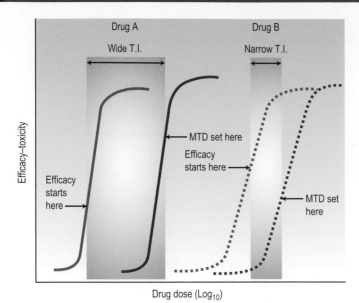

**Figure 55.1** How molecularly targeted therapies may improve therapeutic index (T.I.) compared to standard chemotherapeutic agents. Proposed dose–response curves for two drugs; drug A that is more potent (continued lines) and drug B that is less potent (dashed lines). For each drug, hypothetical efficacy (blue) and toxicity (red) dose–response curves are shown. Measurements of efficacy may be based on a defined pharmacodynamic endpoint, whereas the maximum tolerated dose (MTD) is defined based on standard dose-escalation phase I trials. Drug A could be a molecularly targeted therapy that inhibits a critical protein for melanoma maintenance, progression and survival (e.g. B-Raf V600E), whereas drug B could be a molecularly targeted therapy or chemotherapy that inhibit(s) a critical protein(s) for survival and function of *both* melanoma *and* normal cells (e.g. the anti-apoptotic protein bcl-2 or topoisomerase). Therefore it is anticipated that molecularly targeted therapies are more potent (less drug dose to achieve a measurable effect) and less toxic because they target proteins that are either uniquely expressed in melanoma cells compared to normal host cells (e.g. B-Raf V600E) or proteins that are expressed only in few cells of the human body (for example B-Raf is expressed almost exclusively in cells from the neural crest). On the other side, less potent drugs (location of the dose–response curve at higher numbers along the dose axis) may ultimately have the same greatest attainable response ('ceiling' effect); however, because they have multiple 'off-target' effects, considerable toxicity occurs.

## Targeting melanoma cell surface molecules

Table 55.1 shows clinical trials that are MM-specific or non-selective phase 0–I trials using compounds that target melanoma cell surface proteins. In fact, clinical trials using imatinib (Gleevec®), an inhibitor of c-Kit, were several of the earliest small molecule inhibitor therapies conducted in patients with MM. Both early trials testing imatinib, which were unrestricted for morphotypes, anatomic location, and sun exposure status,[10,11] as well as subsequent trials that actually 'enriched' for patients with specific melanoma sub-types, had disappointing results.[12,13] Similar studies using other small molecule inhibitors of c-Kit, such as sunitinib and dasatinib, alone or in combination with chemotherapy, produced similar disappointing results. The identification of frequent but disparate genetic aberrations of c-KIT in distinct melanoma subtypes,[4] as well as the few anecdotal reports of dramatic clinical responses in melanoma patients to such therapies,[14] has sustained clinical research to further define a subgroup of patients that will most likely respond to c-Kit inhibitors. A recent phase II study of imatinib in 25 Chinese patients with MM and c-Kit gene aberrations was associated with 21% partial response. As has previ-

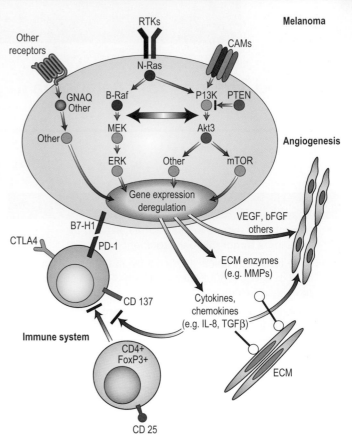

**Figure 55.2** Simplified diagram of several targets in metastatic melanoma of current interest for clinical development. Not all targets are shown. The molecularly targeted targets can be classified as direct, against the melanoma cells, or indirect, targeting tumor-induced angiogenesis, components of the host immune system or components of the extracellular matrix (ECM). Targets can be further classified as those having high incidence of mutations (red letters/cycles), low incidence of mutations (blue letters/cycles) or no mutations (wild-type; grey letters/cycles) or a combination of both (black/red). Only c-Kit, a member of the receptor tyrosine kinase (RTK) family, has high incidence of DNA aberrations (gene amplifications, mutations) whereas receptors for cell adhesion molecules (CAMs; e.g. integrin) have been previously shown to be overexpressed. The role of other receptors (e.g. G-protein-coupled receptors, NOTCH, Wnt) is unclear but higher frequency of mutations in the GRM1 gene (a G-protein-coupled receptor) or other downstream effectors (GNAQ, guanine nucleotide-binding protein alpha-q) have been recently described in melanoma subsets. The Raf-MEK-ERK and PI3K-Akt pathways are constitutively active in the majority of melanoma cases as a result of genetic or epigenetic changes. Such changes in melanoma cells may modulate ECM, host immune response, or angiogenesis. Immune cells (lymphocytes, macrophages, dendritic cells) are frequently dysfunctional within the tumor microenvironment and can be either suppressed (⊥) by melanoma cells themselves or by other lymphocytes (CD4+CD25+FoxP3+ T regulatory cells).

ously been described,[15] no particular mutations and/or gene amplifications were predictors of antitumor response in this study.

Therapeutic targeting of other melanoma cell surface molecules has been less well studied and even less rewarding. Several clinical studies using humanized monoclonal antibodies against integrins have been conducted. Although infrequent objective antitumor responses have been observed, there is a suggestion that such therapies may prolong disease-free and/or overall survival, although the calculated margin of benefit appears to be small enough that only larger phase III trials may establish this. The clinical activity of riluzole, an inhibitor of metabotropic glutamate receptor (GRM1), has

**Table 55.1 Summary of Clinical Trials Using Single Agents that Target Surface Molecules in Melanoma Cells. Clinical Trials Highlighted in Bold Have Reported More than 10% Antitumor Response**

| Drug | Sponsor | Target | Phase | Status | References |
|---|---|---|---|---|---|
| Imatinib | Novartis | c-Abl, p210$^{bcr-abl}$, p185bcr-abl, PDGF-Rβ, c-KIT | II* | Completed | Ugurel (Br J Cancer 2005) Wyman (Cancer 2006) Kim (Br J Cancer 2008) |
| | | | II*, o | Completed | Fiorentini (J Exp Clin Cancer Res 2003) Hofman (Clin Cancer Res 2009) Mouriaux (ASCO 2008, abstr 9061) |
| | | | **II*, m or a/l** | **Ongoing** | **Li (Perspectives in Melanoma XIII, O-0007)** |
| Sunitinib | Pfizer | Flt3, c-kit, VEGF-R2, PDGF-R, RET, CSF-1R | II* | Completed | Chan (ASCO 2008, abstr 9047) |
| | | | II*, m or a/l | Ongoing | N/A |
| Dasatinib | BMS | Bcr-abl, src, c-KIT, ephrin, PDGFβ | II* | Completed | Kluger (ASCO 2009, abstr 9010) |
| Etarasizumab | Medimmune | $\alpha_v\beta_3$ integrin | 0* | Completed | Moschos (J Immunother 2009) |
| | | | rII* | Completed | Hersey (ASCO 2005, abstr 7507) |
| CNTO 95 | Centocor, Janssen-Cilag Farma | αV integrins | rII* | Completed | Loquai (ASCO 2009, abstr 9029) |
| Volociximab | PDL BioPharma Biogen Idec | $\alpha_5\beta_1$ integrin | I | Completed | Ricart (Clin Cancer Res 2008) |
| | | | II* | Completed | Cranmer (ASCO 2006, abstr 8011) |
| KW-2871 | Kyowa Hakko Kirin | Ganglioside GD3 | I* | Completed | Forero (Cancer Bioth Radiopharm 2006) |
| MEDI-547 | Medimmune | EphA2 | I | Ongoing | N/A |
| Pentetreotide$^{In111}$ | Yale University | Somatostatin receptor | I | Ongoing | N/A |
| Riluzone | S-A | GRM1 | 0* | Completed | Yip (Clin Cancer Res 2009) |

BMS, Bristol-Myers Squibb; S-A, Sanofi-Aventis; CSF-1R, colony stimulating factor 1 receptor; FLT3, FMS-like tyrosine kinase 3; GRM1, metabotropic glutamate receptor-1; PDGF-R, platelet-derived growth factor receptor; VEGF-R, vascular endothelial growth factor receptor; *melanoma-specific trials; a/l, acral lentiginous; m, mucosal; o, ocular; r, randomized trials that compare the molecularly targeted agent alone or in combination with chemotherapy; N/A, no results published in peer-reviewed journal or announced at any international medical oncology meeting as of October 2009; ASCO, American Society of Clinical Oncology Annual Meeting.

also recently been suggested in an early biomarker (phase 0) study in patients with MM. The potential importance of this molecule in melanoma was shown in a murine model in which ectopic expression of GRM1 in vivo leads to development of MM that closely resemble the human counterpart but do not usually develop distant metastases.[16] Further clinical development of riluzole is expected to delineate whether targeting this G-protein-coupled receptor of uncertain function provides a true clinical benefit.

## Targeting intracellular molecules

Tables 55.2–55.4 show clinical trials that have focused at least in part upon patients with MM, using molecules that inhibit intracellular targets. Almost 70% of melanomas harbor somatic activating mutations of the B-Raf proto-onco-gene, and up to 20% have activating mutations in N-Ras.[2] Targeting N-Ras has been a challenging task from a drug

discovery standpoint, owing to its different enzymatic type: first, it is a GTPase rather than another ATPase-type kinase; second, when mutated, its enzymatic activity is suppressed as opposed to being constitutively active. Targeting N-Ras first became possible in the clinic by inhibiting farnesylation. A single phase II study of R115777, a farnesyl transferase inhibitor, showed no antitumor activity.

The Raf/MEK/ERK pathway has been extensively targeted in clinical trials for patients with MM, in view of the activating mutations of B-Raf. In fact, B-Raf mutations are not only frequent in melanomas, but also consist of a single substitution (V600E) that results in constitutive activation of its kinase function.[2] This 'signature' B-Raf mutation provides a unique opportunity for targeted therapy of melanoma with a superior therapeutic index, since it is uniquely expressed in melanoma but not normal host cells. Although this B-Raf mutation profile in melanoma has been known for 7 years, highly selective B-Raf kinase inhibitors have only entered the

### Table 55.2 Summary of Clinical Trials in Melanoma and Other Solid Tumors Using Single Agents that Target the Ras-Raf-Mapk-Erk Pathway. Clinical Trials Highlighted in Bold have Reported More than 10% Antitumor Response

| Drug | Sponsor | Target | Phase | Status | Reference |
|------|---------|--------|-------|--------|-----------|
| R115777 | J&J | Farnesyltransferase inhibitor | II* | Completed | Gajewski (ASCO 2006, abstr 8014) |
| RAF265 | Novartis | A-Raf, B-Raf, C-Raf, VEGFR-2 | I/II* | Ongoing | N/A |
| **PLX4032** | **Plexxicon/H-LR** | **B-Raf$^{V600E}$, B-Raf** | **I** | **Ongoing** | **Puzanov (Perspectives in Melanoma XIII)** |
| Sorafenib | Bayer | C-Raf VEGFR2,3, B-Raf/B-Raf$^{V600E}$, FLT-3/c-Kit | I | Completed | Eisen (Br J Cancer 2006) |
| **XL281** | **Exelixis** | **B-Raf, C-Raf, B-Raf$^{V600E}$** | **I** | **Ongoing** | **Schwartz (ASCO 2009, abstr 3513)** |
| AZD6244 | AstraZeneca | MEK1 | rII* | Ongoing | Dummer (ASCO 2008, abstr 9033) |
| PD-325901 | Pfizer | MEK1, MEK2 | I | Completed | Lorusso (ASCO 2005, abstr 3011) |
| RDEA119 | Ardea Biosc | MEK1, MEK2 | I | Ongoing | N/A |

J&J, Johnson & Johnson; H-LR, Hoffman-La Roche; MEK, mitogen-activated protein kinase 1; FLT3, FMS-like tyrosine kinase 3; VEGF-R, vascular endothelial growth factor receptor. *melanoma-specific trials; r, randomized trial that compares the molecularly targeted therapy alone against the standard of care; ASCO, American Society of Clinical Oncology Annual Meeting; N/A, no results published in peer-reviewed journal or announced at any international medical oncology meeting as of October 2009.

### Table 55.3 Summary of Clinical Trials in Melanoma and Other Solid Tumors Using Single Agents that Target the PI3K-Akt-mTOR Pathway

| Drug | Sponsor | Target | Phase | Status | Reference |
|------|---------|--------|-------|--------|-----------|
| PX-866 | ProlX Pharma Oncothyreon | PI3K | I | Ongoing | Jimeno (ASCO 2009, abstr 3542) |
| Perifosine | Keryx Biopharma | Akt, Erk1/2 | II* | Completed | Ernst (Invest New Drugs 2005) |
| BEZ235, BGT226 | Novartis | Dual PI3K and mTOR inhibitor | I | Ongoing | N/A |
| XL765 | Exelixis | Dual PI3K and mTOR1,2 inhibitor | I | Ongoing | Lorusso (ASCO 2009, abstr 3502) |
| GSK1059615 | GSK | Dual PI3K and mTOR inhibitor | I | Ongoing | N/A |
| XL147 | Exelixis | PI3K | I | Ongoing | Shapiro (ASCO 2009, abstr 3500) |
| GDC0941 | Genetech/Piramed/Roche | PI3K | I | Ongoing | Wagner (ASCO 2009, abstr 3501) |
| BKM120 | Novartis | PI3K | I | Ongoing | N/A |
| Triciribine (TCN-PM) | VioQuest Pharma | Akt | I | Ongoing | N/A |
| MK2206 | Merck | Akt | I | Ongoing | N/A |
| UCN-01 | NCI | Pdk1, PKC, chk1, cdk2,4,6 | II* | Ongoing | N/A |
| Everolimus | NCI | mTOR | II* | Completed | Rao (ASCO 2009, abstr 8043) |
| CCI-779 | CCC | mTOR | II* | Completed | Margolin (Cancer 2005) |

GSK, GlaxoSmithKline; NCI, National Cancer Institute; CCC, California Cancer Consortium; mTOR, mammalian target of rapamycin; PI3K, phosphoinositide kinase 3; Pdk1, pyruvate dehydrogenase kinase isoenzyme 1; PKC, protein kinase C; chk, checkpoint kinase; cdk, cyclin-dependent kinase; Erk1/2, extracellular regulated kinase 1, 2; *melanoma-specific trials; ASCO, American Society of Clinical Oncology Annual Meeting; N/A, no results published in peer-reviewed journal or announced at any international medical oncology meeting as of October 2009.

clinic in the past 3 years. Sorafenib, the first clinically available B-Raf inhibitor to be tested in MM, was found to have no antitumor activity,[17] and exhibited very low potency in relation to both wild-type and mutant (V600E) forms of B-Raf (IC$_{50}$ in the micromolar range for cell lines in vitro). Early (phase I) and very recently conducted clinical trials testing highly selective class I (active conformation binder) B-Raf inhibitors have provided encouraging results, indicating that potent inhibition of B-Raf may provide clinical benefit to a majority of MM patients. More specifically, PLX4032, a highly selective inhibitor in melanoma cell lines bearing the B-Raf V600E mutation as opposed to wild-type B-Raf (IC$_{50}$ of wild-type over mutant

**Table 55.4 Summary of Clinical Trials in Melanoma and Other Solid Tumors Using Single Agents that Target Cell Cycle, Apoptosis or Other Intracellular Targets in Melanoma Cells**

| Drug | Sponsor | Target | Phase | Status | References |
|---|---|---|---|---|---|
| SNS-314 | Sunesis Pharma | Aurora kinase A and B | I | Ongoing | Robert (ASCO 2009, abstr 2536) |
| MLN8054 | Millenium Pharma | Aurora kinase A and B | I | Ongoing | Maraculla (ASCO 2009, abstr 2578) |
| AZD1152 | AstraZeneca | Aurora kinase A and B | I | Ongoing | Schellens (ASCO 2006, abstr 3008) |
| BI-2536 | Boehringer Ingelheim | Polo-like kinase 1 | I | Ongoing | Schöffski (ECCO 2009, abstr P-1260) |
| GSK461364 | GSK | Polo-like kinase 1 | I | Ongoing | Olmos (ASCO 2009, abstr 3536) |
| Flavopiridol | NCI | CDK4, CDK6, CDK1, GSK-3β, CDK2 | II* | Completed | Burdette-Radoux (Invest New Drugs 2004) |
| PD-0332991 | Pfizer | CDK4/6 | I | Completed | O'Dwyer (ASCO 2007, abstr 3550) |
| SCH727965 | Schering-Plough | CDK1,2,5,9 | I | Ongoing | Nemunaitis (ASCO 2009, abstr 3535) |
| ALS-357 | Advanced Life Sciences | Intrinsic apoptosis (?) | I-II* | Ongoing | N/A |
| G3139 | Genta Inc | bcl2 | II | Completed | Bedikian (J Clin Oncol 2006) |
| LY573636 | Eli-Lilly | Intrinsic apoptosis (?) | II* | Ongoing | N/A |
| Bortezomib | Millenium Pharma | 26S proteasome | II* | Completed | Markovic (Cancer 2005) |

GSK, GlaxoSmithKline; NCI, National Cancer Institute; CDK, cyclin-dependent kinase; GSK-3β, glycogen synthase kinase 3 beta; bcl2 B-cell lymphoma 2; *melanoma-specific trials; ASCO, American Society of Clinical Oncology Annual Meeting; ECCO, European CanCer Organization Annual Meeting; N/A, no results published in peer-reviewed journal or announced at any international medical oncology meeting as of October 2009.

(V600E) 110 nM and 44 nM, respectively) was administered to 49 patients with MM irrespective of V600E B-Raf mutation status. As of September 2009, PLX4032 was associated with a 70% antitumor response rate by RECIST criteria, although progression-free survival (PFS) was too early to be assessed (Figs 55.3 and 55.4). These early results are a major break-through in the treatment for MM and a proof-of-concept that targeting this oncogenic B-Raf mutation in MM has clinical benefit. Further evidence that selective inhibition of the MAP kinase, the immediate downstream effector of B-Raf, can induce antitumor effects comes from a large phase II study of AZD6244, a MEK1 inhibitor, in patients with MM. In that study, antitumor responses were noted in a small (10%) subset of patients harboring B-Raf mutations.[18] It is currently unknown whether more potent MEK inhibitors that are currently undergoing phase I testing in solid tumors will result in more frequent and impressive clinical responses.

Targeting the PI3K/Akt signaling that is frequently activated in melanoma has been challenging, due to the broader importance of this pathway in normal tissue homeostasis, and the lack of highly selective PI3K inhibitors. To date, targeting of the PI3K pathway in melanoma has been limited to its downstream effectors such as Akt or mammalian target of rapamycin (mTOR). None of the agents relevant to this pathway studied thus far have shown any promising activity. The clinical benefit, if any, that may result from PI3K pathway targeting in melanoma will be more adequately answered in the several ongoing phase I trials using highly selective and more potent inhibitors.

## TARGETING THE MELANOMA TUMOR MICROENVIRONMENT

### Targeting angiogenesis and extracellular matrix

A number of investigations have shown that increased serum levels of angiogenic growth factors, such as vascular endothelial growth factor (VEGF) and basic fibroblast

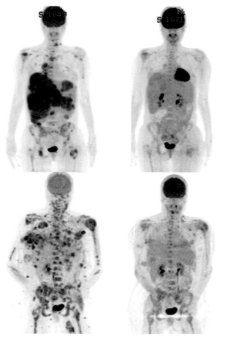

**Figure 55.3** Positron emission tomography (PET) images from two different patients with distant metastatic melanoma expressing the B-Raf[V600E] mutation, before (left) and after 15 days of administration of PLX4032 (right). Noteworthy is the impressive reduction of the tumor's metabolic activity as early as 15 days after administration of the study drug. (Courtesy of Keith T. Flaherty M.D.)

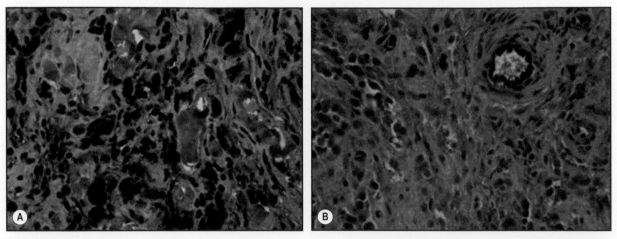

**Figure 55.4** Proof-of-principle that clinical benefit to a molecularly targeted drug is not anticipated unless the drug shows inhibition of its target and its downstream effectors at the tumor site. Melanoma biopsies from a patient with metastatic melanoma before **(A)** and after 15 days of PLX4032 administration (960 mg bid) **(B).** Representative paraffin-embedded tissue sections were immunohistochemically stained with an antibody against the activated-phosphorylated form of ERK. Administration of PLX4032 results in suppression of pERK, the downstream effector of B-Raf (40× magnification). (Courtesy of Katherine Nathanson M.D. and Keith T. Flaherty M.D.)

growth factor (bFGF), are associated with worse prognosis in patients with MM and poor response to standard therapies.[19] Table 55.5 shows clinical trials that have been conducted in, or have included, patients with MM using molecules that target angiogenesis or extracellular matrix components. The phase II trials that targeted angiogenesis, such as those testing TKI258 and aflibercept, have established the principle that targeting angiogenesis may result in clinically significant benefit via disease stabilization. However, no clinical benefit was observed with extracellular matrix inhibitors. Only axitinib (AG-013736), a potent pan-VEGFR and platelet-derived growth factor receptor (PDGFR) kinase inhibitor that was administered in 32 patients with previously treated and adverse prognosis (75% of patients had M1c disease) MM, showed more than 10% objective antitumor response, in addition to prolonged disease stabilization. Potential future phase III clinical trials using these agents will ultimately show whether there is a true clinical benefit for targeting angiogenesis in MM.

### Table 55.5 Summary of Clinical Trials in Melanoma and Other Solid Tumors Using Single Agents That Target Angiogenesis and the Extracellular Matrix. Clinical Trials Highlighted in Bold have Reported More than 10% Antitumor Response

| Drug | Sponsor | Target | Phase | Status | Reference |
|---|---|---|---|---|---|
| **AG-013736** | **Pfizer** | **VEGFR1,2,3, PDGFR, c-Kit** | **II\*** | **Completed** | **Fruehauf (ASCO 2008, abstr 9006)** |
| Bevacizumab | Genetech | VEGF | rII* | Completed | Varker (Ann Surg Oncol 2007) |
| IM1121B | ImClone | VEGFR2 antibody | rII* | Ongoing | N/A |
| ABT-518 | Abbott | Thrombospondin-1 mimetic | II* | Completed | Markovic (Am J Clin Oncol 2007) |
| AZD2171 | Astra Zeneca | VEGFR1,2,3 | II* | Ongoing | N/A |
| TKI258 | Novartis | bFGFR, VEGFR, PDGFR | I/II* | Ongoing | Kim (ASCO 2008, abstr 9026) |
| Rh-Endostatin | Entremed | Endostatin | rII* | Completed | Moschos (Melanoma Res 2007) |
| Aflibercept | Regeneron. CCC | Soluble VEGF | II* | Completed | Tarhini (ASCO 2009, abstr 9028) |
| Marimastat (BB-2516) | British Biotech | MMPs (-2, -3, -9, -12, -13), | II* | Completed | Quirt (Invest New Drugs 2002) |
| Talabostat | Point Therapeutics | Dipeptidyl peptidase | II* | Completed | Redman (ASCO 2005, abstr 7570) |
| Tasidotin (GC1008) | Genzyme | TGF-β | I/II*, renal | Completed | Morris (ASCO 2008, abstr 9028) |
| PI-88 | Progen Pharma | Heparanase | II* | Completed | Lewis (Invest New Drugs 2008) |

GSK, GlaxoSmithKline; NCI, National Cancer Institute; CCC, California Cancer Consortium; bFGFR, basic fibroblast growth factor receptor; VEGF, vascular endothelial growth factor; VEGFR, VEGR receptor; PDGFR, platelet-derived growth factor receptor; MMPs, matrix metalloproteinases; TGF-β, transforming growth factor beta; *melanoma-specific trials; r, randomized trials that compare the molecularly targeted agent alone or in combination with other therapies; ASCO, American Society of Clinical Oncology Annual Meeting; N/A, no results published in peer-reviewed journal or announced at any international medical oncology meeting as of October 2009.

## Targeting immune effector function

Melanoma has long been thought to be a disease that tightly interacts with the host immune system, based on numerous clinical observations of spontaneous or vaccine-induced regression in melanomas, the high incidence of melanomas arising in immunocompromised patients, and the clinical benefit achieved by patients with advanced melanoma following administration of immunomodulatory therapies, such as high-dose interferon-α2b and high-dose bolus interleukin-2 (HDBI2). Over the last decade, clinical trials have been conducted that test molecularly targeted drugs administered as single agents that either antagonize the function of immunosuppressive molecules or activate molecules that augment host immune response (Table 55.6). Most of these trials have established that augmentation of host immune response is feasible by targeting different aspects of the immune system and is associated with clinically significant and durable responses. However, as in the case of HDBI2 therapy, an FDA-approved therapy for MM, this clinical benefit applies to a small (less than 10%) number of patients and is frequently associated with toxic side effects that are linked with autoimmune phenomena. It is unclear at this time whether any of these agents are truly superior to the standard HDBI2 either in terms of toxicity, administration, and/or efficacy, although important research is ongoing to identify predictive biomarkers of drug response.

## COMBINING APPROACHES

The above single-agent studies have provided preliminary insights regarding the side-effect profile, mechanism of action, and the maximum tolerated dose of a variety of study drugs. With the exception of a handful of trials, the clinical benefit is low for a number of reasons. For example, the drug may merely exhibit cytostatic rather than cytotoxic action or have a low therapeutic index. To enhance clinical benefit, molecularly targeted therapies have been combined with other drugs, including chemotherapy. Tables 55.7 and 55.8 summarize clinical trials that have tested the efficacy of one or two molecularly targeted therapies in combination with standard chemotherapeutic agents. Several studies have suggested clinical benefits. Noteworthy is the lack of any significant clinical benefit of sorafenib in combination with chemotherapy, which can now be explained by its lack of specificity and relatively low potency for oncogenic B-Raf. Furthermore, interesting is the borderline clinical benefit in patients with MM and low serum LDH (non-M1c by AJCC criteria) who were treated with agents that target mitochondria in combination with single-agent chemotherapy, such as elesclomol or G3139 (see Table 55.7 for details). This marginal benefit may further substantiate the idea that the chemoresistance observed in MM can be reversed with rational combinations of chemotherapeutic agents and molecularly targeted therapies.

## FUTURE OUTLOOK

Advances in our understanding of the biology of MM along with the ability to develop highly potent and selective molecularly targeted agents against melanoma cells over the last 10 years have recently culminated in early antitumor response in this disease where nearly all prior systemic therapies have failed (Table 55.9). It is unclear at this time whether these objective responses will be durable enough to prolong overall survival. Upcoming *direct* antitumor therapies with clearly defined biomarkers will hopefully identify MM subtypes that are most responsive to a particular therapy and

**Table 55.6 Summary of Clinical Trials in Melanoma and Other Solid Tumors Using Single Agents that Target the Immune System**

| Drug | Sponsor | Target | Phase | Status | Reference |
|---|---|---|---|---|---|
| Ipilimumab (MDX-010) | Medarex-BMS | CTLA-4 | I*<br>rII*<br>rII*b | Completed<br>Completed | Weber (J Clin Oncol 2008)<br>Hamid (ASCO 2008, abstr 9025)<br>Margolin (ECCO 2009, abstr O-9306) |
| Tremelimumab (CP675,206) | Pfizer | CTLA-4 | I*<br>II*<br>rIII* | Completed<br>Completed<br>Ongoing | Ribas (ASCO 2005, abstr 7524)<br>Gomez-Navarro (ASCO 2006, abstr 8032)<br>Chesney (ASCO 2009, abstr 20016)<br>Kirkwood (ASCO 2008, abstr 9023)<br>Ribas (ASCO 2008, abstr 9011) |
| BMS-663513 | BMS | CD137 | I | Ongoing | Sznol (ASCO 2008, abstr 3007) |
| Denileukin Diftitox | Eisai | CD25 | I* | Completed | Chesney (ASCO 2006, abstr 18010) |
| rhIgM12B7 | NCI | PD-L2 cross linking B7-dendritic cells | I* | Ongoing | N/A |
| ADI-PEG20 | Phoenix Pharma | Arginine deaminase | I*<br>II* | Completed<br>Completed | Feun (ASCO 2006, abstr 8045)<br>Ott (ASCO 2009, abstr 9030) |
| 1-methyl-D-tryptophan | Novartis | IDO | I | Ongoing | N/A |
| 852A | 3M Pharma | TLR7, TLR8 | I* | Completed | Dummer (Clin Cancer Res 2008) |

rh, recombinant human; BMS, Bristol-Myers Squibb; NCI, National Cancer Institute; CTLA-4, cytotoxic T-lymphocyte antigen 4; PD-L2, programmed death ligand 2; IDO, indoleamine 2,3-dioxygenase; TLR, Toll-like receptor; *melanoma-specific trials; r, randomized; ASCO, American Society of Clinical Oncology Annual Meeting; ECCO, European CanCer Organization; N/A, no results published in peer-reviewed journal or announced at any international medical oncology meeting as of October 2009.

Table 55.7 Summary of Clinical Trials in Metastatic Melanoma Using Combinations of Agents From Two Different Categories of Anticancer Drugs. Clinical Trials Highlighted in Bold Have Reported More Than 10% Antitumor Response, Whereas Clinical Trials Highlighted in Bold Consist of Two Randomized Arms and Have Reported Progression-Free Survival Benefit in the 'Treatment' Arm as Compared With the 'Control' Arm

| Molecularly targeted Therapy | Other Therapy | Phase | Status | Reference |
|---|---|---|---|---|
| | | | Chemotherapy | |
| **Sorafenib** | **DTIC** | **rII** | **Completed** | **McDermott (J Clin Oncol 2008)** |
| Sorafenib | Temozolomide | I–II, | Completed | Robert (ASCO 2009, abstr 9062) |
| Sorafenib | Carboplatin–paclitaxel | rIII, f-l<br>rIII, s-l | Completed<br>Completed | Flaherty (Perspectives XIII in Melanoma)<br>Hauschild (J Clin Oncol 2009) |
| Sorafenib | Carboplatin-Abraxane™ | II | Ongoing | N/A |
| Sorafenib | Temsirolimus | I–II | Completed | Kim (ASCO 2009, abstr 9026) |
| Imatinib | Temozolomide | II | Completed | Fecher (ASCO 2008, abstr 9059) |
| **Bevacizumab** | **Temozolomide** | **II** | **Completed** | **Von Moos (ECCO 2009, abstr 24LBA)** |
| Bevacizumab | Abraxane™ | II | Ongoing | N/A |
| **Bevacizumab** | **Carboplatin-paclitaxel** | **II rII, f-l** | **Completed**<br>Ongoing | **Perez (Cancer 2009)**<br>**O'Day (ECCO 2009, abstr 23LBA)** |
| Ipilimumab | DTIC | rII | Completed | Hersh (ASCO 2008, abstr 9022) |
| ABT-888 (PARP, Abbott) | DTIC | II | Accruing | N/A |
| AZD2281 (PARP, KuDos Pharma) | DTIC | I | Completed | N/A |
| INO-1001 (PARP, Genetech) | Temozolomide | I | Completed | Wang (ASCO 2006, abstr 12015) |
| Imexon (mitochondrial thiol oxidant, AmpliMed) | DTIC | II | Completed | Samlowski (ASCO 2008, abstr 9066) |
| **Elesclomol** | **Paclitaxel** | **rII**<br>**rIII** | **Completed**<br>**Terminated** | **Gonzalez (ASCO 2008, abstr 9036)**<br>**Hauschild (ASCO, abstr LBA9012)** |
| ATN-224 (SOD, Attenuon) | Temozolomide | II | Ongoing | N/A |
| MPC-6827 (tubulin polym, Myriad Pharma) | Temozolomide | I | Ongoing | N/A |
| G3139 (Antisense Bcl2, Genta) | Carboplatin-Abraxane™ | II | Ongoing | N/A |
| **G3139** | **DTIC** | **rIII** | **Completed** | **Bedikian (J Clin Oncol 2006)** |
| Talabostat | Cisplatin | II | Completed | Cunningham (ASCO 2006, abstr 8040) |
| PI-88 | DTIC | II | Ongoing | N/A |
| Bortezomib | Temozolomide | II | Ongoing | N/A |
| | | | Immunotherapy | |
| KW2871 | IFN-α2b | II | Ongoing | N/A |
| **Tremelimumab** | **IFN-α2b** | **II** | **Ongoing** | **Tarhini (ASCO 2008, abstr 9009)** |
| Bortezomib | IFN-α2b | I | Ongoing | N/A |
| Sorafenib | Pegylated IFN-α2b | II | Ongoing | N/A |

**Table 55.7 Summary of Clinical Trials in Metastatic Melanoma Using Combinations of Agents From Two Different Categories of Anticancer Drugs. Clinical Trials Highlighted in Bold Have Reported More Than 10% Antitumor Response, Whereas Clinical Trials Highlighted in Bold Consist of Two Randomized Arms and Have Reported Progression-Free Survival Benefit in the 'Treatment' Arm as Compared With the 'Control' Arm—Cont'd**

| Molecularly Targeted Therapy | Other therapy | Phase | Status | Reference |
|---|---|---|---|---|
| | **Molecularly Targeted Therapy** | | | |
| Bevacizumab | Ipilimumab | II | Ongoing | N/A |
| Sorafenib | Temsirolimus | rII | Ongoing | N/A |
| Sorafenib | Bevacizumab | II | Suspended | N/A |
| Bevacizumab | Temsirolimus | II | Ongoing | N/A |
| | Everolimus | II | Ongoing | N/A |

PARP, Poly (ADP-ribose) polymerase; SOD, superoxide dismutase; DTIC, dacarbazine; IFN-α2b, interferon alpha 2b; r, randomized; f-l, first-line, no prior chemotherapy is allowed; s-l, second-line, prior chemotherapy is allowed; N/A, no results published in peer-reviewed journal or announced at any international medical oncology meeting as of October 2009.

**Table 55.8 Summary of Clinical Trials in Metastatic Melanoma Using Combinations of Molecularly Targeted Agents with Standard Chemotherapy**

| Molecularly Targeted Therapy 1 | Molecularly Targeted Therapy 2 | Chemotherapy | Phase | Status | Reference |
|---|---|---|---|---|---|
| Sorafenib | Bevacizumab | Oxaliplatin | I | Ongoing | McClay (ASCO 2008, abstr 20020) |
| IFN-α2b | Bevacizumab | Dacarbazine | II, o | Completed | N/A |
| Lenalidomide | Sunitinib | Cyclophosphamide | II, o | Completed | N/A |
| Sorafenib | Bevacizumab | Temozolomide | II, a | Completed | Si (ASCO 2009, abstr e20010) |

IFN-α2b, interferon alpha 2b; o, ocular; a, acral; ASCO, American Society of Clinical Oncology Annual Meeting; N/A no results published in peer-reviewed journal or announced at any international medical oncology meeting.

**Table 55.9 Pitfalls in the Drug Clinical Development for Metastatic Melanoma**

1. Incomplete knowledge about melanoma biology and chemoresistance

2. Melanoma targets
   - Present in melanoma cells but equally important for normal cells (low therapeutic index)
   - Present in melanoma cells but important in earlier rather than later stages of melanoma
   - Irrelevant for melanoma therapy
   - Absent in melanoma cells (lost during cancer progression)

3. Drugs
   - Effective for only a small subset of melanomas (drug benefit is 'diluted')
   - Not rationally combined (empiric treatment combinations)
   - Not potent

4. Clinical trials
   - Endpoints used are less relevant (antitumor response rather than overall survival)
   - Absent biomarkers
   - Drugs were not given at optimal biologic doses

may protect patients from exposure to unnecessary drug toxicity. As in the case of other cancers that have previously benefited from molecularly targeted therapies, such as chronic myelogenous leukemia, drug resistance may be inevitable. Understanding the mechanisms of drug resistance may ultimately guide design of rational combinations.

Targeting multiple different pathways may be required to have clinical effect (horizontal blockade) or, alternatively, multiple components of the same pathway (vertical blockade, Fig. 55.5) within the melanoma cells. In this new era of molecularly targeted therapy the true role of agents that exert an *indirect* antitumor effect, such as those that enhance host immune response or inhibit angiogenesis, may need to be more precisely defined. These agents comprise a relatively stable target pool with low incidence of mutations and therefore low potential for development of drug resistance; and, the approach to simultaneous targeting of melanoma cells, along with efforts to inhibit angiogenesis and potentiate host immune responses, may prove to be synergistic.[20] Overall, advances in drug discovery efforts, understanding of melanoma biology, and higher-quality clinical trials are now more likely to attain significant effects upon this devastating disease (Table 55.10).

**Figure 55.5** Proposed strategies for rational combination of molecularly targeted therapies. If each of two signaling pathways, defined by its extracellular ligand (L), membrane receptor (R) and intracellular signal transduction molecules (A, B, C, etc.), bifurcates, i.e. spreads its signal to the other pathway, then inhibition of cell behavior that each pathway predominantly regulates (e.g. survival, proliferation) will not be effective unless both pathways are targeted (horizontal blockade, panel **A**). If a membrane receptor relays the message to multiple intracellular signal transduction pathways (e.g. c-Kit in melanoma), then blocking its signal at multiple levels should be more effective to inhibit a particular cell behavior (vertical blockade, panel **B**). On several occasions, blocking a particular pathway within a cancer cell (e.g. mammalian target of rapamycin, mTOR) induces counter-regulatory responses (negative feedback loop, e.g. activation of the insulin receptor substrate-1, IRS1) to overcome the blockade by supra-activation of upstream molecules (e.g. Akt). Inhibiting the cell's counter-regulatory response may sustain consistent blockade within the cell (panel **C**).

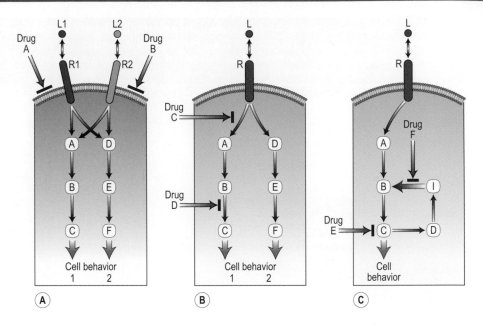

### Table 55.10 Future Challenges in Clinical Drug Development for Metastatic Melanoma

1. Better understand biology of disease and identify more 'B-Raf V600E'-type mutations

2. Develop prognostic and surrogate biomarkers of treatment response

3. Identify patient subgroups that most likely respond to treatment based on drug's mechanism of action

4. Prevent drug resistance to molecularly targeted therapies but applying vertical and horizontal blockade rational drug combinations

5. Develop highly potent drugs with wide therapeutic index

## REFERENCES

1. Korn EL, Liu PY, Lee SJ, et al. Meta-analysis of phase II cooperative group trials in metastatic stage IV melanoma to determine progression-free and overall survival benchmarks for future phase II trials. *J Clin Oncol.* 2008;26:527–534.
2. Davies H, Bignell GR, Cox C, et al. Mutations of the BRAF gene in human cancer. *Nature.* 2002;417:949–954.
3. Van Raamsdonk CD, Bezrookove V, Green G, et al. Frequent somatic mutations of GNAQ in uveal melanoma and blue naevi. *Nature.* 2009;457:599–602.
4. Curtin JA, Busam K, Pinkel D, et al. Somatic activation of KIT in distinct subtypes of melanoma. *J Clin Oncol.* 2006;24:4340–4346.
5. Curtin JA, Fridlyand J, Kageshita T, et al. Distinct sets of genetic alterations in melanoma. *N Engl J Med.* 2005;353:2135–2147.
6. Tsao H, Goel V, Wu H, et al. Genetic interaction between NRAS and BRAF mutations and PTEN/MMAC1 inactivation in melanoma. *J Invest Dermatol.* 2004;122:337–341.

7. Madhunapantula SV, Robertson GP. The PTEN-AKT3 signaling cascade as a therapeutic target in melanoma. *Pigment Cell Melanoma Res.* 2009;22:400–419.
8. Mahabeleshwar GH, Byzova TV. Angiogenesis in melanoma. *Semin Oncol.* 2007;34:555–565.
9. Gajewski TF. Failure at the effector phase: immune barriers at the level of the melanoma tumor microenvironment. *Clin Cancer Res.* 2007;13:5256–5261.
10. Wyman K, Atkins MB, Prieto V, et al. Multicenter phase II trial of high-dose imatinib mesylate in metastatic melanoma: significant toxicity with no clinical efficacy. *Cancer.* 2006;106:2005–2011.
11. Ugurel S, Hildenbrand R, Zimpfer A, et al. Lack of clinical efficacy of imatinib in metastatic melanoma. *Br J Cancer.* 2005;92:1398–1405.
12. Mouriaux F, Delcambre C, Durando X, et al. A Canceropole Nord-Ouest multicenter phase II trial of high-dose imatinib mesylate in metastatic uveal melanoma (abstr 9061). *ASCO Annual Meeting.* 2008;.
13. Fiorentini G, Rossi S, Lanzanova G, et al. Tyrosine kinase inhibitor imatinib mesylate as anticancer agent for advanced ocular melanoma expressing immunohistochemical C-KIT (CD 117): preliminary results of a compassionate use clinical trial. *J Exp Clin Cancer Res.* 2003;22:17–20.
14. Hodi FS, Friedlander P, Corless CL, et al. Major response to imatinib mesylate in KIT-mutated melanoma. *J Clin Oncol.* 2008;26:2046–2051.
15. Hofmann UB, Kauczok-Vetter CS, Houben R, et al. Overexpression of the KIT/SCF in uveal melanoma does not translate into clinical efficacy of imatinib mesylate. *Clin Cancer Res.* 2009;15:324–329.
16. Pollock PM, Cohen-Solal K, Sood R, et al. Melanoma mouse model implicates metabotropic glutamate signaling in melanocytic neoplasia. *Nat Genet.* 2003;34:108–112.
17. Eisen T, Ahmad T, Flaherty KT, et al. Sorafenib in advanced melanoma: a phase II randomised discontinuation trial analysis. *Br J Cancer.* 2006;95:581–586.
18. Dummer R, Robert C, Chapman PB, et al. AZD6244 (ARRY-142886) vs temozolomide (TMZ) in patients (pts) with advanced melanoma: an open-label, randomized, multicenter, phase II study (abstr 9033). *ASCO Annual Meeting.* 2008;.
19. Sabatino M, Kim-Schulze S, Panelli MC, et al. Serum vascular endothelial growth factor and fibronectin predict clinical response to high-dose interleukin-2 therapy. *J Clin Oncol.* 2009;27:2645–2652.
20. Sumimoto H, Imabayashi F, Iwata T, et al. The BRAF-MAPK signaling pathway is essential for cancer-immune evasion in human melanoma cells. *J Exp Med.* 2006;203:1651–1656.

# Imaging Work-up of the Patient with Melanoma

*Hussein Tawbi and John M. Kirkwood*

## Key Points

- Imaging is heavily utilized in the diagnosis and management of melanoma patients but the utility of imaging depends upon the goal in the context of the clinical disease setting.

- For staging purposes, little evidence supports comprehensive body imaging assessment in asymptomatic early-stage melanoma patients.

- High-frequency ultrasound can augment the sensitivity of sentinel lymph node biopsy assessment of regional nodal disease.

- Routine follow-up of melanoma with chest X-ray has not been validated in rigorous studies to date.

- There is no current role for radiologic surveillance, and no rationale for performance of baseline PET or PET/CT studies in stage IIB or III patients.

- Contrast-enhanced MRI is the most sensitive modality for detecting brain metastasis.

## INTRODUCTION

The utility of radiologic imaging at different junctures in the evaluation and management of patients with melanoma continues to increase. With higher-risk deep primary melanoma and melanoma that has spread to regional nodes, surgery with adjuvant therapy reduces local-regional and distant recurrence and the outcome is linked to disease burden. Microscopic nodal disease has a substantially better outcome than gross nodal disease. Imaging technology has evolved rapidly in the past two decades, providing us with new tools to assess the burden of metastatic disease. Imaging at the time of diagnosis of melanoma and for subsequent surveillance plays an important role in management.

## IMAGING AT DIAGNOSIS

The staging of localized primary melanoma is dictated by the microstage (thickness, ulceration, and mitotic index) of the primary lesion. Melanoma metastasis occurs locally through the skin, regionally through the lymphatics, and systemically by hematogenous routes. Sentinel lymph node biopsy (SLNB) is an essential component of staging to be considered for primary melanomas >1 mm Breslow thickness or any primary melanoma with ulceration. Initial staging can employ various imaging modalities, including chest X-ray (CXR), regional nodal ultrasonography, computed tomography (CT), magnetic resonance imaging (MRI), positron emission tomography (PET), and combined (co-registered) PET/CT.

## Chest X-ray (CXR)

Hematogenous dissemination is the third major route of metastasis for melanoma, most commonly afflicting the lung. Modern chest radiography requires small doses of radiation, and is quick, inexpensive, and relatively easy to perform. It therefore seems reasonable as a means to assess the lungs for metastasis although multiple studies have indicated a very low yield for CXR as part of the initial work-up.[1]

In 876 asymptomatic patients with localized melanoma, Terhune et al.[2] found that only 15% had suspicious findings on CXR and only one patient had metastatic melanoma confirmed by biopsy, for a yield of only 0.1%. A similar yield of 0.2% was reported in a study of 524 stage I and II patients, with a sobering 20-fold higher false positive (FP) rate (4.4%).[3] A high FP rate serves to further increase patient anxiety and reduce overall cost-effectiveness.

Yancovitz et al.[4] reported retrospectively on 158 asymptomatic patients with T1b–T3b primary lesions, clinically N0. A total of 344 preoperative imaging studies (CXR, CT, and PET/CT) were performed, resulting in 49 findings suspicious for metastatic melanoma. Only 1 of 344 studies correlated with confirmed metastatic melanoma. No patient was upstaged or had a change in initial surgical management based on preoperative imaging.[4] In addition, no survival benefit from CXR at initial staging or during follow-up has been demonstrated.[2,3,5]

These findings suggest that chest radiography of asymptomatic patients at the time of diagnosis may not be warranted. However, obtaining a chest radiograph in a symptomatic patient or at an advanced T-or N-stage may be reasonable.

## Ultrasound

Ultrasound is a non-invasive, low-cost, portable investigation. It carries a lower risk to patients, given the absence of ionizing radiation. Ultrasound has been used for imaging of skin lesions, abdominal and pelvic organs and staging of regional nodes.

Harland et al.[6] reported 100% sensitivity in distinguishing between basal cell carcinoma and malignant melanoma. Similar sensitivity and specificity (100%) for melanoma were reported in 111 patients among whom 81% of melanomas were correctly identified.[7]

## CT

Computed tomography (CT) is technically more demanding than CXR, more expensive, and imparts a high radiation dose equivalent to 400–500 CXRs. CT is the preferred technique for evaluating the abdomen. Chest CT is superior to chest radiography for evaluation of the hila, mediastinum and pleura (Fig. 56.1).[1] Liver metastases are typically hypervascular and require image acquisition in the correct post-contrast phase (Fig. 56.2).

Heaston et al.[8] found that chest CT detected 19% of metastases in patients with a normal CXR. However, whole-body CT has not been useful in detecting occult metastases in patients with primary melanoma.[9] Miranda et al.[10] showed that CT of the chest, abdomen, pelvis, and brain rarely revealed systemic metastasis at the time of SLNB.[10]

## PET scan

Positron emission tomography (PET) using 18-fluoro-deoxy-D-glucose ([18]FDG) is increasingly popular in staging melanoma. The dynamic nature of imaging using PET enhances the ease of detection compared to CT alone. However, spatial resolution of PET is lower and small or metabolically inactive lesions may be missed (Figs 56.3 and 56.4).[11] The high background activity in normal brain tissue severely limits the use of FDG-PET for brain metastasis.[12] A retrospective study of 101 patients failed to show any metastatic disease when PET was used as initial staging.[13] Clarke et al.[14] showed that PET did not reveal any metastatic lesions in 64 T2–T4 patients. Rinne et al.[15] evaluated PET and CT scanning at primary diagnosis in 52 patients, revealing a sensitivity of 100% and specificity of 94% compared with an

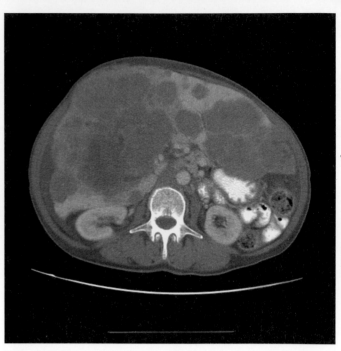

**Figure 56.2** CT scan of the abdomen showing extensive melanoma liver metastases.

accuracy of 68% for conventional imaging. Vereecken et al.[16] also concluded that there was no added value from PET as a baseline staging for primary melanoma, given its low sensitivity and specificity.

A recent systematic review examined the diagnostic performance of PET imaging for initial staging of melanoma in 28 studies involving 2905 patients. The pooled estimates of FDG-PET for the detection of metastasis in the initial staging of melanoma were: sensitivity, 83%; specificity, 85%; positive likelihood ratio (LR), 4.56; negative LR, 0.27; and diagnostic odds ratio, 19.8. Results from eight studies suggested that FDG-PET was associated with disease management changes in 33% (15%–64%). This study concluded that PET is useful as an adjunct for staging patients with higher stages of melanoma, especially stages III and IV, for detection of deep soft tissue, lymph node, and visceral metastases.[17]

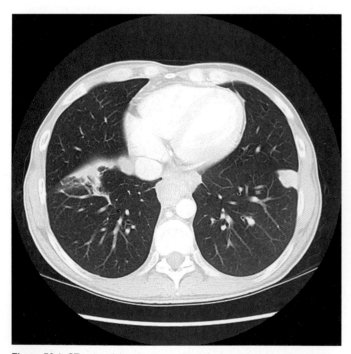

**Figure 56.1** CT scan of the chest revealing left pleural-based melanoma metastasis.

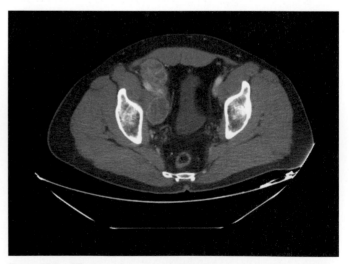

**Figure 56.3** CT scan of the pelvis revealing left external iliac lymph nodes with metastatic melanoma.

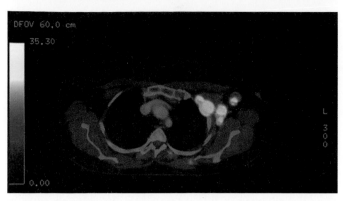

**Figure 56.4** PET/CT with left axillary lymph node metastases with increased FDG uptake consistent with metastatic melanoma, later confirmed with biopsy.

## MRI

Magnetic resonance imaging (MRI) is an excellent modality for delineating soft tissue structures, given a significantly higher contrast resolution than CT. MRI does not employ ionizing radiation; however, it involves complicated, expensive equipment and long image-acquisition times. It is also highly susceptible to artifacts associated with respiration or cardiac movement in the thorax. It is therefore not currently suitable for whole-body scanning and is usually tailored to a single-organ system. T1-weighted images have been shown to give a high signal density for melanoma deposits, which is consistent with the paramagnetic effect of melanin (Fig. 56.5). MRI is more sensitive than CT for detection of metastases that involve the brain, liver and skeleton.[18]

Whole-body MRI was evaluated in 41 stage III and IV melanoma patients and altered the treatment plan in 24% of the patients.[18]

MRI is useful for further characterizing metastasis at certain sites, but at present is not a first-line tool for multi-organ staging due to both availability and cost. MRI has an unequivocal role in the evaluation of the brain, and should be considered for the initial evaluation of patients at high risk for metastatic disease of the CNS or who have symptoms.

## IMAGING FOR SURVEILLANCE OF ADVANCED DISEASE

### Chest X-ray

Despite the low utility of CXR for detection of pulmonary metastases, CXR is routinely obtained as part of postoperative surveillance plans.[19] The National Comprehensive Cancer Network (NCCN) guidelines include CXR every 6–12 months for 2–3 years, although it acknowledges the absence of clear data to support such recommendations.[20] The relatively higher risk of relapse in the first several years following surgery for melanoma has led to the performance of CXR or CT in the context of cooperative group adjuvant studies at 3–4-month intervals through the 2nd–3rd year, and at 6-month intervals to 5 years.

Morton et al.[11] reported their prospective experience with surveillance CXR in patients with microscopically node-positive melanoma. Over a median follow-up period of 52.5 months, 23 of 108 patients had pulmonary metastases. Disease was detected by surveillance CXR in <50% of patients. Worse, a relatively high false-positive rate led to patient anxiety and further work-up associated with additional cost and morbidity.

Dalal et al.[21] reported on 1062 patients who underwent SLNB. A total of 203 (19%) experienced 230 initial sites of recurrence. Symptoms and self-detected physical findings were present in 109 patients (55%). Physician detection occurred in 89 patients (45%), nearly half by a scheduled radiographic test (CXR, 16%; CT, 29%; PET, 1%).

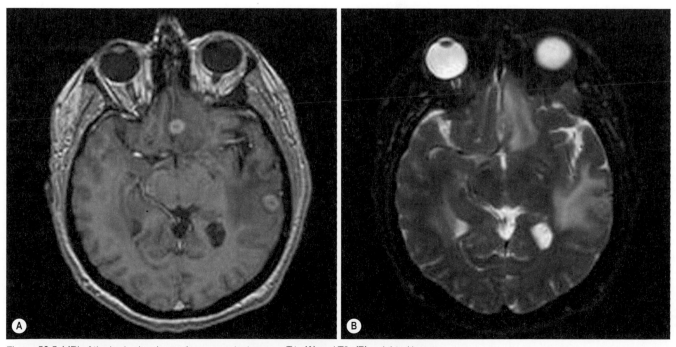

**Figure 56.5** MRI of the brain showing melanoma metastases on T1- **(A)** and T2- **(B)** weighted images.

Mooney et al.[22] conducted a cost-effectiveness analysis of an intensive CXR screening program to detect asymptomatic pulmonary metastases in patients with intermediate-thickness melanoma. The cost of screening was unacceptably high at $165,000 per QALY.

It seems clear that CXR is neither sensitive nor specific enough to serve as an effective surveillance examination for melanoma patients. Even in the absence of certain benefits, it appears that significant cost savings may be possible by decreasing screening frequency in the first 2 years and limiting screening to the first 5 years after diagnosis. The current recommendations for CXR, or other imaging modalities, are non-specific and largely based on a consensus of opinion.

## Ultrasound

A number of recent papers have confirmed ultrasound to be superior to clinical examination in the detection of lymph node metastases based on characteristic appearance; which may help reduce the number of SLNBs.[23] A prospective study of 155 melanoma patients reported 100% sensitivity and 39% specificity of ultrasound coupled with fine-needle aspiration (FNA).[24] Overall, 10% of patients could potentially avoid SLNB and proceed straight to lymphadenectomy. Hocevar et al.[25] had less success, with sensitivity of 71% and specificity of 84%. Garbe et al.,[26] in a 2-year follow-up of over 2000 melanoma patients, found clinical examination and ultrasound had a sensitivity of 68% and 86%, and specificity of 99% and 98.7%, respectively. Machet et al.[27] followed up 373 stage I and II patients for 5 years with regular ultrasound examinations. They found clinical examination and ultrasound to have sensitivity of 71% and 92% and specificity of 99.6% and 97.8%, respectively. The authors concluded that 7.2% of patients benefited from the examination. However, 5.9% of patients were falsely positive and underwent additional procedures such as FNA and excision biopsy. Saiag et al.[28] followed 160 stage III melanoma patients for 6 years. They found clinical examination and ultrasound to have sensitivity of 41% and 77% and specificity of 95.7% and 98.5%, respectively.

Voit et al.[29] recently reported the largest prospective series of 400 patients (median follow-up time of 39 months) scheduled for SLNB who underwent ultrasound examination followed by FNA and cytological/histopathological examination. The presence of peripheral perfusion, loss of central echoes, and balloon-shaped lymph nodes demonstrated the highest sensitivity and positive predictive value (PPV) rates. The combination of these three criteria showed 82% sensitivity and a 52% PPV, with a specificity of 80% and a negative predictive value (NPV) of 94% (P<0.001). In this series, preoperative ultrasound and FNA was able to identify 65% of sentinel nodal metastases and thus reduce the need for surgical SN procedures. This study provides validation for the use of ultrasound in this setting.

## CT

CT scan and MRI did not result in many true-positive findings in SLNB-positive patients studied by Aloia et al.[30] In a study by Buzaid et al.,[9] the benefit of a CT scan in patients with locoregional metastases was also low.

Gold et al.[31] studied a group of 107 patients who received radiologic imaging after a positive SLNB. Distant disease was identified in only 3.7% while different radiologic studies resulted in ambiguous results in 48% of all patients. In this study, CXR did not account for a single discovery of distant metastases. Of all diagnostic procedures ordered, CT scan and PET scan had the highest yield.

In 89 asymptomatic stage III melanoma patients with normal chest radiographs and normal LDH levels, Buzaid et al.[32] found a true-positive (TP) rate of 7% and a FP rate of 22%. Conversely, a TP rate of 16% and FP rate of only 12% were reported in 127 asymptomatic stage III melanoma patients.[33] Miranda et al.,[10] in a retrospective review of 185 stage III patients, found a yield of 0.7% for chest CT with an indeterminate rate of 19%. The brain was assessed with a combination of MRI and CT. The yield was 0%, with a 6.3% indeterminate rate. These findings were mirrored by Aloia et al.[30] in a retrospective study of 270 stage III patients who underwent imaging after diagnosis. The total yield was 1.9%, and 25% of the imaging was abnormal.

## PET and PET/CT

In a rather small series of 39 patients, Akcali et al.[34] reported that FDG-PET/CT scanning had a high sensitivity (91%) and specificity (92%) for detecting metastases.

A meta-analysis of PET imaging for cutaneous melanoma found that PET was more accurate in stage III disease than in stage I or II, although there was generally a poor methodology in the studies.[35] A sensitivity of 87% for PET has been reported in stage III patients.[36] PET sensitivity also varies according to clinical stage of the disease, being 0% in stage I, 24% in stage II, 81% in stage III, and 100% in stage IV.[37]

PET/CT allows mapping of PET images onto CT images acquired simultaneously. The CT images are usually of a lower resolution and without IV contrast as compared to standard CT; nevertheless, this aids more accurate localization of [18]FDG uptake. When combined with CT, the accuracy of PET/CT is synergistic.[38] Reinhardt et al.[39] reported a sensitivity of 98.7% compared to 88.8% for PET alone and 69.7% for CT alone. Iagaru et al.[40] recently reported on 163 patients and showed a sensitivity of 89%, and recommended the use of PET/CT in the evaluation of high-risk melanoma. The PET/CT combination may prove to be an important modality not only in melanoma imaging but also in oncology as a whole.[41,42]

## MRI

For the detection and assessment of cerebral metastases, contrast-enhanced MRI is the most accurate non-invasive imaging technique and has been shown to be superior to contrast-enhanced CT.[43] A recent retrospective review of 100 patients who underwent cerebral MRI for staging of melanoma found that 11% had cerebral metastases. It was therefore recommended that cerebral MRI be performed only in patients with stage IV disease or other stages where the detection of cerebral metastases would alter patient management.[44]

For the assessment of extracranial disease, Ghanem et al.[45] compared FDG-PET and MRI for the detection of hepatic metastases and found that MRI was more sensitive for metastatic lesions than FDG-PET.

There is now rapidly emerging interest in whole-body MRI for cancer staging and recent advances enable whole-body imaging to be performed in less than 1 hour.[46] Three studies compared whole-body MRI with FDG-PET/CT for extracranial tumor staging. The first of these, which included 98 patients, found that overall PET/CT significantly more accurately determined the stage than did MRI (77% vs. 54%) and was significantly more accurate for tumor and node staging, but performed similarly for the detection of metastatic disease. In addition, in 12% of cases, FDG-PET/CT altered patient management compared with MRI.[47] In the second study, MRI detected more metastases in 17% of patients and altered management in 10% of patients.[48] Most recently, in a smaller group of patients, FDG-PET/CT was more accurate than MRI for staging; however, the difference was much smaller (96% vs. 91%).[49]

Nonetheless, tolerability of MRI may be an issue; up to 25% patients in some series were unable to complete the MRI due to metallic implants and claustrophobia.

Whole-body MRI is a promising method for staging in melanoma, but, at present, FDG-PET/CT has greater accuracy overall. Nonetheless, for specific sites, MRI may be superior to FDG-PET/CT, particularly in brain and liver. Regional imaging of these organs with MRI may be of clinical benefit.

## MANAGEMENT SUMMARY

Significant progress has been achieved in the imaging detection, staging and surveillance of melanoma. However, the utility of imaging is mostly dependent on the goal of imaging within the context of the clinical setting.

At diagnosis, high-frequency ultrasound may play a role in identifying and determining the Breslow thickness of primary melanoma. This may reduce unnecessary biopsies and avoid second procedures for wide local excision. Further evaluation of this modality should be encouraged.

For staging purposes, there is very little evidence to support comprehensive body imaging for asymptomatic early-stage melanoma patients. SLNB is the most sensitive and specific assessment of the regional nodes. Patients with macroscopic stage III disease should have a CT scan of the affected lymph basin, chest and abdomen. In addition, the pelvis should be imaged in patients with lower limb lesions and the neck in patients with upper thoracic or head/neck lesions, to encompass both regional and distant disease that may preclude or modify surgical plans. There is little evidence to suggest a value for extensive imaging in asymptomatic stage IIIA microscopic disease. Imaging of the brain in asymptomatic patients is rarely justified, and MRI is the most sensitive modality for detecting brain lesions.

There is no current role for radiologic surveillance and therefore no rationale for baseline PET or CT/PET studies in stage III patients. The role of PET or CT/PET has not yet been fully evaluated, however, and these modalities may have a role in clarifying indeterminate findings on conventional imaging, and measuring the effectiveness of therapy.

Stage III and stage IV melanoma patients have a poorer prognosis. Imaging in symptomatic patients may reveal disease that can be palliated and complex imaging studies should be performed on an individualized basis to guide therapy.

## FUTURE OUTLOOK

Apart from prevention and early detection, the future for improved management of melanoma lies in developing more effective adjuvant therapies. Enhanced imaging will be increasingly important for the assessment of tumor response in melanoma patients and in the evaluation of new treatments and strategies.

## REFERENCES

1. Dancey AL, Mahon BS, Rayatt SS. A review of diagnostic imaging in melanoma. *J Plast Reconstr Aesthet Surg.* 2008;61:1275–1283.
2. Terhune MH, Swanson N, Johnson TM. Use of chest radiography in the initial evaluation of patients with localised melanoma. *Arch Dermatol.* 1998;134:569–572.
3. Hofmann U, Szedlak M, Rittgen W, et al. Primary staging and follow-up in melanoma patients – monocenter evaluation of methods, costs and patient survival. *Br J Cancer.* 2002;87:151–157.
4. Yancovitz M, Finelt N, Warycha MA, et al. Role of radiologic imaging at the time of initial diagnosis of stage T1b-T3b melanoma. *Cancer.* 2007;110:1107–1114.
5. Tsao H, Feldman M, Fullerton JE, et al. Early detection of asymptomatic pulmonary melanoma metastases by routine chest radiographs is not associated with improved survival. *Arch Dermatol.* 2004;140:67–70.
6. Harland CC, Kale SG, Jackson P, et al. Differentiation of common benign pigmented skin lesions from melanoma by high-resolution ultrasound. *Br J Dermatol.* 2000;143:281–289.
7. Bessoud B, Lassau N, Koscielny S, et al. High-frequency sonography and color Doppler in the management of pigmented skin lesions. *Ultrasound Med Biol.* 2003;29:875–879.
8. Heaston DK, Putman CE, Rodan BA, et al. Solitary pulmonary metastasis in high risk melanoma patients: a prospective comparison of conventional and computed tomography. *AJR Am J Roentgenol.* 1983;141:169–174.
9. Buzaid AC, Sandler AB, Mani S, et al. Role of computed tomography in the staging of primary melanoma. *J Clin Oncol.* 1993;11:638–643.
10. Miranda EP, Gertner M, Wall J, et al. Routine imaging of asymptomatic melanoma patients with metastasis to sentinel lymph nodes rarely identifies systemic disease. *Arch Surg.* 2004;139:831–836.
11. Morton RL, Craig JC, Thompson JF. The role of surveillance chest X-rays in the follow-up of high-risk melanoma patients. *Ann Surg Oncol.* 2009;16:571–577.
12. Macapinlac HA. The utility of 2-deoxy-2-fluro-D-glucose positron emission tomography and combined positron emission tomography and computed tomography in lymphoma and melanoma. *Mol Imaging Biol.* 2004;6:200–207.
13. Hafner J, Schmid MH, Kempf W, et al. Baseline staging in cutaneous malignant melanoma. *Br J Dermatol.* 2004;150:677–686.
14. Clark PB, Soo V, Kraas J, et al. Futility of fluorodeoxyglucose F18 positron emission tomography in initial evaluation of patients with T2 to T4 melanoma. *Arch Surg.* 2006;141:284–288.
15. Rinne D, Baum RP, Hor G, et al. Primary staging and follow up of high risk melanoma patients with whole-body 18Ffluorodeoxyglucose positron emission tomography: results of a prospective study of 100 patients. *Cancer.* 1998;82:1664–1671.
16. Vereecken P, Laporte M, Petein M, et al. Evaluation of extensive initial staging procedure in intermediate/high-risk melanoma patients. *J Eur Acad Dermatol Venereol.* 2005;19:66–73.
17. Krug B, Crott R, Lonneux M. Role of PET in the initial staging of cutaneous malignant melanoma: systematic review. *Radiology.* 2008;249:836–844.
18. Muller-Horvat C, Radny P, Eigentler TK, et al. Prospective comparison of the impact on treatment decisions of whole body magnetic resonance imaging and computed tomography in patients with metastatic malignant melanoma. *Eur J Cancer.* 2006;42:342–350.
19. Weiss M, Loprinzi CL, Creagan ET, et al. Utility of follow-up tests for detecting recurrent disease in patients with malignant melanomas. *JAMA.* 1995;274:1703–1705.
20. National Comprehensive Cancer Network. *NCCN Clinical Practice Guidelines in Oncology.* Version 1. <http://www.nccn.org/professionals/physician_gls/PDF/melanoma.pdf > Accessed 18.11.08.

21. Dalal KM, Zhou Q, Panageas KS, et al. Methods of detection of first recurrence in patients with stage I/II primary cutaneous melanoma after sentinel lymph node biopsy. *Ann Surg Oncol*. 2008;15:2206–2214.

22. Mooney MM, Metlin C, Michalek AM, et al. Life-long screening of patients with intermediate-thickness cutaneous melanoma for asymptomatic pulmonary recurrences: a cost-effectiveness analysis. *Cancer*. 1997;80:1052–1064.

23. Kahle B, Hoffend J, Wacker J, et al. Preoperative ultrasonographic identification of the sentinel lymph node in patients with malignant melanoma. *Cancer*. 2003;97:1947–1954.

24. Rossi CR, Mocellin S, Scagnet B, et al. The role of preoperative ultrasound scan in detecting lymph node metastasis before sentinel node biopsy in melanoma patients. *J Surg Oncol*. 2003;83:80–84.

25. Hocevara M, Brackob M, Pogacnikc A, et al. The role of preoperative ultrasonography in reducing the number of sentinel lymph node procedures in melanoma. *Melanoma Res*. 2004;14:533–536.

26. Garbe C, Paul A, Kohler-Spath H, et al. Prospective evaluation of a follow-up schedule in cutaneous melanoma patients: recommendations for an effective follow-up strategy. *J Clin Oncol*. 2003;21:520–529.

27. Machet L, Nemeth-Normand F, Giraudeau B, et al. Is ultrasound lymph node examination superior to clinical examination in melanoma follow-up? A monocentre cohort study of 373 patients. *Br J Dermatol*. 2005;152:66–70.

28. Saiag P, Bernard M, Beauchet A, et al. Ultrasonography using simple diagnostic criteria vs palpation for the detection of regional lymph node metastases of melanoma. *Arch Dermatol*. 2005;141:183–189.

29. Voit C, Van Akkooi AC, Schäfer-Hesterberg G, et al. Ultrasound morphology criteria predict metastatic disease of the sentinel nodes in patients with melanoma. *J Clin Oncol*. 2010;28:847–852.

30. Aloia TA, Gershenwald JE, Andtbacka RH, et al. Utility of computed tomography and magnetic resonance imaging staging before completion lymphadenectomy in patients with sentinel lymph node-positive melanoma. *J Clin Oncol*. 2006;24:2858–2865.

31. Gold JS, Jaques DP, Busam KJ, et al. Yield and predictors of radiologic studies for identifying distant metastases in melanoma patients with a positive sentinel lymph node biopsy. *Ann Surg Oncol*. 2007;14:2133–2140.

32. Buzaid AC, Tinoco L, Ross MI, et al. Role of computed tomography in staging of patients with local-regional metastases of melanoma. *J Clin Oncol*. 1995;13:2104–2108.

33. Prichard RS, Hill AD, Skehan SJ, et al. Positron emission tomography for staging and management of malignant melanoma. *Br J Surg*. 2002;89:389–396.

34. Akcali C, Zincirkeser S, Erbagcy Z, et al. Detection of metastases in patients with cutaneous melanoma using FDG-PET/CT. *J Int Med Res*. 2007;35:547–553.

35. Tyler DS, Onaitis M, Kherani A, et al. Positron emission tomography scanning in malignant melanoma. *Cancer*. 2000;89:1019–1025.

36. Wagner JD. A role for FDG-PET in the surgical management of stage IV melanoma. *Ann Surg Oncol*. 2004;11:721–722.

37. Acland KM, Healy C, Calonje E, et al. Comparison of positron emission tomography scanning and sentinel node biopsy in the detection of micrometastasis of primary cutaneous malignant melanoma. *J Clin Oncol*. 2001;19:2674–2678.

38. Pfannenberga C, Aschoff P, Schanza S, et al. Prospective comparison of 18F-fluorodeoxyglucose positron emission tomography computed tomography and whole-body magnetic resonance imaging in staging of advanced malignant melanoma. *Eur J Cancer*. 2007;43:557–564.

39. Reinhardt MJ, Joe AY, Jaeger U, et al. Diagnostic performance of whole body dual modality 18F-FDG PET/CT imaging for N and M-staging of malignant melanoma: experience with 250 consecutive patients. *J Clin Oncol*. 2006;24:1178–1187.

40. Iagaru A, Quon A, Johnson D, et al. 2-Deoxy-2-[F-18]fluoro-D-glucose positron emission tomography/computed tomography in the management of melanoma. *Mol Imaging Biol*. 2006;8:309–314.

41. Schoder H, Larson SM, Yeung HW. PET/CT in oncology: integration into clinical management of lymphoma, melanoma, and gastrointestinal malignancies. *J Nucl Med*. 2004;45(suppl 1):72S–81S.

42. Strobel K, Dummer R, Husarik DB, et al. High-risk melanoma: accuracy of FDG PET/CT with added CT morphologic information for detection of metastases. *Radiology*. 2007;244:566–574.

43. Davis PC, Hudgins PA, Peterman SB, et al. Diagnosis of cerebral metastases: double-dose delayed CT vs contrast-enhanced MR imaging. *AJNR Am J Neuroradiol*. 1991;12:293–300.

44. Fogarty GB, Tartaguia C, Fogarty GB, et al. The utility of magnetic resonance imaging in the detection of brain metastases in the staging of cutaneous melanoma. *Clin Oncol*. 2006;18:360–362.

45. Ghanem N, Altehoefer C, Hogerle S, et al. Detectability of liver metastases in malignant melanoma: prospective comparison of magnetic resonance imaging and positron emission tomography. *Eur J Radiol*. 2005;54:264–270.

46. Schmidt GP, Haug AR, Schoenberg SO, et al. Whole-body MRI and PET-CT in the management of cancer patients. *Eur Radiol*. 2006;16:1216–1225.

47. Antoch G, Vogt FM, Freudenberg LS, et al. Whole-body dual-modality PET/CT and whole-body MRI for tumor staging in oncology. *JAMA*. 2003;290:3199–3206.

48. Schlemmer HP, Schafer J, Pfannenberg C, et al. Fast whole-body assessment of metastatic disease using a novel magnetic resonance imaging system: initial experiences. *Invest Radiol*. 2005;40:64–71.

49. Schmidt GP, Baur-Melnyk A, Herzog P, et al. High-resolution whole-body magnetic resonance image tumor staging with the use of parallel imaging versus dual-modality positron emission tomography-computed tomography: experience on a 32-channel system. *Invest Radiol*. 2005;40:743–753.

# Treatment of Disseminated Melanoma

*Jason L. Chang, Patrick A. Ott, and Anna C. Pavlick*

## Key Points

- Surgical resection should be considered for all patients with limited numbers of metastatic sites.

- Standard cytotoxic chemotherapy has limited efficacy in metastatic melanoma, with response rates in the 10–20% range and short-lived response durations.

- High-dose IL-2 is associated with a small percentage of complete and durable responses, but is limited to a subgroup of patients with good performance status owing to its toxicity.

- CNS disease is associated with high mortality; surgical resection and stereotactic radiotherapy, if possible, are preferred over whole brain irradiation.

- The clinical activity of PLX4032 validates the concept that the BRAF$^{V600E}$ mutation drives melanoma growth and is a therapeutic target in melanoma.

- CTLA-4 blockade and specific BRAF inhibition are novel treatment approaches that promise to become standard therapeutic options in the near future.

## INTRODUCTION

The tendency for melanoma to spread through the lymphatic system and the bloodstream is in stark contrast to most other skin cancers. Thin melanomas (<1–2 mm) without lymph node involvement is curable in most cases by surgical removal with sufficient margins and adequate staging, which includes assessment of sentinel lymph node involvement if necessary. In contrast, thicker melanomas, ulcerated tumors, or lymph node involvement, although initially mostly amenable to complete surgical resection, confer a much poorer prognosis due to the risk of systemic recurrence, with 5-year survivals ranging from 25% to 75%.[1] Disseminated, locally advanced, or recurrent melanoma is notoriously unresponsive to standard treatment, and is associated with a dismal prognosis, with 5-year survivals of the order of 10–25%.[1]

## EPIDEMIOLOGY

Advanced melanoma has the highest per-death loss of years of potential life expectancy except for adult leukemia. The incidence of melanoma continues to rise worldwide at approximately 3% per year, and in 2009 there were an estimated 68,720 new cases in the United States and 8650 deaths.[1] According to SEER data, roughly 4% of melanomas are already metastatic at time of diagnosis.[2]

## STAGING OF METASTATIC DISEASE

The site of metastatic disease has a direct impact on prognosis and is incorporated within the recent 2009 AJCC staging system, unchanged from 2002. Stage IV melanoma is separated into M1a for skin, soft tissue, or distant lymph node metastases, M1b for pulmonary lesions, and M1c for all other visceral metastases or any distant metastasis with elevated serum LDH levels.[1] Table 57.1 demonstrates the absolute 1-year survival rates of the three M classifications, while Figure 57.1 depicts the relative survival curves generated from the most recent AJCC database.

## MEDICAL THERAPY FOR ADVANCED MELANOMA

### Standard chemotherapy

Systemic chemotherapy for disseminated melanoma has response rates of 6–15% with median progression-free survivals of 2–3 months.[3] Despite its low response rates, the alkylating agent dacarbazine (DTIC) remains the reference standard for metastatic melanoma.[4] Temozolomide is an oral pro-drug that is metabolized to the active moiety of DTIC; it has equivalent efficacy to DTIC but with the advantage of crossing the blood–brain barrier.[5] Temozolomide may also act as a sensitizer for radiotherapy in the setting of brain metastases.[6] Combination chemotherapeutic regimens, such as the dacarbazine-containing Dartmouth regimen (DTIC, vincristine, carmustine, and tamoxifen),[7] have been associated with higher response rates, although usually at the cost of higher toxicity. To date, no combination regimen has demonstrated an improvement in overall survival over single-agent chemotherapy, likely in large part due to the relatively high toxicity of multi-agent therapy.

### Biochemotherapy

Investigators have looked at combinations of interleukin-2 (IL-2)-based immunotherapy and cisplatin- and dacarbazine-based chemotherapy given sequentially or concurrently in patients with metastatic melanoma (Table 57.2). A phase III study comparing the efficacy of chemotherapy (cisplatin, vinblastine, and dacarbazine [CVD]) with sequential biochemotherapy consisting of CVD in combination with IL-2 and interferon alfa-2b showed improvement in response rates (48% vs 25%) and time to progression, and borderline significant improvement in median overall survival.[8] However, this therapy was associated with substantially

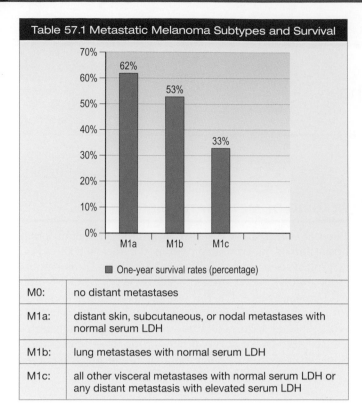

Table 57.1 Metastatic Melanoma Subtypes and Survival

One-year survival rates (percentage): M1a 62%, M1b 53%, M1c 33%

| | |
|---|---|
| M0: | no distant metastases |
| M1a: | distant skin, subcutaneous, or nodal metastases with normal serum LDH |
| M1b: | lung metastases with normal serum LDH |
| M1c: | all other visceral metastases with normal serum LDH or any distant metastasis with elevated serum LDH |

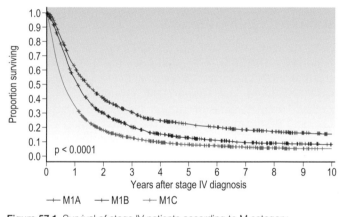

**Figure 57.1** Survival of stage IV patients according to M category.

Table 57.2 Biochemotherapy and Immunotherapy Response Rates

| Regimen | Response Rate | Median Overall Survival |
|---|---|---|
| CVD, interleukin-2, interferon alfa-2b[8] | 48% | 11.9 months |
| CVD, interleukin-2, interferon alfa-2b[9] | 19.5% | 9.0 months |
| Chemotherapy, IL-2, IFN alfa-2b (meta-analysis)[10] | 27% | n/a |
| High-dose IL-2[11,12] | 16% | 11.4 months |
| High-dose IL-2, peptide vaccine gp100:209-217(210M)[13] | 42% | 17.6 months |

CVD: cisplatin, vinblastine, dacarbazine.

greater toxicity. Another recent phase III trial compared concurrent biochemotherapy comprising CVD, IL-2 and interferon alfa-2b, with CVD alone in patients with metastatic melanoma (E3695) and showed no differences in the two groups with regards to overall survival or durable responses.[9] A meta-analysis in more than 2500 patients who received either chemotherapy or biochemotherapy concluded that the complex biochemotherapy regimens consistently improved response rates but not overall survival.[10] Therefore, at this time, biochemotherapy cannot be considered a standard treatment for metastatic melanoma.

## Immunotherapy

In melanoma treatment, it has long been recognized that immune interventions can mediate tumor regression. The most commonly investigated immunotherapy regimens for advanced and unresectable stage IV melanoma include cytokines (IL-2 in particular), vaccines, adoptive cell transfer, and, more recently, monoclonal antibodies.

IL-2, a T-cell growth factor, had been approved by the FDA in 1998 after it was found to have an overall response rate of 16% with a median response duration of 9 months in advanced melanoma patients.[11,12] Perhaps more importantly, the complete response rate was about 6%, and 59% of these patients appear to have durable responses lasting over 7 years. Moreover, visceral metastases and large tumor burdens do not appear to affect the likelihood of response to high-dose IL-2 therapy.[11,12] Recently, the combination of IL-2 with a peptide vaccine (gp100:209-217[210M] peptide + Montanide ISA) was shown to have improved response rates and progression-free survival over IL-2 alone, although the IL-2 arm of the study had lower response rates than would be expected from historical controls.[13]

The main limitation of IL-2 is the severe toxicity that is associated with treatment. Serious adverse events include hypotension, arrhythmias, pulmonary edema, and sepsis, and appear to be mediated by proinflammatory cytokines.[14] Therefore, while this therapy confers a small chance of a complete, durable response, it is limited to patients of good performance status and preserved organ function who have access to specialized treatment centers that can provide the ICU-level care that is often necessary with this therapy.

An experimental treatment in a highly selected patient group utilizing adoptive transfer of tumor infiltrating lymphocytes, in addition to lymphodepletion with chemotherapy and total body irradiation as well as high-dose IL-2, achieved response rates of up to 70% and highlights the potential efficacy of an immune intervention in melanoma.[15]

Increasing knowledge of T-cell regulation has uncovered potential immunologic targets for the treatment of melanoma. The interaction between antigen-presenting cells (APC) and T cells is crucial for inducing melanoma-specific T-cell responses. In addition to the interaction between the HLA-peptide complex on the APC and the T-cell receptor (TCR), several different co-stimulatory and co-inhibitory molecules mediate their respective signals to the T cell. For instance, the T-cell surface molecule CD28 interacts with the B7 receptor on the APC to mediate a co-stimulatory signal, whereas the T-cell cytotoxic T-lymphocyte antigen (CTLA)-4 interacts with B7 to induce an inhibitory signal[16,17] (Fig. 57.2).

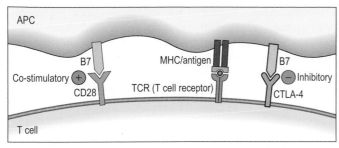

**Figure 57.2** T-cell interactions with antigen-presenting cells (APCs). Binding of the T-cell receptor to the MHC/antigen complex on APCs may be modulated by other cell surface molecules. Binding of the CD28 on the T cell to B7 on the APC provides a co-stimulatory signal that may lead to T-cell activation and IL-2 production. Conversely, binding of CTLA-4 on the T cell to B7 on the APC induces an inhibitory signal that prevents T-cell activation.

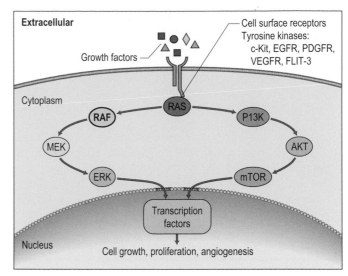

**Figure 57.3** Molecular targets in melanoma: the MAPK and PI3K pathways. Binding of growth factors to cell surface receptors induces their dimerization and activation of the MAPK tyrosine kinase cascade, which includes RAS RAF, MEK and ERK. Activated (phosphorylated) ERK translocates into the nucleus, and phosphorylates transcription factors for genes involved in cell growth and proliferation. This pathway is constitutively activated in many human melanomas. An alternate pathway via PI3K, AKT, and mTOR may also be activated in some melanomas.

This knowledge has led to the development of monoclonal antibodies targeting and blocking CTLA-4 in the attempt to enhance T-cell-mediated antitumor activity, and these agents are currently being evaluated in several clinical trials in melanoma. In the initial phase I study, tremelimumab was relatively well tolerated with mild to moderate toxicity (diarrhea, dermatitis, pruritus, and fatigue), and demonstrated encouraging clinical activity including several complete responses.[18] However, in a randomized phase III study comparing single-agent tremelimumab with either dacarbazine or temozolomide in patients with advanced melanoma, tremelimumab failed to demonstrate a significant improvement in overall survival in comparison to standard chemotherapy.[19]

Ipilimumab is another fully humanized anti-CTLA-4 monoclonal antibody (IgG) that was studied in a phase III trial involving 676 HLA-A*0201-positive patients with unresectable stage III or stage IV melanoma as single agent and in combination with a gp-100 peptide vaccine. All patients had extensive prior therapy and over 70% had M1c disease.[20] Median overall survival was 10.0 months in patients receiving ipilimumab with the gp100 vaccine versus 6.4 months in patients receiving gp100 alone, and was 10.1 months in patients receiving ipilimumab alone. Objective responses were observed in 10.9% of the patients receiving ipilimumab alone; importantly, 60% of these responses were maintained for over 2 years with tumor regression observed in lung, liver, skin, lymph nodes, and brain metastases.

The activity and side-effect profile of anti-CTLA-4 antibodies have several characteristics that likely reflect their immune-mediated mechanism of action. Initial apparent progression of disease, even with emergence of new lesions, and subsequent response over the course of several months has been seen with these therapies. Most importantly, a relatively large proportion of responses have been durable. The characteristic response kinetics has led to the proposal of immune-related response criteria when evaluating treatment responses to these agents.[21]

## Targeted therapies

In recent years, a greater understanding of the molecular biology of melanoma has led to an increase in drugs targeting several molecules that are part of oncogenic signaling pathways (see Chapter 55). The MAP kinase (MAPK) pathway (Fig. 57.3) is a crucial regulator of cell growth and survival, and is activated in many human malignancies.[22] Binding of growth factor ligands to cell surface receptors induces receptor dimerization and activation of tyrosine kinases, leading to a phosphorylation cascade of intracellular tyrosine kinases that include RAS, RAF, MEK, and ERK. Activated ERK then translocates into the nucleus and activates transcription factors for a wide array of genes involved in cellular proliferation and survival.[23] An alternate kinase signaling pathway involves upstream molecules PI3K and AKT activating mTOR, which travels to the nucleus and activates genes involved in cell growth and proliferation.[24]

The MAPK pathway has been of keen interest in melanoma in particular since an initial study by Davies et al. in 2002 which found that over 60% of melanomas harbor a specific missense mutation (V600E) in the BRAF gene.[25] This mutation constitutively activates the MAPK pathway by increasing transcriptional output via ERK and disabling normal feedback inhibition.[26] Sorafenib, which inhibits a number of molecules including BRAF, was initially used in clinical trials to specifically target this pathway, but demonstrated no significant clinical activity as a single agent or in combination with chemotherapeutic drugs.[27–31]

A very promising new drug targeting the MAPK pathway is PLX4032, a specific and potent inhibitor of mutated BRAF. A phase I dose-finding trial and subsequent extension cohort demonstrated a 69% and 81% response rate, respectively, and median progression-free survival greater than 7 months in heavily pre-treated patients carrying tumors with this mutation.[32] The clinical activity associated with this agent validates the concept that the BRAF[V600E] mutation drives melanoma growth and is a therapeutic target in melanoma. A phase III study involving this drug is already underway at multiple institutions.

Imatinib, a kinase inhibitor that has been used with success in other malignancies such as chronic myelogenous leukemia and gastrointestinal stromal tumors, appears to have activity in melanomas that express activation of the c-kit gene. A recent report found that 30–40% of patients with acral or mucosal melanomas have tumors that contain activating mutations or overexpression of the c-kit gene.[33] Case reports have shown occasional impressive responses to imatinib in this subset of patients,[34] and larger studies investigating the role for imatinib are currently in progress.

A number of other agents directed against many different targets, such as MEK, BRAF, mTOR, VEGFR, FGFR, PDGFR and others, are currently in clinical development.[35]

## SURGERY FOR ADVANCED MELANOMA

While surgical resection is the mainstay of treatment for early-stage melanoma, it also has a role in select patients with metastatic disease. In retrospective series, patients with complete surgical removal of metastases (metastasectomy) had higher median and overall survivals than expected from standard non-surgical therapies.[36] For instance, patients with M1a disease (skin, soft tissue, and distant lymph node metastases) ordinarily have a 10–18-month median survival, and this may increase to around 24 months if complete metastasectomy can be performed.[36] Similarly, series have shown that patients with M1b (pulmonary metastases) and M1c (visceral metastases) disease who undergo complete metastasectomies have 5-year survivals of 20–27%, as compared to 3–4% in non-surgical patients (Table 57.3).[36] Although patients in these series were highly selected for limited metastatic disease in anatomical locations amenable to complete surgical resection, it is nevertheless important to consider this option if technically feasible given the potential significant improvement in overall survival. For patients with disseminated disease that cannot be surgically removed, excision is generally reserved for the palliation of symptomatic, accessible metastases, as this modality may offer faster symptom control than other local treatments such as radiotherapy.

## BRAIN METASTASES

Central nervous system (CNS) metastases pose special challenges. They are seen in 10–40% of melanoma patients and represent the first site of recurrence in 15–20% of patients with metastatic disease.[37] After lung and breast carcinomas, melanoma is the third-most common primary tumor among all patients with CNS metastases in the United States.[38]

Brain metastasis portends an extremely poor prognosis, with median survival after diagnosis of only 2–8 months.[37]

Resection is the preferred treatment if the metastases are accessible and low in number, one or two in most cases, and if non-cranial disease burden is low or well controlled. Surgery may also be necessary on an urgent basis if immediate decompression of a critical lesion is required.

Stereotactic radiosurgery (SRS) consists of multiple convergent radiation beams that can deliver high doses of radiation to small fixed areas, thereby limiting toxicity to surrounding brain tissue. SRS has been increasingly used for brain metastases up to 3–4 cm in size that are not readily accessible for surgical resection. The maximum number of brain metastases for SRS has generally been in the 3–5 range; however, depending on the available technology and the operator, up to 10 lesions can be treated. In some patients, recurrent disease, if limited in number, may still be amenable to this treatment modality.[39]

Whole brain radiation (WBRT) is the least favored treatment option for CNS metastases, and is generally reserved for large numbers of brain metastases, lesions that are too large for SRS or surgery, or for lesions located in sensitive locations.[39] Early side effects of WBRT include fatigue, headache, and drowsiness, while long-term toxicities include dementia and ataxia.[39] WBRT may also be used as an adjunct to surgery or SRS to decrease the likelihood of recurrence elsewhere within the brain, although this approach has not been shown to increase overall survival.[39]

## CONCLUSIONS

Advanced melanoma is associated with poor outcomes for most patients. Standard of care systemic treatment remains limited to dacarbazine or temozolomide and, at select institutions, high-dose IL-2. However, response rates are generally low. Alternative treatment approaches such as combination chemotherapy or biochemotherapy yield higher response rates but have not shown improved overall survival.

## FUTURE OUTLOOK

Several novel modalities are in late clinical development and may broaden the armamentarium of clinicians in the near future. Immune-checkpoint blockade with ipilumumab (blocking the negative co-stimulatory molecule CTLA-4 expressed on T cells) is a truly novel immunotherapy approach and acts in a much more specific fashion than cytokines such as IFN-α and IL-2. Although not completely innocuous, anti-CTLA-4 therapy is much better tolerated than cytokine treatment.

Greater understanding of the molecular signaling pathways in melanoma, and most importantly the identification of the BRAF$^{V600E}$ mutation, has led to the development of new agents that specifically block the MAPK pathway; impressive response rates have already been seen in patients with tumors positive for this mutation. Another example is the reported remarkable response rates with imatinib therapy in patients with mucosal, acral, and sun-damaged skin melanomas that harbor mutations in the c-kit gene. These results foreshadow the era of individualized therapy based

| Table 57.3 Survival in Patients Where Complete Metastasectomies can be Performed[36] | | |
|---|---|---|
| Subclass | Median Survival | 5-year Overall Survival |
| M1a | 10–29 months | 5–38% |
| M1b | 11–20 months | 5–27% |
| M1c | 15–49 months | 28–41% |

on specific tumor genotypes, which appears just beyond the horizon in melanoma.

The treatment of advanced melanoma remains a significant clinical challenge. These novel treatments, used singly or in combination with other molecular agents, immunotherapy, or chemotherapy, may lead to improved overall survival for patients with advanced melanoma. In the interim, given the limited efficacy of standard treatments and number of potential new therapeutic targets, eligible patients should be considered for clinical trials.

## REFERENCES

1. Balch CM, Gershenwald JE, Soong S, et al. Final version of 2009 AJCC melanoma staging and classification. *J Clin Oncol.* 2009;27:6199–6206.
2. Horner MJ, Ries LAG, Krapcho M, et al. SEER Cancer Statistics Review, 1975-2006, based on November 2008 SEER data submission, posted to the SEER website 2009.
3. Mays SR, Nelson BR. Current therapy of cutaneous melanoma. *Cutis.* 1999;63:293–298.
4. Serrone L, Zeuli M, Sega FM, et al. Dacarbazine-based chemotherapy for metastatic melanoma: thirty-year experience overview. *J Exp Clin Cancer Res.* 2000;19(1):21–34.
5. Middleton MR, Grob JJ, Aaronson N, et al. Randomized phase III study of temozolomide versus dacarbazine in the treatment of patients with advanced metastatic malignant melanoma. *J Clin Oncol.* 2000;18:158–166.
6. Zhang M, Chakravarti A. Novel radiation-enhancing agents in malignant gliomas. *Semin Radiat Oncol.* 2006;16:29–37.
7. Chapman PB, Einhorn LH, Meyers ML, et al. Phase III multicenter randomized trial of the Dartmouth regimen versus dacarbazine in patients with metastatic melanoma. *J Clin Oncol.* 1999;17:2745–2751.
8. Eton O, Legha SS, Bedikian AY, et al. Sequential biochemotherapy versus chemotherapy for metastatic melanoma: results from a phase III randomized trial. *J Clin Oncol.* 2002;20:2045–2052.
9. Atkins MB, Hsu J, Lee S, et al. Phase III trial comparing concurrent biochemotherapy with cisplatin, vinblastine, dacarbazine, interleukin-2, and interferon α-2b with cisplatin, vinblastine, and dacarbazine alone in patients with metastatic malignant melanoma (E3695): a trial coordinated by the Eastern Cooperative Oncology Group. *J Clin Oncol.* 2008;26:5748–5754.
10. Ives NJ, Stowe RL, Lorigan P, et al. Chemotherapy compared with biochemotherapy for the treatment of metastatic melanoma: a meta-analysis of 18 trials involving 2,621 patients. *J Clin Oncol.* 2007;25:5426–5434.
11. Atkins MB, Lotze MT, Dutcher JP, et al. High-dose recombinant interleukin 2 therapy for patients with metastatic melanoma: analysis of 270 patients treated between 1985 and 1993. *J Clin Oncol.* 1999;17:2105–2116.
12. Atkins MB, Kunkel L, Sznol M, et al. High-dose recombinant interleukin-2 therapy in patients with metastatic melanoma: long-term survival update. *Cancer J Sci Am.* 2000;6(suppl 1):S11.
13. Schwartzentruber DJ, Lawson D, Richards J, et al. A phase III multi-institutional randomized study of immunization with the gp100:209–217(210M) peptide followed by high-dose IL-2 compared with high-dose IL-2 alone in patients with metastatic melanoma. *J Clin Oncol.* 2009;27(18s) Abstr CRA9011.
14. Mier J, Vachino G, Van der Meer J, et al. Induction of circulating tumor necrosis factor (TNF) as the mechanism for the febrile response to interleukin-2 (IL-2) in cancer patients. *J Clin Immunol.* 1988;8:426–436.
15. Dudley ME, Yang JC, Sherry R, et al. Adoptive cell therapy for patients with metastatic melanoma: evaluation of intensive myeloablative chemoradiation preparative regimens. *J Clin Oncol.* 2008;26:5233–5239.
16. Chambers CA, Kuhns MS, Egen JG, et al. CTLA-4-mediated inhibition in regulation of T cell responses: mechanisms and manipulation in tumor immunotherapy. *Annu Rev Immunol.* 2001;19:565–594.

17. Krummel MF, Allison JP. CD20 and CTLA-4 have opposing effects on the response of T cells to stimulation. *J Exp Med.* 1995;182:459–465.
18. Ribas A, Camacho LH, Lopez-Berestein G, et al. Antitumor activity in melanoma and anti-self responses in a phase I trial with the anti-cytotoxic T lymphocyte-associated antigen 4 monoclonal antibody CP-675,206. *J Clin Oncol.* 2005;23:8968–8977.
19. Ribas A, Hauschild A, Kefford R, et al. Phase III, open-label, randomized, comparative study of tremelimumab (CP-675,206) and chemotherapy (temozolomide [TMZ] or dacarbazine [DTIC]) in patients with advanced melanoma. *J Clin Oncol.* 2008;26: LBA 9011.
20. Hodi FS, O'Day SJ, McDermott DF, et al. Improved survival with ipilimumab in patients with metastatic melanoma. *N Engl J Med.* 2010;363:711–723.
21. Wolchok JD, Ibrahim R, DePril V, et al. Antitumor response and new lesions in advanced melanoma patients on ipilimumab treatment. *J Clin Oncol.* 2008;26(May 20 suppl) Abstr 3020.
22. Fecher LA, Amaravadi RK, Flaherty KT, The M.A.P.K. pathway in melanoma. *Curr Opin Oncol.* 2008;20:183–189.
23. Shields JM, Thomas NE, Cregger M, et al. Lack of extracellular signal-regulated kinase mitogen-activated protein kinase signaling shows a new type of melanoma. *Cancer Res.* 2007;67:1502–1512.
24. Stahl JM, Sharma A, Cheung M, et al. Deregulated Akt3 activity promotes development of malignant melanoma. *Cancer Res.* 2004;64:7002–7010.
25. Davies H, Bignell GR, Cox C, et al. Mutations of the BRAF gene in human cancer. *Nature.* 2002;417:949–954.
26. Pratilas CA, Taylor BS, Ye Q, et al. (V600E)BRAF is associated with disabled feedback inhibition of RAF-MEK signaling and elevated transcriptional output of the pathway. *Proc Natl Acad Sci U S A.* 2009;106:4519–4524.
27. Adnane L, Trial PA, Taylor I, et al. Sorafenib (BAY 43-9006, Nexavar), a dual-action inhibitor that targets RAF/MEK/ERK in tumor cells and tyrosine kinases VEGFR/PDGFR in tumor vasculature. *Methods Enzymol.* 2006;407:597–612.
28. Wilhelm SM, Carter C, Tang L, et al. BAY 43-9006 exhibits broad spectrum oral antitumor activity and targets the RAF/MEK/ERK pathway and receptor tyrosine kinases involved in tumor progression and angiogenesis. *Cancer Res.* 2004;64:7099–7109.
29. Eisen T, Ahmad T, Flaherty KT, et al. Sorafenib in advanced melanoma: a phase II randomised discontinuation trial analysis. *Br J Cancer.* 2006;95:581–586.
30. Hauschild A, Agarwala SS, Trefzer U, et al. Results of a phase III, randomized, placebo-controlled study of sorafenib in combination with carboplatin and paclitaxel as second-line treatment in patients with unresectable stage III or stage IV melanoma. *J Clin Oncol.* 2009;27:2823–2830.
31. Ott PA, Hamilton A, Min C, et al. A phase II trial of sorafenib in metastatic melanoma with tissue correlates. *PLos One* 2010;5:e15588.
32. Flaherty KT, Puzanov I, Kim KB, et al. Inhibition of mutated, activated BRAF in metastatic melanoma. *N Eng J Med* 2010;363:809–819.
33. Curtin JA, Busam K, Pinkel D, et al. Somatic activation of KIT in distinct subtypes of melanoma. *J Clin Oncol.* 2006;24:4340–4346.
34. Hodi FS, Friedlander P, Corless CL, et al. Major response to imatinib mesylate in KIT-mutated melanoma. *J Clin Oncol.* 2008;26:2046–2051.
35. Seetharamu N, Ott PA, Pavlick AC. Novel therapeutics for melanoma. *Expert Rev Anticancer Ther.* 2009;9:839–849.
36. Ollila DW. Complete metastasectomy in patients with stage IV metastatic melanoma. *Lancet Oncol.* 2007;7:919–924.
37. Testori A, Rutkowski P, Marsden J, et al. Surgery and radiotherapy in the treatment of cutaneous melanoma. *Ann Oncol.* 2009;20(suppl 6): vi22–vi29.
38. Sampson JH, Carter JH, Friedman AH, et al. Demographics, prognosis, and therapy in 702 patients with brain metastases from malignant melanoma. *J Neurosurg.* 1998;88:11–20.
39. Peacock KH, Lesser GJ. Current therapeutic approaches in patients with brain metastases. *Curr Treat Options Oncol.* 2006;7:479–489.

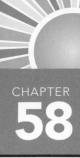
# Management of Skin Cancer in the Immunocompromised Patient

*Thomas Stasko, Allison Hanlon, and Anna Clayton*

---

### Key Points

- Solid organ transplant recipients have an increased risk of developing squamous cell carcinomas.

- Immunocompromised patients can develop aggressive skin cancers with an increased risk for recurrence and metastasis.

- HIV/AIDS patients have an increased risk of human papillomavirus-associated neoplasms, sebaceous carcinoma and Merkel carcinoma.

- Patient education, photoprotection and close surveillance are important aspects of treatment.

## INTRODUCTION

The immune system has the important task of mounting a response against foreign antigens while maintaining self-tolerance. The role of the immune system in surveillance of neoplasms has long been investigated. Tumor-infiltrating lymphocytes are suspected of mounting a specific immune response to tumor antigens.[1] Compromise of the immune system through iatrogenic or infectious means has revealed the importance of immune surveillance in monitoring cutaneous neoplasms. HIV/AIDS patients have a loss of cellular immunity resulting in an increased susceptibility to infection and risk of neoplasms.[2] Solid organ transplant patients requiring long-term immunosuppression have the greatest incidence of non-melanoma skin cancer (NMSC), with an increased risk ranging from 50 to 100 times the general population.[3] Although many factors contribute to the development of skin cancer in these groups, the common theme is this increased risk in the immunocompromised patient.

## SOLID ORGAN TRANSPLANT RECIPIENTS

### Epidemiology

Improved surgical and anesthesia techniques, better understanding of immunological responses, and the development of more specific and potent immunosuppressants have revolutionized solid organ transplant in the past 60 years. Solid organ transplantation has evolved from humble beginnings with early graft rejection to over 173,000 solid organ transplant patients (SOTRs) living in the United States today.[4] With increased success have come increased complications, most notably the development of post-transplant neoplasms. Solid organ transplant recipients have a three- to fivefold increased risk of developing malignancy, providing a unique setting for the identification of

cancers under immunological control. Tumors that are seen more frequently in the transplant population include skin cancer, lymphomas, cervical and anogenital carcinomas, oropharyngeal carcinomas, renal carcinoma, thyroid carcinoma, and various sarcomas.[5]

Skin cancer is by far the most common post-transplant malignancy. It is estimated that 44% of transplant patients will develop multiple skin cancers.[6] Unlike the general population, transplant patients have an alarming rate of squamous call carcinomas (SCC) (Fig. 58.1). The ratio of SCC to basal cell carcinoma (BCC) is 4 to 1 in these patients, a reversal of what is observed in the general population.[7,8] Risk factors associated with the development of post-transplant NMSC are male sex, fair phenotype, ultraviolet radiation (UVR) exposure, degree and type of immunosuppression, age at transplantation and time from transplantation (Table 58.1).[9,10]

The strongest independent risk factor for post-transplantation NSMC is a history of NMSC prior to transplantation.[11] Non-white kidney transplant patients do not have the same risk of developing NMSC, illustrating the importance of the patient's phenotype (Fitzpatrick skin type I–III) in the development of cancer.[12] Most NMSCs are present in sun-exposed sites, making UVR exposure a key risk factor. Older patients with more cumulative exposure to UVR are at a greater risk for developing NMSC post transplant as compared to younger patients.[13]

Transplant-related risk factors include time from transplantation and the intensity and duration of immunosuppression (Table 58.2). Patients 50 years old or greater at transplant have an increased risk of developing skin cancer within the first year of immunosuppression. This risk increases over the next 6 years and then becomes stable. In contrast, younger transplant patients (age <50) have a delay in their relative risk of skin cancers, with the onset almost 10 years post transplant.[3,14] A retrospective cohort study of renal transplant patients has shown that the use of three immunosuppressant medications is associated with an increased incidence of NMSC and a shortened time to NSMC development as compared to patients on two medications.[15] This observation was repeated in the cardiac transplant population, showing that patients with an initial high rejection score and subsequent enhanced immunosuppression were at an increased risk of developing skin cancer.[10] A prospective study revealed that patients with a decreased CD4 count have an increased risk of developing skin cancer.[16] The intensity of immunosuppression varies depending upon the organ transplanted. Cardiac recipients generally require a higher degree of immunosuppression as

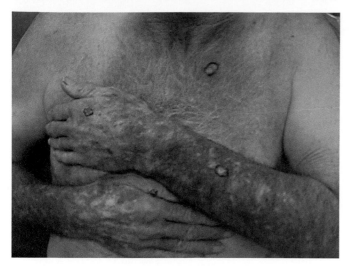

**Figure 58.1** Cardiac transplant patient with a history of multiple squamous cell carcinomas on the chest and extremities. Note the numerous hyperkeratotic papules on the arms. Actinic keratoses, verrucae and squamous cell carcinomas are present.

### Table 58.1 Risk Factors Associated with the Development of Non-Melanoma Skin Cancer[8–10]

- Male sex
- Fair phenotype
- Degree and type of immunosuppression
- Age at transplantation
- Time from transplantation
- History of chronic sun exposure
- Type of organ transplanted
- CD4 lymphopenia
- HPV

compared to kidney patients. The age-adjusted incidence of NMSC is three times higher in heart transplant recipients than kidney transplant recipients, likely reflecting how the degree of immunosuppression correlates with the future development of NMSC.[17]

## Pathogenesis

While there are likely many factors that result in the development of post-transplant neoplasm, two factors that have been the focus of study are immunosuppression and medications that may have a direct oncogenic effect (Table 58.3).

A population-based cohort study of Australian patients with end-stage kidney disease assessed the standardized incidence ratio (SIR) for any cancer (excluding NMSC) in three separate periods: the 5-year period prior to kidney failure, during dialysis, and after transplantation. The SIR for any cancer increased significantly over these three periods, from 1.16 to 1.35 to 3.27.[18] The incidence of cancer after the withdrawal or reduction of immunosuppression can be examined in kidney transplant patients owing to the reinstitution of dialysis following graft failure. In an analysis of Australian kidney transplant patients, the SIR for lip cancer during all periods of dialysis subsequent to transplant failure (SIR 2.16, 95% CI 0.05–12.05) was significantly lower than during periods of transplant function (SIR 52.26, 95% CI 42.57–60.02, p=0.001) and was comparable to that during the period of dialysis prior to transplantation (SIR 3.44, 95% CI 2.23–5.08, p=0.649).[19] The reversal of risk in the development of lip cancer following graft failure may be attributed to the removal of immunosuppressants and reconstitution of the immune system.

Advances in immunology and molecular biology have led to an armamentarium of immunosuppressive medications. Glucocorticoids, the first effective class of anti-rejection drugs, continue to be a mainstay of treatment. Steroids have a broad effect on the immune system by inhibiting antigen presentation, inducing lymphocyte toxicity, and altering cytokine production, but steroid use alone is not sufficient to allow graft survival. Side effects of long-term steroid usage include cutaneous atrophy, increased risk of infection, and impaired wound healing. Chronic steroids are felt to be less important in the induction of skin cancer than are other immunosuppressants.

Antiproliferative agents such as azathioprine and mycophenolate mofetil are an important element of many

### Table 58.2 Management of Other Skin Cancers In Transplant Patients*

| Tumor | Characteristics | Treatment |
|---|---|---|
| Dermatofibrosarcoma protuberans | Low-grade sarcoma<br>High rate of recurrence<br>Scar-like plaque on trunk and extremities | Mohs micrographic surgery or wide local excision[62] |
| Atypical fibroxanthoma | Spindle cell tumor on head and neck of sun-exposed patients<br>Locally aggressive<br>Metastatic potential | Mohs micrographic surgery or wide local excision |
| Malignant fibrous histiocytoma | Soft tissue sarcoma on the extremities of elderly patients<br>Metastasis to lung and lymph nodes | Wide local excision |
| Microcystic adenocarcinoma | Locally aggressive tumor with low rate of metastasis<br>Presents usually in central face and lip | Mohs micrographic surgery or wide local excision |
| Sebaceous carcinoma | Eyelid is common site for presentation<br>Metastasis<br>Associated with Muir–Torre syndrome | Mohs micrographic surgery or wide local excision |

*Rare non-melanoma skin cancers that have been documented in transplant patients. No increased risk for these tumors has been shown in epidemiology studies of transplant patients.

## Table 58.3 Immunosuppressive Medications

| Drug Name | Mechanism | NMSC Risk | Dermatologic Side-Effects |
|---|---|---|---|
| Corticosteroids | Inhibit antigen presentation, induce lymphocyte toxicity, alter cytokine production | + | Acne, striae, skin fragility, ecchymosis |
| OKT3 | Anti-CD3 humanized monoclonal antibody Depletes T lymphocytes | + | Hypersensitivity reaction |
| Thymoglobulin | Polyclonal anti-lymphocyte antibody | Not determined | Rash, pruritus, burning hand and foot pain, urticaria |
| Daclizumab, basiliximab | Chimeric/humanized anti-CD25 monoclonal antibody | Not determined | Impaired wound healing, acne |
| Alemtuzumab | Humanized anti-CD52 antibody | Not determined | Urticaria |
| Azathioprine | Inhibits purine synthesis | +++ | Hypersensitivity reaction including urticaria, maculopapular and vasculitic eruptions |
| Mycophenolate mofetil | Inhibits guanine nucleotide synthesis | +++ | Non-specific rash |
| Cyclosporin | Calcineurin inhibitor Decreases T-cell activation and IL-2 production | ++++ | Hirsutism, sebaceous hyperplasia, gingival hyperplasia |
| Tacrolimus | Calcineurin inhibitor | +++ | Alopecia |
| Sirolimus | Inhibits mammalian target of rapamycin Abrogates IL-2 signal transduction | Anti-carcinogenic effect in limited studies | Impaired wound healing, acne/folliculitis, edema |
| Everolimus | Inhibits mammalian target of rapamycin Abrogates IL-2 signal transduction | No long-term data | Mouth ulcers, stomatitis |

immunosuppressive regimens. Azathioprine is a prodrug that is converted into 6-mercaptopurine, which interferes with DNA replication, limiting the number of B and T lymphocytes. From the early 1960s to the 1980s, azathioprine and corticosteroids in combination was the primary immunosuppressant regimen. Azathioprine is associated with an increased risk of skin cancer and bone marrow suppression.[20] In the past 10 years, azathioprine has been replaced by mycophenolate for new transplant recipients. Mycophenolate inhibits inosine monophosphate dehydrogenase, which is an essential enzyme in the de-novo pathway of purine synthesis. Mycophenolate's main target is lymphocyte proliferation since lymphocytes are deficient in a purine salvage pathway. Mycophenolate has been shown to be superior to azathioprine in the prevention of acute rejection. Mycophenolate is thought to be associated with the development of skin cancer but to a lesser extent than azathioprine.

The calcineurin inhibitors cyclosporine and tacrolimus target T-lymphocyte activation. Ciclosporin binds to cyclophilin, while tacrolimus binds to FK-binding protein. These two protein complexes inhibit calcineurin, a calcium-dependent phosphatase activated following T-cell activation. Inhibition of calcineurin results in abrogation of T-cell activation and interleukin-2 production, an important T-cell growth factor. The role of the calcineurin inhibitors in the development of malignancy has been controversial. In-vitro studies by Yarosh et al. demonstrated that ciclosporin inhibited the removal of cyclobutane dimers and UV-mediated apoptosis.[21] Hojo et al. showed that cyclosporine induced cancer progression by phenotypically

changing cancerous cells to allow for growth and metastasis.[22] Contrasting studies have shown that ciclosporin has an anticarcinogenic effect by inhibiting keratinocyte proliferation in response to epidermal growth factor, TGF-α and interleukin-6.[23,24] Clinical studies indicate a possible dose-dependent carcinogenic effect.[25]

Sirolimus (also known as rapamycin) is an immunosuppressive and anti-angiogenic macrocyclic lactone produced by *Streptomyces hygroscopicus*. Sirolimus and its derivative everolimus target activated T-cell proliferation by binding to FK-binding protein-12 (FKBP-12). Drug-bound FKBP-12 inhibits the activation of the mammalian target of rapamycin (mTOR). mTOR is responsible for phosphorylation of signaling proteins necessary for growth factor-induced transcriptional events. In the absence of active mTOR, lymphocytes are arrested at the G1 to S phase transition of the cell cycle. Renal transplant recipients treated with sirolimus had a significant lower incidence of skin and solid organ cancers than those treated with calcineurin inhibitors.[26] Patients who were changed from a calcineurin inhibitor to sirolimus had a threefold lower incidence of new cancer diagnosis as compared to those who were continued on the calcineurin inhibitor.[27] In patients with a history of malignancy prior to transplant or multiple NMSC post transplant, sirolimus may be considered a first-line immunosuppressant.

It is difficult to pinpoint which immunosuppressive agent is most associated with the development of cutaneous malignancies. Patients are prescribed multiple medications, making it almost impossible to determine the relative role of each agent. Retrospective studies often compare patients from different time periods with different standard treatment regimens. In spite of limited data, the treatment of solid organ transplant patients with multiple NMSC may include mitigating the degree of immunosuppression or changing the regimen from calcineurin inhibitors to an mTOR inhibitor. In patients with advanced cutaneous neoplasms, including in-transit or distant metastasis, the benefit of stopping immunosuppression must be weighed against the risk of subsequent organ rejection. In renal transplant patients, loss of the transplanted organ can be accommodated with dialysis. Cardiac and hepatic transplant recipients do not have the same therapeutic options. A multidisciplinary team approach including transplant physicians, oncologists, surgeons and dermatologists is essential in these advanced cases.

## Cutaneous neoplasms

### Squamous cell carcinoma

Squamous cell carcinoma (SCC) is the most common non-melanoma skin cancer in the transplant population. UVR-induced mutations of keratinocytes, immunosuppression, and fair phenotype are the most likely etiologies for the development of SCC. Human papillomavirus (HPV) has also been implicated, but its role remains uncertain. The ubiquitous presence of HPV in both organ transplant patients and the general population make the contribution of HPV to the development of SCC difficult to elucidate. Transplant patients have a higher prevalence of HPV detection in SCC than non-transplant recipients. Epidermodysplasia verruciformis subtypes (HPV 5, 8) can be isolated more readily from transplant patients.[28]

SCC frequently develops in these patients in sun-exposed skin, often within fields of actinic keratosis and verrucae (Fig. 58.2). In male patients, the most common site of presentation is the head and neck, followed by the upper extremities. Female patients may have more involvement of the trunk.[29] The extensive actinic damage and keratinocyte hyperplasia present in some transplant recipients can make clinical detection difficult. The term transplant hands and scalp has been used to describe this presentation (Fig. 58.3). In severe cases of transplant hands, prophylactic excision of the skin followed by split-thickness skin grafting has been described.[4]

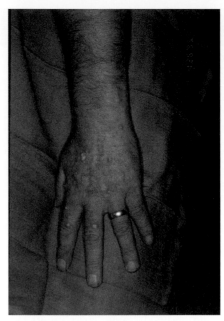

**Figure 58.3** Transplant hand with multiple verrucae, actinic keratoses and hyperkeratotic papules.

SCC in organ transplant patients must be considered a high-risk tumor for invasion and metastasis. In-transit metastases can present months after the excision of a primary aggressive SCC. The most common location is the forehead or scalp (Fig. 58.4). Once regional metastasis has occurred, the overall 3-year survival rate is 48%. Distant metastasis has a worse prognosis, with a 1-year survival rate of 39%.[30] Clinical features associated with invasion and metastases include advanced age, immunosuppression from lymphoma or chemotherapy, and tumor location and size. Tumors greater than 0.6 cm in the mask areas of the face, genitalia or feet; tumors greater than 1 cm on the forehead, neck or scalp; and tumors greater than 2 cm on the trunk or extremities have an increased risk of invasion, local recurrence and metastasis. Tumor features associated with metastasis include indistinct clinical borders, recurrence, ulceration and rapid growth (Table 58.4).

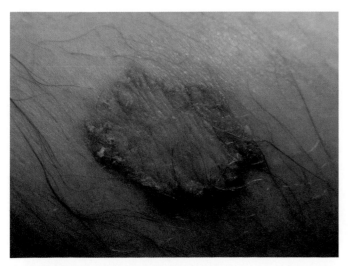

**Figure 58.2** Porokeratosis in a transplant patient.

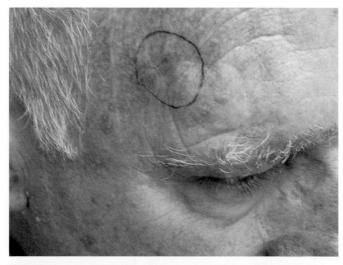

**Figure 58.4** Transplant patient with in-transit squamous cell carcinoma presenting months after excision of primary squamous cell carcinoma on forehead.

## Table 58.4 Features Associated with Metastatic Squamous Cell Carcinomas[31-33]

- Tumor size >0.6 cm on mask areas of face, genitalia, hands and feet
- Tumor size >1.0 cm on cheeks, forehead, neck and scalp
- Tumor size >2.0 cm on trunk and extremities
- Recurrent tumors
- Rapid tumor growth, ulceration, and indistinct clinical borders
- Deep extension into subcutaneous fat and/or perineural invasion on histology
- Tumors within previous radiation fields
- Clinically apparent satellite metastasis

Histological features include tumor depth, deep extension into the subcutaneous fat, poor differentiation, and perineural invasion.[31-33]

Squamous cell carcinomas from transplant patients have distinct histological abnormalities (Fig. 58.5). An examination of SCC histology from transplant and immunocompetent patients showed transplant patients' tumors have HPV-like features, spindle cell morphology, and multinucleated giant cells.[34] The degree of histological atypia does not prognosticate the clinical behavior of the tumor.

The management of SCC in the transplant population can be challenging. While many patients will only develop a few less aggressive SCCs, there are SOTRs who will develop innumerable tumors and/or highly aggressive cancers. The International Transplant Skin Cancer Collaborative and the European Skin Care in Organ Transplant Patients Network have published guidelines for the treatment of SCC.[35] The decision for a particular therapy is determined by tumor characteristics, the presence of metastasis or lymphadenopathy, and the patient's tolerance for treatment. Fundamental to the treatment of squamous proliferations is the classification of lesions as precancerous, lower-risk SCC, or high-risk SCC, as different therapies are implemented based on this categorization (Fig. 58.6).

Precancerous actinic keratosis, verrucae and porokeratosis should be treated to decrease the likelihood of progression to SCC. Cryosurgery or curettage can be used to treat isolated lesions. More involved actinic damage requires field treatment. 5-Fluorouracil, imiquimod, diclofenac, retinoids and photodynamic therapy have been used to decrease the numbers of actinic keratoses. Imiquimod activates the immune system by binding to toll-like receptor 7. Treatment with imiquimod decreased the numbers of actinic keratoses in SOTRs without inducing rejection of the transplanted organ.[36] Importantly, the treatment area was limited to $100 \text{ cm}^2$. In a small trial including renal transplant recipients, diclofenac was beneficial for the treatment of actinic keratosis,[36] but it must be used with caution in these patients due to the risk of systemic absorption. Retinoids, topical and systemic, have been beneficial in decreasing the number of premalignant and malignant lesions. Systemic retinoids are effective in inhibiting tumor development during treatment, but once discontinued, tumor growth continues.[37] Photodynamic therapy has been shown beneficial in reducing the numbers of actinic keratoses in SOTR.[38] Lesions that do not respond to treatment require biopsy to determine if an invasive SCC is present.

SCCs on the extremities and trunk in the absence of metastasis and lymphadenopathy may be considered lower-risk tumors (Fig. 58.7). A deep shave biopsy for tumor debulking and histological examination may be used to classify the tumor. High-risk SCC without metastatic spread or adherence to underlying structures can be treated with surgical excision. Mohs micrographic surgery has the highest cure rate and is the treatment of choice for high-risk tumors in the immunocompromised. Surgical excision with or without intraoperative frozen section analysis can be used. If histological examination shows positive margins or perineural involvement, then adjuvant radiation therapy may be indicated. Primary treatment with radiation may be necessary in tumors in anatomically sensitive areas or in patients who cannot tolerate surgical excision. Aggressive or recurrent SCC may suggest modification of immunosuppression as part of treatment (Fig. 58.8). Oral retinoids, such as acitretin, may be useful as an adjuvant therapy.

SOTRs with a history of SCC require a thorough clinical examination of the draining lymph nodes and skin surrounding the tumor. If metastases are detected clinically, imaging studies are indicated. Clinical or radiographic lymphadenopathy requires histological examination via fine needle aspiration or excision. Studies of the use of sentinel lymph node (SLN) biopsy in SOTRs are very limited and a survival benefit has not been demonstrated. Satellite lesions can be excised or treated with radiation. Satellite and lymph node metastasis may benefit from radiation as a discontinuous tumor has a high rate of developing additional metastasis. Patients with metastasis require a multidisciplinary approach for care, including medical and surgical oncology. Reduction of immunosuppression may be beneficial and should be discussed with the transplant team. Surgical excision and multiagent chemotherapy with cisplatin, 5-fluorouracil, bleomycin and retinoic acid may be considered.

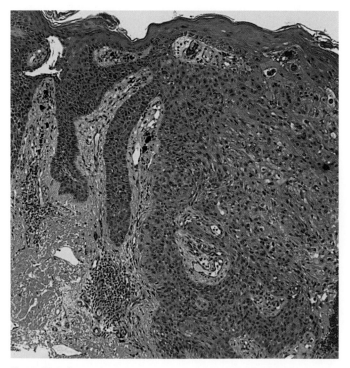

**Figure 58.5** Squamous cell carcinomas in transplant patients have marked cytologic atypia with multiple mitosis and multinucleated giant cells.

**Figure 58.6** Algorithm for the treatment of squamous cell carcinoma in transplant patients.

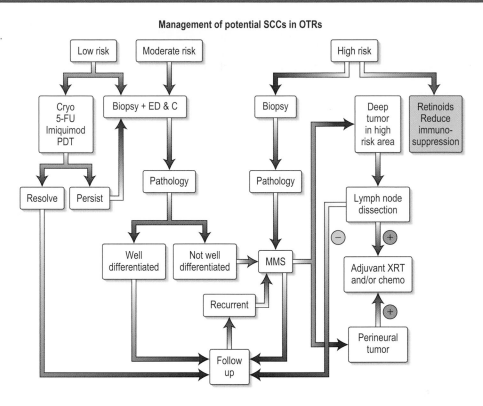

**Management of potential SCCs in OTRs**

Primary prevention of SCC involves daily use of sun protection and regular self and physician examination. Sun avoidance is critical and the routine daily application of an effective sunblock has been shown to reduce the number of keratinocyte malignancies in SOTRs.[39] Monitoring patients at regular intervals is important, as once an SCC has developed, the risk of a subsequent one is 25% during the following year and 50% within 3.5 years. Prior to the development of skin cancer or precancerous lesions, transplant patients should be seen on a yearly basis by a dermatologist. Patients with a history of actinic keratosis or lower-risk NMSC should be seen every 6 months. If they have a history of multiple or high-risk NMSC, then the interval should be shortened to every 3 months. Patients with a history of a rapidly developing, aggressive or metastatic SCC may require even more frequent visits.

Oral retinoids can decrease the development of new tumors in SOTRs, during the treatment period. Side effects of systemic retinoid treatment include mucocutaneous dryness, sticky palms, hypertriglyceridemia, hypercholesterolemia, transaminitis and arthralgias/myalgias (Fig. 58.9). Introducing the retinoid at a low dose, and increasing

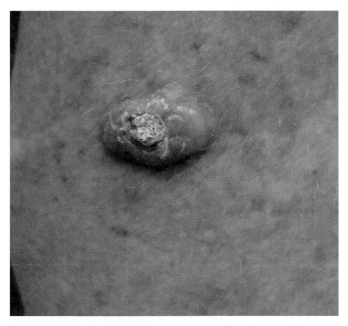

**Figure 58.7** Keratoacanthoma-type squamous cell carcinoma on forearm surrounded by actinically damaged skin.

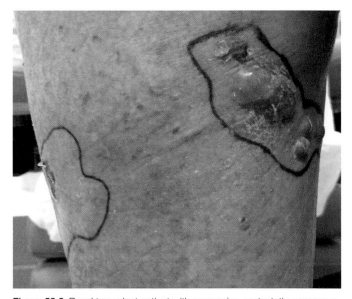

**Figure 58.8** Renal transplant patient with aggressive, metastatic squamous cell carcinoma requiring alteration of immunosuppression and systemic chemotherapy.

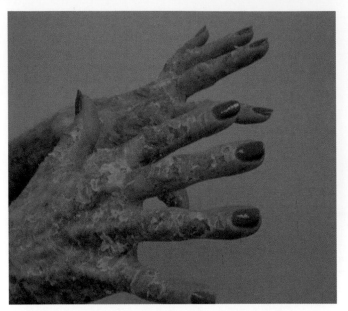

**Figure 58.9** Diffuse xerosis secondary to acitretin use. Dosage was decreased and side effect resolved.

the dosage slowly, may reduce the side effects. The starting dose for acitretin is 10 mg/day, with a target dose between 20 and 25 mg/day. Treatment of women of childbearing potential should generally be avoided, as retinoids are known teratogens. If the benefits of therapy are considered to outweigh the risks, for acitretin, two negative pregnancy tests are required prior to starting treatment and two forms of contraception are required during therapy and for 3 years post treatment.

## Basal cell carcinoma

Basal cell carcinoma (BCC) is the most common form of skin cancer in the general population, but is second to SCC in frequency in the transplant population. SOTRs have an approximately 10-fold increased risk for developing BCC. A history of pre-transplant NMSC is a strong risk factor for post-transplant BCC.[40] The incidence of BCC in Australian renal transplant patients was 21.5% at 5 years, 39.1% at 10 years, 56.2% at 20 years, and 64.3% at greater than 20 years from transplant.[11] Unlike SCC, BCCs in transplant patients are histologically similar to tumors in the general population.[34] There are no specific treatment guidelines for transplant patients. The treatment of BCC depends upon the histological features and location of the tumor. Superficial BCC can be treated with electrodesiccation and curettage, cryosurgery, or a topical immunological modifier (imiquimod).[41] Superficial BCCs located in anatomically sensitive locations may require micrographic surgery for margin control. Infiltrative and nodular BCCs can be treated with surgical excision with or without micrographic margin control as determined by the anatomical location. Case reports and retrospective reviews have shown success of photodynamic therapy with methyl-aminolevulinate (MAL) for superficial and nodular BCCs in the general and transplant populations.[42,43]

## Melanoma

Immunosuppression has not been clearly defined as a risk factor in melanoma. Some studies in the transplant

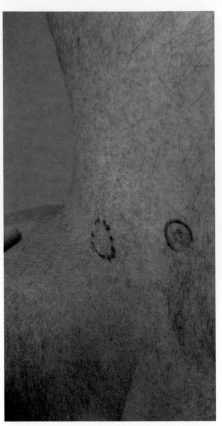

**Figure 58.10** Transplant patient with a history of NMSC presented with melanoma with subcutaneous metastasis.

population have suggested a two- to threefold increased incidence in melanoma, while others have shown no relevant risk. Renal transplant patients have the highest risk of developing melanoma, with the increased risk being between six to eight times that of the general population.[3,44] Transplant organ recipients with a previous history of NMSC have an increased risk of developing melanoma (Fig. 58.10). The incidence of melanoma in African American renal transplant recipients has been reported to be 17.2 times higher than in African Americans in the general population.[45] Histological examination of melanomas arising from nevi in renal transplant patients has shown a scarce tumor inflammatory infiltrate.[44]

Special considerations in the transplant population include patients with a history of melanoma prior to transplant and individuals who received melanoma through transplantation. Patients with a recurrence of melanoma post transplant have a poor prognosis.[46] In a study of 31 SOTRs with a history of melanoma, six patients had a recurrence post transplant. On average, the transplant was 2 years following melanoma treatment. All six patients died from metastatic melanoma, at a mean time of 16 months from recurrence. Melanoma that is obtained through transplantation is highly aggressive. A case series of melanoma transplanted patients had a very poor outcome, with 13 of 21 dying from the disease.[46] Cadaveric donors with death attributed to cerebrovascular accident or a primary brain tumor were responsible for most cases of transmitted melanoma.

In general, transplant patients with thin melanomas (Breslow depth <0.75 mm) have prognosis similar to that of their immunocompetent counterparts.[47,48] The largest study of post-transplant melanoma patients examined the outcome of 177 patients, but had Breslow depths for only 42 cases. Twelve of 29 patients with Breslow depth >0.76 mm died of melanoma. Lymph node metastasis occurred in 20% of patients.[46]

Transplant patients with melanomas less than 0.75 mm in Breslow depth are treated with wide local excision similiar to their immunocompetent counterparts. As the Breslow depth increases, the appropriate management becomes less certain. SLN biopsy is suggested for patients with a Breslow depth greater than 1 mm, but there are no data in the immunocompromised population showing that this changes overall outcome and survival. Further lymph node evaluation and treatment should be considered if SLN biopsy is positive. Adjustments to the immunosuppression regimen should be addressed with the transplant team at all stages of melanoma. In stage IV melanoma and cases of melanoma received during transplant, immunosuppression should be decreased if possible.[49] In cases of melanoma received at transplantation, it is controversial if removal of the transplanted organ will result in a definite cure of the melanoma. A few renal transplant patients with donor-transmitted melanoma have benefited from removal of the allograft followed by immune-mediated treatment of the melanoma.[50] Further studies examining outcomes in transplant patients are necessary in order to establish guidelines of treatment.

## Merkel cell carcinoma

Merkel cell carcinoma (MCC) is a highly aggressive skin cancer with a propensity for early metastasis and local recurrence (Fig. 58.11) (see Chapter 17). Risk factors for the development of MCC include age, sun exposure, history of previous skin cancer, and immune compromised status. Data from the Cincinnati Transplant Registry showed that the ratio of melanoma to MCC was 65 to 1 in the immunocompetent population and 6 to 1 in the transplant population.[51] On average, MCC presented 91 months post transplant.[51] Transplant patients presented with aggressive disease, with 70% developing metastasis and 50% dying from the disease.[51] The increased risk in the immunocompromised

population may be due to decreased immune surveillance or a possible infectious etiology. A new human polyomavirus, named Merkel cell polyomavirus (MCPyV), was discovered when viral DNA was found to be integrated into the tumor chromosomal DNA in 70–80% cases of MCC.[52] Further research efforts have focused on better understanding the effect of the MCPyV in the incidence and outcomes of MCC patients.

The guidelines for the treatment of MCC are evolving. There are no specific recommendations for immunocompromised patients. Wide local excision of the cancer is ideal, but can be difficult in certain anatomic locations. Mohs micrographic surgery has shown high cure rates in immunocompetent patients.[53] Following surgical excision, adjuvant radiation is recommended to the primary site with 3–5 cm margins. If there is no clinically evident lymph node involvement, sentinel lymph node evaluation may be considered. In tumors associated with clinically positive lymph nodes or sentinel node-positive disease, further evaluation of the lymph node basin should be performed. Local and regional diseases are not usually treated with chemotherapy, but disseminated disease requires oncology consultation and evaluation for systemic chemotherapy. Close monitoring and follow-up of these patients is important.

## Kaposi sarcoma

Kaposi sarcoma (KS) is a tumor of endothelial cell origin thought to develop as a response to infection with human herpesvirus-8 (HHV-8). Solid organ transplant-related KS usually presents with involvement of the lower legs but can have other sites involved, including the mucosa.[54] There are numerous treatments for KS, but in all cases reconstitution of the immune system is beneficial. Mitigation of immunosuppression in transplant patients has been associated with resolution of skin lesions. Renal transplant patients whose medication was changed from cyclosporin to sirolimus had clinical regression.[55] If the KS becomes life threatening, discontinuation of immunosuppression and treatment with systemic chemotherapy may be indicated. Localized disease can be treated with cryotherapy, laser surgery, excision, imiquimod, radiation therapy, topical retinoids and intralesional chemotherapy (see Chapter 16).

## HUMAN IMMUNODEFICIENCY VIRUS/ACQUIRED IMMUNODEFICIENCY DISEASE

HIV-infected patients have impaired cellular immunity including a deficiency of CD4+ T lymphocytes, cutaneous anergy and defective cytotoxic T-lymphocyte function. A compromised immune system makes patients more susceptible to virally associated neoplasms, including HHV-8-associated KS and HPV-associated cancers (see Chapter 19).[56] As the patient's CD4 count declines, these virally associated cancers present. Persons with AIDS have a three- to fivefold increased risk of developing an NMSC.[57] Neoplasms in HIV-positive patients are characterized by aggressive clinical behavior with high-grade lesions, more advanced stage, and a shortened survival when compared to those that develop in HIV-negative persons.[56,58] The mechanism underlying the aggressive nature of these tumors has not been determined.

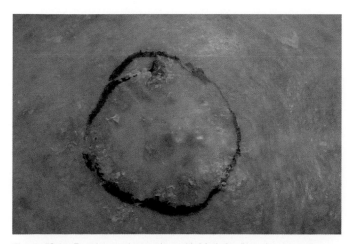

**Figure 58.11** Renal transplant patient with Merkel cell carcinoma on the scalp presenting 3 years following renal transplantation.

Risk factors for the development of NMSC in HIV patients recapitulate those in the general population: fair skin, sun exposure, and a family history of skin cancer. SCC can present following infection with high-risk HPV strains or independent of viral infection. The association between HPV-induced dysplasia and subsequent carcinoma has been established in cervical, genital, anal and oropharyngeal cancers. SCC of the nail unit can also be related to prior HPV infection. SCCs that present outside of these clinical scenarios are much less likely to be HPV associated. Independent of CD4 count, SCC can present more aggressively and at a significantly younger age. The ratio of SCC to BCC is 1:7 in HIV/AIDS patients, similar to that in the general population.[59] Superficial BCC is the most common subtype and the most common location is on the back.

HIV/AIDS patients have an increased incidence of non-keratinocyte-derived cutaneous neoplasms. Data from the US AIDS registry revealed that AIDS patients had an increased risk of melanoma, Merkel cell carcinoma, and sebaceous carcinoma. The increased risk of melanoma was minimal (SIR=1.3) as compared to MCC (SIR=11) and sebaceous carcinoma (SIR= 4.2). Those with the highest incidence of melanoma in the AIDS population were white homosexual men with a history of significant UVR exposure. CD4 count at the time of diagnosis was not associated with the development of melanoma. The total numbers of cases of MCC and sebaceous carcinoma were too small to establish a relationship between CD4 count and the onset of the neoplasms.[60,61]

KS can present with cutaneous and systemic involvement in HIV/AIDS patients. Clinical presentations include non-healing, violaceous plaques and nodules on the head, neck and extremities. Homosexual and bisexual men are disproportionately affected with the neoplasm. The disease is directly related to CD4 count, with more systemic involvement in lymphopenic patients. Treatment options, as discussed previously, include cryotherapy, radiation or excision for local disease. More systemic disease may require chemotherapy. Reconstitution of the immune system with highly active antiretroviral therapy treatment (HAART) has been shown to decrease the burden of the disease and in many cases has been curative.

Since the introduction of HAART, the incidence of cancer in the HIV/AIDS population has decreased overall. Comparison of cancer incidence in Australian AIDS patients during the early (1996–1999) and late (2000–2004) HAART periods with that prior to HAART (1982–1995) showed that the incidence of KS and melanoma decreased significantly.[57] Disappointingly, the incidence of anal cancer was unchanged. Why retroviral therapy and presumed immune reconstitution have an effect on some cancers but not all HIV-associated neoplasms is unclear.

When evaluating an HIV/AIDS patient, there should be high clinical suspicion of a non-healing lesion. Regular skin examinations by the patient and healthcare provider are essential. Patients should be counseled on the signs of skin cancer and the importance of sun protection.

There are no specific guidelines for the treatment of skin cancer in the HIV/AIDS population and the algorithms created for the general population can generally be applied. Case reports and series have shown imiquimod's success in the treatment of HPV and anal intraepithelial neoplasia in HIV/AIDS patients. Despite being immunocompromised, HIV/AIDS patients have sufficient innate immunity to respond to treatment. The burden of verrucae should be decreased in HIV/AIDS patients due to the association with SCC. HPV-associated SCC may be treated with imiquimod prior to surgery, to decrease the size of the tumor in anatomically sensitive sites. Ultimately, excision with adequate margins is the best treatment for SCC. BCC can be treated with electrodesiccation and curettage or excision, depending upon the histological features of the tumor and the anatomical location. Patients with melanoma in situ have outcomes similar to their immunocompetent counterparts. Excision with standard surgical margins is the standard of care. For more invasive melanoma, some physicians have recommended a more extensive search for metastatic disease due to melanoma's more aggressive course in HIV-infected patients.[59] The use of sentinel node biopsy in HIV patients with melanomas with a Breslow depth <0.75 mm is controversial. Ultimately, the standard of care guidelines should determine the surgical margins for re-excision and the evaluation for metastasis.[61] HAART has been shown beneficial in decreasing the incidence of melanoma.[57] In those patients not already on HAART, a referral to an infectious disease physician should be considered.

## FUTURE OUTLOOK

Advances in medical therapies have allowed for increased longevity in both solid organ transplant recipients and HIV/AIDS patients. The increased life expectancy in these two groups will lead to a greater incidence of skin cancer. Education and early detection are at the cornerstone of prevention and treatment. Physicians should begin counseling potential transplant candidates on the importance of daily protection of their skin prior to transplantation. Immunosuppressed patients need to practice a regimen of daily sunblock and protective clothing. In patients practicing strict sun avoidance, supplemental vitamin D may be necessary. The increasing numbers of SOTR and HIV/AIDS patients may allow for larger clinical studies to establish guidelines of care for this at-risk population.

## REFERENCES

1. Loose D, Van der Wiele C. The immune system and cancer. *Cancer Biother Radiopharm.* 2009;24(3):369–376.
2. Vajdic C, van Leeuwen MT. What types of cancers are associated with immune suppression in HIV? Lessons from solid organ transplant recipients. *Curr Opin HIV AIDS.* 2009;4(1):35–41.
3. Moloney FJ Comber H, O'Lorcain P, et al. A population-based study of skin cancer incidence and prevalence in renal transplant recipients. *Br J Dermatol.* 2006;154:498–504.
4. United States, Department of Health and Human Services. Organ Procurement and Transplantation Network. Patient survival rates by transplant. 2009 OPTN / SRTR Annual Report: Transplant Data 1999-2008.
5. Sheil AG, Disney AP, Mathew TH, et al. De novo malignancy emerges as a major cause of morbidity and late failure in renal transplantation. *Transplant Proc.* 1993;25:1383–1384.
6. Vajdic C, van Leeuwen MT. Cancer incidence and risk factors after solid organ transplantation. *Int J Cancer.* 2009;125:1747–1754.
7. Berg D, Otley CC. Skin cancer in organ transplant recipients: epidemiology, pathogenesis, and management. *J Am Acad Dermatol.* 2002;47:1–17.
8. Euvrard S, Kanitakis J, Claudy A. Skin cancers after organ transplantation. *N Engl J Med.* 2003;348:1681–1691.
9. Lampros TD, Cobanoglu A, Parker F, et al. Squamous and basal cell carcinoma in heart transplant recipients. *J Heart Lung Transplant.* 1998;17:586–591.

10. Caforio A, Fortina AB, Piaserico S, et al. Skin cancer in heart transplant recipients: risk factor analysis and relevance of immunosuppressive therapy. *Circulation.* 2000;102(suppl):III 222–III 227.

11. Ramsay HM, Fryer AA, Hawley CM, et al. Factors associated with nonmelanoma skin cancer following renal transplantation in Queensland. Australia. *J Am Acad Dermatol.* 2003;49:397–406.

12. Moosa MR, Gralla J. Skin cancer in renal allograft recipients – experience in different ethnic groups residing in the same geographical region. *Clin Transplant.* 2005;19:735–741.

13. Mithoefer AB, Supran S, Freeman RB. Risk factors associated with the development of skin cancer after liver transplantation. *Liver Transplantation.* 2002;8:939–944.

14. Kelly GE, Meikle W, Sheil AG. Effects of immunosuppressive therapy on the induction of skin tumors by ultraviolet irradiation in hairless mice. *Transplantation.* 1987;44:429–434.

15. Glover MT, Deeks JJ, Raftery MJ, et al. Immunosuppression and risk of non-melanoma skin cancer in renal transplant recipients. *Lancet.* 1997;349:398.

16. Ducloux D, Pellet E, Fournier V, et al. CD4 lymphocytopenia in long-term renal transplant recipients. *Transplant Proc.* 1998;30:2859–2860.

17. Jensen P, Hansen S, Moller B, et al. Skin cancer in kidney and heart transplant recipients and different long-term immunosuppressive therapy regimens. *J Am Acad Dermatol.* 1999;40:177–186.

18. Vajdic CM, McDonald SP, McCredie MR, et al. Cancer incidence before and after kidney transplantation. *JAMA.* 2006;296:2823–2831.

19. van Leeuwen MT, Grulich AE, McDonald SP, et al. Immunosuppression and other risk factors for lip cancer after kidney transplantation. *Cancer Epidemiol Biomarkers Prev.* 2009;18:561–569.

20. Taylor AE, Shuster S. Skin cancer after renal transplantation: the causal role of azathioprine. *Acta Derm Venereol.* 1992;72:115–119.

21. Yarosh DB, Pena AV, Nay SL, et al. Calcineurin inhibitors decrease DNA repair and apoptosis in human keratinocytes following ultraviolet B irradiation. *J Invest Dermatol.* 2005;125(5):1020–1025.

22. Hojo M, Morimoto T, Maluccio M, et al. Cyclosporine induces cancer progression be a cell-autonomous mechanism. *Nature.* 1999;397(6719):530–534.

23. Takahashi T, Kamimura A. Cyclosporin A promotes hair epithelial proliferation and modulates protein kinase C expression and translocation in hair epithelial cells. *J Invest Dermatol.* 2001;117(3):605–611.

24. Karashima T, Hachisuka H, Sasai Y. FK506 and cyclosporin A inhibit growth factor stimulated hair keratinocyte proliferation by blocking G0/G1 phases of cell cycle. *J Dermatol Sci.* 1996;12(3):246–254.

25. Dantal J, Hourmant M, Cantarovich D, et al. Effect of long term immunosuppression in kidney-graft recipients on cancer incidence: randomized comparison of two cyclosporine regimens. *Lancet.* 1998;(351):623–628.

26. Kauffman HM, Cherikh WS, Cheng Y, et al. Maintenance immunosuppression with target of rapamycin inhibitors is associated with a reduced incidence of de novo malignancies. *Transplantation.* 2005;80:883–889.

27. Schena FP, Pascoe MD, Alberu J, et al. Conversion from calcineurin inhibitors to sirolimus maintenance therapy in renal allograft recipients: 24-month efficacy and safety results from the CONVERT trial. *Transplantation.* 2009;87(2):233–242.

28. Boxman IL, Berkhout RJ, Mulder LH, et al. Detection of human papillomavirus DNA in plucked hairs from renal transplant recipients and healthy volunteers. *J Invest Dermatol.* 1997;108:712–715.

29. Lindelof B, Sigurgeirsson B, Gabel H, et al. Incidence of skin cancer in 5356 patients following organ transplantation. *Br J Dermatol.* 2000;143:513–519.

30. Martinez JC, Otley CC, Stasko T, et al. Defining the clinical course of metastatic skin cancer in organ transplant recipients: a multicenter collaborative study. *Arch Dermatol.* 2003;139:301–306.

31. Carucci JA, Martinez JC, Zeitouni NC, et al. In-transit metastasis from primary cutaneous squamous cell carcinoma in organ transplant recipients and non-immunosuppressed patients: clinical characteristics, management, and outcome in a series of 21 patients. *Dermatol Surg.* 2004;30:651–655.

32. Rowe DE, Carroll RJ, Day CL. Prognostic factors for local recurrence, metastasis, and survival rates in squamous cell carcinoma of the skin, ear, and lip. Implications for treatment modality selection. *J Am Acad Dermatol.* 1992;26:976–990.

33. Miller SJ. The National Comprehensive Cancer Network guidelines of care for non-melanoma skin cancer. *Dermatol Surg.* 2000;26:289–292.

34. Harwood CA, Proby CM, McGregor JM, et al. Clinicopathologic features of skin cancer in organ transplant recipients: a retrospective case-control series. *J Am Acad Dermatol.* 2006;54(2):290–300.

35. Stasko T, Brown MD, Carucci JA, et al. Guidelines for the management of squamous cell carcinoma in organ transplant recipients. *Dermatol Surg.* 2004;30:642–650.

36. Ulrich C, Bichel J, BJ, Euvrard S, et al. Topical immunomodulation under systemic immunosuppression: results of a multicentre, randomized, placebo controlled safety and efficacy study of imiquimod 5% cream for the treatment of actinic keratoses in kidney, heart and liver transplant patients. *Br J Dermatol.* 2007;157:25–31.

37. De Graaf YG, Euvrared S, Bouwes Bavnick JN. Systemic and topical retinoids in the management of skin cancer in organ transplant recipients. *Dermatol Surg.* 2004;30:656–661.

38. Dragieva G, Prinz BM, Hafner J, et al. A randomized controlled clinical trial of topical photodynamic therapy with methyl aminolaevulinate in the treatment of actinic keratosis in transplant recipients. *Br J Dermatol.* 2004;151:196–200.

39. Ulrich C, Jurgensen JS, Degen A, et al. Prevention of non-melanoma skin cancer in organ transplant patients by regular use of a sunscreen: a 24 months, prospective, case-control study. *Br J Dermatol.* 2009;161(suppl 3):78–84.

40. Ramsay HM, Fryer AA, Hawley CM, et al. Non-melanoma skin cancer risk in the Queensland renal transplant population. *Br J Dermatol.* 2002;147:950–956.

41. Karve SJ, Feldman SR, Yentzer BA, et al. Imiquimod: a review of basal cell carcinoma treatments. *J Drugs Dermatol.* 2008;7(11):1044–1051.

42. Fai D, Arpaia N, Romano I, et al. Methyl-aminolevulinate photodynamic therapy for the treatment of actinic keratosis and non-melanoma skin cancer: a retrospective analysis of response in 462 patients. *G Ital Dermatol Venereol.* 2009;144(3):281–285.

43. Shokrollahi K, Marsden NJ, Whitaker IS, et al. Basal cell carcinoma treated successfully with combined CO2 laser and photodynamic therapy in a renal transplant patient: a case report. *Cases J.* 2009;11:7920.

44. Le Mire L, Hollowood K, Gray D, et al. Melanomas in renal transplant recipients. *Br J Dermatol.* 2006;154(3):472–477.

45. Hollenbeak CS, Todd MM, Billingsley EM, et al. Increased incidence of melanoma in renal transplantation recipients. *Cancer.* 2005;104(9):1962–1967.

46. Penn I. Malignant melanoma in organ allograft recipients. *Transplantation.* 1996;61:274–278.

47. Greene MH, Young TI, Clark Jr WH. Malignant melanoma in renal transplant recipients. *Lancet.* 1981;8231:1196–1199.

48. Leveque L, Dalac S, Dompmartin A, et al. Melanoma in organ transplant patients. *Ann Dermatol Venereol.* 2000;127(2):160–165.

49. Dapprich DC, Weenig RH, Rohlinger AL, et al. Outcomes of melanoma in recipients of solid organ transplant. *J Am Acad Dermatol.* 2008;59:405–417.

50. Sheil AG. Donor-derived malignancy in organ transplant recipients. *Transplant Proc.* 2001;33:1827–1829.

51. Penn I, First MR. Merkel's cell carcinoma in organ recipients: report of 41 cases. *Transplantation.* 1999;68:1717–1721.

52. Feng H, Shuda M, Chang Y, et al. Clonal integration of a polyomavirus in human Merkel cell carcinoma. *Science.* 2008;319:1096–1100.

53. Gollard R, Weber R, Kosty MP, et al. Merkel cell carcinoma: review of 22 cases with surgical, pathologic and therapeutic considerations. *Cancer.* 2000;88:1842–1851.

54. Zafar SY, Howell DN, Gockerman JP. Malignancy after solid organ transplantation: an overview. *Oncologist.* 2008;13:769–778.

55. Stallone G, Schena A, Infante B, et al. Sirolimus for Kaposi's sarcoma in renal-transplant recipients. *NEJM.* 2005;352(13):1317–1323.

56. Remick SC. Non-AIDS defining cancers. *Hematol Oncol Clin North Am.* 1996;10:1203–1213.

57. Van Leeuwen MT, Vajdic CM, Middleton MG, et al. Continuing declines in some but not all HIV-associated cancers in Australia after widespread use of antiretroviral therapy. *AIDS.* 2009;23(16):183–190.

58. Nguyen P, Vin-Christian K, Ming ME, et al. Aggressive squamous cell carcinomas in persons infected with the human immunodeficiency virus. *Arch Dermatol.* 2002;138:758–763.

59. Wilkins K, Turner R, Dolev J, et al. Cutaneous malignancy and human immunodeficiency virus disease. *J Am Acad Dermatol.* 2004;54(2):189–206.

60. Lanoy E, Dores GM, Madclcine MM, et al. Epidemiology of nonkeratinocytic skin cancers among persons with AIDS in the United States. *AIDS.* 2009;23:385–393.

61. Engels EA, Frisch M, Goedert JJ, et al. Merkel cell carcinoma and HIV infection. *Lancet.* 2002;359:497–498.

62. Coit DG, Andtbacka R, Bichakjian CK, et al. Melanoma. *J Natl Compr Canc Netw.* 2009;7:250–275.

63. van Zuuren EJ, Posma AN, Scholtens RE, et al. Resurfacing of the back of the hand as treatment and prevention of multiple skin cancers in kidney transplant recipients. *J Am Acad Dermatol.* 1994;31(5 Pt 1):760–764.

**643**

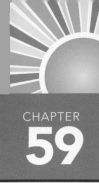

CHAPTER
59

# Indoor Tanning

*James M. Spencer and Darrell S. Rigel*

## Key Points

- Indoor tanning is a US$5 billion a year industry, utilized daily by 1 million Americans.
- It is increasing in popularity.
- Indoor tanning utilizes bulbs that contain UVB amounts similar to the sun and UVA content several multiples higher.
- It is convincingly linked to the development of skin cancer and photoaging.

## INTRODUCTION

The development of indoor tanning over the last 20 years has allowed the public to receive ever greater doses of ultraviolet (UV) radiation, all with the sole purpose of cosmetic tanning. The use of indoor tanning is increasing. At the same time, the incidence of skin cancer has reached epidemic proportions. It is quite likely that the popularity of indoor tanning plays a role in this epidemic and will continue to do so in the future.

## HISTORY OF INTENTIONAL TANNING

During the nineteenth century, fair-skinned populations (particularly those of upper socioeconomic classes) avoided excessive sun exposure.[1] The link between sun exposure and skin cancer was not yet appreciated but the cosmetic results of UV exposure were. Sunburn, suntan, and photoaging were to be avoided. The poor cosmetic outcome of excessive UV exposure was appreciated and acted upon. Sun-protective clothing with broad-brimmed hats and parasols was the norm.

By the end of the nineteenth century, a change in attitudes about tanning began to emerge. This change was driven by the changing status of women and emerging medical information about UV light. First, the status of women improved and offered greater choices in life, including being able to engage in a number of activities that resulted in greater UV exposure. More importantly, medical information was being disseminated that supported the idea of the health benefits of UV radiation. At the beginning of the twentieth century, Neils Finsen received the Nobel prize for reporting the successful use of UV radiation for the treatment of cutaneous tuberculosis.[2] This led to the notion that UV light could treat or even prevent infectious disease, as well as be helpful for a host of medical conditions as diverse as rheumatic diseases, gout, renal disease, diabetes, obesity and respiratory afflictions.[1]

In the 1920s, it was appreciated that UV light stimulated vitamin D production in the skin and thus was both therapeutic and preventative for rickets.[3] These observations led to the widely held view that a tan was healthy and to be encouraged. This feeling that a tan 'looks healthy' persists to this day and is often cited by indoor tanners as a reason for attending indoor tanning salons.[4]

The manufacture and sale of UV lamps for health purposes became big business in the 1930s.[5] These were typically carbon arc or quartz mercury vapor lamps with significant UVC emission (Fig. 59.1) and were available for office and home use with purported systemic health benefits. Ocular damage from shorter-wavelength emission was appreciated, so simple glass filters to block wavelengths below 280 nm were advocated by groups such as the American Medical Association (AMA).[6]

However, by the 1940s, the development of antibiotics and other advances in medicine made the use of UV radiation for systemic disease virtually obsolete. At the same time the medical use of UV light was declining, the period following the Second World War saw a dramatic increase in the popularity of tanning for cosmetic purposes. Tanned skin was seen not only as 'healthy' but also as attractive and beautiful.

Since the 1970s, a growing industry has emerged to fill the public's desire for a tan: the indoor tanning salon. UV-emitting lamps are manufactured and sold to salons, spas and health clubs for the purpose of producing a cosmetically desirable tan. The indoor tanning industry estimates that there are currently over 60,000 indoor tanning facilities and 250,000 indoor tanning units in the US. Almost 30 million North Americans go to an indoor tanning facility each year.[7] As the industry developed and enlarged in the 1980s, it was fueled by the claim that indoor tanning bulbs used 'safe' UVA radiation and thus one could tan without any danger. The bulbs used at that time were never 100% UVA but always contained some amount of UVB. The bulbs in current use contain ever-greater amounts of UVB, increasing potential skin cancer risk.

Today, except for dermatologic conditions such as psoriasis, there is little use for UV light in medicine. However, the cosmetic desirability of a tan has been reinforced by the entertainment and advertising industries, where tanned models and actors are deemed both beautiful and desirable. The idea that a tan is 'healthy' has clearly persisted even if the public is not sure why UV exposure would be healthy. The industry is aggressively promoting

## MECHANISMS OF INDOOR TANNING

The ultraviolet spectrum is defined as electromagnetic radiation with a wavelength from 200 to 400 nm. Although there is some variability in the literature, the most commonly used division of the UV spectrum is that of the International Commission of Illumination (IARC, 1992), which divides the UV spectrum into UVC, UVB and UVA. UVC is defined as 100–290 nm. These wavelengths from the sun are filtered by the ozone layer and do not reach the Earth's surface. UVC is still used in germicidal lamps to kill bacteria, and presumably is the portion responsible for the effects reported by Finsen on cutaneous tuberculosis.[2] The shorter the wavelength, the more energetic the radiation. UVB is 290–320 nm, while UVA is 320–400 nm.

Natural sunlight reaching the Earth's surface contains both UVB and UVA, with the amount of UVA far exceeding that of UVB. The amount of UVA that reaches the Earth's surface is fairly constant, while the amount of UVB is quite variable, depending on such factors as the latitude, the season of the year, the time of day, air pollution, and cloud cover. Nonetheless, natural sunlight most often contains 95% UVA and 5% UVB. Despite being only around 5% of UV radiation, UVB is of shorter wavelength and thus more energetic. For many biologic phenomena, UVB plays a greater role than 5% would suggest.

The action spectrum for tanning has essentially the same shape as the action spectrum for erythema (sunburn) and for the development of squamous cell carcinoma (SCC) in animals: very high in the UVC range then falling through the UVB range to reach a low level in the UVA range (Fig. 59.2). Indoor tanning bulbs utilized in the 1980s were often advertised as 'UVA only' and thus 'safer'. During that time, no bulb was 100% UVA and therefore there was always some amount of UVB.[9] The goal of indoor tanning is to produce a tan and this led to the addition of UVB back into the bulbs. Since UVB is more efficient at inducing a tan, current bulbs typically have a UVB content approximating that of natural sunlight.

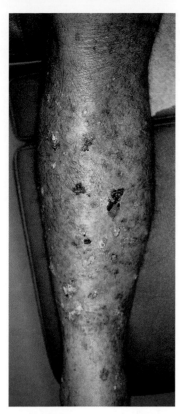

**Figure 59.1** The leg of a patient who built his own carbon arc UV lamp for indoor tanning as a teenager in the 1940s. He used the lamp to tan himself and charged his friends for the same use. He is now literally covered with skin cancers, as is shown on his leg.

indoor tanning as not only safe but actually healthy in a systemic way, much like the claims from 100 years ago. A recent study examining advertising techniques utilized by the indoor tanning industry shows a marked similarity to the tactics used to advertise cigarettes, with a conscious effort to mitigate health concerns while appealing to social acceptance and positive psychotrophoic effects.[8]

**Figure 59.2** The action spectrum for the production of erythema (sunburn) and delayed pigmentation (tanning). MES, Minimum Erythrogenic Stimulus; MED, Minimal Erythema Dose; MMD, Minimum Melanogenic Dose. (From Parrish JA. Erythema and melanogenesis action spectra of normal human skin. *Photochem Photobiol.* 1982;36:187-191. © Allen Press, Inc.)

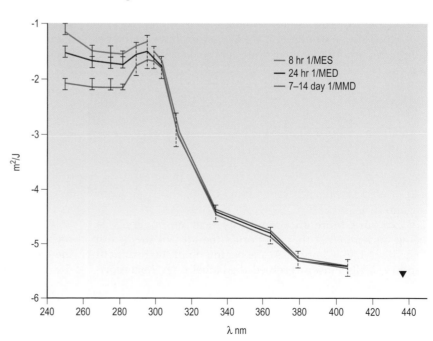

The Quebec Joint Committee of the Ministère de la Santé[10] measured UVA and UVB output from various tanning beds used in tanning salons. UVB output was found to be in the range of 1.1–5.0 W/m², while the sun at its zenith gives off 1.0–2.2 W/m². In contrast, the UVA output from the various models ranged from 150 to 200 W/m², while natural sunlight in Quebec ranges from 46 to 68 W/m². Thus, indoor tanners were receiving UVB doses equivalent to the sun and UVA doses about four times higher than the sun. Similarly, it was found that the most popular indoor tanning bulbs in Switzerland emitted UVB in amounts similar to the sun there, while UVA emission is 10 to 15 times higher than that of the sun.[11] Currently, most bulbs seem to emit UVB ranges similar to natural sunlight with greatly enhanced emissions of UVA.

Thus, the wavelengths that most efficiently induce a tan also induce a burn and may also induce skin cancer. UVA alone can induce a burn or a skin cancer in animals, but much higher doses are required to do so. Today's bulbs contain the same amount of UVB as natural sunlight, and with a UVA content 4–15 times higher. Therefore, tanning salon customers may receive the amount of UVB exposure equal to what would have been received at the beach and several times more UVA exposure.

## EFFECTS OF INDOOR TANNING

The first and most obvious effect of indoor tanning is the development of increased cutaneous melanin, a tan. The preference for tanning was more important in users' decisions to intentionally tan than their perceived risk of developing melanoma, and this finding was consistent among respondents from different countries.[12]

The exact mechanism by which UV radiation causes increased melanin production is being elucidated. Studies have shown that addition of thymidine dinucleotides to cell culture and guinea pig skin can induce melanin production.[13,14] Thymidine dinucleotides mimic UV-induced DNA damage and thus the signal to produce a tan may be DNA damage and the ensuing repair process. This clearly demonstrates that there is no such thing as a safe tan: DNA damage is a prerequisite for tanning.

Acute adverse events of UV exposure include erythema (sunburn), phototoxic reactions, photoallergic reactions, photosensitive disease exacerbation, and corneal burns. The avoidance of these acute complications is something everyone can agree on. It is equally clear that acute adverse events occur with some regularity. A survey of 203 indoor tanners in Quebec showed 26.1% experienced one or more acute adverse events.[10] The survey showed 17.7% had sunburn, 14.8% reported skin dryness, 3% reported ocular burning or itching, and 1.5% reported nausea. Similarly, Rivers et al.[15] reported that 22% of experimental volunteers receiving indoor tanning developed sunburn, 27% had itching, 15% had dry skin, and 4% had nausea.

There is very little regulation of indoor tanning salons, so there is great variability in operator safety. The manufacturers of indoor tanning equipment are regulated at the federal level by the FDA (who at the time of writing of this chapter is considering limitations/bans on usage of tanning beds by minors). Operators of tanning salons are regulated at the state level. Some states have stringent safety regulations while others have minimal to no requirements and little enforcement. Bulb fluence regulations and equipment hygiene are often also not followed. In a survey of indoor tanning salons in New York City, cultures taken from the tanning beds where clients would lie showed that 10 out of 10 salons tested grew pathogens.[16] Other safety standards are often minimally applied or ignored altogether. A survey of ophthalmologists in Wisconsin showed that over a 1-year period, 152 patients were seen for eye burns caused by indoor tanning equipment.[17]

The chronic effects of indoor tanning are of much greater concern. Since the point of indoor tanning is cosmetic enhancement, it is ironic that the long-term effect may be photoaging, which leads to wrinkled, leathery, discolored skin (Fig. 59.3). Human skin exposed to suberythemogenic doses of UVA daily for only 1 month demonstrated many of the histologic changes characteristic of photoaging.[18]

The tanning industry mentions a sense of well-being indoor tanners develop as a benefit of indoor tanning. Seasonal affective disorder (SAD) is a recognized emotional state thought to result from prolonged lack of visible light. However, there is no evidence UV light is effective for SAD. A postulated mechanism for a psychologic effect of UV light in tanners is an elevation in circulating endogenous opioid peptides, which may produce pleasure.[19]

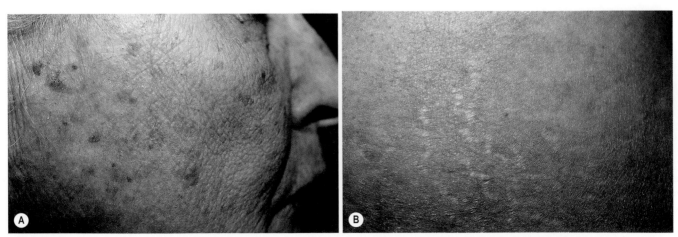

Figure 59.3 **A)** The cheek of an 83-year-old woman showing the changes of photoaging. **B)** The photoprotected buttock cheek of the same woman, showing only the mild changes of intrinsic aging.

real. However, given current market trends, the industry may not need this marketing tool. In a survey of undergraduate and graduate students at a major midwestern university, 47% of students had used indoor tanning equipment in the last 12 months.[38] An extraordinary finding of this survey was that more than 90% of these students were aware that premature aging of the skin and skin cancer were possible complications of indoor tanning.

Young people continue to value a tanned look as desirable and this desire seems to outweigh dangers to their health. As long as tanned skin is perceived as healthy and beautiful, we will probably conintue to see an increase in indoor tanning and a related increase in the development of associated skin cancer.

## REFERENCES

1. Albert MR, Ostheimer KG. The evolution of current medical and popular attitudes toward ultraviolet light exposure: part I. *J Am Acad Dermatol*. 2002;47:930–937.
2. Finsen NR. *Phototherapy*. London: Edward Arnold; 1901.
3. Hess AF, Weinstock M. A study of light waves in their relation to rickets. *JAMA*. 1923;80:687–690.
4. Mawn VB, Fleischer Jr AB. A survey of attitudes, beliefs, and behavior regarding tanning bed use, sunbathing, and sunscreen use. *J Am Acad Dermatol*. 1993;29:959–962.
5. Albert MR, Ostheimer KG. The evolution of current medical and popular attitudes toward ultraviolet light exposure: part II. *J Am Acad Dermatol*. 2003;48(6):909–918.
6. Dr. Spencer. Acceptance of sunlamps. *JAMA*. 1933;100:1863–1864.
7. Humiston D. *Speech. Indoor Tanning Association President*. 2002. Online. Available from: www.tanningtruth.com.
8. Greeman J, Jones DA. Comparision of advertising strategies between the indoor tan and tobacco industries. *J Am Acad Dermatol*. 2010;62(4):685. e1–685.e18.
9. Spencer JM, Amonette RA. Indoor tanning: risks, benefits, and future trends. *J Am Acad Dermatol*. 1995;33(2):288–298.
10. Joint Committee on Exposure to Ultraviolet Rays. *Artificial tanning in Quebec, Government du Quebec, Ministère de la Santé et des Services Sociaux*. Joint Committee on Exposure to Ultraviolet Rays; 1999.
11. Gerber B, Mathys P, Moser M, et al. Ultraviolet emission spectra of sunbeds. *Photochem Photobiol*. 2002;76:664–668.
12. Bränström R, Chang YM, Kasparian N, et al. Melanoma risk factors, perceived threat and intentional tanning: an international online survey. *Eur J Cancer Prev*. 2010;19(3):216–226.
13. Gilchrest BA, Zhai S, Eller MS, et al. Treatment of human melanocytes and S91 melanoma cells with the DNA repair enzyme TV endonuclease enhances melanogenesis after UV irradiation. *J Invest Dermatol*. 1993;101:666–700.
14. Eller MS, Yaar M, Gilchrest BA. DNA damage and melanogenesis. *Nature*. 1994;372:413–416.
15. Rivers JK, Norris PG, Murphy GM, et al. UVA sunbeds: tanning, photoprotection, acute adverse effects, and immunologic changes. *Br J Dermatol*. 1989;120:767–777.
16. Russak JE, Rigel DS. Tanning bed hygiene: microbes found on tanning beds present a potential health risk. *J Am Acad Dermatol*. 2010;62(1):155–157.
17. Leads from the MMWR. Injuries associated with ultraviolet tanning devices. *JAMA*. 1989;261:3519–3520.
18. Lavker RM, Veres DA, Irwin CJ, et al. Quantitative assessment of cumulative damage from repetitive exposures to suberythemogenic doses of UVA in human skin. *Photochem Photobiol*. 1995;62:348–352.
19. Gambichler T, Bader A, Vojvodic M, et al. Plasma levels of opioid peptides after sunbed exposure. *Br J Dermatol*. 2002;147:1207–1211.
20. Mosher CE, Danoff-Burg S. Addiction to indoor tanning: relation to anxiety, depression, and substance use. *Arch Dermatol*. 2010;146(4):412–417.
21. Feldman SR, Liguori A, Kucenic M, et al. Ultraviolet exposure is a reinforcing stimulus in frequent indoor tanners. *J Am Acad Dermatol*. 2004;51(1):45–51.
22. Whitmore SE, Morison WL, Potten CS, et al. Tanning salon exposure and molecular alterations. *J Am Acad Dermatol*. 2001;44(5):775–780.
23. http://www.iarc.fr/en/publications/pdfs-online/wrk/wrk1/ArtificialUVRad&Skin5.pdf accessed Feb 26 2011.
24. Van Weelden H, de Gruijl FR, van der Putte SCJ, et al. The carcinogenic risk of modern tanning equipment: is UVA safer than UVB? *Arch Dermatol Res*. 1988;280:300–307.
25. Swerdlow AJ, Weinstock MA. Do tanning lamps cause melanoma? An epidemiologic assessment. *J Am Acad Dermatol*. 1998;38(1):89–98.
26. Westerdahl J, Ingvar C, Masback A, et al. Risk of cutaneous melanoma in relation to use of sunbeds: further evidence for UV-A carcinogenicity. *Br J Cancer*. 2000;82(9):1593–1599.
27. Ting W, Schultz K, Cac NN, et al. Tanning bed exposure increases the risk of malignant melanoma. *Int J Dermatol*. 2007;46(12):1253–1257.
28. International Agency for Research on Cancer Working Group on artificial ultraviolet (UV) light and skin cancer. The association of use of sunbeds with cutaneous malignant melanoma and other skin cancers: a systematic review. *Int J Cancer*. 2007;120(5):1116–1122.
29. U.S. Department of Health and Human Services, Public Health Service, National Toxicology Program. *10th Report on Carcinogens*. 2002. http://ntp.niehs.nih.gov/index.cfm?objectid=72016262-BDB7-CEBA-FA60E922B18C2540 accessed feb 26 2011.
30. Diffey BL. A quantitative estimate of melanoma mortality from ultraviolet A sunbed use in the U.K. *Br J Dermatol*. 2003;149(3):578–581.
31. Ezzedine K, Malvy D, Mauger E, et al. Artificial and natural ultraviolet radiation exposure: beliefs and behaviour of 7200 French adults. *J Eur Acad Dermatol Venereol*. 2008;22(2):186–194.
32. Karagas MR, Stannard VA, Mott LA, et al. Use of tanning devices and risk of basal cell and squamous cell skin cancers. *J Natl Cancer Inst*. 2002;94(3):224–226.
33. Hemminki K, Zhang H, Czene K. Time trends and familial risks in squamous cell carcinoma of the skin. *Arch Dermatol*. 2003;139:885–889.
34. Sollitto RB, Kraemer KH, DiGiovanna JJ. Normal vitamin D levels can be maintained despite rigorous photoprotection: six years' experience with xeroderma pigmentosum. *J Am Acad Dermatol*. 1997;37(6):942–947.
35. Marks R, Foley PA, Jolley D, et al. The effects of regular sunscreen use on vitamin D levels in an Australian population. Results of a randomized controlled trial. *Arch Dermatol*. 1995;131(4):415–421.
36. Garland CG, Gorham ED, Mohr SB, et al. Vitamin D for cancer prevention: global perspective. *Ann Epidemiol*. 2009;19(7):468–483.
37. Holick MF. Vitamin D deficiency. *N Engl J Med*. 2007;357(3):266–281.
38. Knight JM, Kirincich AN, Farmer ER, et al. Awareness of the risks of tanning lamps does not influence behavior among college students. *Arch Dermatol*. 2002;138(10):1311–1315.

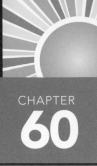

# Vitamin D and UV: Risks and Benefits

*Henry W. Lim, Wenfei Xie, and Darrell S. Rigel*

> ## Key Points
>
> - Vitamin D is important in bone metabolism.
> - Studies have suggested that vitamin D may lower the risk of developing certain cancers and provide benefit in several diseases, although a causal relationship has yet to be established through clinical trials.
> - Adequate vitamin D levels can be maintained with oral supplementation.
> - Because of known side effects of unprotected exposure to natural and artificial UV radiation, using UV exposure as a means of obtaining adequate serum vitamin D levels should be discouraged.

## HISTORY

Vitamin D is a fat-soluble prohormone that plays an important role in calcium and phosphorus homeostasis as well as in many organ systems throughout the body. There are two major physiologically relevant forms of vitamin D: $D_2$ (ergocalciferol) and $D_3$ (cholecalciferol). Vitamin $D_2$, which is present in yeast and mushrooms, is derived from ergosterol, a yeast and plant sterol. Vitamin $D_3$ is produced photochemically in the skin from 7-dehydrocholesterol, a cholesterol precursor.[1]

The modern history of vitamin D began in the mid-1800s, when it was noticed that city children were more likely to have rickets than rural children. Half a century later, Palm reported that children raised in sunny climates virtually never developed rickets. McCollum isolated vitamin D, and Windaus its precursors, receiving the Nobel Prize.[2]

## SOURCES AND METABOLISM OF VITAMIN D

In humans, vitamin D is obtained naturally through two sources, diet and sunlight. Very few foods inherently contain significant amounts of vitamin D. Fatty fish like salmon, tuna, and mackerel, as well as fish liver oils are among the best sources, providing 200 to 1600 IU per serving. Beef liver, cheese, and egg yolks provide small amounts of vitamin D – 12 to 20 IU per serving – and some mushrooms contain variable amounts.[3] The majority of dietary vitamin D in countries like the United States and Canada comes from foods such as milk, milk products, juices, and cereal products that are fortified with vitamin D. One 8 ounce serving of fortified milk or orange juice in the United States provides approximately 100 IU of vitamin D (Table 60.1).

The major natural source of vitamin D in humans is from the exposure of skin to sunlight. UVB radiation is absorbed by cutaneous 7-dehydrocholesterol to form pre-vitamin $D_3$ (Fig. 60.1). This process largely occurs in the stratum basale and stratum spinosum, where 7-dehydrocholesterol is the most concentrated. Pre-vitamin $D_3$ undergoes a temperature-dependent isomerization to form vitamin $D_3$, which is then hydroxylated by the liver to 25-hydroxyvitamin D [25(OH)D] via the 25-hydroxylase enzyme. An additional hydroxylation by the kidney via the 1α-hydroxylase enzyme is necessary to produce the physiologically active vitamin D metabolite, 1α,25-dihydroxyvitamin D [1,25(OH)$_2$D], which is best known for promoting intestinal absorption of calcium and phosphorus, decreasing their clearance from the kidney, and promoting bone mineralization.[4]

In addition to foods and sunlight, vitamin D is also available in supplement form as $D_2$ or $D_3$. Comparisons between the two forms have shown $D_2$ to have a shorter shelf-life, diminished binding of its metabolites to vitamin D binding protein in plasma, and less efficacy in raising and maintaining serum vitamin D metabolite levels.[5,6] Given these findings, vitamin $D_3$ is preferred to $D_2$ for supplementation.

Minimal winter sunlight exposure reaches the lower epidermal layers, and therefore little vitamin D is produced in the wintertime. Melanin, which is produced by melanocytes located in the stratum basale, also affects the quantity of vitamin D produced by absorbing UVB. Melanin concentration determines the amount of UVB that can interact with the 7-dehydrocholesterol in the lower epidermal layers, though it does not change the capacity to produce vitamin D; individuals with darker skin pigmentation may need three to six times longer exposure to produce the same amount of pre-vitamin D as those with fair skin. Skin from older individuals contains less substrate for pre-vitamin D synthesis, and they may produce up to four times less pre-vitamin D than their younger counterparts.[7]

## VITAMIN D IN HEALTH AND DISEASE

Though 25(OH)D has low biological activity, its serum concentration, which can be measured in commercial laboratories, is the most widely used biomarker for an individual's vitamin D status. 25(OH)D levels have been correlated with important health endpoints (Table 60.2);[8–43] the levels are commonly reported as either nmol/L or ng/mL (Table 60.3). One complication in determining vitamin D status is that there is variability among the laboratories that conduct the analyses as well as in the various available assays.[44] However, a new standard reference material for 25(OH)D

## Table 60.1 Common Food Sources of Vitamin D

| Food | International Units (IU) per Serving |
|---|---|
| Atlantic herring, 3.5 ounces | 1600 |
| Cod liver oil, 1 tablespoon | 1360 |
| Mushrooms, enriched with vitamin D, 3 ounces | 400 |
| Salmon, 3.5 ounces | 360 |
| Mackerel, 3.5 ounces | 345 |
| Sardines, canned in oil, drained, 1.75 ounces | 250 |
| Tuna fish, canned in oil, 3 ounces | 200 |
| Orange juice fortified with vitamin D, 1 cup (amount of added vitamin D varies) | 142 |
| Milk, non-fat, reduced fat, and whole, vitamin D fortified, 1 cup | 98 |
| Margarine, fortified, 1 tablespoon | 60 |
| Ready-to-eat cereal, fortified, 0.75–1 cup (amount of added vitamin D varies) | 40 |
| Egg, 1 whole (vitamin D is found in yolk) | 20 |
| Liver, beef, 3.5 ounces | 15 |
| Cheese, Swiss, 1 ounce | 12 |

Source: From US Department of Agriculture, Agricultural Research Service. USDA Nutrient Database for Standard Reference, Release 22. 2009.

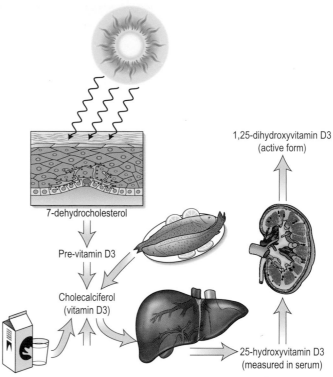

**Figure 60.1** Synthesis of and metabolism of vitamin D. Cutaneous 7-dehydrocholesterol absorbs UVB radiation to form pre-vitamin $D_3$, which then becomes vitamin $D_3$. Vitamin $D_3$ and vitamin $D_2$ are also obtained from the diet. Vitamin D undergoes sequential hydroxylation by enzymes in the liver and kidney to become the physiologically active metabolite, $1\alpha,25$-dihydroxyvitamin D.

became available in July 2009, which should allow for more standardization across laboratories.[45]

## Bone and muscle health

There is a large body of evidence that correlates vitamin D levels to bone health. Several studies show that children in developing countries with rickets have lower serum 25(OH)D concentrations than controls. Some investigators have reported mean or median 25(OH)D concentrations <30 nmol/L in children with rickets, whereas others have reported values between 30 nmol/L and 50 nmol/L. However, there are inconsistent data to determine a threshold serum 25(OH)D level above which rickets does not occur. In adolescents, serum 25(OH)D levels are positively associated with baseline bone mineral density (BMD) as well as change in BMD/bone mineral content (BMC) indices.[8]

A significant positive association between 25(OH)D levels and hip BMD was noted in younger and older whites, younger and older Mexican Americans, and older blacks. There was also a decreased higher-end distribution of 25(OH)D levels in non-white subjects when compared to the white US population.[9]

A meta-analysis of 20 high-quality, double-blinded randomized controlled trials (RCTs) for non-vertebral fractures and hip fractures suggested that there is a dose–response relationship between supplemental vitamin D and fracture prevention among individuals aged 65 years and older.[10] Meta-regression analyses showed a greater reduction in hip fractures with both a higher received dose and with higher achieved 25(OH)D levels.

A prominent symptom of vitamin D deficiency is proximal muscle weakness, supporting a role for vitamin D in muscle health.[7] Human muscle tissue expresses the nuclear vitamin D receptor (VDR), and bound vitamin D may promote de-novo protein synthesis as well as increased diameter and numbers of type II muscle fibers. A meta-analysis of high-quality double-blind RCTs showed that vitamin D in the elderly reduced fall risk by 22% (corrected OR 0.78, 95% CI 0.64–0.92) compared to calcium or placebo.[12]

## Vitamin D and cancers

Vitamin D status has been investigated as a possible explanation for an association between greater sun exposure and lower incidence and mortality for various cancers. A variety of tissues are known to express $1\alpha$-hydroxylase, the enzyme that converts 25(OH)D to $1,25(OH)_2D$, and in-vitro studies have shown that $1,25(OH)_2D$ can inhibit cancer cell line growth. Furthermore, many types of cancer cells are known to express the VDR, giving more support to the notion that vitamin D may play a role in modulating carcinogenesis and/or its progression.[46]

A number of studies have shown an inverse association between serum 25(OH)D levels and the risk of colorectal cancer (CRC). it is estimated that individuals in the high quartile or quintile of 25(OH)D levels (>92.5 nmol/L) have a 50%

**Table 60.2   Summary of Epidemiologic Associations Between Vitamin D and Health and Disease**

| Measurement and Outcome | Study: Findings [reference] |
|---|---|
| Serum 25(OH)D and rickets in children | **Meta-analysis:** Low 25(OH)D levels associated with established rickets [8] |
| Serum 25(OH)D and hip bone mineral density | **NHANES III:** Positive association [9] |
| Supplemental vitamin D and non-vertebral fractures | **Meta-analysis:** Doses below 400 IU/day did not decrease risk (RR 1.02, 95% CI 0.92–1.15); doses above 480 IU/day decreased risk (RR 0.80, 95% CI 0.72–0.89) [10] |
| Supplemental vitamin D and hip fractures | **Meta-analysis:** Doses below 400 IU/day did not decrease risk (RR 1.09, 95% CI 0.90–1.32); doses above 480 IU/day decreased risk (RR 0.82, 95% CI 0.69–0.97) [10] |
| Serum 25(OH)D and lower extremity function | **NHANES III:** Highest 25(OH)D quintile vs. lowest: faster 8-foot walk test ($p < 0.001$) and faster sit-to-stand test ($p = 0.017$) [11] |
| Supplemental vitamin D and falls | **Meta-analysis:** Decreased risk with supplementation (OR 0.78, 95% CI 0.64–0.92) [12] |
| Serum 25(OH)D and colorectal cancer (CRC) | **NHS:** Inverse association* ($p = 0.02$); OR 0.53 for highest 25(OH)D quintile (95% CI 0.27–1.04) [13] <br> **WHI:** Inverse association; OR 2.53 for lowest 25(OH)D quintile (95% CI 1.49–4.32) [14] <br> **EPIC:** Inverse association; OR 1.28 for lowest 25(OH)D quartile (95% CI 1.05–1.56) [15] <br> **NHANES III:** Inverse association for mortality from CRC; RR 0.28 for highest 25(OH)D tertile (95% CI 0.11–0.68) [16] |
| Serum 25(OH)D and prostate cancer | **PHS:** Increased risk of aggressive cancer for low 25(OH)D (OR 2.1, 95% CI 1.2–3.4) [17] <br> **HPFS:** No association ($p = 0.20$) [18] <br> **PLCO:** No association ($p$ trend = 0.05), though higher 25(OH)D may be associated with increased risk of aggressive cancer [19] |
| Serum 25(OH)D and breast cancer | **NHANES III:** Decreased risk of mortality from breast cancer for high 25(OH)D (HR 0.28, 95% CI 0.08–0.93) [16] <br> **Meta-analysis:** Inverse association ($p$ trend < 0.001). OR 0.50 for highest 25(OH)D quintile [20] <br> **Case-control:** Inverse association ($p$ trend < 0.0001). OR 0.31 for highest 25(OH)D quintile (95% CI 0.24–0.42) [21] |
| Serum 25(OH)D and pancreatic cancer | **HPFS:** Inverse association. RR 0.49 for higher 25(OH)D (95% CI 0.28–0.86) [22] <br> **ATBC:** Positive association. OR 2.92 for highest 25(OH)D quintile (95% CI 1.56–5.48) [23] |
| Total vitamin D intake and pancreatic cancer | **Meta-analysis:** Decreased risk for >600 IU/day vs. <150 IU/day (RR 0.59, 95% CI 0.40–0.88) [24] |
| Serum 25(OH)D and non-Hodgkin lymphoma (NHL) | **ATBC:** Inverse association for cases diagnosed less than 7 years from baseline ($p$ trend = 0.01). OR 0.43 for highest vs. lowest 25(OH)D tertile (95% CI 0.23–0.83) [25] <br> **HPFS:** No association [22] <br> **NHANES III:** No association for mortality from NHL [16] |
| Serum 25(OH)D and lung cancer | **Case-control:** Positive association for recurrence-free survival in early-stage non-small cell lung cancer patients ($p$ trend = 0.002). AHR 0.45 for highest 25(OH)D quartile (95% CI 0.24–0.82) [26] <br> **Case-control:** No association for recurrence-free survival in advanced-stage non-small cell lung cancer patients [27] <br> **NHANES III:** No association for mortality from lung cancer [16] <br> **HPFS:** No association [22] <br> **Cohort:** No association overall, but inverse association for women (RR 0.16, 95% CI 0.04–0.59, $p$ trend <0.001) and younger participants (RR 0.34, 95% CI 0.13–0.90, $p$ trend = 0.04) [28] |
| Serum 25(OH)D and total cancer | **HPFS:** Inverse association. RR 0.83 per increase of 25 nmol/L in predicted 25(OH)D (95% CI 0.74–0.92). Inverse association for total cancer mortality. RR 0.71 per increase of 25 nmol/L in predicted 25(OH)D level (95% CI 0.60–0.83) [22] <br> **Cohort:** Inverse association for total cancer mortality. HR 0.66 per increase of 25 nmol/L in 25(OH)D (95% CI 0.49–0.89) [29] <br> **NHANES III:** No association for total cancer mortality [16] |
| Supplemental vitamin D and total cancer | **RCT:** No association [30] <br> **RCT:** No association [31] |

*(Continued)*

**Table 60.2 Summary of Epidemiologic Associations Between Vitamin D and Health and Disease—Cont'd**

| Measurement and Outcome | Study: Findings [reference] |
|---|---|
| Serum 25(OH)D and cardiovascular health | **NHANES III:** Inverse association for cardiac risk factors. For lowest 25(OH)D quartile vs. highest, OR 1.30 for hypertension, OR 1.98 for diabetes mellitus, OR 2.29 for obesity, and OR 1.47 for high serum triglyceride levels ($p < 0.001$ for all) [32]. Low 25(OH)D levels had increased self-reported angina, myocardial infarction, and heart failure (OR 1.20, 95% CI 1.01–1.36) [33]<br>**Cohort:** Inverse association for metabolic syndrome. Inverse association for high hemoglobin A1C, hypertension, and hypertriglyceridemia ($p < 0.004$ for all) [34]<br>**NHS:** Inverse association for incident hypertension. RR 2.67 for low 25(OH)D (95% CI 1.05–6.79) [35]<br>**HPFS:** Inverse association for incident hypertension. RR 6.13 for low 25(OH)D (95% CI 1.00–37.8) [35]<br>**Cohort:** Inverse association for cardiovascular-related death. For low 25(OH)D, HR 2.84 for death due to heart failure (95% CI 1.20–6.74), HR 5.05 for sudden cardiac death (95% CI 2.13–11.97) [36]<br>**Cohort:** Inverse association for cardiovascular-related death. HR 0.76 for highest 25(OH)D quintile (95% CI 0.60–0.95) [37] |
| Supplemental vitamin D and blood pressure | **RCT:** 800 IU/day with 1200 mg/day of calcium decreased SBP by 13 mmHg and heart rate by 4 bpm compared to calcium alone ($p = 0.02$) [38]<br>**Review:** Studies in Denmark, Taiwan, the UK, and the WHI Study in the US showed no association, though lower doses ( 400 IU) of vitamin D were used [39] |
| UVB exposure and blood pressure | **RCT:** UVB exposure decreased both SBP and DBP by 6 mmHg ($p < 0.001$) [40] |
| Serum 25(OH)D and all-cause mortality | **NHANES III:** Inverse association. HR 0.95 per increase of 10 nmol/L in serum 25(OH)D (95% CI 0.92–0.98). AHR 1.83 for lowest 25(OH)D quintile (95% CI 1.14–2.94), AHR 1.47 for second lowest quintile (95% CI 1.09–1.97) [41]<br>**Cohort:** Inverse association. HR 2.08 for lower two 25(OH)D quartiles (95% CI 1.60–2.70) [42] |
| Supplemental vitamin D and all-cause mortality | **Meta-analysis:** Adjusted mean daily dose of 528 IU associated with decreased mortality (RR 0.93, 95% CI 0.87–0.99) [43] |

25(OH)D, 25-hydroxyvitamin D; AHR, adjusted hazard ratio; ATBC, Alpha-Tocopherol, Beta-Carotene Trial; CI, confidence interval; DBP: diastolic blood pressure; EPIC, European Prospective Investigation into Cancer and Nutrition; HPFS, Health Professionals Follow-Up Study; HR, hazard ratio; NHANES III, Third National Health and Nutritional Examination Survey; NHS, Nurses' Health Study; OR, odds ratio; PHS, Physicians' Health Study; PLCO, Prostate, Lung, Colorectal and Ovarian Cancer Screening Trial; RCT, randomized controlled trial; RR, relative risk; SBP, systolic blood pressure; WHI, Women's Health Initiative.
*Inverse association: higher 25(OH)D levels were associated with lower risk.

reduction in colorectal cancer risk compared to those in the lowest group (<15 nmol/L). The optimal level of 25(OH)D for colorectal cancer prevention may be close to 90 nmol/L.[47]

The data on 25(OH)D levels and risk of prostate cancer are equivocal. Some studies suggest a weak inverse association, while others have found an increased risk of prostate cancer in men with the highest levels of 25(OH)D. Similarly, the Prostate, Lung, Colorectal, and Ovarian (PLCO) Cancer Screening Trial did not find a correlation between 25(OH)D levels and prostate cancer risk.[19]

Vitamin D may also reduce breast cancer risk and mortality in women. Cohort data from the NHANES III study found a significant decrease in breast cancer-specific mortality over 9 years of follow-up in women who had 25(OH)D levels >62 nmol/L compared to those with levels ≤62 nmol/L (HR 0.28, 95% CI 0.08–0.93), though the linear trend was not significant (p=0.76).[16] A meta-analysis with pooled data from two cohort studies showed a significant dose–response relationship, with a lower risk among women with higher 25(OH)D levels.[20]

Data from the Health Professionals Follow-up Study (HPFS) and the Nurses' Health Study (NHS) suggest that vitamin D may be protective for the development of pancreatic cancer. A pooled analysis of the HPFS and NHS showed an inverse association between total vitamin D intake and pancreatic cancer (RR 0.59, 95% CI 0.40–0.88 for diet and supplemental vitamin D >600 IU compared with <150 IU).[24]

The Alpha-Tocopherol, Beta-Carotene (ATBC) Cancer Prevention Study indicated an inverse association for cases of non-Hodgkin lymphoma (NHL) diagnosed less than 7 years from baseline, but not for diagnoses made later.[25] An increment of 25 nmol/L of the predicted 25(OH)D level was associated with a risk reduction of NHL, though this association was not significant.[22]

There is little evidence to suggest a correlation between 25(OH)D levels and ovarian, endometrial, renal, or gastric cancers. The risk of esophageal cancer has been shown to be increased in men with higher 25(OH)D levels, and esophageal squamous dysplasia risk has been shown to be increased in individuals of both genders with higher 25(OH)D levels.[46]

## All-cause mortality

All-cause mortality may be reduced in individuals with higher levels of 25(OH)D. Data from NHANES III indicated that in participants aged 65 and older, baseline 25(OH)D levels were inversely associated with all-cause mortality risk (HR 0.95, 95% CI 0.92–0.98, per 10 nmol/L). When comparing subjects with levels <25.0 nmol/L and 25.0–49.9 nmol/L to those with levels of 100 nmol/L or higher, the mortality risk was increased 1.8- and 1.5-fold, respectively.[41]

Many RCTs have investigated the effects of vitamin D supplementation on all-cause mortality but have shown

| Table 60.3 Equivalent Values of Serum 25(OH)D Levels Expressed in Two Different Units | |
|---|---|
| **nmol/L** | **ng/mL** |
| 30 | 12 |
| 50 | 20 |
| 75 | 30 |

To convert nmol/L to ng/mL, divide by 2.496.

little evidence of an association.[8] However, a meta-analysis of 18 RCTs showed that daily vitamin D supplementation of 300 to 2000 IU seemed to be associated with a 7% decreased risk of all-cause mortality (RR 0.93, 95% CI 0.87–0.99).[43]

## OPTIMAL VITAMIN D LEVELS

Suggestions for optimal serum 25(OH)D levels have been published based on the many studies that have investigated vitamin D status and multiple health outcomes. For all endpoints, the target 25(OH)D level was reported to be above 75 nmol/L and optimally between 90 and 120 nmol/L. For fractures, levels above 75 nmol/L are advantageous. For cancer prevention, levels between 90 and 120 nmol/L may be desirable.[48]

Though the amount of vitamin D required to achieve optimal levels of 25(OH)D in most of the population is not clearly established, it has been estimated that 1000 IU/day may increase 50% of adults' 25(OH)D levels to 75 nmol/L.[49,50] Hypercalcemia has been associated only with 25(OH)D levels of above 220 nmol/L. It has been suggested that this value would be reached only by taking oral vitamin D supplementation in excess of 10,000 IU/day.[7] It should be noted that the long-term effect of vitamin D intake of >2000 IU/d is unknown.[15]

Despite many studies that have demonstrated correlations between vitamin D status and health outcomes, it is unclear whether low vitamin D status is a causal factor for increased risk for disease or simply an indicator of impaired health status. Given that there is no current evidence to show that any level of 25(OH)D actually prevents cancer, the World Health Organization International Agency for Research on Cancer (WHO IARC) reports that it is inappropriate to set a lower limit of 'adequate' serum 25(OH)D levels at 20 to 30 ng/mL.[15]

## POPULATIONS AT RISK OF LOW VITAMIN D STATUS

Based on data from NHANES III, only 31% of adult Caucasians in the US aged 20-49 years and less than 9% of older Caucasians have serum 25(OH)D levels of 90 nmol/L or more.[9] Even fewer Mexican American and African American adults meet or exceed that level. Fifty percent of Asians in the UK were found to have levels <12.5 nmol/L.[51] Those who are most vulnerable to low vitamin D levels include the elderly, individuals who live in northern latitudes with prolonged winters, the obese, and African Americans of all ages. Populations with dark skin pigmentation and individuals who practice rigorous photoprotection, and whose religious and cultural beliefs require them to cover most exposed skin with clothing, are also at risk for low vitamin D levels.[48]

## SUN EXPOSURE AND VITAMIN D LEVELS

Given that vitamin D is synthesized in response to UVB irradiation, serum 25(OH)D levels are correlated with sun exposure. Whole body exposure in a fair-skinned individual to 1 minimal erythema dose (MED) of simulated sunlight is equivalent to taking one dose of between 10,000 and 25,000 IU of vitamin D. The response varies by latitude, age, and skin type.[52]

Though studies have shown that noticeable increases in vitamin D levels can be obtained by small, defined UVB doses, data from around the world indicate that living in a sunny climate can still be associated with vitamin D levels below 75 nmol/L. Studies from Chile, Hawaii, India, East Asia, Australia, and New Zealand have found that 21–92% of healthy, fully ambulatory individuals have suboptimal levels of 25(OH)D.[7] Individuals are at increased risk of low vitamin D during the winter season, particularly if they have darkly pigmented skin (Fig. 60.2).[53]

## Risks of sun exposure

The effects of chronic sun exposure on photoaging and photocarcinogenesis have been well documented (see Chapter 9). Sun exposure has been shown to be the main environmental cause of squamous cell carcinoma, and has been well associated with the development of basal cell carcinoma as well as melanoma. The use of tanning beds has also been associated with an increased risk of melanoma and squamous cell carcinoma (see Chapter 59).[54] The World Health Organization has classified UV as a carcinogen, and UV tanning beds as 'carcinogenic to humans'.[55] UV exposure also causes a degenerative process within the skin and skin support system, leading to fine and coarse wrinkling, dryness, roughness, laxity, telangiectasias, pigmentary changes, and loss of tensile strength.

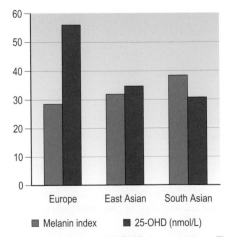

**Figure 60.2** Skin pigmentation and 25(OH)D concentrations. There is an inverse relationship between skin pigmentation or melanin index and serum 25(OH)D levels. *Redrawn from Gozdzik A, Barta JL, Wu H, Wagner D, Cole DE, Vieth R, et al. Low wintertime vitamin D levels in a sample of healthy young adults of diverse ancestry living in the Toronto area: associations with vitamin D intake and skin pigmentation. BMC Public Health. 2008;8:336.*

## Photoprotection and vitamin D

Regular use of a broad-spectrum sunscreen as part of a comprehensive photoprotective regimen has been shown to decrease the risk of the development of actinic keratoses and squamous cell carcinoma.[56-58] However, application of sunscreen with SPF as low as 8 in laboratory settings has significantly suppressed the increase in 25(OH)D levels after exposure to 1 MED of simulated sunlight.[59] Application of SPF 15 sunscreen over 2 years showed higher 25(OH)D levels in the summer for non-sunscreen users and lower levels in the winter in the sunscreen users,[60] although a double-blind RCT comparing daily use of SPF 17 sunscreen against placebo over a summer showed no difference in serum 25(OH)D levels.[61] Most studies show that normal sunscreen usage generally does not result in vitamin D insufficiency, mainly due to inadequacies in application to the skin and because people who use sunscreen may expose themselves to more sun than non-sunscreen users.[62]

## CURRENT VITAMIN D RECOMMENDATIONS

Though many epidemiological studies have demonstrated an association between low serum vitamin D levels and increased risk of a variety of diseases, a causal relationship has yet to be established through clinical trials. It is not known whether low vitamin D status is an indicator of impaired health status and therefore only a predictor of increased risks for disease. The WHO IARC recommends that it is currently inappropriate to set a standard lower limit of 'adequate' serum 25(OH)D levels because no randomized trials have demonstrated that maintenance of any levels truly prevents disease occurrence.[15] In addition, the long-term health effects of daily intake of greater than 2000 IU/day are unknown. Data from NHANES III and the Framingham Heart Study suggest that cardiovascular events and mortality increase linearly with increasing 25(OH)D levels above 100 nmol/L.[15]

The recommendations for vitamin D intake in the United States are established by the Institute of Medicine (IOM). In November 2010, IOM released Recommended Dietary Allowance (RDA) recommendations (Table 60.4).[63,64] These recommendations were made based on data on skeletal health, as the IOM considered that for extraskeletal out-

### Table 60.5 An Example of 600 IU Intake of Vitamin D*

| | |
|---|---|
| Salmon, 3 ounces | 300 IU |
| Vitamin D-fortified orange juice, 1 glass (8 ounces) | 100 IU |
| Vitamin D-fortified milk, 2 glasses (8 ounces each) | 200 IU |
| **Total intake** | **600 *IU*** |

*From National Council on Skin Cancer Prevention. Position Statement on Vitamin D. 2009 [cited 2009 Nov 1]; Available from: http://www.skincancerprevention.org/

comes, evidence was inconsistent, inconclusive as to causality, and insufficient to inform nutritional requirements. Furthermore, the recommendations were made based on an assumption of minimal or no sun exposure, hence eliminating the effects of sun exposure and skin pigmentation in vitamin D levels. IOM also stated that serum 25(OH)D levels of 20 ng/ml (50 nmol/l) to be adequate to cover the requirements of at least 97.5% of the population, and that levels > 50 ng/ml (125 nmol/l) could potentially be associated with adverse effects. An example of 600 IU/day of dietary intake is shown in Table 60.5. Therefore, IOM RDA recommendations for vitamin D can be easily achieved through dietary source, and if need be, in combination with vitamin D supplement. Because of known side effects of unprotected exposure to natural and artificial UV radiation, using UV exposure as a means of obtaining adequate serum vitamin D levels should be discouraged.

## FUTURE OUTLOOK

The history of the role of vitamin D in human health is extensive. Much of that history is yet to be written by scientists through prospective controlled studies that will hopefully elucidate its relationships with many diseases. Alternative methods of maintaining adequate levels beyond UV exposure need to be developed to safely ensure healthy serum levels of vitamin D.

### Table 60.4 Recommended Dietary Allowance (RDA) Recommendations for Vitamin D

| Age | RDA (IU/day) |
|---|---|
| 0–12 months | 400 |
| 1–70 years | 600 * |
| > 70 years | 800 |

Upper Intake Level (UL = the highest daily intake likely to pose no risk):
0- 8 years: 1000-3000 IU/day;
9-71+ years: 4000 IU/day
* Include pregnant and lactating women
Source: 63. Institute of Medicine. *Dietary reference intakes for calcium and vitamin D*. Washington, DC: The National Academies Press; 2011.
64. Ross AC, Manson JE, Abrams SA, et al. The 2011 Report on Dietary Reference Intakes for Calcium and Vitamin D from the Institute of Medicine: What Clinicians Need to Know. *J Clin Endocrinol Metab*. Nov. 29, 2010 [epub].

## REFERENCES

**1.** Institute of Medicine, Food, and Nutrition Board. *Dietary Reference Intakes: Calcium, Phosphorus, Magnesium, Vitamin D, and Fluoride*. Washington, DC: National Academy Press; 1997.
**2.** Mohr SB. A brief history of vitamin D and cancer prevention. *Ann Epidemiol*. 2009;19(2):79–83.
**3.** US Department of Agriculture, Agricultural Research Service. *USDA Nutrient Database for Standard Reference*. Release 22. 2009.
**4.** Holick MF. Vitamin D deficiency. *N Engl J Med*. 2007;357(3):266–281.
**5.** Armas LA, Hollis BW, Heaney RP. Vitamin D2 is much less effective than vitamin D3 in humans. *J Clin Endocrinol Metab*. 2004;89(11):5387–5391.
**6.** Houghton LA, Vieth R. The case against ergocalciferol (vitamin D2) as a vitamin supplement. *Am J Clin Nutr*. 2006;84(4):694–697.
**7.** Bischoff-Ferrari HA, Lim HW. Effect of photoprotection on vitamin D and health. In: Lim HW, Draelos DZ, eds. *Clinical Guide to Sunscreens and Photoprotection*. New York: Informa Healthcare; 2008:117–137.
**8.** Chung M, Balk E, Brendel M, et al. *Vitamin D and Calcium: A Systematic Review of Health Outcomes*. Evidence Report No 183 (Prepared by the Tufts Evidence-based Practice Center under Contract No HHSA 290-2007-10055-I) AHRQ Publication No 09-E015. Rockville, MD: Agency for Healthcare Research and Quality; 2009.
**9.** Bischoff-Ferrari HA, Dietrich T, Orav EJ, et al. Positive association between 25-hydroxy vitamin D levels and bone mineral density: a population-based study of younger and older adults. *Am J Med*. 2004;116(9):634–639.

10. Bischoff-Ferrari HA, Willett WC, Wong JB, et al. Prevention of nonvertebral fractures with oral vitamin D and dose dependency: a meta-analysis of randomized controlled trials. *Arch Intern Med.* 2009;169(6):551–561.

11. Bischoff-Ferrari HA, Dietrich T, Orav EJ, et al. Higher 25-hydroxyvitamin D concentrations are associated with better lower-extremity function in both active and inactive persons aged > or =60 y. *Am J Clin Nutr.* 2004;80(3):752–758.

12. Bischoff-Ferrari HA, Dawson-Hughes B, Willett WC, et al. Effect of vitamin D on falls: a meta-analysis. *JAMA.* 2004;291(16):1999–2006.

13. Feskanich D, Ma J, Fuchs CS, et al. Plasma vitamin D metabolites and risk of colorectal cancer in women. *Cancer Epidemiol Biomarkers Prev.* 2004;13(9):1502–1508.

14. Wactawski-Wende J, Kotchen JM, Anderson GL, et al. Calcium plus vitamin D supplementation and the risk of colorectal cancer. *N Engl J Med.* 2006;354(7):684–696.

15. World Health Organization International Agency for Research on Cancer. *Vitamin D and Cancer. IARC Working Group Reports.* Lyon: International Agency for Research on Cancer; 2008.

16. Freedman DM, Looker AC, Chang SC, et al. Prospective study of serum vitamin D and cancer mortality in the United States. *J Natl Cancer Inst.* 2007;99(21):1594–1602.

17. Li H, Stampfer MJ, Hollis JB, et al. A prospective study of plasma vitamin D metabolites, vitamin D receptor polymorphisms, and prostate cancer. *PLoS Med.* 2007;4(3):e103.

18. Platz EA, Leitzmann MF, Hollis BW, et al. Plasma 1,25-dihydroxy- and 25-hydroxyvitamin D and subsequent risk of prostate cancer. *Cancer Causes Control.* 2004;15(3):255–265.

19. Ahn J, Peters U, Albanes D, et al. Serum vitamin D concentration and prostate cancer risk: a nested case-control study. *J Natl Cancer Inst.* 2008;100(11):796–804.

20. Garland CF, Gorham ED, Mohr SB, et al. Vitamin D and prevention of breast cancer: pooled analysis. *J Steroid Biochem Mol Biol.* 2007;103(3–5):708–711.

21. Abbas S, Linseisen J, Slanger T, et al. Serum 25-hydroxyvitamin D and risk of post-menopausal breast cancer – results of a large case-control study. *Carcinogenesis.* 2008;29(1):93–99.

22. Giovannucci E, Liu Y, Rimm EB, et al. Prospective study of predictors of vitamin D status and cancer incidence and mortality in men. *J Natl Cancer Inst.* 2006;98(7):451–459.

23. Stolzenberg-Solomon RZ, Vieth R, Azad A, et al. A prospective nested case-control study of vitamin D status and pancreatic cancer risk in male smokers. *Cancer Res.* 2006;66(20):10213–10219.

24. Skinner HG, Michaud DS, Giovannucci E, et al. Vitamin D intake and the risk for pancreatic cancer in two cohort studies. *Cancer Epidemiol Biomarkers Prev.* 2006;15(9):1688–1695.

25. Lim U, Freedman DM, Hollis BW, et al. A prospective investigation of serum 25-hydroxyvitamin D and risk of lymphoid cancers. *Int J Cancer.* 2009;124(4):979–986.

26. Zhou W, Heist RS, Liu G, et al. Circulating 25-hydroxyvitamin D levels predict survival in early-stage non-small-cell lung cancer patients. *J Clin Oncol.* 2007;25(5):479–485.

27. Heist RS, Zhou W, Wang Z, et al. Circulating 25-hydroxyvitamin D, VDR polymorphisms, and survival in advanced non-small-cell lung cancer. *J Clin Oncol.* 2008;26(34):5596–5602.

28. Kilkkinen A, Knekt P, Heliovaara M, et al. Vitamin D status and the risk of lung cancer: a cohort study in Finland. *Cancer Epidemiol Biomarkers Prev.* 2008;17(11):3274–3278.

29. Pilz S, Dobnig H, Winklhofer-Roob B, et al. Low serum levels of 25-hydroxyvitamin D predict fatal cancer in patients referred to coronary angiography. *Cancer Epidemiol Biomarkers Prev.* 2008;17(5):1228–1233.

30. Lappe JM, Travers-Gustafson D, Davies KM, et al. Vitamin D and calcium supplementation reduces cancer risk: results of a randomized trial. *Am J Clin Nutr.* 2007;85(6):1586–1591.

31. Trivedi DP, Doll R, Khaw KT. Effect of four monthly oral vitamin D3 (cholecalciferol) supplementation on fractures and mortality in men and women living in the community: randomised double blind controlled trial. *BMJ.* 2003;326(7387):469.

32. Martins D, Wolf M, Pan D, et al. Prevalence of cardiovascular risk factors and the serum levels of 25-hydroxyvitamin D in the United States: data from the Third National Health and Nutrition Examination Survey. *Arch Intern Med.* 2007;167(11):1159–1165.

33. Kendrick J, Targher G, Smits G, et al. 25-Hydroxyvitamin D deficiency is independently associated with cardiovascular disease in the Third National Health and Nutrition Examination Survey. *Atherosclerosis.* 2009;205(1):255–260.

34. Hypponen E, Boucher BJ, Berry DJ, et al. 25-hydroxyvitamin D, IGF-1, and metabolic syndrome at 45 years of age: a cross-sectional study in the 1958 British Birth Cohort. *Diabetes.* 2008;57(2):298–305.

35. Forman JP, Giovannucci E, Holmes MD, et al. Plasma 25-hydroxyvitamin D levels and risk of incident hypertension. *Hypertension.* 2007;49(5):1063–1069.

36. Pilz S, Marz W, Wellnitz B, et al. Association of vitamin D deficiency with heart failure and sudden cardiac death in a large cross-sectional study of patients referred for coronary angiography. *J Clin Endocrinol Metab.* 2008;93(10):3927–3935.

37. Kilkkinen A, Knekt P, Aro A, et al. Vitamin D status and the risk of cardiovascular disease death. *Am J Epidemiol.* 2009;170(8):1032–1039.

38. Pfeifer M, Begerow B, Minne HW, et al. Effects of a short-term vitamin D(3) and calcium supplementation on blood pressure and parathyroid hormone levels in elderly women. *J Clin Endocrinol Metab.* 2001;86(4):1633–1637.

39. Judd SE, Tangpricha V. Vitamin D deficiency and risk for cardiovascular disease. *Am J Med Sci.* 2009;338(1):40–44.

40. Krause R, Buhring M, Hopfenmuller W, et al. Ultraviolet B and blood pressure. *Lancet.* 1998;352(9129):709–710.

41. Ginde AA, Scragg R, Schwartz RS, et al. Prospective study of serum 25-hydroxyvitamin D level, cardiovascular disease mortality, and all-cause mortality in older U.S. adults. *J Am Geriatr Soc.* 2009;57(9):1595–1603.

42. Dobnig H, Pilz S, Scharnagl H, et al. Independent association of low serum 25-hydroxyvitamin D and 1,25-dihydroxyvitamin D levels with all-cause and cardiovascular mortality. *Arch Intern Med.* 2008;168(12):1340–1349.

43. Autier P, Gandini S. Vitamin D supplementation and total mortality: a meta-analysis of randomized controlled trials. *Arch Intern Med.* 2007;167(16):1730–1737.

44. Hollis BW. Editorial: The determination of circulating 25-hydroxyvitamin D: no easy task. *J Clin Endocrinol Metab.* 2004;89(7):3149–3151.

45. National Institute of Standards and Technology. NIST releases Vitamin D Standard Reference Material. *NIST Tech Beat.* July 14, 2009.

46. Rhee HV, Coebergh JW, Vries ED. Sunlight, vitamin D and the prevention of cancer: a systematic review of epidemiological studies. *Eur J Cancer Prev.* 2009; Aug 26 [Epub ahead of print].

47. Gorham ED, Garland CF, Garland FC, et al. Optimal vitamin D status for colorectal cancer prevention: a quantitative meta analysis. *Am J Prev Med.* 2007;32(3):210–216.

48. Bischoff-Ferrari HA. Optimal serum 25-hydroxyvitamin D levels for multiple health outcomes. *Adv Exp Med Biol.* 2008;624:55–71.

49. Reddy KK, Gilchrest BA. What is all this commotion about vitamin D? *J Invest Dermatol.* 2010;130(2):321–326.

50. Bischoff-Ferrari HA. Optimal serum 25-hydroxyvitamin D levels for multiple health outcomes. *Adv Exp Med Biol.* 2008;624:55–71.

51. Young AR, Walker SL. UV radiation, vitamin D and human health: an unfolding controversy introduction. *Photochem Photobiol.* 2005;81(6):1243–1245.

52. Armas LA, Dowell S, Akhter M, et al. Ultraviolet-B radiation increases serum 25-hydroxyvitamin D levels: the effect of UVB dose and skin color. *J Am Acad Dermatol.* 2007;57(4):588–593.

53. Gozdzik A, Barta JL, Wu H, et al. Low wintertime vitamin D levels in a sample of healthy young adults of diverse ancestry living in the Toronto area: associations with vitamin D intake and skin pigmentation. *BMC Public Health.* 2008;8:336.

54. Lim HW, Gilchrest BA, Cooper KD, et al. Sunlight, tanning booths, and vitamin D. *J Am Acad Dermatol.* 2005;52(5):868–876.

55. El Ghissassi F, Baan R, Straif K, et al. A review of human carcinogens – part D: radiation. *Lancet Oncol.* 2009;10(8):751–752.

56. Green A, Williams G, Neale R, et al. Daily sunscreen application and betacarotene supplementation in prevention of basal-cell and squamous-cell carcinomas of the skin: a randomised controlled trial. *Lancet.* 1999;354(9180):723–729.

57. van der Pols JC, Williams GM, Pandeya N, et al. Prolonged prevention of squamous cell carcinoma of the skin by regular sunscreen use. *Cancer Epidemiol Biomarkers Prev.* 2006;15(12):2546–2548.

58. Ulrich C, Jurgensen JS, Degen A, et al. Prevention of non-melanoma skin cancer in organ transplant patients by regular use of a sunscreen: a 24 months, prospective, case-control study. *Br J Dermatol.* 2009;161(suppl 3):78–84.

59. Matsuoka LY, Ide L, Wortsman J, et al. Sunscreens suppress cutaneous vitamin D3 synthesis. *J Clin Endocrinol Metab.* 1987;64(6):1165–1168.

60. Farrerons J, Barnadas M, Rodriguez J, et al. Clinically prescribed sunscreen (sun protection factor 15) does not decrease serum vitamin D concentration sufficiently either to induce changes in parathyroid function or in metabolic markers. *Br J Dermatol.* 1998;139(3):422–427.

61. Marks R, Foley PA, Jolley D, et al. The effect of regular sunscreen use on vitamin D levels in an Australian population. Results of a randomized controlled trial. *Arch Dermatol.* 1995;131(4):415–421.

62. Norval M, Wulf HC. Does chronic sunscreen use reduce vitamin D production to insufficient levels? *Br J Dermatol.* 2009;161(4):732–736.

63. Institute of Medicine. *Dietary reference intakes for calcium and vitamin D.* Washington, DC: The National Academies Press; 2011.

64. Ross AC, Manson JE, Abrams SA, et al. The 2011 Report on Dietary Reference Intakes for Calcium and Vitamin D from the Institute of Medicine: What Clinicians Need to Know. *J Clin Endocrinol Metab.* Nov. 29, 2010 [epub].

# Photography in Skin Cancer Treatment

*Bill Witmer and Peter Lebovitz*

## Key Points

- Photographic documentation is an important adjunct to the care of patients at risk for melanoma.

- The evolution of pigmented lesions can be monitored using standardized procedures of whole body integumentary imaging.

- Individual lesions can be documented using macro-photographic and dermoscopic techniques.

- Photo documentation services can be provided within the practice or through the use of outside services.

## INTRODUCTION

As with most dermatological conditions, visual presentation plays an important role in the diagnosis and treatment of skin cancers. Because of this, clinical photography is a particularly important and powerful adjunct to the care of affected and at-risk patients, and has become a de facto standard of clinical care.[1] The photographic techniques used fall into two categories, depending on whether documentation is being obtained for new occurrences or existing lesions. This chapter will discuss techniques for both, as well as the means for integrating and cross-referencing the results.

Regardless of the intended purpose, there are several standards of clinical photography that are constant. Key among these are posing, lighting and repeatability. In serial photography (i.e. documenting changes over time), repeatability is clearly the most critical factor. Without a standardized method of image capture, the clinical value of a photographic series will be seriously compromised.

## IMAGE CAPTURE OVERVIEW

If one's experience with photography has been limited to everyday 'picture taking', it is possible that the understanding of image capture is to point the camera at the subject and click the shutter. This in essence is the process enabled by today's popular 'point-and-shoot' (PAS) cameras. But while this technique would work well enough in 'vacation' photos, a somewhat higher degree of control is required for meaningful medical documentation.

There are two distinct types of photography typically employed as adjuncts to the treatment of skin cancers. Total body photography (TBP), also referred to as whole body integumentary photography, is a procedure in which the skin covering most of the body is documented in a series of sectional photos. The second type, close-up or macro photography, creates a detailed photograph of a small area of the skin.

Image capture begins, not with the camera, but with the subject. Patient preparation is a simple but important step in the process as it is the first line of defense against the nemesis of good clinical imaging; variability. Simply put, patient preparation means getting rid of anything in the area of interest that is not part of the anatomy. Clothing, jewelry makeup and moisturizers that produce a reflective surface or mask the true appearance, are not only distracting, but can detract from the clinical value of the photographic result. In addition, attention to the background behind the subject is needed. The subject should be posed against a neutral solid color background, preferably blue. A drape sheet may be placed behind the area to obscure the floor, walls and wires commonly in the background of the clinical examination room.

Equally important as preparation is positioning. Maintaining control over both the camera-to-subject distance and the patient pose will assure consistent results, and enable meaningful comparison of photographs taken at different time points. In TBP, the photographer always works at a fixed distance from the subject. The use of a calibrated distance mat, or simply tape marks on the floor, provides a reliable means to assure this consistency. For macro photography, a simple fixture that attaches directly to the camera can greatly simplify the process (Fig. 61.1).

Finally, the importance of correct lighting cannot be overstressed. Lighting can make the difference between an excellent clinical photograph, and one that is worthless.[2] And while it might seem convenient, the camera's built-in flash is seldom the best choice.

Regardless of the type of photography undertaken, there are key issues regarding image storage and retrieval. In the most basic scenario, an image file is captured to a removable memory card inside the camera, where the camera's software assigns a sequential alphanumeric filename to the image. The image file must then be exported to a computer's hard drive, or server, where it can be accessed by a suitable software application. While this process is simple on the front end, it becomes more complex, labor-intensive and error-prone in subsequent stages.

For medical practice, it is far better to implement a system where the images are captured directly into a patient database. In this type of system, the camera is connected to a computer by a cable during the capture sequence, and the image files are automatically stored by image management software.

Using a suitable camera and software, 'tethered capture' with live image overlay offers a number of attractive benefits to the user and is an excellent method of assuring precise, repeatable subject positioning. In this method, a live video image from the camera is superimposed, or 'ghosted',

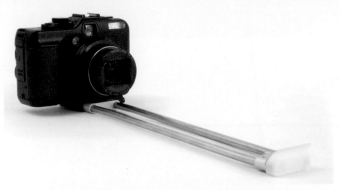

**Figure 61.1** Close-up fixture and scale assures consistent camera distance in macro photography. (Courtesy of Canfield Scientific)

over a previously captured image of the patient. Camera and subject positioning are then adjusted so that the two images exactly coincide when the shutter is actuated. For serial photography comparing different time points, this technique is indispensable.

## TOTAL BODY PHOTOGRAPHY (TBP)

For patients at risk for melanoma, TBP provides the means of establishing a baseline against which to evaluate changes in the patient's presentation.[3] The basis for this type of photography is a multi-section template that divides the body into discrete anatomical areas. This template defines a standardized series of photographs which comprise a 'body map'. A typical body map template consists of 25–30 photographs, and defines both the area of the anatomy to be photographed and the positioning, or pose, of the subject for each picture (Fig. 61.2).

TBP is an objective documentation of the patient's skin surface, and is performed without regard to any lesions that may be visible on the subject. The TBP image series is then burned to a CD along with simple photo viewing software. This software allows the patient to easily navigate the body map and view magnified images if desired. The CD should be password-protected to assure patient privacy. A bound

print book, usually 9×12 or 12×18 inches, may also be provided for the patient to retain.

Physicians who wish to provide TBP within the practice environment need to consider such factors as equipment and physical space requirements as well as staff training. Regarding the latter, it is generally possible to train staff members to a reasonable level of competence, even if they do not have prior photographic skills. Expertise comes with experience, time, and a willingness to learn. The photographer's personal skills and ability to educate the patient about the process will play an important role in assuring patient comfort and compliance.[4]

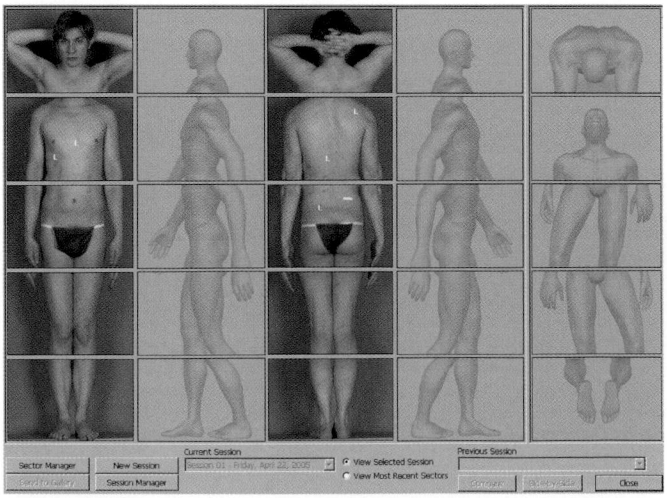

## Studio design and equipment

The first consideration is the amount of space available for photography and whether that space can be dedicated for the purpose. An area of approximately 8 × 10 feet is sufficient for either a permanent or temporary TBP installation (Fig. 61.3). Ideally, this should be in a separate room as you will need to control the ambient light from windows or overhead illumination, and provide privacy for the subject.

For a permanent studio, it is desirable to wall mount the flash units. This assures consistent illumination of the patient and maximizes open floor space. You will also need to assure that the subject is positioned in front of a plain background. A fabric backdrop, seamless background paper, or painted wall will do, with light blue being the color of choice. An indexed posing mat about 2 feet square will aid in consistent anterior, posterior, and lateral subject

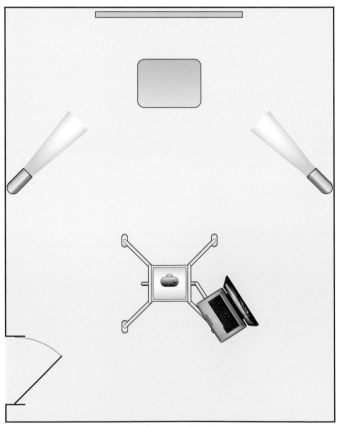

**Figure 61.3** Floor plan for a permanent studio with wall-mounted flash units. (Courtesy of Canfield Scientific)

**Figure 61.2** Body map template guides the imaging series for total body photography. (Courtesy of Canfield Scientific)

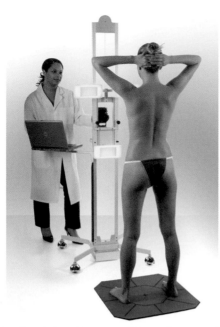

Figure 61.4 Studio solution with camera, lights and computer in a single integrated mobile system. (Courtesy of Canfield Scientific)

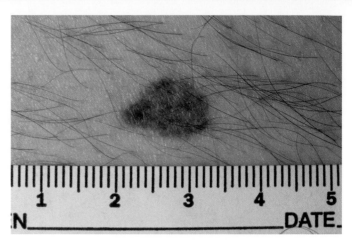

Figure 61.5 Standard macro-photographic view of an atypical nevus. Adhesive scales can be used for reference. (Courtesy of Canfield Scientific)

positioning. The mat can be placed on a stage, or platform, about 8 inches in height to elevate the subject to a convenient level for torso and leg photography.

If space is at a premium, or where a permanent installation is not practical, a compact integrated system can provide an excellent solution. This combines an adjustable camera support, computer platform, and clinical-quality lighting in a sturdy yet mobile fixture. With this type of system, TBP is practical in a space as small as 4 × 6 feet. When not in use, these systems can be rolled out of the way, allowing other uses for the space (Fig. 61.4).

For clinical photography of this type, a single lens reflex (SLR) is the camera of choice. In addition to better image quality, SLRs are more versatile with regard to the available lenses and attachments you will need. Select a lens of medium focal length that will allow imaging an entire torso from a distance of about 6 feet. The lens should also have macro (close-up) capabilities to enable photography of individual lesions, as described in the following section. The camera body and lens are typically purchased separately, as the zoom lenses typically included in camera kits are not well suited to this purpose. A number of SLR designs offer 'live view', a useful feature which enables live image overlay as described above.

## CLOSE-UP PHOTOGRAPHY

A useful adjunct to TBP is close-up photography, sometimes referred to as macro photography. This involves photographing an individual lesion or other small area of interest. There are two methods for this type of image capture, each of which provides a unique and important clinical view. In one method, a standard macro-enabled lens is used to image a close-up view of the lesion. This is typically photographed with a camera-to-subject distance of about

12 inches, corresponding to a reproduction ratio of 1:3 with a 60 mm lens. A millimeter scale is positioned adjacent to the lesion as a visual size reference. This view documents the size, color, margins and surface structure of the lesion and the immediate surrounding area (Fig. 61.5).

As with any clinical photography, correct lighting in close-up work is critical to producing repeatable, meaningful results. Camera-to-subject distance and geometry argue against the use of the camera's built-in flash, which in this application tends to produce overexposed and unevenly lit photographs. Supplementary lighting attachments are available that are calibrated for these close distances, and provide uniform illumination of the subject. Systems can be fitted with polarizing filters to control surface reflections, and also integrate with the camera's through-the-lens metering system (Fig. 61.6).

A more detailed view of structure at the dermal–epidermal junction is acquired with epiluminescence microscopy, or ELM. This imaging is analogous to dermoscopy, and may be implemented with a liquid interface or

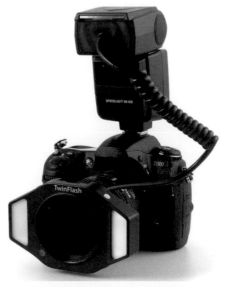

Figure 61.6 Specialized supplementary lighting attachments provide controlled lighting at close distances. (Courtesy of Canfield Scientific)

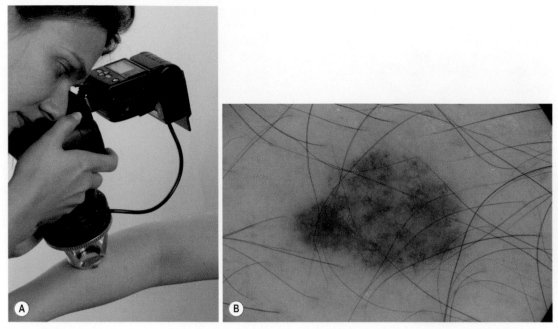

**Figure 61.7** The dermoscopic view reveals detailed structure of the lesion shown in Figure 61.5. (Courtesy of Canfield Scientific)

cross-polarized illumination. Various methods are available to interface a camera and a dermoscope to reveal details that cannot be seen with normal reflected light photography. A convenient solution is provided with a specialized device that integrates a macro camera lens with a contact light source (Fig. 61.7).

When macro photography is used in conjunction with TBP, it is possible to 'tag' the photograph of a specific lesion to its location on the body (Fig. 61.8). In the absence of TBP, it is generally good practice to take a supplementary wider-view photograph that shows the lesion's location on the larger anatomy.

## IMAGE CAPTURE AND MANAGEMENT SOFTWARE

In addition to studio design and equipment, an important component of any clinical photography activity is the software that is used for image management. At a minimum, the software must provide the means to archive and retrieve patient photographs and relevant data. However, for a more robust and seamless solution, look for software that will also help manage the image capture process. This class of software will provide templates for the body map and enables a direct image transfer link between the camera and computer, and is required for tethered capture. Network data sharing, or integration, can directly interface with practice management software. This enables images to be directly saved to, and retrieved from, a central patient database (Fig. 61.9).

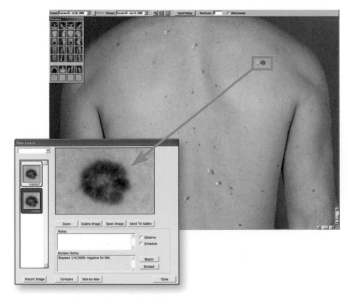

**Figure 61.8** An individual lesion in a TBP series is tagged to a close-up view. (Courtesy of Canfield Scientific)

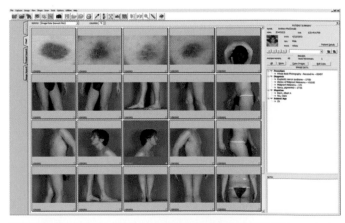

**Figure 61.9** Image management software organizes patient photographs in a central database. (Courtesy of Canfield Scientific)

A secondary benefit offered by such software is the ability to export and repurpose your clinical images for professional presentations and publications. Simple integration with commonly used applications such as PowerPoint®, as well as tools for adding comments, notes and creating layout boards of multiple images, can be useful. It is critical to obtain suitable releases from patients for any such use, and be mindful of HIPAA requirements at all times.

## OUTSIDE SERVICES

Not every practice will have the space, resources or desire to perform clinical photography on the scale described here. There are outside service providers that specialize in TBP as used for the early detection of melanoma. They are typically staffed by experienced medical photographers, and can provide comfortable, confidential and chaperoned photography sessions for your patients. Patients are given their TBP baseline images on a password-protected CD, and, optionally, a digital print portfolio. The patient typically retains the clinical images, which are used as a reference for subsequent self-examinations, and a copy of the CD for the patient records can also be generated.

## REIMBURSEMENT FOR SERVICES

In January 2007, the American Medical Association approved CPT Category I Code 96904 for 'Whole Body Integumentary Photography'. The stated purpose of this classification is 'for the monitoring of high-risk patients with dysplastic nevus syndrome or a history of dysplastic nevi, or patients with a personal or familial history of melanoma'.[5] Under this procedure, the images are to be produced in digital format and delivered with image viewing software and an interactive viewing album.

TBP sessions may be eligible for direct reimbursement. The most common diagnosis codes that are used in prescribing TBP are 238.2 (skin neoplasm of uncertain behavior), 172.9 (melanoma), V10.82 (personal history of melanoma), and v16.8 (family history of melanoma).[6]

## FUTURE OUTLOOK

Clinical imaging allows physicians to clearly document cancerous and precancerous nevi and to track both their development and remediation. The approach will continue to be a valuable adjunct to the detection and treatment of cancers of the skin. Typically, the patient will be imaged using established standards for total body photography, with additional close-up photography of individual lesions of interest. Even with upcoming advances in image collection and storage, the tools and techniques that are required for effective imaging will continue to be within the reach of most practices.

## REFERENCES

**1.** Rhodes AR. Intervention strategy to prevent lethal cutaneous melanoma: use of dermatologic photography to aid surveillance of high-risk persons. *JAMA*. 1998;39(2 Pt 1):262–277.

**2.** DiBernardo B, Pozner J, Codner MA. *Techniques in Aesthetic Plastic Surgery Series: Lasers and Non-Surgical Rejuvenation*. UK: Elsevier Health Sciences; 2009:155–165.

**3.** Halpern AC. The use of whole body photography in a pigmented lesion clinic. *Dermatol Surg*. 2000;26(12):1175–1180.

**4.** Halpern AC, Marghoob AA, Bialoglow TW, et al. Standardized positioning of patients (poses) for whole body cutaneous photography. *J Am Acad Dermatol*. 2003;49:593–598.

**5.** Current Procedural Terminology (CPT®). American Medical Association; 2009.

**6.** Witmer B. *Total Body Photography: A Proven Tool for the Early Detection of Skin Cancer*. DermaTrak Skin Imaging Centers; Fairfield, NJ, USA: 2008 October.

# Psychological Responses and Coping Strategies in Skin Cancer Patients

*Nadine Angele Kasparian and Phyllis Nancy Butow*

## Key Points

- Approximately 30% of all patients diagnosed with melanoma report levels of psychological distress indicative of the need for clinical intervention.

- Psychological distress has been associated with: patient delay in seeking medical advice; decreased adherence to treatment regimens; increased rates of cancer recurrence, morbidity and mortality; lower quality of life; greater medical costs; and reduced engagement in post-treatment screening and preventive behaviors.

- Screening for symptoms of psychological distress in patients with skin cancer should be routinely implemented in clinical practice. Referring patients who have risk factors to specialized psychological services minimizes the likelihood that they will develop significant emotional distress.

## INTRODUCTION

Despite continued progress in the clinical management of malignant skin diseases, the diagnosis of skin cancer, including melanoma and non-melanoma skin cancer (NMSC), remains a difficult time in the lives of many patients and their families. The psychosocial care of a person with skin cancer begins from the time of initial diagnosis, through treatment, recovery and survival, or through the transition from curative to non-curative aims of treatment, initiation of palliative care, death and bereavement. Each patient and their family and friends will experience a range of practical, emotional, physical, and social challenges as a result of their cancer diagnosis and treatment, and these challenges may continue to have an impact on some people long after their initial diagnosis. A diagnosis of skin cancer has the potential to change many aspects of an individual's life, from self-identity, body image, self-esteem, and perceived well-being, to family roles and relationships, sexuality, career opportunities, friendships, and finances. These changes are likely to manifest differently depending on the type of skin cancer diagnosed, as well as a range of other clinical, demographic, and psychosocial factors. Patients experience shock, fear, sadness, and/or anger at the time of diagnosis, and some will also have to face progressive illness and approaching death. Psychological distress has been associated with: patient delay in seeking medical advice; decreased adherence to treatment regimens; increased rates of cancer recurrence, morbidity and mortality; lower quality of life; greater medical costs; and reduced engagement in post-treatment screening and preventive behaviors.[1,2] Understanding the range of emotional, physical and behavioral responses to skin cancer diagnosis (see Table 62.1), as well as effective and sustainable interventions to reduce distress, remain important clinical and research endeavors.

## PSYCHOLOGICAL CHALLENGES ASSOCIATED WITH EARLY-STAGE SKIN CANCERS

The fact that most skin cancers are detected early and are associated with good prognosis, coupled with the often healthy outward appearance of NMSC and early-stage melanoma patients, may contribute to the prevailing belief that such patients have 'little or nothing to worry about'.[3] Despite a good prognosis, however, early-stage melanoma patients deal with both the immediate stress of being diagnosed with a possibly life-threatening disease, as well as the threat of recurrence or systemic spread, which is greatest during the first 2 years after diagnosis but may occur within 10 years of diagnosis. Throughout the diagnostic process, patients with melanoma report significant reductions in emotional functioning and quality of life, as well as greater fatigue and sleep problems.[4] Research suggests that many patients experience the period between detection of a suspicious lesion and skin biopsy as the most stressful time in the diagnostic process, possibly indicating anxiety about the prospect of surgery.[4] Some patients experience an underlying fear of disfigurement caused by surgery, and the visibility of treatment-related scarring may form a constant reminder of the individual's cancer experience.[3] The degree of tissue loss with loss of contour as a consequence of skin grafting rather than primary closure, and the discrepancy between the actual size of a scar and pre-surgery expectations may all contribute to emotional distress.[1] With approximately 20% of melanomas and 80% of NMSCs occurring on the head and neck, disfiguration and change in bodily appearance may threaten patients' self-esteem and self-confidence,[2,5] especially in younger adults. Family, friends, and clinicians may not recognize the need for social and psychological support of seemingly high-functioning NMSC and early-stage melanoma patients (Table 62.2).

## PREVALENCE OF PSYCHOLOGICAL DISTRESS IN PATIENTS WITH SKIN CANCER

Approximately 30% of all patients diagnosed with melanoma report levels of psychological distress indicative of the need for clinical intervention, most commonly in the form of

## Table 62.1 Common Emotional, Physical and Behavioral Responses to the Diagnosis of Skin Cancer

**Emotional responses**

- Shock
- Feeling 'numb'
- Disbelief
- Fear
- Anger
- Confusion
- Uncertainty
- Sadness or depression
- Despair
- Grief
- Anxiety

**Behavioral and physical responses**

- Sleep disturbance
- Appetite changes
- Headaches
- Heart palpitations
- Social withdrawal or an increased need to be around others
- Hypervigilance with regards to sun protection and early detection, or disengagement from health behavior recommendations
- Delays in seeking treatment
- Altered interest in pleasurable activities
- Nausea
- Changes in bowel movements
- Substance use/abuse

## Table 62.2 Common Concerns Expressed by Patients With Skin Cancer[6]

- Dealing with a potentially life-threatening diagnosis
- Managing one's own emotional responses, as well as the responses of others
- Fear of death
- Uncertainty about recurrence and future risk of developing other skin cancers
- Risk of skin cancer in other members of the family
- Fear of bodily disfigurement and scarring, as well as concern about how others may respond to one's changed physical appearance
- Decision-making about clinical management
- Access to the best medical care and most up-to-date information
- Questions about what might have caused the cancer
- Fears about the potential harm caused by future sun exposure
- Impairments in physical functioning and quality of life (such as independence, mobility, activity levels)
- Change to current roles and responsibilities
- Communication to others about cancer experiences
- Social, family and relationship concerns
- Employment, insurance, legal and financial matters

Adapted from Hodgkinson K, Gilchrist J. *Psychosocial Care of Cancer Patients: A health professional's guide to what to say and do.* Melbourne: Ausmed Publications, 2008.

anxiety and/or depression with significant interference in daily life.[7-9] While anxiety and depression commonly coexist, anxiety is uniquely characterized by symptoms of excessive, pervasive and uncontrollable worry or fear, whereas depression is typified by symptoms of low mood, intense and prolonged sadness, increased irritability, social withdrawal, and diminished interest or pleasure in most activities. Gibertini et al.[8] reported that approximately one in five newly diagnosed, non-metastatic melanoma patients have some form of depression. Approximately one in four melanoma patients beginning chemotherapy report clinically relevant levels of anxiety.[10] Overall, anxiety appears to be more prevalent than depression at both the diagnostic and treatment phases, with the proportion of participants within the clinical range for anxiety and depression found to be around 23% and 11%, respectively.[4,11,12]

The proportion of patients with melanoma who report clinically significant levels of distress is equivalent to that identified in breast and colon cancer patients, and demonstrably higher than that reported by patients with gynecological or prostate cancer.[7] There is, however, substantial variability between studies in regard to the prevalence of reported anxiety and depression. Such variation may reflect important differences between study samples in terms of disease stage, time since diagnosis or treatment, involvement in clinical trials, environmental conditions (e.g. areas of high versus low exposure to ultraviolet radiation), or cultural attitudes and beliefs.

## Post-traumatic stress

Psychological responses to skin cancer can also be considered within a post-traumatic stress response framework. From this perspective, two key symptom clusters are considered critical: (a) intrusion, defined as disturbing, persistent and unwanted images, thoughts and feelings, often accompanied by autonomic arousal, hypervigilance and marked anxiety; and (b) avoidance, marked by ignoring the implications of threat, forgetting important problems, and experiencing emotional numbing. In a cross-sectional study of 95 patients with stage I to stage IV melanoma, patients with stage III disease (i.e. nodal metastasis) reported significantly greater post-traumatic stress symptoms compared to patients with stage I disease.[11] Participants with non-metastatic melanoma demonstrated an association between post-traumatic stress and prognostic indication based on tumor thickness.[11] These findings were not replicated using measures of general anxiety and depression, suggesting that post-traumatic stress responses may be more sensitive indicators of the differing psychological concerns emerging across the spectrum of skin cancer progression. Of importance to dermatologists who provide continuing surveillance of melanoma patients, 54% of patients with melanoma attending a routine follow-up appointment at a pigmented lesion clinic reported some degree of anxiety prior to their consultation, with 17% of these patients also reporting physical symptoms of anxiety such as diarrhea, nausea and sleeplessness.[13] These data highlight the need for specific skin cancer-related concerns to be examined as important dimensions of psychological morbidity.

## PSYCHOLOGICAL DISTRESS IN INDIVIDUALS WITH A STRONG FAMILY HISTORY OF SKIN CANCER

Kasparian et al.[14] examined psychological responses reported by Australians who were recently informed of the identification of a family-specific mutation in the *CDKN2A* gene. In Australia, the estimated lifetime risk of melanoma for individuals who carry a pathogenic *CDKN2A* mutation is 91%.[15] Only 1% of participants exhibited clinically relevant levels of post-traumatic stress following notification. Low levels of depressive symptoms were also reported in this cohort, while levels of anxiety were comparable to population norms. In a prospective cohort study designed to examine uptake as well as psychological and behavioral outcomes of genetic testing for melanoma risk, Kasparian et al.[16] found that compared to baseline, individuals identified as *CDKN2A* mutation carriers reported significantly reduced anxiety at 2 weeks, and reduced depression at 2 weeks and 12 months, following receipt of genetic test results. Carriers also reported a significantly greater frequency of clinical skin examination at 12-month follow-up. These data provide preliminary evidence for healthy psychological and behavioral adjustment following participation in genetic testing for melanoma risk. To our knowledge, there are no studies investigating psychological responses among those with a strong family history of NMSC, thus studies in this area would also be a valuable addition to the literature.

## VULNERABILITY FACTORS: DEMOGRAPHIC, CLINICAL, AND PSYCHOSOCIAL CORRELATES OF DISTRESS

A variety of measurable and in some cases relatively stable variables may be predictive of psychological distress in individuals affected by skin cancer (Table 62.3). These include perceptions of skin cancer as threatening, fears of the impact of cancer on the family, limited social support,

**Table 62.3 Demographic, Clinical and Psychosocial Factors Associated With Increased Vulnerability to Emotional Distress in Patients With Skin Cancer**

**Demographic factors**

- Female gender
- Younger age
- Absence of a spouse or committed partner
- Lower education
- Unemployment
- Economic adversity

**Clinical factors**

- Greater physical deterioration
- Tumors on visible parts of the body such as the face or hands
- Reduced physical quality of life

**Psychosocial factors**

- Negative beliefs about skin cancer
- Passive or avoidant coping styles
- Lack of social support
- Concerns about the implications of skin cancer for one's family

and a lack of confidence in one's ability to cope with the situation.[14,17] Subjective beliefs about skin cancer, its treatment, prognosis, and likelihood of recurrence may play a greater role in determining stress responses than the clinical characteristics of the disease, such as disease stage and time since diagnosis.[17] In NMSC, for example, psychosocial concerns tend to be less focused on mortality and disease severity and more on issues relating to disfigurement, discomfort, and illness perception.[5]

Of particular concern is the potential for distress to contribute to a downward spiral in quality of life. Trask et al.[9] found that compared to those experiencing low distress, individuals who reported high distress also reported significantly worse evaluations of current and future personal health, higher ratings of pain intensity, decreased energy ratings, and greater interference from physical and emotional problems. The presence of psychological and depressive symptoms are key predictors of poor quality of life.[18] Substantial decline in an individual's physical quality of life is another important correlate of psychological distress.[19]

## COPING SKILLS AND STRATEGIES

When faced with the diagnosis of skin cancer, each patient will draw on individual coping strategies which have helped in the past, such as specific problem-solving techniques, spiritual faith, or close connections with supportive friends or family. The multidisciplinary care team can also play a key role in strengthening the patient's own resources by providing emotional, educational and practical assistance, and by appropriately fostering a sense of hope or optimism. Coping is defined as the attitudes, beliefs and behaviors that have an adaptive purpose when one is faced with a threatening situation.[2] Thus, coping may be conceptualized as a primary mediator of the impact of stressful events on outcomes. The aims of coping are to safeguard and protect the emotional state of the individual, and to allow for psychological adjustment to aversive conditions. Overall, research suggests that patients who adopt active coping strategies demonstrate better adjustment to skin cancer,[18,20] as well as longer relapse-free periods,[21–23] compared to those who employ avoidant coping styles (see Table 62.4).

### Change in coping and support over the illness trajectory

Clearly, challenges and concerns require the coping skills and support to manage change as the disease progresses.[19,24] Patients with advanced disease face increasing symptoms and side effects of treatment, require more physical care, and face an imminent death. These patients and their families may require more support. In a longitudinal study of coping with metastatic melanoma during the last year of life, Brown et al.[24] found that as terminally ill patients moved closer to death, the use of active coping strategies such as information seeking, meditation and social support increased, despite patients experiencing increasing levels of tiredness and deterioration in mood and daily functioning ability.

| Table 62.4 Coping Styles That May be Utilized by Individuals Affected by Skin Cancer | | |
|---|---|---|
| **Coping Style** | **Description** | **Examples of possible responses** |
| Active-behavioral coping | Overt behavioral attempts to deal directly with skin cancer and its effects | • Enlisting the help and support of others<br>• Adhering to treatment and screening protocols<br>• Information seeking<br>• Use of complementary therapies *in addition to* recommended medical treatment |
| Active-cognitive coping | One's attitudes, beliefs and thoughts about skin cancer | • Accepting the reality of one's illness<br>• Forming realistic expectations and beliefs<br>• Creating time and space to think about one's experiences and the cancer-related information provided |
| Avoidance coping | Attempts to actively avoid the problem or indirectly reduce emotional tension through the use of distraction | • Denial of the diagnosis or the need for treatment<br>• Disengagement from treatment or screening regimens<br>• Substance use or abuse |

## PSYCHOLOGICAL SUPPORT FOR PATIENTS WITH SKIN CANCER

Clinical practice guidelines for the management of melanoma consistently recommend that structured psychosocial interventions and psycho-education be made available to all patients.[25] Broadly, there are three major approaches to psychotherapy with cancer patients: (1) educational techniques; (2) behavioral or skills training; (3) psychotherapy. A supportive care program for patients with skin cancer may feature one or a combination of these approaches and may be tailored to the specific needs of the individual and his or her family. Within these approaches, patients may be offered variations on psychotherapeutic modalities, such as psychodynamic, existential, cognitive-behavioral, supportive-expressive, relaxation, and dialectical behavioral therapies, or approaches that use visualization and guided imagery. Psychosocial support may also be delivered through a variety of modalities, including face-to-face interaction, written materials, web-based or multimedia resources, or telephone-based therapy. Although these varied interventions reflect significant differences in theory and how they are translated into practice, their common goal is to help cancer patients to adjust physically, emotionally, and psychologically to the disease and its treatment.

Five randomized controlled trials (RCT) have been conducted evaluating psychological interventions for patients with melanoma.[20,22,26–30] All of these studies have produced evidence that psychological interventions can improve psychosocial outcomes for melanoma patients, including reductions in general mood disturbance, depression and anxiety. To our knowledge, there are no data on the efficacy of psychological interventions in reducing psychological morbidity and unmet needs in patients with non-melanoma skin cancer.

## COST-EFFECTIVENESS OF PSYCHOSOCIAL INTERVENTIONS

As evidence for the clinical effectiveness of psychological programs continues to grow, studies evaluating the fiscal cost associated with providing supportive care are also necessary to allow for adequate allocation of limited resources. Bares et al.[29] conducted a small RCT of cognitive-behavioral therapy (CBT) for patients with heterogeneous melanomas who were reporting clinically significant levels of distress. CBT was found to be marginally more expensive (49c per minute) than the cost to nursing staff of dealing with distress-driven telephone calls during standard care (41c per minute). However, the cost/benefit ratio (total costs/change in distress) was significantly lower for CBT. The cost to change distress in standard care was >$402 for a one-point change in distress, versus $7.66 for CBT. Including reimbursement for service in the analysis, CBT would generate $1.16 per minute while standard care would cost the hospital $0.40. Thus, CBT was found to be cost-effective.

## COMMUNICATION SKILLS AND STRATEGIES

Qualitative data support a model of psychological intervention in the cancer care setting that takes into consideration patients' needs for a safe place to explore and express their feelings and concerns with a caring professional who can listen attentively and try to understand.[31] When asked, melanoma patients themselves place greatest emphasis on the relational qualities of the therapeutic process (e.g. a sense of emotional connection to someone outside the family whom they trust and with whom they can communicate openly), as opposed to technical, therapy-specific factors.[31] These relational skills or qualities are possessed and can be exercised by all health professionals in a multidisciplinary team as they interact with patients on a daily basis in clinical practice.

The ability of clinicians to communicate with, and relate to, patients and their family is central to optimal cancer care and professional satisfaction. Communication practices at the time of melanoma diagnosis are significantly related to anxiety, depression, and satisfaction with care 13 months later.[32] Further, careful use of strategies to communicate information clearly (such as summarizing, and categorizing information) improves patient recall (Table 62.5).[33] Clearly, sensitivity to the particular needs and emotional experiences of each patient is required, as well as an awareness of issues relating to gender, age, culture, education and socioeconomic status.

## Table 62.5 Interactional Skills and Communication Strategies to Reduce Psychosocial Morbidity and Unmet Needs in Patients With Skin Cancer

- Open and sensitive discussion of the diagnosis, prognosis and life expectancy, as well as how the cancer might affect other aspects of the patient's life
- Use of verbal and non-verbal cues to show empathy and emotional support
- Discussion of the patient's feelings and concerns
- Active listening
- Face-to-face communication in a quiet and private environment
- Allowing time and space for reflection and questions
- Encouraging the patient to be involved in treatment decisions
- Full and clear explanation of all medical terms used
- Checks of the patient's understanding and recall of the information
- Sensitivity to the person's age and cultural background
- Having the people wanted by the patient present in the consultation
- Provision of information about what a patient is likely to experience before, during and after a procedure
- Use of simple diagrams and pictures where appropriate
- Provision of written information 'summarizing' the consultation
- Use of a 'question prompt sheet' to help patients ask relevant and important questions

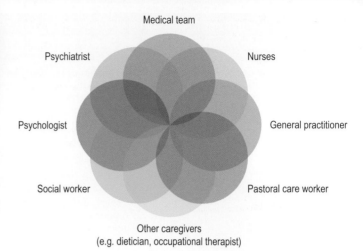

Figure 62.1 Transdisciplinary practice model in the provision of optimal psychosocial care to patients with skin cancer.

## CURRENT CARE AND FUTURE DIRECTIONS

According to the National Institutes of Health in the United States, some of the most basic psychological and social issues affecting cancer patients are not adequately addressed in the clinical setting.[34] All patients with skin cancer who show emotional distress, low social support or tumor-related difficulties in various aspects of daily life should be offered psychological support, irrespective of whether they meet the criteria for psychiatric disorder.[34] Routine psychological screening of patients with melanoma is widely recommended as standard practice in many countries, including Australia, the United States, and the United Kingdom; however, a sensitive brief screening tool for clinical use does not currently exist.[25]

Patients might benefit from increased emotional support and information at the time of initial presentation at a pigmented lesion clinic (prior to biopsy), as the uncertainty associated with this period has been recognized as particularly stressful for some patients.[4] People with skin cancer (and their families and caregivers) may not voice their concerns or even recognize them; often these must be carefully and thoughtfully elicited. Each member of the multidisciplinary treatment team, as well as the person's general practitioner and their family, friends and caregivers, can contribute unique as well as overlapping skills to enhance the psychosocial care of the person with skin cancer (Fig. 62.1).

While a patient-centered approach and empathic communication from the healthcare team can greatly assist patients and their families, recognition and understanding of the emotional issues for health professionals working in this field is also vital. Cancer specialists are at risk of burnout because of the nature of their work, with 28–56% reportedly suffering at least one episode of burnout in their career.[35,36] The development of strategies to address these concerns is

a process likely to lead to improved therapeutic relationships and enhanced professional and patient satisfaction. Other recommendations for the improvement of clinical practice are provided in Table 62.6.

## FUTURE OUTLOOK

There is a need for the development and trial of appropriate, evidence-based psycho-educational resources in a range of formats (e.g. printed, web-based, audiovisual).[4] The planning and development of such resources will include input from clinicians, researchers, patients and their caregivers to ensure that important topics and areas of concern are adequately addressed, as well as to maximize the effective communication of health messages.

## Table 62.6 Summary of Evidence-Based Recommendations for the Psychosocial Care of Patients With Skin Cancer

### Clinical practice recommendations

- Screening for symptoms of psychological distress in patients with skin cancer should be routinely implemented in clinical practice. Referring patients who have risk factors to specialized psychological services minimizes the likelihood of their developing significant emotional distress.
- Clinicians need to consider the increased risk status associated with particular demographic factors. These factors may influence susceptibility to distress, irrespective of patients' medical status or prognosis. The treatment team also needs to be aware that the psychosocial needs of men and women may vary both in extent and how they are expressed. Successful strategies for meeting psychosocial support needs may therefore differ for men and women.
- Access to psychological support should not be limited to patients with poor prognosis. Specialized supportive care should be made available to those experiencing emotional distress or tumor-related difficulties.
- It is essential to ascertain the extent of support available to the patient, to recommend additional support as required, and to provide information about where support is available. A range of therapies, are efficacious in reducing symptoms of psychological distress.

# REFERENCES

1. Cassileth BR, Lusk EJ, Tenaglia AN. Patients' perceptions of the cosmetic impact of melanoma resection. *Plast Reconstr Surg*. 1983;71(1):73–75.
2. Kneier AW. Coping with melanoma: ten strategies that promote psychological adjustment. *Surg Clin North Am*. 2003;83(2):417–430.
3. Sollner W, Zingg-Schir M, Rumpold G, et al. Need for supportive counselling – the professionals' versus the patients' perspective. A survey in a representative sample of 236 melanoma patients. *Psychother Psychosom*. 1998;67(2):94–104.
4. Al-Shakhli H, Harcourt D, Kenealy J. Psychological distress surrounding diagnosis of malignant and nonmalignant skin lesions at a pigmented lesion clinic. *J Plast Reconstr Aesthet Surg*. 2006;59(5):479–486.
5. Rhee JS, Loberiza FR, Matthews BA, et al. Quality of life assessment in non-melanoma cervicofacial skin cancer. *Laryngoscope*. 2003;113(2):215–220.
6. Hodgkinson K, Gilchrist J. *Psychosocial Care of Cancer Patients: A Health Professional's Guide to What to Say and Do*. Melbourne: Ausmed Publications; 2008.
7. Zabora J, Brintzenhofeszoc K, Curbow B, et al. The prevalence of psychological distress by cancer site. *Psycho-Oncol*. 2001;10(1):19–28.
8. Gibertini M, Reintgen DS, Baile WF. Psychosocial aspects of melanoma. *Ann Plast Surg*. 1992;28(1):17–21.
9. Trask PC, Paterson AG, Hayasaka S. Psychosocial characteristics of individuals with non-stage IV melanoma. *J Clin Oncol*. 2001;19(11):2844–2850.
10. Sigurdardottir V, Bolund C, Brandberg Y, et al. The impact of generalized malignant melanoma on quality of life evaluated by the EORTC questionnaire technique. *Qual Life Res*. 1993;2(3):193–203.
11. Kelly B, Raphael B, Smithers M, et al. Psychological responses to malignant melanoma. An investigation of traumatic stress reactions to life-threatening illness. *Gen Hosp Psychiatry*. 1995;17(2):126–134.
12. Brandberg Y, Bolund C, Sigurdardottir V, et al. Anxiety and depressive symptoms at different stages of malignant melanoma. *Psycho-Oncol*. 1992;1(2):71–78.
13. Baughan CA, Hall VL, Leppard BJ, et al. Follow-up in stage I cutaneous malignant melanoma: an audit. *Clinical Oncol*. 1993;5(3):174–180.
14. Kasparian N, Meiser B, Butow PN, et al. Predictors of psychological distress among individuals with a strong family history of malignant melanoma. *Clin Genet*. 2008;73:121–131.
15. Bishop D, Demenais F, Goldstein AM, et al. Geographical variation in the penetrance of CDKN2A mutations for melanoma. *J Natl Cancer Inst*. 2002;94:894–903.
16. Kasparian N, Meiser B, Butow PN, et al. Genetic testing for melanoma risk: a prospective cohort study of uptake and outcomes among Australian families. *Genet Med*. 2009;11(4):265–278.
17. Hamama-Raz Y, Solomon Z, Schachter J, et al. Objective and subjective stressors and the psychological adjustment of melanoma survivors. *Psycho-Oncol*. 2007;16:287–294.
18. Lehto US, Ojanen M, Kellokumpu-Lehtinen P. Predictors of quality of life in newly diagnosed melanoma and breast cancer patients. *Ann Oncol*. 2005;16(5):805–816.
19. Holland JC, Passik S, Kash KM, et al. The role of religious and spiritual beliefs in coping with malignant melanoma. *Psycho-Oncol*. 1999;8(1):14–26.
20. Fawzy FI, Cousins N, Fawzy NW, et al. A structured psychiatric intervention for cancer patients: I. Changes over time and methods of coping in affect of disturbance. *Arch Gen Psychiatry*. 1990;47:720–725.
21. Rogentine Jr GN, van Kammen DP, Fox BH, et al. Psychological factors in the prognosis of malignant melanoma: a prospective study. *Psychosom Med*. 1979;41(8):647–655.
22. Fawzy F, Fawzy N, Hyun CS, et al. Malignant melanoma: effects of an early structured psychiatric intervention, coping, and affective state on recurrence and survival 6 years later. *Arch Gen Psychiatry*. 1993;50(9):681–689.
23. Brown JE, Butow PN, Culjak G, et al. Psychosocial predictors of outcome: time to relapse and survival in patients with early stage melanoma. *Br J Cancer*. 2000;83(11):1448–1453.
24. Brown J, Brown R, Miller RM, et al. Coping with metastatic melanoma: the last year of life. *Psycho-Oncol*. 2000;9:283–292.
25. Australian Cancer Network. *Clinical Practice Guidelines for the Management of Melanoma in Australia and New Zealand*. Canberra, NSW: National Health and Medical Research Council (NHMRC); 2008.
26. Fawzy FI, Kemeny ME, Fawzy NW, et al. A structured psychiatric intervention for cancer patients. II. Changes over time in immunological measures. *Arch Gen Psychiatry*. 1990;47(8):729–735.
27. Boesen EH, Ross L, Frederiksen K, et al. Psycho-educational intervention for patients with cutaneous malignant melanoma: a replication study. *J Clin Oncol*. 2005;23(6):1270–1277.
28. Fawzy NW. A psycho-educational nursing intervention to enhance coping and affective state in newly diagnosed malignant melanoma patients. *Cancer Nurs*. 1995;18(6):427–438.
29. Bares CB, Trask PC, Schwartz SM. An exercise in cost-effectiveness analysis: treating emotional distress in melanoma patients. *J Clin Psycho. Med Settings*. 2002;9(3):193–200.
30. Trask PC, Paterson AG, Griffith KA, et al. Cognitive-behavioral intervention for distress in patients with melanoma: comparison with standard medical care and impact on quality of life. *Cancer*. 2003;98(4):854–864.
31. MacCormack J, Simonian, Lim J, et al. 'Someone who cares': a qualitative investigation of cancer patients' experiences of psychotherapy. *Psycho-Oncol*. 2001;10:52–65.
32. Schofield PE, Butow PN, Thompson JF, et al. Psychological responses of patients receiving a diagnosis of cancer. *Ann Oncol*. 2003;14(1):48–56.
33. Ley P, Whitworth MA, Skilbeck CE, et al. Improving doctor-patient communication in general practice. *J R Coll Gen Pract*. 1976;26(171):720–724.
34. Institute of Medicine. 10-point plan for more comprehensive cancer care. *CA Cancer J Clin*. 2008;58:67–68.
35. Whippen D, Canellos G. Burnout syndrome in the practice of oncology: results of a random survey of 1000 oncologists. *J Clin Oncol*. 1991;9:1916–1920.
36. Ramirez A, Graham J, Richards MA, et al. Burnout and psychiatric disorder amongst cancer clinicians. *Br J Cancer*. 1995;71(6):1263–1269.

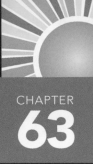

# Medical and Legal Aspects of Skin Cancer Patients

*Abel Torres, Clay Cockerell, Jamison Strahan, and Tanya Nino*

## Key Points

- When practicing innovative therapy for skin cancer treatment, consider which reputable similarly situated skin cancer specialists would support that particular treatment as expert witnesses.

- When a complication occurs during skin cancer treatment, maintaining the patient's trust is the key to successful patient care and is helped by availability and close communication between the dermatologist, the patient, and significant others.

- Enhanced communication between skin cancer specialists and patients can mitigate malpractice pursuit.

- Avoid discussing and making premature conclusions regarding an adverse event/complication in skin cancer care until all the facts are clear.

## INTRODUCTION

As the field of medicine evolves, awareness of the rights and responsibilities of physicians and patients is critically important to healthcare delivery. For the most part, those rights and responsibilities parallel good patient care. Yet, the current medicolegal environment in the United States has created a malpractice climate that is causing doctors to limit the care they provide to patients and sometimes leave the practice of medicine altogether.[1] With an ever-increasing demand for documentation, some providers fall into a habit of practicing defensive medicine, focusing more on what is said than what is done. This approach compromises patient care.[1]

While politics will determine part of the outcome of the current malpractice crisis, dermatologists can effect positive change by better understanding the legal issues involved and managing them appropriately to provide good patient care, minimize malpractice exposure, and avoid having to limit care. This chapter will explore these areas.

It is important to point out that the legal responsibilities of patients and physicians are governed by Federal and State laws and may vary from state to state. Therefore, this chapter is not a substitute for the advice of an attorney when potential or actual medicolegal issues arise.

## MEDICAL MALPRACTICE

One in five dermatologists will face a medical malpractice claim in their career; however, 35% of the claims are either dropped or dismissed in favor of the physician.[2,3] According to an analysis conducted on 78,712 malpractice cases, improper medical performance accounted for one-third of all claims, and the second most common medical misadventure claim was for 'errors in diagnosis'.[2,3] A significant number of claims against dermatologists are related to conditions and procedures dealing with skin cancer management and surgical procedures.[3] Lydiatt performed lawsuit analysis on 99 cases of medical malpractice involving skin cancers.[4] His results are summarized in Figure 63.1.

Regardless of validity, the pursuance of malpractice by a patient requires considerable time and resources from the physician; thus, the astute provider must become familiar with basic malpractice law to minimize the initiation of lawsuits. This section discusses medical malpractice as it relates to the Tort Law of Negligence, which compensates individuals for the losses they suffer due to the unreasonable acts of another person. Negligence is the result of a breach of a duty from the standard of care resulting in harm to another person.[5] In order for a physician to be held liable for negligence, four elements must be satisfied (Table 63.1).

## Duty

How is duty established? Consider Example 1:

### Example 1

You, the skin cancer physician, are at a weekend birthday party when you are approached by another attendee who casually asks you to evaluate a 'funny mole' on his forearm. He asserts that if you can just tell him the mole is okay, then you would save him the hassle of going to the doctor's office, and it would assuage his wife's worries. He shows you the mole, which appears clinically to represent a benign nevus.

The above situation is all too familiar to physicians. A duty to a given patient will generally exist when the physician–patient relationship is established. This usually requires some form of interaction with the patient, which can even consist of gratuitous advice or service, and can even lack physical contact.[6-8] Some may consider the providing of advice to the friend in Example 1 to establish a duty. Therefore, an example of an appropriate response in the above situation would be to confirm the benign-appearing features of this mole, but let the patient know that your assessment is limited by suboptimal lighting, and this mole would be better evaluated in the clinic, where you can perform a full history and physical examination, under proper lighting. This would meet the physician's social obligation

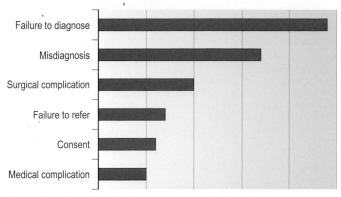

**Figure 63.1** Proportion of skin cancer lawsuits by allegation.

| Table 63.1 Elements of Negligence |
| --- |
| • Duty<br>• Breach of duty<br>• Causation<br>• Damage |

while putting the patient on notice that (s)he should not reasonably solely rely on this interaction.

Duty may also be manifest by a patient simply having an appointment with a physician. Thus, it would be legally prudent for a dermatologist to follow up on appointments missed by patients, especially where the physician is the only one capable of providing the service.

The scope of a physician's duty is usually held to the standard of others in the 'community' in which (s)he practices; however, the boundaries of the community have become blurred by advances in communication technologies.[9,10] It is also important to recognize that physicians are held to the standard of specialists when specialty care is given. If a physician performs a procedure traditionally performed by a specialist, the physician will likely be held to the standard of that specialty.[11]

## Breach of duty

Breach of a duty by a physician requires deviation from the standard of care.[5,9,10] Expert testimony is the main determination for the standard of care. Furthermore, the standard of care is subject to constant change; thus, healthcare providers have a vested interest to keep up to date with evidence-based medicine and current treatments as they evolve.

The community in which one practices influences the standard of care. For example, skin cancer specialists may disagree on the extent of the skin examination required for patients. While some specialists advocate that a full body examination is essential for every patient, others contend this is excessive for the patient presenting with a single benign lesion on the face, and places increasing economic strain on healthcare delivery. If full body skin checks are held to be the standard of care in a particular community, then dermatologists in that community who do not offer this to their patients may fail to meet the standard of care in a court of law, depending on the circumstances.

In the era of evidence-based medicine, the right thing to do for a patient may become less clear. Consider the following real-life example of a lawsuit described in the January 7, 2004 issue of *JAMA* (Example 2):

### Example 2

A physician and residency program were successfully sued for not following the standard of care of the local community despite the disagreement with evidence basis. The patient was seen for routine evaluation and prostate cancer screening was discussed. Given the uncertainty of PSA (prostate-specific antigen) screening, including a high false-positive rate and significant risk to pursuance of procedures in the event of a positive screen, the patient elected not to have this performed. The patient was found to have an aggressive prostate cancer some time after this encounter and he sued this physician for not performing the PSA screen. While the defense argued evidence basis for not screening, including recommendations from the American Academy of Family Physicians, American Urologic Association and American Cancer Society endorsing the physician's approach, the patient ultimately was awarded $1 million because the standard of care of the local community was to perform PSA screening unilaterally without patient input.

This case exemplifies the need for caution when pursuing evidence-based medicine as well as following national guidelines that do not parallel local medical practice. When considering what is the right thing to do, the patient's best interest should come first. Defensive medicine should not dictate a specialist's care, but it should be noted that, should a malpractice suit ensue, it may be easier to find supportive expert witnesses when the specialist conforms to the majority path.

If one is practicing a form of innovative therapy followed by only a few practitioners, finding supportive expert witnesses may be more difficult. The wise practitioner would ensure that the innovative skin cancer approach (s)he uses has been adopted by at least some other reputable practitioners in the community who can be called upon as experts if the need arises.

## Damages

The patient must prove damages have been sustained in order for the physician to be held liable for medical malpractice. This is true even if there was a breach of the duty of care that was the cause of the injury. See Example 3:

### Example 3

Prior to performing a shave biopsy, a practitioner mistakenly injects triamcinolone instead of lidocaine into the biopsy site. He then injects lidocaine into the biopsy site to ensure adequate local anesthesia. He peforms the biopsy without any procedural or post-procedure complications.

In this example, no harm has been suffered by the patient so there is no negligence.

Damage does not necessarily have to be physical, such as a scar; it can be psychological, such as anxiety, depression, and even fear of contracting a disease. Skin cancer is a condition often fraught with many anxieties, fears and misunderstandings. By communicating carefully with patients and addressing their anxieties and fears regarding skin cancer, the astute practitioner provides good patient care while at the same time pre-empting possible legal damages.

Even if a physician is found to be negligent, a malpractice judgment against the physician may be reduced or even nullified if the patient is shown to help cause the injury or not attempt to mitigate the damage him/herself. For example, in skin cancer surgery, postoperative cosmetic and functional outcome is highly dependent on appropriate wound care by the patient. Proper patient education on wound care techniques may help improve the patient's outcome and satisfaction.[12] If a patient does not advise the provider that there is a problem, or fails to follow physician instructions, (s)he may be held accountable for his/her non-compliance.

## Causation

Even if there is a breach of duty by the dermatologist, it only becomes medical negligence if the patient-plaintiff can establish that (s)he was actually damaged (injured) and there was a foreseeable and actual causal link between the breach of the standard of care and the injury to the patient.[13,14] This is where the jury comes in. The jury decides if and how much of a link there was between a physician's breach of standard of care and the patient injury.

### CONSENT/REFUSAL FOR TREATMENT

Obtaining consent for treatment allows patients to participate in decisions regarding their healthcare. A defective or absent consent process is a frequent cause of litigation.[15] Engaging in a consent process is particularly important in the provision of skin cancer care, given the degree of risk from procedures. Consent may be implied, such as performing a simple physical examination in clinic. However, in more complex circumstances and sometimes when examining sensitive areas, relying on implied consent can be risky, since the burden will generally rest on the physician to prove that the patient's conduct implied consent.

### Informed consent

Obtaining informed consent may avoid litigation associated with skin cancer treatment.[16] Whenever possible, patient consent should be documented. Studies show that patients remember only a fraction of what is told to them, with just 35% to 55% information retention after 1 week.[4] For these reasons, written consent and/or documentation of verbal consent provides better evidence, should the veracity of consent be at issue. The advantage of a written consent is that it ensures a framework for addressing the important information, allows for better patient understanding, and constitutes a record in the patient's chart for later documentation.

Informed consent must include the following three elements:

- discussion of the nature of the procedure or treatment, including risks, benefits and alternatives

| Table 63.2 Checklist for Informed Consent/Refusal Requirements |
| --- |
| • Competent adult or authorized decision maker<br>• Common, even if not serious, risks<br>• Uncommon but serious risks<br>• Less need to discuss common knowledge or unlikely, non-material risks<br>• Benefits of a procedure<br>• Alternatives to the given procedure |

- assessment of patient understanding
- acceptance or refusal of the intervention by the patient.

Informed consent and refusal take on special importance in the treatment of skin cancer, since there are so many modalities for treating these neoplasms. Patients should be informed of the diagnosis or potential diagnosis, its progression if untreated, the recommended treatment along with potential benefits and risks, and the alternative viable treatments including their potential benefits and risks.[17] Also, patients may benefit from the opportunity to ask questions and should indicate understanding of the procedure at hand and significant consequences if they refuse. Table 63.2 is a checklist for informed consent.

## MEDICAL RECORDS

Since medical records are the primary credible evidence available in a legal situation,[18] their completeness and accuracy is important not only for patient care, but also for malpractice defense. Table 63.3 shows a checklist for medical record keeping.

The preferred approach by these authors is to maximize the patient's chart use for patient care purposes by recording a brief note in the patient's chart that reflects that the risks (R), benefits (B) and alternatives (A) of a particular diagnosis and/or treatment plan were discussed with the patient and that consent to (or refusal of) treatment was obtained. To avoid the implication that this is a perfunctory note, the authors generally advocate that the brief note indicate that issues particularly relevant to the patient were discussed (see Example 4).

| Example 4 |
| --- |
| A patient with Fitzpatrick type V skin presents for removal of a small congenital mole on the upper chest. After significant discussion of all the issues, you document your discourse in the chart as follows, 'R,B,A, of surgical excision were discussed with the patient, with emphasis on this patient's high risk of scarring and/or pigmentary changes.' |

## ADVERSE EVENTS AND COMPLICATIONS IN SKIN CANCER TREATMENT

In the course of skin cancer treatment, complications are inevitable. However, not all complications lead to an adverse event resulting in patient dissatisfaction and subsequent litigation.[19] The management of a clinical/surgical complication requires that the physician approach the event with an attempt to restore the desired initial clinical outcome and curb any activation of the legal process.

## Table 63.3 Checklist for medical record keeping

- Should be complete but concise
- Avoid self-serving or disapproving comments
- Should be consistent (avoid long notes in response to risk management unless needed for the patient since this may herald unwanted suspicion)
- Describe the facts and make conclusions when essential for patient care (e.g. 'wound separation', but avoid premature conclusion as to why unless pertinent)
- Alter records only if essential for patient care by lining out items, initialing and dating the change or when possible entering a new note that refers to the correction without altering the initial entry
- Only release copy of records after receiving proper authorization and according to HIPAA guidelines
- Consider keeping billing records separate from patient care records
- Always document from a patient care perspective (e.g. if documenting a threat, explain the potential effect on physician–patient relationship, etc.)

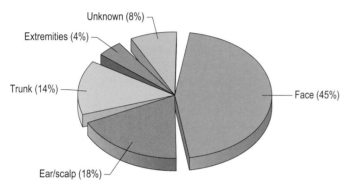

**Figure 63.2** Skin cancer sites in malpractice lawsuits.

Lydiatt performed a lawsuit analysis showing that surgical and medical complications comprised almost 30% of all lawsuits against physicians for skin cancer.[4] Of these complications, tumors originating on the face resulted in the most malpractice claims (Fig. 63.2). Thus, skin cancer care providers should be aware that complications are a potential source of litigation, particularly when they occur on the head and neck.

## Trust building

Erosion of trust can impede patient care and result in litigation.[20] Table 63.4 outlines practice pearls to establishing trust.

## Table 63.4 Practice pearls to mitigate legal risk after a complication

- Maintain honesty with patient
- Show kindness and concern at each encounter
- Validate patient's emotions about complications without conveying blame
- Avoid isolating patient after complication
- Have a remedy planned for the complication
- See patient frequently

In 1996, a survey of patients' attitudes towards physicians' mistakes was published in the *Archives of Internal Medicine*.[21] The survey interviewed 149 responding patients, randomly chosen from among 10,000 patients seen at Loma Linda University Medical Center, a Health Sciences University Medical Center and medical school located in Loma Linda, California. The patients were presented with three hypothetical scenarios of a minor, moderate, and severe mistake made by a doctor. The survey revealed that patients want physicians to acknowledge their mistakes no matter how minor, but would still lose some measure of trust in their physician with this disclosure. Discovery of a mistake by a patient in a physician who failed to disclose was even more damaging, and was more likely to lead the patient to sue or report the doctor. Thus, it is clear that patients value honesty in their interactions with doctors, and physicians would do well to keep honesty foremost as a guide to their actions when dealing with adverse events.

## Remedying an adverse event

It goes without saying that when an adverse event occurs, the clinician needs to take action to minimize the impact of that adverse event on the desired clinical outcome. Empathy with patients' distress is productive in that it communicates concern for their well-being. On the other hand, expressing remorse when the facts have not been fully sorted out may lead to patient distrust and hinder patient care. Physicians should also avoid active problem solving (i.e. differential diagnoses of what went wrong) in the presence of the patient, as persons with a lay background could misunderstand it and possibly interpret this as incompetence.

One of the most important productive positive measures is to make sure that the patient's medical needs are appropriately addressed, including referral for consultations as needed. Putting off a referral is a negative measure that could force the patient to 'shop around' for help, potentially turning to ill-suited physicians to manage his/her complication. Once a patient seeks care elsewhere, his/her new provider may describe your action unfavorably. Comments by other healthcare providers have been documented to be a frequent source for undermining the physician–patient trust and initiating litigation.[19]

## Medical devices

It is conceivable that an adverse event can be the result of a defective device (e.g. lasers). Therefore, advice from a manufacturer or vendor regarding the device should be sought if a complication occurs, but the device used should not be returned until its defect or lack of defect has been properly evaluated and documented in a medical record. A manufacturer may be subject to strict product liability for its devices, which can ease the litigation burden for the provider.[22]

## Communication

Effective communication enhances physician–patient relationships and protects physicians from malpractice litigation.[23] In communicating with a dissatisfied patient (or family member), the discussion should center on factual issues, clearing up misperceptions and clarifying the course of action that will be taken. Premature opinions by the physician should be avoided, and any theories by the patient and his/her family should be acknowledged with the clarification that further data will be gathered and all possibilities explored. Validating a patient's emotion about a given complication without implying culpability is an ideal interaction (see Example 5).

### Example 5

A patient returns with a painful keloid on the back after a skin cancer resection. She is a swimmer and states the wound opened up after a swimming competition 1 week following the surgery. She is tearful and complaining of how horrible the scar looks. An appropriate response would be, 'It's terrible that this happened to you. While thickened scarring sometimes develops, we are always hopeful that this does not occur. I understand how concerned you are about the appearance. We will initiate a scar treatment regimen immediately to improve the look and decrease your pain.' The clinician should note the discussion and temporal relationship between the keloid and the patient's swimming activity and her lack of compliance with instructions if that occurred.

In our haste to communicate honestly with the patient, we must not forget that patients have a right to privacy.[24] HIPAA rules underscore the need to protect confidentiality.[25] Thus, prior to initiating any communication with a patient's family, a physician should procure the patient's consent for this action, with documentation in writing as required by law.

Table 63.5 summarizes the physician's approach to dealing with medicolegal complications.

While the mnemonic in Table 63.5 is an excellent one to remember and recite as a mantra to recall the proper actions to take when a complication occurs, some physicians may find the mnemonic in Table 63.6 to be easier to use. While not as comprehensive, it can still be very helpful.

## SPECIAL MEDICOLEGAL ISSUES IN SKIN CANCER TREATMENT (DERMATOPATHOLOGY)

Although the risk of medicolegal liability in dermatology is limited compared to other specialties, the risk of liability is greatly increased in dermatopathology for the pathologist

### Table 63.5 'Complications' Mnemonic

| C | Be candid, commiserate, acknowledge the complaint |
|---|---|
| O | Discuss facts, not opinion |
| M | Mitigate, address medical needs |
| P | Take positive, not negative, measures |
| L | Accept responsibility, not liability |
| I | Investigate fully |
| C | Clarify, not criticize, and consult |
| A | Accessibility should be facilitated |
| T | Truth leads to trust |
| I | Inform carrier |
| O | Organize meeting to outline risks, benefits and alternatives with patient and significant others respecting HIPAA |
| N | Note and document, not alter the record |
| S | Save evidence, and sincerity above all |

### Table 63.6 'AAA' Mnemonic

| A | Always acknowledge any complaint and express sympathy |
|---|---|
| A | Make sure you or someone you designate is easily 'a'ccessible to the patient making a complaint |
| A | Avoid premature conclusions or comments |

or the dermatologist interpreting his or her own biopsy slides. Dermatologists may also be at risk even when they do not read their own slides.

The most common dermatopathology sources for medicolegal liability are listed in Table 63.7.

1) **Label the biopsy specimen bottle properly and make sure the biopsy specimen is in the formalin in the specimen bottle.**
2) **Fill out the dermatopathology requisition slip appropriately and consider including photographs.**

For biopsies of pigmented lesions, it is helpful to include the age of the patient, location, size of the lesion, and clinical diagnosis and description, including history of previous biopsy, as well as any history of change. If dermoscopy has been performed, include a clinical impression based on dermoscopic evaluation.

The age of the patient is a very important consideration when making a diagnosis of a melanocytic lesion. Melanoma is extremely rare in children, but there are lesions that do occur in children that may simulate melanoma and lead to misdiagnosis. Two of these are congenital nevi biopsied within the first few years of life and Spitz nevi. A 'spitzoid' lesion in an adult is much more likely to represent mela-

### Table 63.7 Common Sources of Medicolegal Liability for Dermatologists as Related to Dermatopathology

- Misdiagnosis of melanocytic neoplasms
- Over-diagnosis and over-aggressive treatment of benign lesions
- Misdiagnosis of non-melanoma skin cancer
- Misdiagnosis of inflammatory skin diseases
- Dermatopathologist renders erroneous diagnosis; claim made against dermatologist secondarily
- Recommendation made to perform additional procedure by dermatopathologist; dermatologist fails to follow recommendation and bad outcome ensues
- Failure of communication between dermatopathologist and dermatologist (i.e. lack of or insufficient clinical information provided)
- Failure to question histologic diagnosis when it does not correlate clinically
- Dermatologist performing histologic interpretation of his or her own biopsies is biased by clinical appearance and gives inaccurate histologic diagnosis
- Dermatologist performing histologic interpretation of his or her own biopsies fails to request second expert opinion in difficult cases
- Dermatologist mandated to submit specimens to laboratory with minimal expertise in dermatopathology
- Vicarious liability for dermatologist with ownership interest in dermatopathology laboratory that renders an erroneous diagnosis
- Vicarious liability for dermatologist who delegates responsibility for office visits and/or procedures to physician extenders who improperly submit a specimen

noma than a benign lesion.[26] Conversely, a 'spitzoid' lesion in a child is more likely to be a Spitz nevus, unless virtually every feature of melanoma is present.

### 3) Ensure that all biopsies performed are representative of the process in question.

The best biopsy is one that provides representative material of the skin disease in question. For inflammatory conditions, take biopsies of the most characteristic lesion, and consider taking more than one biopsy, especially if it is an unusual process or one that exhibits several morphologies. For neoplasms, biopsy the entire lesion or a significant portion of the lesion. Accurate diagnosis of skin neoplasms, especially melanocytic neoplasms, depends on assessment of architectural features, including breadth, symmetry and circumscription, as well as cytologic features.

The National Comprehensive Cancer Network (NCCN) 2009 guidelines recommend excisional biopsy with 1–3 mm margins for melanoma. Per NCCN guidelines, incisional biopsy of the thickest aspect of the lesion is acceptable in certain 'difficult' anatomic areas, including the palms, soles, digits, face and ears, and for large melanomas. However, these guidelines are of limited use to dermatologists because many times, the dermatologist does not know with certainty if the lesion is a melanoma. A biopsy is performed to obtain the diagnosis.[27] Multiple studies have shown that the sensitivity of clinical diagnosis of melanoma is only about 70%.[28] The vast majority of melanocytic neoplasms that are biopsied are benign, and it would be excessive to perform excisional biopsies on all of these lesions. Broad saucerization and incisional biopsies are acceptable alternatives to excision for pigmented lesions that are thought to be benign, such as nevi and lentigines, but have a low likelihood of being melanoma.

It is often stated that for broad pigmented lesions, a punch taken from the darkest or thickest area is a reasonable biopsy to perform when attempting to establish the diagnosis of melanoma. This recommendation is flawed. It is especially problematic when dealing with melanoma in situ, especially on sun-exposed sites. In 2005, Dalton reported that almost 50% of 147 melanomas in situ had contiguous benign pigmented lesions, primarily solar lentigines and pigmented solar keratoses.[29] Darkest areas do not always correlate with malignancy, as nevi may produce more melanin in some cases than melanoma, and areas of hemorrhage into the cornified layer commonly appear jet black. A broad, thin shave gives the pathologist a large and representative area of epidermis to evaluate and does not disfigure the patient (Fig. 63.3).

In addition, punch biopsy of broad melanocytic neoplasms can lead to 'biopsy sculpture' (Fig. 63.4). This refers to the punch producing an artifactually benign appearance. The sampled portion may appear relatively small and symmetric. Melanomas can be 'sculpted' by this method to appear benign when in truth they are not. While multiple punches of the same lesion are better that a single punch, this technique is also suboptimal as it does not allow for assessment of architecture. Some clinicians perform superficial curettage biopsy. These superficial curettage specimens, which barely sample the undersurface of the epidermis and are often fragmented, are extremely diffi-

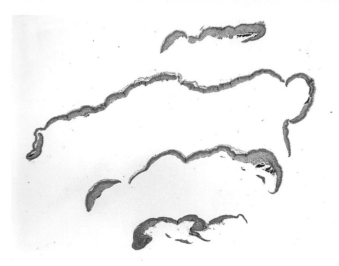

**Figure 63.3** Example of broad shave biopsy – pathologists prefer these types of biopsies when the clinician wants to rule out a diagnosis of lentigo maligna. Punch biopsies, in contrast, are more likely to lead to the wrong diagnosis.

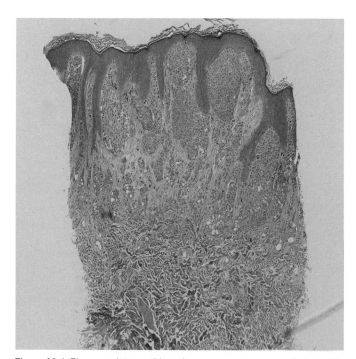

**Figure 63.4** Biopsy sculpture – this melanoma appears symmetrical since it has been 'sculpted' by the partial punch biopsy technique.

cult to interpret and are prone to misdiagnosis (Fig. 63.5). Important architectural features are destroyed and accurate histologic assessment may be impossible.

Finally, clinicians should not freeze or electrodesiccate a specimen before biopsying it for histologic evaluation. These techniques destroy the histologic features and make accurate diagnosis impossible.

### 4) Either submit specimens directly to a dermatopathologist or have ready access to expert dermatopathology consultants.

While the majority of cutaneous neoplasms and pigmented lesions are easily and readily diagnosed, there is

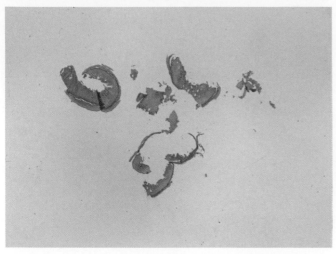

**Figure 63.5** Curettings destroy architecture – these curettings were of melanoma in situ. The diagnosis was missed. The patient ultimately developed a deep melanoma and died. The patient's family sued and the pathology group settled out of court.

a subset that can be very difficult to interpret, and even expert dermatopathologists may have differing opinions about such lesions. One study demonstrated poor consistency between expert pathologists reading melanocytic lesions that were considered difficult to diagnose. There was agreement in diagnosis in only 55% of 143, including a 36% discordance as to whether the lesions were benign or malignant.[30] When one receives a histology report of a challenging or unusual melanocytic lesion, it is prudent to consider seeking a second opinion. One may even want to seek a third opinion. Also, excise the lesion with appropriate margins and consider other techniques such as sentinel lymphadenectomy and imaging studies. Occasionally, it may be impossible to determine the precise nature of some lesions until they metastasize.

While clinicians are aware of the uncertainty in dealing with 'borderline' melanocytic neoplasms, there are no standard recommendations for lessening liability. The most common diagnoses associated with medicolegal liability are listed in Table 63.8.

## Table 63.8 Most Common Diagnoses Associated With Medicolegal Liability for Dermatologists Related to Dermatopathology

- Desmoplastic melanoma misdiagnosed as scar, neurofibroma
- Melanoma confused with nevus: 'dysplastic', Spitz, cellular blue
- Melanoma in situ misdiagnosed as lentigo, solar lentigo
- Melanoma with lichenoid inflammation misdiagnosed as benign lichenoid keratosis
- Solar lentigo misdiagnosed as melanoma in situ leading to overtreatment
- Dermatofibrosarcoma protuberans misdiagnosed as scar, neurofibroma
- Failure to diagnose toxic epidermal necrolysis
- Failure to diagnose non-melanoma skin cancer/basal cell carcinoma due to sampling error
- Merkel cell carcinoma misdiagnosed as basal cell carcinoma
- Pseudocarcinomatous hyperplasia overdiagnosed as squamous cell carcinoma with overly aggressive treatment (i.e. deep mycosis, verrucous lupus erythematosus)

### 5) Perform clinicopathological correlation and be critical of all diagnoses.

Occasionally, a malignant neoplasm may demonstrate histologic features that are less aggressive than those seen clinically. In such cases, we strongly recommend treating the lesion as if it were a malignancy, regardless of what the result of the histologic interpretation of the initial biopsy is. It is not altogether uncommon for an initial biopsy to reveal features characteristic of a 'dysplastic' nevus, yet when a complete excision is performed, it is apparent that there are foci of melanoma arising within the lesion. Clinicians should always ensure that the histologic diagnosis correlates with clinical diagnosis, and, if not, consider that the clinical diagnosis is the more correct one and treat accordingly.

## FUTURE OUTLOOK

Unfortunately, the current legal climate does not promote trust between the physician and patient. Tort reform would be welcome in the future, but, until then, a full understanding of the legal concepts, patient communication, and practice management techniques outlined in this chapter can help reduce a physician's liability while optimizing patient care.

## REFERENCES

**1.** Eisenberg D, Siegger M. The doctor won't see you now. *Time Magazine.* 2003;46–62.
**2.** Altman J. The National Association of Insurance Commissioners' (NIAC) Medical Malpractice Closed Claim Study, 1975–1978. *J Am Acad Dermatol.* 1981;5:721–726.
**3.** Physicians Insurers Association of America. *PIAA Data Sharing Reports.* 1 January, 1985–31 December, 1987. Lawrenceville, NJ: Physicians Insurers Association of America; 1988.
**4.** Lydiatt D. Medical malpractice and cancer of the skin. *Am J Surg.* 2004;187(6):688–694.
**5.** Prosser L, Owen DG, Keeton RE. *Prosser and Keeton on the Law on Torts.* 5th ed. St Paul: West Publishing; 1984: Section 30, 41: 187.
**6.** Hiser v Randolph, 617 P.2d 774 (Ariz 1980).
**7.** Hamil v Bashline, 305 A2d 57 1973.
**8.** Ratushny V, Allen HB. The effect of medical malpractice on dermatology and related specialties. *J Med Sci Res.* 2007;(1):15–20.
**9.** Fiscina FS. *Medical Law for the Attending Physician.* Carbondale, IL: Southern Illinois Press; 1982.
**10.** Sills H. What is the law? *Dental Clin North Am.* 1982;26:256.
**11.** Rapp JA, Rapp RT. *Medical Malpractice: A Guide for the Health Sciences.* St. Louis, MO: CV Mosby; 1988.
**12.** Perlis C, Campbell RM, Perlis RH, et al. Incidence of and risk factors for medical malpractice lawsuits among Mohs surgeons. *Dermatol Surg.* 2006;32:79–83.
**13.** Flamm MB. Medical malpractice: physician as defendant. In: Falk KH, Geisel EB, eds. for the American College of Legal Medicine. *Legal Medicine: Legal Dynamics of Medical Encounters.* 2nd ed. St Louis, MO: CV Mosby; 1991:525–534.
**14.** Prosser L, Owen DG, Keeton RE. *Prosser and Keeton on the Law on Torts.* 5th ed. St Paul: West Publishing; 1984; Ch. 7, Section 44:263–309.
**15.** Meisel A, Kabnick L. Informed consent to medical treatment: an analysis of recent legislation. *U Pitt Law Review.* 1980;407:410.
**16.** Waltz JR, Scheuneman TW. Informed consent to therapy. *Nw U L Rev.* 1970;64(5):628.
**17.** Logan v Greenwich Hosp. Ass'n, 191 Conn. 282 1983.
**18.** Holder AR. The importance of medical records. *JAMA.* 1974;228:118–119.
**19.** Keyes C. Responding to an adverse event. Forum: Risk Management Foundation of the Harvard Medical Institutions Inc. *Adverse Events.* 1997;18(1):2–5.
**20.** Localio AR, Lawthers AG, Brennan TA, et al. Relationship between malpractice claims and adverse events due to negligence. *N Engl J Med.* 1991;325(4):245–251.
**21.** Witman A, Park D, Hardin S. How do patients want physicians to handle mistakes? A survey of internal medicine patients in an academic setting. *Arch Int Med.* 1996;156:2565–2569.

22. *California Jury Instructions 9.003: Products Liability – Strict Liability in Tort – Defect in Manufacture*. vol. 5. 9th ed. BAJI; 2000:324 .

23. Levinson WL, Roter DL, Mullooly JP, et al. Physician-patient communication: the relationship with malpractice claims among primary care physicians and surgeons. *JAMA*. 1997;277:553–559.

24. National Commission for the Protection of Human Subjects of Biomedical and Behavioral Research. *The Belmont Report: Ethical Principles and Guidelines for the Protection of Human Subjects in Research*. DHEW Pub No. (05) 78-0012. Washington DC: US Govt. Printing Office; 1979 .

25. *Health Insurance Portability and Accountability Act of 1996*. Pub. L No.104–191 (Codified at 42 USC Section 1320d 1996.

26. Cesinaro AM, Foroni M, Sighinolfi P, et al. Spitz nevus is relatively frequent in adults: a clinico-pathologic study of 247 cases related to patient's age. *Am J Dermatopathol*. 2005;27(6):469–475.

27. Grant-Kels JM, Bason ET, Grin CM. The misdiagnosis of malignant melanoma. *J Am Acad Dermatol*. 1999;40(4):539–548.

28. Wolf IH, Smolle J, Soyer HP, et al. Sensitivity in the clinical diagnosis of malignant melanoma. *Melanoma Res*. 1998;8(5):425–429.

29. Dalton SR, Gardner TL, Libow LF, et al. Contiguous lesions in lentigo maligna. *J Am Acad Dermatol*. 2005;52(5):859–862.

30. Lodha S, Saggar S, Celebi JT, et al. Discordance in the histopathologic diagnosis of difficult melanocytic neoplasms in the clinical setting. *J Cutan Pathol*. 2008;35(4):349–352.

# INDEX

Note: Page numbers in *italics* refer to illustrations, tables and boxes.

## A

AAA mnemonic *672*
Abbe flap 567
ABCB5 drug transporter 8
ABCD criteria for melanoma
  clinical assessment *262*, 273, *273*, 274, *274*
  dermoscopic scoring system 390, *390*
ABCDE criteria for melanoma 262, 274
abdominal reconstruction 570
ABT-518 *618*
ABT-888 *620*
acanthosis nigricans *371*, 372–373, *373*
N-acetylcysteine, melanoma chemoprevention
  *76*, 77–78
acetylsalicylic acid (ASA; aspirin), melanoma
  chemoprevention *76*, 77
acitretin
  basal cell carcinoma 117
  prevention of non-melanoma skin cancer 74
  transplant recipients 639–640, *640*
Ackerman tumor (oral florid papillomatosis;
  oroaerodigestive verrucous carcinoma)
  96, 129, 202
acquired immune deficiency syndrome *see* HIV
  infection/AIDS
acral myxoinflammatory fibroblastic sarcoma
  (AMFS) 164
acral nevi 345
acral pseudolymphomatous angiokeratoma 215
acral Spitz nevi 345
acrokeratosis paraneoplastica *see* Bazex
  syndrome
acrospirocarcinoma 143, *143*
acrospiroma 143
ACTH
  regulation of melanogenesis 34
  secreting tumors, ectopic 367–369, *370*
actinic cheilitis 91, 128
  imiquimod therapy 491
actinic keratoses (AK) 89–93
  acantholytic 92
  atrophic 92
  bowenoid 92
  chemoprevention studies 74
  clinical appearance 90–91, *90*, 126, *126*
  confocal microscopy 411–413, *411*, *413*
  definition 89
  histopathology and classification 92–93
  hypertrophic 92
  incidence and prevalence 90
  lichenoid 92
  organ transplant recipients 638
  pathogenesis 91
    *CDKN2A* mutations 16
    loss of heterozygosity 16, 91
    p53 gene defects 16, 91
    *RAS* mutations 15
  pigmented 92

progression or transformation 91–92, 126
risk factors 60, 89–90
skin cancer risk 67, 91
treatment 93, *94*
  cryosurgery 93, *94*, 455–456, *457*, *459*
  curettage and electrodesiccation 93, *94*,
    448
  imiquimod 93, *94*, 466, *467*, 484, *485*
  ingenol mebutate *94*, 471–472
  interferons 480
  photodynamic therapy *see under*
    photodynamic therapy
  to prevent progression to cancer 73–74
  resiquimod 468, 491–492
  topical 93, *94*, 462, 464, 473
  topical 5-fluorouracil 93, *94*, 462–464, *464*, *465*
  topical colchicine 93, 471
  topical combinations 473
  topical diclofenac 93, *94*, 468–469, *469*
  topical retinoids 93, *94*, 470
  topical *vs* surgical 463
actinic reticuloid 207–209, *209*
acute febrile neutrophilic dermatoses *see* Sweet
  syndrome
adalimumab, carcinogenic potential 353–354
adaptor protein-1 (AP-1) 26
adaptor protein-3 (AP-3) 26, *26*, 28
adenocarcinoma
  metastatic
    differential diagnosis 190
    *vs* morpheic basal cell carcinoma 110
  sweat glands 530
adenoid cystic carcinoma 141–142, *141*
adenosquamous carcinoma 133, *133*
ADI-PEG20 *619*
adjuvants, melanoma vaccines *607*, 608
adnexal carcinomas 140–149, *530*
  eccrine and apocrine glands 140–146
  epidemiology 140
  hair follicle 146–148
  sebaceous glands 148
  treatment of disseminated 530
adrenocorticotropic hormone *see* ACTH
adult T-cell leukemia/lymphoma (ATLL) 225
adverse events
  legal aspects 670–672, *671*, *672*
  remedying 671
AE1/AE3 antibody staining
  basal cell carcinoma 113
  Mohs micrographic surgery *517*
aflibercept, in melanoma 617–618, *618*
AG-013736 (axitinib), in melanoma 617–618, *618*
age
  basal cell carcinoma management and 118
  diagnosis of melanoma and 275–276
  melanoma prognosis and *285*, *286*, 288
age-related differences
  actinic keratosis incidence 90
  melanoma incidence 45, 46, *46*

melanoma mortality 47, *48*
skin cancer risk *57*, 61, 66–67
aggressive digital papillary adenocarcinoma
  (ADPA) 145–146, *145*
agouti protein (ASIP) 35, *36*
  gene variants 37
AIDS *see* HIV infection/AIDS
air embolism, cerebral 524
AJCC *see* American Joint Commission on
  Cancer
AKT (protein kinase B; PKB) 3, 5
  inhibitors, in melanoma *616*, 617
ALA *see* 5-aminolevulinic acid
alanyl-hydroxyl-benzothiazine 30
alefacept, carcinogenic potential 354
alemtuzumab
  cutaneous T-cell lymphoma *226*, 228
  dermatologic side effects *635*
alitretinoin gel, Kaposi sarcoma 174, 470
alkylating agents
  cancers treated 380
  dermatologic side effects 383
  *see also* dacarbazine; temozolomide
alopecia
  chemotherapy-induced (CIA) 379
  cryosurgery-related 461
  in folliculotropic mycosis fungoides 218–219,
    *219*
  neoplastica, in extramammary Paget's disease
    153
ALS-357 *617*
alternate reading frame (ARF) *see* p14^ARF
altitude, UV radiation and 56
alum *607*
alveolar rhabdomyosarcoma *159*, 165
alveolar soft part sarcoma, genetic alterations *159*
ameboid motility, metastatic cells 5–6, *6*
American Joint Commission on Cancer (AJCC)
  melanoma staging system 282–283, *283*,
    *284*, *309*, 312–315, 318–320, 589–590,
    *590*, *591*
  Merkel cell carcinoma staging system 181,
    *182*
  squamous cell carcinoma staging system 131
5-aminolevulinic acid (ALA) 469, 497
  heme biosynthesis 498, *499*
  lesion specificity and tissue penetration 498
  topical application 500–501, *501*, 502
  *see also* photodynamic therapy
amputation
  digits 540–541, *541*, 573
  ray 541, *542*
amyloid deposition, in basal cell carcinoma 112
amyloidosis, primary systemic *368*, 373–374, *374*
anal cancer 204–205
anal intraepithelial neoplasia, photodynamic
  therapy 505
anaplastic large cell lymphoma, primary
  cutaneous (C-ALCL) 225

anesthesia
for biopsy 435–436, *436*
for cryosurgery 454–455
for topical photodynamic therapy 501
angiogenesis
neoplastic 4–5, *5*
therapeutic targeting in melanoma 617–618, *618*
angiokeratoma, acral pseudolymphomatous 215
angiomatoid fibrous histiocytoma *159*
angiomatous Spitz nevus 342–343
angiopoietin-1 (ang-1) 5
angiopoietin-2 (ang-2) 4, 5
angiosarcomas (AS) 186–195
associated with chronic lymphedema 186–187, 191–192
epidemiology 157–158, 186
epithelioid 190
of face and scalp 186, 191–192
high grade 186, 191–192, *192*
history 186
intermediate grade 189–191
low grade 186, 187–189
Mohs micrographic surgery 522–523
pathogenesis and etiology 186–187
postirradiation 191–192
angiotensin receptor blockers (ARBs), prevention of non-melanoma skin cancers 74
angiotension-converting enzyme (ACE) inhibitors, prevention of non-melanoma skin cancers 74
animal melanoma 305
annular lichenoid dermatitis of youth 215, *215*
anterolateral thigh flap (ALT) *561*, 570, 573, *573, 574*
anthracyclines
cancers treated *380*
dermatologic side effects 379, *380*, 382–383
antibiotics
prophylactic, surgical procedures 508–509, 523–524
topical, cutaneous T-cell lymphoma 226, 227
anticoagulants, cessation prior to surgery 509, 523
anti-epiligrin cicatricial pemphigoid (AECP) *368*, 375, *375*
anti-estrogens, in melanoma 328
antigenic heterogeneity, tumor cells 607
antigens, anti-melanoma vaccines *607*, 606–607
antioxidants, chemoprevention studies 75, *75, 76*
antiretroviral therapy (ART)
in epidemic Kaposi sarcoma 174
skin cancer risk and 642
anti-tumor necrosis factor (anti-TNF) antibodies, carcinogenic potential 63, *350*, 353–354
anxiety
*CDKN2A* mutation carriers 664
skin cancer patients 662–663
*AP3B1* gene mutations *27*
apocrine adenocarcinoma 144–145, *145*
apocrine carcinoma, primary cutaneous cribriform 145, *145*
apocrine epithelioma 110–111
apocrine glands
carcinomas of 140–146
origin of extramammary Paget's disease 153
apomine, melanoma chemoprevention 75–76, *76*

apoptosis *478*
cryosurgery-induced 451, *451*
imiquimod actions 482
melanoma therapies targeting *617*
APUD cell system 367
*ARF* gene product *see* p14<sup>ARF</sup>
ARHGAP22 5–6
arsenical keratoses 95, *95*
arsenic exposure
basal cell carcinoma risk 100, *100*
carcinogenic effects 63, *63*
arthropod bite reactions, persistent nodular 210–211, *212, 213*
ascorbic acid (vitamin C), melanoma chemoprevention *76*
ASIP *see* agouti protein
aspirin (acetylsalicylic acid; ASA), melanoma chemoprevention *76*, 77
ataxia-telangiectasia *368, 370*
*ATF1/EWSR1* gene fusion *143*, 158, 164–165
ATN-224 *620*
atypical fibroxanthoma (AFX) 158, 162–163
clinical features 162, *162*
history 157
organ transplant recipients *635*
pathogenesis and etiology 158, *159*, 162
pathologic diagnosis 162–163, *162*
treatment 163, *517, 521*
atypical melanocytic proliferations 309–311
atypical moles *see* dysplastic nevi
atypical mole syndrome (AMS) *see* dysplastic nevus syndrome
aurora kinase A/B inhibitors *617*
autocrine motility factor (AMF) 5
autoimmunity, in interferon-treated melanoma 599–600
autolumination, in Kaposi sarcoma 172
avobenzone *81, 83*
axial pattern flaps 560, 561, *561*
axillary lymphadenectomy 553–557
axitinib (AG-013736), in melanoma 617–618
azathioprine
carcinogenic potential *350, 352, 635*
organ transplant recipients 635–636
AZD1152 *617*
AZD2171 *618*
AZD2281 *620*
AZD6244 615–617, *616*

**B**

B7 receptor 630, *631*
expression in melanoma 6
bacille Calmette–Guérin (BCG) vaccine *see* BCG vaccine
BAGE/Ba *32*
*Bartonella bacilliformis* 160
basal cell carcinoma (BCC) 99–123
adenocystic 107, 141
adenoid 107, *107*
with aggressive growth pattern 103
surgical excision 512
treatment *114*
anatomic location, treatment aspects 118, 512, *512*
in basal cell nevus syndrome 12, 99–100, *100, 100*, 357, 358–359, *358*
in Bazex syndrome 99–100, *100*, 363
biopsy 113, 441
circumscribed growth pattern 105–108
clinical presentation 101–104, *102*
confocal microscopy 413–415, *413, 414, 415, 416, 417*

cornifying (keratotic) 107, *108*
costs 42–43
cystic 103, 107, *108*
dermoscopy 387–388, *388*
diffuse growth pattern 108–111
disseminated/advanced, treatment 117, 526, *527*
epidemiology 42, 48–49, 99
in epidermolysis bullosa 360
field fire, treatment *114*, 118–119
follicular (infundibulocystic) 107, *108*
genetics 12–14, 61
granular 107
histopathology 104–112
classification 105
evolutionary changes 112
immunohistochemistry 113
ultrastructural features 112
history 99
in HIV-infected patients 204–205, 642
with ill-defined borders 118
incidence 49, *49*
incompletely excised *114*, 119
infiltrating 110, *111*
surgical excision 512
lesion size, and treatment options 118, *118*
local invasion 101
metastatic 101
treatment *114*, 117, 526
micronodular 110, *111*
morpheic (morpheaform) 103, *103*
differential diagnosis 110, *111*
histology 109–110, *110*
surgical excision 512
treatment *114*
mortality 50
multiple lesions, treatment 118, 488
multiple non-syndromic 14
nodular (noduloulcerative; rodent ulcer) 102, *102*
histology 105–108
histopathologic variants 105
treatment *114*, 484–488, 512
non-pigmented, dermoscopy 387–388, *388, 389*
organ transplant recipients 100–101, 634, 640
pathogenesis and etiology 99–101, *100*
perifollicular extension 112, *112*
perineural invasion (neurotropic) 101, 112, *119*
treatment *114, 119*
pigmented 102, *103*, 104
dermoscopy 387, *388, 388*
histology 108, *109*
prevention 53, 66–72
chemoprevention 73–75
efficacy of sunscreens 53, 85
primary 67–69, 73
secondary 69–71, 73–74, *74*
targeting 66–67
recurrence 113, 120
risk factors 113
surgical management 512, 513, 518
treatment *114*, 118, *119*
regression 112
risk factors 52, 56–65, *57*, 99, *100*
indoor tanning 647–648
treatment-related 349–354, *350*
in Rombo syndrome 99–100, 363
sclerosing 103
solid 105–106, *105, 106*
with squamous metaplasia (basosquamous or metatypical) 103
histology 106–107, *106, 107*
treatment *114*

superficial (multicentric) 102–103, *103*
  histology 108, *109*
  surgical excision 512
  treatment *114*
treatment 113–120
  algorithm *113*
  combinations 117–118, 473
  cryosurgery 116, 454, 456, *456, 458, 459*
  curettage and electrodesiccation 113–115, 444–445, 446–447, 448
  disseminated/advanced disease 117, 526, *527*
  factors affecting 118
  follow-up 120
  imiquimod 117, 466–468, *467*, 482, *483, 484–488, 486*
  interferons 117, 479–480, *480*
  Mohs micrographic surgery 115, *115*, 118, *119, 517*, 518
  photodynamic therapy *see under* photodynamic therapy
  radiation therapy 115–116, 578–582, *580, 581*
  reconstructive surgery 560, *565, 566, 568, 569, 572*
  by subtype *114*, 118
  surgical excision 115, 508–514
  topical 5-fluorouracil 117, 464–465
  topical chemotherapy *464*
  topical retinoids 470
unresectable/advanced *114*
in xeroderma pigmentosum 100, *100*, 361
basal cell nevus syndrome (BCNS) 357–359, *364, 368*
  basal cell carcinoma 12, 99–100, *100, 100*, 357, 358–359, *358*
  clinical features 104, *104, 105*, 357–358, *358*
  diagnosis and evaluation 358, *359*
  pathogenesis and etiology 13, 61, 357
  treatment 115, 358–359, 364
basaloid hyperplasia in dermatofibroma 111, *112*
basiliximab *635*
basosquamous carcinoma (metatypical carcinoma) 103
  histology 106–107, *106, 107*
  treatment *114*
Bazex(–Dupré–Christol) syndrome 14, 99–100, *363, 364*
  basal cell carcinoma *100*
  skin signs *371, 373, 373*
BB-2516 *618*
BCC *see* basal cell carcinoma
B-cell lymphoma, cutaneous *see* cutaneous B-cell lymphoma
BCG vaccine
  melanoma therapy 590, *591*
  with melanoma vaccines *607, 608*, 609
bcl-1, in melanoma 347
bcl-2
  in glomangiosarcomas 193
  therapeutic targeting in melanoma *617*
beauty and the beast sign, melanoma 395
behavior, individual
  influencing UV radiation exposure 59
  primary prevention programs targeting 67–69
bemotrizinol *81, 83*
benxyledene malonate polysiloxane (Parsol SLX) *81*, 82–83
benzophenones 83
Ber-EP4, in basal cell carcinoma 113, *517*
beta-carotene
  effects on skin cancer risk 53, 64
  melanoma chemoprevention *76*

beta-catenin 32, 153
bevacizumab
  in Kaposi sarcoma 176
  in melanoma *618, 620, 621*
bexarotene
  oral, cutaneous T-cell lymphoma *226*, 228
  topical *464, 470–471*
    adverse effects 471
    cutaneous T-cell lymphoma *226*, 227, 470–471
BEZ235 *616*
BGT226 *616*
BI-2536 *617*
bilobed flaps, nose reconstruction *567, 568*
biochemotherapy *see* chemobiotherapy
bio-impedance, cellular electrical *401*, 404
biologic agents, carcinogenic potential 353–354
biology, tumor 1–11
bioprosthetic mesh 570
biopsy 434–442
  anesthesia for 435–436, *436*
  basal cell carcinoma 113, 441
  contraindications 436
  curettage and electrodesiccation after 448
  cutaneous T-cell lymphoma 221–222, *223*
  decision-making process 434–436
  dysplastic nevi 242
  equipment 435, *435*
  margins 434
  medico-legal issues 672–674, *672, 673, 674, 674*
  melanoma 284, 298–299, *300*, 318, 439–441
    choice of technique 439–441
    nodal metastasis risk 299
    during pregnancy 330
  non-melanoma skin cancer 441
  post-procedure care 441
  sarcoma 159
  sculpture phenomenon *673, 673*
  squamous cell carcinoma 130, 441
  suspicious pigmented lesions 298–299, *300*, 439–441
  techniques 436–439, *436*
  types 434
  *see also specific types*
Birt–Hogg–Dubé syndrome *368, 369*
bisoctriazole *81*, 83
BKM120 *616*
B-K moles *see* dysplastic nevi
B-K mole syndrome 231
  *see also* dysplastic nevus syndrome
bleeding, postoperative 509
bleomycin
  cancers treated *380*
  dermatologic side effects 380, 383
  squamous cell carcinoma 527, *528*
*BLOC1S3* gene mutations 27
BLOC gene mutations 26
BLOCs *28*
blood pressure, vitamin D and *652*
Bloom syndrome *368, 370*
blue dye, sentinel lymph node biopsy 546, *546*
blue nevus
  cellular 252, *253*, 254
  congenital 252, *253*, 254
  dermoscopy *394*
  malignant 306, *306*
  metastatic melanoma simulating 309, *310*
  progression to melanoma 2–3
blue nevus-like lesions, atypical 309–310
BMS-663513 *619*
body mass index (BMI), increased 64
bone grafts 562–563
bone health, vitamin D and 651, *652*

bone marrow-derived precursor cells
  in premetastatic niches 7
  in tumor angiogenesis 4–5
bone marrow transplantation, melanoma *591*
bone metastases, potential pathways for development 7, *7*
*Borrelia burgdorferi*-associated lymphocytoma cutis 211–212, *213*
bortezomib, in melanoma *617, 620*
bowenoid papulosis (BP) 96, 198–202
  clinical features 199, *199, 200*
  differential diagnosis 126–127, 199, *200*, 201, *201*
  in HIV-infected patients 204–205
  pathogenesis and etiology 96, 199
  pathology 199–201, *201*
  treatment 201–202, 488
Bowen's disease 96–97, *96*, 126–127, *127*
  confocal microscopy *412, 413*
  Merkel cell carcinoma developing within 180
  treatment 137
    cryosurgery 456–457, *459*
    photodynamic therapy 500, 503, *503*
    topical chemotherapy *464, 465*, 488, *489, 490*
  *vs* bowenoid papulosis 201, *201*
  *vs* Paget's disease 152, 155
  *see also* squamous cell carcinoma in situ
B-raf kinase inhibitors
  in melanoma 325, 615–617, *617, 618*, 631
  *see also* sorafenib
*BRAF* mutations
  in benign melanocytic nevi 3, 19, 246–247
  in melanoma 19
    therapies targeting 325, 615–617, *616*, 631
  Spitz nevi 347
brain metastases, in melanoma
  imaging 625, *625, 626*
  management 632
brain tumors, in basal cell nevus syndrome 357–358
breach of duty 669, *669*
breast
  melanoma of 541
  Paget's disease *see* Paget's disease, mammary
breast carcinoma
  cutaneous metastases 142
  mammary Paget's disease 150, 151
  vitamin D and *652*, 653
Breslow thickness 312
  AJCC staging system 282, *283*, 284
  biopsy technique and 299, 439, 440–441
  measurement 284, *286*
  prognostic value 284, *285, 286*
  surgical excision margins and 532
    current recommendations 536–537, *536*
    randomized trials 532–536, *533, 534*
Brooke–Spiegler syndrome 144
bulla formation, after cryosurgery 459
bullous pemphigoid antigen, in basal cell carcinoma 113
burden of disease 40–43
  melanoma 40–42
  non-melanoma skin cancer 42–43
burnout 666
burn scars 64, 95
Buschke–Lowenstein tumor 96, 129, *129*, 202

**C**

cadherins 5
calcification, dystrophic, in basal cell carcinoma 112
calcifying epitheliocarcinoma of Malherbe *see* matrical carcinoma

calcineurin inhibitors 635
  carcinogenic potential 350, 353, 636
  organ transplant recipients 636
  see also ciclosporin; tacrolimus
calcipotriol, topical 472–473
Cam 5.2 517
cameras, for clinical photography 659
camphor derivatives 82–83
cAMP responsive element binding protein
    (CREB) 35
cancer stem cells (CSC) 8, 8
cancer survivors, skin cancer risk 63
Cannon curette 443–444, 445
Canvaxin 608, 609, 610
capecitabine, dermatologic side effects 379
capillaroscopy with Gene Scan, in cutaneous
    T-cell lymphoma 222
carbon dioxide (CO₂) laser, basal cell carcinoma
    116
carboplatin
  basal cell carcinoma 526
  melanoma 620
  Merkel cell carcinoma 530
  squamous cell carcinoma 527
carcinoembryonic antigen (CEA)
  adenosquamous carcinoma 133
  Paget's disease 151–152, 153–154
carcinoid syndrome 370–371, 370
cardiac pacemakers 448, 509
cardiac transplant recipients
  skin cancer risk 634–635
  squamous cell carcinoma risk 124–125, 635
cardiovascular health, vitamin D and 652
carmustine (BCNU), in cutaneous T-cell
    lymphoma 226, 227
carotenoids, melanoma chemoprevention 76
cartilage grafts 567–568, 569
β-catenin 32, 153
causation (legal) 670
CC-chemokine receptor 4 (CCR4), in cutaneous
    T-cell lymphoma 217
CCIU-779 616
CCNU, in melanoma 591
CD4⁺ memory helper T cells, in cutaneous T-cell
    lymphoma 217
CD10 immunohistochemistry, atypical
    fibroxanthoma 517
CD30⁺ lymphoproliferative disorders, primary
    cutaneous 225, 225
CD30⁺ (T-cell) pseudolymphomas 210–211,
    212
CD31 immunohistochemistry, angiosarcomas
    187–188, 190, 191–192
CD34 immunohistochemistry
  angiosarcomas 187–188, 190, 191–192
  dermatofibrosarcoma protuberans 161, 517,
    521
CD63 (NKIC3) immunohistochemistry, in
    melanoma 304
CDC27 32
CDK4 see cyclin-dependent kinase 4
CDK4 gene
  defects in melanoma 2, 16–18, 334
  in mouse models of melanoma 18
CDK inhibitors, in melanoma 617
CDKN2A gene 17, 334
  in melanoma tumorigenesis 2, 16–18
  in mouse models of melanoma 18
  mutations/defects
    behavioral changes in carriers 339
    dysplastic nevus phenotype 233
    genetic testing see genetic testing, for
      melanoma
    management of affected families 339

MC1R genotype interaction 35, 36, 334–335
  in melanoma 2, 16–18, 334–335
  pancreatic cancer risk 2, 16–17, 335
  penetrance 334–335
  psychological impact 664
  promoter methylation, in melanoma 17–18
  signaling pathway 17, 17
  in squamous cell carcinoma tumorigenesis 16
  see also p14ARF; p16INK4A
CDKN2B gene, in melanoma 19–20
celecoxib, in squamous cell carcinoma 528
cellulitis, postoperative 556
cerebral air embolism 524
Cervarix 203
cervical cancer, HIV-infected patients 204–205
cervical intraepithelial neoplasia (CIN), topical
    chemotherapy 464
cervical lymphadenectomy 553–554, 554, 556
cervicofacial rotation advancement flap 565
cetuximab, in squamous cell carcinoma 528
Chédiak–Higashi syndrome 27, 368
chemicals, carcinogenic 57, 63, 63
chemobiotherapy, melanoma 599, 602, 620,
    629–630, 630
chemoprevention 73–79
  history of concept 73
  melanoma 75–78, 76, 77
  non-melanoma skin cancers 73–75, 74, 75
chemotherapy
  adnexal carcinomas 530
  angiosarcomas of face and scalp 191–192
  basal cell carcinoma 117, 526
  carcinogenic potential 63, 351–353
  cutaneous T-cell lymphoma 226, 228
  dermatofibrosarcoma protuberans 162
  dermatologic side effects 379–383
  extramammary Paget's disease 155
  Kaposi sarcoma 174–176
  melanoma 323, 590, 591, 629
    combined with targeted therapies 619, 620,
      621
  Merkel cell carcinoma 184, 530
  squamous cell carcinoma 527–528, 528
  topical see topical chemotherapy
chemotherapy-induced alopecia (CIA) 379
chest reconstruction 568–570
chest X-ray (CXR), in melanoma 623,
    625–626
childhood cancer survivors, skin cancer risk
    63
children
  congenital nevi simulating melanoma
    307–308
  melanoma in 275–276, 307
Chlamydia, in cutaneous T-cell lymphoma
    pathogenesis 217–218
chlorofluorocarbons (CFCs) 57–58
cholecalciferol (vitamin D₃) 650
  biosynthesis 650, 651
  supplements 650
chondrocutaneous flaps 567–568
chondroid syringoma, malignant see malignant
    mixed tumor
chromosome abnormalities (cytogenetics)
  cutaneous sarcomas 158, 159, 160
  cutaneous T-cell lymphoma 218
  Spitz nevus 347
  see also translocations, chromosome
chromosome deletions
  in melanoma 2, 16–17
  in squamous cell carcinoma 16
chronic lymphocytic leukemia (CLL)
  Merkel cell carcinoma risk 179–180
  skin cancer risk 63

chronic myeloid leukemia (CML), skin cancer
    risk 63
CHS1 (LYST) gene mutations 27
chylous leaks, persistent 556
ciclosporin (CsA) 635
  carcinogenic potential 63, 350, 351–352
  organ transplant recipients 636
cidofovir
  bowenoid papulosis 202
  Kaposi sarcoma 176
ciglitazone 493
cinoxate 81, 82
circumferential excision, non-melanoma skin
    cancers 510, 510
cisplatin
  basal cell carcinoma 117, 526
  extramammary Paget's disease 155
  melanoma 620, 629–630, 630
  Merkel cell carcinoma 530
  squamous cell carcinoma 527–528, 528
Clark level of invasion 312, 313
  measurement 287, 287
  prognostic value 285, 286, 287
Clark's nevi see dysplastic nevi
clear cell sarcoma of soft tissue (CCS)
    (melanoma of soft parts) 164–165, 165
  genetic alterations 143, 158, 159, 164–165
  natural history 146, 158
clinical margins 510
clonal heterogeneity, metastatic cells 7–8
Cloquet's node 553
clothing, photoprotective 86, 86
cloud cover 57
CNTO 95, in melanoma 615
cognitive-behavioral therapy (CBT), cost-
    effectiveness 665
cohort effects
  basal cell carcinoma incidence 50
  melanoma incidence 44–45, 45
  melanoma mortality 47–48, 48
COL1A1-PDFGB fusion gene,
    dermatofibrosarcoma protuberans 161,
    161
COL7A mutations, epidermolysis bullosa 359
colchicine, topical 463, 471
  actinic keratosis 93, 471
  indications 464
collagenases, metastatic cells 6
collagen type IV, in basal cell carcinoma 113
colorectal cancer
  hereditary non-polyposis (HNPCC) 362
  in Muir–Torre syndrome 362
  Paget's disease associated with 154–155
  vitamin D status and 651–653, 652
combined Spitz nevus 344, 345, 345
communication, clinician–patient
  medicolegal aspects 671–672, 672
  psychological aspects 665, 666
comparative genomic hybridization (CGH),
    Spitz nevus 347
COMPLICATIONS mnemonic 672
complications of treatment
  legal aspects 670–672, 671, 672
  remedying 671
composite hemangioendothelioma 186,
    188–189, 189
compound nevus 275
  confocal microscopy 416, 421, 422
computed tomography (CT), melanoma 624,
    624, 626, 627
computer-aided diagnosis, for melanoma
    400–406, 401
condyloma acuminatum, vs bowenoid
    papulosis 200, 201, 201

confocal microscopy
  fluorescence 421
  reflectance *see* reflectance confocal
    microscopy
confocal scanning laser microscopy *see*
  reflectance confocal microscopy
congenital blue nevi 252, *253*, 254
congenital melanocytic nevi (CMN) 246–261
  classification 246
  clinical features 247–254, *248*, *249*,
    *250*, *251*
  complications 254–256
  confocal microscopy 417–418, *422*
  dermatoscopic features 254
  desmoplastic hairless hypopigmented variant
    251
  diagnostic evaluation 254
  differential diagnosis 254
  epidemiology 246
  large and giant 246, 247, *247*, *249*
    management 257–259, *258*
    melanoma/malignancy risk 254–256, *255*
  management 256–259, *258*
  melanoma risk 246, 254–256, *255*, *256*
  natural history 247–248, *251*
  neurocutaneous melanocytosis risk 256
  pathogenesis and etiology 246–247
  pathology 254
    simulating melanoma 307–308, *309*
  progression to melanoma 2–3
  psychosocial issues 254
  satellite nevi 247, *249*
    neurocutaneous melanocytosis risk 256
  small and medium-sized 246, 247, *248*
    management 256–257, *257*, *258*
    melanoma risk 254, *255*, 256
  spontaneous regression 248–251
  subtypes 252, *253*
congenital nevus-like nevus (CNLN) 246
  epidemiology 246
  pathogenesis and etiology 247
Connecticut Tumor Registry 44, *45*
consent for treatment 670, *670*
consumption of epidermis 343
contact dermatitis, lymphomatoid 209–210, *209*
coping skills and strategies *663*, *664*
copper, tyrosinase dependence on 30
corticosteroids (glucocorticoids) *635*
  increased skin cancer risk 63
  organ transplant recipients 635
  topical, cutaneous T-cell lymphoma 226–227,
    *226*
*Corynebacterium parvum*, melanoma 590, *591*
cosmetic results
  curettage and electrodesiccation 446, *448*
  radiation therapy 579–582, *580*, *581*, *582*
cost-effectiveness
  chest X-ray screening in melanoma 626
  Mohs micrographic surgery 523
  psychosocial interventions 665
co-stimulatory signals *478*
costs
  of melanoma 41–42, *41*
    effects of early detection 272
  of Mohs micrographic surgery 518
  of non-melanoma skin cancer 42–43
  of skin cancer 40
Cowden syndrome 18, *368*, *369*
crescentic excision
  closure using rule of halves 509–510, *511*
  non-melanoma skin cancers 509–510, *510*
cribriform apocrine carcinoma, primary
  cutaneous 145, *145*
cryochambers 453, *453*, *455*

cryoprobes 453–454, *454*, *455*
cryosurgery 450–461
  actinic keratosis 93, *94*, 455–456, *457*, *459*
  anesthesia 454–455
  basal cell carcinoma 116, 456, *458*, *459*
  chamber or close-cone method 453, *453*, *455*
  clinical applications 455–457, *459*
  close or probe method 453–454, *454*, *455*
  combined with topical chemotherapy 451,
    454, *456*, *458*, *459*, 473
  complications 459–461, *460*
  confined-spray or cone method 453, *455*
  contraindications *460*
  equipment 451–452, *452*
  fractional 457
  history 450
  indications *460*
  Kaposi sarcoma 175, 457, *459*
  open spray method 453, *455*
  patient selection 454–455
  postoperative care and side effects 458–459
  preoperative considerations 454, *456*
  principles 450–451, *451*
  segmental 457, *460*
  squamous cell carcinoma 136, 456–457, *458*,
    *459*, *459*
  techniques 452–454, *452*, *453*, *455*
  *vs* topical chemotherapy *463*
CTLA-4 630, *631*
CTLA-4 blocking antibodies
  in melanoma 323, 602, 603, *619*, 631
  melanoma vaccine therapy with 611
  *see also* ipilimumab
*CTNNB1* gene, in desmoid tumors 158
curcumin, melanoma chemoprevention *76*, *77*
curettage
  biopsy, medico-legal aspects 673, *674*
  combined with imiquimod cream 473
  congenital melanocytic nevi 258
  history 443
  prior to photodynamic therapy 500–501
  techniques 445, *447*
curettage and electrodesiccation (CE) 443–449
  actinic keratosis 93, *94*, 448
  basal cell carcinoma 113–115, 444–445,
    *446*–*447*, 448
  contraindications 448
  cosmetic results 446, *448*
  cure rates 446–447
  equipment 443–444, *445*, *446*
  history 443
  indications 448
  postoperative care 446
  preoperative management 444
  principles 443–444, *445*
  squamous cell carcinoma 136, 444–445, 448
  technique 444–445, *447*
curettes 443–444, *445*, *446*
Cushing syndrome, ectopic ACTH-producing
  tumors 367–369
cutaneous B-cell lymphoma
  in HIV infection 205, *205*
  lymphomatoid drug reactions simulating
    210, *210*
  primary (PCBCL), epidemiology 51
  radiation therapy 586
cutaneous epithelioid angiomatous nodule
  (CEAN) 190
cutaneous horn *90*
cutaneous lymphocyte antigen (CLA), in
  cutaneous T-cell lymphoma 217
cutaneous T-cell lymphoma (CTCL) 217–230
  benign lymphocytic proliferations resembling
    *see* pseudolymphomas, cutaneous

  clinical features 218–220, *218*, *219*
  diagnosis 220–225, *222*, *223*
  differential diagnosis 225
  epidemiology 51, 217
  history 217
  HIV-related 205
  pathogenesis and etiology 217–218
  pathology 221–225, *224*, *225*
  prognosis 225–226
  staging 220–221, *221*, *222*, *223*, *224*
  treatment 226–229, *226*
    imiquimod 491
    interferons *226*, 228, 480–481
    interleukin-2 492
    interleukin-12 493
    photodynamic therapy 504–505
    radiation therapy 227–228, 585–586, *585*
    topical 226–228, *464*, 470–471
  tumor stage 218, *219*, 221–222, *224*
CVD chemotherapy, melanoma 629–630, *630*
cyclic adenosine monophosphate (cAMP), in
  melanin biosynthesis 34–35, *36*
cyclin D1 17
  in melanoma 347
cyclin-dependent kinase 2 (CDK2) 17
cyclin-dependent kinase 4 (CDK4) 17, *32*
  gene *see* *CDK4* gene
  in melanoma pathogenesis 2, 17
  in SCC tumorigenesis 15
cyclin-dependent kinase inhibitor 2A gene
  *see* *CDKN2A* gene
cyclin E 17
cyclo-oxygenase inhibitors
  melanoma chemoprevention *76*, *77*
  topical 74, 468–469
  *see also* diclofenac, topical
cyclophosphamide
  melanoma *621*
  Merkel cell carcinoma 530
cylindrocarcinoma 144
cysteinylDOPA *30*
cytogenetics *see* chromosome abnormalities
cytokeratin 7 (CK7)
  microcystic adnexal carcinoma *141*
  Paget's disease 151–152, 154–155, *517*
cytokeratin 20 (CK20)
  Merkel cell carcinoma 183, *183*, *183*
  Paget's disease 154–155
cytokeratins
  Paget's disease 151–152, 154–155
  squamous cell carcinoma 133
cytokines
  antitumor *478*
  in interferon-treated melanoma 600
cytotoxic T-lymphocyte antigen-4 *see* CTLA-4

**D**

Dabska's tumor *see* endovascular papillary
  angioendothelioma
dacarbazine (DTIC)
  dermatologic side effects 383
  melanoma 323, *591*, *620*, *621*, 629–630,
    *630*
daclizumab *635*
damages (legal) 669–670
darker-skinned individuals
  cutaneous T-cell lymphoma 220
  cutaneous vitamin D synthesis 650
  squamous cell carcinoma 129
  vitamin D levels 654, *654*
  *see also* skin color

Dartmouth regimen, melanoma 323, 629
dasatinib
    dermatologic side effects 383
    melanoma 614, *615*
    squamous cell carcinoma 528
daunorubicin-induced alopecia 379
DCT *see* tyrosinase-related protein 2
deck chair sign 220
deep pelvic lymphadenectomy 553, 556
defibrillators, implanted 448, 509
7-dehydrocholesterol 650, *651*
dendritic cells (DC) *478*
    in-situ vaccine concept 451
    melanoma vaccines and *607*, 608
    response to cryosurgery 451
denileukin diftitox
    cutaneous T-cell lymphoma *226*, 228, 492
    melanoma *619*
depression
    *CDKN2A* mutation carriers 664
    skin cancer patients 662–663
Dermablade® biopsy technique 437, *438*
dermabrasion, actinic keratosis *94*
dermal nevi, confocal microscopy 416
DermaScan C 404
dermatitis herpetiformis 376
dermatofibroma
    basal cell carcinoma arising in 111, *112*
    basaloid hyperplasia in 111, *112*
dermatofibrosarcoma protuberans (DFSP) 157,
        160–162
    clinical features 160–161, *160*
    diagnosis 161, *161*
    epidemiology 51–52, 157–158
    fibrosarcomatous (DFSP-FS) 161–162
    organ transplant recipients *635*
    pathogenesis and etiology 158, *159*, 161, *161*
    reconstructive surgery *563*, *571*
    treatment 161–162, 517, 521
dermatologic side effects of skin cancer
        systemic therapy 379–385
dermatologic therapy-related cutaneous
        carcinogenesis 349–356
    biologic agents 353–354
    chemotherapy and immunosuppressive
        agents 351–353
    potential mechanisms 349
    therapeutic radiation 349–354
dermatomyositis *368*, 376, *376*
dermatopathology, medico-legal issues
        672–674, *672*, *673*, *674*, *674*
dermoepidermal junction (DEJ)
    atypical melanocytes at 295, *296*
    in-vivo confocal microscopy 409, *410*, *410*
DermoGenius Ultra 401
dermoscopes
    non-polarized (NPD) 386, *387*, *387*
    polarized (PD) 386, *387*, *387*
dermoscopy 386–399
    basal cell carcinoma 387–388
    benign melanocytic nevi 392, 393, *393*, *394*,
        *395*
    computer-based algorithms 400–401
    congenital melanocytic nevi 254
    cryosurgery follow-up 454, *456*
    dysplastic (atypical) nevi
        diagnosis 241–242
        pattern analysis 395, *398*
        surveillance 242
    equipment 386
    image capture 659–660, *660*
    melanoma 70, 390, *390*
        7-point checklist 390–391, *391*
        ABCD rule 390, *390*

CASH algorithm 391, *391*
        Menzies method 392, *392*
        pattern analysis 392–395, *396*, *396*, *397*, *398*
        primary care physicians 70–71
    multispectral digital image analysis 401–404,
        *402*
    squamous cell carcinoma 388–389
desmin 164
desmoid tumors (desmoid fibromatosis) 158, *159*
desmoplastic melanoma (DMM) 302–304
    clinical features *264*, 302, *303*
    histopathology 302–303, *303*, *304*
    immunohistochemistry 303–304, *304*
    perineural involvement 302–303, *304*
    surgical excision 538
desmoplastic small round cell tumor *159*
desmoplastic Spitz nevus 342–343
desmoplastic trichoepithelioma 110, *111*, 140
desmosomes, in basal cell carcinoma 105–106, 113
DETOX (detoxified Freund's adjuvant) *607*,
        *608*, 610
dewars, liquid nitrogen 452, *452*
Dewar valence isomer 59
DFMO (α-difluoromethyl-DL-ornithine)
    chemoprevention studies 75, *76*
    topical therapy 472
diacylglycerol (DAG), in melanogenesis 33
diclofenac, topical *463*, 468–469
    actinic keratoses 93, *94*, 468–469, *469*
    adverse effects 469
    chemoprevention of non-melanoma skin
        cancers 74
    combined with cryosurgery 473
    indications *464*
    organ transplant recipients 469, *638*
diet
    skin cancer risk and 57, *64*
    sources of vitamin D 650, *651*
diethylamino hydroxybenzoyl hexylbenzoate
        (Univil A Plus) *81*, 83
diethylhexyl butamido triazone (Uvasorb HEB)
        *81*, 82–83
α-difluoromethyl-DL-ornithine *see* DFMO
digits, surgical excision of melanoma 540–541,
        *541*
5,6-dihydroxyindole (DHI) *30*
5,6-dihydroxyindole-2-carboxylic acid (DHICA)
        *30*, *30*
5,6-dihydroxyindole-2-carboxylic acid
        (DHICA)-melanin 30, *30*
5,6-dihydroxyindole (DHI)-melanin 30, *30*
dihydroxyphenylalanine *see* DOPA
1,25-dihydroxyvitamin D (1,25(OH)$_2$D),
        biosynthesis 650, *651*
dioxybenzone *81*, 83
diphenhydramine 435–436
disodium phenyl dibenzimidazole
        tetrasulfonate (Neo Helioplan T) *81*, 83
disseminated melanoma, treatment 629–633
disseminated non-melanoma skin cancers,
        treatment 526–531
*DKC1* gene mutations 363
DNA damage, UV-induced 59, *59*
    actinic keratoses 91
    indoor tanning devices 646, 647, *647*
    squamous cell carcinoma 125
DNA repair, defects 61
docetaxel
    basal cell carcinoma 526
    dermatologic side effects 379
    extramammary Paget's disease 155
    Kaposi sarcoma 176
DOPA (dihydroxyphenylalanine) 30, *30*
DOPAchrome 30, *30*

DOPAquinone 30
doxorubicin
    basal cell carcinoma 117
    cutaneous T-cell lymphoma *226*, 228
    dermatologic side effects 379, 380, 382–383
    Kaposi sarcoma 175–176
    Merkel cell carcinoma 530
    squamous cell carcinoma 527, *528*
drains, surgical 556
drug reactions, lymphomatoid 210–216, *210*,
        *211*, *211*
drug-related cutaneous carcinogenesis
    biologic agents 353–354
    chemotherapy and immunosuppressive
        agents 351–353
    potential mechanisms 349
DTIC *see* dacarbazine
*DTNBP1* gene mutations 27
duty of care 668–669, *668*
    breach of 669, *669*
dyskeratosis congenita (DKC) 363, *364*
dysplastic nevi (DN) (atypical moles; Clark's
        nevi) 231–245, 276
    clinical features 234–238, *234*, *235*, *236*, *237*,
        *238*, 276, *276*
    confocal microscopy 417–418, *422*, *423*
    dermoscopy *see under* dermoscopy
    EGIR genomic characterization 430–431, *430*
    epidemiology 232
    etiology and pathogenesis 232–233
    histology 238–240
        architectural features 239–240, *239*, *240*
        atypical features 240, *240*, *241*
        cytological features 240
    history 231–232
    management 240–243
    melanoma arising within *234*, 240, *241*, 276,
        *277*, 324
    melanoma risk 232, *232*, 276
        assessment 241
    patient evaluation 241–242
    pregnancy-related changes 330
    progression to melanoma 2–3, *4*, 233, 298
    surveillance 242–243
    terminology 231–232
    treatment 242, 243
    *vs* acquired melanocytic nevi *238*
    *vs* early melanoma 234, *235*
dysplastic nevus syndrome (DNS) (atypical
        mole syndrome; AMS)
    diagnostic criteria 237–238, *238*
    melanoma *270*
    melanoma screening 70
    surveillance 242–243
        during pregnancy 330
    use of term 238


E

E2F transcription factor 17
ear
    melanoma of outer helix 540, *541*
    radiation therapy 579, *581*
    reconstruction 567–568, *570*
    squamous cell carcinoma 128, *128*
early detection of skin cancer 69–71
E-cadherin 5
    in Paget's disease 153
ecamsule *81*, 83
eccrine epithelioma 110–111
eccrine glands, carcinomas of 140–146
eccrine hidradenitis, neutrophilic 380, 383
ectopic ACTH-producing tumors 367–369, *370*

edema, cryosurgery-related 459
educational interventions 67, 68
EGIR™ see epidermal genetic information retrieval
852A 619
elderly
    basal cell carcinoma management 118
    cryosurgery 454
    melanoma incidence 45
    melanoma mortality 40–41, 47
    musculoskeletal benefits of vitamin D 651
    squamous cell carcinoma mortality 50
    vitamin D synthesis 650
electrical bio-impedance (resistance), cellular 401, 404
electrical impedance spectroscopy (EIS) 404
electrodesiccation 443
    and curettage see curettage and electrodesiccation
    principles 443, 445
    technique 445, 447
electromagnetic spectrum 56, 57
electron beam therapy 576
    Kaposi sarcoma 175
electron microscopy
    basal cell carcinoma 112
    cutaneous sarcoma 160
electro-stimulative implants, electrosurgery and 448, 509
electrosurgery
    implanted cardiac devices and 448, 509
    principles of 443, 444, 444, 445
elesclomol 619, 620
emotional distress see psychological distress
endometrial stroma sarcoma 159
endoplasmic reticulum (ER), proteins destined for melanosomes 26, 26
endothelin-3 (EDN3) 24, 24
endothelin B receptors (EDNRB) 24, 24
endothelium, adherence of tumor cells 7
endovascular papillary angioendothelioma (EPE) (Dabska's tumor) 186, 187–188, 187
ensulizole 81, 82
ephelides 275–276
epidemiology 44–55
    analytic 52
    descriptive 44–52
    future outlook 53
    historical aspects 44
    interventional 52–53
epidermal genetic information retrieval (EGIR™) 429–433
    characterization of melanoma and nevi 430–431, 430
    detection of melanoma 431
    further development 431–432, 432, 433, 433
epidermal growth factor receptor (EGFR)
    inhibitors (EGFRIs)
        cancers treated 380
        dermatologic side effects 380–382, 381, 382
        squamous cell carcinoma 528
    pathway 529
epidermal melanin unit 25, 25
epidermis, consumption of 343
epidermodysplasia verruciformis (EV) 196–198, 362, 364
    clinical features 197, 197
    diagnosis 197–198, 198
    pathogenesis and etiology 61–62, 96, 196–197
    pathology 198, 198
epidermolysis bullosa (EB) 359–360, 360, 364, 376

epidermotropism, in cutaneous T-cell lymphoma 221–222, 224–225, 224
epigenetic modification 12
epiluminescence microscopy (ELM) 659–660, 660
    see also dermoscopy
epithelial membrane antigen (EMA), Paget's disease 151–152
epitheliocarcinoma of Malherbe, calcifying see matrical carcinoma
epithelioid angiomatous nodule, cutaneous (CEAN) 190
epithelioid angiosarcoma 190
epithelioid hemangioendothelioma 189–191, 190
epithelioid sarcoma 158, 159
epithelioma
    apocrine 110–111
    eccrine 110–111
    sebaceous 107
epithelioma cuniculatum 129, 130, 202, 202
epitopes
    anti-melanoma vaccines 606
    heteroclitic 606
epitrochlear lymphadenectomy 554–555, 555
equivalent dose, radiation therapy 577–578
ergocalciferol (vitamin D₂) 650
    supplements 650
ERK pathway see Raf/MEK/ERK pathway
erlotinib, squamous cell carcinoma 528
erythema ab igne 64, 64
erythema gyratum repens 368, 377, 377
erythroderma, in Sézary syndrome 219–220, 219
erythroplasia of Queyrat 96, 97, 126–127
    photodynamic therapy 503
eschar, after cryosurgery 459
Estlander flap 567
estrogen receptor β (ERβ), expression in melanoma 327–328
estrogen therapy, in melanoma survivors 331
etanercept, carcinogenic potential 353–354
etaracizumab, in melanoma 615
ethnic differences
    cutaneous T-cell lymphoma 217
    melanoma incidence 40, 45
    melanoma mortality 47
    primary cutaneous B-cell lymphoma 51
    skin cancer risk 57
ethylhexyl triazone (Univil T 150) 81, 82–83
etiologic factors in skin cancers 56–65
etoposide
    extramammary Paget's disease 155
    Merkel cell carcinoma 530
etretinate, basal cell carcinoma 117
eumelanin 29–30
    biosynthesis 30, 30, 31
        regulation 35, 36
    pheomelanin ratio, factors affecting 33
eumelanosomes 27, 29–30
EVER1/EVER2 genes 196–197
everolimus 635
    chemoprevention of non-melanoma skin cancers 74–75
    in melanoma 616
    organ transplant recipients 636
evidence-based medicine, legal aspects 669, 669
Ewing sarcoma 143, 165
    genetic alterations 159
EWSR1 gene fusions, in clear cell sarcoma 143, 158, 164–165
excisional biopsy 434, 436
    medico-legal aspects 673
    suspicious pigmented lesions 299, 439
    techniques 436–439, 437, 438, 439
extracellular matrix, therapeutic targeting in melanoma 617–618, 618

extracellular-related kinase (ERK) pathway see Raf/MEK/ERK pathway
extracorporeal photopheresis (ECP), cutaneous T-cell lymphoma 226, 227–228
extravasation, metastatic tumor cells 7
eye
    adverse effects of indoor tanning 646
    effects of sun exposure 86
    photoprotection 86–87
eyelid tumors
    cryosurgery 455, 457
    radiation therapy 579, 580, 581
    reconstructive surgery 565

## F

facial reconstruction 563, 565, 566
factor XIIIa, dermatofibrosarcoma protuberans 161
familial atypical mole-melanoma syndrome (FAMMM) 231–232, 364
    genetics 233
familial cancer syndromes, with dermatological features 367, 368
familial melanoma 334
    behavioral changes in mutation carriers 339
    genes involved 2, 16–18, 19–20, 334
    genetic testing 325, 334–340
    management of affected families 325, 339
    molecular pathogenesis 2, 16–18
    prevalence 334, 335
    psychological responses of gene carriers 664
family history
    of skin cancer 57, 67
        psychological impact 664
    taking a 336
Fanconi's anemia 363
farnesyltransferase inhibitors 615, 616
fascial flaps 570
fasciocutaneous flaps 572, 573
FDA see Food and Drug Administration
febrile neutrophilic dermatoses, acute see Sweet syndrome
fenretinide, topical 470
Ferguson–Smith syndrome 130, 362
fetal metastases, melanoma 330
fibroblast growth factor-β (FGF-β; basic fibroblast growth factor; bFGF)
    therapeutic targeting in melanoma 617–618
    tumor angiogenesis and lymphangiogenesis 4, 5
fibroblastoma, giant cell 161
fibroepithelioma of Pinkus 103
    histology 107, 109
fibromyxoid sarcoma, low-grade 159
fibrosarcoma, infantile 159
fibrous histiocytoma, angiomatoid 159
fibroxanthoma, atypical see atypical fibroxanthoma
field cancerization
    concept 64, 73–74
    cryosurgery 454, 456
    topical treatment 462
fingers
    melanoma in webspace 541, 542
    surgical excision of melanoma 541, 541
flag sign, hypertrophic actinic keratosis 92
flaps
    axial pattern 560, 561, 561
    free see free tissue transfer, microvascular
    local 560, 561
    pedicle 570, 572
    random 561, 562

flavonoids, melanoma chemoprevention 76
flavopiridol 617
floxuridine, dermatologic side effects 379
fluorescence in-situ hybridization (FISH),
    cutaneous sarcomas 160
fluorescence navigation, extramammary Paget's
    disease 155
5-fluorouracil (5-FU)
    dermatologic side effects 379
    extramammary Paget's disease 155
    squamous cell carcinoma 527, 528
    topical 462–466
        actinic keratosis 93, 94, 462–464, 463,
            464, 465
        basal cell carcinoma 117, 464–465
        basal cell nevus syndrome 358–359
        combinations 454, 456, 473
        extramammary Paget's disease 465
        indications 464
        squamous cell carcinoma 136–137, 465
flushing, in carcinoid syndrome 370–371
folded luggage pattern 220
follicular mucinosis
    in folliculotropic mycosis fungoides 222–223
    idiopathic (IFM) 223
    lymphoma-associated (LAFM) 223
folliculotropism, in folliculotropic mycosis
    fungoides 222–223, 224
Fontana–Masson stain 311
Food and Drug Administration (FDA)
    monograph on sunscreens 81, 82, 83
    regulation of indoor tanning 646
    sunscreen labeling 84
    Time and Extend Application (TEA) process 83
foot reconstruction 573–575, 574
forehead reconstruction 563–566, 566, 567
foscarnet, Kaposi sarcoma 176
Fowler's solution 95
Fox curette 443–444, 445
freckles 275–276
free tissue transfer, microvascular 560, 561
    prior radiation therapy and 560
freeze–thaw cycle, cryosurgery 451, 452
freezing
    direct cellular injury caused by 450, 451
    see also cryosurgery
French Cooperative Group Trial 533, 533, 534
Freund's adjuvant, detoxified (DETOX) 607,
    608, 610
fusiform ellipse
    excisional biopsy 434, 436
        suspicious pigmented lesions 439
        technique 438–439, 439, 440
    surgical excision of melanoma 539
    surgical excision of non-melanoma skin
        cancers 509, 510

G

G3139 617, 619, 620
GAGE1/2/MZ2-F 32
galea aponeurosis 562
gamma probes, sentinel lymph node biopsy
    546, 546
ganciclovir, Kaposi sarcoma 176
Gardasil 203
Gardner syndrome 362, 368, 369
gastrointestinal carcinoma, cutaneous
    metastases 142
GC1008 618
GDC-0499
    in basal cell carcinoma 117, 526, 527
    in basal cell nevus syndrome 364

GDC0941 616
gefitinib, squamous cell carcinoma 528, 528, 529
gemcitabine
    cutaneous T-cell lymphoma 226, 228
    dermatologic side effects 379, 380
gender differences
    actinic keratoses 90
    basal cell carcinoma incidence 49, 50
    melanoma incidence 40, 45–46, 46, 46, 647, 648
    melanoma mortality 47, 47, 48
    melanoma prognosis 285, 286, 288
    skin cancer risk 57, 61, 66–67
    squamous cell carcinoma incidence 49, 49,
        124
    squamous cell carcinoma mortality 50
gene expression profiling see microarray-based
    gene expression profiling
Gene Scan 222
GeneTests 336, 336
genetic counselling 336
genetic disorders predisposing to skin cancer
    357–366, 364
Genetic Information Nondiscrimination Act
    (GINA) 336
genetics 12–22, 60–61
    basal cell carcinoma 12–14
    cutaneous sarcomas 158, 159
    future outlook 20
    melanoma 16–20, 61
    squamous cell carcinoma 15–16
genetic testing, for melanoma 325, 334–340
    in clinical practice 335–339
    counselling and informed consent 336, 337
    gene identification 334–335
    management of positive results 339
    online resources 336
    patient behavioral changes after 339
    patient selection 335–336, 336
    procedure 336–339
genistein, melanoma chemoprevention 76
GenoMEL 335, 336
genomics, clinical, for melanoma detection
    429–433
geographical variations
    melanoma incidence 46–47, 46
    melanoma mortality 47–48
    penetrance of CDKN2A mutations 334–335
giant cell fibroblastoma 161
giant condyloma of Buschke–Lowenstein see
    Buschke–Lowenstein tumor
giant mucocutaneous papillomatosis see oral
    florid papillomatosis
Gleevec® see imatinib mesylate
Gli proteins 13, 14, 349
Global Solar UV Index 58–59
glomangiosarcomas (malignant glomus tumors)
    192–193, 193
glucagonoma syndrome 371, 371
glucocorticoids see corticosteroids
glutamate receptors, metabotropic (GRM1), in
    melanoma 614–615
glutathione 31
GMK vaccine 596, 597, 598, 608, 609–610
GNAQ mutations
    in melanoma 3, 19
    targeted therapy 325
Golgi phosphoprotein 3 (GOLPH3) 19
Gorlin syndrome see basal cell nevus syndrome
Gottron's papules 376, 376
gp75 see tyrosinase-related protein 1
gp100/Pmel17 27, 30, 32
    melanoma vaccine 608, 610, 630, 630
    regulation of activity 33
    see also HMB-45 immunostaining

graft-versus-host disease (GVHD), cutaneous
    T-cell lymphoma 228–229
granular cell tumor 523
granulocyte macrophage colony-stimulating
    factor (GM-CSF) 492
    melanoma therapy 599
    in melanoma vaccines 607, 608
granuloma annulare 200
granulomatous slack skin 219, 223
Grays 577
Griscelli syndrome 27–28, 27, 368
groin lymphadenectomy, superficial 553, 556
gross cystic disease fluid protein 15 (GCDFP-
    15), in Paget's disease 154–155
growth, tumor
    local extension 5–6
    mechanisms of 1–8
    radial to vertical transition 5
Grzybowski syndrome 130, 362
GSK461364 617
GSK1059615 616
GTDC-0449, prevention of non-melanoma skin
    cancers 75
guanine nucleotide exchange factors (GEFs) 5–6

H

hair
    loss see alopecia
    photoprotective effects 86
    preoperative removal 508
hair follicles
    basal cell carcinoma extending around 112, 112
    carcinomas of 146–148
    melanocytes 25
halo dermatitis, congenital melanocytic nevi
    249–251
halo phenomenon
    congenital melanocytic nevi 249–251, 251
    Spitz nevus 341, 345, 345
hand–foot skin reaction (HFSR), sorafenib-
    induced 382
hand–foot syndrome, chemotherapy-induced
    379, 380, 382–383
hands
    reconstructive surgery 573, 573, 574
    transplant 637, 637
hats, photoprotective effects 86
head and neck
    melanoma, excision margins 537–538
    reconstructive surgery 561–568
heat shock proteins, melanoma vaccine with
    608, 610
hedgehog signaling pathway
    in cutaneous carcinogenesis 13–14, 14, 349, 357
    inhibitors
        in basal cell carcinoma 117, 526, 527
        chemoprevention role 75
helper T cells, memory CD4+, in cutaneous
    T-cell lymphoma 217
hemangioendothelioma 186
    composite 186, 188–189, 189
    epithelioid 189–191, 190
    polymorphous 188–189
    retiform (RH) 186, 187–188, 188
hematological malignancies
    in HIV-infected patients 205
    skin cancer risk 63
    see also chronic lymphocytic leukemia;
        lymphoma
hematopoietic precursor cells (HPCs)
    in neoplastic angiogenesis 4
    in premetastatic niches 7

hematoxylin and eosin (H&E) 515–517
heme biosynthesis 498, *499*
hemophagocytic syndrome 225
hepatic metastases *see* liver metastases
hepatocyte growth factor (HGF) 5
  dermal melanocytes and 25
  overexpression in congenital melanocytic
    nevi 246–247
Her2/Neu, Paget's disease 151–152
hereditary leiomyomatosis renal cell cancer
    syndrome *368*
hereditary melanoma *see* familial melanoma
hereditary non-polyposis colorectal cancer
    (HNPCC) 362
Hermansky–Pudlak syndrome (HPS) 26, *27, 27*
herpes simplex 210
herpes zoster 210
hexachlorobenzene *63*
hidradenoma, Mohs micrographic surgery 523
highly active antiretroviral therapy (HAART)
    in epidemic Kaposi sarcoma 174
    skin cancer risk and 642
hip fractures, vitamin D and 651
Hirschsprung disease 24
histologic margins 510–511
histone deacetylase (HDAC) inhibitors,
    cutaneous T-cell lymphoma 228
HIV infection/AIDS 196, 203–205
  Kaposi sarcoma *see* Kaposi sarcoma (KS),
    epidemic
  lymphoreticular malignancies 205
  management of skin cancer 641–642
  Merkel cell carcinoma risk 179–180
  skin cancer risk 63, 204–205, 642
HLA haplotypes
  cutaneous T-cell lymphoma 217–218
  melanoma vaccine therapy and 607, 610
HMB-45 immunostaining
  clear cell sarcoma 165
  melanoma 303–304, *304*, 311
  Mohs micrographic surgery *517*
  *see also* gp100/Pmel17
Hodgkin disease, cutaneous, in HIV infection
    205
homosalate *81*, 82
hormone replacement therapy (HRT), in
    melanoma survivors 331
hormone-secreting tumors, skin changes
    367–371
Howel–Evans syndrome *368*
*HPS1–6* gene mutations *27*
HPV *see* human papillomaviruses
*H-RAS* gene
  in melanoma pathogenesis 18
  mutations in Spitz nevi 3, 347
  in squamous cell carcinoma tumorigenesis 15
Human Genome Project 429
human herpesvirus 8 (HHV8) 61–62, 168, 203–204
  latency-associated nuclear antigen (LANA)
    173
  serology 173
human immunodeficiency virus infection *see*
    HIV infection/AIDS
human papillomaviruses (HPV) 196
  alpha 196
  beta 61–62, 196
  bowenoid papulosis and 96, 199
  epidermodysplasia verruciformis-associated
    (EVHPVs) 96, 196–197
  neoplastic disorders associated with 96,
    196–203
  phylogenetic tree *62*
  skin cancer in transplant recipients and
    61–62, 637

in squamous cell carcinoma development
    61–62, 96, 126
  vaccination for 203
  verrucous carcinoma and 96, 202
human T-cell leukemia virus 1 (HTLV-1) 225
Huriez syndrome 363–364, *364*
Hutchinson's melanotic freckle *see* lentigo maligna
Hutchinson's sign *270, 277*
hydrogen peroxide radiosensitization,
    extramammary Paget's disease 155
25-hydroxyvitamin D (25(OH)D) 650
  serum levels 650–651, *654*
    health and disease associations 650–654, *652*
    optimal 654
    sun exposure and 654–655
hyperpigmentation
  after cryosurgery 461
  ectopic ACTH-producing tumors 367–369, *370*
  familial progressive 24
hyperthermic isolated limb perfusion (HILP) 323
hypertrichosis, congenital melanocytic nevi
    247, *251*
hypertrichosis lanuginosa acquisita 371–372,
    *371, 372*
hypopigmentation, after cryosurgery 460

**I**

ifosfamide, dermatologic side effects 383
IκBα 15
*IL9* gene 334–335
ilioinguinal (deep pelvic) lymphadenectomy
    553, 556
IM1121B *618*
imaging, radiological
  cutaneous T-cell lymphoma 220, *223*
  Kaposi sarcoma 173
  melanoma 320, 623–628
    at diagnosis 623–625
    follow-up 324, 625–627
    during pregnancy 330–331
  Merkel cell carcinoma 181–182
  Paget's disease 151, 153–154
  sarcomas 161, 164
  squamous cell carcinoma 130–131
imatinib mesylate
  dermatofibrosarcoma protuberans 162, 521
  dermatologic side effects 383
  Kaposi sarcoma 176
  melanoma 325, 614, *615, 620*, 632
imexon *620*
imiquimod *463*, 466–468, 482–491
  actinic cheilitis 491
  actinic keratosis 93, *94*, 466, *467*, 484, *485*
  adverse effects 491
  basal cell carcinoma 117, 466–468, *467*, 482,
    *483*, 484–488, *486*
  Bowenoid papulosis 488
  Bowen's disease 488, *489, 490*
  combined with cryosurgery 451, 454, *458,
    459*, 473
  combined with curettage 473
  cutaneous T-cell lymphoma 491
  drug interactions 491
  extramammary Paget's disease 155, 491
  indications *464*, 484–491
  Kaposi sarcoma 176, 468
  mechanism of action 482–483, *483*
  melanoma 489–490
  organ transplant recipients 468, 484, 638
  squamous cell carcinoma 136–137, 466–468,
    482–483, *486*, 488, *490*
  use in pregnancy 491

immune reconstitution inflammatory syndrome
    (IRIS), Kaposi sarcoma-associated 174
immune response modifiers 477–496
  basal cell carcinoma 117, 479–480
  cancers treated *380*
  combined with cryosurgery 451
  dermatologic side effects 383
  mechanisms of action *478*
  melanoma 323, 479, 489–490, 492
  squamous cell carcinoma 527–528
  *see also* imiquimod; ingenol mebutate;
    interferon(s); interleukin-2;
    interleukin-12; resiquimod
immune system
  antimelanoma responses 606, *607*
  antitumor mechanisms 477, *478*, 634
  effects of cryosurgery 451, *451*
  melanoma therapies targeting 619, *619*, 630,
    631, *631*
  tumor evasion 6–7, 477, *478*
immunobullous disorders 375–376
immunocompromised patients *see*
    immunosuppressed patients
immunocryosurgery 451
immunohistochemistry (IHC)
  acral myxoinflammatory fibroblastic sarcoma
    164
  angiosarcomas 187–188, 190, 191
  atypical fibroxanthoma 163
  basal cell carcinoma 113
  clear cell sarcoma of soft tissue 165
  cutaneous T-cell lymphoma 223
  dermatofibrosarcoma protuberans 161
  glomangiosarcomas 193
  Kaposi sarcoma 173
  melanoma 303–304, *304*, 311, *311*
  Merkel cell carcinoma 183, *183*
  Mohs micrographic surgery 516–517, *517*
  Paget's disease 151–152, 154–155
  pleomorphic hyalinizing angiectatic tumor 165
  sarcomas 159–160, 161
  Spitz nevus *vs* melanoma 347
  squamous cell carcinoma 133–134
  superficial leiomyosarcoma 164
immunostimulants, non-specific, in melanoma
    590, *591*
immunosuppressed patients 634–643
  actinic keratosis 90
  basal cell carcinoma 100–101, *100*
  epidermodysplasia verruciformis 198, *198*
  HPV-associated squamous cell carcinoma 96
  increased skin cancer risks 62–63, 67
  Kaposi sarcoma 172
  Merkel cell carcinoma 179–180
  Mohs micrographic surgery 517
  squamous cell carcinoma 124–125
  *see also* HIV infection/AIDS; organ transplant
    recipients
immunosuppression, sunlight-induced 91
immunosuppressive agents *635*
  carcinogenic potential *350*, 351–353, *635*
  dermatologic side effects *635*
  organ transplant recipients 635–637, *635*
immunotherapy
  melanoma 630–631, *630*
  *see also* immune response modifiers; vaccine
    therapy
implantable cardioverter-defibrillators (ICDs)
    448, 509
incisional biopsy 434, *436*
  medico-legal aspects 673
  melanoma 318, 440–441
  suspicious pigmented lesions 299, 439–441, *441*
  technique 436–439, *437*

incyclinide (Metastat), Kaposi sarcoma 176
indinavir, Kaposi sarcoma 176
indole-5,6-quinone *30*
indole-5,6-quinone-2-carboxylic acid *30*
indoleamine-2,3-dioxygenase (IDO) 6–7
indoor tanning *see* tanning, indoor
infections
   chronic, skin cancer risk 95, *125*
   complicating cryosurgery 460
   postoperative wound
     management 509
      prevention 508–509, 523–524
      regional lymphadenectomy 556
inflammation, chronic 64, 95, 125–126, *125*
inflammatory dermatoses associated with
     internal malignancy 371–377, *371*
inflammatory myofibroblastic tumor *159*
infliximab, carcinogenic potential 353–354
informed consent 670, *670*
infrared radiation (IR) 56
   protection from biologic effects 85
ingenol mebutate (ingenol-3-angelate; Ing3A)
     471–472, 492
   actinic keratoses *94*, 471–472
   basal cell carcinoma 117
inguinofemoral (superficial groin)
     lymphadenectomy 553, 556
*INK4A* gene product *see* p16^INK4A
innovative therapy, legal aspects 669
INO-1001 *620*
insect bite reaction, exaggerated *368*, 377, *377*
in-situ hybridization, cutaneous sarcomas 160
integrins 5
   αVβ3 5
   therapeutic targeting in melanoma 614–615
interferon(s) (IFNs) 477–482
   mechanisms of action 477–479, *478*, 592–593, *593*
   types 592–593, *593*
interferon-α (IFN-α) 592–593, *593*
   actinic keratoses 480
   adverse effects 481–482, *481*
   basal cell carcinoma 117, 479–480, *480*
   contraindications 481
   cutaneous T-cell lymphoma *226*, 228, 480–481
   dermatologic side effects 383
   drug interactions 482
   imiquimod actions 482
   indications 479–481
   Kaposi sarcoma 175, 481
   keratoacanthoma 480
   mechanisms of action 477–479, *478*, 593, *593*
   melanoma 322, 479, 590–603
     alternatives to standard high-dose regimen
      601–602
     biomarkers of therapeutic benefit 599–600
     clinical trials 593–598, *594*, *595*, *596*
     combination therapies 602, *620*, *621*,
      629–630, *630*
     contraindications and cautions 600, *600*
     duration of therapy 599
     high-dose regimens 594–597, *596*, *597*,
      598–599
     indications 600, *600*
     intermediate-dose regimens *596*, 598
     low-dose regimens 594–597, *596*, 598
     quality-of-life studies 601
     role of induction phase 602
     specific patient subgroups 602
     standard of care 599
     toxicity 600–601, *601*
     very-low-dose regimens 598
     *vs* completion lymph node dissection 599
     *vs* ipilimumab 602, 603
     *vs* vaccine therapy *596*, *597*, 598, *608*, 609–610

pegylated *see* pegylated interferon-α2b
   squamous cell carcinoma 480, 527–528, *528*
   use in pregnancy 482
interferon-β (IFN-β) 477–479, 592–593, *593*
   dermatologic side effects 383
interferon-γ (IFN-γ) 477–479, 592–593, *593*
Intergroup Melanoma Surgical Trial *533*, *534*,
     535–536, *535*
interleukin-1 (IL-1), regulation of
     melanogenesis 34
interleukin-2 (IL-2) *478*, 492
   adverse effects 492, 630
   contraindications 492
   cutaneous T-cell lymphoma 492
   dermatologic side effects 379, 383
   indications 492
   mechanism of action *478*, 492
   melanoma 323, 492, 630
     combined with chemotherapy 629–630,
      *630*
     melanoma vaccination with *607*, 608, *608*,
      610, 630, *630*
   *see also* denileukin diftitox
interleukin-8 (IL-8) 4, 5
interleukin-12 (IL-12) *478*, 493
   cutaneous T-cell lymphoma 493
   Kaposi sarcoma 175
   mechanism of action *478*, 493
   melanoma 493
international normalized ratio (INR) 509
intradermal nevus 275
invasion, tumor 5–6
in-vitro diagnostic multivariate index
     (IVDMIA), melanoma risk score 431–432,
     *433*, 433
ipilimumab, melanoma 323, 602, 603, *619*, *620*,
     631
*IRF4* gene variants 37
isobutylmethylxanthine 35
isotherms, cryosurgical site 452, *452*
isotretinoin
   basal cell carcinoma 117
   in basal cell nevus syndrome 117, 359
   prevention of non-melanoma skin cancer 74,
     359, 362
   topical, actinic keratosis 470

**J**

junctional nevi 275
   confocal microscopy 416, *419*

**K**

Kamino bodies 342, 344
Kaposi sarcoma (KS) 168–178
   classic 169–170, *170*
     radiation therapy *583*, 584
     staging *170*
     treatment 174
   clinical features 168–169, *169*, 169
   diagnostic evaluation 172–174
   differential diagnosis 172, *173*
   endemic 172, *172*, 174
   epidemic (AIDS-related) 170–171, 203–204
     AIDS Clinical Trials Group classification
      171, *172*
     clinical features 170–171, *171*, 203–204,
      *204*
     pathogenesis 168
     radiation therapy 584–585, *584*
     treatment 174, 642

epidemiology 52
future outlook 176
histopathology 172–173, *173*
history 168
non-epidemic, in men who have sex with
     men 171
pathogenesis 168
post-transplant (iatrogenic) 172, 352, *352*
   management 174, 641
treatment 174–176, *176*
   cryosurgery 175, 457, *459*
   interferons 175, 481
   radiation therapy 175, 204, 583–585, *583*, *584*
   topical chemotherapy 174–175, 176, *464*,
     468, 470
Kaposi sarcoma-associated herpesvirus (KSHV)
   *see* human herpesvirus 8
Kaposi sarcoma-associated immune
     reconstitution inflammatory syndrome
     (KS-IRIS) 174
Karapandzic flap 567
keloid-prone patients, curettage and
     electrodesiccation 448
keratinocyte carcinomas (KC)
   epidemiology 48–49
   precursor lesions 89–98
   risk factors 52
   social impact 50–51
   *see also* basal cell carcinoma; squamous cell
     carcinoma
keratinocytes, transfer of melanosomes to
     27–28, *29*
keratinocytic intraepidermal neoplasia (KIN)
     92–93, *93*
keratoacanthoma (KA) 130, *130*
   centrifugum marginatum 130
   in Muir–Torre syndrome 130, 362
   multiple 130, *130*, 362
   pathology 133, *133*
   transplant recipients *639*
   treatment
     cryosurgery 456–457, *459*
     interferons 480
     topical chemotherapy 465
keystone flaps 572–573
Ki-67
   melanoma 312
   Spitz nevus 347
kinase inhibitors, multitargeted *see* multikinase
     inhibitors
KIT
   neural crest cell requirements 24, *24*
   neural crest cells *24*
*KIT* gene mutations
   in melanoma 19, 613
     therapies targeting 325, 614, 632
   in pigmentary disorders 24
*KITLG* gene
   mutations 24
   variants 37
KIT ligand (steel factor; stem cell factor)
   genes *see* *KITLG* gene; *steel* gene
   neural crest cell requirements 24, *24*
   soluble (sKitL) 4–5
*K-RAS* mutations, in squamous cell carcinoma 15
*KRT5* mutations, epidermolysis bullosa 359
*KRT14* mutations, epidermolysis bullosa 359
KW-2871 *615*, *620*

**L**

laboratory tests, melanoma 320
   follow-up 324

lactic dehydrogenase (LDH), serum
  initial melanoma work-up 320
  melanoma staging 283, *283*, 291, 292
laminin, in basal cell carcinoma 113
laminin 332 mutations 359
Lancaster, H.O 44
Langer, lines of 509–510, *510*
laser treatment
  actinic keratosis *94*
  basal cell carcinoma 116
  congenital melanocytic nevi 257, 258–259
  dysplastic nevi 243
  Kaposi sarcoma 176
lateral arm flap 573
lateral calcaneal flap 574–575
latissimus dorsi flaps *564*, 569, 570, *572*
latitude effects
  melanoma incidence 47
  squamous cell carcinoma incidence 50
  UV radiation 56
legal aspects 668–675
leiomyomatosis renal cell cancer syndrome,
      hereditary *368*
leiomyosarcoma, superficial (SLMS) 157, 164
  pathogenesis and etiology 158
lenalidomide *621*
lentigines
  gene expression profiling 430, 431
  PUVA-related *351*
  simple 275
  solar 275
lentiginous nevi, speckled (SLN) 252, *253*
lentigo maligna (melanoma) 301, *301*
  confocal microscopy 419–420, *427*
  genomic detection 431
  treatment 320, *322*
    cryosurgery 457, *459*
    imiquimod 468, 489–490
    interferon-α 479
    Mohs micrographic surgery 518–519
    surgical excision 536–537, *538*
    topical chemotherapy *464*
  *see also* melanoma in situ
Leser–Trélat sign *371*, 373, *373*
leukocytoclastic vasculitis, cutaneous 376
leukoplakia, oral 128, *464*
levamisole, melanoma *591*
lichen aureus 212–214, *214*
lichenoid (lymphomatoid) keratosis 212–214, *214*
lichenoid pigmented purpuric dermatitis
      212–214, *214*
lichen planus *200*
lichen sclerosus on genital skin 212–214
lidocaine
  local anesthesia 435–436
  toxicity 523
Li–Fraumeni syndrome 158
lighting, for clinical photography 657, 658–659, *659*
light sources, for photodynamic therapy 499–500
limb
  perfusion, isolated, melanoma 323, *591*
  reconstruction 572–575
lion-like facies, in Sézary syndrome 220, *220*
lip
  actinic cheilitis 91, 128
  reconstruction 567
  squamous cell carcinoma 128
  switch flaps 567
lipomatous tumor, atypical 165
liposarcoma
  molecular mechanisms 158
  myxoid/round cell *159*
  well-differentiated *159*, 165

liposomes, melanoma vaccines *607*, 608
β-lipotropin 367–369
liquid nitrogen (LN) 451, 452
  delivery system 451, *452*
  methods of delivery 453–454, *453*, *454*
  storage containers 452, *452*
  *see also* cryosurgery
liver metastases
  melanoma 624, *624*, 627
  potential pathways for development 7, *7*
liver spot 275
local anesthesia
  for biopsy 435–436, *436*
  cryosurgery 454–455
local anesthetic toxicity 523
loss of heterozygosity (LOH)
  in actinic keratoses 16, 91
  in squamous cell carcinoma 16
lower extremity reconstruction 572–575
lung cancer, vitamin D and *652*
lupus profundus (lupus panniculitis)
      214–215
LY573636 *617*
lycopene, melanoma chemoprevention 76
lymphadenectomy *see* lymph node dissection
lymphangiogenesis, neoplastic 5, *5*, 7
lymphatic mapping, in melanoma 320–321, 545–546
  in pregnancy 330
  reconstructive surgery and 559
  scientific basis 545–546, *545*
  staging 283, 289
  techniques 546–547, *546*
  *see also* sentinel lymph node biopsy
lymphedema
  chronic, angiosarcoma associated with
      186–187, 191–192
  complicating regional lymphadenectomy 556
lymph node biopsy
  cutaneous T-cell lymphoma 220, *223*
  melanoma 544–552
  sentinel *see* sentinel lymph node biopsy
lymph node dissection (lymphadenectomy)
  completion (CLND) 321, 551, 599
  elective (ELND) 544–545, 548–549
  regional 552–553
    extent and technique 552
    indications 552
    in multiple lymph node basins 556–557
    postoperative care and morbidity 556
    pre-surgical planning 552–553
    techniques 553–557
  selective 545–546, 548–549, *549*
  therapeutic (TLND) 544–545, 549
lymph node metastases, melanoma 544
  biopsy-related risk 299
  histopathologic diagnosis 295–297
  management 322–323
  number of involved nodes 289, *289*
  pathways of development 7
  prognostic implications 321, *322*
  submicroscopic 291
  surgical management *see* lymph node
      dissection
  tumor burden 289, *289*
  from unknown primary site 283, 292
  *see also* melanoma, stage III
lymph node surgery, regional, in melanoma
      544–558
lymphocytes, tumor-infiltrating *see* tumor-
      infiltrating lymphocytes
lymphocytoma cutis 211–212, *213*, *214*
lymphoepithelial-like carcinoma 216

lymphoma
  benign lymphocytic proliferations mimicking
      207–216, *208*
  drug therapy-related 350, 351–352, 353, 354
  HIV infection 205, *205*
  *see also* cutaneous B-cell lymphoma;
      cutaneous T-cell lymphoma; non-
      Hodgkin lymphoma
lymphomatoid contact dermatitis 209–210, *209*
lymphomatoid drug reactions 210–216, *210*, *211*, 211
lymphomatoid (lichenoid) keratosis 212–214, *214*
lymphomatoid papulosis (LyP) 225, *225*
lymphoscintigraphy, cutaneous 546, *546*
*LYST (CHS1)* gene mutations 27

## M

macrophages, tumor-associated *478*, 478
MAGE1/MZ2-E 32
MAGE3/MZ2-D 32
  vaccine 325, 610–611
magnetic resonance imaging (MRI)
  dermatofibrosarcoma protuberans 521
  melanoma 404, 625, *625*, 626–627
  neurocutaneous melanocytosis 256, 259
malignancies
  congenital melanocytic nevus-related 254–256
  extramammary Paget's disease-related
      152–153, 376
  skin signs of internal 367–378
    criteria for analyzing 367
    hormone-secreting tumors 367–371
    inherited syndromes 367, *368*
    proliferative and inflammatory dermatoses
      371–377, *371*
malignant fibrous histiocytoma *see*
      undifferentiated pleomorphic sarcoma/
      malignant fibrous histiocytoma
malignant mixed tumor 143–144, *144*
malpractice, medical 668–670
  lawsuit analyses 669, 671, *671*
  preventing litigation 671–672, *672*
mammalian target of rapamycin (mTOR) 636
  inhibitors *see* mTOR inhibitors
mammary Paget's disease *see* Paget's disease,
      mammary
MAP kinase *see* mitogen-activated protein
      kinase
margins
  clinical 510
  histologic 510–511
  Mohs micrographic surgery 515
  radiation therapy 576–577
  surgical *see* surgical margins
marimastat *618*
Marjolin's ulcer 95, 125–126
  clinical features 129, *129*
MART-1/MelanA
  melanoma *32*, 303–304, *304*, 307, 311, *311*
  Mohs micrographic surgery *517*, 520, *520*
MART2 32
matrical carcinoma 147–148, *148*
matrix metalloproteinase-2 (MMP-2) 5
matrix metalloproteinase-9 (MMP-9) 4–5, 7
MC1R *see* melanocortin-1 receptor
*MC1R* genotypes 35, *35*, 37, 61
  interaction with *CDKN2A* mutations 35, *36*, 334–335
  melanoma risk 19, 35
  red hair phenotype 23, 35, 61
  response to UV radiation and 38

*MC2R* gene mutations 34
*MC4R* gene mutations 34
*MDM2* gene, in liposarcoma 158
MDM2 protein
  cellular function *17*
  in melanoma pathogenesis 2, 17
MDX-010 *see* ipilimumab
MEDI-547, in melanoma *615*
medial plantar flap 574–575
medical conditions, prior, cryosurgery and 454
medical devices, complications due to 671
medical records 670, *670*, *671*
medicolegal aspects 668–675
Medpor implants, ear reconstruction 568
medulloblastoma 14, 357–358
megestrol, in melanoma 590, *591*
MEK *see* mitogen-activated protein kinase
MEL-5 *see* tyrosinase-related protein 1
Melacine *608*, 610
MelaFind *401*, 402, *402*, *403*
MelanA *see* MART-1/MelanA
melanin 29–38
  biosynthesis 30–31, *30*
    regulation 33–35
    UVR-induced 33, 34, 36–38, 646
  deposition in melanosomes 27, *29*
  photoprotective effects 38
melanoblasts 23–24
  congenital proliferation 308
melanocortin-1 receptor (MC1R) 23, *32*, 34–35, *34*, *35*, 61
  agouti protein actions 35, *36*
  genotypes *see* MC1R genotypes
  regulation of melanogenesis 33, 34
  signal transduction 34–35, *36*
melanocortin-2 receptor (MC2R) *34*
melanocortin-3 receptor (MC3R) *34*
melanocortin-4 receptor (MC4R) *34*
melanocortin-5 receptor (MC5R) *34*
melanocortin receptors (MCRs) 34–35, *34*
melanocortins
  functions 34
  regulation of melanogenesis 34
melanocyte-differentiation antigens 31, *32*
  role in melanoma-associated leukoderma 31, *33*
melanocytes 23–39
  atypia of single cells 519
  dermal 25
  effects of UV radiation 36–38
  epidermal 25, *25*
  hair follicles 25
  historical studies 23
  migration during development 23–24, *24*, *25*
  single cell proliferations simulating melanoma *304*, 308, *309*
  structure and function 23–26
  upward migration within epidermis *309*
α-melanocyte-stimulating hormone (α-MSH)
  antagonism by agouti protein 35, *36*
  regulation of melanogenesis 33, 34
melanocytic lesions
  atypical 309–311
  confocal microscopy 415–420, *418*
  surgical excision of atypical 538–539
  *see also* pigmented lesions
melanocytic nevi
  atypical/dysplastic *see* dysplastic nevi
  confocal microscopy 416–418, *418*, *419*, *421*, *422*, *423*
  congenital *see* congenital melanocytic nevi
  dermoscopic patterns 392, *393*, *393*, *394*, *395*
  factors affecting development 60

persistent (recurrent), simulating melanoma 308, *308*
signature nevus pattern 241, 298–299
of special sites, simulating melanoma 307, *307*
ugly duckling sign 241, 274
*vs* bowenoid papulosis 200
*vs* dysplastic nevi *238*
*see also* pigmented lesions
melanocytic tumors of unknown malignant potential (MELTUMP) 309–310, 346–347
  surgical excision 538–539
melanogenesis *see* melanin, biosynthesis
melanogenesis-related proteins 31, *32*
melanoma
  ABCD criteria
    clinical assessment 262, 273, *273*, 274, *274*
    dermoscopic scoring system 390, *390*
  ABCDE criteria 262, 274
  acrolentiginous 298, 301, *302*
  adjuvant therapy 322–323, 589–605
    identifying patients at risk for relapse 589–590
    prior approaches 590, *591*
    present concepts 590–602
    next phases of development 602–603
    *see also* interferon(s)
  advanced *271*, 629–633
    epidemiology 629
    medical therapy 629–632
    surgery 632, *632*
  advancing 265
  amelanotic 269, 273–274
    confocal microscopy 419–420
  anatomic sites
    clinical appearances 269, *270*, *271*
    diagnostic difficulties in certain 307, *307*
    prognostic value 285, *286*, 288
  animal 305
  arising within dysplastic nevi *234*, 240, *241*, 276, 277, 324
  arising within pre-existing nevi 264, 297, *298*
  biomarkers 292, 320
  biopsy *see under* biopsy
  blue nevus-like 306, *306*
  breast, surgical excision 541
  burden of disease 40–42
  cancer stem cells 8
  in children 275–276, 307
  Clark level of invasion *see* Clark level of invasion
  clinical examination 276–277
  clinical genomics for detection 429–433
  clinical presentations 262–271, *262*, *263*, *264*, *265*, *266*, *267*, *268*, *269*, *270*, *271*
  computer-aided diagnosis 400–406, *401*
  confocal microscopy *401*, *403*, 404, 418–420, *418*, *424*, *425*, *426*, *427*
  costs 41–42, *41*
    effects of early detection 272
  dermoscopy *see under* dermoscopy
  desmoplastic *see* desmoplastic melanoma
  digital, surgical excision 540–541, *541*
  disseminated, treatment 629–633
  ear, surgical excision 540, *541*
  early detection 272–281
    clinical characteristics 262, 273–275, *273*, *273*
    clinical genomics 429–433
    computer-aided methods 400–406, *401*
    confocal microscopy *401*, *403*, 404, 418–420, *418*, *424*, *425*, *426*, *427*
    drawbacks of current methods 429
    history 272–273, *273*

    importance 272
    knowledge requirements 273
    mass screenings 280
    physician examination 70–71, 276–277
    potential precursor lesions 276
    self-examination 69–70, 277–280
    *vs* common benign pigmented lesions 275–276
  epidemiology 40–42, 44–48
  in epidermolysis bullosa 360
  epidermotropic metastases 295–297
  familial *see* familial melanoma
  genetics 16–20, 61
  genetic testing *see* genetic testing, for melanoma
  Glasgow checklist 274
  head and neck, excision margins 537–538
  histopathologic diagnosis 295–315
    biopsy technique 298–299
    challenges in 307–311
    criteria for 299–301, *300*
    different clinical forms 301–307
    immunohistochemistry 303–304, *304*, 311, *311*
    medico-legal issues 672–674, *672*, *673*, *674*, *674*
    natural history and 295–298, *296*, *297*, *298*
    proliferation markers 312
    special stains 311
    techniques for improving accuracy 311–312
  HIV-infected patients 642
  imaging work-up 320, 623–628
  immune response modifiers 322, 323, 479, 489–490, 492, 493
  incidence 40, 44–48, *45*, *46*
    age-related trends 45, *46*
    cohort effects 44–45, *45*
    gender differences 45–46, *46*
    secular trends 44, 262, 272
  interferon therapy *see under* interferon(s)
  in-transit metastases 290, *290*
    management 323
    microscopic 291
    sentinel node biopsy and risk 551
    *versus* local recurrence 291
  invasive 272
    clinical features *263*
  ipilimumab therapy 323, 602, 603
  lifetime risk 262, *262*, 272
  localized *see* melanoma, stage I and II
  local recurrence 291
    excision margin trials 533–536, *534*
  lymph node metastases *see* lymph node metastases, melanoma
  management 318–326
    adjuvant therapy 322–323, 589–605
    extent of work-up 320
    follow-up 323–325
    guidelines 318, *319*
    improved risk stratification 325
    initial assessment 318–320
    metastatic disease 323
    pitfalls in drug development *615*
    surgical 320–322
  mechanisms of growth and metastasis 1–8, *2*, *3*
    angiogenesis and lymphangiogenesis 4–5
    entry into venolymphatic channels 6
    establishing metastatic sites 7–8
    immune system evasion and survival in circulation 6–7
    initial transformation and propagation 2–4, *4*, 233, 298
    local extension 5–6

metastatic 629–633
    clinical features *271*
    epidemiology 629
    histopathology 295–297, *298*, 309, *310*
    imaging 623–625
    management 323, 629–633
    staging 629
    surgery 632, *632*
    survival rates *630, 630*
    targeted therapies 613–622
    vaccine therapy 608–609
    *see also* melanoma, stage III; melanoma,
        stage IV
minimum deviation, of Spitz type 346–347
mitotic rate 314
    AJCC staging system 282, *283*, 314
    hot spot method of assessment 287
    prognostic value *285, 287, 287*
Mohs micrographic surgery *517, 518*,
    520–521, 541
mortality 40–41, 47–48, *47, 48*
natural history, histologic aspects 295–298,
    *296, 297, 298*
nevoid 305, *305*
nodal metastases *see* lymph node metastases,
    melanoma
nodular *267*
    confocal microscopy 419–420
    histopathology 301, *302*
ocular/uveal, screening in dysplastic nevus
    syndrome 243
organ transplant recipients 640–641, *640*
pathology 295–317
photodynamic therapy 505
pregnancy after 331
pregnancy-associated *see* pregnancy-
    associated melanoma
prevention 66–72
    chemoprevention 75–78, *76, 77*
    efficacy of sunscreens 85
    primary 67–69
    secondary 69–71
    selenium and 53
    targeting 66–67
prognosis and staging 282–294, 589–590
    distant metastases 291–292
    future outlook 292–293
    histologic evaluation 312–315
    initial assessment 318–320
    localized disease 283–288, *285*
    regional disease 288–291
    survival rates by stage 283, *284, 285*, 320, *321*
    *see also* lymphatic mapping; sentinel lymph
        node biopsy
psychological impact 41–42, 662–663
psychological support 325, 665
radial growth phase (RGP) 4, 5, 288, *288*, 297,
    298
radiation therapy 322–323, 582–583
reconstructive surgery 560, *566, 570, 574*
regional lymph node surgery 544–558
regression 266, 288
    histopathology 308, *309*
    prognostic value 314
risk factors 52, 56–65, *57*, 335
    common nevi 232, *232*
    congenital melanocytic nevi 246, 252,
        254–256, *255, 256*
    dermatologic treatment-related 349–354,
        *350*
    dysplastic nevi 232, *232*, 276
    indoor tanning 647, *648*
risk stratification 318–320, 325
satellite metastases 290, *290*

histology 309, *310*, 314–315
    microscopic *290*, 291, 314–315
    *versus* local recurrence 291
self-examination of skin 277–280
spindle cell 306–307, *307*
spitzoid 306, *306*, 345, 347
stage I and II (localized disease)
    criteria 282, *283*
    groupings (T classification) *284*, 288
    management 320–321, 544–545
    prognosis 283–288, *285, 285, 286, 286*
stage III (regional disease)
    criteria 282, 283, *283, 284*
    evolution 289
    groupings *284*, 291
    N classification 288–291
    prognosis *285*, 288, *289*
    satellite and in-transit disease 290
    *see also* lymph node metastases,
        melanoma
stage IV (distant metastases) 283
    criteria 283, *283, 284*
    management 323
    prognosis *285, 286*, 291–292
staging *see* melanoma, prognosis and
    staging
staging system 282–283, *283, 284*, 309,
    312–315, 589–590, *590, 591*
superficial spreading (SSM) 301
surgical excision *see under* surgical excision
survival rates *see under* melanoma, prognosis
    and staging
targeted therapies 325, 613–622, 631–632
tumor-infiltrating lymphocytes 288,
    *288*, 314
tumor thickness *see* Breslow thickness
ulceration 284–286, 312
    AJCC staging system 282, *283*, 287, 290,
        *309*
    clinical appearance *268*
    histology *286*, 312, *314*
    interferon-α therapy and 602
    prognostic value 284–287, *285, 286, 286*,
        290, 312
ungual *270*
from unknown primary (MUP) 283, 292
vaccine therapy *see* vaccine therapy, for
    melanoma
verrucous 304–305, *305*
vertical growth phase (VGP) 4, 5, 288, *288*,
    297, 298, 550
*vs* dysplastic nevi 234, *235*
*vs* Paget's disease 152, 155
*vs* Spitz nevus 311, 346–347, *346*
webspace, surgical excision 541, *542*
in xeroderma pigmentosum 361
melanoma-associated antigens (MAAs) 31, *32*
melanoma-associated leukoderma (MAL) 31,
    *33*
melanoma chondroitin sulfate proteoglycan
    (MCSP) 5
melanoma in situ 272
    clinical features *263*
    confocal microscopy *424, 427*
    within desmoplastic melanoma 302–303,
        *303*
    evolving within dysplastic nevi 234, *240,
        241*
    histopathologic diagnosis 295, *296*,
        301, *301*
    Mohs micrographic surgery 518–521, *519,
        519, 520*
    surgical excision 536–537
    *see also* lentigo maligna

melanoma of soft parts *see* clear cell sarcoma of
    soft tissue
melanonychia striata 277, *277*
melanophilin 27–28
melanosomes 26–29
    degradation 28–29
    development 25
    effects of UV radiation 36–38
    stages of melanization 27, *29*
    synthesis and processing of proteins 26, *26*
    targeting of proteins to 26, *26, 28*
    transfer to keratinocytes 27–28, *29*
    variations with skin color 28–29, *29, 29*
MELTUMP *see* melanocytic tumors of unknown
    malignant potential
membrane-associated transporter protein
    (MATP) 31
memory CD4+ helper T cells, in cutaneous T-cell
    lymphoma 217
Menkes kinky hair syndrome 30
men who have sex with men (MSM)
    epidemic (AIDS-related) Kaposi sarcoma
        168, 171
    non-epidemic Kaposi sarcoma 171
meradimate *81*, 83
Merkel cell carcinoma (MCC) 179–185
    clinical features 180, *181*
    disseminated, treatment 529–530
    epidemiology 51, 179
    history 179
    HIV infected patients 642
    new specific diagnostic codes 182, *182*
    organ transplant recipients 179–180, 641,
        *641*
    pathogenesis and etiology 179–180
    pathology 182–183, *183, 183, 184*
    patient evaluation and diagnosis 180–182
    prognosis and staging 180
    radiation therapy 184, *185*, 586
    reconstructive surgery 560
    staging system 181, *182*
    treatment 183–184, *185*, 522, 586
Merkel cell polyomavirus (MCPyV) 62, 180
    T antigens 180, 183, *184*
    vaccine development 530
Merkel cells 179, 180, *180*
mesenchymal motility, metastatic cells 5–6, *6*
metals, heavy 63
metastases, cutaneous
    adenocarcinoma 190
    cryosurgery 457, *459*
    mucinous carcinoma 142
    potential pathways for development 7, *7*
    sarcoma 165
metastasis, tumor
    cell arrest, extravasation and proliferation in
        new sites 7–8
    entry into venolymphatic channels 6
    immune system evasion 6–7
    local tumor extension 5–6
    mechanisms of 1–8
    multistep process 1, *2*
    organ and tissue specific 7, *7*
    role of cancer stem cells 8, *8*
    survival in general circulation 6–7
metatypical basal cell carcinoma *see* basal
    cell carcinoma (BCC), with squamous
    metaplasia
meteorological conditions, local 57
methchlorethamine hydrochloride *see* nitrogen
    mustard
methotrexate (MTX)
    carcinogenic potential *350*, 351
    cutaneous T-cell lymphoma 226, 228

methylaminolevulinate (MAL) 469, 497, *499*
  lesion specificity and tissue penetration 498
  topical application 500–501, *501*, *502*
  *see also* photodynamic therapy
1-methyl-D-tryptophan *619*
*MET* proto-oncogene, in congenital melanocytic nevi 246–247
Mexoryl XL (silatriazole) *81*, 83
Meyerson phenomenon, congenital melanocytic nevi 249–251
microarray-based gene expression profiling 429–430
  characterization of melanoma and nevi 430–431, *430*, *431*
  detection of melanoma 431, *431*
microcystic adenocarcinoma, organ transplant recipients *635*
microcystic adnexal carcinoma (MAC) 140, 530
  Mohs micrographic surgery 521–522
  pathology 140, *141*
microophthalmia-associated transcription factor (MITF) *32*
  immunohistochemistry, in melanoma *304*
  in melanocyte survival 24
  in melanoma pathogenesis 19
  Mohs micrographic surgery *517*
  regulation of activity *33*
microRNAs 12
microsatellite instability, in Muir–Torre syndrome 362
milker's nodule 210, *212*
milk-fat-globule membrane protein (MFGM-gp 155), in Paget's disease 154–155
mineral oils 63
miR-17~19 cluster family of microRNAs 14
miRNA-205 16
MIRROR DermaGraphix 400
MITF *see* microophthalmia-associated transcription factor
mitogen-activated protein kinase (MAPK; MEK)
  in melanoma pathogenesis 18–19
  melanoma therapies targeting 615–617, *616*
  signaling pathway *see* Raf/MEK/ERK pathway
mitomycin C, extramammary Paget's disease 155
mitotic rate
  melanoma *see under* melanoma
  Spitz nevi 343–344
mixed tumors
  benign 143–144
  malignant 143–144, *144*
MK2206 *616*
MLN8054 *617*
*MLPH* mutations 27–28, *27*
Mohs micrographic surgery (MMS) 515–525
  angiosarcoma 522–523
  atypical fibroxanthoma *517*, 521
  basal cell carcinoma 115, *115*, 118, *119*, *517*, 518
  contraindications 517–518
  current controversies 523
  dermatofibrosarcoma protuberans *517*, 521
  extramammary Paget's disease 155, *517*, 522
  granular cell tumor 523
  hidradenoma 523
  indications 517
  malignant fibrous histiocytoma 521
  melanoma *517*, 518, 520–521, 541
  melanoma in situ 518–521, *519*, *519*, *520*
  Merkel cell carcinoma 522, 586
  microcystic adnexal carcinoma 521–522
  procedure 515–517, *516*

safety 523–524
  sebaceous carcinoma *517*, 522
  special stains 516–517, *517*
  squamous cell carcinoma 137, *137*, *517*, 518
  transplant recipients 638
molecularly targeted therapies *see* targeted therapies
molecular mechanisms 60–61
MoleMapCD 400, *402*
MoleMate 404
MoleMax *401*
molluscum contagiosum 210
morbilliform eruption, chemotherapy-induced 380
morphea, inflammatory 215
mortality
  all cause, vitamin D and *652*, 653–654
  basal cell carcinoma 50
  cutaneous T-cell lymphoma 51
  melanoma 40–41, 47–48, *47*, *48*
  Merkel cell carcinoma 51
  squamous cell carcinoma 50
motility, tumor cell 5–6, *6*
  ameboid 5–6, *6*
  mesenchymal 5–6, *6*
MPC-6827 *620*
M-plasty 509–510, *510*
MRI *see* magnetic resonance imaging
mTOR *636*
mTOR inhibitors *635*
  melanoma *616*, 617
  organ transplant recipients 636
  post-transplant Kaposi sarcoma 174
  prevention of non-melanoma skin cancers 74–75
  *see also* sirolimus
mucin-1 (MUC1), Paget's disease 151–152
mucinous carcinoma
  metastatic 142
  primary cutaneous 142, *142*
mucositis, chemotherapy-induced 379–380
Muir–Torre syndrome (MTS) 361–362, *364*, *368*, *369*
  diagnostic criteria 362, *362*
  keratoacanthoma 130, 362
  sebaceous carcinoma 148, 362
mule spinner's disease 63
Multicenter Selective Lymphadenectomy Trial-1 (MSLT-1) 548–549, *548*, *549*
Multicenter Selective Lymphadenectomy Trial-2 (MSLT-2) 551
multicentric reticulohistiocytosis *368*, 376
multikinase inhibitors
  cancers treated *380*
  dermatologic side effects 382, *383*
  Kaposi sarcoma 176
  *see also* imatinib mesylate; sunitinib
multiple endocrine neoplasia (MEN)
  type 1 *368*
  type 2a *368*
  type 2b (multiple mucosal neuromas) *368*, *370*
multiple mucosal neuroma syndrome *368*, *370*
multispectral digital dermoscopy image analysis 401–404, *402*
multispectral imaging 401–404
multitargeted kinase inhibitors *see* multikinase inhibitors
MUM1–3 *32*
muscle health, vitamin D and 651, *652*
Mustarde flap 565
mycophenolate mofetil (MMF) *635*
  carcinogenic potential *350*, 352–353
  organ transplant recipients 635–636

mycosis fungoides (MF) 217–230
  benign lymphocytic proliferations resembling *see* pseudolymphomas, cutaneous
  clinical features 218–220, *218*, *219*
  diagnosis 220–225, *222*, *223*
  differential diagnosis 225
  epidemiology 217
  erythrodermic 219–220, *219*
  folliculotropic (FMF) 218–219, *219*, 222–223, *224*
  history 217
  palmaris et plantaris (MFPP) 218
  pathogenesis and etiology 217–218
  pathology 221–223, *224*, *225*
  prognosis 225–226
  staging 220–221, *221*, *222*, *223*, *224*
  treatment 226–229, *226*
    imiquimod 491
    interferons 480–481
    radiation therapy 585–586, *585*
  tumor stage 218, *219*, 221–222, *224*
  *see also* cutaneous T-cell lymphoma
myeloid suppressor cells, in melanoma 6
*MYO5A* mutations 27–28, *27*
myosin Va 27–28, *29*
myxoid chondrosarcoma, extraskeletal *159*
myxoid/round cell liposarcoma *159*

## N

NA17-A *32*
N-acetylcysteine, melanoma chemoprevention 76, 77–78
nails
  chemotherapy-induced changes 380
  melanoma within *270*
nasolabial flap 567
National Cancer Institute Cancer Genetics Service Directory *336*
National Comprehensive Cancer Network (NCCN), melanoma guidelines 318, *319*, 673
National Society of Genetic Counselors *336*
natural killer (NK) cells *478*, *478*
neck reconstruction 568, *571*
necrobiotic xanthogranuloma *368*, 377
necrolytic migratory erythema 371, *371*
necrosis, in basal cell carcinoma 112
NEDD9 19
negligence, medical 668–670, *669*
Neo Helioplan T *81*, 83
neonates
  congenital nevi simulating melanoma 307–308
  melanoma 330
neural crest cells
  melanocyte origins 23–24, *24*
  receptor–ligand interactions 24, *24*
neurocristic hamartomas 252
neurocutaneous melanocytosis (NCM) 246, 256
  asymptomatic 256
  screening for/management 259, *259*
  symptomatic 256
neurofibromatosis type I *368*
neurotization, of congenital melanocytic nevi 247–248, *251*, 254
neutrophilic eccrine hidradenitis 380, *383*
nevi
  acral 345
  with architectural disorder 231–232, 238
  atypical/dysplastic *see* dysplastic nevi
  benign, progression to melanoma 2–3, *4*
  compound *see* compound nevus
  epidermal *200*
  genomic characterization 430–431, *430*

genomic detection of melanoma 431, *431*
intradermal 275
junctional 275
melanoma arising within *264*, 297, *298*
melanoma risk 232, *232*
pregnancy-related changes 330
skin cancer risk *57*
of special sites, simulating melanoma 307, *307*, 345
*see also specific types*
nevoid basal cell carcinoma syndrome *see* basal cell nevus syndrome
nevoid melanoma 305, *305*
nevus sebaceous, basal cell carcinoma arising in 100
nimesulide, chemoprevention studies *75*
9p21 chromosome deletions
in melanoma 2, 16–17
in squamous cell carcinoma 16
9q22.3 chromosome locus 13
nitric oxide (NO), regulation of melanogenesis *33*
nitrogen
gas insufflation 460
liquid *see* liquid nitrogen
nitrogen mustard (methchlorethamine), topical *464*, 471
adverse effects 471
cutaneous T-cell lymphoma *226*, 227, 471
NKIC3 (CD63) immunohistochemistry, in melanoma *304*
nodular fasciitis, *vs* cutaneous sarcoma 160
*NOLA2/NOLA3* gene mutations 363
nominal standard dose (NSD), radiation therapy 577
non-Hodgkin lymphoma (NHL)
classic Kaposi sarcoma and 170
cutaneous, in HIV infection 205, *205*
vitamin D and *652*, 653
*see also* cutaneous T-cell lymphoma
non-melanoma skin cancer (NMSC)
biopsy techniques 441
burden of disease 42–43
chemoprevention 73–75, *74*, *75*
confocal microscopy 409–415, *413*
costs 42–43
curettage and electrodesiccation 443–449
disseminated, treatment 526–531
epidemiology 42, 48–52
in epidermolysis bullosa 360
incidence 42, 48–50, *49*, 124
indoor tanning and 647–648
prevention 66–72, 73–75, *74*
risk factors 56–65, *57*
surgical excision 508–514, *511*
terminology 48
treatment-related risks 349–354
in xeroderma pigmentosum 361
*see also* basal cell carcinoma; squamous cell carcinoma. *other specific types*
non-steroidal anti-inflammatory drugs (NSAIDs)
melanoma chemoprevention *76*, 77
topical 74, 468–469
nose
reconstruction 566–567, *568*, *569*
tumors, radiation therapy 579, *580*
*N-RAS* mutations
in benign nevi 3
in congenital melanocytic nevi 246–247
in melanoma 18
therapies targeting 615
in squamous cell carcinoma 15

nucleotide excision repair (NER), defective 360–361
nutrients, skin cancer risk and *57*, 64
NY-ESO1 *32*

O

occupational risk factors *57*
octinoxate *81*, 82
octisalate *81*, 82
octocrylene *81*, 82
oculocutaneous albinism (OCA) *364*
type 1 23, 25
type 1A *27*, 30
type 1B *27*
type 2 *27*, 31
type 3 *27*, 30
type 4 *27*
odontogenic keratocysts, in basal cell nevus syndrome 357
oil-red-O stain 516–517, *517*, 522
OKT3 monoclonal antibody *635*
oncogene-induced cell senescence 3
oncogenes 12, *13*
Oncophage/Vitespen *608*, 610
optical coherence tomography (OCT) *401*, 405
oral contraceptive pill (OC), melanoma and 328, 331
oral florid papillomatosis (oroaerodigestive verrucous carcinoma; Ackerman tumor) 96, 129, 202
orf 210
organ transplant recipients (OTR) 634–641
basal cell carcinoma 100–101, 634, 640
chemoprevention of non-melanoma skin cancers 74–75
epidemiology 634–635
HPV-related skin cancers 61–62, 637
imiquimod therapy 468, 484, 638
Kaposi sarcoma *see* Kaposi sarcoma (KS), post-transplant
melanoma 640–641, *640*
Merkel cell carcinoma 179–180, 641, *641*
pathogenesis of skin cancer 635–637
photodynamic therapy 505, 638
risk factors for non-melanoma skin cancers 634–635, *635*
skin cancer risk 62–63, 67, 351–353, 634
skin cancers *635*, 637–641
squamous cell carcinoma 637–640
clinical presentations 637, *637*
histopathology 638, *638*
increased risk 124–125, 634, *635*, 637
management 638, *639*
metastatic risk *635*, 637–638, *637*
prevention 639–640
topical diclofenac 469, 638
oxaliplatin, in melanoma *621*
oxybenzone *81*, 83
ozone layer 57–59, *58*

P

p14ARF 2, 17, 334
function in cell cycle 2, 17, *17*
in melanoma pathogenesis 2, 17, 18
*p14ARF* gene defects, in melanoma 17, 334
p15 *32*
p16INK4A 17, 334
function in cell cycle 2, 17, *17*
in melanoma pathogenesis 2, 17, 18
Spitz nevus 347
*p16INK4A* gene defects, in melanoma 17, 19, 334

p19ARF
in melanoma pathogenesis 18
in SCC pathogenesis 16
p21CIP1 17, *17*
p27KIP1 18
*p53* gene *see TP53* gene
p53 protein 2
in basal cell carcinoma pathogenesis 14
in extramammary Paget's disease 153
function 16, *17*
in melanoma pathogenesis 17, 61
in squamous cell carcinoma pathogenesis 16
p73 protein, in extramammary Paget's disease 153
pacemakers, cardiac 448, 509
paclitaxel
basal cell carcinoma 526
dermatologic side effects 379, 382
Kaposi sarcoma 176
melanoma *620*
squamous cell carcinoma 527
padimate O *81*, 82
pagetoid dyskeratosis of nipple epidermis 152
pagetoid reticulosis 219, 223
Paget's disease 150–156
extramammary (EMPD) 150, *151*, 152–155, *368*
clinical features 153, *153*, *154*, *377*
imiquimod therapy 155, 491
Mohs micrographic surgery *517*, 522
pathology 154–155, *154*
photodynamic therapy 155, 505
topical chemotherapy *464*, 465
treatment 155
underlying malignancies 152–153, *376*
mammary (MPD) 150–152, *151*
clinical features 151, *151*
pathology 151–152, *152*
treatment 152
pain, cryosurgery-related 459
palifermin 379–380
palisading, in basal cell carcinoma 105–106, *106*
palliative cryosurgery 457, *459*
palmoplantar erythrodysesthesia, chemotherapy-induced 379, *380*
pancreatic cancer
*CDKN2A* mutations and risk 2, 16–17, 335
criteria for genetic testing 335–336, *336*
screening in *CDKN2A* mutation carriers 339
vitamin D and *652*, 653
papillary adenocarcinoma, aggressive digital (ADPA) 145–146, *145*
para-aminobenzoic acid (PABA) *81*, 82
paramedian forehead flap 567
paraneoplastic pemphigus (PNP) *368*, 375
parents, primary prevention role 68–69
Parsol SLX *81*, 82–83
partner-assisted skin examination 69–70, *70*
patched-1 (PTCH1) protein 13, 14, *14*, 349, 357
*see also PTCH1* gene
pathology, medico-legal issues 672–674, *672*, *673*, *674*, *674*
Pautrier's microabscesses 221–222
*PAX3* gene 24
PD-325901 *616*
PD-0332991 *617*
pearly penile papule *200*
pectoralis major flap *561*, 568, 569
peels, actinic keratosis 94
pegylated interferon-α2b (PEG-IFN-α2b), melanoma 479, *596*, 601–602
Pellacani scoring system 420
pelvic area reconstruction 570–571
pelvic lymphadenectomy, deep 553, 556
pemphigoid, anti-epiligrin cicatricial (AECP) *368*, 375, *375*

pemphigus, paraneoplastic (PNP) *368*, 375
penis
  pearly papule *200*
  squamous cell carcinoma 128, *129*
pentetreotide, in melanoma *615*
PEP005 *see* ingenol mebutate
peptide vaccines, anti-melanoma 606, 607
perifosine *616*
perillyl alcohol 472
  melanoma chemoprevention 75–76, *76*
perineum area reconstruction 570–571
perineural invasion
  adenoid cystic carcinoma 141, *141*
  basal cell carcinoma 101, 112, *114*, 119, *119*
  desmoplastic melanoma 302–303, *304*
  limiting extent of surgery 524
  squamous cell carcinoma 134, *134*
    radiation therapy 582
periungual squamous cell carcinoma 128, *129*
Peutz–Jeghers syndrome *368*, 369
*P* gene variants 27, 31, 37
pheomelanin 29–30
  biosynthesis *30*, 31
    regulation 35, *36*
  effects of UV radiation 38
  eumelanin ratio, factors affecting 33
pheomelanosomes 27, 29–30
phorbol esters 63
phosphoglucose isomerase 5
phosphoinositide 3-kinase (PI3K)/Akt signaling
    pathway 631, *631*
  in melanoma pathogenesis 613, *614*
  melanoma therapies targeting *616*, 617
  *see also* AKT; mTOR
photoaging, induced by indoor tanning 646,
    *646*
photodynamic therapy (PDT) *463*, 469–470,
    497–507
  absorption spectrum 499, *500*
  actinic keratosis 93, *94*, 470, 502–503, *502*
    light sources 500
    photosensitizers compared 498
    procedure 500–501, *501*, 502
  advantages and disadvantages 497, *498*
  adverse effects 469–470, 505
  ambulatory 500
  basal cell carcinoma 117, 503–504, *504*
    penetration of photosensitizer 498
    procedure 500–501, 502, *502*
  Bowen's disease 500, 503, *503*
  combination therapy 473
  contraindications *498*
  cutaneous T-cell lymphoma 504–505
  extramammary Paget's disease 155, 505
  fractionation 500
  history 497
  indications *464*, 497, *498*, 502–505
  Kaposi sarcoma 176
  mechanism of action 498–500, *499*
  melanoma 505
  organ transplant recipients 505, 638
  prevention of skin cancer 75, 505
  principles 498–500, *499*
  procedure 500–502, *501*
  pulsed light 500
  squamous cell carcinoma 137, 503
  therapeutic effect 500
photography 657–661
  close-up (macro) 657, 659–660, *659*
    image capture 657, *658*
    total body photography combined with
      660, *660*
  image capture overview 657–658
  image management software 660–661, *660*

outside services 661
  positive margins of Mohs defects 524
  total body *see* total body photography
photoprotection 80–88
  adjunctive measures 85–87
  families at high-risk of melanoma 339
  history 80
  interventions to modify behavior 67–69, 73
  levels of utilization 59
  melanoma patients 323–324
  oral preparations 87
  organ transplant recipients 639
  sunscreens *see* sunscreens
  vitamin D status and 655
  in xeroderma pigmentosum 361
phototherapy
  cutaneous T-cell lymphoma *226*, 227, *227*
  increased skin cancer risk 349–351
physician surveillance 70–71
PI-88 *618*, 620
piebaldism, human 24
pigmentary dilution, diffuse 27
pigmentary disorders, molecular pathogenesis 24
pigmentation
  anatomic variations 25
  genes associated with physiologic variation 37
  physiology of 23–39
  UV-induced 24, 646
  *see also* darker-skinned individuals;
    hyperpigmentation; melanin
pigmented lesions
  ABCD criteria *see* ABCD criteria for melanoma
  biopsy 298–299, *300*, *436*, 439–441
  common benign 275–276
  EGIR genomic characterization 430–431, *430*,
    *431*
  genomic detection of melanoma 431, *431*
  medico-legal issues 672–674, *673*, *674*, *674*
  surgical excision of atypical 538–539
  *see also* melanocytic nevi; melanoma; early
    detection
pigmented spindle cell nevus (Reed nevus) 341,
    344, *344*
pilomatricoma, malignant *see* matrical
    carcinoma
pimecrolimus, topical, carcinogenic potential 353
*pink-eyed dilution* gene 31
pits, palmoplantar, in basal cell nevus
    syndrome *104*, 357, *358*
placenta
  examination, pregnant women with
    melanoma 331
  metastases, in melanoma 330
placental growth factor (PlGF) 4, 328
plakoglobin, in Paget's disease 153
platelet-derived growth factor (PDGF) 4, 5
platelet-derived growth factor (PDGF)-β
  overexpression in dermatofibrosarcoma
    protuberans 161, *161*
  targeted therapy 162
platelet-derived growth factor receptor
    (PDGFR) inhibitors, in melanoma
    617–618, *618*
pleomorphic hyalinizing angiectatic tumor
    (PHAT) 165
pleural melanoma, imaging assessment 624,
    *624*
PLX4032, in melanoma 615–617, *616*, *617*, *618*,
    631
podoplanin, in angiosarcomas 188, 191–192
poikiloderma
  in dermatomyositis 376, *376*
  in mycosis fungoides/Sézary syndrome
    218, *219*

pollutants, carcinogenic 57, 63
polo-kinase 1 inhibitors *617*
polychlorinated biphenyls (PCBs) 63
polycyclic aromatic hydrocarbons (PAHs) 63,
    *63*
polymerase chain reaction (PCR)
  in cutaneous T-cell lymphoma 222
  melanoma cell detection 31
polyomaviruses 62
polypodium leucotomos (PL) 87
POMC *see* proopiomelanocortin
*POMC* gene mutations 34, 61
popliteal lymphadenectomy 555, *555*, *556*
porocarcinoma 142–143, *142*, *143*
positron emission tomography (PET),
    melanoma 624, *625*, *626*, *627*
post-traumatic stress 663
Potts, Percival 44, 56
P protein 31, *31*, *32*
  regulation of activity 33
PRAME (preferentially expressed antigen in
    melanoma) 32
pregnancy
  interferon therapy during 482
  in melanoma survivors 331
pregnancy-associated melanoma 288, 327–333
  clinical features 330
  epidemiology 327
  history 327
  pathogenesis and etiology 327–328
  pathology 331
  patient evaluation and diagnosis 330–331
  placental and fetal metastases 330
  prognosis 328–330, *328*, *329*
  treatment 331, *331*
premetastatic niches 7
prevention of skin cancer 66–72
  history 66
  primary 67–69
    efficacy of sunscreens 53, 85
    *see also* photoprotection
  secondary 69–71
  targeting 66–67, *68*
  *see also* chemoprevention
previous history of skin cancer 64, 67
  basal cell carcinoma risk *100*
  chemoprevention studies 74
primary care physicians, skin cancer detection
    70–71
primary closure 560
primary cutaneous B-cell lymphoma (PCBCL),
    epidemiology 51
primitive neuroectodermal tumor (PNET),
    genetic alterations *159*
programmed death-1 (PD-1) 6
programmed death ligand-1 (PD-L1) 6
progression, tumor 2–4, *4*
prokinectin-2 4–5
proliferating cell nuclear antigen (PCNA), in
    verrucous carcinoma 133
proliferating tricholemmal cystic carcinoma
    147, *147*
proliferating tricholemmal tumor 147
proliferative dermatoses associated with
    internal malignancy 371–377, *371*
promontory sign, in Kaposi sarcoma 172
proopiomelanocortin (POMC) 34, 61
  post-translational processing *34*
  regulation of melanogenesis 33, 34
prostate cancer, vitamin D status and *652*, 653
proteasomes, degradation of aberrant proteins
    26, *26*
protein kinase A (PKA) 35
protein kinase B (PKB) *see* AKT

proto-oncogenes 12, *13*, 60–61
protoporphyrin IX (PpIX) 498, *499*
pseudoepitheliomatous hyperplasia (PEH) 132
    after cryosurgery 461
pseudolymphomas, cutaneous 207–216
    CD30+ (T-cell) 210–211, *212*
    classification 207, *208*
pseudomelanoma 308, *308*
psoralen and ultraviolet A (PUVA) therapy 59–60
    cutaneous T-cell lymphoma 227, *227*
    increased skin cancer risk 95, 350–351, *350, 351*
    induced keratoses 95
    Merkel cell carcinoma risk 179
psoriasis, *vs* bowenoid papulosis *200*
psychological distress
    individuals with strong family history 664
    prevalence 662–663
    screening for 666
    vulnerability factors 664, *664*
psychological responses 662–667
    congenital melanocytic nevi 254
    diagnosis of skin cancer 662, *663*
    early-stage skin cancer 662
    indoor tanning 646, *647*
    melanoma 41–42, 662–663
psychological support 325, 665, 666
    communication skills and strategies 665, *666*
    cost-effectiveness 665
    current provision and recommendations 666, *666*
*PTCH1* gene 13, *14*, 357
    mutations 13, 14, 61, 357
    protein product *see* patched-1
*PTCH2* gene 13–14, 357
PTEN, in melanoma pathogenesis 3, 18
*PTEN* gene defects 18
pulmonary metastases, melanoma 323
    imaging assessment 623, 625–626
    surgical excision 632
punch biopsy 434, *436*
    curettage and electrodesiccation after 448
    device *435*
    medico-legal aspects 673, *673*
    non-melanoma skin cancer 441
    suspicious pigmented lesions 299, *300*, 439
    technique 436–439, *437*
PUVA therapy *see* psoralen and ultraviolet A therapy
PX-866 *616*
pyoderma gangrenosum 368, 375, *375*
pyrimidine dimers *59*

## Q

QS-21 *607*
quality of life (QoL)
    defined 41
    impact of melanoma 41–42
    impact of non-melanoma skin cancer 43
    psychological distress and 664
quantitative reverse transcriptase polymerase chain reaction (qPCR), detection of melanoma 431–432, *432*

## R

R115777 615, *616*
RAB27A 27–28

*RAB27A* mutations 27–28, *27*
Rac1, in metastatic motility 5–6
racial differences *see* ethnic differences
radial forearm flaps *566, 567, 567*, 573
radial growth phase (RGP), melanoma 4, 5, 288, *288*, 297, 298
radiation
    ionizing 57, 60
        *see also* radiation-induced malignancy
    non-ionizing 56
        *see also* ultraviolet (UV) radiation
radiation dermatitis *382*, 383
radiation-induced dermatoses (ionizing) 94–95
radiation-induced malignancy (ionizing) 56, *57*, 94–95
    angiosarcomas 191–192
    basal cell carcinoma 60, 100, 118–119
    potential mechanisms 349
    squamous cell carcinoma 60, 129
radiation recall phenomenon 383
radiation therapy (RT) 576–588
    anatomic site 577
    basal cell carcinoma 115–116, 578–582, *580, 581*
    biologic effects 577–578
    cutaneous B-cell lymphoma 586
    cutaneous T-cell lymphoma 227–228, 585–586, *585*
    dermatofibrosarcoma protuberans 162
    electron beam 576
    equivalent dose concept 577–578
    extramammary Paget's disease 155
    field size 576–577
    Kaposi sarcoma 175, 204, 583–585, *583, 584*
    malignancies induced by *see* radiation-induced malignancy
    melanoma 322–323, 582–583
        brain metastases 632
    Merkel cell carcinoma 184, *185*, 586
    physical factors 576–577
    principles 576–578
    reconstructive surgery and 560, *566*
    squamous cell carcinoma 136, 578–582, *580, 581, 582*
    superficial-quality X-rays 576
radioisotope navigation, extramammary Paget's disease 155
radiological imaging *see* imaging, radiological
RAF265 *616*
*RAF* gene defects, in melanoma 18–19
Raf/MEK/ERK pathway (MAPK pathway) 15, 614, 631, *631*
    in melanoma pathogenesis 3, 5, 18–19, 613
    melanoma therapies targeting 615–617, *616*, 631
RAF proteins 15, 18–19
rapamycin *see* sirolimus
*RAS* gene defects
    in actinic keratoses 15
    in melanoma 18–19
    in squamous cell carcinoma 15, 16
RAS signaling pathway 15, 614, 631, *631*
    melanoma chemoprevention targeting 75–76
    in melanoma pathogenesis 18, 246–247, 613
    melanoma therapies targeting 615–617, *616*
    in squamous cell carcinoma pathogenesis 15
ray amputation 541, *542*
RB1 protein, cellular function 17, *17*
RCM *see* reflectance confocal microscopy
RDEA119 *616*
reactive oxygen species (ROS), in melanoma progression 5

reconstructive surgery 559–575
    head and neck 561–568
    pelvis/perineum area 570–571
    planning 559–560, *560*
    selection of techniques 560–561
    trunk 568–570
    upper and lower extremities 572–575
records, medical 670, *670, 671*
red hair phenotype 23, 35, 61
Reed nevus (pigmented spindle cell nevus) 341, 344, *344*
reflectance confocal microscopy (RCM)
    ex vivo 407
    history 407
    in vivo 407
    margin mapping and treatment monitoring 421
    melanocytic neoplasms 415–420, *418*
    melanocytic nevi 416–418, *418, 419, 421, 422, 423*
    melanoma *401, 403, 404*, 418–420, *418, 424, 425, 426, 427*
    non-melanoma skin cancers 409–415, *413*
    normal skin 409, *410, 410*
    principles 407–408, *408, 409*
reflex transmission imaging (RFI) 404
refusal of treatment 670
registries, cancer 44
renal transplant recipients
    basal cell carcinoma 640
    melanoma 640, 641
    pathogenesis of skin cancers 635
    skin cancer risk 352–353, 634–635
    squamous cell carcinoma 124–125, *639*
resiquimod 468, 491–492
    indications *464*
resveratrol, melanoma chemoprevention *76*
reticulohistiocytosis, multicentric 368, 376
retiform hemangioendothelioma (RH) 186, 187–188, *188*
9-cis-retinoic acid, Kaposi sarcoma 174
13-*cis*-retinoic acid, squamous cell carcinoma 527–528, *528*
retinoids
    basal cell carcinoma 117
    melanoma chemoprevention *76*
    non-melanoma skin cancer prevention 74
    side effects 639–640, *640*
    topical *463*, 470–471
        actinic keratoses 93, *94*, 470
        in basal cell nevus syndrome 358–359
        chemoprevention trial 74
        indications *464*
        non-melanoma skin cancers 470
    transplant recipients 638, 639–640
    *see also individual agents*
reverse transcription polymerase chain reaction (RT-PCR)
    cutaneous sarcomas 160
    melanoma 291
rhabdomyosarcoma, alveolar *159*, 165
Rh-Endostatin *618*
rheumatoid arthritis (RA) 63, 351, 353–354
rhIgM12B7 *619*
RhoA 5–6
Rho-GTPases, in metastatic motility 5–6
rhomboid flaps *562*, 570
rickets 650, *651, 652*
riluzole, in melanoma 614–615, *615*
risk factors 56–64, *57*
    primary prevention interventions 67–69
    for targeting prevention efforts 66–67, *68*
rodent ulcer *see* basal cell carcinoma (BCC), nodular

Rombo syndrome 14, 99–100, 363, *364*
rotation flaps 539–540, *564*
Rothmund–Thomson syndrome *368*
rule of halves, closure using 509–510, *511*

# S

S100B protein, serum, in melanoma 292, 320
S100 protein immunostaining
  clear cell sarcoma 165
  melanoma 303–304, *304*, 311, *311*
  Mohs micrographic surgery *517*
salicylates, used in sunscreens *81*, 82
sarcoidosis 63
sarcomas, cutaneous 157–167, *158*
  diagnosis 159–160
  epidemiology 157–158
  follow-up and surveillance 165–166
  history 157
  metastatic 160, 165
  natural history 158
  pathogenesis and etiology 158
  reconstructive surgery *573*
  *see also* angiosarcomas; *specific types*
saucerization biopsy 434, *436*
  suspicious pigmented lesions 299, *300*, 439
  technique 438, *438*
scabies, persistent nodular 210–211, *212, 213*
scalp reconstruction 562–563, *563, 564*
scars 95, 125–126, *125*
SCC *see* squamous cell carcinoma
SCH727965 *617*
schools, primary prevention interventions 68
scleroatrophic syndrome of Huriez
    (sclerotylosis) 363–364, *364*
scleroderma, localized 215
scleromyxedema *368*, 374, *374*
screening, skin cancer 70–71, 280
scrotal cancer, soot exposure and 44, 56
seasonal affective disorder (SAD) 646
sebaceous carcinoma 148, *148*
  HIV-infected patients 642
  Mohs micrographic surgery *517*, 522
  in Muir–Torre syndrome 148, 362
  organ transplant recipients *635*
  treatment of disseminated 530
sebaceous epithelioma 107
sebaceous glands, carcinomas of 148
seborrheic keratosis *200*, 275–276, *276*
  sign of Leser–Trélat 373, *373*
second malignancies
  in classic Kaposi sarcoma 170
  in cutaneous T-cell lymphoma 220
selenium, and melanoma 53, *76*
self-examination of skin (SSE) 69–70, 277–280
  melanoma patients 323–324
  partner-assisted 70, *70*
  procedure *278, 279*, 280
senescence 3–4
  oncogene-induced cell 3
sentinel lymph node biopsy (SLNB) 548
  atypical melanocytic proliferations 310
  melanoma 283, 289, 320–321, 322, 545–551, *552*
    biologic and prognostic relevance 290,
      547–548, *547, 547, 548*
    completion dissection after 551
    complications and morbidity 551
    increased risk of in-transit metastasis 551
    Mohs micrographic surgery and 518
    patient selection 550–551
    pattern of recurrence after 324
    during pregnancy 330
    rationale 548

regional disease control 549
  scientific basis 545–546, *545, 546*
  survival benefits 548–549, *549*
  techniques 546–547, *546*
Merkel cell carcinoma 180
Spitz nevus 347
squamous cell carcinoma 130–131
sentinel lymph nodes (SLNs)
  clinical relevance of submicroscopic disease
    291
  histologic examination 315, 549–550
  interval, in-transit or ectopic 547, *547*
  intraoperative identification *289*,
    546–547, *546*
seroma, postoperative 556
Sézary cells 221–222, 223–224, *224*
Sézary syndrome (SS) 217–230
  clinical features *218*, 219–220, *219, 220*
  diagnosis 220–225, *223*
  epidemiology 217
  history 217
  pathogenesis and etiology 217–218
  pathology 221–222, 223–225
  prognosis 225–226
  staging 220–221, *221, 222, 223, 224*
  treatment 226–229, *226*, 480–481
  *see also* cutaneous T-cell lymphoma
shade, seeking 85–86
shave biopsy 434, *436*
  curettage and electrodesiccation after 448
  medico-legal aspects 673, *673*
  melanoma 318
  non-melanoma skin cancer 441
  suspicious pigmented lesions 299, 439
  technique 437, *438*
side effects of skin cancer systemic therapy,
    dermatologic 379–385
signature nevus pattern 241, 298–299
silatriazole *81*, 83
silver *see* gp100/Pmel17
silymarin 75
Sipple syndrome *368*
sirolimus (rapamycin) *635*
  chemoprevention of non-melanoma skin
    cancers 74–75
  extramammary Paget's disease 155
  organ transplant recipients 636
  post-transplant Kaposi sarcoma 174
skin color
  melanocyte activity determining 25–26
  melanosome variations with 28–29, *29, 29*
  *see also* darker-skinned individuals
skin examination
  early diagnosis of melanoma 277
  partner-assisted 69–70, *70*
  *see also* self-examination of skin
skin grafts 560–561
  hands *573*
  head and neck 563–565, *563, 564, 566, 570*
  pelvis/perineum area *571*
  resected melanomas 539–540
skin phenotype
  actinic keratosis risk and 89
  cancer risk and 61, 67
skin self-examination *see* self-examination of
    skin
skin tension lines, relaxed 509–510, *510*
skin type
  basal cell carcinoma risk and *100*
  effects of UV radiation and 38
  skin cancer risk and 57
  variations in melanogenesis by 33
*SLC24A4* gene variants 37
*SLC24A5* gene variants 37

*SLC45A2 (MATP)* gene variants 27, *37*
*SMOH* gene mutations 61
smoking, cigarette 63, 170
smoothened (Smo; SMOH) 13, *14*, 61, 349,
    357
  small-molecule inhibitor 117, 364
smooth muscle actin (SMA) 113, 164, 188
SNS-314 *617*
social impact, keratinocyte carcinomas 50–51
solar elastosis, melanoma in situ with 301,
    *301*
solar keratoses *see* actinic keratoses
solar lentigo 275
SolarScan *401*, 403
solid organ transplant recipients *see* organ
    transplant recipients
solitary small- to medium-sized pleomorphic
    T-cell nodule of undetermined
    significance 215, *216*
sonic hedgehog (SHH) 13, 14, *14*
soot exposure, scrotal cancer and 44, 56
sorafenib
  dermatologic side effects 382
  Kaposi sarcoma 176
  melanoma 615–617, *616, 619, 620, 621*, 631
SOS response 33
sotirimod 468
*SOX10* gene 24
Sp1, in extramammary Paget's disease 153
speckled lentiginous nevi (SLN) 252, *253*
spectrophotometric intracutaneous analysis
    (SIAscopy) *401*, 403–404
spinal accessory nerve, surgical damage 556
spindle and epithelioid cell nevus *see* Spitz
    nevus
spindle cell melanoma 306–307, *307*
spiradenocarcinoma 144, *144*
Spitz nevus 275–276, 341–348
  acral 345
  angiomatous 342–343
  clinical features 341, *342*
  combined 344, 345, *345*
  compound 342–344, *343*
  confocal microscopy 417–418
  dermal 343
  desmoplastic 342–343
  halo reaction 341, 345, *345*
  history 341
  junctional 342, 343–344, *343*
  malignant 346
  management 348
  molecular features 3, 347
  pagetoid 341
  pathology 341–346, *343*
  persistent or recurrent 345, 346
  variants 344–346, *344*
  *vs* melanoma 311, 346–347, *346*
spitzoid melanocytic lesions, atypical 309–311,
    346–347
spitzoid melanoma 306, *306*, 347
  of childhood *345*
Spitz tumor 346–347
S-plasty, non-melanoma skin cancers 509–510,
    *510*
squamous cell carcinoma (SCC) 124–139
  adenoid or acantholytic 133
  adenosquamous 133, *133*
  anogenital region 128, *129*
  associated primary dermatoses *125*
  biopsy 130, 441
  clinical features 126–130, *127*
  confocal microscopy 411–413, *411, 412, 413,
    413*
  costs 42–43

dermoscopy 388–389, *389*
desmoplastic 134
differential diagnosis 130
disseminated/advanced, treatment 526–529, *528, 529*
in dyskeratosis congenita 363
ear 128, *128*
epidemiology 42, 48–49, 124–125
epidermodysplasia verruciformis-associated 196, 197, *197*, 198, *198*
in epidermolysis bullosa 360, *360*
future outlook 138
genetics 15–16
histologic grading 132–133, *132*
in HIV-infected patients 204–205, 642
human papillomavirus-associated 61–62, 96, 126
incidence 49–50, *49, 49*, 124
intraoral 128
invasive
    clinical features 127–128, *127*
    pathology 132, *132*
    treatment 137
keratoacanthoma type *see* keratoacanthoma
lip 128
Merkel cell carcinoma developing within 180
metastatic 135, *135, 136*
    clinical features 127–128, *128*
    prognostic factors 135, *135*
    transplant recipients *635*, 637–638, *637*
    treatment 526–529
mortality 50, 124
organ transplant recipients *see under* organ transplant recipients
pathogenesis 125–126
pathology 131–135
patient evaluation and diagnosis 130–131, *131*
perineural invasion 134, *134*
    radiation therapy 582
periungual 128, *129*
precursor lesions 89–98
prevention 53, 66–72, 137
    chemoprevention 73–75, 137
    efficacy of sunscreens 53, 85
    primary 67–69, 73
    secondary 69–71, 73–74, *74*
    targeting 66–67
progression of actinic keratoses to 91–92, 126
reconstructive surgery *564, 567, 574*
recurrence
    clinical features *131*
    risk factors *135*
    surgical management 513
risk factors 52, 56–65, *57*, 124–126, *125*
    indoor tanning 647–648, *647*
    treatment-related 349–354, *350, 351*
in scleroatrophic syndrome of Huriez 363–364
spindle cell 133–134, *134*
staging 131
treatment 135–137
    cryosurgery 136, 456–457, 458, 459, *459*
    curettage and electrodesiccation 136, 444–445, 448
    imiquimod 136–137, 466–468, 482–483, *486, 488, 490*
    interferons 480
    Mohs micrographic surgery 137, *137*, 517, 518
    photodynamic therapy 137, 503
    radiation therapy 136, 578–582, *580, 581, 582*
    surgical excision 137, *137*, 508–514

topical 5-fluorouracil 136–137, 465
topical chemotherapy 136–137, *464*
tumor depth 134–135
in xeroderma pigmentosum 361
squamous cell carcinoma in situ (SCCIS) 96–97, 126–127
confocal microscopy 411, 412–413, *412, 413*
dermoscopy 388–389, *389*
pathology 132, *132*
treatment 136–137
    cryosurgery 456–457, *459*
    curettage and electrodesiccation 448
    imiquod cream 466–468
    topical chemotherapy *464*, 465
    topical retinoids 470
*see also* Bowen's disease
stains, tissue, for Mohs micrographic surgery 516–517
standard of care, legal aspects 669, *669*
*Staphylococcus aureus*, in cutaneous T-cell lymphoma pathogenesis 217–218
statins, melanoma chemoprevention 75–77, *76*
steel factor *see* KIT ligand
*steel* gene mutations 24
stem cell factor *see* KIT ligand
stem cell transplant, cutaneous T-cell lymphoma 226, 228–229
stereotactic radiosurgery (SRS), brain metastases 632
Stewart–Treves syndrome (angiosarcomas associated with chronic lymphedema) 186–187, 191
stroma-derived factor-1 (SDF-1) 4–5
stromolysin 3, in basal cell carcinoma 113
subcutaneous panniculitis-like T-cell lymphoma 225
SUFU 13, *14*
sulindac, melanoma chemoprevention 77
sulisobenzone *81*, 83
sun, position of 57
sunburn 646
    UV action spectrum for 645, *645*
sunburn cells 59
sun exposure
    dysplastic nevus induction 233
    keratinocyte carcinoma risk and 52
    protection from *see* photoprotection
    risks 654
    skin cancer risk and 56–64, *57, 67*
    squamous cell carcinoma risk and 125
    timing and character 60
    vitamin D levels and 654–655
    vitamin D synthesis 650
    *see also* ultraviolet (UV) radiation
sunglasses 86–87
sunitinib
    dermatologic side effects 383
    Kaposi sarcoma 176
    melanoma 614, *615, 621*
sunlight
    ultraviolet spectrum 56, 645
    *see also* visible light
sun protection factor (SPF) 83, 84
    equivalence of constitutive pigmentation 38
    role in practical use 84–85
    UV filters in sunscreens 81
sunscreens 80–85
    application 84–85
    broadspectrum UVA and UVB filters 83
    commonly used agents 81, *81, 82*
    future outlook 87
    history 80
    inorganic UV filters 80–81, 83–84
    measuring efficacy 84

mechanisms 80–81
organic UV filters 80, 82–83
    UVA 83
    UVB 82–83
    protection from visible light and infrared radiation photodamage 85
    skin cancer prevention 53, 85
    vitamin D sufficiency and 655
    water resistant 85
SunSphere 87
superficial groin lymphadenectomy 553, 556
superficial spreading melanoma (SSM) 301
surgical excision
    atypical fibroxanthoma 163
    atypical melanocytic lesions 538–539
    basal cell carcinoma 115, 508–514
    congenital melanocytic nevi 256, 257–258, *257, 258*
    dermatofibrosarcoma protuberans 161–162
    dysplastic nevi 242, 243
    extramammary Paget's disease 155
    Kaposi sarcoma 176
    melanoma 320–322, *321, 321, 322*, 532–543
        excision margin trials 532–536, *533, 534*
        head and neck 537–538
        histologic variants 538–539
        history 532
        metastatic disease 323, 632, *632*
        during pregnancy 330
        recommended margins *321*, 536–537
        techniques 539, *539, 540*
        wound closure techniques 539–541, *539*
    melanoma in situ 536–537
    Merkel cell carcinoma 184
    non-melanoma skin cancer 508–514, *511*
        clinical, surgical and histologic margins 510–513
        incomplete, and tumor recurrence 513
        perioperative management 508–509
        planning 509–510, *510*
    squamous cell carcinoma 137, *137*, 508–514
        transplant recipients 638
    *vs* topical chemotherapy *463*
    *see also* Mohs micrographic surgery
surgical margins
    basal cell carcinoma 115, 511–512
    confocal microscopy for mapping 421
    defined 510–511
    melanoma 320, 532–539
        current recommendations *321*, 536–537, *536*
        head and neck 537–538
        histologic variants 538–539
        randomized clinical trials 532–536, *533, 534*
    melanoma in situ 518–519
    Mohs micrographic surgery 515
    non-melanoma skin cancer 511–513
    reconstructive surgery and 559, 560
    squamous cell carcinoma 137, *137*, 512–513
Surveillance, Epidemiology and End Results (SEER) program 40, 44, 45
Swedish Melanoma Group Trial *533, 534*, 535
Sweet syndrome 368, 374–375, *374, 375*
syncope, complicating cryosurgery 460
synovial sarcoma *159*
syphilis, secondary 215
syringocystadenocarcinoma papilliferum 146, *146*
syringoma
    differential diagnosis 140
    malignant chondroid *see* malignant mixed tumor
    *vs* morpheic basal cell carcinoma 110

systemic lupus erythematosus (SLE) 63
systemic oncologic therapy, dermatologic side
    effects 379–385

# T

T4 endonuclease 75, *464*, 472
tacrolimus *635*
    organ transplant recipients 636
    topical, carcinogenic potential 353
talabostat *618*, *620*
tamoxifen, eccrine carcinoma 530
tanning
    action spectrum for 645, *645*
    attitudes and beliefs 69, 644–645
    history of intentional 644–645, *645*
    indoor 644–649
        carcinogenic effects 59–60, 69, 647–648
        effects 646–647, *646*
        health benefit claims 648, *648*
        history 644–645
        mechanisms 645–646
        primary prevention programs 69
        vitamin D synthesis 648
    mechanisms of *33*, 36–38, 646
    *see also* ultraviolet (UV) radiation
tanning industry, indoor 644–645, 648–649
tanning salons 644
    safety standards 646
tape stripping, for EGIR genomic
        characterization 430, *430*
targeted therapies
    melanoma 325, 613–622, *615*, 631–632
        angiogenesis and extracellular matrix
            617–618, *618*
        cell surface molecules 614–615, *615*
        combined approaches 619, *620*, *621*
        future strategies 619–621, *622*
        immune effector function 619, *619*, 630,
            631, *631*
        intracellular molecules 615–617, *616*, *617*
        targets 613, *614*, *631*
        therapeutic index 613, *614*
        tumor microenvironment 617–619
    squamous cell carcinoma 528
tar keratoses 95
tasidotin *618*
tattoos, pseudolymphomatous reactions 214, *215*
taxanes
    cancers treated *380*
    dermatologic side effects 379, 380, 382
tazarotene, topical 470
T-cell antigens, in cutaneous T-cell lymphoma
        222, *222*
T-cell lymphoma
    cutaneous *see* cutaneous T-cell lymphoma
    subcutaneous panniculitis-like 225
T-cell modulators, carcinogenic potential *350*, 354
T-cell receptor gene rearrangements, in
        cutaneous T-cell lymphoma 220–221, *222*
T cells
    CD30⁺ pseudolymphomas 210, *212*
    cryosurgery-mediated activation 451
    effector *478*, *478*
    inhibition by melanoma cells 6–7
    nodular scabies 210–211
tea, melanoma chemoprevention 76
teletherapy 576
telomerase, in melanoma progression 3–4
temozolomide
    dermatologic side effects 383
    melanoma 323, *620*, *621*, 629
temsirolimus, melanoma *620*

*TERC* gene mutations 363
*TERT* gene mutations 363
thalidomide, Kaposi sarcoma 176
therapeutic index, molecularly targeted
        therapies 613, *614*
thermal stress, long-term 64, *64*
thermocouples 452
thorax, reconstruction 568–570
thumb, melanoma 541, *541*
thymoglobulin *635*
*TINF2* gene mutations 363
Tinosorb M (bisoctriazole) *81*, 83
Tinosorb S (bemotrizinol) *81*, 83
tissue expansion 561
tissue transfer, microvascular free *see* free tissue
        transfer, microvascular
titanium dioxide *81*, 83–84
TKI258 617–618, *618*
tobacco use 63, 528
alpha-tocopherol 76
    topical 472
toes
    melanoma 540
    webspace melanoma 541
Toker cells 150, 152, 153
toluidine blue 515–517
topical calcineurin inhibitors (TCI), carcinogenic
        potential *350*, 353
topical chemotherapy 462–476
    actinic keratosis 93, *94*, 462, *463*, *464*
    basal cell carcinoma 117, *464*
    combination therapy 473
    cyclooxygenase inhibitors 468–469
    DNA analog antimetabolites 462–466
    emerging agents 471–473
    head-to-head trials 473
    imidazoquinolones 466–468
    indications *464*
    squamous cell carcinoma 136–137, *464*
    *vs* surgical treatment 463
    *see also* photodynamic therapy; *specific agents*
topotecan, Merkel cell carcinoma 530
total body photography (total body digital
        imaging; TBPI) 657, 658–659
    close-up views combined with 660, *660*
    computer-enhanced 400, *402*
    image capture 657–658
    image management software 660–661, *660*
    melanoma follow-up 324, *324*
    outside services 661
    reimbursement 661
    studio design and equipment 658–659,
        *658*, *659*
    surveillance of dysplastic nevi 242
    template 658, *658*
total skin electron beam (TSEB) therapy,
        cutaneous T-cell lymphoma *226*, 227–228
*TP53* gene (*p53* gene) 60–61
    mutations
        actinic keratoses 16, 91
        atypical fibroxanthoma 162
        basal cell carcinoma 14, 61, 100, 101
        dermatologic therapies inducing 349
        indoor tanning-related 647
        sarcomas 158
        squamous cell carcinoma 16
        UV signature 59
    protein product *see* p53 protein
*TPCN2* gene variants 37
transdifferentiation, of cancer stem cells 8, *8*
transfer factor, melanoma 590, *591*
transformation, malignant 2–4
trans-Golgi network (TGN) 26, *26*
translocations, chromosome

clear cell sarcoma of soft tissue *143*, 158, 164–165
cutaneous sarcomas 158, *159*
dermatofibrosarcoma protuberans 158, 161, *161*
transplant hands and scalp 637, *637*
transplant recipients, solid organ *see* organ
        transplant recipients
transposition flap *562*
transverse rectus abdominis myocutaneous
        (TRAM) flap 570
trapezius flap 568, 569, *571*
trapezius weakness, postoperative 556
trauma, benign proliferation of blasts
        simulating lymphoma 215
treatment
    adverse events and complications, legal
        aspects 670–672, *671*, *672*
    consent to/refusal of 670, *670*
    medico-legal issues in dermatopathology
        672–674, *672*
treatment-related cutaneous carcinogenesis *see*
        dermatologic therapy-related cutaneous
        carcinogenesis
trees, shade provided by 85–86
T regulatory cells (Tregs), in melanoma 6
tremelimumab, in melanoma *619*, *620*, 631
tretinoin, topical
    actinic keratoses 470
    in basal cell nevus syndrome 358–359
    chemoprevention study 74
trichoepithelioma
    in Bazex syndrome 363
    desmoplastic 110, *111*, 140
    in Rombo syndrome 363
    *vs* follicular basal cell carcinoma 107
tricholemmal cystic carcinoma, proliferating
        147, *147*
tricholemmal tumor, proliferating 147
tricholemmomal (or tricholemmal) carcinoma
        146–147, *146*
triciribine 616
tripe palms *371*, 372–373
troglitazone 493
trolamine salicylate *81*, 82
trunk reconstruction 568–570
trust building, after complications 671, *671*
tumor-infiltrating lymphocytes (TILs)
    adoptive transfer, in melanoma 630
    melanoma 288, *288*, 314
tumor necrosis factor-α (TNF-α) blockers,
        carcinogenic potential 63, *350*, 353–354
tumor progression 2–4, *4*
tumor suppressor genes 12, *13*, 60–61
tumor/testis-specific antigens 31, *32*
*TYR* gene variants *27*, 37
tyrosinase 32
    function 30, *31*
    immunostaining, in melanoma *304*, 311
    processing and trafficking 31
    regulation of activity *33*
    synthesis and processing *26*, *26*
    targeting to melanosomes *26*, *26*
tyrosinase-related protein 1 (TYRP1) 30, *31*, *32*
    regulation of activity *33*
    synthesis and processing 26
tyrosinase-related protein 2 (TYRP2) 30, *31*, *32*
    regulation of activity *33*
tyrosine 30, *30*
tyrosine kinase inhibitors (TKI), squamous cell
        carcinoma 528
*TYRP1* gene
    mutations *27*, 30
    variants 37
TYRP proteins *see* tyrosinase-related protein 1;
        tyrosinase-related protein 2

# U

UCN-01 *616*
ugly duckling sign 241, 274, 395
ulceration
  chronic, squamous cell carcinoma and 95
  melanoma *see under* melanoma
  pigmented skin lesions 274
ulcers, biopsy technique 441
ultrasound imaging
  cryosurgery evaluation 454
  melanoma 623–624, 626, 627
    early detection *401*, 404
ultraviolet A (UVA) 56, 80, 645
  -1 therapy, cutaneous T-cell lymphoma 227
  biological effects 83
  carcinogenic effects 59, *59*
  cutaneous effects 645, *645*
  indoor tanning lamps 645, 646
  non-solar sources 59–60
  phototherapy *see* psoralen and ultraviolet A
      (PUVA) therapy
  protection with sunscreens 80, 84
    available agents *81*, 83
    measuring efficacy 84, *84*
  in squamous cell carcinoma pathogenesis
      125
ultraviolet B (UVB) 56, 80, 645
  broadband (BB-UVB) therapy
    carcinogenic risks *350*, 351
    cutaneous T-cell lymphoma 227
  carcinogenic effects 59, *59*
  cutaneous effects 645, *645*
  indoor tanning lamps 645, 646
  narrowband (NB-UVB) therapy
    carcinogenic risks *350*, 351
    cutaneous T-cell lymphoma 227
  non-solar sources 59–60
  protection with sunscreens 80, 84
    available agents *81*, 82–83
    measuring efficacy 84
  signature mutations 59
  squamous cell carcinoma pathogenesis 125
ultraviolet C (UVC) 56, 80, 645
  cutaneous effects 645, *645*
ultraviolet protection factor (UPF) 86
ultraviolet (UV) radiation (UVR) 56–60, *57*, 80,
      645
  in actinic keratosis development 89–90, 91
  acute adverse effects 646
  atypical fibroxanthoma risk 162
  in basal cell carcinoma pathogenesis 99, 100
  carcinogenic effects 59, *59*, 349
  in dysplastic nevus pathogenesis 233
  extreme sensitivity to, actinic reticuloid 207,
      209
  factors affecting intensity 56, *57*–59
  medical use
    history 644
    increased skin cancer risk 349–351
    *see also* phototherapy; psoralen and
        ultraviolet A (PUVA) therapy
  Merkel cell carcinoma risk 179
  ocular effects 86
  pigmentary response 33, 34, 36–38, 646
    *see also* tanning
  protection from *see* photoprotection
  in squamous cell carcinoma tumorigenesis
      16, 125
  transplant-related skin cancers and 634
  *see also* sun exposure
undifferentiated pleomorphic sarcoma/
      malignant fibrous histiocytoma (UPS/
      MFH) 158, 163–164, *163*

epidemiology 157–158
  organ transplant recipients *635*
  treatment 164, 521
  *vs* atypical fibroxanthoma 162
United Kingdom (UK) Melanoma Study Group
      *533*, *534*, 536
Univil A Plus *81*, 83
Univil T 150 *81*, 82–83
upper extremity reconstruction 572–575
US Preventive Service Task Force (USPSTF), on
      screening for skin cancer 71
UV *see* ultraviolet
Uvasorb HEB *81*, 82–83

# V

vaccination
  human papillomaviruses 203
  prevention of non-melanoma skin
      cancers 75
vaccines, anti-melanoma
  adjuvants *607*, 608
  allogeneic whole-cell *607*, *608*, 610
  autologous whole-cell 608, *608*, 610
  defined-antigen 606–607
  dendritic cell-based *607*, 608
  requirements for effective 606
  tumor escape phenomenon 607
  types 606–608
  whole-cell *607*, 608
vaccine therapy, for melanoma 322–323, 590,
      *591*, 606–612
  clinical trials *608*, 609–610, 630, *630*
  current trials 610–611
  patient selection 608–609
  potentially harmful effects 610
  rationale 606, *607*
  *vs* interferon-α *596*, 597, 598
vascular endothelial growth factor (VEGF) 4
  in angiosarcomas 186
  in extramammary Paget's disease 153
  therapeutic targeting in melanoma 617–618,
      *618*
vascular endothelial growth factor (VEGF)-A 7
vascular endothelial growth factor (VEGF)-C 5
vascular endothelial growth factor (VEGF)-D
      5, 186
vascular endothelial growth factor receptor-3
      (VEGFR-3) 5, 191
vascular endothelial growth factor receptor
      (VEGFR) inhibitors, in melanoma
      617–618, *618*
vascular injury, cryosurgical 450, *451*
vascular leak syndrome, treated cutaneous
      T-cell lymphoma 228
vascular malignancies 186–195
  topical chemotherapy *464*
  *see also* angiosarcomas; Kaposi sarcoma
vasculitis, cutaneous leukocytoclastic 376
VEGF *see* vascular endothelial growth factor
venolymphatic channels, tumor cell entry
      into 6
verrucous carcinoma 202–203
  anogenital (Buschke–Lowenstein variant) 96,
      129, *129*, 202
  clinical features 129, *129*, *130*
  oroaerodigestive (Ackerman tumor) 96, 129,
      202
  palmoplantar *see* epithelioma cuniculatum
  pathogenesis and etiology 96, 202
  pathology 133, *133*, 202–203, *203*
  treatment 203
verrucous melanoma 304–305, *305*

verruga peruana, *vs* cutaneous sarcoma 160
vertical growth phase (VGP), melanoma 4, 5,
      288, *288*, 297, 298
vertical rectus abdominis myocutaneous
      (VRAM) flap 570
vesicles, after cryosurgery 459
vinblastine
  intralesional, Kaposi sarcoma 174–175
  melanoma 629–630, *630*
vincristine, Merkel cell carcinoma 530
vindesine, melanoma 590
vinorelbine, dermatologic side effects 379
viruses
  carcinogenic 61–62
  CD30+ (T-cell) pseudolymphomas 210
  in cutaneous T-cell lymphoma pathogenesis
      217–218
  neoplastic disorders associated with
      196–206
  *see also specific viruses*
visible light 56
  protection from biologic effects 85
  *see also* sunlight
vitamin A
  chemoprevention studies 74
  melanoma 590, *591*
  *see also* retinoids
vitamin D 64, 650–656
  all-cause mortality and *652*, 653–654
  bone and muscle health and 651, *652*
  cancers and 651–653, *652*
  current recommendations 655, *655*
  health and disease associations 650–654,
      *652*
  indoor tanning and 648
  melanoma chemoprevention *76*, 78
  risk factors for insufficiency 654
  serum levels *see* 25-hydroxyvitamin D
      (25(OH)D), serum levels
  sources 650, *651*
  sun exposure and 654–655
  synthesis and metabolism 650, *651*
vitamin D receptor (VDR) polymorphisms 64
vitamin E *see* alpha-tocopherol
Vitespen/Oncophage *608*, 610
VLA-4 7
volociximab, in melanoma *615*
vorinostat, cutaneous T-cell lymphoma *226*,
      228
vulvar intraepithelial neoplasia (VIN)
  photodynamic therapy 505
  topical chemotherapy *464*, 466–467
V-Y flaps 572

# W

Waardenburg syndrome
  type I 24
  type II 24
  type III 24
  type IV 24
warfarin, cutaneous surgery and 509
warts, flat *200*
webspace melanomas, surgical resection 541,
      *542*
Wermer syndrome *368*
Werner syndrome *368*
whole body integumentary photography *see*
      total body photography
wide local excision
  melanoma 539, *539*, *540*
  *see also* surgical excision
Wiskott–Aldrich syndrome *368*

Wood's light examination
  Mohs micrographic surgery 519, *520*
  photodynamic therapy 497, 500–501, *502*
  suspicious pigmented lesions 439
World Health Organization (WHO) Melanoma
        Program Trial No. 10 533–535, *533, 534*
wound closure, surgical
  biopsy defects *437*, 439, *440*
  primary 560
  resected melanomas 539–541, *539*
  rule of halves 509–510, *511*
  *see also* reconstructive surgery
wounds, chronic 64

**X**

xanthogranuloma, necrobiotic *368*, 377
xenon chloride laser therapy, cutaneous T-cell
        lymphoma 227
xeroderma pigmentosum (XP) 360–361,
        *364*
  basal cell carcinoma 100, *100*, 361
  chemoprevention of skin cancer 74, 75, 361,
        472
  skin cancer risk 61, 361
  squamous cell carcinoma pathogenesis 125
XL147 *616*

XL281 *616*
XL765 *616*
X-rays, for radiation therapy 576

**Z**

zinc chloride paste 515
zinc oxide *81*, 83–84
Zinsser-Engman-Cole syndrome *see*
        dyskeratosis congenita
Z-plasty *562*